Hypoxemia, 5, 222

Idiopathic thrombocytopenic purpura, 116
Infections, catheter-related, 114
Infections, cytomegalovirus, 98
Infections, fungal, 95, 96
Infections, Gram-negative, 94
Infections, Gram-positive, 93
Infections, herpes, 97
Infections, human immunodeficiency virus, 99
Infections, in bone marrow transplant patients, 102
Infections in neutropenic cancer patient, 101
Infections, in solid organ transplant patients, 103
Infections, oropharyngeal, 107
Infections, soft tissue, 112
Intracerebral hemorrhage, 81
Intracranial hypertension, 84
Insect stings, 78, 150
Isopropanol intoxication, 68

Jelly fish sting, 59

Ketoacidosis, 49, 50, 68
Kidney transplantation, 147

Lactic acidosis, 48
Left ventricular failure, 24
Lightening injury, 146
Lithium overdose, 64
Lower gastrointestinal hemorrhage, 131
Loxosceles envenomation, 78

Magnesium imbalances, 43, 44
Malignant hyperthermia, 86
Massive transfusion, 116
Meningitis, 108
Metabolic acidosis, 47-50
Metabolic alkalosis, 47
Methanol intoxication, 59, 68
Methemoglobinemia, 72, 218
Mucormycosis, 96
Mushroom poisoning, 59
Myasthenia gravis, 87
Myocardial contusion, 23
Myocardial infarction, acute, 20
Myocardial infarction, mechanical complications, 22
Myocardial infarction, right ventricular, 21
Myxedema coma, 56

Narcotic overdose, 62
Near drowning, 151
Necrotizing soft tissue infections, 112
Neuroleptic drug overdose, 73
Neuroleptic malignant syndrome, 86
Neutropenia, infectious complications, 101

Nosocomial sinusitis, 111

Obstetric catastrophes, 156
Ogilvie's syndrome, 124
Oliguria, 3
Organophosphate poisoning, 77
Organ transplantation, infectious complications, 103

Pancreatitis, 124, 125
Penetrating trauma, 137, 138
Perforated peptic ulcer, 124
Pericardial tamponade, 30, 196
Pericarditis, 29
Peripartum cardiomyopathy, 156
Peripheral arterial occlusion, 143
Peripheral vascular bypass, post-operative management, 142
Peritonitis, 124
Phenothiazine overdose, 73
Pheochromocytoma, 57
Phosphorus imbalances, 45, 46
Pneumocystis carinii pneumonia 99, 100
Pneumonia, 12
Pneumothorax, 9, 202
Poisoning, 59
Polyuria, 53
Post-cardiac surgery management, 141
Post-craniotomy management, 140
Postpartum hemorrhage, 156
Post-peripheral vascular bypass management, 142
Potassium imbalances, 39, 40
Pre-operative assessment, 136
Pressure ulcers, 157
Pulmonary edema, 7, 8
Pulmonary edema, cardiogenic, 24
Pulmonary embolism, 10
Pulseless electrical activity, 34

Radiation toxicity, 181
Rattlesnake, 59, 78
Renal failure, acute, 134
Renal failure, chronic, 135
Respiratory distress, 5, 8
Respiratory failure, 5, 6
Rhabdomyolysis, 153
Ruptured ectopic pregnancy, 124

Salicylate overdose, 61
Salpingitis, 124
Scorpion envenomation, 59, 78
Sedative-hypnotic overdose, 62
Seizures, 79
Sepsis, 91
Septic abortion, 156
Septic shock, 92
Serotonin syndrome, 76
Shock, anaphylactic, 150
Shock, cardiogenic, 27
Shock, septic, 92
Sickle cell crisis, 122

Sinusitis, 111
Smoke inhalation, 16, 70, 71, 145
Snake envenomation, 78
Sodium imbalance, 37, 38, 54
Spinal cord compression, 85
Status asthmaticus, 11
Status epilepticus, 79
Stroke (infarction), 80
Subarachnoid hemorrhage, 82
Subdural hematoma, 83
Superior vena cava syndrome, 155
Supraventricular tachycardia, 33
Syndrome of inappropriate antidiuresis, 54
Systemic inflammatory response syndrome, 91

Tachycardia, supraventricular, 33
Tachycardia, ventricular, 35
Tachypnea, 5
Tamponade, 30, 196
Tetanus, 90
Theophylline overdose, 63
Thrombocytopenia, 116
Thromboembolism, arterial, 143
Thromboembolism, venous, 10, 118
Thrombotic thrombocytopenic purpura, 116
Thermal burn injury, 145
Thyroid storm, 55
Thyrotoxicosis, 55
Toxic megacolon, 133
Toxicology, 59
Toxic shock syndrome, 110
Transfusion reaction, 121
Transplantation, kidney 147
Trauma, abdominal, 138
Trauma, chest, 137
Trauma, head, 139
Traumatic brain injury, 139
Tricyclic antidepressant overdose, 74
Tuberculosis, 104
Tuberculosis, pharmacotherapy 186
Tumor lysis syndrome, 154

Ulcers, pressure, 157
Unstable angina, 19
Upper gastrointestinal hemorrhage, 130
Urinary tract infection, 106
Urosepsis, 106
Uterine rupture, 156

Valvular heart disease, 28
Venom injuries, 78
Venous thromboembolism, 10, 118
Venous thrombosis, 118
Ventricular fibrillation, 35
Ventricular tachycardia, 35
Viral hepatitis, 128, 129

Withdrawal, alcohol, 69

Saunders
Manual of
Critical Care

Saunders
Manual of
Critical Care

James A. Kruse, M.D.
Professor of Medicine
Wayne State University School of Medicine
Director, Medical Intensive Care Unit
Chief, Pulmonary/Critical Care Medicine
Detroit Receiving Hospital
Detroit, Michigan

Mitchell P. Fink, M.D.
Professor and Chairman
Department of Critical Care Medicine and
Watson Professor of Surgery
University of Pittsburgh Medical School
Pittsburgh, Pennsylvania

Richard W. Carlson, M.D., Ph.D.
Professor of Medicine
Mayo Medical School
Scottsdale, Arizona
Professor of Clinical Medicine
University of Arizona
Chair, Department of Medicine
Maricopa Medical Center
Phoenix, Arizona

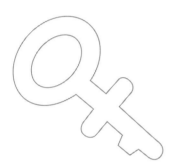

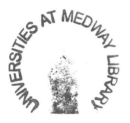

Saunders
An Imprint of Elsevier Science
Philadelphia   London   Toronto   Montreal   Sydney   Tokyo

SAUNDERS
An Imprint of Elsevier Science

The Curtis Center
Independence Square West
Philadelphia, Pennsylvania 19106

SAUNDERS MANUAL OF CRITICAL CARE ISBN 0–7216–9419–5

Notice

Medicine is an ever-changing field. Standard safety precautions must be followed, but as new research and clinical experience broaden our knowledge, changes in treatment and drug therapy may become necessary or appropriate. Readers are advised to check the product information currently provided by the manufacturer of each drug to be administered to verify the recommended dose, the method and duration of administration, and contraindications. It is the responsibility of the treating physician, relying on experience and knowledge of the patient, to determine dosages and the best treatment for each individual patients. Neither the Publisher nor the editors assume any liability for any injury and/or damage to persons or property arising from this publication.

THE PUBLISHER

Library of Congress Cataloging-in-Publication Data

Saunders manual of critical care / James A. Kruse—[et al.].—1st ed.
  p. cm.
    Includes bibliographical references and index.
    ISBN 0–7216–9419–5
    1. Critical care medicine—Handbooks, manuals, etc. I. Title: manual of critical care.
II. Kruse, James A.
RC86.8.S28 2003
616′.028—dc21

2003021153

Publishing Director, Surgery: Richard H. Lampert
Senior Acquisitions Editor: Allan Ross
Senior Developmental Editor: David Orzechowski

PIT/CCW

Printed in the United States of America

Last digit is the print number: 9 8 7 6 5 4 3 2 1

Contributors

GEORGE J. ALANGADEN, M.D.
Associate Professor, Division of Infectious Diseases, Department of Internal Medicine, Wayne State University School of Medicine, Detroit, Michigan
Infections in Neutropenic Cancer Patients

ALI H. AL-KHAFAJI, M.D.
Assistant Professor of Medicine, University of North Dakota; Staff Physician, Critical Care Medicine, MeritCare Health System, Fargo, North Dakota
Oliguria; Continuous Renal Replacement Therapy

MICHAEL J. APOSTOLAKOS, M.D.
Associate Professor of Medicine, University of Rochester; Director, Adult Critical Care, Strong Memorial Hospital, Rochester, New York
Status Asthmaticus; COPD Exacerbation

ELI AZZI, M.D.
Fellow, Pulmonary Medicine, State University of New York–Downstate, New York, New York
Pulmonary Edema

REMZI BAG, M.D.
Assistant Professor of Medicine, Section of Pulmonary and Critical Care Medicine, Department of Medicine, Baylor College of Medicine; Staff Physician, The Methodist Hospital and St. Luke's Episcopal Hospital, Houston, Texas
Life-Threatening Infections of the Oropharynx; Deep Venous Thrombosis; Fat Embolism

MARIE R. BALDISSERI, M.D.
Associate Professor of Critical Care Medicine, University of Pittsburgh Medical School; Co-Director, Neurovascular ICU, and Medical Director, Magee-Womens Hospital ICU, University of Pittsburgh Medical Center, Pittsburgh, Pennsylvania
Subarachnoid Hemorrhage; Subdural Hematoma

PERRY A. BALL, M.D.
Associate Professor of Surgery and Anesthesiology, Dartmouth Medical School, Hanover; Staff Neurosurgeon and Intensivist, Dartmouth-Hitchcock Medical Center, Lebanon, New Hampshire
Spinal Cord Compression

VENKATA BANDI, M.D.
Assistant Professor of Medicine, and Associate Director, Medical Intensive Care Unit, Baylor College of Medicine; Director, Medical Intensive Care Unit, Ben Taub General Hospital, Houston, Texas
Neuroleptic Malignant Syndrome and Malignant Hyperthermia; Tetanus

STEVEN BORZAK, M.D.
Assistant Professor (Tenure Track), Case Western Reserve University, Cleveland, Ohio; Florida Cardiovascular Research, LC, Florida Cardiology Group, Atlantis, Florida
Transcutaneous Pacing; Cardioversion and Defibrillation

ARTHUR J. BOUJOUKOS, M.D.
Associate Professor, Critical Care Medicine, University of Pittsburgh Medical School; Medical Director, Cardiothoracic Intensive Care Unit, University of Pittsburgh Medical Center, Pittsburgh, Pennsylvania
Left Ventricular Failure; Atrial Fibrillation and Flutter

STEPHEN A. BOWLES, M.D.
Assistant Professor of Medicine, Department of Anesthesiology and Critical Care Medicine, University of Pittsburgh Medical Center, Pittsburgh, Pennsylvania
Kidney Transplantation

T.J. BUNT, M.D., F.A.C.S.
Chairman, Department of Surgery, Maricopa Medical Center, Phoenix; Clinical Professor of Surgery, University of Arizona, Tucson, Arizona
Acute Peripheral Arterial Occlusion

MARGARET L. CAMPBELL, R.N., M.S.N., F.A.A.N.
Assistant Professor of Medicine, Wayne State University; Nurse Practitioner, Palliative Care Service, Detroit Receiving Hospital, Detroit, Michigan
Do Not Resuscitate Orders

RICHARD W. CARLSON, M.D., Ph.D.
Professor of Medicine, Mayo Medical School, Scottsdale, Arizona; Professor of Clinical Medicine, University of Arizona; Chair, Department of Medicine, Maricopa Medical Center, Phoenix, Arizona
Cor Pulmonale; Smoke Inhalation; Calcium Channel and β-Blocker Drug Overdoses; Alcohol Withdrawal Syndrome; Venom Injuries: Snake and Arthropod; Urosepsis; Nosocomial Sinusitis; Epiglottitis; Acute Renal Failure; Chronic Renal Failure; Near Drowning; Hemodialysis; Intrahospital Transport; Sedation Monitoring

CHARLES M. CARPATI, M.D.
Chief, Medical Intensive Care Unit, Saint Vincents Hospital and Medical Center, New York, New York
Pulmonary Edema

PRANATHARTHI H. CHANDRASEKAR, M.D.
Professor of Medicine and Infectious Diseases, and Program Director, Infectious Diseases Fellowship, Wayne State University School of Medicine; Harper University Hospital, Detroit, Michigan
Herpes Infections; Infections in Bone Marrow Transplant Patients

CHAI JIE CHANG, M.D.
Fellow, Department of Anesthesiology, University of Florida, Gainesville, Florida; Former Resident, Maricopa Medical Center, Phoenix, Arizona
Smoke Inhalation

SEEMANT CHATURVEDI, M.D.
Associate Professor of Neurology, Wayne State University School of Medicine; Associate Director of Stroke Program, Wayne State University, Detroit, Michigan
Coma; Cerebral Infarction

LAKSHMIPATHI CHELLURI, M.D., M.P.H
Associate Professor, University of Pittsburgh School of Medicine; Associate Professor, Department of Anesthesiology/Critical Care Medicine, University of Pittsburgh Medical Center, Pittsburgh, Pennsylvania
Intracerebral, Hemorrhage; Post-Craniotomy Management

MARK S. CHESTNUTT, M.D.
Assistant Professor of Medicine, Pulmonary and Critical Care Medicine, and Director, Medical Critical Care, Oregon Health and Science University Hospital, Oregon Health and Science University, Portland, Oregon
Respiratory Failure

KEITH D. CLANCY, M.D.
Former Assistant Professor of Surgery and Anesthesiology, Department of Anesthesiology/Critical Care Medicine, University of Pittsburgh Medical Center, Pittsburgh, Pennsylvania
Chest Trauma

STACY J. CLARK, D.O.
Staff Physician, Southern California Permanente Medical Group, Kaiser Permanente, Santa Clarita, California
Epiglottitis

VIVIAN L. CLARK, M.D.
Senior Staff Physician, Interventional Cardiology, Henry Ford Hospital, Detroit, Michigan
Unstable Angina; Acute Myocardial Infarction; Right Ventricular Myocardial Infarction; Mechanical Complications of Acute Myocardial Infarction; Cardiogenic Shock; Pericardial Tamponade; Aortic Dissection; Glycoprotein IIb/IIIa Receptor Antagonists; Antidysrhythmic Agents; Pericardiocentesis; Intra-Aortic Balloon Counterpulsation

REBECCA L. COREY, PHARM.D.
Pharmacy Special Resident, Solid Organ Transplantation, Strong Memorial Hospital, University of Rochester Medical Center, Rochester, New York
Macrolides

HOWARD L. CORWIN, M.D.
Professor of Medicine and Anesthesiology, Dartmouth Medical School, Hanover; Section Chief, Critical Care Medicine, and Medical Director, Intensive Care Unit, Dartmouth Hitchcock Medical Center, Lebanon, New Hampshire
Oliguria; Continuous Renal Replacement Therapy

LAWRENCE R. CRANE, M.D.
Professor of Medicine, Division of Infectious Diseases, and Director, HIV/AIDS Program, Wayne State University; Director, HIV/AIDS Program, Detroit Medical Center, Detroit, Michigan
Cytomegalovirus Infections; Acquired Immune Deficiency Syndrome; Pneumocystis carinii Pneumonia

SUSAN E. DANTONI, M.D.
Clinical Instructor, Department of Obstetrics and Gynecology, University of Rochester; Clinical Adjunct Professor, Department of Health Science, Rochester Institute of Technology; Attending Physician, Department of Obstetrics and Gynecology, Jordon Health Center, Rochester, New York
Toxic Shock Syndrome

JOSEPH M. DARBY, M.D.
Associate Professor, Department of Critical Care Medicine, University of Pittsburgh School of Medicine; Medical Director, Trauma ICU, University of Pittsburgh Medical Center, Pittsburgh, Pennsylvania
Traumatic Brain Injury

JOHN W. DEVLIN, PHARM.D.
Adjunct Assistant Professor of Pharmacy, Wayne State University College of Pharmacy; Clinical Pharmacist Specialist, Surgery/Critical Care, Detroit Receiving Hospital and University Health Center, Detroit, Michigan
Digoxin Overdose; Acid-Inhibiting Agents and Sucralfate; Neuromuscular Blocking Drugs; Narcotic Agonists and Naloxone; Digoxin

ROBERT DiCENZO, PHARM.D., B.C.P.S.
Clinical Assistant Professor, School of Pharmacy and Pharmaceutical Sciences, University at Buffalo, Buffalo; Research Professor, University of Rochester Medical Center, Rochester, New York
Aminoglycosides

MARK A. DOUGLASS, PHARM.D.
Adjunct Assistant Clinical Professor, Wayne State University College of Pharmacy; Clinical Pharmacy Specialist, Internal Medicine, Detroit Receiving Hospital and University Health Center, Detroit Medical Center, Detroit, Michigan
Anticoagulants

MURRAY N. EHRINPREIS, M.D.
Professor of Medicine, Division of Gastroenterology, Department of Internal Medicine; Wayne State University School of Medicine; Attending Gastroenterologist, Harper University Hospital, Detroit, Michigan
Lower Gastroenteral Hemorrhage; Diarrhea; Toxic Megacolon

MITCHELL P. FINK, M.D.
Chairman, Department of Critical Care Medicine and Watson Professor of Surgery, University of Pittsburgh Medical School, Pittsburgh, Pennsylvania
Necrotizing Soft-Tissue Infections; Acute Abdominal Pain; Acute Pancreatitis; Acute Cholecystitis; Upper Gastroenteral Hemorrhage; Chest Trauma; Post-Cardiac Surgery Management; Filgrastim; Fluoroquinolone Antibiotics

TISHA FUJII, D.O.
Attending Physician, Section of Critical Care Medicine, Saint Francis Medical Center, Honolulu, Hawaii
Pulmonary Embolism

ADEL GHULOOM, M.D.
Instructor, Department of Medicine, Baylor College of Medicine, Houston, Texas
Tetanus

GENEEN M. GIBSON, PHARM.D., M.S.
Clinical Associate Professor, Department of Pharmacy Practice, University at Buffalo, Buffalo; Clinical Pharmacy Specialist, Infectious Diseases, Strong Memorial Hospital, University of Rochester Medical Center, Rochester, New York
Penicillins and Cephalosporins

KALPALATHA K. GUNTUPALLI, M.D.
Professor of Medicine, Pulmonary/Critical Care, Baylor College of Medicine; Associate Chief of Medicine, Chief, Pulmonary/Critical Care Section, and Director, Medical Intensive Care Unit, Ben Taub General Hospital, Houston, Texas
Acute Respiratory Distress Syndrome; Massive Hemoptysis; Botulism; Conventional Mechanical Ventilation; Newer Modes of Mechanical Ventilation; Discontinuing Mechanical Ventilation

ELIZABETH S. GUY, M.D., F.C.C.P.
Assistant Professor of Medicine, Baylor College of Medicine; Ben Taub General Hospital, Houston, Texas
Air Embolism

JORGE A. GUZMAN, M.D.
Assistant Professor of Medicine, Wayne State University; Director, Medical Intensive Care Unit, Harper University Hospital, Detroit, Michigan
Hypertensive Crisis; Hypocalcemia; Hypercalcemia; Hypomagnesemia; Hypermagnesemia; Fenoldopam; Nitroglycerin; Nitroprusside; Enteral Feeding; Parenteral Nutrition; Nutritional Assessment; Monitoring Oxygen Transport; Capnography; Gastric Tonometry

ALI A. HAMDAN, M.D.
Clinical Instructor in Medicine, Department of Medicine, Strong Memorial Hospital, University of Rochester School of Medicine and Dentistry
Organophosphate Poisoning; Positive End-Expiratory Pressure

NICOLA A. HANANIA, M.D., F.C.C.P., F.R.C.P.(C)
Assistant Professor of Medicine, Pulmonary and Critical Care Medicine, Baylor College of Medicine, Houston, Texas
Hypothermia

MARILYN T. HAUPT, M.D.
Professor, Department of Internal Medicine, Oregon Health and Science University; Medical Director, Critical Care Services, Oregon Health and Science University Hospital, Portland, Oregon
Anaphylaxis

STEPHEN O. HEARD, M.D.
Professor of Anesthesiology and Surgery, and Executive Vice-Chair, University of Massachusetts Medical School; Director, Surgical Intensive Care Units, Department of Anesthesiology, University of Massachusetts Memorial Medical Center, Worcester, Massachusetts
Catheter-Related Bloodstream Infection; Preoperative Evaluation of the Critically Ill Patient

JEFF D. HUNTRESS, PHARM.D.
Clinical Associate Professor, State University of New York at Buffalo School of Pharmacy, Buffalo; Associate Director, Clinical Pharmacy Services, and Critical Care Clinical Pharmacy Specialist, University of Rochester Medical Center, Rochester, New York
Dantrolene; Inhaled Bronchodilators; Miscellaneous Antibiotics

MEENA KAKARALA, M.D.
Staff Physician, Department of Medicine, Maricopa Medical Center, Phoenix, Arizona
Nosocomial Sinusitis

SALMAAN KANJI, PHARM.D.
Fellow, Critical Care Pharmacotherapy, Wayne State University College of Pharmacy; Post-Doctoral Critical Care Pharmacotherapy Fellow, Detroit Receiving Hospital and University Health Center, Detroit, Michigan
Digoxin Overdose; Digoxin

LINDA KIRSCHENBAUM, D.O.
Chief, Respirator Unit, Saint Vincents Hospital and Medical Center, New York, New York
Pulmonary Embolism

DANA G. KISSNER, M.D., M.S.
Associate Professor of Medicine, Division of Pulmonary, Critical Care Medicine; Attending Physician, Harper University Hospital, Detroit Medical Center, Detroit, Michigan
Tuberculosis; Antituberculosis Drugs

DAVID J. KRAMER, M.D.

Adjunct Associate Professor, Department of Critical Care Medicine, University of Pittsburgh Medical School, Pittsburgh, Pennsylvania; Senior Associate Consultant, Transplant Critical Care, Mayo Clinic Jacksonville, Jacksonville, Florida
Acute Alcoholic Hepatitis; Viral Hepatitis; Fulminant Hepatic Failure

WILLANE S. KRELL, M.D.

Associate Professor of Medicine, Wayne State University; Medical Director, Respiratory Therapy, Detroit Receiving Hospital, Detroit, Michigan
Tachypnea and Hypoxemia; Fiberoptic Bronchoscopy

JAMES A. KRUSE, M.D.

Professor of Medicine, Wayne State University School of Medicine; Chief, Pulmonary Critical Care Medicine, and Director, Medical Intensive Care Unit, Detroit Receiving Hospital, Detroit, Michigan
Cardiogenic Shock; Aortic Dissection; Hyponatremia; Hypernatremia; Hypokalemia; Hyperkalemia; Hypocalcemia; Hypercalcemia; Hypomagnesemia; Hypermagnesemia; Hypophosphatemia; Hyperphosphatemia; Acid-Base Disturbances; Lactic Acidosis; Alcoholic Acidosis; Diabetic Ketoacidosis; Hyperosmolar Nonketotic Coma; Hypoglycemia; Diabetes Insipidus; Syndrome of Inappropriate Antidiuresis; Thyroid Storm; Myxedema Coma; Pheochromocytoma; Adrenal Insufficiency; Acetaminophen Overdose; Salicylate Intoxication; Sedative-Hypnotic and Narcotic Drug Overdose; Theophylline Overdose; Lithium Overdose; Cocaine Intoxication; Alcohol and Glycol Intoxications; Cyanide Poisoning; Methemoglobinemia; Cyclic Antidepressant Drug Overdose; Status Epilepticus; Electrical and Lightning Injuries; Rhabdomyolysis; Intravenous Fluids; Amrinone and Milrinone; Vasoactive Catecholamines; Acid-Inhibiting Agents and Sucralfate; Neuromuscular Blocking Drugs; Benzodiazepines and Flumazenil; Anticoagulants; Endotracheal Intubation; Central Venous Catheterization; Arterial Catheterization; Pulmonary Artery Catheterization; Temporary Transvenous Pacemaker; Lumbar Puncture; Paracentesis; Thoracentesis; Chest Tube Thoracostomy; Brain Death Determination; Fluid Challenge; Sengstaken-Blakemore Tube Placement; Transnasal and Transoral Gastroenteric Intubation; Hemodynamic Monitoring; Fast Flush Test; Blood Gas and Oximetry Monitoring; Oxygen Therapy

BURKHARD LACHMANN, M.D., Ph.D.

Professor of Anesthesiology and Director of Anesthesia Research, Department of Anesthesiology, Erasmus University, Rotterdam, The Netherlands
Atelectasis

STEVEN J. LAVINE, M.D.

Associate Professor of Internal Medicine, and Director, Noninvasive Laboratory, University of Florida/Jacksonville, Jacksonville, Florida
Pericarditis

DONALD P. LEVINE, M.D.

Professor of Medicine, and Chief, Division of General Internal Medicine, Wayne State University; Chief of Staff and Vice-Chief of Medicine, Detroit Receiving Hospital, Detroit, Michigan
Gram-Positive Infections; Gram-Negative Infections; Endocarditis

RICHARD A. LEWIS, M.D.

Professor and Associate Chairman, Department of Neurology, Wayne State University School of Medicine; Vice Chief of Neurology and Director of Clinical Neurophysiology, Harper University Hospital, Detroit Medical Center, Detroit, Michigan
Guillain-Barré Syndrome

HO-YIN ADRIAN LI, M.B., Ch.B., F.F.A., B.A.O., M.B.A.

Chairman, Department of Anesthesiology, Putnam Community Medical Center, Palatka, Florida
Neuroleptic Drug Overdose

RANDY A. LIEBERMAN, M.D.

Assistant Professor of Internal Medicine, Wayne State University; Director, Cardiac Electrophysiology, Harper University Hospital, Detroit Medical Center, Detroit, Michigan
Supraventricular Tachycardia; Pulseless Electrical Activity; Ventricular Tachycardia and Fibrillation; Conduction Disturbances

DOUGLAS F. LINDAHL, D.O.

Senior Resident, Department of Medicine, Maricopa Medical Center, Phoenix, Arizona
Urosepsis

PETER K. LINDEN, M.D.

Associate Professor of Critical Care Medicine, University of Pittsburgh School of Medicine; Director, Abdominal Organ Transplant ICU, University of Pittsburgh Medical Center, Pittsburgh, Pennsylvania
Candidal Infections; Non-Candidal Fungal Infections; Infections in Solid Organ Transplant Patients; Antifungal Therapy

ROBERT P. LISAK, M.D.

Professor and Chair of Neurology, and Professor of Immunology and Microbiology, Wayne State University School of Medicine; Neurologist-in-Chief, Detroit Medical Center; Chief of Neurology, Harper University Hospital; Attending Neurologist, Detroit Receiving Hospital, Detroit, Michigan
Myasthenia Gravis

ALAN LISBON, M.D.

Harvard Medical School; Chief, Division of Critical Care, Department of Anesthesia and Critical Care, Beth Israel Deaconess Medical Center, Boston, Massachusetts
Post-Cardiac Surgery Management; Post-Peripheral Vascular Bypass Management

G. DANIEL MARTICH, M.D.
Associate Professor of Critical Care Medicine, University of Pittsburgh Medical School; Executive Director, Electronic Health Record, University of Pittsburgh Medical Center Health Science; Medical Director, Critical Care Information System, and Co-Director, Cardiothoracic Intensive Care Unit, University of Pittsburgh Medical Center–Presbyterian University Hospital, University of Pittsburgh Medical Center Health Systems, Pittsburgh, Pennsylvania
Valvular Heart Disease

BRIAN A. MASON, M.D.
Associate Professor, Wayne State University School of Medicine, Detroit, Michigan
Pregnancy-Induced Hypertension; Obstetric Crises

JOAN MATTHEWS, M.D.
Adjunct Associate Professor of Clinical Anesthesia, University of Cincinnati, Cincinnati, Ohio
Hypotension

KENNETH R. McCURRY, M.D.
Assistant Professor of Surgery, University of Pittsburgh Medical Center; Director of Adult Lung Transplantation, University of Pittsburgh Medical Center–Presbyterian, Pittsburgh, Pennsylvania
Valvular Heart Disease

MARC D. MEISSNER, M.D., C.M., F.A.C.C., F.A.C.P.
Clinical Associate Professor of Internal Medicine, Wayne State University; Cardiovascular Education Coordinator, Staff Cardiologist, and Electrophysiologist, Sinai-Grace Hospital, Detroit, Michigan
Supraventricular Tachycardia; Pulseless Electrical Activity; Ventricular Fibrillation and Tachycardia; Conduction Disturbances

MARY M. MEYER, M.D.
Associate Professor, Division of Pulmonary and Critical Care Medicine, and Division of Nephrology and Hypertension, Oregon Health and Science University, Portland, Oregon
Diuretics

DANIEL B. MICHAEL, M.D., Ph.D., F.A.C.S.
Associate Professor of Neurological Surgery, Anatomy, and Cell Biology, Department of Neurological Surgery, Wayne State University School of Medicine; Chief of Neurosurgery, and Surgical Director, William R. Darmody M.D. Neurotrauma ICU, Detroit Receiving Hospital, Detroit, Michigan
Intracranial Hypertension; Intracranial Pressure Monitoring

M. SHERIF MOKHTAR, M.D.
Professor of Cardiology, and Chief, Department of Critical Care Medicine, Cairo University, Cairo, Egypt
Sedation Monitoring

LISA MUELLER, M.D.
Assistant Professor, Division of Hematology and Oncology, Department of Pediatrics, State University of New York at Stony Brook, Stony Brook, New York
Graft Versus Host Disease; Tumor Lysis Syndrome; Superior Vena Cava Syndrome; Complications of Chemotherapeutic Agents

ANH TU DUY NGUYEN, M.D.
Baylor College of Medicine, Houston, Texas
Botulism

DANE J. NICHOLS, M.D.
Assistant Professor of Medicine, Division of Pulmonary/Critical Care, Oregon Health Sciences University, Portland, Oregon
Sepsis and SIRS; Septic Shock

VIVEK PADEGAL, M.D.
Fellow, Pulmonary—Critical Care, Baylor College of Medicine, Houston, Texas
Neuroleptic Malignant Syndrome and Malignant Hyperthermia

PETER J. PAPADAKOS, M.D., F.C.C.M.
Associate Professor of Anesthesiology and Surgery, and Director, Division of Critical Care Medicine, University of Rochester School of Medicine, Rochester, New York
Respiratory Failure; Atelectasis; Neuroleptic Malignant Syndrome and Malignant Hyperthermia; Positive End-Expiratory Pressure

MARGARET M. PARKER, M.D.
Professor of Pediatrics, State University of New York at Stony Brook; Director, Pediatric Intensive Care Unit, University Medical Center, Stony Brook, New York
Meningitis; Encephalitis

ROBERT I. PARKER, M.D.
Associate Professor and Vice Chairman for Academic Affairs, and Director, Pediatric Hematology/Oncology, Department of Pediatrics, State University of New York at Stony Brook School of Medicine; Director, Pediatric Hematology/Oncology, University Hospital at Stony Brook, Stony Brook, New York
Hypercoagulable States; Thrombolytic Agents

DEVINA PRAKASH, M.D., M.B.B.S.
Assistant Professor, School of Medicine; Assistant Professor, Pediatric Hematology/Oncology, Department of Pediatrics, University Hospital, State University of New York at Stony Brook, Stony Brook, New York
Anemia; Acute Hemolytic Disorders; Transfusion Reactions; Sickle Cell Crises

JAI K. PRASAD, M.D., F.R.C.S., F.A.C.S.
Associate Professor of Surgery, Wayne State University School of Medicine; Medical Director, Burn Center, Detroit Receiving Hospital, Detroit, Michigan
Thermal Burn Injury; Electrical and Lightning Injuries; Pressure Ulcers

JAYA M. RAJ, M.D.
Clinical Instructor in Medicine, Mayo Graduate School of Medicine, Rochester, Minnesota, and University of Arizona College of Medicine, Tucson; Attending Physician, Maricopa Medical Center, Phoenix, Arizona
Alcohol Withdrawal Syndrome; Nosocomial Sinusitis

PAUL L. ROGERS, M.D.
Professor of Critical Care Medicine, and Director, Multidisciplinary Critical Care Medicine Training Program, University of Pittsburgh Medical School; Director, SICU, VA Pittsburgh Healthcare System, Pittsburgh, Pennsylvania
Fever; Barotrauma

MICHAEL J. RUFFING, PHARM.D.
Adjunct Assistant Professor, Wayne State University College of Pharmacy and Allied Health Professions, Detroit; Clinical Assistant Professor, University of Michigan College of Pharmacy, Ann Arbor; Clinical Coordinator, Pharmacy Services, and Clinical Specialist, Critical Care Medicine, Detroit Receiving Hospital, Detroit, Michigan
Benzodiazepines and Flumazenil; Propofol; Anticonvulsants; Antidysrhythmic Agents

FAYYAZ H. SAGARWALA, M.D., M.R.C.P.
Staff Nephrologist, Department of Medicine, Maricopa Medical Center, Phoenix, Arizona
Hemodialysis

SYED K. SHAHRYAR, M.D.
Chief, Medical Critical Care, and Director, Medical Intensive Care Unit, Maricopa Medical Center, Phoenix, Arizona
Cor Pulmonale; Smoke Inhalation; Venom Injuries: Snake and Arthropod; Near Drowning

MUKARRAM A. SIDDIQUI, M.D.
Fellow, Cardiology, Wayne State University School of Medicine, Detroit, Michigan
Pulseless Electrical Activity

ALLISON L. SOMERVILLE, PHARM.D.
Adjunct Assistant Professor of Pharmacy, Wayne State University; Clinical Pharmacist Specialist, Medicine/Critical Care, Detroit Receiving Hospital and University Health Center, Detroit, Michigan
Amrinone and Milrinone; Antihypertensives

FRANCISCO J. SOTO, M.D.
Baylor College of Medicine; Chief and Fellow, Pulmonary/Critical Care, Ben Taub General Hospital, Houston, Texas
Discontinuing Mechanical Ventilation

SHEILA SUDHAKAR, M.D., M.S.
Chief Resident, Maricopa Medical Center, Phoenix, Arizona
Intrahospital Transport

JAMES SULLIVAN, D.O.
Fellow, Department of Nephrology, Medical College of Georgia, Augusta, Georgia
Acute Renal Failure; Chronic Renal Failure

JANE E. SUNDBERG, PHARM.D., B.C.P.P.
Associate Professor in Psychiatry, University of Rochester Medical Center; Clinical Specialist—Psychopharmacology, Strong Memorial Hospital, Rochester, New York
Serotonin Syndrome

JAMES E. SZALADOS, M.D., M.B.A., M.H.A.
Vice-Chairman, Department of Anesthesiology, Associate Director, Adult Critical Care Medicine, and Associate Professor of Anesthesiology and Medicine, University of Rochester, University of Rochester School of Medicine, University of Rochester Medical Center; Adjunct Clinical Faculty, Rochester Institute of Technology, Rochester, New York
Pneumonia in Adults; Aspiration Pneumonitis and Pneumonia

PER THORBORG, M.D., Ph.D.
Associate Professor of Anesthesiology, Division of Critical Care Medicine, Oregon Health Sciences University, Portland, Oregon
Coagulopathy; Thrombocytopenia

SAMUEL A. TISHERMAN, M.D.
Associate Professor of Surgery and Critical Care Medicine, University of Pittsburgh Medical School, Pittsburgh, Pennsylvania
Myocardial Contusion; Abdominal Trauma; Abdominal Aortic Aneurysm

ALAIN TREMBLAY, M.D.
Baylor College of Medicine; Fellow, Ben Taub General Hospital, Houston, Texas
Acute Respiratory Distress Syndrome; Massive Hemoptysis; Conventional Mechanical Ventilation; Newer Modes of Mechanical Ventilation

ADRIANA H. WECHSLER, M.D.
Assistant Professor of Medicine, Department of Medicine, Baylor College of Medicine; Attending Emergency Physician, Emergency Center, Ben Taub General Hospital, Houston, Texas
Calcium Channel and β-Blocker Drug Overdoses; Heat Stroke

SUZANNE R. WHITE, M.D.
Associate Professor, Emergency Medicine and Pediatrics, Wayne State University School of Medicine; Medical Director, Children's Hospital of Michigan Regional Poison Control Center, Detroit, Michigan
Approach to Poisoning and Drug Overdose; Carbon Monoxide Poisoning; Anticholinergic Poisonings

Preface

The **Saunders Manual of Critical Care** is intended for intensivists and other acute care practitioners, including medical subspecialists, surgeons, emergency medicine physicians, trainees, clinicians, and nurses involved in the management of critically ill patients in the intensive care unit. The **Manual** provides a rapid review of common as well as infrequently encountered disorders, including diagnostic tips and a step-by-step approach to therapy. Both seasoned intensivists and house officers rotating on an ICU service will find a concise summary of the key facts needed for diagnosis, monitoring, and treatment.

The **Manual** is organized into sections, beginning with several problem-based chapters covering management approaches for some common physiologic derangements seen in critically ill patients. The main section contains 146 disease-oriented chapters grouped by organ system or discipline, covering common and uncommon diseases, syndromes, and disturbances of homeostasis from the perspective of the ICU setting. Acute derangements of the circulatory, respiratory, renal, gastrointestinal, and central nervous systems, as well as metabolic and hematologic disorders, are covered, as are those involving surgery, infectious diseases, and other disciplines. Accordingly, these chapters provide concise information regarding etiology, differential diagnosis, clinical manifestations, laboratory findings, diagnostic methods, and therapeutic approaches. Although prognostic information is given in many chapters, aspects of outpatient follow-up and long-term care are not included. A miscellaneous subsection deals with various disorders that are not readily classified by discipline or organ system, such as hypothermia, fat embolism syndrome, rhabdomyolysis, pressure ulcers, and air embolism.

Other sections deal with trauma and postoperative topics, procedures, monitoring, and critical care pharmacology. The pharmacology section provides key actions, indications, contraindications, and drug interactions, as well as standard doses and side effects for a wide variety of agents used in the ICU. The procedures section reviews the elements of common bedside diagnostic and therapeutic techniques, including their indications, technical aspects of their performance, and where appropriate, basic interpretation of findings. Figures illustrate selected procedural devices and relevant anatomic landmarks.

The section on monitoring covers the derivation and interpretation of numerical hemodynamic and oxygen transport data, describes techniques for intravascular and intracranial pressure measurement, and contains chapters on capnography, blood gas and oximetry interpretation, gastric tonometry, and nutritional assessment. Common pitfalls in applying some of these monitoring methods are also discussed. A final section on mechanical ventilation and respiratory techniques includes specific chapters on conventional and newer modes of positive pressure ventilation, oxygen therapy, positive end-expiratory pressure, and discontinuing mechanical ventilation.

Each chapter is a distillation of practical information required for bedside ICU management. When there is no clear consensus on therapeutic options, more than one approach to management is provided. Each chapter is encompassed within a few pages using an outline format along with boxed and bulleted key points and, where appropriate, tables and captioned graphics. Within each section, chapter-to-chapter conformity is maintained by drawing on a common pool of headings to provide a consistent approach and style. To allow for both brevity and the clarity required for the diversity of topics within the scope of critical care practice, only those headings deemed essential for a given chapter are used. Selected chapters contain flow diagrams that depict algorithmic approaches to diagnosis or management.

The reader who wishes to explore details of pathophysiologic mechanisms, examine controversial aspects of patient management, or delve deeply into pharmacokinetics is encouraged to consult standard comprehensive textbooks. For further reference or an in-depth review of specific aspects of a particular topic, a brief bibliography is listed at the end of each chapter.

The **Saunders Manual of Critical Care** focuses on useful and practical information that can be applied at the bedside of the critically ill or injured patient.

James A. Kruse, M.D.
Mitchell P. Fink, M.D.
Richard W. Carlson, M.D., Ph.D.

Contents

Part I
Frequently Encountered Problems in
the ICU 1

Part II
Pulmonary Disorders 17

Part III
Cardiac Disorders 59

Part IV
Electrolyte and Acid-Base Disturbances..... 119

Part V
Endocrine Emergencies...................... 164

Part VI
Toxicologic Emergencies 194

Part VII
Neurologic Crises 277

Part VIII
Infectious Diseases 317

Part IX
Hematologic Problems 406

Part X
Intra-Abdominal Disorders 439

Part XI
Renal Disorders 477

Part XII
Surgical, Traumatic, Postoperative
Conditions 484

Part XIII
Miscellaneous Disorders 525

Part XIV
Pharmacology 564

Part XV
Procedures 677

Part XVI
Monitoring...................................... 770

Part XVII
Respiratory Care and Mechanical
Ventilation 803

Index 823

Detailed table of contents begins on following right hand page

Part I
Frequently Encountered Problems in the ICU

1 Fever 1
Paul L. Rogers

2 Hypotension 5
Joan Matthews

3 Oliguria 8
Ali H. Al-Khafaji and Howard L. Corwin

4 Coma 11
Seemant Chaturvedi

5 Tachypnea and Hypoxemia 14
Willane S. Krell

Part II
Pulmonary Disorders

6 Respiratory Failure 17
Mark S. Chesnutt and Peter J. Papadakos

7 Pulmonary Edema 20
Eli Azzi and Charles M. Carpati

8 Acute Respiratory Distress Syndrome 23
Alain Tremblay and Kalpalatha K. Guntupalli

9 Barotrauma 28
Paul L. Rogers

10 Pulmonary Embolism 30
Tisha Fujii and Linda Kirschenbaum

11 Status Asthmaticus 34
Michael J. Apostolakos

12 Pneumonia in Adults 37
James E. Szalados

13 Aspiration Pneumonitis and Pneumonia 42
James E. Szalados

14 COPD Exacerbation 46
Michael J. Apostolakos

15 Cor Pulmonale 48
Syed K. Shahryar and Richard W. Carlson

16 Smoke Inhalation 51
Syed K. Shahryar, Chai Jie Chang, and
Richard W. Carlson

17 Massive Hemoptysis 53
Alain Tremblay and Kalpalatha K. Guntupalli

18 Atelectasis 57
Burkhard Lachmann and Peter J. Papadakos

Part III
Cardiac Disorders

19 Unstable Angina 59
Vivian L. Clark

20 Acute Myocardial Infarction 64
Vivian L. Clark

21 Right Ventricular Myocardial Infarction 69
Vivian L. Clark

22 Mechanical Complications of Acute Myocardial Infarction 71
Vivian L. Clark

23 Myocardial Contusion 73
Samuel A. Tisherman

24 Left Ventricular Failure 75
Arthur J. Boujoukos

25 Hypertensive Crisis 80
Jorge A. Guzman

26 Pregnancy-Induced Hypertension 83
Brian A. Mason

27 Cardiogenic Shock 88
Vivian L. Clark and James A. Kruse

28 Valvular Heart Disease 90
Kenneth R. McCurry and G. Daniel Martich

29 Pericarditis 96
Steven J. Lavine

30 Pericardial Tamponade 100
Vivian L. Clark

31 Aortic Dissection 102
Vivian L. Clark and James A. Kruse

32 Atrial Fibrillation and Flutter 104
Arthur J. Boujoukos

33 Supraventricular Tachycardia 107
Marc D. Meissner and Randy A. Lieberman

34 Pulseless Electrical Activity 111
Randy A. Lieberman, Marc D. Meissner, and
Mukarram A. Siddiqui

35 Ventricular Fibrillation and Tachycardia .. 114
Randy A. Lieberman and Marc D. Meissner

36 Conduction Disturbances 116
Marc D. Meissner and Randy A. Lieberman

Part IV
Electrolyte and Acid-Base Disturbances

37 Hyponatremia 119
James A. Kruse

38 Hypernatremia 124
James A. Kruse

39 Hypokalemia 129
James A. Kruse

40 Hyperkalemia 132
James A. Kruse

41 Hypocalcemia 135
Jorge A. Guzman and James A. Kruse

42 Hypercalcemia 139
Jorge A. Guzman and James A. Kruse

43 Hypomagnesemia 143
Jorge A. Guzman and James A. Kruse

44 Hypermagnesemia 146
Jorge A. Guzman and James A. Kruse

45 Hypophosphatemia 147
James A. Kruse

46 Hyperphosphatemia 151
James A. Kruse

47 Acid-Base Disturbances 154
James A. Kruse

48 Lactic Acidosis 158
James A. Kruse

49 Alcoholic Ketoacidosis 161
James A. Kruse

Part V
Endocrine Emergencies

50 Diabetic Ketoacidosis 164
James A. Kruse

51 Hyperosmolar Nonketotic Coma 168
James A. Kruse

52 Hypoglycemia 171
James A. Kruse

53 Diabetes Insipidus 174
James A. Kruse

54 Syndrome of Inappropriate Antidiuresis .. 178
James A. Kruse

55 Thyroid Storm 181
James A. Kruse

56 Myxedema Coma 184
James A. Kruse

57 Pheochromocytoma 187
James A. Kruse

58 Adrenal Insufficiency 191
James A. Kruse

Part VI
Toxicologic Emergencies

59 Approach to Poisoning and Drug Overdose 194
Suzanne R. White

60 Acetaminophen Overdose 201
James A. Kruse

61 Salicylate Intoxication 205
James A. Kruse

62 Sedative-Hypnotic and Narcotic Drug Overdose 209
James A. Kruse

63 Theophylline Overdose 213
James A. Kruse

64 Lithium Overdose 216
James A. Kruse

65 Cocaine Intoxication 219
James A. Kruse

66 Calcium Channel and β-Blocker Drug Overdoses 223
Adriana H. Wechsler and Richard W. Carlson

67 Digoxin Overdose 229
Salmaan Kanji and John W. Devlin

68 Alcohol and Glycol Intoxications 233
James A. Kruse

69 Alcohol Withdrawal Syndrome 240
Richard W. Carlson and Jaya M. Raj

70 Cyanide Poisoning 244
James A. Kruse

71 Carbon Monoxide Poisoning 249
Suzanne R. White

72 **Methemoglobinemia** 253
James A. Kruse

73 **Neuroleptic Drug Overdose** 256
Ho-Yin Adrian Li

74 **Cyclic Antidepressant Drug Overdose** 259
James A. Kruse

75 **Anticholinergic Poisonings** 263
Suzanne R. White

76 **Serotonin Syndrome** 267
Jane E. Sundberg

77 **Organophosphate Poisoning** 269
Ali A. Hamdan

78 **Venom Injuries: Snake and Arthropod** 272
Syed K. Shahryar and Richard W. Carlson

Part VII
Neurologic Crises

79 **Status Epilepticus** 277
James A. Kruse

80 **Cerebral Infarction** 281
Seemant Chaturvedi

81 **Intracerebral Hemorrhage** 284
Lakshmipathi Chelluri

82 **Subarachnoid Hemorrhage** 287
Marie R. Baldisseri

83 **Subdural Hematoma** 291
Marie R. Baldisseri

84 **Intracranial Hypertension** 293
Daniel B. Michael

85 **Spinal Cord Compression** 298
Perry A. Ball

86 **Neuroleptic Malignant Syndrome and Malignant Hyperthermia** 301
Vivek Padegal, Venkata Bandi, and
Peter J. Papadakos

87 **Myasthenia Gravis** 304
Robert P. Lisak

88 **Guillain-Barré Syndrome** 307
Richard A. Lewis

89 **Botulism** 311
Anh Tu Duy Nguyen and
Kalpalatha K. Guntupalli

90 **Tetanus** 314
Adel Ghuloom and Venkata Bandi

Part VIII
Infectious Diseases

91 **Sepsis and SIRS** 317
Dane J. Nichols

92 **Septic Shock** 321
Dane J. Nichols

93 **Gram-Positive Infections** 327
Donald P. Levine

94 **Gram-Negative Infections** 333
Donald P. Levine

95 **Candidal Infections** 339
Peter K. Linden

96 **Non-Candidal Fungal Infections** 344
Peter K. Linden

97 **Herpes Infections** 350
Pranatharthi H. Chandrasekar

98 **Cytomegalovirus Infections** 354
Lawrence R. Crane

99 **Acquired Immune Deficiency Syndrome** .. 356
Lawrence R. Crane

100 *Pneumocystis carinii* **Pneumonia** 359
Lawrence R. Crane

101 **Infections in Neutropenic Cancer Patients** 362
George J. Alangaden

102 **Infections in Bone Marrow Transplant Patients** 365
Pranatharthi H. Chandrasekar

103 **Infections in Solid Organ Transplant Patients** 369
Peter K. Linden

104 **Tuberculosis** 374
Dana G. Kissner

105 **Endocarditis** 379
Donald P. Levine

106 **Urosepsis** 384
Douglas F. Lindahl and Richard W. Carlson

107 Life-Threatening Infections of the Oropharynx 387
Remzi Bag

108 Meningitis 390
Margaret M. Parker

109 Encephalitis 392
Margaret M. Parker

110 Toxic Shock Syndrome 394
Susan E.Dantoni

111 Nosocomial Sinusitis 397
Meena Kakarala, Jaya M. Raj, and Richard W. Carlson

112 Necrotizing Soft-Tissue Infections 399
Mitchell P. Fink

113 Epiglottitis 402
Stacy J. Clark and Richard W. Carlson

114 Catheter-Related Bloodstream Infection .. 404
Stephen O. Heard

Part IX
Hematologic Problems

115 Coagulopathy 406
Per Thorborg

116 Thrombocytopenia 409
Per Thorborg

117 Hypercoagulable States 413
Robert I. Parker

118 Deep Venous Thrombosis 416
Remzi Bag

119 Anemia 421
Devina Prakash

120 Acute Hemolytic Disorders 425
Devina Prakash

121 Transfusion Reactions 429
Devina Prakash

122 Sickle Cell Crises 433
Devina Prakash

123 Graft Versus Host Disease 436
Lisa Mueller

Part X
Intra-Abdominal Disorders

124 Acute Abdominal Pain 439
Mitchell P. Fink

125 Acute Pancreatitis 446
Mitchell P. Fink

126 Acute Cholecystitis 450
Mitchell P. Fink

127 Acute Alcoholic Hepatitis 452
David J. Kramer

128 Viral Hepatitis 455
David J. Kramer

129 Fulminant Hepatic Failure 458
David J. Kramer

130 Upper Gastroenteral Hemorrhage 463
Mitchell P. Fink

131 Lower Gastroenteral Hemorrhage 466
Murray N. Ehrinpreis

132 Diarrhea 470
Murray N. Ehrinpreis

133 Toxic Megacolon 474
Murray N. Ehrinpreis

Part XI
Renal Disorders

134 Acute Renal Failure 477
James Sullivan and Richard W. Carlson

135 Chronic Renal Failure 481
James Sullivan and Richard W. Carlson

Part XII
Surgical, Traumatic, Postoperative Conditions

136 Preoperative Evaluation of the Critically Ill Patient 484
Stephen O. Heard

137 Chest Trauma 488
Keith D. Clancy and Mitchell P. Fink

138 Abdominal Trauma 491
Samuel A. Tisherman

139 Traumatic Brain Injury 494
Joseph M. Darby

140 Post-Craniotomy Management 498
Lakshmipathi Chelluri

141 Post-Cardiac Surgery Management 500
Alan Lisbon and Mitchell P. Fink

142 Post-Peripheral Vascular Bypass Management 504
Alan Lisbon

143 Acute Peripheral Arterial Occlusion 507
T.J. Bunt

144 Abdominal Aortic Aneurysm 509
Samuel A. Tisherman

145 Thermal Burn Injury 512
Jai K. Prasad

146 Electrical and Lightning Injuries 517
Jai K. Prasad and James A. Kruse

147 Kidney Transplantation 521
Stephen A. Bowles

Part XIII
Miscellaneous Disorders

148 Hypothermia 525
Nicola A. Hanania

149 Heat Stroke 530
Adriana H. Wechsler

150 Anaphylaxis 534
Marilyn T. Haupt

151 Near Drowning 537
Syed K. Shahryar and Richard W. Carlson

152 Fat Embolism 539
Remzi Bag

153 Rhabdomyolysis 542
James A. Kruse

154 Tumor Lysis Syndrome 546
Lisa Mueller

155 Superior Vena Cava Syndrome 549
Lisa Mueller

156 Obstetric Crises 552
Brian A. Mason

157 Pressure Ulcers 557
Jai K. Prasad

158 Air Embolism 561
Elizabeth S. Guy

Part XIV
Pharmacology

159 Intravenous Fluids 564
James A. Kruse

160 Amrinone and Milrinone 568
Allison L. Somerville and James A. Kruse

161 Vasoactive Catecholamines 571
James A. Kruse

162 Antihypertensives 575
Allison L. Somerville

163 Fenoldopam 583
Jorge A. Guzman

164 Nitroglycerin 585
Jorge A. Guzman

165 Nitroprusside 587
Jorge A. Guzman

166 Diuretics 589
Mary M. Meyer

167 Acid-Inhibiting Agents and Sucralfate 593
John W. Devlin and James A. Kruse

168 Neuromuscular Blocking Drugs 597
John W. Devlin and James A. Kruse

169 Narcotic Agonists and Naloxone 602
John W. Devlin

170 Benzodiazepines and Flumazenil 605
Michael J. Ruffing and James A. Kruse

171 Propofol 609
Michael J. Ruffing

172 Anticonvulsants 611
Michael J. Ruffing

173 Anticoagulants 617
Mark A. Douglass and James A. Kruse

174 Thrombolytic Agents 622
Robert I. Parker

175 **Glycoprotein IIb/IIIa Receptor Antagonists** 624
Vivian L. Clark

176 **Digoxin** 626
Salmaan Kanji and John W. Devlin

177 **Antidysrhythmic Agents** 629
Michael J. Ruffing and Vivian L. Clark

178 **Dantrolene** 634
Jeff D. Huntress

179 **Inhaled Bronchodilators** 636
Jeff D. Huntress

180 **Filgrastim** 639
Mitchell P. Fink

181 **Complications of Chemotherapeutic Agents** 641
Lisa Mueller

182 **Penicillins and Cephalosporins** 645
Geneen M. Gibson

183 **Aminoglycosides** 650
Robert DiCenzo

184 **Fluoroquinolone Antibiotics** 653
Mitchell P. Fink

185 **Macrolides** 655
Rebecca L. Corey

186 **Antituberculosis Drugs** 660
Dana G. Kissner

187 **Miscellaneous Antibiotics** 665
Jeff D. Huntress

188 **Antifungal Therapy** 671
Peter K. Linden

Part XV
Procedures

189 **Endotracheal Intubation** 677
James A. Kruse

190 **Central Venous Catheterization** 683
James A. Kruse

191 **Arterial Catheterization** 687
James A. Kruse

192 **Pulmonary Artery Catheterization** 690
James A. Kruse

193 **Temporary Transvenous Pacemaker** 694
James A. Kruse

194 **Transcutaneous Pacing** 699
Steven Borzak

195 **Cardioversion and Defibrillation** 701
Steven Borzak

196 **Pericardiocentesis** 704
Vivian L. Clark

197 **Intra-Aortic Balloon Counterpulsation** 706
Vivian L. Clark

198 **Fiberoptic Bronchoscopy** 709
Willane S. Krell

199 **Lumbar Puncture** 713
James A. Kruse

200 **Paracentesis** 716
James A. Kruse

201 **Thoracentesis** 719
James A. Kruse

202 **Chest Tube Thoracostomy** 724
James A. Kruse

203 **Hemodialysis** 729
Fayyaz H. Sagarwala and Richard W. Carlson

204 **Continuous Renal Replacement Therapy** 733
Ali H. Al-Khafaji and Howard L. Corwin

205 **Intrahospital Transport** 737
Sheila Sudhakar and Richard W. Carlson

206 **Do Not Resuscitate Orders** 739
Margaret L. Campbell

207 **Brain Death Determination** 742
James A. Kruse

208 **Fluid Challenge** 746
James A. Kruse

209 **Sengstaken-Blakemore Tube Placement** .. 749
James A. Kruse

210 **Transnasal and Transoral Gastroenteric Intubation** 754
James A. Kruse

211 **Enteral Feeding** 760
Jorge A. Guzman

212 **Parenteral Nutrition** 764
Jorge A. Guzman

Part XVI
Monitoring

213 Nutritional Assessment 770
Jorge A. Guzman

214 Hemodynamic Monitoring 774
James A. Kruse

215 Fast Flush Test 778
James A. Kruse

216 Monitoring Oxygen Transport 781
Jorge A. Guzman

217 Capnography 784
Jorge A. Guzman

218 Blood Gas and Oximetry Monitoring 788
James A. Kruse

219 Gastric Tonometry 793
Jorge A. Guzman

220 Intracranial Pressure Monitoring 796
Daniel B. Michael

221 Sedation Monitoring 800
M. Sherif Mokhtar and Richard W. Carlson

Part XVII
Respiratory Care and Mechanical Ventilation

222 Oxygen Therapy 803
James A. Kruse

223 Conventional Mechanical Ventilation 808
Alain Tremblay and Kalpalatha K. Guntupalli

224 Newer Modes of Mechanical Ventilation 813
Alain Tremblay and Kalpalatha K. Guntupalli

225 Positive End-Expiratory Pressure 817
Ali A. Hamdan and Peter J. Papadakos

226 Discontinuing Mechanical Ventilation 820
Francisco J. Soto and Kalpalatha K. Guntupalli

Index 823

1 Fever

Paul L. Rogers

Definition and Pathophysiology

A. Definition
1. Fever is defined as an increase in body temperature exceeding the normal circadian variation.
2. Normal core body temperature is $36.8° \pm 0.4°C$ ($98.2° \pm 0.7°F$) and varies in a circadian fashion by approximately $0.6°C$ ($1°F$), being lowest in the morning.

B. Pathophysiology
1. Endogenous pyrogens (including the cytokines interleukin-1, and tumor necrosis factor) are released by monocytes and macrophages in response to inflammation, injury, or infection.
2. These cytokines regulate temperatures in the hypothalamus by releasing prostaglandin E_2 (PGE_2).
3. Fever may enhance the immune response to infection; mediated, in part, by augmenting T and B cell responses.

Etiology

A. Common infectious causes of fever: the differential diagnosis is influenced by the patient population (medical vs. surgical, immunocompromised vs. immunocompetent, community vs. nosocomial)
1. Central nervous system (CNS)
   a. Meningitis
   b. Encephalitis
   c. Abscess
2. Cardiovascular
   a. Vascular-catheter related
   b. Endocarditis
3. Pulmonary
   a. Pneumonia
   b. Empyema
4. Gastrointestinal
   a. Intra-abdominal abscess
   b. Cholecystitis (calculous or acalculous)
   c. Antibiotic-related colitis
   d. Peritonitis
   e. Perirectal abscess
5. Renal
   a. Cystitis
   b. Pyelonephritis
   c. Perinephric abscess
6. Cutaneous
   a. Cellulitis
   b. Wound infection
   c. Necrotizing soft-tissue infection
7. Sinusitis

B. Noninfectious causes of fever
1. Central nervous system
   a. Hemorrhage (subarachnoid or intracerebral)
   b. Infarction
2. Cardiovascular
   a. Myocardial infarction
   b. Pericarditis
3. Pulmonary
   a. Atelectasis
   b. Pulmonary embolism
   c. Fibroproliferative phase of acute respiratory distress syndrome
4. Gastrointestinal
   a. Acalculous cholecystitis
   b. Pancreatitis
5. Rheumatologic or autoimmune
   a. Vasculitis (e.g., polyarteritis nodosa, temporal arteritis, Wegener's granulomatosis)
   b. Collagen vascular disease (e.g., systemic lupus erythematosus, rheumatoid arthritis, Sjögren's syndrome)
6. Endocrine
   a. Hyperthyroidism
   b. Adrenal insufficiency
   c. Pheochromocytoma
7. Miscellaneous
   a. Drug fever (e.g., antibiotics, methyldopa, procainamide, phenytoin)
   b. Transfusion reactions (packed red blood cells or platelets)
   c. Neoplasm (e.g., lymphoma, renal cell carcinoma, hepatoma)
   d. Malignant hyperthermia (due to genetic predisposition and exposure to succinylcholine or inhaled anesthetic agents)

e. Neuroleptic malignant syndrome (due to decreased levels of dopamine in the CNS in response to antidopaminergic antipsychotic neuroleptic drugs or rapid withdrawal of levodopa)

f. Serotonin syndrome

g. Withdrawal syndromes (e.g., opioids, alcohol)

h. Procedures associated with transient bacteremia or endotoxemia (e.g., hemodialysis, endoscopy)

Key Evaluation

- Perform a focused history and physical examination to exclude noninfectious etiologies and identify the most likely source.

- Obtain two sets of blood cultures (10 to 15 mL of blood each) for patients with a new fever.

- If infection is thought to be the most likely cause of the new fever, perform a thorough, site-specific evaluation (see Management).

Management

A. General considerations

1. A key problem for physicians caring for the febrile patients in the ICU is that the differential diagnosis includes numerous infectious as well as noninfectious etiologies.

2. Unless the clinician's response to the evaluation and treatment of patients with fever is thoughtful, many patients will be treated unnecessarily with expensive antibiotics, driving up the cost of health care and promoting the emergence of resistant microbes.

3. Temperatures exceeding 38.3°C should initiate an evaluation of possible infectious sources.

4. Oral, rectal, or central (via intravascular thermistor) measurements of temperature are acceptable; axillary and groin measurements should not be considered reliable.

5. Because fever may enhance the immune response to infection, most patients should not routinely receive empiric antipyretic medications.

6. Antipyretics are indicated for the control of fever in the following groups of patients:

   a. Patients with coronary artery disease, in whom tachycardia can result in increased myocardial oxygen consumption

   b. Patients with intracranial trauma

   c. Children with previous febrile or nonfebrile seizures

7. Cyclo-oxygenase inhibitors, such as ibuprofen and aspirin, exert antipyretic effects by inhibiting PGE_2 synthesis

8. Acetaminophen has antipyretic effects because it is oxidized in the CNS to a cyclo-oxygenase inhibitor

B. Infectious etiologies

1. CNS

   a. Meningitis is more common in medical patients, but it should be considered in patients after neurosurgery or instrumentation of the CNS (e.g., placement of an intraventricular pressure monitor).

   b. Although CNS infections are usually associated with focal neurologic findings, sedatives and opioids may alter the examination.

   c. If the patient has evidence of focal neurologic findings, computed tomography (CT) of the head (without contrast) should be performed prior to diagnostic lumbar puncture.

   d. Cerebrospinal fluid studies should be sent for glucose and protein concentrations, total and differential white cell count, Gram stain, and culture.

   e. If CNS infection is considered likely, antibiotics should not be withheld while awaiting computed tomography and lumbar puncture.

2. Vascular catheter-related fever

   a. Non-cuffed catheters have a higher risk for catheter-related bloodstream infection.

   b. Inflammation or purulence at the insertion site suggests catheter-related infection.

   c. Two blood cultures should be obtained from peripheral sites.

   d. Catheters should be removed and the catheter tip sent for semi-quantitative culture (an intracutaneous segment of the catheter may also be sent for culture).

   e. The finding of positive blood cultures along with growth of the same organism from the catheter culture (>15 colony forming units) is consistent with the diagnosis of catheter-related bloodstream infection.

3. Pulmonary infections

   a. Pulmonary infections are often difficult to diagnose in intubated patients in the intensive care unit (ICU).

   b. When history, physical examination, and chest x-ray are suggestive of pneumonia, sputum should be sampled by deep suctioning and processed within 2 hours.

   c. Bronchoscopy should be considered for immunosuppressed patients when *Pneumocystis carinii,* cytomegalovirus, or *Mycobacterium* species are possible pathogens.

d. Consider diagnostic thoracentesis if pleural effusion is present.

   (1) Not all patients with fever and pleural effusion require diagnostic thoracentesis.

   (2) Patients with hypoalbuminemia, congestive heart failure, or subphrenic postoperative processes, for example, do not need thoracentesis unless infection is considered likely and the pleural fluid can be safely aspirated.

   (3) Fluid should be sent to the laboratory for protein and glucose concentration, total and differential cell counts, pH, Gram stain, culture, and cytology.

4. Antibiotic-associated colitis

  a. The most common cause of fever with concomitant diarrhea in the ICU is colitis caused by a toxin released from *Clostridium difficile.*

  b. *C. difficile* colitis should be considered in any patient with these symptoms who received antibiotics within the previous 3 weeks.

  c. Stool specimens should be analyzed for the presence of *C. difficile* toxin.

  d. If two specimens are negative, flexible sigmoidoscopy can be performed to exclude the diagnosis.

  e. If the diagnosis of *C. difficile* colitis is strongly suspected, then metronidazole (500 mg every 6 hours) should be given until laboratory results are available.

5. Urinary tract infection

  a. Most patients in the ICU with catheters have bacteriuria; whether it is the cause of fever is often difficult to determine.

  b. Urine should be collected from a sampling port (rather than from the Foley collection bag) and sent for chemical and microscopic urinalysis, Gram stain, and quantitative bacterial culture.

  c. If pyuria (>10 white blood cells per high-power field) and more than 10^5 CFU/mL are present, antibiotic treatment for urinary tract infection should be initiated.

6. Skin

  a. Surgical wound infections occur in 3% to 6% of patients postoperatively.

  b. The likelihood of infection increases if the operative site was contaminated or dirty.

  c. Wounds should be examined for erythema and purulence.

  d. If the site is suspected as a source of fever, the wound should be opened and any purulent material sent for culture.

7. Sinusitis

  a. Patients with nasotracheal or nasogastric tubes are at greatest risk for development of sinusitis.

  b. Patients with facial pain, orbital edema, or purulent nasal drainage should be evaluated with CT.

  c. Ultrasonography is sensitive but not specific.

  d. Treatment includes removal of the nasogastric or nasotracheal tube, decongestant sprays, and appropriate antibiotic therapy.

  e. If clinically indicated, the sinuses should be drained and the aspirate sent for culture.

C. Noninfectious etiologies

1. Postoperative patients

  a. Fever after an operation is usually benign and self-limited if it occurs within 4 days of surgery.

  b. Early fever is likely related to pulmonary atelectasis and responds to pulmonary toilet and incentive spirometry; no other intervention is required unless alternative infectious etiologies are identified.

  c. Early wound infections are rare; however, sites should be evaluated for signs of group A streptococcal or clostridial myonecrosis.

2. Drug fever

  a. The onset of fever after drug administration is variable.

  b. The diagnosis is confirmed by the resolution of fever after discontinuation of the medication.

  c. Resolution of fever after discontinuation of the offending drug may take days.

3. Transfusion reactions

  a. Most reactions are mild and consist of fever secondary to inflammatory mediators released in response to alloantigens present on white blood cells.

  b. If the patient develops a fever during transfusion, blood products should be discontinued and an antihistamine (e.g., diphenhydramine) administered.

  c. Severe hemolytic reactions due to ABO incompatibility occur in 1 of 6,000 transfusions and result in hemolysis as well as fever.

4. Malignant hyperthermia

  a. Body temperature increases rapidly, along with muscle rigidity, tachycardia, and increasing end-tidal PCO_2.

b. Typical laboratory results include acidosis, hyperkalemia, and elevated myoglobin levels.

c. If the diagnosis is suspected, it is crucial to discontinue surgery and stop all anesthetic agents.

d. Pharmacotherapy consists of dantrolene, 2 mg/kg every 5 minutes for a total dose of 10 mg/kg.

e. After the event, myoglobinuria and renal failure may develop.

5. Neuroleptic malignant syndrome

a. Symptoms include fever, muscle rigidity, and hypercapnea (similar to those observed with malignant hyperthermia).

b. Treatment includes discontinuation of potentially offending neuroleptic agent or reinstitution of levodopa (if it had been abruptly discontinued), and administration of dantrolene (see above).

6. Serotonin syndrome

a. Occurs with psychiatric drugs that increase serotonin levels, including serotonin reuptake inhibitors and monoamine oxidase inhibitors.

b. The symptoms are similar to those described above.

c. Treatment includes removal of the likely agent.

PEARLS

- Not all fevers are caused by infection.
- The clinician should make every effort to distinguish infectious from noninfectious causes of fever in order to minimize the unecessary admininstration of antibiotics.
- Review all medications: if one is considered a likely cause of a drug-related fever, discontinue it and replace it with another drug (if possible).

Bibliography

Chuma BA. Fever in the critical care unit. Crit Care Clin 1998;14:1–14.

Circiumaru B, Bladdock G, Cohen J. A prospective study of fever in the intensive care unit. Intensive Care Med 1998;25:668–673.

O'Grady NP, Barre PS, Bartlett JG, et al. Practice guidelines for evaluating new fever in critically ill patients. Clin Infect Dis 1998;26:1042–1059.

2 Hypotension

Joan Matthews

Arterial blood pressure (BP) can be measured using a variety of noninvasive or invasive methods. Commonly used noninvasive methods include manual measurements using a sphygmomanometer and a stethoscope as well as a variety of automated approaches, such as oscillometry and photoplethysmography. Direct (invasive) measurement of blood pressure is almost always performed by using fluid-filled tubing connecting an intra-arterial catheter to an external strain-gauge transducer. The signal generated by the transducer is electronically amplified and displayed as a continuous waveform. Digital values for systolic, diastolic, and mean arterial pressure (MAP) are also displayed by the monitor. When using direct measurements of intra-arterial pressure to monitor patients, clinicians should be in the habit of using MAP readings as the basis for making decisions. In contradistinction to systolic and diastolic BP, MAP is not affected by under- or over-damping of the catheter-tubing-transducer system.

Key Definitions

- Hypotension can be defined as a decrease in MAP to less than 80% of the resting baseline value.

- When the baseline value is unknown, common operational definitions are systolic BP less than 90 or MAP less than 70 mm Hg.

Etiology

A. MAP is determined by a physiological version of Ohm's law.
1. $MAP = CVP + (CO \times SVR/80)$, where CVP is central venous pressure (mm Hg), CO is cardiac output (L/min), and SVR is systemic vascular resistance (dyne $\cdot$ sec/cm^5)
2. Because CO = heart rate (beats/min) $\times$ stroke volume (mL), $MAP \approx$ heart rate $\times$ stroke volume $\times$ SVR.
3. Therefore, hypotension (low MAP) can be caused by low SVR, low stroke volume (SV), low heart rate, or a combination of any of these factors.

B. Causes of low SVR
1. Sepsis
2. Systemic inflammatory response syndrome
3. Vasodilating drugs
4. Spinal or epidural anesthetics
5. Other drugs (e.g., narcotics, benzodiazepines, propofol)
6. Spinal or neurogenic shock due to trauma

C. Causes of low stroke volume
1. The determinants of stroke volume are cardiac preload, afterload, contractility, and valvular competence.
2. Preload is determined by ventricular end-diastolic volume (V), which is a function of intracavitary pressure (P_i), extramural pressure (P_e), and ventricular compliance (C), such that $V \propto (P_i - P_e) \times C$. Therefore, causes of low preload include
   a. Low filling pressure
      (1) Hypovolemia
      (2) Tachydysrthythmia or loss of atrial systole (NOTE: in these conditions left ventricular end-diastolic pressure may be low despite normal or elevated central venous pressure or pulmonary artery occlusion pressure.)
   b. High extramural pressure
      (1) Cardiac tamponade
      (2) Positive end-expiratory pressure (PEEP)
      (3) Dynamic hyperinflation (intrinsic PEEP)
      (4) Tension pneumothorax
   c. Decreased myocardial compliance (e.g., due to left ventricular hypertrophy)
3. High (right ventricular) afterload
   a. Pulmonary embolism
   b. Pulmonary hypertension
4. Decreased myocardial contractility
   a. Right ventricular (RV)
   b. Left ventricular (LV)
   c. Biventricular
5. Acute valvular dysfunction: valvular insufficiency diminishes net forward flow.

D. Low heart rate (i.e., bradydysrhythmia)

Diagnostic Evaluation

A. Noninvasive methods
1. Electrocardiogram
   a. Rhythm disturbance

b. Ischemia

c. Infarction

d. Right ventricular strain (indicative of pulmonary hypertension or embolism)

e. Decreased voltage (decreased myocardial mass)

f. Right ventricular hypertrophy

g. Left ventricular hypertrophy

2. Chest x-ray

a. Pneumothorax

b. Pulmonary congestion

3. Echocardiography

a. Tamponade

b. Valvular dysfunction

c. Systolic dysfunction

d. Diastolic dysfunction (i.e., poor diastolic filling)

B. Invasive methods

1. Central venous pressure (CVP) monitoring

a. Central venous pressure provides an estimate of RV filling pressure.

b. If CVP is low (i.e., <4 mm Hg), the most likely diagnosis is hypovolemia.

c. If CVP is very high (i.e., >15 mm Hg), then the clinician should suspect problems associated with high extramural pressure (e.g., tamponade, tension pneumothorax).

d. If CVP is intermediate (i.e, >4, but <15 mm Hg), then the diagnosis is uncertain and virtually any of the above causes of hypotension could be present.

e. Monitoring using a central venous catheter is helpful when large shifts in intravascular volume are anticipated in a patient without risk factors for other causes of hypotension.

2. Pulmonary artery (PA) catheterization

a. The following parameters can be monitored using a conventional thermodilution PA catheter: CVP; systolic, diastolic, and mean PA pressure; PA occlusion pressure (PAOP); CO; mixed venous oxygen saturation ($S\bar{v}O_2$).

b. It is important to collect and analyze the available data in a systematic step-wise fashion; evaluate CO first.

c. If CO is high or normal, treat for low SVR state.

d. If CO is low, determine whether the problem is bradycardia or low SV.

e. If SV is low, assess left ventricular filling (PAOP).

f. If PAOP is high (>18 mm Hg), look for evidence of LV systolic dysfunction (ECG and echocardiography) or causes of increased extracardiac pressure (tamponade, pneumothorax) or decreased compliance.

3. If PAOP is low (<8 mm Hg), examine right ventricular filling (CVP) and afterload (PA pressure).

4. If CVP is low, treat for hypovolemia.

5. If CVP is high and PA pressure is low, look for evidence of RV systolic dysfunction (using ECG and echocardiography).

6. If CVP and PA pressure are high, look for pulmonary causes of pulmonary hypertension (pulmonary embolism, acute respiratory distress syndrome).

Treatment

A. Low SVR

1. Administer a vasoconstrictor.

a. Phenylephrine is a pure α-adrenergic agonist.

b. Dopamine exhibits predominantly α-adrenergic effects when infused at higher doses (i.e., >8 μg/kg per minute)

c. Norepinephrine is a mixed agonist that exhibits both α- and β-adrenergic effects, but it causes a net increase in SVR and inotropic state.

2. Treat the underlying problem; e.g., administer antibiotics for sepsis and discontinue vasodilating drugs.

B. Bradycardia

1. Transvenous or transcutaneous electrical pacing

2. Positive chronotropic drugs (e.g., epinephrine, atropine, isoproterenol)

C. Low or inadequate stroke volume

1. Treat hypovolemia by rapid infusion of IV fluids.

a. Crystalloids (normal saline or Ringer's lactate solution)

b. Colloids (e.g., 5% albumin or 6% hetastarch)

c. Packed red blood cells (if hematocrit is low)

2. Treat impaired diastolic filling due to a dysrhythmia by using pharmacologic or electrical cardioversion.

3. Treat LV systolic dysfunction.

a. Inotropic agents (e.g., epinephrine, dobutamine, milrinone, amrinone)

b. Agents to improve myocardial perfusion (cautious doses of a coronary vasodilator like nitroglycerine)

c. Devices to provide mechanical assistance for a failing ventricle
   (1) Intra-aortic balloon counterpulsation
   (2) Ventricular assist device
4. Treat RV systolic dysfunction.
   a. Inotropic agents
   b. Agents to improve myocardial perfusion (cautious doses of a coronary vasodilator like nitroglycerine)
   c. Pulmonary vasodilators (inhaled nitric oxide, inhaled prostacyclin)
5. Treat causes of high extramural pressure.
   a. For tamponade, perform pericardiocentesis, create a pericardial window, or (in the early postoperative period after median sternotomy and cardiac surgery) reopen the chest incision.
   b. For tension pneumothorax, use needle decompression (second intercostal space in the midclavicular line), then place a chest tube.
   c. For dynamic hyperinflation, administer bronchodilators and adjust ventilator settings to permit adequate time for expiration.

B Bibliography

Dorman T, Breslow MJ, Lipsett PA, et al. Radial artery pressure monitoring underestimates central arterial pressure during vasopressor therapy in critically ill surgical patients. Crit Care Med 1998;26:1646–1649.

Melo J, Peters JI. Low systemic vascular resistance: differential diagnosis. Crit Care 1999;3:71–77.

3 Oliguria

Ali H. Al-Khafaji
Howard L. Corwin

Definition

A. Urine output less than 400 mL/day
B. Often viewed as the hallmark of acute renal failure.
C. Can result from either functional or structural renal abnormalities.

Etiology

A. Pre-renal causes (volume depletion or decreased effective circulatory volume)
  1. Hypovolemia due to
    a. Hemorrhage
    b. Gastrointestinal volume losses
    c. Renal volume losses
    d. Cutaneous volume losses
  2. Volume redistribution due to
    a. Sequestration of fluid into the third space (e.g., the peritoneal cavity)
    b. Hypoalbuminemia
    c. Vasodilation (e.g., as occurs in sepsis)
  3. Decreased cardiac function due to
    a. Congestive heart failure
    b. Cor pulmonale
    c. Circulatory shock
    d. Valvular heart disease
    e. Pericardial tamponade
  4. Renal vascular disease
B. Renal causes—abnormalities of the renal parenchyma
  1. Glomerular damage or dysfunction due to
    a. Primary glomerulonephritis
    b. Glomerulonephritis secondary to systemic disease
  2. Tubulointerstitial damage or dysfunction due to
    a. Ischemia or reperfusion injury (acute tubular necrosis)
    b. Nephrotoxins (e.g., aminoglycosides, amphotericin B)
    c. Drug-induced allergic interstitial nephritis
    d. Immune complex formation (non-drug-related)
    e. Metabolic toxins (e.g., uric acid, calcium)
  3. Vascular damage or dysfunction due to
    a. Renal atheroemboli
    b. Small-vessel disease (e.g., diabetes mellitus, scleroderma)
    c. Disseminated intravascular coagulopathy
    d. Thrombotic thrombocytopenic purpura
    e. Renal vascular occlusion
C. Post-renal causes (obstruction to urine output)
  1. Ureteral obstruction
    a. Intra-ureteral
      (1) Calculi
      (2) Papillary necrosis
      (3) Crystalluria
      (4) Tumor
      (5) Blood clots
    b. Extra-ureteral
      (1) Tumor
      (2) Retroperitoneal fibrosis
  2. Bladder obstruction
    a. Prostatic hypertrophy or malignancy
    b. Bladder tumor
    c. Functional neuropathy
    d. Calculus
    e. Blood clot
  3. Urethral obstruction
    a. Stricture
    b. Meatal stenosis
    c. Phimosis or paraphimosis
  4. Foley catheter occlusion

Laboratory Tests

A. Urinalysis
  1. Dipstick test
    a. Strongly positive test for protein suggests intrinsic renal disease with glomerular damage.
    b. Conditions other than glomerular lesions tend to be associated with lower levels of proteinuria.
    c. Proteinuria should be quantified using a 24-hour collection.
  2. Microscopic examination of centrifuged urine for the presence of cells, casts, cellular debris in the resulting sediment (the most important part of the urinalysis)

a. Pre-renal
   (1) Rare cells
   (2) Hyaline casts
b. Tubular injury
   (1) Epithelial cells, cellular debris
   (2) Pigmented granular casts
c. Interstitial nephritis
   (1) White blood cells (WBCs)
   (2) WBC casts
   (3) Eosinophils
d. Glomerulonephritis
   (1) Red blood cells (RBCs)
   (2) RBC casts
e. Postrenal
   (1) Variable (can be bland sediment)
   (2) Crystals, RBCs, or WBCs possible

B. Sulfosalicylic acid precipitation test
   1. A dipstick test may be negative or weakly positive in patients with multiple myeloma.
   2. The sulfosalicylic acid assay will yield a positive result in these cases.

C. Urine diagnostic indices
   1. Most useful for distinguishing pre-renal causes from renal causes of oliguria
   2. However, considerable overlap exists and there are exceptions (e.g., acute glomerulonephritis may have urine indices similar to pre-renal oliguria).

Imaging Studies

A. Primarily useful for identifying obstruction
B. Can provide clues to the presence of renal disease
C. May also be used to assess renal blood flow abnormalities
D. Specific modalities

1. Renal ultrasonography: the simplest initial test to detect evidence of obstruction
2. Computed tomography: useful for detecting obstruction once a urinary catheter is placed or, if present, has been flushed to make certain that catheter is not clogged
3. Antegrade or retrograde contrast radiography
4. Intravenous pyelography: no role in the evaluation of oliguria
5. Arteriography
6. Duplex sonography
7. Radionuclide scan
8. Magnetic resonance imaging

Other Tests

A. Renal biopsy
   1. Usually not necessary for the evaluation of oliguria
   2. May be useful to establish the diagnosis of certain intrinsic renal diseases (e.g., acute glomerular or interstitial nephritis)
B. Hemodynamic monitoring: occasionally may be necessary to assess intravascular volume status, cardiac function, and effective circulating volume

> **PEARL**
>
> Evaluation of the patient with oliguria should focus on early identification of functional and potentially reversible causes.

Treatment

A. General
   1. Optimize intravascular volume status and cardiac function.
   2. Avoid additional renal insults.

Key Laboratory Findings

Urine Diagnostic Index	Pre-renal Cause	Renal Cause
• Urine sodium concentration	<20 mmol/L	>40 mmol/L
• Fractional excretion of sodium	<1%	>1%
• Urine osmolality	>500 mOsm/kg H_2O	<350 mOsm/kg H_2O
• Urine/plasma creatinine	>40	<40
• Blood urea nitrogen/creatinine ratio	>20	<10
• Urine/plasma urea	>8	<3 (post-renal cause)

Key Treatment

- Initial evaluation of a patient with acute oliguria is directed to differentiating among pre-renal, renal, and post-renal causes.

- Examination of the urine sediment and measurement of urine sodium, fractional excretion of sodium, and osmolality are the most useful initial diagnostic studies.

- Renal ultrasonography is the best initial imaging study to exclude obstruction.

- Oliguria from pre-renal factors is often reversible.

- Oliguria from intrinsic renal disease often requires renal replacement therapy.

B. Diuretics

1. Scant data to support the contention that mannitol or loop diuretics can prevent or ameliorate the course of established renal failure

2. Continuous infusion of loop diuretic (e.g., up to 40 mg/hour furosemide) may be more effective than IV bolus dosing in inducing a diuresis in otherwise diuretic-resistant patients.

C. Low-dose dopamine

1. Has diuretic and natriuretic properties in the functioning kidney

2. Few data support its use in preserving renal function.

D. Renal replacement therapy

1. Intermittent hemodialysis, (continuous arterio-venous hemofiltration, or continuous veno-venous hemofiltration

2. Continuous therapy is particularly effective for controlling volume status.

Bibliography

Corwin HL, Bonventre JV. Acute renal failure in the intensive care unit. Intensive Care Med 1998;14:10–16.

Klahr S, Miller SB. Acute oliguria. N Engl J Med 1998; 338:671–675.

Marik PE, Iglesias J. Low-dose dopamine does not prevent acute renal failure in patients with septic shock and oliguria. Am J Med 1999;107:387–390.

Thadhani R, Pascual M, Bonventre JV. Acute renal failure. N Engl J Med 1996;334:1448–1460.

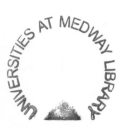

4 Coma

Seemant Chaturvedi

Coma is a clinical diagnosis. It arises from brain dysfunction involving disruption of either the brainstem reticular activating system or the two cerebral hemispheres. In evaluating the patient with coma, the clinician should first try to determine whether the mechanism is bihemispheric brain dysfunction or brainstem dysfunction, and then attempt to define the precise etiology of the decreased level of consciousness (LOC).

Etiologies

A. Vascular
   1. Pontine infarction
   2. Pontine hemorrhage
   3. Subarachnoid hemorrhage
   4. Cerebellar infarction or hemorrhage with brainstem compression
   5. Hemispheric infarction or hemorrhage with brainstem compression
B. Infection
   1. Meningitis
   2. Encephalitis
C. Metabolic
   1. Hypoglycemia
   2. Hyperosmolar coma
   3. Hypoxic encephalopathy
   4. Uremia
   5. Hepatic coma
   6. Hyponatremia
   7. Hypercalcemia
   8. Myxedema coma
   9. Hypothermia or hyperthermia
D. Intoxication or iatrogenic etiology
   1. Opiate/narcotic overdose
   2. Alcohol intoxication (e.g., ethanol, methanol, ethylene glycol)
   3. Sedative/hypnotic drug overdose (e.g., benzodiazepines, barbiturates)
   4. Other drug overdoses and poisonings (e.g., salicylates, carbon monoxide)
E. Trauma
   1. Subdural hematoma
   2. Diffuse axonal injury
F. Status epilepticus

Terminology

A. Drowsiness: decreased LOC with response elicitable by verbal stimulation
B. Stupor: decreased LOC with response elicitable only with tactile or painful stimulation
C. Coma: decreased LOC with no meaningful response to verbal or tactile stimulation and no awareness or interaction with the outside environment
D. Persistent vegetative state: decreased LOC with no interaction with the outside environment, but with preserved brainstem function
E. Brain death: decreased LOC with no interaction with the outside environment plus no brainstem function

Physical Findings

A. Evaluate brainstem reflexes (presence or absence).
   1. Pupillary light response: evaluates cranial nerves II and III
   2. Corneal reflex: evaluates cranial nerves V and VII
   3. Oculocephalic reflex (doll's-eyes maneuver): evaluates cranial nerves III, VI, and VIII
   4. Gag reflex: evaluates cranial nerves IX and X
   5. Spontaneous respirations: evaluates medullary respiratory centers
B. Evaluate level of responsiveness (see Table 4–1).
   1. Purposeful, volitional movement
   2. Withdrawal response to noxious stimuli
   3. Stereotyped responses
      a. Decorticate posturing

TABLE 4–1. GLASGOW COMA SCALE*

EYE OPENING		VERBAL RESPONSE		MOTOR RESPONSE	
Spontaneous	4	Oriented	5	Obeys commands	6
To voice	3	Confused	4	Localizes pain	5
To pain	2	Inappropriate	3	Withdraws from pain	4
None	1	Incomprehensible	2	Abnormal flexion	3
		None	1	Abnormal extension	2
				None	1

*Total score can range from 3 (worst) to 15 (normal). Coma defined as ≤8.

      b. Decerebrate posturing

      c. Triple flexion response

C. Evaluate vital signs for fever, hypotension, hypertension, tachycardia, bradycardia, abnormal respiratory patterns.

D. Evaluate other physical findings.

    1. Pupillary asymmetry (can signal brainstem compression)

    2. Pinpoint pupils (seen with opiate overdose or pontine lesions)

    3. Preretinal hemorrhage (seen in subarachnoid hemorrhage)

    4. Nuchal rigidity (sign of meningitis or subarachnoid hemorrhage)

    5. Battle's sign (indicative of basilar skull fracture, or subdural or epidural hemorrhage)

    6. Hyperthermia (can be secondary to infection or status epilepticus)

    7. Persistent nystagmus (may be seen in status epilepticus)

Key Findings

- Pupillary response
- Corneal reflex
- Oculocephalic reflex
- Gag reflex
- Spontaneous respiration
- Motor response

Laboratory Tests

A. Serum or blood glucose (to exclude hypoglycemia or hyperglycemia)

B. Serum electrolytes (to exclude hyposodium and hypercalcium)

C. Arterial blood gases or pulse oximetry (to exclude hypoxemia)

D. White blood cell count (to exclude leukocytosis as a sign of sepsis)

E. Liver function tests (to exclude hepatic coma)

F. Serum urea nitrogen and creatinine (to exclude uremic encephalopathy)

G. Toxicology screen (to exclude intoxication from ethanol, opiates, benzodiazepines, barbiturates, salicylates, and other agents)

Imaging Studies

A. Brain computed tomography

    1. Cerebral infarction

    2. Cerebral hemorrhage

    3. Cerebral edema (e.g., due to meningitis or hepatic encephalopathy)

    4. Loss of gray matter/white matter differentiation (hypoxia, edema)

    5. Subdural hematoma

    6. Subarachnoid hemorrhage

    7. Skull fracture

B. Magnetic resonance imaging is better for visualizing

    1. Brainstem infarction

    2. Cerebellar infarction

    3. Temporal lobe pathology (herpes encephalitis)

C. Imaging studies may be normal with

    1. Diffuse axonal injury

    2. Hypoxic encephalopathy

    3. Status epilepticus

    4. Metabolic processes

Key Tests

- Complete blood count
- Biochemical profile
- Arterial blood gases
- Toxicology screen
- Brain computed tomography
- Electroencephalography

Treatment

A. Unexplained coma

    1. Intravenous dextrose

    2. Intravenous or intramuscular thiamine

    3. Naloxone

B. Explained coma (treat underlying pathology)

    1. Brainstem compression: consider immediate decompressive surgery

    2. Pontine hemorrhage: surgery is rarely undertaken because of the poor prognosis

    3. Subarachnoid hemorrhage: fluid and blood pressure management; consider surgery or angiographic coiling for aneurysms depending on patient condition

    4. Meningitis/encephalitis: treat according to cerebrospinal fluid and blood culture results

5. Metabolic processes: correct underlying problem if possible (e.g., hypoglycemia)

6. Subdural hematoma: consider hematoma evacuation

7. Ethanol intoxication: fluid management, withdrawal prophylaxis

8. Opiate overdose: naloxone, respiratory support

9. Benzodiazepine overdose: flumazenil

10. Status epilepticus: lorazepam followed by phenytoin, fosphenytoin, or phenobarbital

 Bibliography

Adams RD, Victor M. Principles of Neurology, 5th ed. New York: McGraw-Hill, 1993, pp 300–318.

Levy DE, Bates D, Caronna JJ. Prognosis in nontraumatic coma. Ann Intern Med 1981;94:293–301.

Maiese K, Caronna JJ. Coma after cardiac arrest: clinical features, prognosis, and management. In: Ropper AH, Neurological and Neurosurgical Intensive Care, 3rd ed. New York: Raven, 1993, pp 331–350.

Plum F, Posner JB. Diagnosis of Stupor and Coma, 3rd ed. Philadelphia: F.A. Davis, 1980.

Towne AR, Waterhouse EJ, Boggs JG, et al. Prevalence of nonconvulsive status epilepticus in comatose patients. Neurology 2000;54:340–345.

5 Tachypnea and Hypoxemia

Willane S. Krell

Because of the ubiquitous availability of pulse oximetry in the intensive care unit (ICU), physicians are quickly alerted to changes in a patient's oxyhemoglobin saturation. Care must be taken, however, to give clinical meaning to any alterations observed. Tachypnea is observed frequently in ICU patients but is often underappreciated. Although it is a nonspecific finding, it is a very sensitive indicator of changes in patient status and deserves attention. Tachypnea and hypoxemia may occur simultaneously or separately, depending on the etiology and other circumstances. The finding of either phenomenon should prompt examination and evaluation of the patient.

Hypoxemia

Etiology

A. Respiratory causes
  1. Hypoventilation
    a. Reduced alveolar ventilation and hypercarbia
    b. Common causes
      (1) Sedative-hypnotic or narcotic drugs
      (2) Central nervous system trauma
      (3) Severe obstructive lung disease
      (4) Chest wall problems (pain, deformity)
  2. Low ventilation-perfusion ratio
    a. Most common cause of hypoxemia
    b. Commonly encountered in obstructive lung disease due to perfusion of poorly ventilated lung areas
    c. Hypoxemia correctable by increasing fractional concentration of inspired oxygen (FIO_2)
  3. Intrapulmonary right-to-left shunt
    a. Pulmonary perfusion without ventilation: represents a special case of low ventilation–perfusion ratio in which the ratio is zero
    b. Common in pulmonary edema (cardiogenic or noncardiogenic)
    c. Hypoxemia is refractory to increases in FIO_2; hypoxemia does not correct even with an FIO_2 of 1.00
  4. High ventilation–perfusion ratio
    a. Caused by increased dead space ventilation
    b. Occurs commonly with pulmonary embolism
  5. Low inspired oxygen tension
    a. High-altitude hypoxemia
    b. Low FIO_2 (i.e., <0.21)

      (1) Equipment malfunction: e.g., low oxygen pressure alarm on mechanical ventilator disabled
      (2) Inadvertent varying of gas mixtures: e.g., mixtures containing oxygen plus anesthetic gases or helium

B. Cardiovascular causes
  1. Circulatory shock or severe heart failure
  2. Extrapulmonary right-to-left shunt
    a. Intracardiac right-to-left shunt: e.g., atrial or ventricular septal defect in conjunction with severe pulmonary hypertension
    b. Systemic arteriovenous malformation or fistula; e.g., iatrogenic peripheral shunt for hemodialysis

C. Other abnormalities of oxygen carrying capacity
  1. Severe anemia
  2. Carbon monoxide poisoning
  3. Methemoglobinemia

Diagnosis

A. Confirm hypoxemia.
  1. Review clinical scenario.
  2. Check pulse oximetry function.
    a. Check for appropriate probe position, absence of nail polish, and adequacy of peripheral perfusion.
    b. Assure valid signal waveform.
    c. Check that pulse rate by oximeter agrees with that by palpation.
  3. Consider arterial blood gas to confirm hypoxemia.

B. Historical context
  1. If sudden onset, consider
    a. Airway problems
    b. Embolic phenomena
    c. Pneumothorax
    d. Cardiogenic pulmonary edema
  2. If subacute or progressive onset, consider
    a. Pulmonary edema, cardiogenic shock, or the acute respiratory distress syndrome (ARDS)
    b. Infectious process
    c. Inflammatory process
    d. Progression of initial disease

C. Examination
  1. Vital signs
     a. Tachypnea or hypoventilation
     b. Tachycardia
     c. Hypo- or hypertensive
  2. Upper airway patency
     a. Endotracheal tube malposition
     b. Secretions or mucus plugging
     c. Other airway or endotracheal tube obstruction
  3. Chest examination
     a. Exclude tracheal shift.
     b. Palpate for crepitations (subcutaneous emphysema) or tenderness.
     c. Perform percussion.
        (1) Hyperresonance suggests pneumothorax.
        (2) Areas of dullness suggest fluid or consolidation.
     d. Auscultation
        (1) Absent breath sounds
        (2) Bronchial breath sounds
        (3) Wheezing
        (4) Rales
  4. Cardiac examination
     a. Signs of right or left heart failure
     b. Tachydysrhythmias
     c. New heart murmur
     d. Peripheral cyanosis or signs of poor perfusion
D. Immediate testing
  1. Obtain arterial blood gases.
  2. Obtain chest x-ray.
  3. Check ventilator settings.
  4. If invasive monitoring is in place, assess cardiac filling pressures.
E. Further testing
  1. Assess response to FIO_2 of 1.00.
  2. Obtain echocardiogram.
  3. Evaluate sputum.
     a. White blood cells
     b. Microorganisms
     c. Hemoptysis
  4. Obtain complete peripheral blood cell count.
  5. Consider thromboembolism.
     a. Doppler studies of lower extremities
     b. Radionuclear pulmonary ventilation-perfusion scan or helical computed tomography
     c. Quantitative D-dimer level
     d. Pulmonary angiogram

PEARL

Pulse oximetry readings may be inaccurate if the oximeter's pulse rate readout does not agree with the electrocardiographic heart rate, or (for devices having plethysmographic capability) the plethysmographic waveform is noisy, flat, or otherwise unacceptable.

Treatment

A. Confirm hypoxemia.
  1. Recheck oxyhemoglobin saturation by pulse oximetry (SpO_2).
  2. Consider arterial blood gas analysis.
     a. Assess response to supplemental oxygen; i.e., by arterial oxyhemoglobin saturation by CO oximetry (SaO_2) and PaO_2
     b. Assess ventilation by $PaCO_2$
B. Increase FIO_2 and note response.
C. Check airway patency.
D. Adjust ventilator as needed.
E. Based on patient evaluation, order initial studies and perform specific treatment as indicated.
  1. Airway suctioning
  2. Adjustment of ventilator settings to improve oxygenation and ventilation
  3. Chest tube insertion
  4. Diuresis
  5. Antibiotics
  6. Anticoagulants
  7. Fluid resuscitation
  8. Blood transfusion
F. Consider maneuvers to decrease oxygen requirement.
  1. Sedation
  2. Therapeutic paralysis

Tachypnea

Etiology

A. Pulmonary
  1. Obstructive airway disease
     a. Upper airway, including endotracheal tube, obstruction
     b. Intrapulmonary airways
        (1) Mucus
        (2) Edema
        (3) Bronchospasm
  2. Restrictive
     a. Infectious causes (e.g., pneumonia)

  b. Acute respiratory distress syndrome
  c. Inflammatory, fibrosis, or scarring
    (1) Auto-immune diseases
    (2) Bronchiolitis obliterans with organizing pneumonia
    (3) Drug toxicity
    (4) Radiation injury
    (5) Idiopathic
  3. Pneumothorax
  4. Atelectasis
B. Chest wall
  1. Pleural space
    a. Effusion
    b. Inflammation
  2. Rib cage
    a. Trauma
    b. Chest wall distortion
  3. Diaphragm
    a. Direct trauma
    b. Phrenic nerve injury
    c. Muscle fatigue or dysfunction
C. Cardiovascular
  1. Cardiogenic pulmonary edema
  2. Low cardiac output
  3. Pulmonary vascular occlusion
  4. Pericardial disease
D. Abdominal
  1. Pain
  2. Distension
    a. Intraluminal
    b. Ascites
E. Central nervous system
  1. Pain
  2. Anxiety
  3. Central hyperventilation

Diagnosis

A. Assess airway patency.
  1. Mucus plug or other airway secretions
  2. Other upper airway obstruction
  3. Malposition of endotracheal tube
B. Assess lungs.
  1. Percussion dullness
  2. Absent breath sounds
  3. Wheezing
  4. Rales
  5. Pleural friction rub
C. Perform cardiovascular evaluation.
  1. Tachydysrhythmias

2. New murmur
3. Signs of heart failure
4. Pericardial friction rub
D. Perform general assessment.
  1. Evaluate abdomen.
  2. Assess pain management.
  3. Evaluate level of anxiety.

Treatment

A. Alter or add therapy based on examination and testing.
  1. Airway suctioning or chest physiotherapy
  2. Use of artificial airway; e.g., endotracheal tube, nasal trumpet, oral airway
  3. Pharmacotherapy; e.g., bronchodilators, diuretics, anticoagulation
B. Adjust ventilator sensitivity and output to patient.
C. Provide adequate analgesia.
D. Provide adequate anxiety control.
  1. Reassurance
  2. Pharmacotherapy

Key Management

- Check vital signs.
- Measure SpO$_2$, consider arterial blood gas analysis.
- Evaluate upper and lower airway patency and secretions.
- Perform cardiopulmonary and abdominal examination.
- Assess for anxiety, pain, and adequacy of pain management.
- Increase FIO$_2$ and note response.
- Ascertain mechanical ventilator settings, pressures, and volumes.
- Obtain chest x-ray, if indicated.

Bibliography

Glauser FL, Polaty P, Sessler CN. Worsening oxygenation in the mechanically ventilated patient: Causes, mechanisms and early detection. Am Rev Respir Dis 1988;138: 458–474.

Hansen-Flachen JH. The agitated patient in respiratory failure. In: Fishman AP (ed). Update: Pulmonary Diseases and Disorders. New York: McGraw-Hill, 1992; pp 38–400.

Marini JJ, Rodriquez RM, Lamb VJ. The inspiratory workload of patient-initiated mechanical ventilation. Am Rev Respir Dis 1986;134:902–909.

Tobin MJ. State of the art: respiratory monitoring in the intensive care unit. Am Rev Respir Dis 1988;148:1625–1642.

6 Respiratory Failure

Mark S. Chesnutt
Peter J. Papadakos

Key Definitions

- Respiratory failure: gas exchange abnormalities severe enough to deprive vital organs of oxygen or cause acidosis secondary to hypercapnia

- Hypoxemic respiratory failure: PaO_2 lower than 60 torr

- Hypercarbic respiratory failure: $PaCO_2$ higher than 50 torr

Pathophysiology

A. Mechanisms of hypoxemia (reduced PaO_2)
1. Reduced FIO_2
2. Reduced barometric pressure
3. Hypoventilation
4. Ventilation–perfusion mismatch
5. Right-to-left shunt
6. Diffusion block
7. Low $P\bar{v}O_2$

B. Mechanisms of hypoventilation
1. Decreased tidal volume without a compensatory increase in respiratory rate
2. Decreased respiratory rate without a compensatory increase in tidal volume
3. Increased dead space ventilation without a compensatory increase in minute ventilation
4. Increased CO_2 production without a compensatory increase in minute ventilation

Etiology

A. Airway disorders
1. Obstruction of large central airway (pharynx, larynx, trachea, mainstem bronchus, or lobar bronchus)
    a. Mucus plug
    b. Foreign body
    c. Edema
       (1) Allergic reaction
       (2) Infection (e.g., epiglottitis)
       (3) Smoke or toxic gas inhalation
       (4) Aspiration
       (5) Toxin exposure
       d. Tumor mass
       e. Laryngospasm
2. Asthma
3. Acute exacerbation of chronic bronchitis or emphysema

B. Pulmonary edema
1. Increased hydrostatic pressure edema
    a. Left ventricular dysfunction (e.g., from acute myocardial ischemia or chronic heart failure)
    b. Mitral regurgitation
    c. Left atrial outflow obstruction (e.g., from mitral stenosis, thrombus, or tumor)
    d. Volume overload states
    e. Overperfusion of pulmonary vascular bed
2. Increased pulmonary capillary permeability
    a. Acute respiratory distress syndrome (ARDS)
    b. Acute lung injury
3. Pulmonary edema of unclear etiology
    a. Neurogenic
    b. Negative pressure (inspiratory airway obstruction)
    c. Re-expansion
    d. Tocolytic-associated

C. Other parenchymal lung disorders
1. Pneumonia
2. Interstitial lung diseases
3. Diffuse alveolar hemorrhage syndromes
4. Alveolar proteinosis
5. Carcinoma: bronchogenic, metastatic
6. Lung contusion

D. Pulmonary vascular disorders
1. Thromboembolism
2. Air embolism
3. Amniotic fluid embolism
4. Intrinsic pulmonary vascular diseases

E. Pleural disorders
1. Pneumothorax
2. Pleural effusion
3. Pleural fibrosis

F. Chest wall and diaphragm disorders
1. Flail chest
2. Rib fractures with splinting
3. Kyphoscoliosis

4. Massive ascites

5. Morbid obesity

6. Abdominal distension and abdominal compartment syndrome

G. Neuromuscular and related disorders

1. Primary neuromuscular diseases: Guillain-Barré syndrome, myasthenia gravis, poliomyelitis, muscular dystrophy, amyotrophic lateral sclerosis, polymyositis

2. Drug or toxin-induced: botulism, organophosphates, neuromuscular blocking agents, aminoglycosides

3. Spinal cord injury

4. Phrenic nerve injury or dysfunction

5. Electrolyte disturbances: hypokalemia, hypermagnesemia, hypophosphatemia

6. Miscellaneous: myxedema, malnutrition, fatigue, hypoxemia, periodic paralysis

H. Central nervous system disorders

1. Drugs: sedative-hypnotic, narcotic, or anesthetic agents

2. Brain stem respiratory center disorders: trauma, tumor, vascular disorders, hypothyroidism

3. Sleep-disordered breathing: central sleep apnea, obesity-hypoventilation syndrome

4. Intracranial hypertension

5. Central nervous system infections

6. Idiopathic hypoventilation syndrome

I. Increased CO_2 production

1. Fever

2. Infection

3. Hyperalimentation with excess caloric and carbohydrate intake

4. Hyperthyroidism

5. Seizures

6. Rigors

Clinical Findings

A. Symptoms

1. Related to hypoxemia: dyspnea

2. Related to hypercapnia: dyspnea and headache

3. Those associated with the underlying disease

B. Physical findings

1. Related to hypoxemia: cyanosis, tachycardia, tachypnea, hypertension, restlessness, anxiety, confusion, delirium, tremor, dysrhythmias

2. Related to hypercapnia: tachycardia, tachypnea, hypertension, peripheral and conjunctival hyperemia, impaired consciousness, asterixis, papilledema

Key Tests

- Arterial blood gas analysis
- Chest x-ray
- Other testing directed by history and physical examination findings

Treatment

A. Treatment of underlying disorder

B. General supportive care

C. Supplemental oxygen administration to correct hypoxemia

D. Noninvasive positive pressure ventilation

1. Useful in selected patients who can protect and maintain the patency of their airway, handle their own secretions, and tolerate the mask apparatus

2. May use nasal or full-face masks

3. Bi-level positive pressure ventilation mode is preferred for both hypoxemic and hypercarbic respiratory failure in selected patients.

E. Criteria for endotracheal intubation and mechanical ventilation (no hard-and-fast rules)

1. Apnea

2. Loss of airway protective mechanisms

3. Induction of deep sedation or co-administration of paralytic agents

4. Inability to clear secretions

5. Upper airway obstruction

6. Progressive hypoventilation and worsening respiratory acidosis

7. Progressive hypoxemia despite supplemental oxygen

8. Progressive general fatigue, tachypnea, use of accessory respiratory muscles, or mental status deterioration

9. Patient's own sense of exhaustion

Key Treatment

- Treatment of underlying disorder
- Supplemental oxygen administration to correct hypoxemia
- Noninvasive positive pressure ventilation (selected cases)
- Endotracheal intubation and mechanical ventilation, if needed
- General supportive care

Prognosis

A. When cause is uncomplicated narcotic or sedative overdose: excellent

B. When cause is chronic obstructive lung disease without need for intubation and mechanical ventilation: good

C. When cause is chronic obstructive lung disease with need for intubation and mechanical ventilation: fair

D. Survival rates for adults requiring mechanical ventilation for all causes of acute respiratory failure

    1. To weaning: 62%

    2. To hospital discharge: 43%

    3. To 1 year after hospital discharge: 30%

E. Survival rates for adults with ARDS: 60% to 65%

Key Prognosis

Prognosis in respiratory failure is related to the underlying etiology, reversibility and severity of the gas exchange abnormalities, and presence of other organ system dysfunction.

Bibliography

Chesnutt MS, Prendergast TJ. Lung. In: Tierney LM, McPhee SJ, Papadakis MA (eds). Current Medical Diagnosis & Treatment 2002, 41st ed. New York: Lange Medical Books, McGraw-Hill, 2002; pp 269–362.

Jasmer RM, Luce JM, Matthay MA. Noninvasive positive pressure ventilation for acute respiratory failure: underutilized or overrated? Chest 1997;111:1672–1678.

Miletin MS, Detsky AS, Lapinsky SE, Mehta S. Non-invasive ventilation in acute hypoxemic respiratory failure. Intensive Care Med 2000;26:242–245.

Raju P, Manthous CA. The pathogenesis of respiratory failure: an overview. Respir Clin North Am 2000;6:195–212.

Shapiro MB, Anderson HL III, Bartlett RH. Respiratory failure. Surg Clin North Am 2000;80:871–883.

Tremblay A, Gursahaney A. Adult respiratory failure. Chest Surg Clin North Am 1998;8:557–583.

Wood LDH, Schmidt GA, Hall JB. Principles of critical care of respiratory failure. In: Murray JF, Nadel JA, Mason RJ, Boushey HA (eds). Textbook of Respiratory Medicine, 3rd ed. Philadelphia: WB Saunders, 2000, pp 2377–2411.

7 Pulmonary Edema

Eli Azzi
Charles M. Carpati

Pathophysiology

A. Pulmonary edema results when the flux of fluid entering the pulmonary interstitium and alveoli is greater than the flux back into the bloodstream and removal by the lymphatic system.

B. These fluid fluxes are described by Starling's equation:

1. $Q = K_f [(P_{cap} - P_{int}) - \sigma(\pi_{cap} - \pi_{int})]$, where

2. Q = fluid flux from pulmonary capillaries to interstitium

3. K_f = coefficient of filtration across the capillary wall

4. P_{cap} and P_{int} = capillary and interstitial hydrostatic pressure, respectively

5. σ = reflection coefficient

6. π_{cap} and π_{int} = capillary and interstitial colloid oncotic pressure, respectively

C. Cardiogenic pulmonary edema

1. Caused by increased pulmonary capillary hydrostatic pressure

2. Secondary to left-sided heart failure

D. Noncardiogenic pulmonary edema

1. Caused by an increase in pulmonary capillary permeability

2. Mechanism does not involve heart failure, although concomitant heart failure can occur and potentially lead to edema formation

E. Pulmonary edema formation is abetted by decreased capillary colloid osmotic pressure in cardiogenic and noncardiogenic forms.

Etiology

A. Cardiogenic pulmonary edema

1. Systolic ventricular dysfunction

   a. Ischemic heart disease, acute myocardial infarction (MI)

   b. Dilated cardiomyopathy

   c. Valvular stenosis or regurgitation

2. Diastolic ventricular dysfunction

   a. Ischemic heart disease, acute MI

   b. Hypertensive cardiomyopathy

   c. Hypertrophic cardiomyopathy

   d. Restrictive cardiomyopathy

B. Noncardiogenic pulmonary edema (acute lung injury and acute respiratory distress syndrome)

1. Aspiration of gastric or oropharyngeal contents

2. Sepsis

3. Pancreatitis

4. Trauma

5. Burns

6. Transfusion reactions

7. Re-expansion pulmonary edema

8. Neurogenic pulmonary edema

9. Inhalation injury

10. Near-drowning

11. Drug-induced pulmonary edema (e.g., opiates)

Clinical Findings

A. Vital signs

1. Hypotension or hypertension

2. Tachycardia

3. Tachypnea

B. Pulmonary

1. Copious watery sputum

2. Rales

3. Expiratory wheezing

4. Dullness to percussion (pleural effusion)

C. Cardiovascular

1. Cardiogenic

   a. Distended neck veins

   b. S_3 or S_4 gallop

   c. Valvular murmur

   d. Hepatojugular reflux

   e. Peripheral edema at presentation

2. Noncardiogenic

   a. Flat neck veins

   b. Gallop not typical

   c. Flow murmur

   d. No hepatojugular reflux

   e. Peripheral edema after resuscitation

D. Abdomen

1. Hepatomegaly (cardiogenic)

2. Ascites (cardiogenic)

E. Central nervous system

1. Anxiety

2. Confusion

3. Disorientation

F. Urinary tract: oliguria

G. Skin

  1. Cool, clammy extremities (cardiogenic pulmonary edema)

  2. Warm extremities (often in noncardiogenic pulmonary edema, after resuscitation)

  3. Pallor

  4. Cyanosis

  5. Diaphoresis

Key Clinical Findings

- Respiratory distress
- Pulmonary rales
- Tachypnea
- Hypoxemia
- Tachycardia
- Diffuse bilateral pulmonary infiltrates

Laboratory and Other Tests

A. Serum biochemical tests

  1. Hyponatremia

  2. Hypokalemia

  3. Azotemia

    a. Caused by poor renal perfusion (pre-renal) in cardiogenic pulmonary edema

    b. Caused by acute tubular necrosis in noncardiogenic pulmonary edema

  4. Elevated bilirubin concentration and transaminase and alkaline phosphatase activity in congestive hepatopathy

  5. Elevated cardiac markers in cardiogenic pulmonary edema after MI

B. Arterial blood tests

  1. Blood gases

    a. Hypoxemia (PaO_2/FIO_2 typically <300 torr)

    b. Early: respiratory alkalosis

    c. Late: respiratory acidosis

  2. Increased arterial lactate concentration

C. Urine specific gravity: high

D. Electrocardiography: possible ischemic changes in cardiogenic pulmonary edema

E. Chest x-ray

  1. Cardiogenic etiology

    a. Bilateral perihilar ("butterfly distribution") infiltrates, or diffuse bilateral interstitial and alveolar infiltrates

    b. Kerley B lines

    c. Base-to-apex vascular redistribution

    d. Possible pleural effusion

  2. Noncardiogenic etiology: diffuse bilateral interstitial and alveolar infiltrates

F. Echocardiography

  1. Cardiogenic pulmonary edema: may show poor left ventricular contraction (systolic dysfunction) or hypertrophy (diastolic dysfunction)

  2. Noncardiogenic pulmonary edema: may show hyperdynamic function

Monitoring

A. Continuous electrocardiographic monitoring

B. Continuous pulse oximetry

C. Respiratory mechanics during positive pressure ventilation

  1. Airway pressures (peak and plateau) elevated

  2. Pulmonary and chest wall static compliance decreased

D. Pulmonary artery catheterization

  1. Cardiogenic

    a. Central venous pressure may be elevated.

    b. Pulmonary artery occlusion pressure elevated (>18 mm Hg)

    c. Cardiac index typically low (except in high output heart failure)

    d. Mixed venous oxyhemoglobin saturation low (<65%)

  2. Noncardiogenic

    a. Central venous pressure may be low.

    b. Pulmonary artery occlusion pressure <18 mm Hg

    c. Mixed venous oxyhemoglobin saturation typically normal or high

Treatment

A. General measures

  1. Bed rest

  2. Supplemental oxygen

  3. Endotracheal intubation and mechanical ventilation for respiratory failure

B. Cardiogenic pulmonary edema

  1. Preload reduction

    a. Salt restriction

    b. Loop diuretic

    c. Morphine sulfate

    d. Nitrates (options)

      (1) Continuous IV infusion of nitroglycerin

      (2) Dermal patch nitroglycerin

      (3) Sublingual nitroglycerin

(4) Oral isosorbide dinitrate or mononitrate

(5) Continuous IV infusion of nitroprusside

e. Goal is to lower pulmonary artery occlusion pressure to less than 18 mm Hg.

2. Afterload reduction

a. Continuous IV infusion of nitroprusside, nitroglycerin, or dobutamine

b. Alternatives: intermittent IV hydralazine, angiotensin converting enzyme inhibitor

c. Not feasible if concomitant hypotension (see Chapter 26, Cardiogenic Shock)

3. Noninvasive continuous positive airway pressure ventilation

a. Decreases left ventricular systolic wall tension (afterload) by increasing the pressure gradient between the left ventricle and extrathoracic arteries.

b. May obviate necessity for endotracheal intubation, allowing time for pharmacotherapy to reverse respiratory failure.

4. Augmentation of contractility

a. Dobutamine

b. Milrinone: inotropic and potent vasodilator properties

c. Dopamine

(1) Inotropic properties

(2) Vasodilator properties at low doses

(3) Vasoconstrictor properties at high doses, which can increase afterload; avoid except in the pressure of hypotension

d. Digoxin

C. Noncardiogenic pulmonary edema

1. Mechanical ventilation using low tidal volume (e.g., 6 mL/kg ideal body weight)

2. Limit plateau pressures to 30 to 35 cm H_2O

a. Limits barotrauma and volutrauma

b. Facilitated by use of sedation and pressure control ventilation

c. Consider use of permissive hypercapnia if necessary to lower plateau pressure.

3. Positive end-expiratory pressure (PEEP)

a. Titrate to allow reduction of FIO_2 to 0.50 or less, if possible.

b. PEEP-induced hypotension usually responds to fluid loading.

4. Target: lowest pulmonary artery occlusion pressure that does not result in compromised organ perfusion

5. Prone positioning may improve gas exchange in patients with refractory hypoxemia.

6. Treat underlying disease.

Key Treatment

- Supplemental oxygen
- Positive pressure ventilation
- Specific pharmacotherapy for cardiogenic etiologies
- Specific ventilator strategies for noncardiogenic etiologies
- Supportive measures

Bibliography

Artigas A, Bernard GR, Carlet J, et al. The American-European Consensus Conference on ARDS, part 2: ventilatory, pharmacologic, supportive therapy, study design strategies, and issues related to recovery and remodeling. Acute respiratory distress syndrome. Am J Respir Crit Care Med 1998;157:1332–1347.

Curley MA. Prone positioning of patients with acute respiratory distress syndrome: a systematic review. Am J Crit Care 1999;8:397–405.

Kosowsky JM, Storrow AB, Carleton SC. Continuous and bilevel positive airway pressure in the treatment of acute cardiogenic pulmonary edema. Am J Emerg Med 2000; 18:91–95.

Pang D, Keenan SP, Cook DJ, et al. The effect of positive pressure airway support on mortality and the need for intubation in cardiogenic pulmonary edema: a systematic review. Chest 1998;114:1185–1192.

Sacchetti AD, Harris RH. Acute cardiogenic pulmonary edema. What's the latest in emergency treatment? Postgrad Med 1998;103:145–162.

Ware LB, Matthay MA. The acute respiratory distress syndrome. N Engl J Med 2000;342:1334–1349.

8 Acute Respiratory Distress Syndrome

Alain Tremblay
Kalpalatha K. Guntupalli

Acute respiratory distress syndrome (ARDS) is a disorder commonly seen in the intensive care unit (ICU), often in conjunction with multiple organ failure. Its pathophysiologic hallmarks are pulmonary inflammation and increased capillary permeability leading to pulmonary edema. Acute respiratory distress syndrome is recognized by a constellation of clinical, radiologic, and physiologic abnormalities that cannot be explained by, but that can coexist with, left atrial or pulmonary capillary hypertension. Patients with ARDS can have any of a wide variety of inciting or complicating severe pulmonary and extrapulmonary illnesses, which makes management extremely challenging. Although supportive care remains the mainstay of management, research into the pathophysiology of ARDS has led to the development of potential specific interventions, some of which are now in clinical trials.

Key Diagnostic Criteria for Acute Lung Injury and ARDS

- Acute onset of respiratory dysfunction

- Bilateral diffuse pulmonary infiltrates on chest x-ray

- Pulmonary artery occlusion pressure lower than 18 mm Hg or absence of clinical signs of left ventricular failure

- Pao_2/Fio_2 ratio lower than 300 (acute lung injury) or lower than 200 (ARDS) torr

Risk Factors

A. Pulmonary
1. Pneumonia
2. Aspiration pneumonitis
3. Pulmonary contusion
4. Toxic gas inhalation
5. Fat, air, or amniotic fluid embolism
6. Drug toxicity

B. Extrapulmonary
1. Sepsis
2. Circulatory shock

3. Pancreatitis
4. Central nervous system injury
5. Trauma
6. Thermal burn injury
7. Blood transfusion
8. Extracorporeal circulation

Key Pathophysiology

- Increased pulmonary capillary permeability

- Decreased lung compliance

- Large right-to-left shunt (typically 25% to 50%)

- Inhomogeneity of affected lung units

- Pulmonary hypertension

Pathophysiology

A. Initial injury
1. Direct injury to lung (e.g., infection, aspiration)
2. Inflammatory response to injury (direct or indirect)
   a. Cellular infiltration: neutrophils, macrophages
   b. Cytokine expression
   c. Prostaglandin release
   d. Increased protease activity
   e. Oxygen free-radical generation

B. Early exudative phase (days 1 to 3)
1. Increased pulmonary capillary permeability
2. Alveolar filling with proteinaceous exudate
3. Diffuse alveolar damage with hyaline membrane formation and alveolar edema seen histologically
4. Severe hypoxemic respiratory failure with large intrapulmonary right-to-left shunt

C. Intermediate proliferative phase (days 3 to 10)
1. Inflammatory cellular infiltration of interstitium
2. Thickened alveolar walls, proliferating fibroblasts, and cellular exudates seen histologically

23

3. Decreasing lung compliance, increasing alveolar dead space

D. Late fibrotic phase (beyond 10 days)

1. Resolution of cellular alveolar infiltrates

2. Progressive collagen deposition in interstitium

3. Diffuse interstitial fibrosis and bullae formation

4. Decreased lung compliance, increased dead space, improvement in hypoxemia, high risk of pneumothorax

Key Clinical Findings

- Dyspnea and respiratory distress

- Tachycardia

- Tachypnea

- Pulmonary rales

- Findings associated with inciting event

Laboratory, Imaging, and Other Tests

A. Chest x-ray

1. Initially may be normal

2. Diffuse bilateral alveolar infiltrates evolve.

B. Computed tomography of chest

1. Inhomogeneity of infiltration is more apparent than on plain x-rays.

2. Infiltrates are gravity dependent.

a. In supine patients, infiltrates are posterior and anterior lung fields appear less affected.

b. Infiltrates migrate with body position changes.

c. Reversal of the above pattern can occur in patients maintained in the prone position.

C. Arterial blood gases

1. Respiratory alkalosis

2. Hypoxemia

D. Bronchoalveolar lavage: shows prevalent polymorphonuclear leukocytes

Key Differential Diagnosis

- Cardiogenic pulmonary edema

- Bilateral pneumonia

- Diffuse alveolar hemorrhage

- Acute eosinophilic pneumonia

Key Monitoring

- Blood pressure and continuous electrocardiography

- Continuous pulse oximetry monitoring

- Intermittent arterial blood gas measurements

- Lung mechanics and airway pressure

- Fluid balance

- Pulmonary artery catheterization in selected patients

Treatment

A. Mechanical ventilation

1. Maintain adequate arterial oxygen saturation and avoid pulmonary oxygen toxicity: minimize FIO_2 as long as a PaO_2 of 55 to 80 torr or SaO_2 0.88 to 0.95 is maintained.

2. Employ positive end-expiratory pressure (PEEP).

a. Use PEEP to allow further reduction of FIO_2; PEEP prevents end-expiratory collapse of small airways and alveoli and redistributes edema fluid to non–gas-exchanging areas of the lung, thereby improving oxygenation and lung compliance in the early phases of ARDS.

b. Positive end-expiratory pressure use may be limited by adverse hemodynamic effects; therefore, titrate PEEP to a level that improves oxygenation without causing hemodynamic instability.

c. See Chapter 225, Positive End-Expiratory Pressure.

3. Prevent ventilator-induced lung injury by minimizing barotrauma and volutrauma.

a. Limit tidal volume to approximately 6 mL/kg.

b. Maintain plateau pressure ($P_{plateau}$) less than 30 cm H_2O (note that conditions that decrease chest wall compliance will also increase $P_{plateau}$, but are of less concern, as transpulmonary pressure is not increased).

c. Use PEEP in conjunction with the above measures to minimize cyclic recruitment–derecruitment injury and prevent end-expiratory small airway and alveolar collapse.

d. This approach is associated with a lower mortality rate than conventional ventilatory strategies.

4. Permissive hypercapnia (also see Chapter 224, Newer Modes of Mechanical Ventilation)

a. Maintain adequate ventilation, if possible; however, consider permissive hypercapnia if high tidal volumes or airway pressures are required to avoid respiratory acidosis.

b. Acceptance of respiratory acidosis allows use of lower tidal volumes and airway pressures and minimizes risks of barotrauma and volutrauma.

c. Tolerated in most patients, but may require deep sedation and, in some cases, neuromuscular paralysis

d. Use of a buffering agent (usually sodium bicarbonate) may be required for severe respiratory acidosis (pH <7.2).

e. Contraindicated in the presence of increased intracranial pressure

5. Inverse ratio ventilation

a. A ventilation strategy employing an increased inspiratory:expiratory (I:E) ratio from the usual 1:3 to 1:1 or more

b. The resulting increase in mean alveolar pressure may improve lung recruitment and oxygenation without increasing PEEP or peak alveolar pressure.

c. Sustained inflation may recruit alveoli with slow time constants as well as allow better gas mixing, leading to improved ventilation–perfusion ratios.

d. Short expiratory times may lead to dynamic hyperinflation or intrinsic PEEP.

e. Achieved by adding end-inspiratory pause or decreasing inspiratory flow rate in volume-controlled ventilation, or changing inspiratory time on pressure-controlled ventilation

6. Recruitment maneuvers

a. Imposition of a sustained high-volume, high-pressure breath to recruit lung units ("open the lung"), used in conjunction with PEEP to prevent derecruitment (maintain lung open)

b. There is no standardized method, but one approach is to sustain a single inflation for 30 to 60 seconds using an inflation pressure of 40 to 60 cm H_2O.

c. The maneuver can be repeated after each disconnection from the ventilator (e.g., for suctioning).

d. Monitor hemodynamics during the procedure.

7. Pressure–volume curves

a. Monitor pressure–volume curves in selected patients to tailor ventilatory settings.

b. Pressure–volume curves should be assessed during inflation with a super-syringe or during a low-flow (10 to 15 L/minute) inspiratory maneuver.

c. Set PEEP above the lower inflection point to maximize recruitment while maintaining $P_{plateau}$ below the upper inflection point to minimize hyperinflation (see Chapter 225, Positive End-Expiratory Pressure).

d. Caveats: inflection points are not always seen and the influence of chest wall compliance on inflection points can be substantial

8. Investigational approaches to ventilation in ARDS

a. High-frequency jet ventilation

b. Tracheal gas insufflation

c. Partial liquid ventilation

d. Airway pressure release ventilation

e. Extracorporeal oxygenation and CO_2 removal

f. Noninvasive positive pressure ventilation

9. Tracheostomy

a. Timing is controversial; consider if long-term (beyond 2 weeks) mechanical ventilation is likely.

b. Both surgical tracheostomy and the bedside percutaneous approach are used.

B. Nonpharmacologic therapies

1. Fluid management

a. Negative fluid balance is associated with improved outcome in observational studies.

b. Lower filling pressures should limit edema formation for a given degree of capillary permeability.

c. Avoid hypervolemia; consider fluid restriction or diuresis in hemodynamically stable patients.

d. In unstable patients, consider fluid therapy and vasopressors; ensure continuous renal replacement.

2. Prone positioning

a. Repositioning from the supine to the prone position may improve oxygenation by altering gravity-dependent lung infiltrates and ventilation–perfusion relationships.

b. May improve functional residual capacity, diaphragmatic function, and secretion clearance

c. Procedure is labor intensive, risks dislodgement of catheters and tubes, and makes routine and emergency care more difficult.

d. There are currently no standardized protocols.

e. A randomized trial of 304 patients showed improved oxygenation but no survival benefit.

3. Nutrition
   a. Whenever possible, employ early enteral feeding with adequate protein and caloric dosing.
   b. Possible benefit of "immunonutrition formulas," containing eicosapentaenoic acid, γ-linolenic acid, antioxidants, continues to be investigated.
C. Pharmacological therapies
   1. Antibiotics
      a. There is no role for routine empiric antibiotics, unless underlying pneumonia or sepsis is the cause of the ARDS.
      b. Treat nosocomial infections.
      c. Pneumonia can be difficult to diagnose because fever, purulent sputum, and pulmonary infiltrates may be seen in ARDS without pneumonia, and tracheal secretions are often colonized with bacteria.
      d. Bronchoscopy with bronchoalveolar lavage or protected brush sampling may improve the accuracy of diagnosis.
   2. Neuromuscular blockade
      a. Not routinely used in ARDS, but occasionally employed to facilitate ventilation and improve oxygenation
      b. No documented improvement in respiratory mechanics or oxygenation compared to deep sedation alone
      c. Can be associated with significant complications, including prolonged paralysis, myopathy, delayed weaning, and pressure ulcerations
   3. Corticosteroids
      a. High-dose steroid therapy in the early stages of ARDS has had neutral or negative effects in controlled trials and is not recommended.
      b. Possible benefit for patients with persistent late-phase ARDS with no infections (or receiving appropriate antibiotic treatment); multicenter trial in process
      c. Recommended dose in late ARDS: IV methylprednisolone, 2 mg/kg per day in 4 divided doses for 14 days, then taper to 1 mg/kg per day for 7 days, 0.5 mg/kg per day for 7 days, 0.25 mg/kg per day for 2 days, and 0.125 mg/kg per day for 2 days; oral equivalent can be used and the taper started after extubation
   4. Inhaled nitric oxide
      a. Nitric oxide is a potent pulmonary vasodilator and the inhaled route improves perfusion to ventilated lung zones.

   b. Improvements in oxygenation and pulmonary vascular resistance have been observed in some patients, but this effect may be transient.
   c. No demonstrated improvement in outcome, although potential utility as a salvage therapy in severely hypoxemic patients
   5. Inhaled surfactant
      a. May improve lung function, but no demonstrated outcome improvement in sepsis-induced ARDS
      b. Newer formulations are under development to optimize composition and delivery.

Key Treatment

- Use mechanical ventilation with tidal volumes of approximately 6 mL/kg.
- Maintain $P_{plateau}$ below 30 cm H_2O, if possible.
- Use the lowest FIO_2 that maintains adequate SaO_2.
- Titrate PEEP to allow reduction of FIO_2 to less than 0.50, if possible.
- Provide supportive care, enteral nutrition, and treatment for infections.
- Employ careful fluid restriction as long as perfusion is not compromised.

Key Complications

- Nosocomial infection and sepsis, especially pneumonia
- Pneumothorax
- Multisystem organ failure
- Pulmonary fibrosis
- Prolonged ICU stay

Key Prognosis

- The overall in-hospital mortality rate is 30% to 50%.
- Mortality in patients with ARDS and multiple organ failure is 75% to 80%.
- In general, survivors have good functional recovery.
- Lung function improvement occurs mainly during the first 3 months, but can continue for up to 6 to 12 months.

Bibliography

Artigas A, Bernard GR, Carlet J, et al. The American-European Consensus Conference on ARDS, Part 2. Ventilatory, pharmacologic, supportive therapy, study design strategies, and issues related to recovery and remodeling. Am J Respir Crit Care Med 1998;157:1332–1347.

Bernard GR, Artigas A, Brigham KL, et al. The American-European Consensus Conference on ARDS: definitions, mechanisms, relevant outcomes, and clinical trial coordination. Am J Respir Crit Care Med 1994;149:818–824.

Brower RG, Matthay MA, Morris A, et al. Ventilation with lower tidal volumes as compared with traditional tidal volumes for acute lung injury and the acute respiratory distress syndrome. N Engl J Med 2000;342:1301–1308.

Dreyfuss D, Saumon G. Ventilator-induced lung injury. Lessons from experimental studies. Am J Respir Crit Care Med 1998;157:294–323.

Hirschl RB, Pranikoff T, Wise C, et al. Initial experience with partial liquid ventilation in adult patients with the acute respiratory distress syndrome. JAMA 1996;275:383–389.

Humphrey H, Hall J, Sznajder I, et al. Improved survival in ARDS patients associated with a reduction in pulmonary capillary wedge pressure. Chest 1990;97:1176–1180.

McIntyre RC Jr, Pulido EJ, Bensard DD, et al. Thirty years of clinical trials in acute respiratory distress syndrome. Crit Care Med 2000;28:3314–3331.

Meduri GU, Headley AS, Golden E, et al. Effect of prolonged methylprednisolone therapy in unresolving acute respiratory distress syndrome: a randomized controlled trial. JAMA 1998;280:159–165.

Steinberg KP, Hudson LD. Acute lung injury and acute respiratory distress syndrome. The clinical syndrome. Clin Chest Med 2000;21:401–417.

Ware LB, Matthay MA. The acute respiratory distress syndrome. N Engl J Med 2000;342:1334–1349.

9 Barotrauma

Paul L. Rogers

Definitions

A. Barotrauma refers to any air that has leaked outside the tracheobronchial tree.
1. Pneumothorax
2. Pneumomediastinum
3. Subcutaneous emphysema
4. Pneumopericardium
5. Pulmonary interstitial emphysema
6. Subpleural air cysts

B. Volutrauma refers to over-distention and excessive mechanical shearing of alveoli.
1. There is no frank leakage of air from the tracheobronchial tree.
2. Can contribute to lung injury

Key Epidemiology

- Barotrauma is the most common complication of positive pressure ventilation, occurring in 7% to 25% of patients receiving mechanical ventilation.

- Mortality from barotrauma may be as high as 31% if the diagnosis is delayed.

- The incidence of barotrauma can be as high as 50% in patients with acute respiratory distress syndrome (ARDS), presumably due to higher pressures generated during ventilation of lung parenchyma with reduced compliance.

Pathophysiology

A. Over-distention of alveoli
1. Occurs when excessively large tidal volumes or levels of positive end-expiratory pressure (PEEP) are employed and lung compliance is not homogeneous.
2. Disproportionate volume is delivered to unaffected or compliant areas of the diseased lung because of the low compliance of the affected regions.

B. Over-distention and rupture of alveoli permits air to leak into the pulmonary interstitium and along the perivascular sheath, resulting in interstitial emphysema.

C. Air in the perivascular interstitium can enter the mediastinum and dissect into the subcutaneous tissues of the neck, chest, and extremities.

D. Air can also dissect into the peritoneum or the pericardium, or rupture the mediastinal pleural and create a pneumothorax.

E. Air may track along the perivascular sheath to the pleura and create subpleural cysts.
1. Cysts may either resolve, become secondarily infected, or rupture and create a pneumothorax.
2. Subpleural cysts are more common in younger patients, presumably because they have looser connective tissue in the interstitium.

Key Risk Factors

- Acute respiratory distress syndrome
- Necrotizing pneumonias
- Over-distention of alveoli (high tidal volumes)
- High (plateau) airway pressure

Clinical Findings

A. Subcutaneous emphysema (palpable crepitus)
B. Tension pneumothorax
1. Tachypnea
2. Tachycardia
3. Increased peak and plateau airway pressure
4. Hypotension
5. Pulseless myocardial electrical activity

PEARL

Anterior pneumothorax may be unrecognized on a supine chest x-ray.

X-ray Findings

A. Pneumothorax
1. Anterior pneumothorax may be unrecognized on a supine radiograph.
2. The deep sulcus sign: visualization of a deep costophrenic sulcus
3. The double diaphragm sign

B. Pneumomediastinum: air may outline the left subclavian artery, the left and right common carotid arteries, and into the neck.

C. Subcutaneous emphysema: air dissects the muscle bundles.

D. Pulmonary interstitial emphysema
1. Mottled radiolucencies within consolidated lung parenchyma
2. Non-branching radiolucencies from the hila to the peripheral regions of the lung
3. Subpleural air cysts

Key Treatment

- Patients with cardiopulmonary compromise due to tension pneumothorax require emergent evacuation of air, either with a large-bore needle inserted into the pleural cavity via the second intercostal space anteriorly or with immediate thoracostomy tube placement.

- An immediate release of air, reduction in airway pressures, and return of blood pressure indicate successful treatment of tension pneumothorax.

- The leak may stop in minutes or persist for days.

Prevention

A. Recommendations to minimize the incidence of barotrauma have included limiting peak inspiratory pressure (PIP) and PEEP.
1. However, recent studies have been unable to demonstrate a correlation between PIP, PEEP, and barotrauma.
2. Peak inspiratory pressure represents the proximal airway pressure and is influenced by resistance and flow rate.
3. Plateau airway pressure represents the static pressure required to generate a given tidal volume; thus, it may be more important to limit plateau pressure.

B. In patients with severe ARDS and reduced compliance, a lung-protective ventilator strategy (LPVS) is recommended.
1. A LPVS consists of using low tidal volumes and limiting plateau airway pressure.
   a. Pressure-control ventilation
   b. Limiting tidal volume (V_T) to 6 mL/kg ideal body weight
   c. Using sufficient PEEP to recruit collapsed alveoli but limiting over-distention
   d. Limiting the plateau airway pressure to 30 cm H_2O, if possible
2. Compared to conventional ventilation (V_T of 12 mL/kg ideal body weight, respiratory rate to maintain $PaCO_2$ ~35 torr, and PEEP to maintain PaO_2 >80 torr with an FIO_2 <0.60), this LPVS has been shown to reduce the incidence of barotrauma from 42% to 7%.

C. There is no role for prophylactic chest tube thoracostomy.

PEARL

Patients with ARDS should be ventilated using low tidal volumes ("lung-protective ventilator strategy"), limiting tidal volume to 6 mL/kg or less (ideal body weight), if necessary, to maintain plateau airway pressure lower than 30 cm H_2O.

Bibliography

The Acute Respiratory Distress Syndrome Network. Ventilation with lower tidal volumes as compared with traditional tidal volumes for acute lung injury and the acute respiratory distress syndrome. N Engl J Med 2000;342: 1301–1308.

Amato MBP, Barbon CSV, Medeiror DM, et al. Effect of a protective-ventilator strategy on mortality in the acute respiratory distress syndrome. N Engl J Med 1995;338: 347–354.

Gammon RB, Shin MS, Grover RH, et al. Clinical risk factors for pulmonary barotrauma. Am J Respir Crit Care Med 1995;152:1235–1240.

Haake R, Schlichtig R, Ulstad DR, et al. Barotrauma: Pathophysiology, risk factors, and prevention. Chest 1987;91: 608–613.

Stewart TE, Meade MO, Cook DJ, et al. Evaluation of a ventilation strategy to prevent barotrauma in patients at high risk for acute respiratory distress syndrome. N Engl J Med 1998;338:355–361.

Tocino I, Westcott JL. Barotrauma. Radiol Clin North Am 1996;34:59–81.

Weg JG, Anzueto A, Balk RA, et al. The relationship of pneumothorax and other air leaks to mortality in the acute respiratory distress syndrome. N Engl J Med 1998; 338:341–346.

10 Pulmonary Embolism

Tisha Fujii
Linda Kirschenbaum

With an estimated incidence of more than 600,000 cases per year in the United States, pulmonary thromboembolism (PE) remains a major health problem. Furthermore, despite the availability of various diagnostic modalities, its identification continues to elude physicians and generate much controversy. Because the mortality of untreated PE is 18% to 30% (vs. 2.5% for treated PE), a high degree of clinical suspicion is required.

Key Pathophysiology (Virchow's triad)

- Venous stasis
- Vascular wall injury
- Alterations in coagulation

Risk Factors

A. Acquired
 1. Immobilization
 2. Postoperative period (<3 months)
 3. Thrombophlebitis
 4. Congestive heart failure
 5. Chronic obstructive lung disease
 6. Obesity
 7. Malignancy
 8. Prior venous thromboembolism
 9. Estrogen therapy or oral contraceptive use
 10. Pregnancy or postpartum period
 11. Trauma
 12. Indwelling vascular devices
B. Inherited
 1. Activated protein C resistance
 2. Hyperhomocysteinemia
 3. Antiphospholipid antibody syndrome (anticardiolipin antibody lupus anticoagulant)
 4. Antithrombin III deficiency
 5. Protein C and S deficiency
 6. Plasminogen & tissue plasminogen activator abnormalities
 7. Factor VII deficiency
 8. Thrombocytopenia
 9. Factor V Leiden (prothrombin gene variation)
 10. Prothrombin gene variation 20210G → A

Key Risk Factors For Hemodynamic Instability in PE

- Size of embolus (especially if >40% of pulmonary vasculature obstructed)
- Pre-existing cardiopulmonary disease

Clinical Findings

A. History
 1. Dyspnea
 2. Pleuritic or angina-like chest pain
 3. Apprehension
 4. Cough
 5. Hemoptysis
 6. Syncope
 7. Leg pain
 8. Risk factors
B. Physical examination
 1. Tachypnea
 2. Tachycardia
 3. Hypotension
 4. Jugular vein distension
 5. Wheezing or rales
 6. Leg swelling
 7. Homan's sign
 8. S4 gallop
 9. Increased pulmonary component of second heart sound

Key History

- Dyspnea
- Apprehension
- Cough
- Pleuritic chest pain
- Syncope
- Risk factor for PE

Laboratory and Other Tests

A. Arterial blood gases
 1. Lack specificity and sensitivity
 2. Abnormal PaO_2, $PaCO_2$, or $PA-aO_2$ are compatible with PE, but normal values do not exclude the diagnosis.

B. D-dimer test using quantitative enzyme-linked immunosorbent assay (ELIZA)

   1. Detects endogenous fibrinolysis of cross-linked fibrin

   2. Pulmonary thromboembolism unlikely if less than 500 $\mu g/L$

   3. D-dimer by ELIZA is more than 500 $\mu g/L$ in over 90% of patients with PE, but elevated levels are nonspecific.

   4. High incidence of false positives expected in intensive care unit (ICU) populations

C. Electrocardiogram (abnormal in >70% of patients, but findings lack specificity)

   1. Sinus tachycardia

   2. Atrial tachydysrhythmias

   3. Nonspecific ST segment and T wave changes

   4. QRS axis deviation

   5. Right bundle branch block

   6. $S_1Q_3T_3$ patterns (uncommon)

D. Electrical impedance plethysmography

   1. Noninvasive test that identifies proximal lower extremity deep vein thrombosis

   2. Variable reported sensitivity; 90% specificity

   3. Largely supplanted by duplex ultrasonography

Imaging Studies

A. Chest x-ray

   1. General

      a. May be unremarkable in previously healthy patient

      b. Findings are nonspecific.

      c. May be dominated by findings of the underlying critical illness

   2. Focal atelectasis

   3. Pleural effusion

   4. Consolidation

   5. Prominent central pulmonary artery

   6. Focal oligemia (Westermark's sign)

   7. Hampton's hump

      a. Wedge-shaped, pleural-based opacity

      b. Signifies pulmonary infarction

   8. Hemidiaphragm elevation

B. Ventilation–perfusion (V/Q) scintigraphy (Fig. 10–1)

   1. Normal: no perfusion defects

   2. Very low probability: 3 small or less (<25% of segment) segmental perfusion defects and normal chest x-ray

   3. Low probability

      a. Single moderate (25% to 74%) segmental perfusion defect without matching ventilation defect (i.e., unmatched) and normal chest x-ray

      b. Large (≥75%) or moderate segmental defects with 4 or fewer segments in one lung and 3 or fewer segments in one lung area with matching ventilation defects of equal or larger size, and no or smaller corresponding abnormalities on chest x-ray

      c. Any perfusion defect with a larger chest x-ray abnormality

      d. More than three small segmental perfusion defects with a normal chest x-ray

      e. Nonsegmental perfusion defects

   4. High probability

      a. Two or more large segmental unmatched perfusion defects

      b. Two or more moderate segmental unmatched perfusion defects plus one large unmatched segmental perfusion defect

      c. Four or more moderate segmental unmatched perfusion defects

   5. Intermediate probability (i.e., indeterminate)

      a. Not fitting into one of the above categories

      b. Difficult to categorize

C. Duplex doppler ultrasonography

   1. Noninvasive test that identifies peripheral deep vein thrombosis

      a. Employs B-mode ultrasonography to image veins

      b. Employs doppler ultrasound to determine venous blood velocity

   2. Sensitivity and specificity for detecting deep-vein thrombosis approach 100% (sensitivity lower in asymptomatic patients).

D. Radiocontrast venography

   1. Thrombi visualized as in situ filling defects

   2. Largely supplanted by alternative noninvasive tests

E. Helical computed tomography

   1. May identify clot within pulmonary arteries

   2. Negative study may not exclude PE.

F. Magnetic resonance imaging

   1. Capable of demonstrating clot in deep veins and pulmonary arteries

   2. Not as sensitive as pulmonary angiography

   3. Diagnostic role still under evaluation

G. Doppler echocardiography

   1. May show signs of right ventricular (RV) dysfunction and pulmonary hypertension (not specific for PE)

      a. Right ventricular dilation and hypokinesis

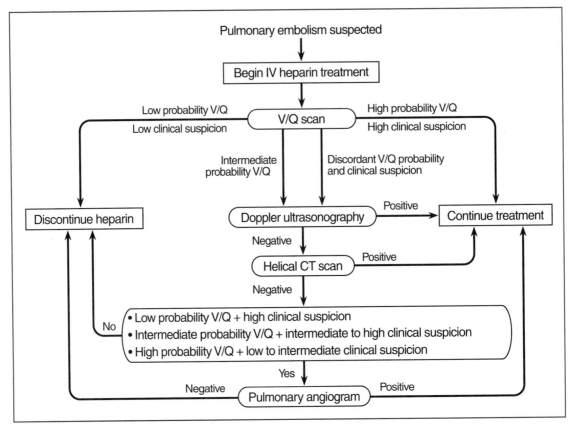

Figure 10–1 Algorithm for diagnosis and treatment of pulmonary embolism.

b. Pulmonary artery dilation

c. Tricuspid regurgitation

d. Septal flattening

e. Increase in estimated pulmonary artery pressure

2. May show clot within RV or pulmonary artery

H. Pulmonary angiography

1. Invasive procedure requiring pulmonary artery catheterization and radiocontrast injection

2. Criterion standard test for PE

3. Morbidity risk: less than 1% (e.g., bleeding, contrast-induced renal dysfunction)

4. Mortality risk: less than 0.01%; markedly increased with severe pulmonary hypertension

Treatment

A. Unfractionated heparin (see Chapter 173, Anticoagulants)

1. Initial IV loading dose of 80 U/kg, followed by a continuous IV infusion at 18 U/kg per hour

2. Monitor using activated partial thromboplastin time (PTT)

3. Goal is PTT of 1.5 to 2.5 times normal.

B. Low molecular weight heparin (see Chapter 173, Anticoagulants)

1. Alternative to unfractionated heparin

2. Enoxaparin dose: 1 mg/kg subcutaneously every 12 hours

C. Warfarin

1. Oral anticoagulant for long-term anticoagulation

2. Withheld until stable anticoagulation is achieved with heparin; warfarin can induce a procoagulant state during the early stage of therapy

3. Therapy initiated at 5 mg/day orally

4. Dose titrated using daily international normalized ratio (INR) test to achieve INR goal of 2 to 3

5. Heparin discontinued once INR goal achieved and stable

6. Warfarin may not be appropriate in the intensive care unit for unstable patients because of its long duration of action and potential need for rapid but temporary reversal of anticoagulation for procedures.

D. Thrombolytic therapy (also see Chapter 174, Thrombolytic Agents)

1. Consider in patients with acute, massive PE who are hemodynamically unstable (Fig. 10–2).

2. Discontinue heparin until PTT is less than 1.5 times control.

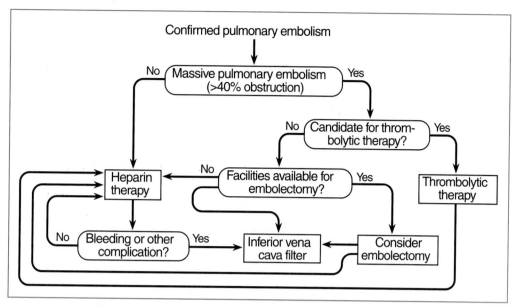

Figure 10-2 Algorithm for treatment of massive pulmonary embolism.

3. Dosing regimens (IV)

   a. Streptokinase: 250,000 unit loading dose, then 100,000 U/hour for 24 hours

   b. Urokinase: 4,400 U/kg loading dose, then 2,200 U/kg per hour for 12 hours

   c. Recombinant tissue plasminogen activator: 100 mg (56 million units) over 2 hours

4. Restart heparin after thrombolytic therapy is completed, once PTT has returned to less than 1.5 times control.

E. Inferior vena caval filter placement recommendations

   1. Contraindication to or complication of anticoagulation in a patient with or at high risk for venous thromboembolism

   2. Documented recurrent thromboembolism despite therapeutic anticoagulation

   3. Chronic recurrent embolism with pulmonary hypertension

   4. Concurrent surgical pulmonary embolectomy or pulmonary endarterectomy procedures

F. Pulmonary embolectomy

   1. Controversial therapeutic modality

   2. May be considered in certain circumstances at centers experienced with the technique

   a. Massive PE

   b. Hemodynamic instability despite anticoagulation and resuscitation efforts

   c. Failure of or contraindication to thrombolytic therapy

B Bibliography

American College of Chest Physicians Consensus Committee on Pulmonary Embolism. Opinions regarding the diagnosis and management of venous thromboembolic disease. Chest 1998;113:499–504.

Grenier PA, Beigelman C. Spiral computed tomographic scanning and magnetic resonance angiography for the diagnosis of pulmonary embolism. Thorax 1998;53(Suppl 2):S25–S31.

Hyers TM, Agnelli G, Hull RD, et al. Antithrombotic therapy for venous thromboembolic disease. Chest 2001; 119(1 Suppl):176S–193S.

Janssen MC, Wollersheim H, Verbruggen B, et al. Rapid D-dimer assays to exclude deep venous thrombosis and pulmonary embolism: current status and new developments. Semin Thromb Hemost 1998;24:393–400.

The PIOPED Investigators. Value of the ventilation/perfusion scan in acute pulmonary embolism. Result of the prospective investigation of pulmonary embolism diagnosis (PIOPED). JAMA 1990;263:2753–2759.

Weg JG. Venous thromboembolism—pulmonary embolism and deep vein thrombosis. Irwin and Rippe's Intensive Care Medicine, 4th ed. Philadelphia: Lippincott-Raven, 1999; pp 650–672.

11 Status Asthmaticus

Michael J. Apostolakos

Asthma is a disease characterized by wheezing, dyspnea, and cough resulting from airway hyperreactivity and inflammation. All patients with this disorder are in danger of developing a severe attack of asthma that places them at risk of developing respiratory failure, a disorder referred to as *status asthmaticus*. This condition, which may be triggered by infection, allergens, or nonspecific irritants, can occur suddenly or, more often, over several days. The progression of airway inflammation and edema can result in ventilatory failure and death. Cornerstones of treatment include β_2-adrenergic agonists, corticosteroids, low-flow supplemental oxygen and, if necessary, mechanical ventilation.

Key Pathogenesis

- Bronchial wall thickening from edema and inflammation secondary to allergens or nonspecific irritants

- Hypertrophy and hyperplasia of bronchial smooth muscle and submucosal glands

- Deposition of collagen beneath epithelial basement membrane

- Intermittent airflow obstruction caused by the above mechanisms

Clinical Findings

A. Symptoms
1. Breathlessness
2. Preoccupation with the task of breathing
3. Preference for an upright posture
4. Anxiety
5. Fatigue

B. Physical findings
1. Pulmonary
   a. Diffuse expiratory wheezing
   b. Tachypnea (>30 breaths/minute)
   c. Use of accessory muscles
   d. Increased inspiratory:expiratory ratio (>1:3)
2. Cardiovascular
   a. Tachycardia (>120 beats/minute)
   b. Pulsus paradoxus (>15 mm Hg)

Laboratory Findings and Other Tests

A. Pulmonary function tests
1. Reduced peak expiratory flow rate: less than 120 L/minute signifies a severe exacerbation
2. Reduced forced expiratory volume in 1 second (FEV_1): less than 1 L signifies severe exacerbation
3. Usually not possible to obtain in patients with status asthmaticus because of the severity of dyspnea

B. Arterial blood gases
1. To assess level of hypoxemia and acid-base status
2. Correlate findings with pulse oximetry.

C. Chest radiography
1. Usually shows hyperexpanded lungs
2. Evaluate for signs of barotrauma.

Key Differential Diagnosis

- Upper airway obstruction (e.g., tumor or foreign body)

- Functional laryngospasm

- Chronic obstructive pulmonary disease

- Left ventricular failure (pulmonary edema)

Key Monitoring

- Serial peak expiratory flow rates or FEV_1

- Serial arterial blood gases

- Frequent clinical reassessment for signs of impending respiratory failure

Treatment

A. Pharmacotherapy
1. Bronchodilators
   a. β_2-Adrenergic agonists (e.g., albuterol, metaproterenol): drugs of choice for smooth-muscle–mediated bronchoconstriction
      (1) Initial treatment: 2.5 mg albuterol (0.5 mL of 0.5% solution in 2.5 mL saline)

by nebulization every 20 minutes × 3, then hourly

  (2) May also administer continuously by nebulization

  (3) Metered dose inhalers combined with a spacing device may be as effective.

  (4) Doses are limited by tachycardia, dysrhythmias, or tremors.

  b. Ipratropium bromide

    (1) An anticholinergic drug that produces less bronchodilation than β_2-adrenergic agonists

    (2) Consider if poor response to β_2-adrenergic agonists and corticosteroids.

    (3) Usual dose is 0.25 mg to 0.5 mg by nebulization every 20 minutes × 3 doses initially, then every 4 to 6 hours.

  c. Theophylline

    (1) Use is controversial; consider if poor or incomplete response to other bronchodilators and steroids.

    (2) Loading dose is 5 mg/kg (6 mg/kg for aminophylline) over 30 minutes, followed by continuous infusion of 0.4 mg/kg per hour (0.5 mg/kg per hour for aminophylline).

    (3) Check plasma levels frequently, targeting 8 to 12 μg/mL.

2. Corticosteroid (e.g., methylprednisolone)

  a. Treats airway inflammation and decreases mucus production

  b. Potentiates effects of β-agonists and decreases β-agonist tachyphylaxis

  c. Initial dose of methylprednisolone ranges from 40 to 125 mg IV every 6 hours; if improving, reduce to 60 to 80 mg daily in divided doses, tapered over 10 to 14 days.

3. Magnesium sulfate

  a. Not routinely recommended

  b. Mechanism of bronchodilation is unknown.

  c. Usual dose is 1 to 2 g IV over 20 minutes.

4. Antibiotics

  a. No role for routine use; most infections that trigger asthma are viral.

  b. Use is directed toward patients with fever, leukocytosis, and neutrophils (not eosinophils) in sputum, those with pneumonia, and those with acute sinusitis.

B. Supplemental oxygen

1. Hypoxemia is generally mild and secondary to ventilation–perfusion mismatch.

2. Administration of 1 to 3 L/minute by nasal prongs is usually sufficient for patients who do not require endotracheal intubation.

3. Assess effectiveness with arterial blood gas or pulse oximetry monitoring.

4. If refractory hypoxemia, search for additional pathological features such as pneumonia or barotrauma.

C. Mechanical ventilation

1. Noninvasive positive pressure ventilation (positive pressure by mask)

  a. May be considered in patients not responding adequately to pharmacological intervention but not requiring immediate intubation

  b. Patient must be alert, cooperative, and able to maintain the airway.

  c. Typical setting for continuous positive airway pressure is 5 to 10 cm H_2O.

  d. Typical settings for bilevel positive airway pressure are inspiratory pressure of 8 to 15 cm H_2O and expiratory pressure of 3 to 8 cm H_2O to offset intrinsic positive airway pressure.

2. Invasive (i.e., endotracheal intubation and mechanical ventilation)

  a. Required for patients who fail the above therapy

  b. No mode of mechanical ventilation is proven superior.

  c. Avoid hyperinflation.

  d. Recommended initial settings

    (1) Tidal volume of 8 mL/kg

    (2) Respiratory rate 11 to 14 breaths/minute

    (3) Inspiratory : expiratory ratio of 1 : 3, 1 : 4, or 1 : 5 (shortens inspiratory time and lengthens expiratory time)

    (4) No positive end-expiratory pressure

  e. Adjust ventilator settings to maintain plateau pressure below 30 cm H_2O.

  f. May require permissive hypercapnia

  g. Also see Chapters 223, 224, and 226 on Mechanical Ventilation.

Key Treatment

- β_2-Adrenergic agonists administered frequently

- Corticosteroids to treat airway inflammation

- Supplemental oxygen to treat hypoxemia

- Avoid hyperinflation in failing patients who require intubation and mechanical ventilation; keep plateau pressures below 30 cm H_2O.

Complications

A. Barotrauma

1. Forms

   a. Pneumothorax

   b. Subcutaneous emphysema

   c. Pneumomediastinum

2. Mechanism is rupture of alveoli caused by high plateau pressure and hyperinflation.

3. Manifestations

   a. Chest pain

   b. Mediastinal crunch

   c. Crepitus (subcutaneous emphysema)

   d. Asymmetric breath sounds

4. Prevention: occurrence minimized by extending expiratory time (lowering plateau pressure)

B. Hypotension

1. Hypovolemia

2. Hyperinflation

3. Tension pneumothorax

4. Oversedation

Key Prevention

- Patient education

- Elimination of triggers

- Compliance with anti-inflammatory maintenance therapy

- Vaccinations (influenza and pneumococcal)

Bibliography

Corbridge TC, Hall JB. The assessment and management of adults with status asthmaticus. Am J Respir Crit Care Med 1995;151:1296–1316.

Graham VA, Milton AF, Knowles GK, et al. Routine antibiotics in hospital management of acute asthma. Lancet 1982;1(8269):418–420.

Haskell RJ, Wong BM, Hansen JE. A Double-blind, randomized clinical trial of methylprednisolone in status asthmaticus. Arch Intern Med 1983;143:1324–1327.

Meduri GU, Cook TR, Turner RE, et al. Non-invasive positive pressure ventilation in status asthmaticus. Chest 1996;110:767–774.

Tuxen DV. Permissive hypercapnic ventilation. Am J Respir Crit Care Med 1994;150:870–874.

12 Pneumonia in Adults

James E. Szalados

Epidemiology

A. Incidence is approximately 2.5 million cases per year in the United States.

B. Hospital-acquired pneumonia (HAP) occurs at a frequency of 0.5% to 1.0% of hospital admissions, but the incidence increases 6- to 20-fold with the use of mechanical ventilation.

C. The cumulative incidence of pneumonia associated with the use of mechanical ventilation statistically approximates 1% to 5% per day.

D. In the intensive care unit (ICU), 50% of cases of pneumonia are caused by Gram-negative bacilli and 10% by Gram-positive cocci.

E. A significant change in the oropharyngeal bacterial flora, due to antibiotic-driven selection pressure and colonization can be documented in almost 100% of ICU patients within 24 hours of admission.

Etiology

A. Aspiration of oropharyngeal secretions or gastric contents (the most common cause of pneumonia)
   1. Depressed consciousness
      a. Sedation (e.g., anesthesia, alcohol intoxication, drug overdose)
      b. Central nervous system dysfunction (e.g., cerebrovascular accident, seizure, dementia)
   2. Disorders of deglutition
      a. Neuromuscular disorders
      b. Gastroesophageal reflux
      c. Nasogastric intubation and gastric colonization
   3. Secretion retention
      a. Zenker's diverticulum
      b. Sinus drainage
   4. Disorders of mucociliary clearance
      a. Cystic fibrosis
      b. Tobacco smoke
      c. Endotracheal intubation

B. Inhalation of infected aerosol
   1. Droplet infection
   2. Contaminated ventilator tubing or humidifiers

C. Inoculation
   1. Contaminated suction devices
   2. Dental plaque
   3. Sinusitis
   4. Contaminated hardware (e.g., bronchoscope, endotracheal tube)

D. Hematogenous spread
   1. Translocation and migration from ischemic splanchnic viscera
   2. Migration from remote abscess site, infected foreign body, or prosthesis

Risk Factors

A. Pathogen factors
   1. Organism identity
   2. Virulence
   3. Inoculum dose

B. Host factors
   1. Altered mucosal integrity
      a. Oral protease release
      b. Fibronectin loss
      c. Epithelial injury (viral "priming")
      d. Recent aspiration
   2. Impaired immunity
      a. Steroid exposure
      b. Immunosuppressive therapy
      c. Cytotoxin exposure
      d. Cancer
      e. Diabetes mellitus
      f. Viral infection
      g. Renal failure
      h. Liver disease
   3. Aspiration risk
   4. Atelectasis
   5. Tobacco use
   6. Impaired volitional cough
   7. Malnutrition
   8. Underlying lung disease (e.g., cystic fibrosis, restrictive lung disease)
   9. Chronic obstructive lung disease
   10. Post-obstructive pneumonia

Classification

A. By site of acquisition and host factors
   1. Community acquired pneumonia (CAP)

a. Onset is within 96 hours of hospital admission.

b. Common pathogens are *Streptococcus pneumoniae*, *Haemophilus influenza*, and *Moraxella catarrhalis*.

c. Although only 20% to 30% of patients with CAP require hospital admission, and most do not need ICU care, CAP constitutes about 10% of all medical ICU admissions.

 (1) About 50% of ICU patients with CAP will require mechanical ventilation.

 (2) Mortality in ICU patients with CAP may be as high as 25% to 50%.

d. Risk stratification, prognosis, and empiric therapy are based on existing comorbid conditions and the setting of the initial presentation.

e. Not all patients with severe CAP can be recognized at admission.

2. Hospital acquired pneumonia

 a. Onset occurs more than 96 hours after hospital admission.

 b. Encompasses ventilator-associated pneumonia (VAP)

 c. Common pathogens include aerobic Gram-negative bacilli, including *Escherichia coli*, *Klebsiella pneumoniae*, *Enterobacter* spp., *Acinetobacter* spp., and *Pseudomonas aeruginosa*.

3. Immunocompromised host

 a. Transplant recipients

 b. Human immunodeficiency virus

 c. Cancer

 d. Chemotherapy

B. By pathogen

 1. Typical pathogens

 a. Gram-positive cocci: *Streptococcus pneumoniae* (the most common pathogen in CAP), *Staphylococcus aureus*, *Enterococcus faecalis*, and *Enterococcus faecium*

 b. Gram-positive bacilli: *Bacillus anthracis* and *Corynebacterium diphtheriae*

 c. Gram-negative diplococci: *Moraxella catarralis*

 d. Gram-negative bacilli: *H. influenzae* and *K. pneumoniae*, Enterobacteriaceae, *Pseudomonas aeruginosa*, *E. coli*, *Proteus mirabilis*, *Proteus morgagni*, and *Serratia marcescens*

 2. Atypical pathogens

 a. *Legionella pneumophilia* (Gram-negative bacilli)

 (1) The causative agent of Legionnaire's disease

 (2) More common in patients treated with corticosteroids

 b. *Mycoplasma pneumoniae* ("walking pneumonia")

 c. Chlamydia: *Chlamydia pneumoniae* (previously known as "TWAR" agent) and *Chlamydia psittaci* (the causative agent of psittacosis)

 d. Viruses: influenzae, parainfluenzae, adenovirus, respiratory syncytial virus, varicella-zoster, Epstein-Barr virus, herpesvirus, pulmonary hantavirus syndrome

3. Other pathogens

 a. Mycobacteria: *Mycobacterium tuberculosis* and *Mycobacterium avium-intracellulare* complex

 b. *Tularensis*: causative agent of tularemia

 c. *Coxiella burnettii*: causative agent of Q fever

 d. Potential agents for biowarfare or bioterrorism: *Yersinia pestis* (causative agent of pneumonic plague) and *Bacillus anthracis* (causative agent of anthrax)

4. Fungi

 a. *Candida* spp.: common in patients who are immunosuppressed or receiving antibacterial therapy

 b. *Aspergillus*: pathogenic in disorders of cellular immunity

 c. *Histoplasma*

 (1) Endemic to Ohio and Mississippi Valleys

 (2) Can lead to acute overwhelming pulmonary infection

 (3) Chronic upper lobe cavitary lesions can occur.

 (4) Progressive disseminated histoplasmosis can lead to fibrosing mediastinitis.

 (5) Diagnosis is by enzyme immunoassay (on serum or urine).

 d. Blastomycoses

 (1) Endemic to midwest and south-central United States

 (2) Presentations include acute, chronic, and disseminated forms.

 (3) Diagnosis facilitated by 10% KOH preparation

 e. Coccidioidomycosis: endemic to southwest United States

 f. *Pneumocystis carinii*

 (1) Human immunodeficiency virus infection

(2) Lymphoma

(3) High-dose corticosteroid therapy

(4) Human immunodeficiency virus infection

   g. *Nocardia*

Diagnosis

A. Symptoms
   1. Fever
   2. Chills
   3. Cough (productive or nonproductive)
   4. Dyspnea

B. Physical findings
   1. Fever (may be absent in immunocompromised patients)
   2. Rigors
   3. Tachypnea
   4. Tachycardia
   5. Cyanosis
   6. Wheezing, rhonchi, egophony
   7. Other signs of sepsis or septic shock

Key Diagnostic Findings

Community-Acquired Pneumonia

- Cough

- Purulence or increased volume of sputum

- Sputum microscopic examination showing <10 squamous cells and >25 polymorphonucleocytes per low-power field

- Infiltrate on chest x-ray

- Isolation of pathogen(s) from sputum

Ventilator-Associated Pneumonia

- Purulence or increased volume of tracheal secretions

- Temperature >38.5° or <36°C

- Peripheral white blood cell count <4,000 or >11,000 cells/mm³

- Abnormal oxygenation

- New, progressive, or persistent infiltrate on chest x-ray

- Isolation of pathogen(s) from tracheal aspirate

Laboratory Tests

A. White blood cell count

   1. Leukopenia or leukocytosis
   2. Differential cell count
      a. Increased numbers of immature white cell forms are associated with bacterial infection.
      b. Absence of excessive immature forms is more commonly seen with viral, fungal, and other "atypical" pathogens.

B. Blood cultures
   1. Low sensitivity for diagnosis, but of value prognostically and for guiding antibiotic therapy
   2. Help identify severely ill patients

C. Sputum microbiologic tests
   1. Gram stain: false-negative rate is 50%.
   2. Sputum culture and susceptibility profile
   3. Special stains
      a. Acid-fast bacillus stains for Mycobacteria
      b. Potassium hydroxide preparation for fungi
      c. Elastin fiber stain

D. Serology tests and advanced sputum analysis (epidemiological utility)
   1. Pneumococcal antigen
      a. Counter-immunoelectrophoresis
      b. Latex agglutination test
      c. Coagglutination test
      d. Enzyme immunoassay test
   2. *Legionella*
      a. Sputum or urine direct fluorescent antigen detection test
      b. Sputum polymerase chain reaction test
      c. Sputum indirect immunofluorescence antibody test
      d. Serum enzyme immunoassay test
   3. *Mycoplasma*
      a. Serum immunoglobulin M antibody ("cold agglutinins") test
      b. Serum polymerase chain reaction test
      c. Serum complement fixation test
   4. *Chlamydia*
      a. Serum polymerase chain reaction test
      b. Serum complement fixation test
      c. Serum microimmunofluorescence test
      d. Serum enzyme immunoassay test
   5. Q fever: serum indirect immunofluorescence test
   6. Viruses
      a. Serum immunofluorescence test
      b. Serum tissue culture

E. Urine tests
   1. Counter-immunoelectrophoresis for pneumococcus

2. Enzyme-linked immunosorbent assay for Legionella serogroup 1

Key Chest X-ray Findings

- Alveolar or lobar consolidation: usually demonstrate air bronchograms

- Bronchopneumonia: manifests as segmental and patchy infiltrates

- Interstitial, reticular pattern: suggests infection with atypical organism (e.g., *Legionella, Mycoplasma*)

- Nodular infiltrates: suggests infection with histoplasmosis or tuberculosis

- Cavitation: suggests infection with *Staphylococcus* or *Aspergillus*

Invasive Diagnostic Testing

A. Bronchoscopy (see Chapter 198, Fiberoptic Bronchoscopy)
   1. Protected brush specimen
      a. High specificity and sensitivity only if prior to antibiotic therapy
      b. May be performed with or without bronchoscopy
   2. Bronchoalveolar lavage
   3. Protected bronchoalveolar lavage
B. Transthoracic needle aspiration (contraindicated if positive pressure ventilation used)
C. Thoracentesis (see Chapter 201)
   1. Diagnostic: for pleural fluid analysis
   2. Therapeutic: for symptomatic relief of pleural effusion
D. Tube thoracostomy for therapeutic drainage of parapneumonic effusion or empyema (see Chapter 202, Chest Tube Thoracostomy)
E. Transtracheal needle aspiration (infrequently used)

Key Treatment

- Empiric antibiotic regimens for CAP must provide effective coverage for *Streptococcus pneumoniae*; and empiric coverage of *Mycoplasma* and *Legionella* should be strongly considered.

- Appropriate initial empiric antibiotic therapy is associated with improved survival in severe pneumonia.

Treatment

A. Antibiotic therapy
   1. Empiric regimens
      a. Treatment of CAP: ceftriaxone or cefotaxime, plus either a macrolide (e.g., azithromycin) or a fluoroquinolone
      b. Early-onset HAP: provide coverage against CAP core pathogens ± methicillin-sensitive *Staphylococcus aureus*
         (1) Ceftriaxone, cefuroxime, or cefotaxime; ± a macrolide
         (2) β-Lactam + β-lactamase inhibitor, ± a macrolide
         (3) Newer generation fluoroquinolone
         (4) Cefepime
         (5) Add vancomycin to any of the above regimens if methicillin-resistant *Staphylococcus aureus* is suspected.
      c. Late-onset HAP and VAP: provide coverage against CAP core pathogens with high index of suspicion for *Pseudomonas aeruginosa, Acinetobacter* spp.
         (1) Aminoglycoside + either cefepime, ceftazidime, cefoperazone, or an antipseudomonal penicillin (± β-lactamase inhibitor)
         (2) Newer generation fluoroquinolone + an aminoglycoside
         (3) Add vancomycin to either of the above if methicillin-resistant *Staphylococcus aureus* is suspected.
         (4) Add erythromycin ± rifampin if *Legionella* is suspected
      d. Aspiration pneumonia or anaerobic pneumonia: either clindamycin or a combination β-lactam + β-lactamase inhibitor
   2. Other treatment alternatives
      a. "Typical" pneumonia
         (1) β-Lactam antibiotic with a β-lactamase inhibitor
         (2) Second-generation cephalosporin (e.g., cefuroxime)
         (3) Third-generation cephalosporin (e.g., ceftriaxone, ceftazidime, or cefotaxime)
         (4) Fourth-generation cephalosporin (i.e., cefepime)
         (5) Monobactam (i.e., aztreonam: provides aerobic Gram-negative coverage only)
         (6) Carbapenem (i.e., imipenem-cilastin or meripenem)

(7) Vancomycin (for coverage of methicillin-resistant staphylococci)

b. "Atypical" pneumonia

(1) Macrolide (e.g, erythromycin or azithromycin)

(2) Doxycycline

(3) Rifampicin

(4) Fluoroquinolone (e.g., levofloxacin, moxifloxacin, gatifloxacin)

c. Tuberculosis (see Chapter 186, Antituberculosis Drugs)

d. Viral

(1) Amantadine

(2) Acyclovir

(3) Ribavarin

(4) Ganciclovir

3. Resistance issues

a. Gram-positive bacteria

(1) Methicillin-resistant *Staphylococcus aureus*, vancomycin-intermediate (glycopeptide) sensitive *Staphylococcus aureus*, and vancomycin-resistant enterococci

(2) Potential antimicrobial therapy: quinupristin-dalfopristin, linezolid

b. Gram-negative bacteria

(1) Inducible β-lactamase production (e.g., by *Pseudomonas*, *Enterobacter*, or *Klebsiella*)

(2) Extended spectrum β-lactamase production (e.g., *Klebsiella*)

4. Duration of antibiotic therapy

a. Duration of antibiotic therapy for core pathogens: 7 to 10 days

b. For *Pseudomonas* and *Acinetobacter* the average duration of antibiotic therapy is 10 to 14 days.

B. Adjunctive therapy (none are routine)

1. Supplemental oxygen

2. Positive pressure ventilation

a. Noninvasive ventilation

b. Endotracheal intubation and mechanical ventilation

3. Bronchodilators

4. Chest physical therapy

5. Subglottic suctioning

6. Fiberoptic bronchoscopy for mucus plug removal (selected cases)

7. See Chapter 91, Sepsis and SIRS, and Chapter 92, Septic Shock.

C. Supportive therapy

1. Address fluid and electrolyte imbalances.

2. Fluid resuscitation

3. Intensive monitoring

4. Nutritional support

5. Prophylaxis against deep venous thrombosis

6. Prophylaxis against stress-induced gastritis or ulceration

Key Prognosis

- Pneumonia constitutes the leading cause of death from infectious diseases and the sixth leading cause of death overall in the United States.

- The mortality with HAP is approximately 50%.

- Ventilator-associated pneumonia carries the highest mortality rate of all hospital-acquired infections, ranging from 50% to 70%, and is polymicrobial in up to 50% of cases.

Bibliography

American Thoracic Society. Guidelines for the management of adults with community-acquired pneumonia. Diagnosis, assessment of severity, antimicrobial therapy, and prevention. Am J Respir Crit Care Med 2001;163:1730–1754.

Bartlett JG, Breiman RF, Mandell LA, File TM Jr. Community-acquired pneumonia in adults: guidelines for management. Clin Infectious Dis 1998;26:811–838.

Campbell GD, Niederman MS, Broughton WA, et al. Hospital-acquired pneumonia in adults: diagnosis, assessment of severity, initial antimicrobial therapy and preventive strategies. Am J Respir Crit Care Med 1995;153:1711–1725.

Fine MJ, Auble TE, Yealy DM, et al. A prediction rule to identify low-risk patients with community-acquired pneumonia. N Engl J Med 1997;336:243–250.

Girou E, Schortgen F, Delclaux C, et al. Association of noninvasive ventilation with nosocomial infections and survival in critically ill patients. JAMA 2000;284:2361–2367.

Higgins TL. Nosocomial pneumonia. Clin Intensive Care 2000;12:115–126.

McEachern R, Campbell GD Jr. Hospital-acquired pneumonia: epidemiology, etiology, and treatment. Infect Dis Clin North Am 1998;12:761–779.

13 Aspiration Pneumonitis and Pneumonia

James E. Szalados

Aspiration is underdiagnosed and should be considered as a possible cause of any acute pulmonary decompensation. Aspiration of secretions is the leading cause of pneumonia, especially in the presence of dysphagia. Fully inflated endotracheal tube and tracheostomy tube cuffs do not prevent aspiration. Aspiration occurs in approximately 38% of patients with small-bore feeding tubes, and the risk is only marginally greater with large-bore nasogastric tubes.

Subclinical (silent) aspiration occurs in approximately 45% of healthy people, in 70% of patients with depressed consciousness, and in as many as 1% of patients undergoing uneventful general anesthesia. Clinical aspiration syndrome is uncommon in otherwise healthy patients and depends on the character and volume of the aspirate. In the presence of active regurgitation, the incidence of aspiration increases to 20%.

> **PEARL**
>
> Aspiration is a major cause of acute respiratory illness, including community-acquired pneumonia (10%), acute respiratory distress syndrome (up to 35%) and acute lung injury.

Terminology

A. Aspiration pneumonitis: pulmonary chemical injury induced by aspiration of gastric contents, oropharyngeal secretions, or inflammatory exogenous liquids

B. Aspiration pneumonia: an infectious process caused by aspiration of material colonized with bacteria

C. Mendelson's syndrome
   1. A parenchymal inflammatory syndrome progressing to acute lung injury (ALI) or acute respiratory distress syndrome (ARDS) after aspiration of acidic gastric contents (>25 mL or 0.4 mL/kg, with pH <2.5)
   2. Mortality ranges from 35% to 60%.

D. Foreign body or particulate aspiration
   1. Obstructive ("café coronary")
      a. Results from complete tracheal or bronchial obstruction

   b. Attempts at positive pressure ventilation lead to high airway pressures and unsuccessful ventilation.
   c. Negative pressure pulmonary edema may result.

2. Partially obstructive
   a. Partial tracheal obstruction results in sudden respiratory distress and stridor.
   b. Complete bronchial obstruction results in respiratory distress and may lead to distal hyperinflation and pneumothorax if ball-valve air-trapping occurs.

> **Key Classification**
>
> - Chemical: gastric acid, hydrocarbons (lipoid pneumonia), meconium, water (freshwater or saltwater near-drowning)
>
> - Bacterial: oropharyngeal secretions, purulent material (e.g., pharyngeal abscess or empyema)
>
> - Inert substances: foreign bodies, blood

Risk Factors

A. Depressed level of consciousness
   1. Sedation
   2. Drug overdose or alcohol intoxication
   3. General anesthesia (especially emergency surgery with "full stomach")
   4. Head injury
   5. Encephalopathy or coma
   6. Seizures

B. Impaired gag reflex
   1. Nasogastric intubation
   2. Topical or regional anesthesia affecting the larynx or pharynx
   3. Presence of nasogastric tube, endotracheal tube, or posterior nasal packing
   4. Bulbar dysfunction (e.g., due to cerebrovascular accident or degenerative neurologic disease)

C. Alimentary tract disorders
   1. Tracheoesophageal fistula
   2. Zenker's diverticulum

3. Esophageal motility disorders (e.g., achalasia, scleroderma, stricture)

4. Gastroesophageal reflux disease, hiatal hernia

5. Gastrointestinal hemorrhage

6. Diabetic or posttraumatic gastroparesis

7. Intestinal obstruction and ileus

D. Drugs that decrease lower esophageal (gastroesophageal) sphincter tone

1. Anticholinergics (e.g., atropine, glycopyrrolate)

2. Adrenergic agents (e.g., epinephrine, dopamine)

3. Nitrates (e.g., nitroprusside, nitroglycerin)

4. Phosphodiesterase inhibitors (e.g., caffeine, theophylline)

5. Calcium channel receptor antagonists

6. Estrogen

E. Other

1. Obesity

2. Parturition

Key Risk Factors

- Depressed sensorium

- Laryngeal dysfunction

- Altered upper gastrointestinal physiology

Pathophysiology

A. Trachea

1. Early epithelial denudation

2. Late desquamation

B. Bronchi: late inflammatory bronchiolitis

C. Alveoli

1. Inflammatory exudates, microhemorrhage, interstitial edema

2. Pneumocyte (types I and II) degeneration

3. Neutrophil infiltration

4. Hyaline membrane formation

5. Fibroblast proliferation

D. Pulmonary hypertension

1. Results from elevated pulmonary vascular resistance

2. May lead to acute right heart failure

E. Hypoxemia

1. Ventilation–perfusion mismatch and intrapulmonary shunting

2. Surfactant loss and atelectasis

3. Development of pulmonary edema (ARDS)

4. Bronchospasm (mediated by vagal reflexes)

F. Superinfection

1. Epithelial denudation and loss of ciliary clearance 2 to 10 days after aspiration

2. Mortality increased threefold

G. Microbiology

1. Older studies suggested that anaerobic organisms predominate.

2. Newer studies indicate infecting organisms are related to the setting, temporal features, host, and other factors, with recovery of aerobic organisms more likely.

Key Microbiologic Etiologies

- Aerobic Gram-positive organisms: *Streptococcus pneumoniae*, other streptococci, *Staphylococcus aureus*

- Aerobic Gram-negative organisms: *Haemophilus influenzae* and Enterobacteriaceae (e.g., *Klebsiella*, *Escherichia coli*, and *Pseudomonas aeruginosa*)

- Anaerobic Gram-positive organisms: *Peptostreptococcus, Lactobacillus, Clostridium, Eubacterium* spp.

- Gram-negative organisms: *Fusobacterium nucleatum, Prevotella melaninogenica, Bacteroides fragilis, Bacteroides ureolyticus*

Prevention

A. Rapid-sequence airway intubation

1. Gastric intubation prior to induction (will not remove large particles)

2. Avoid positive airway pressure without definitely secured airway.

3. Rapid induction of anesthesia and neuromuscular blockade

4. Cricoid pressure (Sellick's maneuver)

B. High-volume, low-pressure endotracheal tube cuff

C. Positioning (for patients at risk)

1. Semi-recumbent or upright position

2. Reverse Trendelenburg (head-up) position

3. Avoid supine position.

D. Decrease gastric volume.

1. Nothing per os, when possible

2. Gastrokinetic agents (e.g., metclopramide, erythromycin, domperidone)

3. Nonparticulate antacids (e.g., sodium citrate)

4. H_2-receptor antagonists to reduce volume and increase pH of gastric contents (e.g., ranitidine, famotidine, cimetidine)

5. Proton-pump inhibitors (e.g., omeprazole)

E. Anti-emetic administration (e.g., ondansetron, droperidol)

F. Emergency airway back-up (e.g., Combitube)

G. Gastric volume monitoring

H. Deglutition studies (i.e., barium pharyngo-esophagography)

I. Continuous or intermittent aspiration of subglottic secretions

Clinical and Laboratory Findings

A. Symptoms and physical findings
   1. History of witnessed regurgitation and aspiration
   2. Expectorated food particles
   3. Particulate matter in hypopharynx and upper airways
   4. Respiratory distress, tachypnea, cough, cyanosis, pulmonary edema
   5. Stridor, laryngospasm, bronchospasm, respiratory arrest
   6. Purulent sputum
   7. New adventitial breath sounds

B. Laboratory findings
   1. Arterial hypoxemia by pulse oximetry or arterial blood gas analysis
   2. Polymorphonuclear leukocytes in sputum

C. Chest x-ray
   1. Infiltrate(s) (changes may be delayed for up to 48 hours)
   2. Atelectasis

D. Clinical course
   1. Typically there is a short latent interval to onset of symptoms (less than 1 hour) with subsequent rapid progression.
   2. There may be rapid clinical and radiologic improvement (60%), progressive deterioration and death (10%), or rapid initial improvement and deterioration (30%).

PEARL

The particular infecting organism is related to the setting (hospital, ICU, community), time of sampling (early vs. late), technique (tracheal aspirate, expectorated sputum, protected brush, transthoracic needle), and host factors (alcoholic, nursing home resident, anesthesia recipient).

Treatment

A. Emergency management
   1. Protect airway, using endotracheal intubation if necessary.
   2. Position patient to prevent further aspiration.
   3. Suction oropharynx and trachea.
   4. Provide supplemental oxygen.
   5. Insert nasogastric tube for gastric decompression.
   6. Continuous positive airway pressure or positive end-expiratory pressure can be helpful to improve oxygenation.
   7. See also Chapter 6, Respiratory Failure and Chapter 8, Acute Respiratory Distress Syndrome.

B. Antibiotics* (not indicated routinely for aspiration pneumonitis)
   1. Community-acquired aspiration pneumonia: levofloxacin 500 mg/day or ceftriaxone 1 to 2 g/day
   2. Nursing home resident or patient with gastric colonization or small bowel obstruction: levofloxacin 500 mg/day or ciprofloxacin 400 mg every 12 hours or piperacillin-tazobactam 3.375 g every 6 hours or ceftazidime 2 g every 8 hours
   3. Severe periodontal disease or alcoholism: piperacillin-tazobactam 3.375 g every 6 hours, imipenem 500 mg every 8 hours to 1 g every 6 hours, or a combination of a quinolone or ceftriaxone (1 to 2 g/day) plus either clindamycin 600 mg every 8 hours or metronidazole 500 mg every 8 hours

C. Bronchospasm can be treated with inhaled bronchodilators, ipratropium, and corticosteroids (see Chapter 179, Inhaled Bronchodilators).

D. Fluid resuscitation for patients with hypotension or other signs of perfusion failure (see Chapter 91, Sepsis and SIRS, Chapter 92, Septic Shock, and Chapter 208, Fluid Challenge)

E. Unproven or controversial therapy
   1. Systemic corticosteroids are of no proven benefit for aspiration pneumonitis or pneumonia.
   2. Lavage of the airways is ineffective.
   3. Attempts to neutralize acid aspiration are not indicated (potential for exothermic reactions that can produce airway burns).
   4. Bronchoscopy is reserved for particulate aspiration and atelectasis not responsive to positive

---

* Doses given are for patients with normal renal function.

pressure ventilation with continuous positive airway pressure or positive end-expiratory pressure.

Bibliography

Boysen PG, Modell J. Pulmonary aspiration. In: Shoemaker WC, Ayres SM, Grenvik A, Holbrook PR (eds). Textbook of Critical Care, 4th ed. Philadelphia: WB Saunders 2000, pp 1432–1439.

Franquet T, Gimenez A, Roson N, et al. Aspiration diseases: findings, pitfalls, and differential diagnosis. Radiographics 2000;20:673–685.

Kluger MT, Short TG. Aspiration during anaesthesia: a review of 133 cases from the Australian Incident Monitoring Study (AIMS). Anaesthesia 1999;54:19–26.

Lundy DS, Smith C, Colangelo L, et al. Aspiration: cause and implications. Otolaryngol Head Neck Surg 1999; 120:474–478.

Marik PE. Aspiration pneumonitis and aspiration pneumonia. N Engl J Med 2001;334:665–671.

Marik PE, Careau P. The role of anaerobes in patients with ventilator-associated pneumonia and aspiration pneumonia: a prospective study. Chest 1999;115:178–183.

Tietjan PA, Kaner RJ, Quinn CE. Aspiration emergencies. Clin Chest Med 1994;15:117–124.

14 COPD Exacerbation

Michael J. Apostolakos

Chronic obstructive pulmonary disease (COPD) is a major medical problem and the fourth leading cause of death in the United States. Cigarette smoking remains the single leading risk factor. Acute exacerbations are manifested by increased dyspnea, wheezing, coughing, sputum production, and impaired gas exchange. The major precipitants are infectious, although air pollution and changes in temperature play a role.

Risk Factors

A. Cigarette smoking
B. Infections
   1. Viruses: rhinoviruses, influenza virus, parainfluenza virus, coronavirus
   2. Bacteria: *Haemophilus influenzae, Streptococcus pneumoniae, Moraxella catarrhalis, Mycoplasma pneumoniae, Chlamydia pneumonia*
C. Pollutants
D. Chemical irritants
E. α_1-Antitrypsin deficiency

Symptoms

A. Increased cough
B. Changes in volume, tenacity, and purulence of sputum
C. Increased breathlessness
D. Wheezing
E. Chest tightness

Physical Findings

A. Use of accessory muscles for breathing
B. Paradoxical breathing
C. Changes in mentation

Laboratory Findings (also see Chapter 218, Blood Gas and Oximetry Monitoring)

A. Hypoxemia
B. Hypercarbia
C. Respiratory acidosis
D. Reduced peak expiratory flow rate
E. White blood cells in sputum

Imaging Studies

A. Chest radiography
   1. Hyperinflation
   2. Increased anterior–posterior thoracic diameter
   3. Flattened diaphragm
   4. Increased retrosternal airspace
   5. Long, narrow cardiac shadow
   6. Bullae
   7. Hilar vascular prominence
   8. Pneumonia if cause of exacerbation
B. Computed tomography of chest
   1. Greater sensitivity and specificity than chest radiography
   2. May predict benefit from pulmonary resection and identify bronchiectasis

Key Monitoring

- Arterial blood gases
- Peak expiratory flow rate
- Mental status
- Signs of respiratory fatigue

Treatment

A. Bronchodilator therapy
   1. β_2-adrenergic agonists (albuterol, metaproterenol, terbutaline): give every 2 to 4 hours via nebulization or metered dose inhaler with a spacer
      a. Continuous nebulization required in some cases
      b. Dosing often limited by tremulousness and tachydysrhythmias
   2. Anticholinergics (ipratropium bromide): give every 4 to 6 hours via nebulization or metered dose inhaler with spacer
      a. Bronchodilator effects similar to β_2-adrenergic agonists; may be synergistic
      b. Fewer side effects than β_2-adrenergic agonists
   3. Theophylline or aminophylline: role is limited because of high toxic to therapeutic index; lim-

ited proof of efficacy when combined with bronchodilators.

B. Anti-inflammatory agents

1. Corticosteroids: methylprednisolone 120 to 240 mg/day intravenously or equivalent in divided doses for 3 days, followed by once a day oral prednisone 60 mg, tapering to 20 mg by day 14

2. Use is associated with an increased rate of improvement in oxygenation, spirometry, and decreased treatment failure rate; hyperglycemia may result.

C. Antibiotic therapy

1. Cotrimoxazole, amoxicillin, or doxycycline; use second- or third-generation cephalosporins, fluroquinolone, newer macrolide, or broad-spectrum penicillin for resistant organisms or severely ill patient

2. Use is associated with increased symptom resolution, improvement of peak expiratory flow rate, and decreased treatment failure rate.

D. Supplemental oxygen (also see Chapter 222, Oxygen Therapy)

1. Low-flow oxygen at 1 to 2 L/minute via nasal prong or 28% venturi mask for modest hypoxemia

2. Goal is to achieve arterial oxygen saturation of approximately 90%.

3. Serial blood gases to assess oxygenation, hypercarbia, and acidosis

E. Mechanical ventilation

1. Indication: progressive fatigue and respiratory or ventilatory failure

2. Noninvasive ventilation

a. Continuous positive airway pressure mask with supplemental oxygen

(1) Criteria: cooperative, hemodynamically stable, alert or only mildly obtunded, no significant upper gastrointestinal problems, able to maintain airway and clear secretions, adequate fitting mask

(2) Setting: 5 to 10 cm H_2O

b. Noninvasive mechanical ventilation: bi-level positive airway pressure device or conventional ventilator

(1) Initial settings: inspiratory pressure approximately 8 to 15 cm H_2O, expiratory pressure approximately 5 to 10 cm H_2O

(2) Monitor closely, assess for mask-induced facial trauma.

(3) Avoid peak pressures greater than 30 cm H_2O.

(4) Blood gas changes may lag behind clinical improvement.

(5) Provide intervals of unassisted breathing.

3. Invasive mechanical ventilation (see Chapters 223, 224, 226, on Mechanical Ventilation)

a. Indications include persistent hypoxemia, progressive respiratory acidosis, fatigue, deteriorating mental status, inability to protect airway or clear secretions.

b. No proven superiority of any specific mode of mechanical ventilation

c. Ensure long expiratory times to decrease hyperinflation.

d. Utilize permissive hypercapnia to avoid high plateau pressures and intrinsic (auto-) positive end-expiratory pressure to reduce risk of barotrauma.

Key Treatment

- Antibiotics
- Anti-inflammatory agents
- Bronchodilators
- Supplemental oxygen
- Frequent reassessment of need for assisted ventilation

Prevention

A. Smoking cessation

B. Pulmonary rehabilitation

C. Improved nutrition

D. Early medical intervention during exacerbation

E. Pneumococcal and influenza vaccines

F. Chemoprophylaxis (amantadine) in unvaccinated patients exposed to influenza

 Bibliography

American Thoracic Society. Standards for the diagnosis and care of patients with chronic obstructive pulmonary disease. Am J Respir Crit Care Med 1995;152:S77–S120.

Barnes PJ. Chronic obstructive pulmonary disease. N Engl J Med 2000;343:269–280.

Brochard L, Mancebo J, Wisocki M, et al. Noninvasive ventilation for acute exacerbations of chronic obstructive pulmonary disease. N Engl J Med 1995;333:817–822.

Ferguson GT. Recommendations for the management of COPD. Chest 2000;117:23S–28S.

Madison JM, Irwin RS. Chronic obstructive pulmonary disease. Lancet 1998;352:467–473.

Niewoehner DE, Erbland ML, Deupree RH, et al. Effect of systemic glucocorticoids on exacerbations of chronic obstructive pulmonary disease. N Engl J Med 1999;340:1941–1947.

Sayiner A, Aytemur ZA, Cirit M. Systemic glucocorticoids in severe exacerbations of COPD. Chest 2001;119:726–730.

15 Cor Pulmonale

Syed K. Shahryar
Richard W. Carlson

Key Definition

Cor pulmonale refers to alterations in the structure and function of the right ventricle of the heart with hypertrophy or dilation due to pulmonary hypertension secondary to disease of the lung or its vasculature.

Pathophysiology

A. Mechanisms may be acute or chronic

B. Hypoxemia induces pulmonary vasoconstriction. Production and levels of endothelin-1, nitric oxide, prostaglandins, and leukotrienes may correlate with hypoxic pulmonary vasoconstriction and be operative in the development of cor pulmonale.

C. The major cause of right ventricular (RV) overload is an increase in pulmonary vascular resistance.

D. The right ventricle is normally a low-pressure, high-volume pump.
   1. Acute processes that increase RV systolic pressure to 55 to 60 mm Hg (mean 40 mm Hg) lead to acute cor pulmonale.
   2. Chronic processes are associated with higher RV pressures.

E. Acute cor pulmonale: dilatation predominates

F. Chronic cor pulmonale: dilatation and hypertrophy increase RV size

G. Accounts for 20% of hospitalizations for heart failure

Etiology

A. Chronic obstructive pulmonary disease (COPD, the leading cause of chronic cor pulmonale)

B. Interstitial lung disease

C. Collagen vascular diseases
   1. Systemic lupus erythematosus
   2. Progressive systemic sclerosis
   3. Variant syndromes

D. Acute and chronic pulmonary thromboembolism

E. Primary pulmonary hypertension

F. Pulmonary venous obstruction
   1. Neoplastic: carcinoma, lymphoma
   2. Infectious
      a. Tuberculosis
      b. Histoplasmosis
   3. Inflammatory and fibrotic
      a. Sarcoidosis
      b. Radiation therapy
      c. Sickle cell disease

G. Drugs (e.g., certain anorectic drugs)

H. Alveolar hypoventilation
   1. Ineffective respiratory muscle pump
      a. Myasthenia gravis
      b. Guillain-Barré syndrome
      c. Muscular dystrophy
      d. Other neuromuscular disorders
   2. Impaired central respiratory drive
      a. Sleep apnea syndrome
      b. Cerebral vascular events
   3. Thoracic cage defects (e.g., kyphoscoliosis)
   4. Severe obesity

Key Symptoms (Generally Nonspecific)

- Fatigue
- Dyspnea
- Cough
- Leg edema
- Syncope
- Palpitations

Physical Examination

A. Tachycardia

B. Tachypnea

C. Jugular venous distention
   1. Early *a* wave prominence
   2. *v* wave enlarges later.
   3. Rapid *y* descent

D. Cardiac findings
   1. Parasternal lift
   2. Systolic ejection click
   3. Loud P_2
   4. S_3 or S_4 gallop
   5. Diastolic murmur of pulmonary insufficiency (Graham-Steell murmur)
   6. Systolic murmur of tricuspid insufficiency

E. Hepatomegaly

F. Asterixis

G. Clubbing

H. Somnolence

I. Cyanosis

J. Peripheral edema

Imaging Studies

A. Chest x-ray

1. Large central pulmonary arteries

2. Widening of descending pulmonary arteries

3. Distal pruning

B. Echocardiogram and echo-Doppler

1. Increased RV wall thickness

2. Enlarged RV cavity

3. Leftward displacement of the interventricular septum

4. Increased RV systolic pressure

5. Increased mean pulmonary artery pressure

C. Magnetic resonance imaging: also allows assessment of RV dimensions

D. Computed tomography of chest

1. Assesses the parenchyma

2. Detects malignancy or fibrosis

E. Ventilation–perfusion scan or pulmonary angiogram: performed to exclude pulmonary embolic disease

---

PEARL

Pulmonary embolism must be excluded, especially in acute cor pulmonale.

Other Tests

A. Electrocardiogram

1. Evidence of RV hypertrophy

2. P pulmonale

3. Rightward QRS axis

4. ST segment depression in leads II, III, and aVF

5. Right bundle branch block

B. Laboratory tests

1. Arterial blood gases

a. Hypoxemia, often with poor response to increasing FIO_2

b. Hypocarbia or hypercarbia

2. Serologic studies for collagen vascular diseases and sarcoidosis

C. Pulmonary function tests

D. Sleep studies

E. Right heart catheterization

Treatment

A. Correct hypoxemia (PaO_2 higher than 60 mm Hg; SaO_2 higher than 90%).

B. Identify and treat COPD or pulmonary embolism (see Chapters 10 and 14).

C. Administer diuretics for edema.

1. Use cautiously to avoid critically decreasing RV preload.

2. Avoid exacerbating metabolic alkalosis.

D. Give digitalis; helpful in the presence of left ventricular failure.

E. Consider slow phlebotomy if the hematocrit is above 55%.

F. Attempt treatment of cardiac dysrhythmias.

G. Consider anticoagulation (targeted international normalized ratio is 2 to 3).

H. Consider corticosteroids for severe COPD.

I. Consider vasodilator therapy.

1. Must be used cautiously

2. First, document pulmonary vasodilator reserve with acute vasodilator challenge during right heart catheterization.

3. Drug choices

a. Calcium channel blockers: nifedipine or diltiazem

b. Epoprostenol (analogue of prostaglandin I_2) by IV infusion

c. Inhaled nitric oxide (investigational)

J. Consider transplantation for progressive disease.

Key Treatment

• Correct hypoxemia.

• Treat underlying disorder.

Prognosis

A. Prognosis is related to the underlying disorder.

B. Pulmonary hypertension is rapidly progressive and usually is fatal within years.

C. Secondary pulmonary hypertension is associated with shortened survival, except for certain treatable disorders such as pulmonary thromboembolism.

Bibliography

Cargill RI, Kiely DG, Clark RA, et al. Hypoxaemia and release of endothelin-1. Thorax 1995;50:1308–1310.

Clini E, Cremona G, Campana M, et al. Production of endogenous nitric oxide in chronic obstructive pulmonary disease and patients with cor pulmonale. Correlates with echo-Doppler assessment. Am J Respir Crit Care Med 2000;162(2 pt 1):446–450.

MacNee W. Pathophysiology of cor pulmonale in chronic obstructive pulmonary disease. I. Am J Respir Crit Care Med 1994;150:833–852.

MacNee W. Pathophysiology of cor pulmonale in chronic obstructive pulmonary disease. II. Am J Respir Crit Care Med 1994;150:1158–1168.

Rich S, Seidlitz M, Dodin E, et al. The short-term effects of digoxin in patients with right ventricular dysfunction from pulmonary hypertension. Chest 1998;114:787–792.

Vizza CD, Lynch JP, Ochoa LL, et al. Right and left ventricular dysfunction in patients with severe pulmonary disease. Chest 1998;113:576–583.

16 Smoke Inhalation

Syed K. Shahryar
Chai Jie Chang
Richard W. Carlson

Smoke is a suspension of particles in hot air and a mixture of toxic gases. Smoke inhalation results from outdoor or indoor fires, occupational exposures, industrial accidents and military applications. More than 2 million fires occur annually in the United States, a high proportion of which are residential fires, and the annual death rate exceeds 4,000. The composition of burning materials affects the components of the smoke produced, but it may include carbon monoxide, carbon dioxide, phosgene, aldehydes, benzene, hydrogen chloride, and hydrogen cyanide, among other toxic gases. Direct thermal airway injury, with burns involving the larynx and the upper and lower airways, occurs in many fire victims and increases mortality.

Pathophysiology

A. Direct thermal injury to the airway as well as effects of inhalation of toxic gases
B. Pulmonary injury occurs in two phases.
   1. A cellular and exudative phase with production of inflammatory mediators and leukocyte infiltration
   2. A repair and proliferative phase with cellular hyperplasia, fibrosis, and hyaline membrane formation

---

PEARL

Most deaths from fires result from smoke inhalation, rather than direct thermal injuries (burns) or other trauma.

Diagnosis

A. Clinical clues
   1. Victim trapped in confined space
   2. Altered mental status
   3. Facial or upper cervical burns
   4. Singed eyebrows or nasal vibrissae
   5. Bronchial breath sounds
   6. Wheezing, rales, cyanosis
   7. Expectoration of carbonaceous sputum
B. Initial evaluation
   1. Clinical assessment
      a. Vital signs
      b. Sensorium and mentation
      c. Presence of respiratory distress
      d. Direct laryngoscopy
   2. Key laboratory tests
      a. CO-oximetry is necessary to quantify carboxyhemoglobin and assess oxygenation.
      b. Carboxyhemoglobin levels higher than 20% are associated with increased morbidity and mortality.
      c. Use blood lactate level and presence of metabolic acidosis to assess for critical hypoxia, carbon monoxide, and cyanide toxicity.
      d. Cardiac marker assays to assess for myocardial ischemia or infarction
   3. Electrocardiogram
   4. Chest x-ray
      a. The initial chest x-ray is insensitive for detecting inhalation injury and is often normal.
      b. Focal or patchy infiltrates typically evolve within 24 to 36 hours.
      c. Diffuse pulmonary edema with progressive injury can occur.
      d. Evaluate for pneumothorax, hydrothorax, and hemothorax, pulmonary contusion, and fractures.
   5. Assess for other injuries and surface burns.
C. Subsequent evaluation
   1. Perform bronchoscopy within 24 hours.
      a. Detects large airway injury, mucosal damage, edema, erosions, hemorrhage, necrosis, and particulate material
      b. Helpful to identify late complications such as tracheobronchial stenosis and polyps
      c. Normal bronchoscopic examination does not exclude small airway injury.
   2. Computed tomography scan of chest: helpful for identifying other injuries and to detect sequelae such as bronchiectasis, bronchiolitis obliterans, and fibrosis.
   3. Xenon 133 ventilation–perfusion scan useful to evaluate pulmonary injury

---

PEARL

Hypoxemia caused by carboxyhemoglobinemia is not detectable by pulse oximetry or by blood gas panels that do not include multi-wavelength CO-oximetry.

Treatment

A. Initial management
1. Maintain airway
2. Potential indications for endotracheal intubation
   a. Stridor
   b. Upper airway–laryngeal edema
   c. Respiratory distress
   d. Altered sensorium with inability to protect airway
   e. Hypercarbia
   f. Refractory hypoxemia
3. Oxygenate
   a. Provide FIO_2 of 1.00 initially to all patients.
   b. Maintain FIO_2 of 1.00 if there is metabolic acidosis, high carboxyhemoglobin level, hyperlactatemia, cyanide intoxication, or shock.
4. Assess and treat surface burns (see Chapter 145, Thermal Burn Injury).
5. Assess and treat other injuries.
   a. Provide volume resuscitation.
   b. Assess cervical spine if there is neurologic impairment.
6. Coordinate management of smoke inhalation with that for surface burns and other injuries.

B. Intensive care unit management
1. Mechanical ventilation with FIO_2 of 1.00 is employed for all cases of significant carbon monoxide or cyanide toxicity (see Chapter 70, Cyanide Poisoning, and Chapter 71, Carbon Monoxide Poisoning).
2. Positive end-expiratory pressure (PEEP) and other maneuvers to maintain oxygenation (see Chapters 223, 224, and 226 on mechanical ventilation and Chapter 225 PEEP)
3. High-frequency percussive ventilation employed by some burn centers
4. Inhaled bronchodilator therapy
5. Racemic epinephrine may be helpful in patients with upper airway changes or stridor who do not require intubation.
6. Aggressive pulmonary toilet, bronchoscopic removal of casts, nebulization
7. Corticosteroids
   a. Use is controversial, but has been recommended for patients without thermal surface burns who have findings of upper airway edema or severe bronchospasm unresponsive to bronchodilators, and for treatment of bronchiolitis obliterans.
   b. Dose: 2 mg/kg per day of methylprednisolone (or equivalent) for 24 to 48 hours
8. Pain control, sedation
9. Nutritional support
10. Antibiotics
    a. Risk of infection increases within 48 to 72 hours of inhalational injury.
    b. Reserve antibiotics for documented infection (fever, purulent sputum, leukocytosis with developing infiltrates on chest x-ray).

CAUTION

- Because of the increased risk of infection, corticosteroids are not routinely indicated for inhalational injury associated with surface burns.

- Antibiotics do not influence survival rates and should not be used routinely.

Complications

A. Hyperreactivity of airways
B. Recurrent chronic bronchitis and pneumonia
C. Chronic obstructive pulmonary disease
D. Tracheal stenosis
E. Bronchiectasis
F. Bronchiolitis obliterans
G. Interstitial fibrosis
H. Endobronchial polyposis

Bibliography

Demling RH. Smoke inhalation injury. New Horizons 1993;1:422–434.

Fitzpatrick JC, Cioff WG. Diagnosis and Treatment of Inhalation Injury. In: Herndon DN (ed). Total Burn Care. Philadelphia: WB Saunders, 1996, pp 184–192.

Hantson P, Butera R, Clemessy JL, et al. Early complications and value of initial clinical and paraclinical observations in victims of smoke inhalation without burns. Chest 1997;111:671–675.

Haponik EF. Smoke inhalation injury: Some priorities for respiratory care professionals. Respir Care 1992;37:609–613.

Orzel RA. Toxicological aspects of firesmoke: polymer pyrolysis and combustion. Occup Med 1993;8:414–429.

Weiss SM, Lakshminarayan S. Acute inhalation injury. Clin Chest Med 1994;15:103–116.

17 Massive Hemoptysis

Alain Tremblay
Kalpalatha K. Guntupalli

Massive hemoptysis can be defined as 500 mL or more of gross bleeding from the tracheobronchial tree in a 24-hour period. It is a life-threatening condition, demanding prompt stabilization and a management strategy to prevent asphyxiation. Often, prompt treatment must be performed prior to definitive determination of the etiology. Despite its relative frequency, especially in large referral hospitals, no controlled trials are available to guide optimal management. Therefore, therapeutic recommendations employ expert opinion and uncontrolled case series. Management is often dependent on local resources as well as physician preference and expertise. Successful management requires communication and cooperation between multiple specialists.

Etiology

A. Tuberculosis
   1. Active
      a. Bronchiolar necrosis
      b. Rupture of Rasmussen's aneurysm (pseudo-aneurysm of the pulmonary artery)
   2. Healed
      a. Bronchiectasis
      b. Fungus ball
      c. Rasmussen's aneurysm
      d. Broncholith erosion of calcified node into bronchial artery
      e. Scar carcinoma
B. Bronchiectasis
   1. Postinfectious
   2. Cystic fibrosis
C. Pulmonary infections
   1. Fungal mycetoma
      a. *Aspergillus fumigatus* is most common; seen with other fungi as well.
   2. Lung abscess
   3. Invasive fungal infection
      a. *Aspergillus*
      b. Mucormycosis
   4. Other bacterial infections
   5. Septic pulmonary emboli
   6. Paragonimiasis
D. Carcinoma (particularly squamous cell carcinoma)
E. Iatrogenic
   1. Post-bronchoscopy
   2. Right heart catheterization (pulmonary artery rupture)
   3. Transthoracic needle biopsy
F. Alveolar hemorrhage syndromes
   1. Anti-basement membrane antibody syndrome
   2. Systemic lupus erythematosus and other correc-tive tissue distress
   3. Rapidly progressive glomerulonephritis
   4. Systemic vasculitides
   5. Post–bone marrow transplant
   6. Wegener's granulomatoses
G. Airway trauma
H. Coagulopathy
I. Mitral stenosis (less common cause; resolves with valve replacement)
J. Vascular malformations
   1. Hereditary hemorrhagic telangiectasia
   2. Arteriovenous malformations
K. Pulmonary embolism
   1. Pulmonary infarction
   2. From anticoagulant or thrombolytic therapy

Key Etiologies

- Tuberculosis
- Bronchiectasis
- Cancer
- Mycetoma
- Other infectious causes
- Iatrogenic causes
- Alveolar hemorrhage
- Trauma
- Vascular malformations
- Pulmonary embolism

Pathophysiology

A. Lung vasculature
   1. Bronchial circulation
      a. High (systemic) pressure circulation
      b. Drains into right atrium (extrapulmonary bronchi)
      c. Also drains into pulmonary veins (intrapul-monary bronchi)
      d. Anterior spinal artery may originate from bronchial artery (5% of cases).

53

2. Pulmonary circulation
   a. Low-pressure circulation
   b. Multiple anastomoses exist between bronchial and pulmonary circulations.

Clinical Findings

A. Symptoms
   1. Hemoptysis, dyspnea, cough, anxiety
   2. Patient's subjective localization of side of bleeding is suggestive.
   3. Elicit symptoms of possible underlying etiologies (examples):
      a. Fever and weight loss in tuberculosis
      b. Hematuria in vasculitides
   4. Smoking and travel history may be revealing.

B. Physical findings
   1. Bloody sputum
      a. Frothy blood–sputum mixture
      b. Bright red
      c. Alkaline
   2. Tachypnea, respiratory distress
   3. Findings specific to etiology (examples)
      a. Localized wheezing (if endobronchial source)
      b. Apical rales (tuberculosis)
      c. Poor dentition (in lung abscess)
      d. Digital clubbing (in malignancy or bronchiectasis)

Key Differential Diagnosis

- Upper gastrointestinal bleeding: suggested by presence of dark blood, food particles, or acid pH; consider endoscopy to confirm
- Upper airway bleeding: perform thorough examination of mouth, nose, and pharynx

Laboratory Tests

A. There are no specific laboratory abnormalities, unless associated with the underlying disease.

B. Sputum tests
   1. Microbiologic stains and cultures for bacteria (Gram stain and acid-fast bacilli testing) and fungi
   2. Cytologic examination

C. Blood tests
   1. Complete blood cell count (hemoglobin is rarely low as a direct result of hemoptysis)
   2. Platelet count

   3. Coagulation tests: prothrombin and partial thromboplastin times
   4. Type and cross match
   5. Arterial blood gases

D. Urinalysis

E. 12-Lead electrocardiogram

Imaging Studies

A. Chest x-ray
   1. May suggest etiology
   2. Normal x-ray suggests endobronchial or extrapulmonary source.
   3. Potentially misleading radiographic findings
      a. Aspirated blood with infiltrate distant from source
      b. Chronic changes unrelated to acute event

B. Chest computed tomography scan
   1. Useful in stable patients; not indicated in actively bleeding, unstable patients
   2. High-resolution scans are useful to detect bronchiectasis.
   3. Similar caveats to chest x-ray

C. Other tests as clinically indicated, e.g., nuclear ventilation–perfusion scan, echocardiography

D. Angiography: see later under Treatment section.

Key Monitoring

- Admit to intensive care unit.
- Respiratory and airway monitoring
- Continuous pulse oximetry
- Continuous electrocardiography
- Blood pressure monitoring

Treatment

A. General measures
   1. Place patient with bleeding site (if known) down to prevent aspiration into contralateral lung.
   2. Provide supplemental oxygen, as needed.
   3. Mild cough suppression may be given; aggressive cough suppression will impair airway clearance of blood.
   4. Avoid sedation.
   5. Correct coagulopathy and thrombocytopenia, if present.
   6. Consultation

a. Early critical care and thoracic surgery consultation

b. Consider early involvement of anesthesiologist and interventional radiologist.

B. Primary goal is airway control.

1. Asphyxiation, not blood loss, is the cause of death.

2. Only stable patients with ability to clear their own airway should be managed without endotracheal intubation.

3. Endotracheal intubation

a. Intubation should be performed by experienced personnel.

b. Large tube (≥8 Fr) should be used to permit bronchoscopy and suctioning.

c. Consider bronchial blocker tube or double lumen endotracheal tube if site of bleeding is known.

C. Secondary goal is localization of bleeding.

1. Bronchoscopy is required in most patients.

2. Endotracheal intubation is recommended prior to bronchoscopy.

3. Rigid bronchoscopy

a. Recommended by some authors to facilitate airway control and allow better suctioning of blood

b. Disadvantages include inability to visualize beyond main stem bronchi and lack of physician trained in the procedure.

D. Bronchoscopic interventions

1. Endobronchial blockade

a. Bronchial-blocker endotracheal tube or Fogarty balloon catheter to occlude bleeding lung, lobe, or segment

2. Topical coagulants: fibrin or fibrinogen–thrombin solution may be helpful if injected beyond bronchial blockage.

3. Consider Nd:YAG laser coagulation, electrocoagulation, or argon plasma coagulation if a bleeding lesion is visible.

4. Lavage with iced saline may be effective.

5. Topical epinephrine is helpful for bleeding after bronchoscopic lung biopsy.

E. Unilateral lung ventilation

1. If bleeding is from left lung, a single-lumen endotracheal tube can be advanced into the right main stem bronchus.

2. Disadvantage is loss of access to left lung

3. Right upper lobe (RUL) obstruction and collapse is a frequent complication.

F. Use of double-lumen endotracheal tube

1. Protects the non-bleeding lung from large-volume aspiration

2. "Left-sided" tube should be used in most cases to avoid RUL obstruction.

3. Difficult to position tube properly

4. Individual lumens are too small for bronchoscope (pediatric bronchoscope may fit) and may obstruct easily with blood clots or secretions.

5. Airway obstruction is the most frequent practical problem.

6. Displacement of the tube can lead to sudden asphyxiation.

7. Patient should be therapeutically paralyzed and not moved.

G. Bronchial arteriography and embolization

1. The favored initial approach if facilities and expertise are available

2. High success rate: approximately 90% when a bleeding bronchial vessel is identified

3. Recurrence rate ranges from 10% to 27%.

4. Approximately 10% of patients bleed from the pulmonary circulation (usually from tuberculosis or mycetoma), which should be examined if no bronchial bleeding is identified.

5. Serious complications include occlusion of anterior spinal artery with paraplegia, and embolic infarction of distal organs.

H. Early surgical treatment

1. Offers definitive treatment

2. Indicated for lateralized massive life-threatening hemoptysis, or failure or recurrence after other interventions

3. Preoperative evaluation must be expedited, but could include spirometry and quantitative lung scanning.

4. Contraindications

a. Poor baseline respiratory function

b. Inoperable lung carcinoma

c. Inability to localize bleeding site

d. Diffuse lung disease (relative contraindication), e.g., cystic fibrosis

5. Mortality is higher if bleeding is acute.

I. Late surgical treatment

1. Indicated for definitive treatment of underlying lesion, once bleeding has subsided

2. Indications may include mycetoma, resectable carcinoma, and localized bronchiectasis.

Key Treatment

- Control of airway
- Localization of bleeding (bronchoscopy)
- Bronchial artery embolization
- Definitive surgical therapy

Prognosis

A. Factors likely affecting outcome
  1. Etiology of hemoptysis
  2. Underlying co-morbid illnesses
  3. Surgical versus medical treatment
B. Mortality
  1. Estimated medical mortality: 17% to 85%
  2. Estimated early surgical mortality: 0% to 50%
  3. Most case series reports preceded the development of angiographic embolization.

Bibliography

Brinson GM, Noone PG, Mauro MA, et al. Bronchial artery embolization for the treatment of hemoptysis in patients with cystic fibrosis. Am J Respir Crit Care Med 1998;157(6 Pt 1):1951–1958.

Cahill BC, Ingbar DH. Massive hemoptysis. Assessment and management. Clin Chest Med 1994;15:147–167.

Dweik RA, Stoller JK. Role of bronchoscopy in massive hemoptysis. Clin Chest Med 1999;20:89–105.

Knott-Craig CJ, Oostuizen JG, Rossouw G, et al. Management and prognosis of massive hemoptysis. Recent experience with 120 patients. J Thorac Cardiovasc Surg 1993;105:394–397.

Ost D, Corbridge T. Independent lung ventilation. Clin Chest Med 1996;17:591–601.

Remy J, Arnaud A, Fardou H, et al. Treatment of hemoptysis by embolization of bronchial arteries. Radiology 1977;122:33–37.

18 Atelectasis

Burkhard Lachmann
Peter J. Papadakos

Collapse of alveolar beds is a common finding in critically ill patients. This process can lead to atelectasis, which is associated with a variety of physiologic disturbances that can affect patient management and outcome.

Etiology

A. Respiratory fatigue

B. Increased work of breathing

C. Mucous plugging or foreign body

D. Cyclic opening and closing of alveoli with mechanical ventilation

E. Low levels of tidal volume or positive end-expiratory pressure (PEEP) during mechanical ventilation

F. Pulmonary contusion

G. Postoperative state, especially after thoracic or upper abdominal procedures

Pathophysiology

A. Surfactant depletion

B. Decreased functional residual capacity

C. Hypoxemia, caused by increased right-to-left shunting

D. Barotrauma

E. Bacterial transmigration with pneumonitis

F. Cytokine modulation and release

Clinical Findings

A. Respiratory distress, dyspnea

B. Poor inspiratory effort, low tidal volume

C. Increased respiratory rate

D. Increased work of breathing

E. Crackles on physical examination (from opening and closing of alveolar beds)

F. Dullness to percussion and decreased fremitus (lobar collapse)

G. Decreased breath sounds (occluded bronchus); tubular breath sounds and egophony (central airway patency)

H. Fever is an unreliable finding of atelectasis.

Key Findings

- Dyspnea
- Tachypnea
- Low tidal volume
- Dullness to percussion
- Decreased or tubular breath sounds
- Pulmonary rales

Laboratory and Other Tests

A. Arterial blood gas analysis

B. End-tidal CO_2 monitoring

C. Pressure–volume curve on ventilator graphics

D. Ventilator opening pressure

E. Chest radiography

F. Computed tomography scanning of the chest

Key Radiographic Findings

- Radiographic findings of atelectasis may be absent (microatelectasis), moderate (plate-like), or massive (lobar collapse).

- Air bronchograms in atelectasis correlate with central airway patency and tubular breath sounds on examination.

Differential Diagnosis

A. Pulmonary embolism

B. Pneumonia

C. Pulmonary edema, including the acute respiratory distress syndrome

D. Ventilatory failure

E. Cardiovascular collapse

F. Aspiration

Treatment

A. Supplemental oxygen

B. Pulmonary toilet

  1. Suctioning and chest percussion

  2. Deep breathing, frequent turning

  3. Upright posture, if possible; lateral decubitus with collapsed region uppermost

4. Mucolytic agents are often administered, but their efficacy is not well substantiated.

C. Bronchodilator therapy

D. Treat pain, avoid excessive sedation.

E. Bronchoscopy

 1. Controversial

 2. Consider if physical therapy maneuvers cannot be tolerated, failure of 1 to 2 days of conservative measures, massive atelectasis, lack of central air bronchograms, or presence of foreign body.

F. Ventilator management (also see Chapters 223, 224, and 226, on Mechanical Ventilation and Chapter 225, PEEP)

 1. Open lung concept

  a. Use short intervals of peak pressure of 40 to 60 cm H_2O with end-inspiratory pauses; decline in plateau pressure suggests re-expansion.

  b. Splint the lung with PEEP to recruit lung units.

  c. Adjust peak inspiratory pressure.

 2. Consider rotational bed therapy or prone positioning during mechanical ventilation.

Key Treatment

- Supplemental oxygen
- Pulmonary toilet
- Open lung concept

Prevention

A. Preoperative

 1. Smoking cessation at least 3 weeks prior to procedure

2. Bronchodilators for obstructive disease

3. Treat bronchopulmonary infection.

B. Postoperative

 1. Early mobilization

 2. Deep breathing, cough exercises

 3. Upright posture if possible

 4. Consider use of continuous positive airway pressure.

 5. Respiratory therapy maneuvers; suctioning, incentive spirometry, chest physiotherapy

 6. Avoid excessive sedation.

 7. Relief of pain; consider intercostal or epidural blocks.

 Bibliography

Brooks-Brunn JA. Postoperative atelectasis and pneumonia: risk factors. Am J Crit Care 1995;4:340–349.

Engoren M. Lack of association between atelectasis and fever. Chest 1995;107:81–84.

Kallet RH, Siobal MS, Alonso JA, et al. Lung collapse during low tidal volume ventilation in acute respiratory distress syndrome. Respir Care 2001;46:49–52.

Lachmann B. Open up the lung and keep the lung open. Intensive Care Med 1992;18:319–321.

Marini JJ, Pierson DJ, Hudson DL. Acute lobar atelectasis: a prospective comparison of fiberoptic bronchoscopy and respiratory therapy. Am Rev Respir Dis 1979;119:971–978.

Massard G, Wihlm JM. Postoperative atelectasis. Chest Surg Clin North Am 1998;8:503–528.

Papadakos PJ. Artificial ventilation. In: Hemmings HC, Hopkins PM (eds). Foundations of Anesthesia: Basic and Clinical Science. St. Louis: Mosby, 2000, pp 507–514.

Papadakos PJ, Lachmann B. The open lung concept of alveolar recruitment can improve outcome in respiratory failure and ARDS. Mt Sinai J Med 2002;69:73–77.

Raoof S, Chowdhrey N, Raoof S, et al. Effect of combined kinetic therapy and percussion therapy on the resolution of atelectasis in critically ill patients. Chest 1999;115:1658–1666.

Uzieblo M, Welsh R, Pursel SE, et al. Incidence and significance of lobar atelectasis in thoracic surgical patients. Am Surgeon 2000;66:476–480.

Wood LDH, Schmidt GA, Hall JB. Principles of critical care of respiratory failure. In: Murrary JF, Nadel JA (eds). Textbook of Respiratory Medicine, 3rd ed. Philadelphia: WB Saunders, 2000, pp 2377–2411.

19 Unstable Angina

Vivian L. Clark

Definition

A. Angina occurring at rest or prolonged
B. New onset angina with severity of at least class III, based on the Canadian Classification System (Table 19–1)
C. Change in anginal pattern
  1. Increasing frequency
  2. Increasing severity
  3. Occurring at a lower threshold of activity

Etiology

A. Atherosclerotic plaque rupture with formation of a nonocclusive thrombus
B. Coronary vasospasm
C. Mismatch between myocardial oxygen supply and demand
  1. Increased myocardial oxygen demand
    a. Fever
    b. Tachycardia
    c. Increased systemic metabolic demand (e.g., thyrotoxicosis, beriberi)
    d. Myocardial hypertrophy (e.g., hypertrophic cardiomyopathy, longstanding hypertension)
  2. Reduced myocardial blood flow due to hypotension
  3. Reduced myocardial oxygen supply due to decreased arterial blood oxygen content
    a. Anemia
    b. Hypoxemia

Clinical Features and Diagnostic Testing

A. Chest discomfort
  1. Chest pain or discomfort is typically substernal, often described as pressure-like or squeezing.
    a. May radiate into the neck, jaw, shoulders, or arms
    b. Discomfort may occur only in the neck, jaw, shoulder, or arms.
  2. Duration is usually less than 20 minutes.
  3. Usually relieved by rest or sublingual nitroglycerin (NTG)
  4. Often accompanied by other symptoms (these symptoms may occur in place of chest discomfort)
    a. Dyspnea
    b. Diaphoresis
    c. Epigastric discomfort or heartburn
  5. Presence of risk factors for coronary artery disease increases the likelihood that pain is of ischemic origin.
    a. Age 70 years or older
    b. Male sex
    c. Hypertension
    d. Diabetes mellitus
    e. Cigarette smoking
    f. Extracardiac vascular disease
  6. Chest discomfort not characteristic of ischemia includes
    a. Pleuritic pain
    b. Discomfort located in the mid or lower abdomen
    c. Highly localized pain, particularly over the left ventricular apex
    d. Discomfort reproduced by movement or palpation
    e. Discomfort that persists for many hours
    f. Very brief episodes of pain (i.e., lasting a few seconds)
    g. Discomfort radiating into the lower extremities
B. Physical findings
  1. Physical examination may be completely normal.
  2. Blood pressure may be normal or elevated.
  3. Jugular venous pressure is usually normal.
  4. Pulmonary rales may be present if ischemia is associated with significant left ventricular dysfunction.
  5. Cardiac examination may be completely normal or may reveal
    a. S_4 gallop, which is indicative of decreased left ventricular compliance
    b. Murmur of mitral insufficiency, if there is associated papillary muscle dysfunction
C. Electrocardiographic (ECG) findings include
  1. ST segment depression

TABLE 19–1. GRADING ANGINA PECTORIS*

CLASS	DESCRIPTION
I	Angina occurs with more than ordinary activity (i.e., strenuous, rapid, or prolonged exertion at work or during recreation).
II	Angina occurs during ordinary activity (i.e., walking or climbing stairs rapidly; walking uphill; walking or stair climbing after meals, in wind, or under emotional stress; or only during the few hours after awakening).
III	Ordinary activity is significantly limited (e.g., angina occurs with walking 1 to 2 blocks on level ground and climbing 1 flight of stairs at a normal pace).
IV	Angina occurs during any activity or at rest.

*Based on the Canadian Cardiovascular System.

Key Symptoms

- Substernal pressure, chest pain, or chest discomfort occurs in most patients.

- Pain may localize or radiate to neck, jaw, shoulders, or arms.

- Pain is usually of less than 20 minutes' duration.

- Pain is relieved by rest or sublingual nitroglycerin.

- Dyspnea, diaphoresis, or heartburn may accompany pain or occur in place of pain.

- For patients with chronic angina, pain is more frequent or occurs at rest.

2. Localized symmetrical T wave inversion
3. Dysrhythmias
   a. Sinus tachycardia
   b. Premature atrial or ventricular contractions (PVCs)
   c. Atrial fibrillation or other tachydysrhythmias may occur or may be the cause of the unstable angina.
4. Conduction disturbances
   a. First-, second-, or third-degree atrioventricular (A-V) block may occur.
   b. New fascicular or bundle branch block may occur.
5. Electrocardiographic abnormalities are usually transient and subside with resolution of ischemia; persistent ECG abnormalities suggest acute myocardial infarction (MI).
6. May be completely normal, particularly if the ischemic zone is posterior

D. Echocardiographic findings
   1. Segmental wall motion abnormalities generally corresponding to the ECG location of the ischemia; wall motion abnormalities should improve with resolution of ischemia.
   2. Compensatory hyperdynamic function may be present in non-involved segments.
   3. Doppler examination may show evidence of decreased left ventricular (LV) compliance or transient mitral insufficiency.

E. Chest radiograph
   1. May be completely normal unless the patient has preexisting cardiovascular disease
   2. Pulmonary congestion, if there is associated congestive heart failure (CHF)
   3. Pleural effusion, if there is associated CHF

F. Nuclear imaging: reversible perfusion defects on thallium 201 or technetium 99m sestamibi perfusion scanning

Differential Diagnosis

A. Acute MI (see Chapter 20, Acute Myocardial Infarction)
B. Aortic dissection
   1. Pain is more often sharp or tearing in quality, localized to the back and usually decreases in intensity after onset.
   2. Usually distinguished by ECG, chest x-ray, and echocardiography findings
C. Pericarditis
   1. Pain is generally pleuritic and affected by position and inspiration.
   2. Can usually be distinguished by ECG, chest x-ray, and echocardiography
D. Pulmonary disease
   1. Pulmonary embolism
   2. Pneumothorax
   3. Pleurisy
E. Gastrointestinal disorders
   1. Esophageal spasm
   2. Cholecystitis
   3. Peptic ulcer disease
   4. Pancreatitis
F. Chest wall pain
G. Psychogenic chest pain

Triage

Initial management of patients with suspected unstable angina often occurs in the emergency department or a dedicated chest pain unit and focuses on distinguishing patients with true ischemic pain from those without. This generally includes an observation period of several hours during which serial ECGs and serum biochemical markers are obtained.

A. If the patient remains pain free, serial ECGs are normal, and there is no increase in biochemical markers, but there remains a suspicion that the pain is ischemic, stress testing should be performed.

1. Select the type of stress test.
   a. A treadmill exercise test should be obtained in patients without baseline ECG abnormalities who are able to exercise.
   b. Exercise testing with associated imaging studies should be performed if there are baseline ECG abnormalities (e.g., left ventricular hypertrophy, nonspecific ST segment or T wave changes).
   c. In patients unable to exercise because of co-morbid conditions (e.g., severe arthritis or chronic obstructive pulmonary disease) a pharmacologic stress test should be performed.
2. Patients with a negative stress test may be discharged and managed on an outpatient basis.

B. Indications for admission include
1. An abnormal stress test
2. Ongoing pain, particularly when associated with ECG changes
3. Abnormal serum biochemical markers

C. Early risk stratification for patients with definite or probable ischemic chest pain
1. Factors associated with high risk for death or nonfatal MI
   a. Accelerating ischemic symptoms over the previous 48 hours
   b. Prolonged (>20 min), ongoing pain
   c. Pulmonary edema secondary to ischemia
   d. New or worsening mitral insufficiency, pulmonary rales, or S_3 gallop
   e. Age 75 years or older
   f. Angina at rest with transient ST segment changes or new bundle branch block
   g. Sustained ventricular tachycardia
   h. Elevated serum troponin levels
2. Factors associated with an intermediate risk of death or nonfatal MI
   a. Concomitant cerebrovascular or peripheral vascular disease, prior MI or coronary artery bypass surgery, or prior aspirin use
   b. Prolonged (>20 min) rest pain, now resolved, or relieved by sublingual NTG
   c. T wave inversion greater than 0.2 mV
   d. Pathologic Q waves
   e. Slightly elevated serum troponin levels

Treatment

A. Monitoring and testing
1. Continuous ECG monitoring to detect rhythm or conduction disturbances
2. Vital signs; urine output, if CHF is present
3. 12-lead ECG obtained during an episode of chest pain (useful in patients who have a normal ECG on initial presentation)
4. Serial serum cardiac marker studies (including creatine phosphokinase [CK]-MB isoenzymes, and cardiac troponin levels) to exclude acute MI

B. Aspirin 160 mg PO daily
1. Contraindications
   a. Allergy
   b. Active bleeding
   c. Hemophilia
   d. Severe untreated hypertension
   e. Peptic ulcer disease
2. Alternative platelet inhibitors for patients with aspirin intolerance or contraindications
   a. Ticlopidine: loading dose of 500 mg PO, followed by 250 mg every 12 hours
   b. Clopidigrel: 300 to 600 mg PO loading dose followed by 75 mg PO daily
   c. Monitoring of platelets during treatment is required because there is a small risk of thrombotic thrombocytopenic purpura (greater for ticlopidine than for clopidigrel).

C. Sublingual NTG followed by continuous IV infusion at 10 μg/min and titrated to symptoms, maintaining mean arterial blood pressure ≥70 mm Hg

D. Morphine sulfate 1 to 4 mg intravenously when symptoms are not relieved by NTG or are accompanied by acute pulmonary congestion

E. Supplemental oxygen for patients with respiratory distress, cyanosis, or arterial oxyhemoglobin desaturation

F. β-Adrenergic receptor antagonists, unless contraindicated
1. See Chapter 20, Acute Myocardial Infarction, for IV dosing for ongoing chest pain.
2. Oral preparations (e.g., metoprolol 25 to 50 mg twice daily or atenolol 50 mg daily)
3. Contraindications to β-blockers
   a. Heart rate 60 beats/min or lower
   b. Systolic blood pressure lower than 110 mm Hg
   c. Second- or third-degree A-V block
   d. Electrocardiographic PR interval more than 0.23 seconds
   e. Uncompensated congestive heart failure
   f. Asthma
   g. Severe chronic obstructive pulmonary disease
   h. Insulin-dependent diabetes mellitus, particularly in patients prone to hypoglycemia

G. Calcium channel blockers may be considered in lieu of β-blockers if the latter are ineffective or contraindicated.

1. Verapamil 40 to 80 mg PO every 8 hours

2. Diltiazem 30 to 60 mg PO every 8 hours

3. Avoid dihydropyridine preparations (e.g., nifedipine).

4. Contraindications include CHF, LV dysfunction, and A-V block.

H. Angiotensin converting enzyme (ACE) inhibitors are indicated for patients who have persistent hypertension in spite of NTG and β-blocker therapy, particularly those with LV dysfunction or diabetes mellitus.

1. Start with short-acting agents administered at a low dose.

   a. Captopril 6.25 mg every 6 hours

   b. Enalapril 2.5 to 5.0 mg every 12 hours

2. If tolerated, can subsequently substitute longer-acting agents such as lisinopril (10 to 20 mg daily) or ramipril (2.5 to 20 mg daily).

3. Use with caution in patients with renal insufficiency.

I. Heparin

1. Unfractionated heparin: initiate with 60 to 70 U/kg bolus (up to 4000 U) IV followed by an infusion at 12 to 15 U/kg per hour (up to 1000 U/hr) and titrate to maintain partial thromboplastin time 1.5 to 2 times normal.

2. Low molecular weight heparin (e.g., enoxaparin 1 mg/kg subcutaneously every 12 hours)

J. Glycoprotein IIb/IIIa inhibitors are indicated for patients considered to be at high risk and for those in whom percutaneous intervention is planned. (For specific drugs and dosing, see Chapter 175 Glycoprotein IIb/IIIa Receptor Antagonists.)

K. Intra-aortic balloon counterpulsation (IABP) for patients who have ongoing symptoms and ECG changes in spite of intensive medical therapy or for patients with hemodynamic instability

1. Generally, IABP insertion is performed in the catheterization laboratory before or after diagnostic coronary angiography (see later under Cardiac Catherization).

2. Contraindications

   a. Aortic insufficiency

   b. Peripheral vascular disease

   c. Abdominal aortic aneurysm

   d. Aortic dissection

L. Anxiolytic agents (e.g., lorazepam 1 mg PO every 4 to 12 hours)

Key Treatment

- Continuous electrocardiographic monitoring

- Aspirin

- Sublingual or IV nitroglycerin

- Supplemental oxygen

- β-Adrenergic receptor antagonist

- Heparin (unfractionated or low molecular weight)

- Glycoprotein IIb/IIIa inhibitor (if high-risk or percutaneous intervention planned)

- Angiotensin converting enzyme inhibitor (if persistent hypertension)

Risk Stratification Using Noninvasive Testing

Patients who have been admitted and stabilized on medical treatment can be further risk stratified based on results of noninvasive testing.

A. Timing

1. Low-risk patients (i.e., those with no clinical features indicative of high or intermediate risk) may undergo noninvasive testing if free of ischemia at rest or with low-level activity for 12 to 24 hours.

2. Intermediate-risk patients may undergo noninvasive testing after freedom from ischemia at rest or with low-level activity for 2 to 3 days.

B. Options

1. Standard treadmill exercise test: for patients who are able to exercise and who have normal baseline ECG

2. Treadmill exercise testing with imaging (either nuclear or echocardiographic): used in patients who are able to exercise but who have baseline ECG abnormalities

3. Pharmacologic stress testing: dobutamine echocardiography or adenosine nuclear imaging should be used for patients who are unable to exercise because of other medical conditions

Cardiac Catheterization

A. Indications for cardiac catheterization

1. Recurrent ischemic chest pain at rest or with low-level activity while on intensive medical therapy

2. Recurrent ischemic chest pain associated with CHF or new or worsening mitral insufficiency

3. High-risk findings on noninvasive testing

a. Resting LV dysfunction: ejection fraction (EF) less than 40%

b. Exercise-induced LV dysfunction: EF less than or equal to 35%

c. Large perfusion defect or multiple perfusion defects

d. Large, fixed perfusion defect associated with LV dilation or increased ^{201}Tl lung uptake

e. Exercise-induced perfusion defect associated with LV dilation or increased ^{201}Tl lung uptake

f. Echocardiographic wall motion abnormalities involving 2 or more segments induced by low-dose dobutamine infusion or exercise with heart rate of 120 beats/min or less

g. Evidence of extensive ischemia by stress echocardiography

4. Hemodynamic instability

5. Sustained ventricular tachycardia

6. Percutaneous intervention within the previous 6 months

7. Previous coronary artery bypass surgery

8. Repeated presentations for unstable angina despite medical management

B. Possible indications for cardiac catheterization

1. Age 65 years or older

2. ST segment depression at presentation

3. Elevated serum troponin levels at presentation

Bibliography

Ambrose JA, Dangas G. Unstable angina: current concepts of pathogenesis and treatment. Arch Intern Med 2000; 160:25–37.

Braunwald E, Antman EM, Beasley JW, et al. ACC/AHA guidelines for the management of patients with unstable angina and non-ST segment elevation myocardial infarction: a report of the American College of Cardiology/American Heart Association Task Force on Practice Guidelines (Committee on the Mangement of Patients with Unstable Angina). J Am Coll Cardiol 2000;36:970–1062.

Lange RA, Hillis LD. Aggressive versus conservative therapy in unstable angina. Cardiol Clin 1999;17:387–399.

White HD. Optimal treatment of patients with acute coronary syndromes and non-ST-elevation myocardial infarction. Am Heart J 1999;138:S105–S114.

Yeghiasarians Y, Braunstein JB, Askari A, et al. Unstable angina pectoris. N Engl J Med 2000;342:101–114.

20 Acute Myocardial Infarction

Vivian L. Clark

Definition

A. Acute myocardial infarction (MI)

1. Typical temporal pattern of serum biochemical markers of myocardial necrosis (cardiac troponin or creatine phosphokinase [CK]-MB)

   a. Maximal concentration of troponin T or I exceeding the ninety-ninth percentile for a reference control group

   b. Maximal CK-MB activity

      (1) Exceeding the ninety-ninth percentile for a reference control group on two successive samples, or

      (2) Exceeding twice the upper limit of normal on one occasion during the hours following the index clinical event

      (3) Values for CK-MB should rise and fall; levels that are elevated and remain elevated are rarely due to MI.

   c. Total CK of more than twice the upper limit of normal (if troponin or CK-MB levels are unavailable)

2. In addition to biochemical markers, at least one of the following must be present.

   a. Ischemic symptoms

   b. Development of pathologic Q waves on electrocardiogram (ECG)

   c. Electrocardiographic changes indicative of ischemia (ST segment elevation, ST segment depression, or T wave abnormalities)

   d. Setting of coronary intervention (e.g., percutaneous transluminal coronary angioplasty)

3. Pathological changes of acute MI on post-mortem examination

B. An established MI is based on the following criteria.

1. Development of new pathologic Q waves on the ECG

   a. The patient may not recall previous symptoms.

   b. Serum biochemical markers of myocardial necrosis may have normalized, depending on the time elapsed since the infarction developed.

2. Pathological findings of a healed or healing MI on post-mortem examination

Clinical Findings

A. History

1. Chest discomfort

   a. Typically pain is substernal, often described as pressure-like or squeezing and may radiate into the neck, jaw or shoulders.

   b. Duration is usually longer than 20 minutes.

   c. Painless MI can occur (more commonly in patients with diabetes).

2. Other symptoms that may accompany or occur in place of chest discomfort

   a. Dyspnea

   b. Diaphoresis

   c. Nausea, emesis, or urge to defecate

   d. Anxiety or a feeling of impending doom

B. Physical findings

1. Blood pressure and pulse may be normal, elevated, or decreased.

2. Jugular venous pressure is usually normal, but it may be increased if there is right ventricular involvement or cardiogenic shock.

3. Pulmonary rales or frank pulmonary edema may be present.

4. Cardiac auscultatory findings

   a. S_4 gallop, which is indicative of decreased left ventricular compliance

   b. Murmur of mitral insufficiency (if there is associated papillary muscle dysfunction)

   c. Pericardial friction rub (if there is associated pericarditis)

Electrocardiographic Findings

A. ST segment elevation or Q waves in at least two contiguous leads

B. New left bundle branch block (LBBB)

C. ST segment depression or localized T wave inversions may be seen in non–Q wave MI.

1. Changes should be present on at least two contiguous leads.

2. Changes should be present on at least two consecutive ECGs obtained several hours apart.

D. Myocardial infarction involving the circumflex distribution may have precordial lead ST segment de-

64

pression, increased R wave amplitude in leads V_1 and V_2, or no significant ECG findings.

E. Cardiac dysrhythmias
  1. Sinus tachycardia
  2. Premature atrial or ventricular contractions (PVCs)
  3. Atrial fibrillation
  4. Ventricular tachycardia or fibrillation (may occur in the absence of PVCs)
  5. Conduction disturbances
     a. First-, second-, or third-degree atrioventricular (A-V) block may occur.
     b. New fascicular or bundle branch block may occur.

Diagnostic Imaging

A. Echocardiographic findings
  1. Segmental wall motion abnormalities, generally corresponding to the ECG location of the infarction
  2. Compensatory hyperdynamic function may be present in non-involved segments.
  3. Pericardial effusion (if there is associated pericarditis)
  4. Doppler examination may show evidence of decreased left ventricular compliance or mitral insufficiency.

B. Chest x-ray
  1. May be completely normal
  2. Cardiac size is usually normal in first acute MI unless the patient has preexisting cardiovascular disease.
  3. Pulmonary congestion (if there is associated congestive heart failure [CHF])
  4. Pleural effusion (if there is associated CHF)

C. Nuclear imaging
  1. Perfusion defect on thallium 201 or technetium 99m sestamibi single-photon emission computed tomographic (SPECT) perfusion imaging
  2. Increased uptake at infarct site using ^{99m}Tc pyrophosphate scintigraphy

Differential Diagnosis

A. Aortic dissection
  1. Pain is more often sharp or tearing in quality, localized to the back and usually decreases in intensity after onset.
  2. Usually distinguished by ECG, chest x-ray, and echocardiographic findings
  3. Since dissection may be complicated by acute MI, a high index of suspicion is required.

B. Pericarditis
  1. Pain is generally pleuritic and affected by position and inspiration.
  2. Distinguishable by biochemical markers, ECG, chest x-ray, and echocardiography

C. Chest pain secondary to mismatch in myocardial supply and demand (not due to coronary artery disease)
  1. Hypertension with severe left ventricular hypertrophy
  2. Hypertrophic cardiomyopathy
  3. Aortic stenosis
  4. Other conditions associated with right ventricular hypertrophy such as primary pulmonary hypertension or mitral stenosis

D. Pulmonary disease
  1. Pulmonary embolism
  2. Pneumothorax
  3. Pleurisy

E. Gastrointestinal disorders
  1. Esophageal spasm
  2. Cholecystitis
  3. Peptic ulcer disease
  4. Pancreatitis

F. Chest wall pain

G. Psychogenic chest pain

Key Risk Stratification

Clinical factors associated with an increased risk of morbidity and mortality in acute MI

- Advanced age

- Female gender

- Tachycardia and hypotension

- Evidence of CHF

- Anterior MI

- Echocardiographic evidence of severe left ventricular dysfunction (ejection fraction less than 40%)

- Co-morbid conditions: diabetes mellitus, renal insufficiency, previous MI, peripheral vascular disease

Monitoring

A. Continuous ECG monitoring to detect rhythm or conduction disturbances

B. Serial vital signs; urine output, if CHF is present or patient is at high risk

C. Continuous pulse oximetry to ensure adequate oxygenation in high-risk patients

D. Pulmonary artery catheterization may be indicated in patients with CHF or mechanical complications for hemodynamic monitoring and assessment of mixed venous oxygenation.

E. Daily 12-lead ECG (more frequently if there is recurrent chest pain)

F. Serial serum cardiac marker studies, including total CK, CK-MB isoenzyme activities and cardiac troponin levels

G. Echocardiographic evaluation is useful to assess global left ventricular (LV) function in selected patients who may require angiotensin converting enzyme inhibitors or prolonged anticoagulation.

Key Monitoring

Continuous ECG monitoring is mandatory for patients with acute MI.

Treatment

A. Reperfusion therapy (Fig. 20–1)

B. Aspirin: 325 mg chewed stat; then orally each day thereafter

C. Nitroglycerin: 0.3 to 0.4 mg, sublingually; for ongoing pain initiate a continuous IV infusion at 10 μg/minute and titrate to relief of ischemic symptoms, maintaining mean arterial blood pressure of at least 70 mm Hg

D. Supplemental oxygen
   1. For overt pulmonary congestion
   2. For hypoxemia (SaO$_2$ ≤0.90)
   3. For uncomplicated patients with acute MI, but acceptable SaO$_2$, supplemental oxygen is recommended only during the first few hours.

E. β-Adrenergic receptor antagonist (unless contraindicated)
   1. Metoprolol
      a. Administer a 5 mg IV bolus every 2 minutes (while monitoring heart rate, blood pressure, and ECG) to a total of 15 mg, if tolerated.
      b. If full IV dose is tolerated, give 50 mg orally every 6 hours, starting 15 minutes after the last IV dose and continue for 48 hours.
      c. Thereafter, give 100 mg orally every 12 hours.
   2. Atenolol
      a. Administer 5 mg IV over 5 minutes (while monitoring heart rate, blood pressure, and

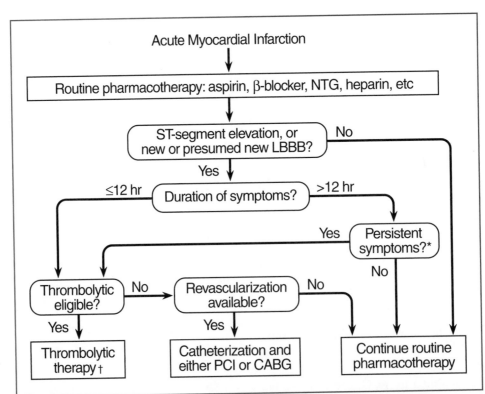

Figure 20–1 Algorithm for reperfusion therapy in patients with acute myocardial infarction. CABG = coronary artery bypass grafting, LBBB = left bundle branch block, NTG = nitroglycerin, PCI = percutaneous coronary intervention. *In addition to persistent symptoms, development of cardiogenic shock in patients younger than 75 years old is an indication to consider late reperfusion therapy performed within 18 hours of the onset of shock. †Catheterization followed by either primary PCI or CABG is an acceptable alternative to thrombolytic therapy.

ECG) and repeat 10 minutes later, if tolerated.

   b. If full IV dose is tolerated, give 50 mg orally 10 minutes after the last IV dose.

   c. Thereafter, give 50 mg orally each day.

3. Contraindications to β-blockers

   a. Marked bradycardia; i.e., 60 beats/minute or less

   b. Systolic blood pressure lower than 110 mm Hg

   c. Second- or third-degree A-V block

   d. PR interval more than 0.23 seconds

   e. Uncompensated CHF

   f. Asthma

   g. Severe chronic obstructive pulmonary disease

   h. Insulin-dependent diabetes mellitus (particularly patients prone to hypoglycemia)

F. Calcium channel blockers can be given in lieu of β-blockers if ineffective or contraindicated.

1. For ongoing ischemia

2. To control rapid ventricular response in atrial fibrillation

3. Contraindications include CHF, LV dysfunction, and A-V block.

G. Angiotensin converting enzyme inhibitors are indicated for patients with large anterior MI or with CHF who have no contraindications.

1. Start with short-acting agents administered at a low dose.

   a. Captopril 6.25 mg orally every 6 hours

   b. Enalapril 2.5 to 5.0 mg orally every 12 hours

2. If tolerated, switch to longer-acting agents (e.g., lisinopril at 10 to 20 mg orally every day or ramipril at 2.5 to 20 mg orally every day).

3. Use with caution in patients with renal insufficiency.

H. Heparin

1. Indications

   a. During the first 48 hours after thrombolytic therapy with alteplase or retaplase

   b. Non-ST segment elevation MI

   c. Postinfarction angina pectoris

   d. Left ventricular thrombus or high risk for LV thrombus (large anterior MI, ejection fraction less than 40%)

   e. Atrial fibrillation

   f. Patients in whom indications for long-term anticoagulation exist (e.g., previous deep vein thrombosis [DVT], prosthetic heart valve)

2. Dosing for above indications

   a. Unfractionated heparin: initiate with 60 U/kg (up to 4000 U) IV bolus followed by IV infusion of 12 U/kg per hour (up to 1000 U/hour) and titrate to maintain partial thromboplastin time (PTT) at 50 to 70 seconds

   b. Low molecular weight heparin: e.g., enoxaparin 1 mg/kg subcutaneously every 12 hours (no need to follow PTT)

3. Dosing for patients not included in above indications (i.e., use for DVT prophylaxis only)

   a. Unfractionated heparin: 5000 to 7500 U subcutaneously every 12 hours, until patient is ambulatory

   b. Low molecular weight heparin: e.g., enoxaparin 1 mg/kg subcutaneously every 12 hours, until patient is ambulatory

I. Diuretics for patients with pulmonary congestion or CHF

J. Stool softener

K. Anxiolytic drugs (e.g., lorazepam 1 mg orally every 4 to 12 hours)

L. Atropine

1. Indications

   a. Symptomatic sinus bradycardia

   b. Ventricular asystole

   c. Symptomatic A-V block occurring at the A-V nodal level (i.e., Mobitz type I second-degree or third-degree with narrow-complex escape rhythm)

2. Dosage: increments of 0.5 mg IV to achieve desired heart rate, up to 2.0 mg

M. Indications for placement of transcutaneous electrode patches and transcutaneous pacing

1. Sinus bradycardia (≤50 beats/min) with hypotension that is unresponsive to drug treatment

2. Mobitz type II second-degree A-V block

3. Third-degree A-V block

4. As a bridge to temporary transvenous pacing (see below)

N. Temporary transvenous pacing indications

1. Asystole

2. Symptomatic bradycardia unresponsive to atropine

3. Bilateral bundle branch block (RBBB with alternating fascicular block, or alternating RBBB and LBBB) of any age

4. New or indeterminate age bifascicular block (RBBB with fascicular block or LBBB) with first-degree A-V block

5. Mobitz type II second-degree A-V block

6. Third-degree A-V block

7. Incessant ventricular tachycardia, for atrial or ventricular overdrive pacing

8. Recurrent sinus pauses of at least 3 seconds unresponsive to atropine

O. For treatment of patients with right ventricular MI, mechanical complications of acute MI, or cardiogenic shock, see Chapters 21, 22, and 27.

Key Treatment

- Aspirin

- Sublingual or IV nitroglycerin

- Supplemental oxygen

- Reperfusion therapy (thrombolytic therapy or revascularization)

- β-Adrenergic receptor antagonist

- Heparin (unfractionated or low molecular weight)

- Angiotension converting enzyme inhibitors (large MI or CHF, and no contraindication)

Bibliography

Gersh BJ. Optimal management of acute myocardial infarction at the dawn of the next millennium. Am Heart J 1999;138(2 Pt 2):188–202.

Michaels AD, Goldschlager N. Risk stratification after acute myocardial infarction in the reperfusion era. Prog Cardiovasc Dis 2000;42:273–309.

Myocardial infarction redefined: a consensus document of the Joint European Society of Cardiology/American College of Cardiology Committee for the Redefinition of Myocardial Infarction. J Am Coll Cardiol 2000;36:959–969.

Ryan TJ, Anderson JL, Antman EM, et al. ACC/AHA guidelines for the management of patients with acute myocardial infarction: a report of the American College of Cardiology/American Heart Association Task Force on Practice Guidelines (Committee on Mangement of Acute Myocardial Infarction). J Am Coll Cardiol 1996; 28:1328–1428.

Ryan TJ, Antman EM, Brooks NH, et al. 1999 update: ACC/AHA guidelines for the management of patients with acute myocardial infarction: a report of the American College of Cardiology/American Heart Association Task Force on Practice Guidelines (Committee on Mangement of Acute Myocardial Infarction). J Am Coll Cardiol 1999;34:890–911.

Zeymer U, Neuhaus KL. Clinical trials in acute myocardial infarction. Curr Opinion Cardiol 1999;14:392–402.

21 Right Ventricular Myocardial Infarction

Vivian L. Clark

Incidence

A. Right ventricular (RV) infarction occurs primarily in the setting of inferior myocardial infarction (MI) as a result of occlusion of the proximal right coronary artery.

B. Approximately 40% of patients with an inferior MI have RV involvement, but only a small proportion have significant clinical consequences.

C. Isolated RV MI (i.e., without left ventricular involvement) occurs in about 3% of cases of MI.

Key Clinical Features

- Hypotension that responds to IV fluids
- Increased jugular venous pressure
- Clear lung fields
- Pericarditis

Clinical Features and Diagnostic Testing

A. Hypotension that may respond to IV fluid administration

B. Increased jugular venous pressure

C. Clear lung fields; however, rales can occur if there is significant concomitant left ventricular involvement.

D. Pericardial friction rub; pericarditis occurs more commonly in the setting of RV MI.

E. Electrocardiographic (ECG) evidence of inferior MI; other findings include ST segment elevation in V_1 or in the right-sided chest leads, particularly V_3R or V_4R (Fig. 21–1).

F. Echocardiography often shows RV dilation and dysfunction, as well as inferior wall motion abnormalities.

Hemodynamic Features

A. Elevated right atrial (RA) pressure generally exceeds pulmonary artery occlusion pressure (PAOP), although not if PAOP is markedly increased.

B. Evidence of poor RV compliance
   1. Prominent x descent in RA waveform
   2. Dip and plateau pattern of RV waveform

C. RV and pulmonary artery systolic pressures are often normal.

D. Reduced cardiac output

Differential Diagnosis

A. Pulmonary embolism
   1. May have similar clinical presentation, physical signs, and hemodynamic findings
   2. Right ventricular MI often can be distinguished by ECG; radionuclide ventilation-perfusion scanning, helical computed tomography, and echocardiography are useful adjuncts.

B. Pericardial tamponade
   1. Similar hemodynamic findings to RV MI; however, tamponade shows equalization of diastolic pressures and blunting of x and y descents on right heart catheterization.
   2. Can be distinguished by ECG, chest x-ray, and echocardiography

C. Pericardial constriction
   1. Similar hemodynamic findings to RV MI; however, right heart catheterization shows equalization of diastolic pressures and a prominent y descent.
   2. Constriction generally has a more subacute presentation and different ECG findings.

Key Treatment

- Aspirin, oxygen, morphine, β-blocker
- Volume loading
- Reperfusion therapy
- Dual chamber pacing for heart block

Treatment

A. Usual medical therapy for acute MI: e.g., aspirin, oxygen, morphine, β-blocker (see Chapter 20, Acute Myocardial Infarction)

B. If RV MI is suspected as cause of hypotension, pulmonary artery catheterization can confirm the diagnosis and aid in management.

C. Reperfusion with thrombolytic therapy or primary angioplasty

D. Volume loading
   1. Increases right heart filling and restores systemic perfusion
   2. If significant left ventricular involvement is present, fluid must be given cautiously.

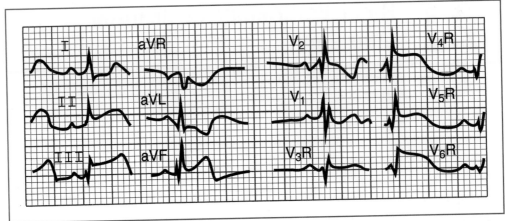

Figure 21-1 Electrocardiogram in patient with RV MI showing right-sided chest leads with ST segment elevation in leads V_3R through V_6R.

E. An inotropic agent or intra-aortic balloon counterpulsation may be indicated in patients who do not respond to fluid or in whom there is significant pulmonary congestion.

F. In patients who develop heart block, dual chamber pacing will maintain cardiac output more effectively than ventricular pacing alone.

Bibliography

Bowers TR, O'Neill WW, Grines C, et al. Effect of reperfusion therapy on biventricular function and survival after right ventricular infarction. N Engl J Med 1998;338: 933–940.

Bueno H, Lopez-Palop R, Perez-David E, et al. Combined effect of age and right ventricular involvement in acute inferior myocardial infarction prognosis. Circulation 1998;98:1714–1720.

Goldstein JA. Right ventricular ischemia: pathophysiology, natural history and clinical management. Prog Cardiovasc Dis 1998;40:325–341.

Santamore WP, Dell'Italia LJ. Ventricular interdependence: significant left ventricular contributions to right ventricular systolic function. Prog Cardiovasc Dis 1998;40:289–308.

Zeymer U, Neuhaus KL, Wegsheider K, et al. Effects of thrombolytic therapy in acute inferior myocardial infarction with or without right ventricular involvement. HIT-4 Trial Group. Hirudin for Improvement of Thrombolysis. J Am Coll Cardiol 1998;32:876–881.

22 Mechanical Complications of Acute Myocardial Infarction

Vivian L. Clark

Definition

Mechanical complications of acute myocardial infarction (MI) include papillary muscle dysfunction or rupture, ventricular septal rupture and ventricular free wall rupture.

> **CAUTION**
>
> Early recognition and treatment of these complications is critical as they can result in cardiogenic shock and are frequently fatal.

Ventricular Free Wall Rupture

Epidemiology

A. Rupture of the free wall results in rapid development of pericardial tamponade or, less frequently, development of ventricular pseudoaneurysm.

B. Incidence is 1% to 3% in acute MI, although it has decreased in the era of thrombolytic therapy and primary angioplasty.

C. Rupture generally occurs within the first week after MI; 30% occur within the first 24 hours.

D. A relatively common cause of in-hospital death in acute MI

E. Risk factors include hypertension, anterior MI, first infarction, advanced age, and transmural MI; risk may also be increased in patients who are taking anti-inflammatory drugs or have received thrombolytic therapy.

Clinical Findings

A. Rupture most often presents with sudden onset of circulatory shock or pulseless electrical activity.

B. Free wall rupture may be preceded by persistent or recurrent chest pain and tachycardia.

C. Rupture resulting in pseudoaneurysm often presents as an incidental finding on echocardiography or left ventriculography.

D. Electrocardiogram usually shows evidence of a recent transmural MI.

Key Diagnosis and Treatment of Ventricular Free Wall Rupture

- Free wall rupture should be suspected in any patient with recent transmural MI who suddenly develops severe hypotension unresponsive to fluids and vasopressors.

- Emergency echocardiography and pericardiocentesis can confirm the diagnosis and must be followed by emergency surgery.

Ventricular Septal Rupture

Epidemiology

A. Rupture of the interventricular septum usually occurs in the setting of transmural anteroseptal or inferior MI; blood supply to the septum is from septal branches of the left anterior descending and the posterior descending coronary arteries.

B. Septal rupture is more common in the setting of anterior MI than inferior or posterior MI.

C. Rupture usually occurs within the first 7 days; up to 30% occur within 24 hours of onset of acute MI.

Key Clinical Findings of Ventricular Septal Rupture

- Usual presentation is with congestive heart failure or cardiogenic shock.

- A loud holosystolic murmur is heard at the lower left sternal border, often accompanied by a thrill.

Diagnosis and Treatment

A. Transthoracic echocardiography with color-flow doppler ultrasonography shows a left-to-right shunt at the level of the interventricular septum; abnormal septal motion is also observed.

B. Oxyhemoglobin saturations obtained during right heart catheterization show a step-up at the level of the right ventricle.

C. The diagnosis can also be confirmed in the catheterization laboratory by left ventriculography in the left anterior oblique projection; this also allows the coronary anatomy to be defined.

D. Initial treatment includes blood pressure support and afterload reduction, pharmacologically or by intra-aortic balloon counterpulsation.

E. Emergency surgery to repair the defect, with or without coronary artery bypass, should be performed in patients who fail to respond to medical therapy.

F. Delayed repair should be considered in patients who can be stabilized medically.

Mitral Valve Dysfunction

Clinical Findings

A. Mitral valve dysfunction with associated mitral insufficiency occurs as a result of papillary muscle ischemia, infarction, or rupture.

B. Mitral insufficiency can occur intermittently in patients with papillary muscle dysfunction secondary to ischemia.

C. Mitral insufficiency usually occurs in the setting of inferior or posterior wall MI, because the posterior papillary muscle has a single blood supply, whereas two vessels frequently supply the anterior papillary muscle.

D. Patients frequently present with acute pulmonary edema and hypotension.

E. Physical examination reveals a loud holosystolic murmur at the apex and along the left sternal border; this may be accompanied by a thrill and an S_3 gallop.

Diagnosis

A. Two-dimensional echocardiography and color-flow doppler ultrasonography will confirm the diagnosis in most cases; findings include
   1. Left atrial enlargement
   2. Prolapse of a mitral leaflet into the left atrium

   3. A large Doppler regurgitant flow jet into the left atrium
B. Right heart catheterization
   1. Elevated pulmonary artery occlusion pressure
   2. Large, pathologic v waves
C. Left heart catheterization is generally required to assess the coronary anatomy.

Treatment

A. Pharmacologic treatment
   1. Loop diuretics
   2. Afterload reduction
   3. Inotropic support
B. An alternative to pharmacologic afterload reduction is the use of intra-aortic balloon counterpulsation.
C. If ischemia is suspected, IV nitroglycerin, β-blockers, and heparin should be administered.
D. Urgent surgery with mitral valve repair or replacement and coronary artery revascularization is required in most cases.
E. Percutaneous coronary intervention may be effective if papillary muscle dysfunction is ischemic in origin.

B Bibliography

Becker RC, Gore JM, Lambrew C, et al. A composite view of cardiac rupture in the United States National Registry of myocardial infarction. J Am Coll Cardiol 1996;27:1321–1326.

Crenshaw BS, Granger CB, Birnbaum Y, et al. Risk factors, angiographic patterns, and outcomes in patients with ventricular septal defect complicating acute myocardial infarction. GUSTO-1 (Global Utilization of Streptokinase and TPA for Occluded Coronary Arteries) Trial Investigators. Circulation 2000;101:27–32.

Di Summa M, Actis Dato GM, Centofanti P. Ventricular septal rupture after a myocardial infarction: clinical features and long term survival. J Cardiovasc Surg 1997;38:589–593.

Yamanishi H, Izumoto H, Kitahara H. Clinical experiences of surgical repair for mitral regurgitation secondary to papillary muscle rupture complicating acute myocardial infarction. Ann Thorac Cardiovasc Surg 1998;4:83–86.

23 Myocardial Contusion

Samuel A. Tisherman

Chest trauma is a common cause of death in victims of blunt trauma, being the direct cause of death in about 25% of cases and contributing to mortality in another 25%. Blunt myocardial injury or myocardial contusion is caused by a direct blow to the sternum, often when the chest strikes the steering wheel during a motor vehicle crash. The right ventricle is the most frequently affected chamber due to its anterior location. Cardiac dysrhythmias are the most common manifestation. Fortunately, myocardial contusions rarely cause significant hemodynamic changes, cardiac failure, valvular injury, or rupture of a cardiac chamber. The diagnosis and management of this injury remains controversial.

Key Risk Factors

- Front-end vehicular crash at speeds higher than 15 mph
- Deformed steering wheel
- Multiple injuries

Clinical Findings

A. Symptoms
   1. Chest pain
   2. Shortness of breath
   3. Palpitations
B. Signs
   1. Chest wall contusions or ecchymosis
   2. Irregular pulse
   3. Hypotension (rare)
   4. Multiple injuries

Laboratory Findings

A. Serum creatine phosphokinase activity
   1. Elevations are nonspecific.
   2. Increased levels are often secondary to skeletal muscle injury.
B. Serum troponin I or T
   1. Assays should be obtained on admission and at 24 hours.
   2. May be too sensitive an assay
   3. May detect indirect cardiac injury due to circulatory shock

Key Imaging Study

- Echocardiography is a sensitive test for myocardial contusion.
- Can manifest as wall motion abnormalities or valvular injury
- Wall motion abnormalities spontaneously resolve within weeks (often not clinically significant).

Electrocardiographic Findings

A. Dysrhythmias and other changes on the electrocardiogram (ECG) are usually apparent within first 12 hours.
B. Sinus tachycardia
   1. Most common dysrhythmia with blunt myocardial injury
   2. Nonspecific finding
C. Premature atrial contractions
D. Atrial flutter/fibrillation
E. Premature ventricular contractions
F. Right bundle branch block
G. Acute injury pattern
   1. ST segment elevation
   2. T wave flattening or inversion

Key Findings

- Pertinent mechanism of injury (e.g., deformed steering wheel)
- Dysrhythmias or ST segment and T wave changes by ECG
- Wall motion abnormalities by echocardiography

Treatment

A. Indications for continuous ECG monitoring
   1. Hemodynamic instability
   2. Baseline ECG abnormality
B. Indications for echocardiography
   1. Hemodynamic instability
   2. Persistent dysrhythmias or ECG abnormalities
C. Supportive monitoring and treatment

73

Key Complications

- Life-threatening dysrhythmias

- Congestive heart failure

- Cardiogenic shock

- Papillary muscle injury or valvular injury

- Myocardial rupture

1. Repeat ECG
2. Hemodynamic monitoring for 24 to 48 hours
3. Inotropic support as needed
4. Antidysrhythmic drugs as needed

D. Noncardiac surgical procedures

   1. Should not be considered contraindicated

2. Invasive hemodynamic monitoring or intraoperative transesophageal echocardiography may be indicated.

Bibliography

Biffl WL, Moore FA, Moore EE, et al. Cardiac enzymes are irrelevant in the patient with suspected myocardial contusion. Am J Surg 1994;169:523–528.

Edouard AR, Benoist JF, Cosson C, et al. Circulating cardiac troponin I in trauma patients without cardiac contusion. Intensive Care Med 1998;24:569–573.

Fabian TC, Cicala MS, Croce MA, et al. A prospective evaluation of myocardial contusion: Correlation of significant arrythmia and cardiac output with CPK-MB measurements. J Trauma 1991;31:653–659.

Frazee RC, Mucha P Jr, Farnell MB, et al. Objective evaluation of blunt cardiac trauma. J Trauma 1999;26:510–519.

Karalis DG, Victor MF, Davis GA, et al. The role of echocardiography in blunt chest trauma: A transthoracic and transesophageal echocardiographic study. J Trauma 1994;36:53–58.

24 Left Ventricular Failure

Arthur J. Boujoukos

Dysfunction of the left ventricle of the heart can be systolic or diastolic in nature. Systolic dysfunction is characterized by an ejection fraction (EF) lower than 45% as a result of either global or regional myocardial hypokinesis. Diastolic dysfunction is characterized by decreased compliance of the left ventricle, leading to impaired diastolic filling. Patients can have both systolic and diastolic dysfunction. Left ventricle (LV) failure can lead to symptoms on the basis of pulmonary congestion or low cardiac output or both.

In the intensive care unit (ICU), the most refractory cases of LV failure are in patients with cardiogenic shock after cardiac surgery or myocardial infarction (MI). With aggressive support, 25% of patients with cardiogenic shock after cardiac surgery will survive. Cardiogenic shock after MI is associated with a mortality rate of 80% to 90%. However, patients who are successfully revascularized fare better, and current approaches to management are based on the concept of emergency revascularization.

Etiology

A. Systolic dysfunction
   1. Ischemia causing "myocardial hibernation" (reversible)
   2. Ischemic cardiomyopathy without reversible component
   3. Post-cardiotomy LV dysfunction
   4. Alcoholism
   5. Chronic hypertension
   6. Infectious myocarditis
      a. Viral
      b. Toxoplasmosis
      c. Trichinosis
      d. Trypanosomiasis
      e. Lyme disease
   7. Inflammatory conditions
      a. Giant cell arteritis
      b. Polyarteritis
      c. Scleroderma
      d. Dermatomyositis
   8. Valvular heart disease
      a. Aortic insufficiency
      b. Mitral insufficiency
   9. Peripartum cardiomyopathy
   10. Hypothyroidism
   11. Pheochromocytoma
   12. Adriamycin
   13. Cardiac allograft rejection
   14. Idiopathic
B. Diastolic dysfunction
   1. Chronic hypertension
   2. Aortic stenosis
   3. Post-cardiotomy LV dysfunction
   4. Sarcoidosis
   5. Amyloidosis
   6. Radiation fibrosis
   7. Hypereosinophilic cardiomyopathy

Symptoms

A. Congestive symptoms
   1. Peripheral edema
   2. Paroxysmal nocturnal dyspnea
   3. Exertional dyspnea
   4. Orthopnea
B. Low output symptoms
   1. Chronic
      a. Weakness
      b. Fatigue
      c. Weight loss
   2. Acute
      a. Confusion
      b. Sense of impending doom
      c. Dyspnea
      d. Abdominal pain

Physical Findings

A. Chronic LV failure
   1. Jugular venous distention
   2. S_3 gallop
   3. Rales
   4. Hepatojugular reflux
   5. Hepatomegaly
   6. Edema
B. Acute LV failure
   1. Tachycardia

2. Diaphoresis

3. Tachypnea

4. Low blood pressure (not always present)

5. Cool extremities

6. Mottling of skin (livedo reticularis)

7. Oliguria

PEARL

Development of oliguria, hypotension, or lactic acidosis should be assumed to be due to a low output state until proven otherwise.

Tests and Imaging Studies

A. Chest x-ray

1. Pulmonary edema

2. Apical redistribution

B. Echocardiography

1. The best diagnostic modality

2. Provides data regarding etiology (e.g., valvular heart disease, wall motion abnormalities).

3. Evidence for dilated cardiomyopathy is low EF (<40%) and ventricular dilation.

4. Isolated wall motion abnormalities suggest coronary artery disease.

5. Evidence for restrictive cardiomyopathy is small ventricular volume, relative normal systolic function, impaired LV filling during diastole, and (in some cases) thickened LV walls.

C. Right heart (pulmonary artery) catheterization

1. Should be performed when the diagnosis is uncertain

2. In cardiogenic pulmonary edema, pulmonary artery occlusion pressure (PAOP) is higher than 18 mm Hg.

3. Under certain conditions (e.g., oliguric renal failure), patients can develop pulmonary edema on the basis of intravascular volume overload in the absence of cardiomyopathy; these patients typically are hypertensive and hyperdynamic.

4. Low output states are characterized by cardiac index (CI) lower than 2.1 L/minute per m².

   a. Some patients (notably those with chronic LV dysfunction or obesity) can appear to have adequate perfusion when CI is higher than 1.7 L/minute per m².

b. Typically, PAOP is higher than 18 mm Hg.

c. Arteriovenous oxygen content difference ($a\bar{v}DO_2$) is greater than 5 mL/dL.

d. Mixed venous oxygen saturation ($S\bar{v}O_2$) typically is lower than 0.60, although low values can be caused by factors (e.g., arterial hypoxemia and anemia) in addition to or in lieu of low cardiac output.

D. Laboratory findings when cardiac output is low

1. Elevated arterial lactate concentration

2. Widened $a\bar{v}DO_2$

3. Serum urea nitrogen concentration is increased to a greater extent than serum creatinine concentration.

4. Urine sodium concentration is lower than 10 mmol/L.

5. Urinary fractional excretion of filtered sodium is less than 1%.

Key Imaging Study

- Echocardiography should be performed early in the evaluation of suspected LV failure of recent onset.

- Echocardiography should be obtained on an emergency basis in all hemodynamically unstable patients to guide therapy and rule out potentially reversible causes.

Diagnosis

A. Pulmonary edema

1. Cardiogenic pulmonary edema is probably over-diagnosed in the ICU setting.

2. Pulmonary edema is often noncardiogenic, due to acute lung injury or infection rather than impaired cardiac output.

3. Nevertheless, in patients with hypoxemia and evidence of adequate cardiac output, a trial of diuretic therapy is generally warranted.

4. Obtain a 12-lead electrocardiogram (ECG) to exclude acute myocardial ischemia; if myocardial ischemia is present, make efforts to correct the problem.

5. Basilar rales are present and do not resolve with coughing.

6. Characteristic findings are present on the chest x-ray.

7. If the patient is hypotensive or has worsening renal function, then right heart catheterization

may be useful to verify the presence of elevated PAOP and to evaluate the adequacy of cardiac output.

8. Right heart catheterization is usually not indicated in pulmonary edema if the patient appears to be adequately perfused based on clinical findings (e.g., normal capillary refill and temperature, adequate urine output) and laboratory findings (normal lactate concentration).

B. Low output syndrome (clinical evidence of hypoperfusion)

1. Obtain a 12-lead ECG to exclude myocardial ischemia.

2. Seek to determine if myocardial ischemia is the cause or the result of systemic arterial hypotension; if ischemia is the cause of the hypotension, then emergency cardiac catheterization and revascularization or placement of an intra-aortic balloon pump (IABP) should be considered.

3. Arterial blood lactate concentration is elevated.

4. $a\bar{v}DO_2$ is widened.

5. Consider right heart catheterization to assess adequacy of preload and to exclude inadequate resuscitation of unsuspected vasodilated state.

6. Consider echocardiography to exclude potentially reversible but unsuspected causes of low output, such as pericardial tamponade or right ventricular failure.

Treatment

A. Pulmonary edema (all cases)

1. Provide supplemental oxygen as needed to maintain SaO_2.

   a. Face mask or nasal prongs

   b. Use of noninvasive bilevel positive airway pressure may obviate the need for endotracheal intubation in selected cases.

   c. Endotracheal intubation should be carried out and mechanical ventilation instituted as guided by saturation monitoring and response to therapy.

2. Insert Foley catheter and monitor urine flow.

B. Pulmonary edema (when cardiac output and peripheral perfusion are deemed to be adequate based on clinical findings or measurements)

1. Induce diuresis with furosemide (40 mg IV)

   a. If net negative fluid balance is greater than 200 mL over the succeeding 2 hours, continue intermittent doses of furosemide (20 to 40 mg IV) every 6 to 8 hours until symp-

toms and signs of pulmonary congestion resolve.

   b. If net negative fluid balance is less than 200 mL over the succeeding 2 hours, administer a second dose of furosemide (80 mg IV) and reassess over the next 2 hours.

   c. If net negative fluid balance is greater than 400 mL since beginning diuretic therapy, administer furosemide (40 to 80 mg IV) every 6 to 8 hours until symptoms and signs of pulmonary congestion resolve.

   d. If net negative fluid balance is less than 400 mL since beginning diuretic therapy, then consider one of the following alternative diuretic regimens.

      (1) Metolazone 10 mg orally 30 minutes prior to each dose of furosemide (40 to 80 mg IV every 6 to 8 hours)

      (2) Furosemide given as a 100 mg IV loading dose followed by a continuous IV infusion at 5 to 20 mg/hour

      (3) Bumetanide 5 to 10 mg IV every 6 to 8 hours

      (4) Torsemide 20 to 50 mg IV every 6 to 8 hours

Key Treatment Points Regarding Diuresis

- A reasonable target for diuresis in the patient with pulmonary edema is a net negative fluid balance of 1 to 1.5 L per 24-hour period.

- In patients undergoing a brisk diuresis induced with a potent loop diuretic (e.g., furosemide), be sure to monitor serum potassium and magnesium levels and supplement these electrolytes as needed.

- Diuresis seldom improves cardiac output or peripheral perfusion; its main value is to improve pulmonary function and arterial oxygenation.

2. If systolic blood pressure (BP_S) is higher than 100 mm Hg and mean arterial pressure (MAP) is higher than 65 mm Hg, then relief of pulmonary congestion may be facilitated by adding

   a. Nitroglycerine paste (0.5 to 1.0 inch topically) every 6 hours (remove at 10 PM), or

   b. Nitroglycerine infusion (0.5 to 1.0 μg/kg per minute intravenously) titrated to reduce BP_S to 100 to 105 mm Hg or MAP of approximately 70 mm Hg

3. Consider adding dobutamine (5 to 10 μg/kg per minute) if diuretic therapy fails to provide adequate improvement in symptoms and signs.

    a. Treatment with dobutamine, however, can increase the myocardial oxygen requirement substantially and precipitate myocardial ischemia in patients with fixed coronary blood flow; caution, therefore, is advised.

    b. Tachycardia, ventricular dysrhythmias, and increased intrapulmonary shunting may also occur.

4. Afterload reduction may be beneficial in some patients; appropriate agents for this purpose include

    a. Captopril 6.25 mg orally every 8 hours, or other angiotensin converting enzyme inhibitor

    b. Hydralazine 5 to 20 mg intravenously every 4 hours

    c. Sodium nitroprusside 0.5 to 2.0 μg/kg per minute titrated to reduce BP_s to 100 mm Hg and MAP to 65 to 70 mm Hg

5. Digoxin, 1 mg loading dose, with additional doses based on renal function, may be helpful in some cases.

C. Low cardiac output and MAP lower than 65 mm Hg (i.e., cardiogenic shock)

1. If PAOP is lower than 18 mm Hg (or there is no evidence of pulmonary edema), perform fluid challenge with normal saline or colloid until PAOP is above 20 mm Hg or there is evidence of pulmonary edema or hemodynamic status is adequate (defined by a CI higher than 2.1 L/minute per m^2 and MAP higher than 65 mm Hg).

2. If PAOP is at least 18 mm Hg (or there is evidence of pulmonary congestion), then infuse an inotropic agent.

    a. Dobutamine, 2 to 5 μg/kg per minute initially and titrated up to 20 μg/kg per minute based on serial determinations of CI, is usually the agent of choice.

    b. Add a vasoconstrictor catecholamine if low systemic vascular resistance is contributing to the development of hypotension.

        (1) Dopamine 2 to 20 μg/kg per minute

        (2) Norepinephrine 0.04 to 0.4 μg/kg per minute; less likely to cause excessive tachycardia and may therefore be preferable to dopamine

    c. Milrinone 50 μg/kg IV loading dose followed by 0.2 to 0.75 μg/kg per minute (or lower doses with renal failure); an effective inotropic agent, but it is also a potent vaso-

dilator and therefore can induce or exacerbate hypotension

    d. Epinephrine 0.05 to 0.1 μg/kg per minute may be useful in revascularized patients with cardiogenic shock after cardiac surgery; however, this agent can promote lactic acidosis and hyperglycemia.

3. If PAOP is at least 18 mm Hg and the patient remains in cardiogenic shock despite infusion of an inotropic agent, then IABP should be considered early for the following conditions.

    a. Low output state after cardiac surgery (LV function often improves if the patient can be supported for 48 to 72 hours).

    b. Low output state after MI if early revascularization is part of the therapeutic plan

    c. Low output state in a cardiac transplant candidate

    d. Potentially reversible low output state (e.g., β-adrenergic blocker overdose or cardiac allograft rejection episode)

4. Insertion of a ventricular assist device may be a consideration in patients with severe, potentially reversible LV dysfunction after cardiac surgery or as a bridge to cardiac transplantation.

5. Mechanical ventilation should be routine to decrease oxygen consumption associated with the work of breathing.

D. Low cardiac output and MAP higher than 65 mm Hg

1. If PAOP is lower than 18 mm Hg, then infuse isotonic saline or colloid.

2. Milrinone 50 μg/kg IV loading dose followed by 0.2 to 0.75 μg/kg per minute continuous IV infusion

3. Afterload reduction using one of the following agents:

    a. Captopril 6.25 mg orally every 8 hours, or other angiotensin converting enzyme inhibitor

    b. Hydralazine 5 to 20 mg IV every 4 hours

    c. Sodium nitroprusside 0.5 to 2.0 μg/kg per minute titrated to reduce BP_s to 100 mm Hg and MAP to 65 to 70 mm Hg

E. Diastolic LV dysfunction

1. Increasing PAOP higher than 24 mm Hg may be acceptable in some cases, as long as pulmonary edema is not evident.

2. Afterload reduction

3. Control heart rate with β-adrenergic blocker or diltiazem and, for patients with atrial fibrillation, convert to normal sinus rhythm; tachydys-

rhythmias limit the time available for diastolic filling and markedly compromise cardiac output.

PEARL

In patients with LV failure and hypotension, mechanical devices (IABP or a ventricular assist device) are the only ways to improve cardiac output without increasing myocardial work and oxygen demand.

Bibliography

Boujoukos AJ, Martich GD. Mechanical circulatory assist devices. J Intensive Care Med 1996;11:23–26.

Califf RM, Bengtson JR. Cardiogenic shock. N Engl J Med 1994;330:1724–1730.

The CONSENSUS Trial Study Group. Effects of enalapril on mortality in severe congestive heart failure. N Engl J Med 1987;316:1429–1435.

Dec GW, Fuster V. Idiopathic dilated cardiomyopathy. N Engl J Med 1994;331:1564–1575.

Kushwaha SS, Fallon JT, Fuster V. Restrictive cardiomyopathy. N Engl J Med 1997;336:267–276.

25 Hypertensive Crisis

Jorge A. Guzman

Definitions

A. Hypertensive crisis: any severe elevation in systemic arterial blood pressure that is potentially life-threatening

B. Hypertensive emergency
1. Acute elevation in blood pressure accompanied by signs of acute or progressive end-organ damage
2. Requires immediate lowering of the blood pressure (not necessarily to normal)

C. Hypertensive urgency
1. Acute elevation in blood pressure without accompanying signs of acute or progressive end-organ damage
2. Does not require immediate lowering of blood pressure, but lowering can be safely accomplished over approximately 12 to 24 hours

---

PEARL

Clinical differentiation of hypertensive emergencies from urgencies is based on the presence of end-organ dysfunction, not the level of blood pressure.

Pathophysiology

A. Systemic arterial blood pressure is a function of cardiac output and systemic vascular resistance.

B. Mechanisms of acute blood pressure elevation
1. Plasma volume expansion
   a. Fluid overload
   b. Renal dysfunction
   c. Hyperaldosterone states
2. Increased myocardial contractility
   a. β-Adrenergic catecholamines
   b. Thyrotoxicosis
3. Increased systemic vascular resistance
   a. α-Adrenergic catecholamines
   b. Activation of the renin–angiotensin system
   c. Vasopressin
   d. Mild hypovolemia
   e. Vascular disease
   f. Neurogenic mechanisms

C. Major end-organ effects
1. Central nervous system effects
   a. Cerebral blood flow is maintained constant over a wide range of blood pressure by an autoregulatory process.
   b. Acute rises in blood pressure above the upper limit of autoregulation increase cerebral blood flow, which can result in brain injury and cerebral edema.
   c. Ischemic brain damage can occur if blood pressure falls by more than 30% of the subject's resting baseline mean arterial blood pressure (MAP), the lower limit of cerebral autoregulation for both normotensive and hypertensive individuals.
2. Cardiovascular effects
   a. Increased myocardial oxygen demand can precipitate ischemia.
   b. Increased left ventricular afterload can precipitate heart failure and secondary pulmonary edema, hypoxemia, and respiratory failure.
3. Renal effects
   a. Acute microangiopathy can precipitate or worsen renal failure.
   b. Activation of the renin–angiotensin system and oliguria can further increase blood pressure and renal vascular injury.

Etiology

A. Abrupt increase in blood pressure in patients with chronic hypertension, including essential hypertension (most common)

B. Renovascular hypertension

C. Parenchymal renal disease

D. Acute glomerulonephritis

E. Withdrawal from antihypertensive drugs

F. Drugs (e.g., cocaine, amphetamines, diet pills)

G. Head injury

H. Pregnancy-induced hypertension

I. Collagen vascular diseases and vasculitis

J. Autonomic hyperactivity (e.g., Guillain-Barré or spinal cord syndromes)

K. Hyperaldosterone states (e.g., primary aldosteronism, renin-secreting tumor, Cushing's syndrome)

L. Pheochromocytoma

M. Hypercalcemia

N. Coarctation of the aorta

Complications

A. Associated with hypertensive emergency
1. Hypertensive encephalopathy
2. Acute left ventricular failure with pulmonary edema
3. Aortic dissection
4. Post-coronary artery bypass
5. Acute intracranial events
   a. Hypertensive intracranial bleeding
   b. Acute subarachnoid hemorrhage
   c. Thrombotic cerebrovascular accident
6. Eclampsia
7. Acute coronary syndromes
   a. Unstable angina
   b. Myocardial infarction
8. Excess catecholamine states
   a. Pheochromocytoma crisis
   b. Antihypertensive withdrawal
   c. Monoamine oxidase–tyramine interaction
B. Associated with hypertensive urgencies (overlap with hypertensive emergency occurs)
1. Severe diastolic hypertension without acute end-organ damage
2. Malignant hypertension without acute end-organ damage
3. Some cases of perioperative hypertension
4. Some cases of hypertension associated with increased circulating catecholamines

Symptoms

A. Nonspecific and related to the underlying disease or to end-organ sequelae
1. Neurologic
   a. Headache
   b. Nausea and vomiting
   c. Visual disturbances
   d. Confusion
   e. Seizures
   f. Weakness or other focal neurologic deficits
2. Cardiovascular
   a. Angina pectoris
   b. Dyspnea
   c. Palpitations
   d. Fatigue
3. Renal
   a. Generalized weakness
   b. Oliguria
   c. Polyuria
   d. Hematuria

Physical Findings

A. Vital signs
1. Hypertension
2. Tachycardia
B. Funduscopic findings (Keith-Wagener-Barker classification)
1. Grade I: narrowed arteriovenous ratio
2. Grade II: focal arteriolar spasm
3. Grade III: hemorrhages and exudates
4. Grade IV: papilledema
C. Cardiovascular
1. Diaphoresis
2. Jugular vein distention
3. Pulmonary rales
4. Third heart sound
5. Murmurs
6. Pericardial friction rub
7. Pulse deficits
D. Renal
1. Pedal edema
2. Hematuria
3. Oliguria
E. Neurologic
1. Alterations in sensorium
2. Focal neurologic deficits

Key Tests

- Complete blood count and peripheral blood smear
- Serum electrolytes, urea nitrogen, creatinine levels
- Serum creatine phosphokinase and troponin levels
- Urinalysis, including microscopic sediment examination
- Quantitative urine protein determination
- 12-Lead electrocardiogram
- Chest x-ray
- Computed tomography (CT) scan of brain
- Specific tests according to clinical scenario; e.g., chest CT (if aortic dissection considered), toxicology screen, echocardiography, renal ultrasonography

Treatment

A. Hypertensive emergencies

1. The goal of treatment of hypertensive crisis should be to reduce MAP by 20% to 25%, over a period of minutes to hours, depending on the nature of the emergency.

2. Parenteral antihypertensive therapy is indicated. (For drug selection, dosing, and related information, see Chapter 162, Antihypertensives, and chapters on specific antihypertensive agents.)

3. Precipitous reductions in blood pressure or reductions to values below normotensive levels can cause acute end-organ hypoperfusion.

4. Monitoring

   a. Frequent blood pressure monitoring in an ICU or equivalent setting is required.

   b. Invasive arterial blood pressure monitoring is necessary in critically ill patients, those requiring nitroprusside infusion, and selected other patients with hypertensive emergencies.

5. Following immediate reduction of blood pressure by approximately 20%, further reductions should be gradual; normalization may be achieved over a period of 24 to 72 hours or more.

6. Special considerations in specific conditions

   a. Cerebrovascular disorders

      (1) Cerebral infarction

         (a) Caution is recommended in the treatment of elevated blood pressures, because rapid reductions can cause cerebral hypoperfusion.

         (b) Consider treatment for severe diastolic hypertension (e.g., >130 mm Hg).

         (c) Mild to moderate hypertension is acceptable (e.g., diastolic pressure of 100 to 120 mm Hg).

      (2) Subarachnoid hemorrhage

         (a) There is increased risk of rebleeding if MAP remains elevated immediately after the event.

         (b) After several days, the likelihood of vasospasm increases, and excessive reductions in blood pressure may worsen neurologic status.

   b. Hypertensive encephalopathy: MAP should be reduced gradually by 20% to 25% over a period of approximately 2 hours.

   c. Cardiovascular disorders

      (1) Reduction of MAP improves left ventric-
ular function and relieves myocardial ischemia.

      (2) The limits of myocardial blood flow autoregulation are wider than those for the brain; thus, in absence of neurological manifestations a more rapid decrease in MAP is beneficial and well tolerated.

      (3) In aortic dissection, blood pressure should be rapidly decreased to the lowest level that allows adequate vital organ perfusion (see Chapter 31, Aortic Dissection).

   d. Pheochromocytoma (see Chapter 57, Pheochromocytoma)

   e. Pregnancy (see Chapter 26, Pregnancy-Induced Hypertension)

B. Hypertensive urgencies

1. Patients with hypertensive urgencies may not require ICU admission.

2. Noninvasive blood pressure monitoring suffices in most cases.

3. Choice of pharmacotherapy

   a. Blood pressure reduction can generally be achieved with oral antihypertensive drugs.

   b. Parenteral medications can be employed, but are usually not necessary.

   c. For dosing and related information, see Chapter 162, Antihypertensives, and chapters on specific antihypertensive agents.

Key Treatment

- Reduce MAP immediately in hypertensive emergencies, but not by more than 25% of the presenting value.

- The subsequent blood pressure target depends on the patient's chronic baseline blood pressure and the nature of the associated emergency.

- Treatment of hypertension in the setting of acute cerebrovascular events should be undertaken with caution because it can lead to critical reductions in cerebral blood flow and further neurologic damage.

Bibliography

Gifford RW. Management of hypertensive crisis. JAMA 1991;266:829–835.

Heyka RJ. Evaluation and management of hypertension in the intensive care unit. In: Irwin RS, Cerra FB, Rippe JM (eds). Intensive Care Medicine. Philadelphia: Lippincott-Raven, 1999, pp 559–568.

Strandgaard S, Paulson OB. Cerebral autoregulation. Stroke 1984;15:413–416.

Varon J, Marik PE. The diagnosis and management of hypertensive crisis. Chest 2000;118:214–227.

26 Pregnancy-Induced Hypertension

Brian A. Mason

Hypertensive disorders complicate up to 8% of all pregnancies and can lead to potentially lethal complications including renal failure, cerebral hemorrhage, disseminated intravascular coagulation, and abruptio placentae. Collectively, hypertensive disorders in pregnancy are the second leading cause of maternal death in the United States. In addition to maternal complications, the hypertensive disorders are major contributors to neonatal morbidity and death. More specifically, a hypertensive condition unique to pregnancy known as preeclampsia accounts for a disproportionate share of both maternal and fetal maladies.

Preeclampsia is distinct from simple gestational hypertension and is a systemic syndrome with a variety of pathophysiologic effects. A number of its nonhypertensive effects may be life-threatening in the face of minimal blood pressure elevations. The pathophysiologic effects of this disorder are primarily related to vasospasm and the resultant ischemia, which can affect a variety of organ systems individually or collectively. While the causes of preeclampsia are unknown, most investigators consider the placenta to be in some way responsible, because delivery is the only cure for this condition. An inflammatory-like response appears to be an important mediator of the physical manifestations of preeclampsia, and much research is being devoted to this area. Until the disease is better understood mechanistically, treatment is centered on supportive care and limiting morbidity to mother and fetus until sufficient fetal maturity has been achieved for delivery to be undertaken.

> **PEARL**
>
> Because of the profound implications of maternal and fetal risk weighed against the potential complications of premature delivery, it is important to distinguish between preeclampsia and the other more benign disorders of blood pressure regulation in pregnancy.

Classification

A. Chronic hypertension (blood pressure at least 140 mm Hg systolic or 90 mm Hg diastolic)
  1. Present before pregnancy, or
  2. Present before 20 weeks gestation, or
  3. Diagnosed in pregnancy and does not resolve postpartum

B. Gestational hypertension
  1. A nonspecific diagnosis
  2. Blood pressure elevation detected for first time after 20 weeks gestation in the absence of proteinuria
  3. Includes patients with preeclampsia who have not yet developed proteinuria
  4. Final determination that patient does not have preeclampsia can only be made postpartum.
    a. If blood pressure elevation persists postpartum, patient has chronic hypertension.
    b. If preeclampsia never develops and blood pressure returns to normal by 12 weeks postpartum, patient had transient hypertension of pregnancy.

C. Eclampsia and preeclampsia
  1. Pregnancy-specific syndromes
  2. Usually occur after 20 weeks gestation (may present earlier if trophoblastic disease present)
  3. Defined as gestational blood pressure elevation plus proteinuria
    a. Gestational blood pressure elevation defined as higher than 140 mm Hg systolic or 90 mm Hg diastolic after 20 weeks gestation in previously normotensive patient
    b. If no proteinuria present, still suspect the disease in patient with hypertension plus:
      (1) Visual disturbance
      (2) Right upper quadrant abdominal pain
      (3) Headache
      (4) Thrombocytopenia ($<100,000$ platelets/mm^3)
      (5) Elevated serum transaminase activity (aspartate aminotransferase >100 IU/L)
      (6) Hyperuricemia (serum uric acid level greater than 6 mg/dL)
  4. Blood pressure increases more than 30 mm Hg systolic or 15 mm Hg diastolic should be closely observed for developing signs or symptoms or preeclampsia, but these findings alone no longer serve as criteria to define the condition.
  5. Proteinuria
    a. Defined in pregnancy as urinary protein excretion of at least 3 g/24 hours
      (1) Correlates roughly with at least 30 mg/

dL or 1+ on urine dipstick in a random urine sample

(2) Exclude other etiologies of proteinuria; e.g., urinary tract infection

b. Because of the variable nature of urine protein excretion, a 24 hr urine sample is advisable; shorter timed collection may be used if corrected for creatinine excretion and a 24-hour sample cannot be obtained.

6. Other factors suggesting preeclampsia

a. Persistent headache

b. Visual or other cerebral disturbances

c. Persistent epigastric pain

d. Thrombocytopenia

e. Elevated serum activities of hepatic enzymes

f. Elevated serum creatinine level (>1.2 mg/dL)

g. Microangiopathic hemolytic anemia (evidenced by increased serum lactic acid dehydrogenase activity and findings on peripheral blood smear)

h. Edema is no longer considered a marker symptom for preeclampsia because it is ubiquitous in pregnancy.

7. Eclampsia is defined as otherwise unexplained seizure activity in a patient with preeclampsia.

D. Superimposed preeclampsia

1. Preeclampsia that occurs in women with chronic hypertension

2. Carries a worse prognosis than either condition individually

3. Difficult to distinguish from worsening chronic hypertension

4. Suspect if

a. Hypertensive patient without proteinuria develops new-onset proteinuria

b. Sudden increase in proteinuria develops in a patient with proteinuria prior to 20 weeks gestation

c. Thrombocytopenia

d. Increase in serum hepatic transaminase activity

e. Sudden increase in previously well-controlled blood pressure

Differential Diagnosis

A. Hypertension prior to 20 weeks gestation

1. Probable chronic hypertension

2. Obtain baseline urine protein excretion study (significant increase in proteinuria suggestive of superimposed preeclampsia).

3. Pre-pregnancy or first-trimester blood pressure readings are most useful, because the normal physiologic mid-trimester drop in blood pressure may mask underlying chronic hypertension.

B. Hypertension after 20 weeks gestation

1. Suggestive of gestational hypertension or preeclampsia

2. Measure urine protein excretion.

a. Proteinuria higher than 1+ on clean-catch spot specimen needs follow-up with 24-hour urine collection.

b. Proteinuria higher than 300 mg/24 hours suggests renal involvement consistent with preeclampsia.

c. Pregnancy-associated hypertension plus proteinuria is preeclampsia until proven otherwise.

3. Serum uric acid elevation is suggestive of preeclampsia.

4. Thrombocytopenia suggests severe preeclampsia.

5. Serum transaminase activity elevation suggests severe preeclampsia.

6. Hemoconcentration is consistent with preeclampsia, but hematocrit may be decreased if hemolysis is present.

7. Other tests have been examined (e.g., urinary calcium excretion, urinary kallikrein concentration, plasma fibronectin, and platelet activation), but these lack sufficient predictive value to be applied to individual patients.

Key Findings

- Pregnancy of more than 20 weeks duration
- Proteinuria
- Hypertension (blood pressure greater than 140/90 mm Hg)
- Thrombocytopenia
- Headache
- Hyperuricemia
- Visual disturbances
- Elevated serum transaminases
- Right upper quadrant abdominal pain
- Microangiopathic hemolytic anemia
- Seizures
- Elevated serum creatinine

Treatment of Chronic Hypertension in Pregnancy

A. In most cases blood pressure elevation is mild to moderate (<180/110 mm Hg).

B. Most morbidity results from superimposed preeclampsia.

C. Treatment remains controversial.

1. There is limited evidence of improved outcome with treatment of hypertension lower than <180/110 mm Hg.

2. Antihypertensive therapy does not limit propensity to develop superimposed preeclampsia.

3. Antihypertensive drug therapy is commonly employed for diastolic blood pressure less than 110 mm Hg despite the lack of evidence of improved clinical outcome.

D. Antihypertensive agents

1. α-Methyldopa

   a. Traditional drug of choice

   b. Documented fetal safety in studies following children to 7 years of age

   c. Documented stability of uteroplacental blood flow and fetal hemodynamics

   d. Relatively weak antihypertensive

   e. Somnolence is a common side effect.

   f. Compliance is a problem due to daily dosing.

2. Labetalol

   a. Both α- and β-adrenergic blocking effects

   b. Appears to be both safe and efficacious for mother and fetus, but long-term follow-up studies are lacking

   c. Legitimate concerns over β-blockade component of this drug

      (1) Pure β-blockers (e.g., atenolol) given early in pregnancy have been confirmed to cause intrauterine growth restriction and oligohydramnios.

      (2) β-blocker effect of labetalol dominates its α-blockade effect.

3. Nifedipine

   a. Vasodilator effect dominates negative inotropic effect, thereby maintaining perfusion to placenta.

   b. Once-a-day dosing using a sustained-release formulation is preferred.

   c. Several robust multicenter trials demonstrate

      (1) No evidence of attributable problems when begun in the second trimester

      (2) No evidence of teratogenicity from use in the first trimester

4. Diuretics

   a. Traditionally avoided in pregnancy

      (1) Disrupt natural blood volume expansion associated with pregnancy

      (2) Problematic in cases where intravascular volume is already decreased (e.g., preeclampsia)

      (3) May exacerbate placental hypoperfusion and worsen intrauterine growth restriction

   b. Recent meta-analysis of nine randomized controlled trials revealed no increase in adverse outcome to fetuses and efficacy in mothers.

   c. May be given with caution, if indicated, but avoid in preeclampsia and conditions associated with uterine hypoperfusion

E. Fetal monitoring in chronic or gestational hypertension

1. Estimate fetal growth and amniotic fluid volume when diagnosis made; if normal, repeat testing only if there is a change in maternal condition.

2. Perform non-stress test at 28 to 32 weeks gestation as baseline.

   a. If nonreactive, perform biophysical profile (and if result is 8 of 8, repeat testing only if there is a change in maternal condition).

   b. If nonstress test is reactive, repeat testing only if there is a significant change in maternal condition.

Treatment of Preeclampsia

A. Basic principles of management

1. Goal of therapy is to prevent complications of preeclampsia.

2. Delivery is always an appropriate therapy from the maternal standpoint.

   a. May have negative effects on fetus

   b. Determination of delivery timing is based on maternal condition and whether fetus may survive outside the uterus without significant neonatal complications.

3. Delay of delivery is indicated to allow fetal maturation or to allow the cervix to become more favorable for induction (if not detrimental to mother or fetus).

4. Poor perfusion is central to maternal and fetal morbidity and mortality; attempts to "treat" preeclampsia by antihypertensive therapy or diuresis may worsen the physiologic derangement.

B. Assessment of the mother

1. Goals are to recognize preeclampsia early on, and to monitor progress of condition to determine when timing of delivery is optimal for mother and fetus.

2. Hospitalization is indicated when signs or

symptoms of severe preeclampsia become manifest.

    a. Hospitalization is continued for duration of pregnancy.

    b. Decision to continue pregnancy is determined by daily assessment.

    c. Frequent determinations of platelet count, serum liver enzyme activities, renal function, and urine protein excretion should be undertaken.

    d. Close attention should be given to central nervous system symptoms (e.g., headache and visual changes) and progression of hypertension.

  3. Therapeutic efforts other than delivery are only palliative.

    a. May limit symptoms and permit continuation of pregnancy to achieve greater fetal maturity, but do not affect the underlying physiologic derangement

    b. Although efficacy not proven, restricting activity is usually recommended.

    c. Sodium restriction and diuretic therapy are not indicated.

C. Fetal indications for delivery

  1. Decision to deliver is based on maternal and fetal condition as well as gestational age.

  2. Severe fetal growth restriction, especially if oligohydramnios present

  3. Non-reassuring fetal heart rate testing

  4. Suspected abruptio placentae

  5. Any patient with even mild disease and a favorable cervix should be delivered at 38 weeks gestation (34 weeks if severe disease is present).

D. Maternal indications for delivery

  1. Gestational age at least 38 weeks with mild disease or 34 weeks with severe disease

  2. Thrombocytopenia (<100,000 platelets/mm^3)

  3. Deterioration in renal function

  4. Deterioration in hepatic function

  5. Persistent severe headache

  6. Visual changes

  7. Severe epigastric pain, nausea, or vomiting

E. Preferred route of delivery

  1. Vaginal delivery is preferred over cesarean delivery (avoids the additional stress of surgery).

  2. Aggressive induction indicated to accomplish delivery within 24 hours of the decision to deliver

  3. Cesarean delivery is indicated for usual obstetrical indications or if vaginal delivery cannot be achieved in a timely fashion.

F. Analgesia

  1. Intravenous opioids may be used as in any delivery.

  2. Epidural analgesia is safe and effective if properly applied.

    a. Dilute infusions of local anesthetic plus opioid

    b. Judicious volume loading with 500 to 1000 mL of IV crystalloid prior to placement of epidural catheter

    c. Slow, controlled induction followed by continuous infusion

  3. For cesarean delivery

    a. Carefully applied spinal anesthesia is the method of choice after appropriate volume expansion (relatively contraindicated if coagulopathy present).

    b. General endotracheal anesthesia is to be avoided.

      (1) Airway edema increases risk of failed intubation.

      (2) Significant increase in hypertension at time of intubation and extubation (blood pressure may double during these events)

G. Invasive hemodynamic monitoring

  1. Useful in monitoring fluid balance in cases of severe preeclampsia

  2. In many cases, volume status is a delicate balance between pulmonary edema (due to capillary leak) and hypoperfusion (due to depleted intravascular volume).

  3. May be particularly useful in cases of

    a. Pulmonary edema

    b. Intractable hypertension

    c. Persistent oliguria unresponsive to volume challenge

    d. Monitoring fluid balance in patients requiring plasma volume expansion

    e. Coexisting cardiovascular disease

H. Anticonvulsants

  1. Should be used in all cases of preeclampsia during labor and continued for 24 hours after delivery of the fetus

  2. Drug of choice is magnesium sulfate.

    a. Superior to phenytoin for seizure prophylaxis

    b. Demonstrated safety for mother and fetus

    c. Normal regimen is 6 g $MgSO_4$ intravenously over 20 minutes followed by a continuous IV infusion of 2 g/hour.

    d. Must be used with caution in patients with renal dysfunction (dose adjustment may be required)

e. Monitor serum level carefully; maintain between 5 and 7 mg/dL.

f. Monitor for signs of toxicity (lethargy, loss of deep tendon reflexes, respiratory depression).

I. Antihypertensive therapy for acute blood pressure management

1. Generally used when diastolic blood pressure exceeds 105 mm Hg

2. Ideal agent would

   a. Lower pressure in a controlled fashion

   b. Have rapid onset

   c. Reverse uteroplacental vasoconstriction

   d. Not reduce cardiac output

   e. Have no adverse fetal or maternal side effects

3. Agents most often used in acute management of hypertension in preeclampsia

   a. Hydralazine

      (1) Considered a drug of first choice

      (2) Begin with 5 to 10 mg intravenously.

      (3) Repeat at 20-minute intervals until desired blood pressure level achieved.

      (4) Repeat as needed (typically every 2 to 3 hours) to maintain desired blood pressure.

      (5) Consider trying an alternate agent if control is not achieved after giving 20 to 30 mg.

   b. Labetalol

      (1) Begin with 20 mg IV dose.

      (2) If no response after 10 minutes, give a 40 mg IV dose.

      (3) If control still not achieved, may give up to two additional IV doses of 80 mg each.

      (4) If not controlled after a total of 220 mg is given, consider alternative agent.

      (5) Avoid in cases where β-blockers are contraindicated (e.g., congestive heart failure, asthma, etc.).

   c. Sodium nitroprusside

      (1) Used in severe cases not responsive to drugs listed above

      (2) Fetal cyanide poisoning may occur if used longer than 4 hours

      (3) Begin continuous IV infusion at 0.25 μg/kg per minute and titrate to desired blood pressure.

      (4) Do not exceed 5 μg/kg per minute.

WARNING

Angiotensin-converting enzyme inhibitors are contraindicated in pregnancy; adverse fetal effects include oligohydramnios, embryopathy, and neonatal renal failure.

 Bibliography

American College of Obstetricians and Gynecologists. Hypertension in pregnancy. ACOG Technical Bulletin No. 219. Washington, DC: American College of Obstetricians and Gynecologists, 1996:1–8.

Caritis S, Sibai B, Hauth J, et al. Low-dose aspirin to prevent preeclampsia in women at high risk. National Institute of Child Health and Human Development Network of Maternal-Fetal Medicine Units. N Engl J Med 1998;338:701–705.

Lindheimer MD, Roberts JM, Cunningham FG (eds). Hypertensive Disorders in Pregnancy. Stamford, CT: Appleton-Lange, 1999:349–374.

Magee LA, Ornstein MP, von Dadelszen P. Fortnightly review: management of hypertension in pregnancy. BMJ 1999;318:1332–1336.

National High Blood Pressure Education Program. Working Group Report on High Blood Pressure in Pregnancy. NIH Publication No. 00-3029. Bethesda, MD: National Institutes of Health, 2000.

North RA, Taylor RS, Schellenberg JC. Evaluation of a definition of preeclampsia. Br J Obstet Gynaecol 1999; 106:767–773.

27 Cardiogenic Shock

Vivian L. Clark
James A. Kruse

Cardiogenic shock is a state of circulatory failure, of cardiac origin, associated with inadequate organ perfusion in the presence of adequate intravascular volume.

Etiology

A. Large acute myocardial infarction (MI)

B. Acute myocardial infarction in the setting of preexisting left ventricular dysfunction

C. Myocardial ischemia, particularly if superimposed on preexisting left ventricular dysfunction

D. Valvular heart disease

E. Cardiomyopathy

F. Acquired ventricular septal defect

G. Myocarditis

H. Acute cardiac transplant rejection

I. Pericardial tamponade

Pathophysiology

A. Critically decreased systemic oxygen delivery due to low cardiac output

B. Usually precipitated by MI or ischemia

C. Decreased contractility and stroke volume due to myocardial dysfunction can further reduce coronary perfusion, resulting in worsening ischemia and dysfunction.

D. Compensatory responses such as vasoconstriction and fluid retention can exacerbate ischemia by increasing afterload, increasing filling pressures, and contributing to hypoxemia.

Differential Diagnosis

A. Septic shock, which is characterized by signs of sepsis and, typically, increased cardiac output and low systemic vascular resistance

B. Hypovolemic shock, which is characterized by low cardiac filling pressures

C. Shock due to ventricular dysfunction should be distinguished from that related to mechanical complications such as ventricular septal rupture and mitral valve dysfunction, which can be discerned by physical examination, echocardiography, and right heart catheterization.

Manifestations

A. Hypotension: systolic blood pressure lower than 90 mm Hg or necessitating vasopressors to maintain at 90 mm Hg or higher

B. Signs of pulmonary congestion on clinical examination or chest x-ray

C. Evidence of inadequate organ perfusion: oliguria; cool, clammy skin; abnormal sensorium

D. Chest pain typical of angina may be present if there is underlying ischemia.

E. Electrocardiogram

   1. Sinus tachycardia is typical.

   2. Bradycardia may be present in shock when associated with inferior MI complicated by heart block.

   3. Electrocardiographic ST segment and T wave changes may be present if there is underlying ischemia.

   4. Ventricular dysrhythmias are common.

   5. Tachydysrhythmias may lead to shock in the setting of underlying ventricular dysfunction; rate control or cardioversion is mandatory.

F. Chest x-ray

   1. Signs of pulmonary vascular congestion are frequently present.

   2. Cardiac size may be normal in shock when associated with acute MI.

G. Echocardiography

   1. Regional wall motion abnormalities are present in cases of ischemic heart disease.

   2. Global left ventricular dysfunction suggests an underlying cardiomyopathic process or myocarditis.

   3. Essential for diagnosis of mechanical complications such as ventricular septal defect or mitral valve dysfunction

H. Hemodynamic findings

   1. Pulmonary artery occlusion pressure greater than 18 mm Hg

   2. Cardiac index less than 2.2 L/m^2

   3. Systemic vascular resistance index higher than 2400 dyne·sec·m^2/cm^5

   4. Cardiac ejection fraction is usually markedly impaired, although it may be normal in shock

secondary to valvular dysfunction, ventricular septal defect, or pericardial tamponade.

I. Laboratory findings

1. Elevated arterial blood lactate concentration, which is an indicator of global hypoperfusion

2. Cardiac enzymes are elevated in shock related to acute MI, often markedly so.

3. Hyponatremia is common, particularly in patients with chronic underlying left ventricular dysfunction.

4. Blood urea nitrogen and creatinine may be normal early in course.

Key Findings

- Systemic hypotension and pulmonary congestion

- Signs of inadequate organ perfusion (e.g., oliguria, impaired mentation)

- Right heart catheterization confirms diagnosis and excludes other causes of shock.

Monitoring

A. Continuous electrocardiographic monitoring to detect rhythm or conduction disturbances

B. Clinical signs of hypoperfusion: vital signs, sensorium, urine output

C. Continuous pulse oximetry to insure adequate oxygenation

D. Arterial blood lactate concentration

E. Arterial blood gases and pH to assess for impaired gas exchange and acid-base derangements

F. Systemic arterial catheterization to allow continuous blood pressure monitoring, frequent serial blood tests, and to facilitate titration of vasoactive drug infusions

G. Pulmonary artery catheterization for hemodynamic monitoring and assessment of mixed venous oxygenation

H. Serial 12-lead electrocardiographic examinations to detect cardiac ischemia, injury, or inflammation

I. Serial cardiac marker studies (creatine phosphokinase, including MB isoenzymes, and cardiac troponin levels)

Treatment

A. Vasopressors to maintain systolic blood pressure above 90 mm Hg or mean arterial pressure above 70 mm Hg; dopamine or a combination of dopamine and dobutamine

B. Diuretics for pulmonary congestion; intubation and mechanical ventilation may be required if there is significant hypoxemia.

C. Nitrates for ischemia; after initiation of vasopressors

D. Intra-aortic balloon counterpulsation

1. Decreases afterload

2. Increases myocardial perfusion

3. Can be used as a bridge to revascularization or myocardial transplant, but probably is of little benefit alone

E. In the setting of acute MI, revascularization by primary angioplasty or coronary artery bypass; thrombolytic therapy may reduce the incidence of shock but does not improve mortality.

F. Surgery: if shock is secondary to ventricular septal defect, free wall rupture, or valvular disease

G. Left ventricular assist device: as a bridge to transplantation

Key Treatment

- Coronary revascularization should be considered for most patients with cardiogenic shock due to acute ischemic syndromes.

- Intra-aortic balloon counterpulsation may be an effective bridge to revascularization but has little impact on survival alone.

Prognosis

A. Treated medically, the mortality is more than 80%.

B. With coronary revascularization, mortality is 50% to 60%; mortality advantage with revascularization may be limited to patients under age 75.

Bibliography

Bates ER, Stomel RJ, Hochman JS, et al. The use of intra-aortic balloon counterpulsation as an adjunct to reperfusion therapy in cardiogenic shock. Int J Cardiol 1998; 65(Suppl 1):S37–S42.

Hochman JS, Sleeper LA, Webb JG, et al. Early revascularization in acute myocardial infarction complicated by cardiogenic shock. SHOCK Investigators. Should we emergently revascularize occluded coronaries for cardiogenic shock? N Engl J Med 1999;341:625–634.

Hochman JS, Sleeper LAD, Godfrey E, et al. Should we emergently revascularize occluded coronaries for cardiogenic shock: an international randomized trial of emergency PTCA/CABG-trial design? The SHOCK Trial Study Group. Am Heart J 1999;137:313–321.

Hollenberg SM, Kavinsky CJ, Parillo JE. Cardiogenic shock. Ann Intern Med 1999;13:47–59.

Santoro GM, Buonamici P. Reperfusion therapy in cardiogenic shock complicating acute myocardial infarction. Am Heart J 1999;138:126–131.

28 Valvular Heart Disease

Kenneth R. McCurry
G. Daniel Martich

Overview

A. Aortic stenosis (AS)
1. Normal adult aortic valve area is 3.0 to 4.0 cm^2.
   a. Mild AS: 1.5 to 2.9 cm^2
   b. Moderate AS: 1.0 to 1.52 cm^2
   c. Severe AS: less than 1.0 cm^2
2. Anatomic classification
   a. Subvalvular
      (1) 8% to 10% of congenital AS is due to a fibromuscular ring around the outflow tract of the left ventricle (LV).
      (2) Idiopathic hypertrophic subaortic stenosis
   b. Supravalvular (congenital tubular narrowing of ascending aorta)
   c. Valvular (by far the most common in adults)
3. In patients with AS, cardiac output is relatively fixed.
4. Patients with sepsis or other hyperdynamic states may not be able to increase cardiac output to compensate for the loss of peripheral vasomotor tone.
5. Loss of atrial systole can decrease cardiac output by 25% in patients with AS.
6. If left untreated, AS leads to death 2, 3, or 5 years after the onset of symptoms of congestive heart failure (CHF), syncope, or angina, respectively

B. Aortic regurgitation (AR)
1. Classically, chronic AR is characterized by an insidious course of progressive LV dilatation, ultimately leading to severe LV dysfunction and late onset of symptoms.
2. Acute AR results in a catastrophic increase in LV filling pressure with a concomitant decrease in cardiac output, producing CHF and cardiogenic shock.

C. Mitral stenosis (MS)
1. Normal mitral valve area is 4.0 to 6.0 cm^2.
2. Symptoms develop only after narrowing to less than 2.5 cm^2.
3. Symptoms typically do not develop until 20 to 40 years after rheumatic fever (most common cause).

D. Mitral regurgitation (MR)
1. Much like chronic AR, chronic MR is associated with an insidious course of progressive LV dilatation with ultimate LV dysfunction and late onset of symptoms.
2. Acute, severe MR typically produces acute CHF and variable degrees of cardiogenic shock.

E. Tricuspid valve (TV) disease
1. Acquired TV disease is very uncommon in adults.
2. Most cases are secondary to trauma or bacterial endocarditis in IV drug abusers.

PEARL

Even with no anticoagulation, the risk of stroke for patients with a St. Jude mechanical valve in the aortic position, in sinus rhythm, is 8% to 12% per year.

Etiology

A. Aortic stenosis etiology is dependent on age at the time of diagnosis.
1. Younger than 50 years
   a. Bicuspid: 50%
   b. Rheumatic: 25%
   c. Degenerative: 25%
2. Older than 50 years
   a. Degenerative: 50%
   b. Rheumatic: 25%
   c. Bicuspid: 25%

B. Aortic regurgitation
1. Acute
   a. Aortic dissection
   b. Infective endocarditis
   c. Trauma
2. Chronic
   a. Rheumatic fever
   b. Bicuspid aortic valve
   c. Infective endocarditis
   d. Marfan's syndrome
   e. Ehlers-Danlos syndrome
   f. Syphilitic aortitis

g. Giant cell arteritis

h. Ankylosing spondylitis

C. Mitral stenosis

1. Rheumatic (mainly)

2. Congenital (occasional cases)

D. Mitral regurgitation

1. Acute MR typically occurs as a result of endocarditis, papillary muscle rupture several days after a myocardial infarction, or acute rupture of a chordae tendineae in a chronically diseased (typically myxomatous) mitral valve.

2. Chronic MR can occur as a result of an abnormality of the mitral annulus, mitral leaflets, chordae tendineae or the papillary muscles.

3. Acute MR

a. Disorders of the valve leaflets

(1) Infective endocarditis

(2) Trauma

(3) Left atrial myxoma

b. Disorders of chordae tendineae

(1) Infective endocarditis

(2) Trauma

(3) Rheumatic valvulitis

(4) Acute rheumatic fever

(5) Idiopathic ("spontaneous rupture")

c. Dysfunction of papillary muscle

(1) Myocardial ischemia or infarction

(2) Left ventricular dilation

(3) Left ventricular aneurysm

d. Rupture of papillary muscle

(1) Trauma

(2) Myocardial infarction

(3) Myocardial abscess

e. Prosthetic valve malfunction

(1) Deterioration of disc

(2) Lodging of the ball or disc in the open position

(3) Dislodgement of the ball or disc

(4) Ring or strut fracture

(5) Paravalvular leak

(6) Suture or pledge dislodgement

(7) Deterioration of leaflet(s) of bioprosthetic valve

4. Chronic MR

a. Inflammatory

(1) Infective endocarditis

(2) Rheumatic heart disease

(3) Scleroderma

b. Degenerative

(1) Myxomatous degeneration of mitral leaflets

(2) Marfan's syndrome

(3) Ehlers-Danlos syndrome

(4) Pseudoxanthoma elasticum

(5) Calcification of mitral valve annulus

c. Infective endocarditis

d. Structural

(1) Rupture of chordae tendineae

(2) Rupture or dysfunction of papillary muscle

(3) Dilation of mitral valve annulus and LV cavity

(4) Hypertrophic cardiomyopathy

(5) Paravalvular prosthetic valve leak

e. Congenital

(1) Mitral valve clefts or fenestrations

(2) Parachute abnormality

(3) Abnormalities in association with endocardial cushion defects, endocardial fibroelastosis, transposition of the great arteries, or anomalous origin of the left coronary artery

E. Tricuspid valve disease

1. Cases of both tricuspid stenosis (TS) and tricuspid regurgitation (TR) have been associated with rheumatic fever and carcinoid syndrome.

2. Marfan's syndrome, Ebstein's anomaly (inferior displacement of the septal and posterior leaflets of the tricuspid valve into the right ventricle), and some anorectic drugs may cause TR.

3. Tricuspid stenosis is mostly rheumatic in origin and almost never is an isolated valvular lesion.

F. Pulmonic valve disease

1. Pulmonic regurgitation is most commonly caused by valve ring dilatation secondary to pulmonary hypertension.

2. Pulmonic stenosis is most commonly congenital.

Diagnosis

A. Aortic stenosis

1. Symptoms

a. Angina pectoris: 50% of patients with AS who experience angina also have concomitant coronary artery disease

b. Syncope

c. Congestive heart failure

2. Signs and laboratory evaluation

a. Physical examination reveals a systolic ejection murmur at the base.

b. Electrocardiogram (ECG) shows LV hypertrophy in 85% of cases with severe AS.

c. Chest x-ray: calcification is found in almost all adults with AS; cardiac size is usually normal.

d. Cardiac catheterization is needed to evaluate the coronary arteries in adults prior to valve-replacement surgery, since many patients will require simultaneous coronary artery bypass grafting.

B. Aortic regurgitation

1. Symptoms of acute AR

   a. Pulmonary edema

   b. Cardiogenic shock

2. Symptoms of chronic AR

   a. Paroxysmal nocturnal dyspnea

   b. Exertional dyspnea

   c. Orthopnea

3. Physical examination

   a. Diastolic high-pitched murmur beginning immediately after S_2

   b. Severity of disease correlates with the duration of the murmur rather than its intensity.

   c. The murmur is augmented by anything that increases vasomotor tone.

   d. Water-hammer pulses with widened pulse pressure

   e. Findings may be absent in acute AR.

4. Electrocardiogram

   a. Left axis deviation with intraventricular conduction delay are findings that occur late in the course of the disease.

   b. Electrocardiographic findings may be absent in acute AR.

5. Chest x-ray: cardiomegaly (heart size correlates with the chronicity and severity of AR)

6. Echocardiography is used to establish the diagnosis and calculate regurgitant fraction.

C. Mitral stenosis

1. Symptoms are nonspecific; dyspnea and fatigue are common complaints.

2. Physical examination

   a. Frank pulmonary edema, atrial fibrillation, hemoptysis, or an embolic event may be the first signs of MS.

   b. Low-pitched diastolic rumble best heard at the apex

3. Electrocardiogram

   a. Left atrial enlargement if sinus rhythm

   b. Right ventricular (RV) hypertrophy if pulmonary hypertension is present.

D. Mitral regurgitation

1. Symptoms

   a. Fatigue and weakness are caused by chronically low cardiac output.

   b. Later in the course of the disease, symptoms related to pulmonary edema become more prominent.

2. Physical examination

   a. Heart sounds in MR are characterized by a soft S_1 followed by a holosystolic murmur.

   b. The murmur of MR is differentiated by examination from the murmur of AS; the former decreases with standing, exercise, or administration of isoproterenol.

   c. The heart sounds of mitral valve prolapse (MVP) are characterized by a midsystolic click representing sudden tensing of the mitral valve apparatus as the leaflets prolapse into the left atrium during systole.

3. Electrocardiogram

   a. In acute MR, the ECG is normal.

   b. In chronic MR, there is left atrial enlargement (LAE) and atrial fibrillation.

4. Chest x-ray

   a. In acute MR, the chest film is usually normal.

   b. In chronic MR, there is LAE, cardiomegaly, and/or a calcified annulus.

5. Echocardiography

   a. In acute MR, left atrial size is usually normal, and a demonstrable source of acute MR (e.g., flail leaflet, ruptured chordae, vegetations) can be identified.

   b. In chronic MR, there is LAE, the LV is dilated, and the cause may be identified (e.g., MVP, rheumatic valvular disease).

E. Tricuspid valve disease

1. Symptoms due to low cardiac output, edema, and hepatomegaly are prominent findings in patients with either or both TS or TR.

2. Physical examination

   a. In TS, tall sharp *a* waves are present in the jugular venous pulse.

   b. In TR, there is jugular venous distention with prominent *y* descent.

3. Electrocardiogram

   a. In TS, there is right atrial enlargement or atrial fibrillation.

   b. In TR, incomplete right bundle branch block and atrial fibrillation are common.

4. Echocardiography

a. In TS, there is diastolic doming of leaflets.

b. In TR, echocardiography demonstrates the cause of TR (e.g., tricuspid annular dilatation, RV dilatation, tricuspid valvular prolapse, or Ebstein's anomaly).

5. Pulmonary artery (PA) catheterization

   a. Useful for determining if pulmonary hypertension is the cause of the TR

   b. Thermodilution cardiac output measurements may be artifactually decreased or increased; accordingly, this method should not be used to monitor cardiac output in patients with TR.

F. Pulmonic regurgitation

   1. Physical examination

      a. Hyperdynamic right ventricle

      b. When PA pressure exceeds 60 mm Hg, the regurgitant jet causes a Graham-Steel murmur.

   2. Electrocardiography, echocardiography, and chest x-ray all reveal evidence of RV enlargement and possibly PA enlargement.

Key Diagnosis

- Auscultation remains the most widely used method for assessing cardiac murmurs and possible heart valve disease.

- Echocardiography should be employed to evaluate murmurs unless the murmur is low-grade (<III/VI) and mid-systolic in nature.

Treatment

A. Aortic stenosis

   1. Indications for aortic valve replacement

      a. Onset of symptoms related to severe AS (angina, dyspnea, CHF, or syncope)

      b. Moderate AS (mean pressure gradient ≥30 to 50 mm Hg) in a patient undergoing coronary artery bypass surgery

      c. Absence of symptoms but presence of severe AS with progressive LV systolic dysfunction or abnormal response to exercise (e.g., hypotension)

   2. Medical management

      a. Medical management and follow-up are indicated for asymptomatic patients irrespective of severity of AS as graded by echocardiography (except as noted above).

      b. Frequency of follow-up examinations and echocardiography should depend on the severity of AS and on the presence of comorbid conditions.

      c. Follow-up is generally yearly for mild AS and more frequent for moderate or severe AS.

      d. Balloon valvuloplasty may be used as a "bridge" to surgery in moribund patients, or in patients with symptomatic AS who are deemed to not be surgical candidates, or in patients with severe AS who require urgent noncardiac surgery.

      e. With balloon valvuloplasty, the restenosis rate at 6 months is 50%.

   3. Choice of replacement valve (in general)

      a. Stented bioprosthetic valves should be used for patients older than 75 years of age or those older than 65 to 70 years of age who have coronary artery disease (CAD) or those who cannot undergo long-term anticoagulation (Table 28–1).

      b. Mechanical valves should used for all other patients, except as noted below.

      c. Ross procedure (use is controversial)

         (1) Replacement of the aortic valve with the patient's native pulmonic valve and use of a homograft for pulmonic valve replacement

         (2) Used in young patients; 3 months of anticoagulation

      d. Indications for stentless bioprosthetic valves are controversial and evolving.

TABLE 28–1. RECOMMENDED INTERNATIONAL NORMALIZED RATIO (INR) RANGES FOR WARFARIN ANTICOAGULATION IN PATIENTS WITH PROSTHETIC HEART VALVES

PATIENT CHARACTERISTICS	INR RANGE
Mechanical prosthetic valves	
Bileaflet valve in aortic position, normal left atrial size, normal sinus rhythm, normal ejection fraction	2.0 to 3.0
Tilting disk or bileaflet valve in mitral position	2.5 to 3.5
Bileaflet aortic valve and atrial fibrillation	2.5 to 3.5
Caged ball or caged disk	2.5 to 3.5 (and aspirin, 80 mg/day)
Bioprosthetic heart valves	
Mitral or aortic position, normal sinus rhythm	2.0 to 3.0 for 3 months after surgery
Atrial fibrillation	2.0 to 3.0
Permanent pacemaker	2.0 to 3.0 (optional)
History of systemic embolism	2.0 to 3.0 for 3 to 12 months
Left atrial thrombus	2.0 to 3.0 for lifetime

B. Aortic regurgitation

1. Acute AR

   a. Early surgical intervention

   b. Use of intra-aortic balloon counterpulsation is absolutely contraindicated.

2. Chronic AR

   a. Indications for aortic valve replacement (AVR)

      (1) Generally indicated in patients with severe AR as assessed by echocardiography or cardiac catheterization

      (2) Presence of symptoms (exertional dyspnea, fatigue, orthopnea)

      (3) Mild or moderate LV dysfunction (ejection fraction 0.25 to 0.49) with or without associated symptoms

      (4) Severe LV dilatation (end-diastolic dimension >75 mm or end-systolic dimension >55 mm) with or without symptoms (even with normal LV systolic function)

      (5) Presence of angina with or without CAD

      (6) A LV ejection fraction lower than 0.25 is generally a contraindication to AVR.

   b. Medical management

      (1) Vasodilating agents, diuretics, and digitalis

      (2) Frequency of follow-up should be based on the degree of AR, degree of LV dilatation, and the LV ejection fraction.

3. Choice of replacement valve is the same as for AS.

C. Mitral stenosis

1. Medical management

   a. Digoxin is used to control ventricular rate for patients with atrial fibrillation.

   b. β-Adrenergic blockers may improve exercise tolerance, even for patients in sinus rhythm.

2. Invasive management

   a. Indications for balloon valvotomy are New York Heart Association (NYHA) functional class II to IV symptoms or pulmonary hypertension (PA systolic pressure >50 mm Hg at rest) associated with moderate or severe stenosis (<1.5 cm^2) and valve morphology favorable for balloon valvotomy.

   b. Indications for surgical repair or replacement (valve morphology not favorable for balloon valvotomy)

      (1) NYHA functional class III to IV/VI and moderate or severe MS

      (2) NYHA functional Class I to II symptoms and severe MS with severe pulmonary hypertension (PA systolic pressure >60 mm Hg)

      (3) Moderate or severe MS with thromboembolism despite adequate anticoagulation

   c. Surgical options

      (1) Closed commissurotomy (now used only in underdeveloped countries)

      (2) Open commissurotomy (during cardiopulmonary bypass); as is the case for balloon valvotomy, there is a requirement for favorable valve morphology for good outcome

      (3) Mitral valve replacement (MVR) is used when repair (open commissurotomy) is not feasible; bioprosthetic and mechanical valves are both options, but the use of bioprosthetic valves is generally contraindicated in patients with a small or normal-sized left ventricle (high risk of LV perforation due to the high profile of bioprosthetic valves).

D. Mitral regurgitation

1. Medical

   a. Afterload-reducing agents as well as digoxin and diuretics in MR patients with cardiomegaly and sinus rhythm

   b. Digoxin and anticoagulation (Table 28–1) in MR patients with atrial fibrillation

2. Surgical

   a. Acute MR following papillary muscle rupture in the setting of ischemic heart disease requires prompt placement of an intra-aortic balloon catheter for afterload reduction followed by emergent surgery.

   b. Indications for surgical intervention in patients with chronic MR

      (1) Acute severe MR

      (2) NYHA functional class at least II

      (3) Left ventricular dysfunction (ejection fraction <0.6) with or without symptoms

      (4) Left ventricular dilatation (end-diastolic dimension >45 mm) with or without symptoms

      (5) Atrial fibrillation

      (6) Pulmonary hypertension (PA systolic pressure >50 mm Hg at rest or >60 mm Hg with exercise)

   c. Surgical options

      (1) Repair of the native valve apparatus depends on the presence of favorable valve morphology and disease process.

(2) Operative mortality and long-term thromboembolism rates are lower, and LV function is better preserved with repair than with replacement.

(3) A variety of repair techniques can be employed, depending on pathology (e.g., annuloplasty rings, partial leaflet resection, chordal transposition, creation of "neochords," patch repair).

(4) Mitral valve replacement is associated with the development of LV dysfunction (independent of the type of valve used), which contributes to early and late morbidity.

(5) The patient with a prosthetic valve is also at risk for thromboembolism or hemorrhage (mechanical prosthesis), mechanical dysfunction (bioprosthesis), or infective endocarditis (any type of prosthesis).

E. Tricuspid valve disease

1. Medical management consists of dietary sodium restriction and diuretics.

2. Surgical intervention is reserved for medical therapy failures or in conjunction with surgery on another cardiac valve (typically the mitral valve).

   a. In TS, surgical correction is performed with MVR when the TV orifice is smaller than 2.0 cm² and the mean diastolic pressure gradient is greater than 5 mm Hg.

   b. In TR, surgical correction is performed only if the patient has severe pulmonary hypertension.

   c. Valve repair is frequently possible with an annuloplasty ring.

   d. Tricuspid valve replacement in severe TR is controversial and reserved for primary disease of the valve, as in Ebstein's anomaly and carcinoid syndrome.

3. Valve replacement options

   a. Bioprosthetic valves are generally preferred when TV replacement is necessary.

   b. The risk of thromboembolism or valve thrombosis was high with previous generations of mechanical valves in the TV position, but newer mechanical valves appear to have a lower incidence of complications and are being used with increasing frequency.

F. Pulmonic regurgitation

1. Surgical intervention is seldom necessary.

2. Digoxin for right heart failure symptoms

Key Prevention

Endocarditis prophylaxis is recommended for the following conditions:

- Most congenital heart malformations

- Acquired valvular dysfunction

- Previous bacterial endocarditis

- All prosthetic heart valves

- Surgically constructed systemic-pulmonary shunts

- Mitral valve prolapse with mitral regurgitation or thickened leaflet(s)

 Bibliography

Christ G, Zehetgruber M, Mundigler, et al. Emergency aortic valve replacement for critical aortic stenosis. A life-saving treatment for patients with cardiogenic shock and multiple organ failure. Intensive Care Med 1997;23:297–300.

Heerdt PM, Blessios GA, Beach ML, et al. Flow dependency of error in thermodilution measurement of cardiac output during acute tricuspid regurgitation. J Cardiothorac Vasc Anesth 2001;15:183–187.

Lin JC, Ott RA. Acute traumatic mitral valve insufficiency. J Trauma 1999;47:165–168.

Stouffer GA, Uretsky BF. Hemodynamic changes of aortic regurgitation. Am J Med Sci 1997;314:411–414.

Tiede DJ, Nishimura RA, Gastineau DA, et al. Modern management of prosthetic valve anticoagulation. Mayo Clin Proc 1998;73:665–680.

29 Pericarditis

Steven J. Lavine

Etiology

A. Idiopathic (most common)

B. Uremic

C. Neoplastic

D. Drug induced: procainamide, hydralazine, minoxidil

E. Post-myocardial infarction (MI)

F. Post-pericardiotomy

G. Infection: viral, bacterial, tuberculous, fungal

H. Connective tissue disorders: systemic lupus erythematosus (SLE), scleroderma, rheumatoid arthritis

I. Myxedema

J. Trauma

K. Radiation

Symptoms

A. Acute pericarditis
  1. Chest pain
     a. Central pain or discomfort (worsens with recumbency)
     b. Pleuritic pain
     c. Angina-like pain
  2. Constitutional symptoms (e.g., fever, malaise)
  3. Symptoms attributable to the etiology of pericarditis

B. Pericardial effusion
  1. May be asymptomatic
  2. Hoarseness, dysphagia, dyspnea (if the effusion is large enough to compress adjacent structures)
  3. Symptoms attributable to the etiology of the pericardial effusion

C. Pericardial tamponade (see Chapter 30, Pericardial Tamponade)

Physical Findings

A. Pericardial friction rub
  1. May be present with or without accompanying effusion or tamponade
  2. Three-component rub is most common (systolic, early diastolic, and late systolic component); with tachycardia, only two components may be heard (one systolic and one diastolic).
  3. Can be evanescent

B. Distant heart sounds (if significant pericardial effusion or tamponade)

C. Bronchial breath sounds at left lower scapula (compressive effect on the left lower lobe)

D. Ascites and leg edema may occur with neck vein distention if the compressive effect of the effusion is chronic or if there is constrictive pericarditis.

E. Pericardial knock (constrictive pericarditis)

F. Atrial fibrillation (constrictive pericarditis)

G. Pulsus paradoxus
  1. May be present with significant pericardial effusions, especially with tamponade
  2. Can be absent with aortic regurgitation, atrial septal defect, severe left ventricular dysfunction and heart failure, hypotension
  3. Difficult to evaluate in atrial fibrillation

H. See Chapter 30, Pericardial Tamponade, for other findings seen in tamponade.

Key Physical Findings

- Pericardial friction rub
- Pulsus paradoxus
- Ascites and leg edema (effusion or constriction)
- Pericardial knock
- Distant heart sounds (pericardial effusion)
- Hypotension (tamponade)

Differential Diagnosis

A. Myocarditis

B. Acute MI or ischemia

C. Valvular heart disease (tricuspid regurgitation) or ventricular septal defect

D. Congestive heart failure (ischemic and nonischemic cardiomyopathy)

E. Restrictive cardiomyopathy (constrictive pericarditis)

Laboratory Tests

A. Blood tests
  1. Cardiac markers (normal unless myocarditis or acute MI)
  2. White blood cell count (elevated in infectious etiologies)

3. Elevated sedimentation rate and acute phase reactants

4. Serum biochemical abnormalities (e.g., urea nitrogen, creatinine, and electrolyte concentrations; thyroid function tests; antinuclear antibodies); findings vary with etiology

B. Pericardial fluid analysis

1. Cytology to detect neoplasm

2. Biochemical tests: glucose and protein concentration

3. Microbiological stains and cultures

4. Serologic (viral) tests

Imaging Tests

A. Chest x-ray

1. Increased size of the cardiac silhouette (if pericardial fluid volume exceeds 250 mL)

2. "Water bottle" appearance of the heart (pericardial effusion; see Figure 30–2)

3. Clear lung fields

4. Pleural effusion

5. Irregular cardiac silhouette (constrictive pericarditis)

6. Pericardial calcification, by fluoroscopy (constrictive pericarditis)

B. Echocardiography

1. Pericardial effusion

2. Loculation behind the right atrium (postoperatively)

3. Swinging of the heart

4. Signs of hemodynamic compromise or tamponade

   a. Right atrial invagination during more than 33% of the cardiac cycle (late diastole through early ventricular systole)

   b. Right ventricular early-diastolic collapse that does not reexpand until late diastole

   c. Both right atrial and right ventricular findings may be ameliorated with tricuspid regurgitation, right ventricular hypertrophy, or pulmonary hypertension.

   d. Respiratory variations of transmitral flow (>25% change in the E wave), transtricuspid flow (>50% change in the E wave), and transaortic flow (>25% change in the peak velocity or time velocity integral) by pulsed Doppler ultrasound

   e. Increase in right ventricular size with inspiration with corresponding decrease in left ventricular size on M-Mode echocardiogram

5. Signs suggesting constriction

   a. Pericardial thickening or calcification

   b. Fibrous strands in the pericardial fluid connecting visceral and parietal pericardium

   c. Restrictive filling pattern on transmitral Doppler ultrasound with respiratory variations of transmitral flow above 25%, transtricuspid flow above 50%, or transaortic flow above 25%

   d. Rapid expansion of LV cavity on M-mode echocardiogram and flattening of the posterior wall late in diastole

   e. Septal bounce on M-mode echocardiogram

   f. LV walls are not speckled and atrial septum is of normal thickness.

C. Computed tomography or magnetic resonance imaging

1. Thickened or calcified pericardium (constrictive pericarditis)

2. Pericardial effusion

D. Cardiac catheterization

1. Pericardial tamponade (see Chapter 30, Pericardial Tamponade)

2. Constrictive pericarditis

   a. Equalization of right- and left-sided intracardiac pressures

   b. RV systolic pressures lower than 50 mm Hg

   c. Dip and plateau pattern on the LV pressure tracing

   d. Prominent x and y descents of the right atrial tracing

   e. Increased distance between the catheter against the right atrial wall and the edge of the cardiac silhouette on fluoroscopy

Key Tests

Electrocardiogram (see Figure 29–1)	Echocardiogram (see Figure 29–2)
• Diffuse, concave ST segment elevation	• Pericardial effusion
• PR segment depression	• Right atrial invagination (tamponade)
• Low voltage (pericardial effusion)	• Diastolic RV collapse (tamponade)
• Electrical alternans	• Respiratory variations of transmitral pulsed Doppler ultrasound greater than 25% (tamponade)

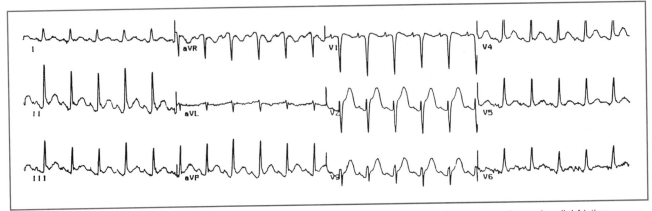

Figure 29–1 A 12-lead ECG from a patient with acute pericarditis manifested by chest pain and a pericardial friction rub. There is diffuse ST segment elevation (primarily J point elevation), and PR segment depression best seen in lead II.

Monitoring

A. Once the presence of an effusion is established, follow-up Doppler echocardiography is necessary.

B. Frequency of follow-up depends on the likelihood or extent of hemodynamic compromise.

C. Finding significant respiratory variation of Doppler velocities across the cardiac valves necessitates repeating the study daily, along with consideration for pericardiocentesis.

  1. Variations approaching or higher than 25% for left-sided valves

  2. Variations approaching or higher than 50% for the tricuspid valve

D. Following pericardiocentesis, daily and then weekly follow-up echocardiographic studies are needed until the effusion either disappears, is small, or becomes stable.

Treatment

A. Nonsteroidal anti-inflammatory drugs (NSAIDs)

  1. Aspirin 900 mg every 6 hours PO, or

  2. Indomethacin 25 mg every 6 hours PO

  3. Some NSAIDs other than aspirin may cause thinning of myocardial scars if the pericarditis is from recent MI.

B. Treatment of the underlying cause of pericardial disease (e.g., thyroid hormone replacement for hypothyroidism, corticosteroids for SLE)

C. Pericardiocentesis: may be diagnostic and therapeutic (see Chapter 196, Pericardiocentesis)

D. Pericardial resection

  1. Pericardial window

    a. Surgically created from the subxiphoid approach

    b. Performed to obtain fluid and tissue for evaluation

    c. Obliteration of the pericardial space may occur.

    d. Drainage needs to be established either to the pleural or intraperitoneal cavities, otherwise fluid will continue to accumulate.

  2. Larger areas of the pericardium can be resected; useful if pericardial constriction is present.

  3. Pericardiectomy

    a. Usually reserved for the treatment of constrictive pericarditis

    b. Removal of both the visceral pericardium and the parietal pericardium is necessary.

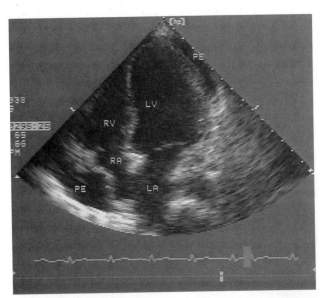

Figure 29–2 Apical 4-chamber view of 2-dimensional echocardiogram showing pericardial fluid (PE), with evidence of right atrial (RA) invagination (*arrowheads*). RV = right ventricle, LV = left ventricle, LA = left atrium.

c. This is an extensive procedure with significant blood loss, morbidity, and mortality.

Key Treatment

- NSAIDs for chest pain
- Treat the underlying cause
- Assess need for pericardiocentesis
- Assess need for pericardial resection

Complications

A. Complications of pericardiocentesis (see Chapter 196, Pericardiocentesis)

B. Complications of NSAIDs: e.g., renal dysfunction, gastric bleeding, intrapericardial bleeding

C. Postoperative complications following pericardial resection

1. Atelectasis
2. Pneumonia
3. Atrial and ventricular dysrhythmias
4. Postoperative MI

Prognosis

A. Acute pericarditis: prognosis depends on etiology

1. Idiopathic: excellent prognosis, unless recurrent pericardial effusions
2. Uremic: may require pericardial window or resection

3. Other underlying etiologies may determine the prognosis (e.g., SLE, scleroderma, etc.)

B. Pericardial effusion: prognosis depends on etiology

1. Idiopathic: excellent prognosis
2. If uremic, then a pericardial window or resection may be required.
3. If neoplastic, prognosis depends on the disease progression, which is extensive in most cases; prognosis is likely poor.
4. For other etiologies, prognosis depends on the course of the disease (e.g., SLE).

C. Pericardial tamponade

1. Relief of tamponade usually resolves the emergency.
2. The etiology of the pericardial effusion then determines the prognosis.

D. Constrictive pericarditis: prognosis generally good if pericardial resection normalizes hemodynamics

Bibliography

Lavine SJ. Right-sided heart and pericardial disease. In: Carlson RW, Geheb MA (eds). Principles and Practice of Medical Intensive Care. Philadelphia: WB Saunders, 1993, pp 1025–1038.

Mehta A, Mehta C, Jain AC. Constrictive pericarditis. Clin Cardiol 1999;22:334–344.

Oh JK, Hatle LK, Seward JB, et al. Diagnostic role of Doppler echocardiography in constrictive pericarditis. J Am Coll Cardiol 1994;23:154–162.

Otto C. Pericardial disease: two-dimensional echocardiographic and Doppler findings. In: Otto C (ed). Textbook of Clinical Echocardiography. Philadelphia: WB Saunders, 1999, pp 213–228.

Sagrista-Sauleda J, Angel J, Permanyer-Miralda G, et al. Long-term follow-up of idiopathic chronic pericardial effusion. N Engl J Med 1999;341:2054–2059.

30 Pericardial Tamponade

Vivian L. Clark

Pericardial tamponade is a state of reduced cardiac output and inadequate organ perfusion secondary to accumulation of fluid in the pericardial sac. The size of an effusion required to cause tamponade is dependent on the rapidity with which the effusion develops.

Etiology

A. Acute pericarditis, particularly of infectious or malignant origin, is the most common cause of pericardial tamponade.
B. Proximal aortic dissection with extension into the pericardial space; this is a frequent cause of death among patients with dissection.
C. Blunt or penetrating chest trauma
D. Iatrogenic: post-pericardiotomy or associated with catheter insertion
E. Myocardial free wall rupture after acute myocardial infarction (MI)

Clinical Findings

A. Chest discomfort and shortness of breath, usually improved by assuming an upright position
B. Hypotension: systolic blood pressure 90 mm Hg or lower, or requiring vasopressors to maintain 90 mm Hg or higher
C. Tachycardia; generally sinus, although atrial fibrillation or flutter can occur
D. Pulsus paradoxus of 10 mm Hg or more
E. Quiet precordium; muffled heart sounds
F. Jugular venous distention
G. Absence of pulmonary congestion
H. Pericardial friction rub
I. Dullness to percussion below the left scapula (Ewart's sign)

J. Evidence of inadequate organ perfusion: decreased urine output, cool clammy skin, abnormal mental status
K. Tamponade occurring in the setting of ventricular free wall rupture often presents as cardiac arrest with pulseless electrical activity.

Hemodynamic Findings

A. Elevation and equalization of diastolic cardiac filling pressures (Fig. 30–1)
B. Narrowed right- and left-sided pulse pressures
C. Pulsus paradoxus
D. Reduced cardiac index

 Key Findings

- Hypotension with pulsus paradoxus and neck vein distention
- Enlarged cardiac silhouette without pulmonary congestion on chest x-ray
- Echocardiographic evidence of a large pericardial effusion, plus right atrial and right ventricular free wall collapse during diastole

Differential Diagnosis

A. Dilated cardiomyopathy with shock can present with similar findings, but pulmonary congestion is usually present; it is readily distinguished by echocardiography.
B. Pericardial constriction has similar physical and hemodynamic findings, but the course is usually more insidious; echocardiography shows a thickened pericardium.

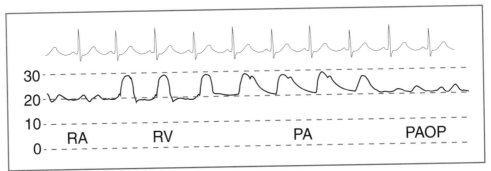

Figure 30–1 Pressure sweep during right heart catheterization showing equalization of diastolic pressures.

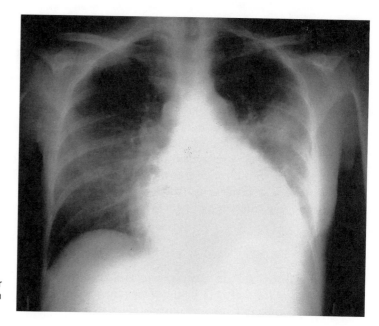

Figure 30–2 Chest radiograph showing enlarged, globular cardiac silhouette ("water-bottle heart") in a patient with tamponade due to a malignant effusion.

C. Right ventricular MI may have similar physical and hemodynamic findings; symptoms, electrocardiographic evidence of infarction, and elevated cardiac serum markers are distinguishing features.

Laboratory and Other Tests

A. Electrocardiogram: sinus tachycardia, low voltage, electrical alternans, diffuse ST segment elevation, and PR segment depression

Key Treatment

- Intravenous fluids, vasopressors, and inotropic agents: may be used temporarily to increase blood pressure and perfusion

- Pericardiocentesis: performed under echocardiographic or electrocardiographic guidance (removal of as little as 50 mL of fluid can result in dramatic hemodynamic improvement)

- Surgical pericardiotomy: preferred approach for treating bacterial or malignant effusions and those due to perforation

B. Chest x-ray: enlarged, globular cardiac silhouette, absence of pulmonary congestion (Fig. 30–2)

C. Echocardiogram: large pericardial effusion, right atrial and right ventricular free wall collapse (see Fig. 29–2)

D. Laboratory tests: none are specific for pericardial tamponade, but laboratory abnormalities may point to the underlying etiology of the effusion

Bibliography

Ameli S, Shah PK. Cardiac tamponade: pathophysiology, diagnosis and management. Cardiol Clin 1991;9:665–674.

Chong HH, Plotnick GD. Pericardial effusion and tamponade: evaluation, imaging modalities, and management. Compr Ther 1995;21:378–385.

Larose E, Ducharme A, Mercier LA, et al. Prolonged distress and clinical deterioration before pericardial drainage in patients with cardiac tamponade. Can J Cardiol 2000;16:331–336.

Merce J, Sagrista-Sauleda J, Permanyer-Miralda G, et al. Correlation between clinical and Doppler echocardiographic findings in patients with moderate and large pericardial effusion: implications for the diagnosis of cardiac tamponade. Am Heart J 1999;138:759–764.

Spodick DH. Pathophysiology of cardiac tamponade. Chest 1998;113:1372–1378.

Tsang TS, Oh JK, Seward JB. Diagnosis and management of cardiac tamponade in the era of echocardiography. Clin Cardiol 1999;22:446–452.

31 Aortic Dissection

Vivian L. Clark
James A. Kruse

Aortic dissection results from a tear in the intimal layer of the aorta, and it leads to communication of the true aortic lumen with an intramural false lumen containing either thrombus or free-flowing blood. The clinical course is dependent on the site at which the tear originates and the affected tributaries.

Classification

A. Type A: proximal dissections originating in the ascending aorta that may be limited to the ascending aorta and arch or extend around the aortic arch and involve the descending aorta (Fig. 31–1). This category includes both type I and type II dissections of the older DeBakey classification.

B. Type B: distal aortic dissections originating distal to the left subclavian artery and potentially extending throughout the descending aorta (Fig. 31–1). This type is equivalent to type III of the DeBakey classification.

Key Etiologies and Clinical Associations

- Hypertension

- Trauma; primarily blunt chest trauma

- Pregnancy

- Syphilitic aortitis

- Connective tissue disease with cystic medial necrosis; particularly related to Marfan's syndrome

Clinical Findings

A. Chest and back pain: often described as tearing in character; asymptomatic dissections are possible

B. Pain is usually most severe at its onset.

C. Hypertension is common at presentation.

D. Pulse deficits or differences in arterial blood pressure between extremities

E. Neurologic deficits secondary to carotid, innominate, vertebral, or spinal cord artery involvement

F. Aortic insufficiency: can occur in proximal dissections involving the aortic root

G. Acute myocardial infarction (MI): can occur in proximal dissections involving a coronary artery ostium

H. Circulatory shock: can occur secondary to hemorrhage, pericardial tamponade, or acute MI

Diagnostic Testing

A. Electrocardiography
   1. There are no diagnostic electrocardiographic findings.
   2. Sinus tachycardia and left ventricular hypertrophy are often seen.
   3. Findings of acute MI may be seen if a coronary artery is affected.

B. Chest x-ray
   1. Widening of the mediastinum is often seen in proximal dissections.
   2. Separation of intimal calcification in the aortic knob from the adventitial border may be present.
   3. Hemothorax can occur.

C. Echocardiography
   1. Transesophageal echocardiography
      a. Has a high sensitivity for detecting proximal dissection
      b. May show aortic root dilation
      c. A linear shadow (intimal flap) dividing the true and false lumens may be seen.
   2. Transthoracic echocardiography
      a. Useful for identifying complications of dissection such as aortic insufficiency or pericardial tamponade
      b. May reveal an intimal flap in proximal dissections originating in the aortic root

D. Computed tomography
   1. Has a high sensitivity and specificity
   2. Usually the initial diagnostic study of choice because of its widespread availability

E. Magnetic resonance imaging
   1. High sensitivity and specificity
   2. Use is hampered by limited availability and difficulty in monitoring unstable patients.

F. Aortic angiography
   1. Considered the gold standard
   2. Invasive and may not be rapidly available

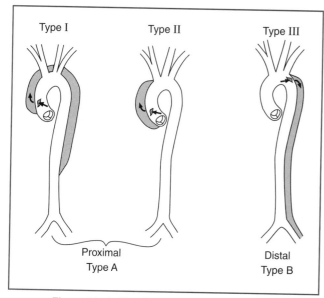

Figure 31–1 Classification of aortic dissections.

Treatment

A. Medical therapy should be initiated when type A or B aortic dissection is suspected, even before the definitive diagnosis is made. The goals of therapy are to reduce mean aortic pressure (MAP) to 60 to 75 mm Hg and reduce aortic shear forces.

1. Sodium nitroprusside should be initiated at 0.5 μg/min and titrated to the targeted MAP; this agent should always be combined with a β-blocker.

2. β-adrenergic blocking agents

   a. Propranolol

      (1) Used in combination with nitroprusside

      (2) Loading dose is given by IV injection; e.g., 0.5 to 1.0 mg every 5 minutes (up to 3 mg) to achieve the desired degree of blockade, which may be judged by effect on heart rate.

      (3) Follow by IV maintenance doses (e.g., 1 mg every 4 hours) or oral maintenance doses (typically 20 to 80 mg every 6 hours).

   b. Esmolol

      (1) Can be used as an alternative to propranolol

      (2) Used in conjunction with nitroprusside

      (3) Loading dose is 1 mg/kg followed by an infusion ranging from 150 to 300 μg/kg per minute to achieve desired MAP.

   c. Labetolol

      (1) Load with 20 mg intravenously over 2 minutes (and may repeat).

      (2) Follow with a continuous infusion of 0.5 to 2 mg/minute.

      (3) Because labetolol possesses α-adrenergic antagonist effects, it has been used without nitroprusside.

3. Trimethaphan

   a. A ganglionic blocking agent

   b. Initiated at 1.0 mg/minute

   c. Can be used alone in lieu of the nitroprusside/β-blocker combination

   d. Patient should be placed in a reverse Trendelenburg position.

   e. Risk of significant autonomic side effects (e.g., urinary retention)

B. Type A dissections: emergency surgery is the treatment of choice

C. Type B dissections: treated conservatively with chronic antihypertensive therapy unless one of the following conditions is present

1. Progression of the dissection

2. Compromise of an extremity or vital organ

3. Rupture or impending rupture

4. Marfan's syndrome

5. Retrograde extension to the ascending aorta

Key Treatment

- Initiate medical therapy while obtaining diagnostic tests.

- Combine nitroprusside with a β-blocker to reduce MAP and decrease aortic shear stress.

- Urgent surgery is the treatment of choice for type A dissections.

 Bibliography

Coady MA, Rizzo JA, Goldstein LJ, et al. Natural history, pathogenesis, and etiology of thoracic aortic aneurysms and dissections. Cardiol Clin 1999;17:615–635.

David TE, Armstrong S, Ivanov J, et al. Surgery for type A aortic dissections. Ann Thorac Surg 1999;67:1999–2001.

Elefteriades JA, Lovoulos CJ, Coady MA, et al. Management of descending aortic dissection. Ann Thorac Surg 1999;67:2002–2005.

Hagen PG, Nenaber CA, Isselbacher EM, et al. The international registry of acute aortic dissection: new insights into an old disease. JAMA 2000;283:897–903.

Sebastia C, Pallisa E, Quioga S, et al. Aortic dissections: diagnosis and follow-up with helical CT. Radiographics 1999;19:45–60.

Von Kodolitsch Y, Schwartz AG, Nienaber CA. Clinical prediction of acute aortic dissection. Arch Intern Med 2000;160:2977–2982.

32 Atrial Fibrillation and Flutter
Arthur J. Boujoukos

Atrial fibrillation and flutter are among the most common dysrhythmias in patients with cardiorespiratory disease. In the critically ill patient, new-onset atrial fibrillation generally reflects a combination of cardiorespiratory disease plus adrenergic stress. In postcardiotomy patients, new-onset atrial fibrillation is so common (30% to 40%) that looking for secondary etiologies is not required. In thoracotomy, major vascular and abdominal surgery patients, excluding perioperative myocardial ischemia and pulmonary emboli should be considered.

Key Etiologies

- Myocardial ischemia
- Cardiomyopathy
- Pericarditis
- Tricuspid valve disease
- Mitral valve disease
- Hyperthyroidism
- Postcardiotomy
- Respiratory failure
- Chronic obstructive lung disease
- Pulmonary embolism

Diagnosis

A. Symptoms
  1. Palpitations
  2. Dyspnea
  3. Lightheadedness
B. Signs
  1. Atrial fibrillation
    a. Irregular pulse
    b. Usually tachycardic
    c. Variable intensity of the first heart sound
  2. Atrial flutter
    a. Pulse is regular, but tachycardic (usually 145 to 155 beats/min).
    b. Flutter waves may be evident in the jugular venous pulse.
C. Electrocardiogram (ECG)
  1. Atrial fibrillation
    a. Fibrillatory waves are often seen preceding the QRS complex.
    b. Baseline may appear flat.
    c. Ventricular response is irregularly irregular, with rates ranging up to as high as 200 beats/minute.

d. High ventricular rates can make the RR intervals appear regular, thereby making recognition more difficult.
    e. The ventricular response may be as low as low as 40 beats/minute if the atrioventricular (A-V) node is affected by drugs or disease.
    f. A regular rhythm or regular grouped beating in the absence of discernible P waves may reflect atrial fibrillation with A-V block (e.g., digoxin toxicity).
  2. Atrial flutter
    a. Saw-toothed flutter waves, usually best seen in inferior leads
    b. Atrial rate is usually between 250 to 350 beats/minute, most commonly approximately 300 beats/minute.
    c. Atrioventricular conduction is usually 2:1 or 4:1, but may be a higher ratio (i.e., 8:1); odd ratios, such as 3:1, are rare.
D. Carotid sinus massage
  1. May be a useful maneuver in rare cases to distinguish re-entrant supraventricular tachycardia (SVT) from atrial fibrillation or atrial flutter when the ECG reveals a regular narrow-complex tachycardia with difficult-to-discern P waves
  2. May block A-V conduction and terminate re-entrant SVT
  3. May unmask flutter waves by slowing AV conduction
E. Adenosine
  1. Pharmacological equivalent of carotid sinus massage
  2. Use of adenosine should be reserved for those rare cases where re-entrant SVT is strongly suspected but sequential carotid sinus massage fails to block the A-V node, or where carotid sinus massage is contraindicated.
  3. Administration of adenosine to a patient with atrial fibrillation results in fibrillatory waves or a (transiently) flat-line ECG tracing with recurrence of atrial fibrillation after a short interval.
F. If atrial epicardial pacemaker wires are in place after cardiotomy, these leads can be connected to an ECG V-lead for diagnosis and monitoring of atrial flutter.

Treatment

A. All patients

1. Minimize adrenergic stress.

   a. Provide mechanical ventilatory support if work of breathing is excessive.

   b. Provide adequate pain control.

2. If there is evidence of low cardiac output (cool, clammy, mottled extremities, hypotension) or angina, proceed with synchronized cardioversion, beginning with 100 joules.

3. Atrial fibrillation or flutter associated with critical illness will likely recur as long as the patient remains critically ill; maintenance therapy should be instituted.

4. Optimize the metabolic milieu (e.g., administer magnesium sulfate and correct hypokalemia).

B. Atrial fibrillation

1. Rate control should be achieved first, if the patient is hemodynamically stable; goal should be <120 beats/minute.

   a. If possible, reduce the rate of catecholamine infusions (epinephrine, dobutamine, dopamine).

   b. Institute therapy with a β-adrenergic antagonist, a calcium channel antagonist, or digoxin; β-blockade alone may lead to conversion to normal sinus rhythm (NSR).

      (1) Metoprolol: 5 mg intravenously every 5 minutes

      (2) Esmolol: IV loading dose of 500 μg/kg over 1 minute, then 50 μg/kg per minute by continuous infusion; may administer a second bolus as above and increase infusion rate by 50 μg/kg per minute every 5 minutes up to 400 μg/kg per minute

      (3) Diltiazem: 5 to 10 mg IV boluses; infusion at 5 to 20 mg/hour

      (4) Verapamil: 5 to 10 mg IV boluses; plus $CaCl_2$ 1 g slowly over 8 minutes to prevent development of hypotension

      (5) Digoxin: 0.5 mg IV, then 0.25 mg IV 4 hours and 8 hours later, if the patient has not been on digoxin previously and has normal renal function

2. The ultimate goal is conversion to NSR unless the patient has a history of chronic atrial fibrillation.

   a. Chemical cardioversion should be attempted once the ventricular rate is <120 beats/minute after one of the therapeutic interventions above.

   b. If the patient does not have chronic lung disease, then the agent of choice is amiodarone.

      (1) Oral regimen: 600 to 800 mg orally every 8 hours for 4 days, then 200 mg orally daily (stop digoxin, because bradycardia can occur)

      (2) Intravenous regimen (significantly more expensive): 150 mg over 10 minutes, then 1 mg/minute for 6 hours, then 0.5 mg/minute

   c. If left ventricular function is good and there is no evidence of active bronchospasm, then sotalol is an acceptable alternative to amiodarone.

      (1) Standard dose is 80 mg orally every 12 hours.

      (2) Dose should decreased for renal dysfunction or bradycardia.

      (3) Monitor the QTc interval; if higher than 500 msec, hold the next dose of the drug and reduce the dosage thereafter.

   d. Second-line drugs for pharmacological cardioversion of atrial fibrillation

      (1) Procainamide

         (a) Loading dose: 1000 mg intravenously over 1 hour

         (b) Maintenance dose: 12.5 mg/kg orally every 6 hours using the sustained-release formulation of procainamide (Procan SR)

         (c) Decrease maintenance dose if renal function is impaired.

         (d) If QTc interval is less than 500 msec in 24 hours and fibrillation persists, give an additional 500 mg over 30 minutes and increase maintenance dose by 250 mg orally every 6 hours.

         (e) Heart rate must be controlled prior to loading with procainamide, since A-V conduction, and hence ventricular rate, may otherwise increase.

      (2) Ibutelide

         (a) 1 mg over 10 minutes; may repeat once

         (b) 0.01 mg/kg for patients weighing less than 60 kg

         (c) Drawbacks associated with this agent are a 4% incidence of ventricular tachycardia and the lack of an available oral formulation.

3. Synchronized cardioversion

a. Indications

(1) Hemodynamic instability

(2) Failure to respond to pharmacological approaches for 48 hours

b. Start with 100 joules.

c. Paroxysmal atrial fibrillation should be cardioverted only after augmenting antidysrhythmic drug levels or suppressing sympathetic stimulation.

C. Atrial flutter

1. Compared to atrial fibrillation, it is more difficult to achieve ventricular rate control but easier to convert to NSR.

2. Synchronized cardioversion may be tried starting at 50 joules using appropriate short-acting conscious sedation (e.g., methohexitol).

3. If the patient converts to atrial fibrillation, try to convert as above, starting with 100 joules.

4. If the resulting rhythm is still atrial fibrillation, achieve ventricular rate control and use pharmacological agents as described above to convert to NSR.

5. For cases of refractory or recurrent atrial flutter, achieve ventricular rate control with metoprolol, esmolol, diltiazem, or verapamil as above.

6. In atrial flutter, therapy with digoxin may produce toxicity before ventricular rate control of flutter.

7. Once ventricular rate is controlled, institute therapy with amiodarone, sotalol, procainamide as above.

8. If patient remains in flutter at 48 to 72 hours, reattempt synchronized cardioversion after loading with an antidysrhythmic drug.

9. If atrial pacing leads are present, such as after cardiac surgery, consider rapid atrial pacing to convert to NSR.

10. If, despite the above, there still is failure to convert to NSR, electrophysiologic evaluation should be requested for consideration for radiofrequency ablation.

Key Treatment

- Seek to ameliorate excessive sympathetic stimulation by correcting the underlying causes.

- Obtain ventricular rate control prior to attempting pharmacological or electrical cardioversion unless there is hemodynamic instability, evidence of low cardiac output, or angina.

- Attempt pharmacological cardioversion early.

- Consider synchronized cardioversion if attempts at pharmacological conversion to NSR are still unsuccessful with 48 hours of therapy; otherwise, anticoagulation with heparin should be instituted.

Bibliography

Kowey PR, Marinchak RA, Rials SJ, et al. Acute treatment of strial fibrillation. Am J Cardiol 1998;81(5A):16C–22C.

Pritchell EL. Management of atrial fibrillation. N Engl J Med 1992;326:1264–1271.

Reiffel JA. Selecting an antiarrythmic agent for atrial fibrillation should be a patient-specific, data-driven decision. Am J Cardiol 1998;81:72N–81N.

33 Supraventricular Tachycardia

Marc D. Meissner
Randy A. Lieberman

Supraventricular tachycardia (SVT) may be defined as tachycardia (rate >100 beats/minute) in which the origin is not in the ventricle (i.e., not ventricular tachycardia or ventricular fibrillation). This definition includes atrial fibrillation and flutter (discussed in Chapter 32, Atrial Fibrillation and Flutter) and sinus tachycardia. SVT most commonly originates from atrial tissue or the atrioventricular (AV) junction and may or may not require the AV junction to sustain the dysrhythmia. Supraventricular tachycardias that require the AV node to sustain the dysrhythmia are generally responsive to adenosine. Supraventricular tachycardias other than sinus tachycardia are usually abrupt in onset and termination, and they usually have a regular P-P interval (exceptions are multifocal atrial tachycardia and atrial fibrillation).

Classification

A. Sinus tachycardia

   1. Atrial rate: ≥100 beats/minute

   2. Not adenosine sensitive (i.e., not AV node dependent)

   3. P waves on 12-lead electrocardiogram (ECG) are identical to those of baseline sinus rhythm.

   4. May be seen with exercise, fever, thyrotoxicosis, heightened sympathetic states

B. Unifocal atrial tachycardia

   1. Approximate atrial rate: 120 to 220 beats/minute

   2. Most cases are not adenosine sensitive (i.e., not AV node dependent).

   3. Approximately 10% are adenosine responsive

C. Multifocal atrial tachycardia (MAT)

   1. Approximate atrial rate: 100 to 220 beats/minute

   2. Not adenosine sensitive (i.e., not AV node dependent)

   3. Multiple (≥3) different P wave morphologies present

   4. Common associations

      a. Hypoxemia (e.g., due to acute pulmonary or cardiac problems)

      b. Exacerbation of chronic obstructive lung disease

      c. Increased sympathetic tone

      d. Electrolyte abnormalities (e.g., hypokalemia, hypomagnesemia)

      e. Theophylline toxicity

D. Atrial fibrillation (see Chapter 32, Atrial Fibrillation and Flutter)

   1. Approximate atrial rate: 400 to 700 beats/minute

   2. Not adenosine sensitive (i.e., not AV node dependent)

E. Atrial flutter (see Chapter 32, Atrial Fibrillation and Flutter)

   1. Atrial rate: approximately 300 beats/minute

   2. Not adenosine sensitive (i.e., not AV node dependent)

F. Atrioventricular node re-entry

   1. Approximate atrial rate: 120 to 220 beats/minute

   2. Adenosine sensitive (i.e., AV node dependent)

G. Accessory pathway-related AV re-entry (e.g., Wolff-Parkinson-White syndrome)

   1. Approximate atrial rate: 140 to 230 beats/minute

   2. Adenosine sensitive (i.e., AV node dependent)

   3. Classification

      a. Narrow complex (orthodromic)

      b. Wide complex (pre-excited): see Chapter 35, Ventricular Fibrillation and Tachycardia (VF/VT)

H. Junctional tachycardia

   1. Approximate atrial rate: 70 to 130 (but may be as high as 200) beats/minute

   2. Adenosine sensitive (i.e., AV node dependent)

   3. Evaluate in context (e.g., acute myocardial infarction, post-valvular surgery, digoxin toxicity).

I. Paroxysmal atrial tachycardia with second-degree heart block

   1. Approximate atrial rate: 120 to 220 beats/minute

   2. Most cases are not adenosine sensitive (i.e., not AV node dependent).

   3. Highly suggestive of digoxin toxicity (see Chapter 67, Digoxin Overdose)

Clinical Features

A. Common underlying problem in intensive care unit (ICU) setting
   1. Hypertension
   2. Pulmonary processes (e.g., pneumonia or chronic obstructive lung disease)
   3. Postoperative state
   4. Cardiac decompensation
   5. Sepsis
B. Symptoms (can vary widely)
   1. Asymptomatic
   2. Palpitations
   3. Fluttering sensation in the chest
   4. Chest pressure
   5. Dyspnea
   6. Fatigue
   7. Dizziness or lightheadedness
   8. Syncope or near-syncope
C. Physical examination
   1. May be unremarkable, except for rapid heart rate
   2. Hemodynamic status depends on multiple factors (e.g., SVT rate, ventricular function, systemic vascular resistance).
   3. Findings suggesting AV dissociation (e.g., cannon *a* waves, variable S1, nonrespiratory variation in blood pressure)
      a. Favor VT rather than SVT
      b. Not always present in VT, and when present may be easily overlooked on physical examination

Diagnosis

A. Classification of SVT, if possible, facilitates its management, even though many of the same principles and treatments apply to different SVT types.
B. Recognize that a history of myocardial infarction or other heart disease makes VT a more likely diagnosis than SVT in wide complex tachycardias.
C. Electrocardiographic findings
   1. Invaluable for diagnosis and correct classification of SVT
   2. Make careful comparison with previous ECGs.
   3. QRS complex width may be narrow or wide.
      a. Wide QRS complex tachydysrhythmias can be due to SVT with aberrancy or pre-excitation, or can be due to VT.
      b. Distinguishing these two mechanisms can be important in optimizing management; how-

ever, a definitive distinction cannot always be made.
      c. Potentially helpful differentiating clues are shown in Table 33–1.
   4. Consider use of nonstandard leads to facilitate identification of P waves.
      a. Esophageal lead: the electrode contacts the area of the esophagus that is adjacent to the left atrium
      b. Epicardial leads (e.g., if left in place after open-heart surgery)
      c. Transvenous intracardiac electrogram
      d. CR lead: bipolar lead with negative electrode on the right arm and positive electrode on the chest as an exploring electrode
      e. Modified CL lead (MCL 1): positive electrode at V1 and negative electrode under outer third of left clavicle. The ground wire is placed under the outer third of the right clavicle. Advantages include ability to see P waves, distinguish right from left bundle branch block, and allowing mid- and left precordium free for defibrillation or cardiopulmonary resuscitation.
   5. Consider Wolff-Parkinson-White syndrome or digitalis toxicity if ECG shows multiple (beat-to-beat) "bundle branch block"-type morphologies.
D. Adenosine: diagnostic use
   1. Can induce transient AV block, thereby unmasking P waves and aiding differentiation of wide complex SVT from VT
   2. Infrequently, VT may be adenosine sensitive, and electrophysiologic studies may be necessary to differentiate VT from SVT with aberrancy.
   3. Can acutely terminate SVT, potentially consistent with SVT etiology (see above)
   4. Dosing given under Treatment section below
E. Blood tests
   1. Measure serum electrolytes, especially potassium.
   2. Consider arterial blood gas analysis.
   3. Perform digoxin assay, if toxicity is a possibility.
   4. Consider toxicologic screening if drug overdose (e.g., cyclic antidepressant) is a possibility.
F. Echocardiography to assess atrial mechanical activity and ventricular function
G. Electrophysiologic studies

TABLE 33–1. FEATURES POTENTIALLY HELPFUL IN DISTINGUISHING WIDE COMPLEX SVT FROM VT*

FEATURE	FAVORS VT	FAVORS SVT
QRS duration	≥140 msec	<140 msec (except with pre-excitation)
QRS axis	Superior (especially extreme right or left)	Normal
AV dissociation	Yes	No
Capture beats	Yes	No
Fusion beats	Yes	No
Bundle branch block pattern identical to that in sinus rhythm	No	Yes
Abrupt change in wide QRS morphology	Yes	No
More QRS complexes than P waves	Yes	No
Precordial QRS concordance	Yes	No
Precordial morphology		
Right bundle branch block pattern	V1 rS (r < S) or QS in V6	V1 triphasic; R > s in V6
Left bundle branch block pattern	V1 showing initial r wave of >30 msec, notch in downslope of S wave, and ≥70 msec interval from QRS onset to nadir of QS or S wave	V1: R amplitude in tachycardia <R amplitude in sinus rhythm
	V6: any Q wave	
RS precordial pattern	No	Yes
RS interval >100 msec in ≥1 precordial lead	Yes	No
QRS polarity in leads V4 to V6	Predominantly negative	Predominantly positive
QR complex in any lead from V2 to V6	Yes	No
History of myocardial infarction or other heart disease	Yes	No

* These are general guidelines; exceptions occur.

Key Diagnostic Points

- Ventricular tachycardia and SVT are not reliably distinguished on the basis of blood pressure, mental status, or heart rate.

- History of myocardial infarction or left ventricular dysfunction favors VT over SVT.

- Either SVT or VT can have mild variability in heart rate (i.e., R-R interval).

- When in doubt, the working diagnosis should be VT.

Treatment

A. General principles: management of ICU patients with SVT requires familiarity with current advanced cardiac life-support protocols and algorithms

B. Narrow QRS complex SVT (not relevant for sinus tachycardia)

1. If significant hemodynamic compromise, follow current advanced cardiac life-support recommendations, which generally include

   a. Assurance of an adequate airway (endotracheal intubation, if necessary)

   b. Supplemental oxygen and, if necessary, positive pressure ventilation

   c. Cardiopulmonary resuscitation, if necessary

   d. Vascular access

   e. Electrical cardioversion, following sedation, if and as appropriate

2. If no significant hemodynamic compromise

   a. Attempt vagal maneuvers

      (1) Carotid sinus massage for 5 seconds, if no carotid arterial disease

      (2) Valsalva maneuver

      (3) Head-down tilt maneuver

      (4) Do not use eyeball massage.

   b. Adenosine

      (1) Give 6 mg as rapid IV bolus, followed immediately by rapid flush with normal saline.

      (2) Transient side effects may include flushing, chest tightness, asystole, ectopy.

      (3) If SVT does not terminate in 1 to 2 minutes, give 12 mg of adenosine as a rapid IV bolus.

      (4) Adenosine is less effective in the presence of theophylline.

      (5) Avoid adenosine in patients receiving dipyridamole because it can potentiate the

effect of adenosine by blocking cellular uptake.

c. Persistent SVT

(1) 18 mg dose of adenosine intravenously

(2) 0.25 mg/kg diltiazem intravenously; or, if not hypotensive, 1.5 to 5 mg verapamil intravenously

d. If SVT persists, consider the following (not mutually exclusive, but patient's heart rate, blood pressure, and clinical status must be carefully reassessed before adding any agent).

(1) Repeat diltiazem using 0.35 mg/kg intravenously; or, if not hypotensive, repeat verapamil using 5 to 10 mg intravenously.

(2) Consider β-adrenergic blocker. Dosage of calcium channel blocker should generally be reduced or the drug discontinued once β-blocker is optimized (unless heart rate is still uncontrolled).

(3) Consider digoxin.

(4) Consider membrane-active drugs (e.g., procainamide, amiodarone).

C. Wide QRS complex tachycardia

1. If significant hemodynamic compromise, follow current advanced cardiac life-support algorithm for VT treatment.

2. If no significant hemodynamic compromise

a. Adenosine: 6 mg as rapid IV bolus followed immediately by rapid IV flush with normal saline

b. If wide complex tachycardia not terminated in 1 to 2 minutes, give 12 mg adenosine as rapid IV bolus and flush IV catheter.

3. Options if dysrhythmia persists

a. Lidocaine

(1) 1 to 1.5 mg/kg IV loading dose

(2) Follow with a continuous IV infusion at 0.5 to 0.75 mg/minute, to a maximum total of 3 mg/kg. Discontinue immediately if signs of toxicity.

b. Procainamide

(1) Maximum of 15 mg/kg at 20 to 50 mg/minute until any one of the following occurs: hypotension, dysrhythmia suppression, QRS interval widening by more than 50% (watch QT interval also)

(2) Follow with a maintenance IV infusion at 1 to 4 mg/minute, if renal function is normal.

(3) Check serum procainamide and N-acetyl-procainamide levels if drug is continued.

c. Synchronous cardioversion

D. Special considerations for MAT

1. May respond to correction of hypoxemia and treatment of underlying lung disease

2. May respond to non-dihydropyridine calcium channel blocker (e.g., verapamil)

3. Avoid digitalis, antidysrhythmic agents, and β-adrenergic blockers.

E. Address any underlying disorders or exacerbating factors (e.g., electrolyte derangements, hypoxia, myocardial ischemia, hypovolemia, drug intoxication).

F. Longer-term options

1. Radiofrequency ablation

2. Implantable cardioverter-defibrillator, if VT

Key Treatment

- Provide basic and advanced cardiac life-support measures, as indicated.

- Secure IV access and give supplemental oxygen.

- Determine clinical status: cardiovert promptly if hemodynamically compromised

- When possible, obtain 12-lead ECG.

- If wide complex SVT and hemodynamically stable, try vagal maneuvers first, then adenosine, then other A-V nodal blockers, then amiodarone or procainamide (see text).

- If unable to exclude VT, adenosine may be used, but do not use calcium channel blockers.

Bibliography

DiMarco JP, Miles W, Akhtar M, et al. Adenosine for paroxysmal supraventricular tachycardia. Dose ranging and comparison with verapamil: assessment in placebo-controlled, multicenter trials. The Adenosine for PSVT Study Group. Ann Intern Med 1990;113:104–110.

Hazinski MF, Cummins RO, Field JM (eds). 2000 Handbook of Emergency Cardiovascular Care for Healthcare Providers. Dallas, TX: American Heart Association, 2000.

Meissner MD, Lessmeier TJ, Steinman RT, et al. Hemodynamically tolerated sustained ventricular tachycardia: clinical features and risk of sudden death during follow up. In: Akhtar M (ed). Sudden Cardiac Death. Baltimore: Williams and Wilkins, 1994; pp 496–512.

Miller JM, Hsia HH, Rothman SA, et al. Ventricular tachycardia versus supraventricular tachycardia with aberration: electrocardiographic distinctions. In: Zipes DP, Jalife J (eds). Cardiac Electrophysiology—From Cell to Bedside. Philadelphia: WB Saunders, 2000; pp 696–705.

Weiss J, Stevenson WG. Narrow QRS ventricular tachycardia. Am Heart J 1986;112:843–847.

Wellens HJ. The electrocardiographic diagnosis of arrhythmias, In: Topol EJ (ed). Textbook of Cardiovascular Medicine. Philadelphia: Lippincott-Raven, 1998; pp 1591–1609.

34 Pulseless Electrical Activity

Randy A. Lieberman
Marc D. Meissner
Mukarram A. Siddiqui

Definition

A. Pulseless electrical activity (PEA) is the presence of electrical cardiac activity on the surface electrocardiogram (ECG) in the absence of a detectable pulse.

B. Formerly known as electromechanical dissociation

C. Results in critical systemic hypoperfusion

D. May manifest as various surface ECG rhythms, including the following

1. Narrow complex QRS rhythm (the most common)

2. Idioventricular rhythm (including post-defibrillation idioventricular rhythms)

3. Ventricular escape rhythm

4. Bradyasystolic rhythms

Key Etiologies

- Hypovolemia
- Hypoxia
- Cardiac tamponade
- Hyperkalemia
- Acute myocardial infarction
- Tension pneumothorax
- Pulmonary embolism
- Drug overdose
- Acidosis
- Hypothermia

Clinical Findings and Tests

Clinical findings and diagnostic tests that suggest specific potential causes of PEA are given in Table 34–1.

Treatment

Familiarity with cardiopulmonary resuscitation (CPR) and advanced life-support guidelines is essential for proper management of patients with PEA. Refer to current American Heart Association guidelines for details. Key management points, in the context of specific etiologies, are summarized in Table 34–2.

Key Treatment

- Properly attach and operate ECG monitor and recognize PEA by ECG and physical examination.

- Confirm absence of pulse and initiate CPR after assuring airway and ventilation.

- Secure IV access.

- Seek and treat specific causes (see Tables 34–1 and 34–2).

- Administer IV epinephrine, atropine, and possibly bicarbonate.

- Use specific measures, where appropriate: e.g., defibrillation (for ventricular fibrillation or pulseless ventricular tachycardia), pericardiocentesis, needle decompression for pneumothorax.

Bibliography

Charlap S, Kahlan S, Lichstein E, et al. Electromechanical dissociation: diagnosis, pathophysiology and management. Am Heart J 1989;118:355–360.

Hazinski MF, Cummins RO, Field JM (eds). 2000 Handbook of Emergency Cardiovascular Care for Healthcare Providers. Dallas: American Heart Association, 2000.

Ornato JP, Peberdy MA. Cardiopulmonary resuscitation, In: Topol EJ (ed). Textbook of Cardiovascular Medicine. Philadelphia: Lippincott-Raven, 1998; pp 1779–1805.

Stueven HA, Aufderheide T, Waite EM, et al. Electromechanical dissociation: six years prehospital experience. Resuscitation 1989;17:173–182.

TABLE 34-1. DIAGNOSTIC CLUES TO POTENTIAL CAUSES OF PEA

CAUSE OF PEA	CLUES	COMMON ECG FINDINGS	DIAGNOSTIC AIDS*
Cardiac tamponade	History (e.g., thrombolytic use, indwelling right heart catheter or pacemaker wire, trauma, cancer, renal failure) Examination (e.g., venous distention, no pulse with CPR)	Sinus tachycardia	Echocardiogram; pulmonary artery catheter; cardiac catheterization
Hypovolemia	History (e.g., gastrointestinal hemorrhage) Examination (e.g., flat neck veins)	Sinus tachycardia	Hematocrit; serum electrolyte levels; serum urea nitrogen and creatinine levels
Hypothermia	History Central body temperature	Bradycardia	ECG showing Osborn waves
Hypoxia	History Cyanosis	Wide QRS complex	Pulse oximetry; arterial blood gases
Drug overdose (e.g., β-blocker, calcium channel blocker, cyclic antidepressant, digoxin)	History Pill counts Pupillary abnormalities	Depends on specific drug; May include bradycardia; bizarre, wide QRS complexes; QT prolongation	Drug and toxicology screening; serum electrolyte levels; arterial blood gases
Hyperkalemia	History (e.g., renal failure, diabetes mellitus, medication use)	Tall, narrow, peaked T waves; intraventricular conduction defects; absent or diminished P waves; ST segment changes simulating injury current; atrioventricular block; ventricular tachycardia or fibrillation	Serum electrolyte levels; arterial blood gases
Massive pulmonary embolism	History (e.g., venous thrombosis) Examination (e.g., neck vein distention, no pulse with CPR)	S1Q3 pattern; rightward QRS axis; right bundle branch block; T-wave inversions in right precordial leads	Ventilation/perfusion lung scan; helical computed tomography; echocardiography; pulmonary angiography
Tension pneumothorax	History (e.g., post-percutaneous subclavian or jugular venous access) Examination (e.g., tracheal deviation, diminished ipsilateral air entry, no pulse with CPR)	Rightward QRS axis shift; decreased voltage in lead 1 and left precordial leads; T wave inversions in precordial leads; may have sinus tachycardia	Chest x-ray Fluoroscopy (diminished heart motion, especially ipsilaterally); echocardiography
Acidosis	Preexisting acidosis Renal failure	Depends on other electrolyte abnormalities (e.g., hyperkalemia or hypokalemia) and underlying cause	Arterial blood gases; serum electrolyte concentrations
Acute massive myocardial infarction, with or without myocardial rupture	History (e.g., chest pain, risk factors)	ST segment changes (usually elevation); T wave changes; Q waves (depending on timing)	ECG; cardiac marker (serum creatine phosphokinase and troponin) levels; echocardiogram

* Treatment for PEA must be initiated immediately, while diagnostic studies are arranged for promptly.

TABLE 34-2. ETIOLOGIES AND KEY MANAGEMENT POINTERS IN PEA

ETIOLOGY OF PEA	KEY MANAGEMENT
Pericardial tamponade	Pericardiocentesis
Hypovolemia	Fluid resuscitation
Hypothermia	Rewarming measures
Hypoxemia	Supplemental oxygen
	Positive pressure ventilation
Drug overdose	Drug screening
	Gastric lavage
	Hemodialysis or hemoperfusion, where appropriate
	See chapters on specific drugs (e.g., Chapter 67, Digoxin Overdose for use of antibody fragment treatment).
Hyperkalemia	IV $CaCl_2$ or calcium gluconate (first-line)
	IV insulin and dextrose
	Sodium bicarbonate
	Cation exchange resin
	Diuresis (e.g., with furosemide)
	Hemodialysis
Pulmonary embolism	Thrombolytic or anticoagulant therapy
	Embolectomy
Tension pneumothorax	Needle decompression followed by chest tube thoracostomy
Acute myocardial infarction	See Chapter 20, Acute Myocardial Infarction
Acidosis	Hyperventilation (for hypercapnia)
	Sodium bicarbonate (for selected indications)

35 Ventricular Fibrillation and Tachycardia

Randy A. Lieberman
Marc D. Meissner

To adequately manage patients with ventricular fibrillation (VF) and ventricular tachycardia (VT) in the intensive care unit (ICU), familiarity with advanced cardiac life-support (ACLS) protocols is essential. This chapter assumes familiarity with ACLS and focuses on management features that tend not to be emphasized in standard critical care textbooks.

Ventricular tachycardia can be subclassified on the basis of various parameters, such as mechanisms (e.g., re-entry, automaticity), location, duration, drug responsiveness, catecholamine sensitivity, or relation to exercise. Most broadly, the electrocardiogram (ECG) can distinguish monomorphic VT from polymorphic VT.

Key Definitions

- Ventricular fibrillation: rapid, disorganized and asynchronous contractions of cardiac ventricular muscle, also reflected by a "chaotic" ECG appearance

- Ventricular tachycardia: three or more complexes of ventricular origin at ≥100 beats/minute
    - Sustained VT: ≥30 second duration, or resulting in hemodynamic compromise
    - Monomorphic VT: presence of a single, uniform QRS morphology within each lead
    - Polymorphic VT: presence of multiple QRS morphologies within any given lead

Etiology

A. Coronary artery disease and ischemia
B. Acute myocardial infarction
C. Nonischemic cardiomyopathy (e.g., dilated cardiomyopathy, hypertrophic cardiomyopathy)
D. Dysrhythmogenic right ventricular dysplasia
E. Congenital heart disease
F. Primary valvular heart disease
G. Inflammatory (e.g., myocarditis)
H. Idiopathic (primary electrical disease)
I. Congenital long QT syndromes (ion "channelopathy")
    1. Brugada syndrome
    2. Romano-Ward syndrome
    3. Jervell and Lange-Nielsen syndrome
J. Wolff-Parkinson-White syndrome (WPW) and atrial fibrillation, simulating or degenerating into VT
K. Post-cardiac surgery
L. Pacing during the "vulnerable" period (e.g., R on T phenomenon)
M. Metabolic
    1. Electrolyte disturbances
        a. Hypokalemia
        b. Hyperkalemia
        c. Hypomagnesemia
        d. Hypocalcemia
        e. Acidemia or alkalemia
    2. Hypoxia
N. Drug-related (drugs that can prolong the QT interval)
    1. Antidysrhythmic drugs
        a. Class IA agents: e.g., quinidine, procainamide, disopyramide
        b. Class III agents: e.g., sotalol, bretylium, amiodarone, dofetilide
        c. Note that dofetilide is absolutely contraindicated in combination with any of the following drugs because VT can be the result: verapamil, ketoconazole, cimetidine, trimethoprim, megestrone, prochlorperazine
    2. Antimicrobial drugs: e.g., trimethoprim-sulfamethoxazole, erythromycin, ketoconazole, fluconazole, pentamidine
    3. Antihistamines: e.g., terfenadine, astemizole
    4. Psychoactive drugs: phenothiazines, cyclic antidepressants, lithium
    5. Miscellaneous: cisapride, probucol, bepridil

Clinical Findings

Patients may be asymptomatic or minimally symptomatic, or they may experience palpitations, chest fluttering, chest discomfort, shortness of breath, or multiple symptoms. More serious presentations include loss of consciousness, seizures, cyanosis, absent pulse, and death.

Key Management

- Ensure "ABCDs" of advanced cardiac life support.

- Obtain 12-lead ECG (performed pre-, during, and post-dysrhythmia, whenever possible).

- Echocardiography

- Laboratory tests (serum electrolyte concentrations, toxicologic screening, antidysrhythmic drug levels)

- Exclude cardiac ischemia.

Treatment

A. Acute management follows the current ACLS guidelines of the American Heart Association.

B. Intravenous amiodarone is the first-line pharmacological agent for the treatment of ventricular tachydysrhythmias associated with hemodynamic compromise and clinical instability, including when left ventricular ejection fraction is less than 40% or in the presence of congestive heart failure. Other agents (e.g., procainamide) may be considered in some situations.

C. In the ICU setting, further acute management is based primarily on the pathophysiology and hemodynamic status of the patient.

D. Pointers for specific management (beyond ACLS) of VT that is not associated with hemodynamic compromise or clinical instability, in specific clinical contexts or with specific ECG patterns

1. Polymorphic VT without WPW
   a. Exclude ischemia.
   b. Exclude drug proarrhythmia.
   c. Exclude cocaine toxicity.

2. Wolff-Parkinson-White syndrome with pre-excited atrial fibrillation
   a. Cardioversion, if unstable
   b. Intravenous procainamide
   c. Avoid drugs that block the atrioventricular node.
   d. Radiofrequency ablation

3. Prolonged QT interval
   a. Correct hypokalemia, hypomagnesemia, hypocalcemia.
   b. Discontinue offending agent (e.g., procainamide), if any.
   c. If pause related, raise heart rate pharmacologically or using temporary pacing.

4. Monomorphic VT and structurally normal heart
   a. Left bundle branch block, usually with inferior axis (idiopathic right ventricular outflow tract)
      (1) Consider β-adrenergic blocker.
      (2) Consider calcium channel blocker.
      (3) Radiofrequency ablation
   b. Right bundle branch block with left ventricular posterior fascicular hemiblock (superior axis)
      (1) Verapamil or diltiazem
      (2) Radiofrequency ablation

5. Nonsustained VT (e.g., post-coronary artery bypass surgery)
   a. Exclude ischemia (e.g., from graft closure).
   b. Correct electrolyte disturbances.
   c. Avoid antidysrhythmic agents.
   d. Consult electrophysiologist.

6. Implantable cardioverter-defibrillator shocks
   a. Without VT or VF
      (1) Suspect atrial fibrillation or other form of supraventricular tachycardia.
      (2) Consider using β-adrenergic blocker or calcium channel blocker.
      (3) Consult electrophysiologist.
   b. With VT or VF: manage as recurrent VT or VF

E. Optimal long-term management of VT is directed by the specific etiology and ECG patterns of the dysrhythmia, and by the underlying disorder.

Bibliography

Ewy GA, Ornato JP. 31st Bethesda Conference. Emergency cardiac care. J Am Coll Cardiol 2000;35:825–880.

Hazinski MF, Cummins RO, Field JM (eds). 2000 Handbook of Emergency Cardiovascular Care for Healthcare Providers. Dallas, TX: American Heart Association, 2000.

Kudenchuk PJ, Cobb LA, Copass MK, et al. Amiodarone for resuscitation after out-of hospital cardiac arrest due to ventricular fibrillation. N Engl J Med 1999;341:871–878.

Meissner MD. Proarrhythmia: how to assess and manage it. Am Coll Cardiol Curr J Rev 1998;7:16–22.

Meissner MD, Akhtar M, Lehmann MH. Nonischemic sudden tachyarrhythmic death in atherosclerotic heart disease: pathophysiologic and clinical correlates. Circulation 1991;84:905–912.

Meissner MD, Lehmann MH, Steinman RT et al. Ventricular fibrillation in patients without significant structural heart disease: a multicenter experience with implantable cardioverter-defibrillator therapy. J Am Coll Cardiol 1993;21:1406–1412.

Siddoway LA. Pharmacologic principles of antiarrhythmic drugs, In: Podrid P, Kowey PR (eds). Cardiac Arrhythmia—Mechanisms, Diagnosis, and Management. Baltimore: Williams and Wilkins;1995, pp 355–368.

36 Conduction Disturbances

Marc D. Meissner
Randy A. Lieberman

Definitions

A. First-degree atrioventricular (AV) block: conduction of atrial electrical activity to the ventricles with a 1:1 relationship between P wave and QRS and a PR interval greater than 200 msec

B. Second-degree AV block: intermittent conduction of atrial electrical activity to the ventricles with an intermittent and possibly varying relationship between P waves and QRS complexes

   1. Mobitz type I second-degree AV block

      a. If typical, a periodic, repeating rhythm pattern evident on the electrocardiogram (ECG), showing progressive PR prolongation and shortening of R-R intervals, followed by a nonconducted P wave ("dropped" QRS) and appearance of "grouped" beating.

      b. Also known as Wenckebach phenomenon

      c. The conduction abnormality is within the AV node.

   2. Mobitz type II second-degree AV block

      a. Intermittently nonconducted P waves ("dropped" QRS) without antecedent PR interval changes

      b. The conduction abnormality is below the AV node.

C. Third-degree AV block

   1. Failure of all P waves to conduct to the ventricle, resulting in complete dissociation of P waves and QRS complexes

   2. The ventricular rhythm is maintained by a subsidiary pacemaker (e.g., junctional or idioventricular).

   3. The ventricular rate is typically slower than the atrial rate.

   4. QRS complex may be narrow (if junctional escape mechanism) or wide.

Etiology or Contributing Factors

A. Sick sinus syndrome (associated with hypertension, coronary artery disease, and other forms of heart disease)

B. Drugs

   1. Cardiac glycosides

   2. β-Adrenergic blockers (including eye drop formulations)

   3. Calcium channel blockers

   4. Antidysrhythmic drugs (e.g., sotalol, amiodarone)

   5. α-Methyldopa

   6. Lithium carbonate

   7. Cimetidine

   8. Clonidine

C. Myocardial ischemia and infarction, particularly inferior wall involvement

D. Hypoxia

E. Hypothermia

F. Metabolic abnormalities

   1. Acidemia

   2. Hyperkalemia

   3. Hypokalemia

   4. Hypothyroidism

G. Neurocardiogenic

H. Heightened vagal tone

   1. Related to sleep, pain, or tracheal stimulation

   2. May be present in well-conditioned athletes

I. Cardiac surgery

   1. Post-coronary artery bypass surgery

   2. Post-aortic or mitral valve surgery

   3. Other open-heart operations

J. Sleep apnea

K. Cerebrovascular accident

L. Congenital heart block

Clinical Features

A. May be minimally symptomatic or asymptomatic

B. Fatigue

C. Palpitations

D. Dizziness, lightheadedness, faintness, presyncope

E. Frank syncope

F. Increasing angina

G. Signs and symptoms of congestive heart failure

H. Hypotension and/or bradycardia (not universally present)

Diagnosis

A. Compatible history

   1. Symptoms

   2. Past medical history

3. Drug history

B. Physical examination

1. Bradycardia may be evident.

2. Consider carotid sinus massage.

   a. May be helpful if there is a history of syncope

   b. There is a small risk of stroke if performed in patients with signs of carotid arterial disease (e.g., carotid bruit).

   c. Perform under continuous ECG monitoring.

3. Attempt to reproduce symptoms if related to a specific activity.

C. Electrocardiography (see Table 36–1)

1. 12-lead ECG

2. Long rhythm strip

D. Toxicologic screening, including drug levels (e.g., digoxin) when appropriate

E. Serum thyrotropin assay

F. Echocardiography

Treatment

A. Management varies according to patient's clinical status (symptoms and hemodynamics) in relation to ECG findings.

B. Urgent intervention

1. Necessary for patients with hemodynamic compromise and persistent or recurrent A-V block, profound bradycardia, or asystole

2. Initiate treatment following American Heart Association advanced cardiac life-support guidelines, including atropine, dopamine, or both, in an attempt to increase heart rate. At times, epinephrine may be necessary and helpful.

3. Cardiac pacing (refer to American College of Cardiology/American Heart Association Guidelines)

   a. Temporary transvenous cardiac pacing (see Chapter 193, Temporary Transvenous Pacemaker)

      (1) May be more reliable and more comfortable (for conscious patients) than external pacing

      (2) Takes longer to place than external pacemaker

      (3) Risks involved with obtaining vascular access; potential provocation of cardiac dysrhythmias and cardiac perforation

      (4) Risk of serious consequences of cardiac perforation are increased if patient has received thrombolytic or anticoagulant therapy.

   b. External cardiac pacing (see Chapter 194, Transcutaneous Pacing)

      (1) May be less reliable and less comfortable than transvenous pacing

      (2) Potentially useful applications

         (a) Patients at high risk of serious complications from transvenous pacing

         (b) Use while readying for placement of transvenous pacing catheter.

         (c) Back-up in the stable patient

   c. Placement of permanent cardiac pacemaker

      (1) No role in acute emergency setting

      (2) Usually required ultimately in patients with high-grade (i.e., second-degree Mobitz type II and third-degree) AV block (see Table 36–1)

C. Non-urgent intervention

1. Patients with transient conduction disturbances, normotension, and minimal or no symptoms

2. Specific measures

   a. Discontinue potential offending drug.

   b. Employ continuous ECG monitoring.

   c. Give atropine and dopamine for chronotropic effects, as needed.

   d. Place transcutaneous pacemaker, set to standby mode.

   e. Cardiology or electrophysiology consultation

   f. Consider transvenous pacemaker placement for persistent or recurrent conduction disturbances or recurrent transient symptomatic episodes.

TABLE 36–1. BEDSIDE CLUES TO THE LEVEL OF BLOCK IN SECOND-DEGREE AV BLOCK*

PARAMETER	FAVORS MOBITZ TYPE I BLOCK	FAVORS MOBITZ TYPE II BLOCK
QRS complex	Narrow	Wide
Escape rate (beats/min)	>40	≤40
Heart rate response to carotid sinus massage	May slow	No change or may increase
Heart rate response to atropine, dopamine, or exercise	Increase	No change or may decrease
Location of acute myocardial infarction	Inferior	Anterior

* These represent guidelines, not invariate findings; e.g., block within the bundle of His can occur with a narrow QRS complex.

Key Treatment

- Ensure adequacy of airway, ventilation, and perfusion.

- Monitor ECG continuously; etiologic and diagnostic evaluation (see text).

- Discontinue unnecessary rate-slowing medications (see above list).

- Administer IV chronotropic drug(s) if necessary (atropine, dopamine).

- Place external pacemaker electrodes, set at least to standby mode.

- Individualize approach regarding need for temporary transvenous pacemaker.

Bibliography

Cummins RO, Graves JR, Larsen MP, et al. Out-of-hospital transcutaneous pacing by emergency medical technicians in patients with asystolic cardiac arrest. N Engl J Med 1993;328:1377–1382.

Gregoratos G, Cheitlin MD, Conill A, et al. ACC/AHA Guidelines for implantation of cardiac pacemakers and antiarrhythmia devices, a report of the American College of Cardiology/American Heart Association Task Force on Practice Guidelines (Committee on Pacemaker Implantation). Circulation 1998;97:1325–1335 or J Am Coll Cardiol 1998;31:1175–1209.

Hazinski MF, Cummins RO, Field JM (eds). 2000 Handbook of Emergency Cardiovascular Care for Healthcare Providers. Dallas, TX: American Heart Association, 2000.

Prystowsky EN, Klein GJ. Cardiac Arrhythmias—An Integrated Approach for the Clinician. New York: McGraw-Hill, 1994.

Sra J, Jazayeri M, Avitall B, et al. Comparison of cardiac pacing with drug therapy in the treatment of neurocardiogenic syncope with bradycardia or asystole. N Engl J Med 1993;328:1085–1090.

37 Hyponatremia

James A. Kruse

Hyponatremia is common in hospitalized patients and has a wide variety of causes. In most cases, the mechanism is not a deficiency in sodium but rather an excess of total body water due to an inability to elaborate adequately diluted urine. Symptoms are generally absent until the plasma sodium concentration is well below 120 mmol/L, but they tend to manifest sooner in rapidly developing hyponatremia. There has been considerable controversy regarding the optimal methods and rate of correction of the disorder, and no absolute consensus. This reflects the dangers of both undertreatment and overly rapid correction of hyponatremia. The latter can lead to the osmotic demyelination syndrome, also known as *central pontine myelinolysis*. This iatrogenic complication can potentially result in severe and sometimes permanent neurologic sequelae.

Differential Diagnosis

A. First consider serum osmolality

  1. Iso-osmolar hyponatremia

    a. Severe hyperproteinemia (multiple myeloma or macroglobulinemia) or hyperlipidemia

      (1) This form of hyponatremia is artifactual.

      (2) A result of volumetric laboratory assays that do no account for the decreased water content of hyperlipidemic or hyperproteinemic serum

      (3) Also known as *spurious hyponatremia* or *pseudohyponatremia*

      (4) Methods of identification

        (a) Measured osmolality is normal.

        (b) Osmole gap (measured osmolality − calculated osmolality) is increased (see Chapter 68, Alcohol and Glycol Intoxications).

        (c) In severe hyperlipidemia the serum is grossly lactescent.

        (d) Serum water content (W_s) is decreased; can be determined gravimetrically (normal ~93%).

        (e) Derive W_s from measured serum lipid (L_s) and protein (P_s) contents (g/dL) by

$$W_s = (99.1 − 1.03 \times L_s − 0.73 \times P_s) \div 100$$

        (f) Derive corrected serum sodium concentration ($Na_{corrected}$) from measured sodium level ($Na_{measured}$) and W_s by

$$Na_{corrected} = Na_{measured} \times 93 \div W_s$$

        Can similarly correct other spurious volumetric assay results

    b. Infusion of isotonic mannitol, glucose, sorbitol, glycerol, glycine

    c. Presence of non-sodium cation: immunoglobulin G myeloma, tromethamine infusion, lithium

  2. Hyperosmolar hyponatremia

    a. Hyperglycemia

      (1) Results in true hyponatremia due largely to dilution by osmosis-induced water flux from intracellular space to extracellular space

      (2) Can determine expected change in serum sodium concentration (ΔNa, mmol/L) by a given degree of hyperglycemia (glucose, mg/dL) using

$$\Delta Na = 0.016 \times (glucose − 100)$$

    b. Infusion of hypertonic mannitol, glycerol, sorbitol, glycine

  3. Hypo-osmolar hyponatremia (see B, below)

B. If hypo-osmolar, clinically assess extracellular (ECF) volume status (e.g., pulse, orthostatic blood pressure, jugular venous distension, edema, central venous pressure).

  1. Hypervolemic hypo-osmolar hyponatremia (edematous)

    a. Urine sodium concentration lower than 10 mmol/L

      (1) Congestive heart failure

      (2) Cirrhosis

      (3) Nephrotic syndrome

      (4) Hypothyroidism

      (5) Hypoalbuminemia due to malnutrition

      (6) Pregnancy

      (7) Idiopathic

b. Urine sodium concentration greater than 20 mmol/L

   (1) Acute renal failure

   (2) Chronic renal failure

2. Hypovolemic hypo-osmolar hyponatremia (clinical signs of volume depletion; nonedematous)

   a. Gastrointestinal (GI)

      (1) Causes: vomiting, nasogastric suction, diarrhea, pancreatitis, GI fistula fluid loss

      (2) Urine sodium and chloride concentrations less than 20 mmol/L (>20 mmol/L early on)

   b. Renal disease

      (1) Causes: non-oliguric renal failure, partial urinary tract obstruction, renal tubular acidosis, tubulointerstitial nephritis, other salt-wasting nephropathies

      (2) Urine sodium concentration greater than 20 mmol/L

   c. Diuretics

      (1) Hyponatremia occurs in conjunction with excess free water intake.

      (2) Urine sodium concentration greater than 20 mmol/L during diuretic use; lower than 10 mmol/L after discontinuation

   d. Cerebral salt wasting

      (1) Caused by central nervous system (CNS) disorders

      (2) May be mediated in part by atrial or brain natriuretic peptides

      (3) Urine sodium concentration greater than 20 mmol/L

      (4) Responds to salt or saline administration

   e. Cutaneous water loss: urine sodium concentration lower than 10 mmol/L

      (1) Burn injury

      (2) Excessive sweating

   f. Mineralocorticoid deficiency: urine sodium concentration greater than 20 mmol/L

   g. Third space fluid sequestration

      (1) Peritonitis

      (2) Pancreatitis

      (3) Bowel obstruction

      (4) Rhabdomyolysis

3. Clinically isovolemic, hypo-osmolar hyponatremia (ECF volume generally is slightly expanded, but not sufficient to cause edema)

   a. Water intoxication (urine osmolality lower than 100 mOsm/kg H_2O)

      (1) Psychogenic polydipsia: a psychiatric disorder, also known as compulsive water drinking or psychogenic diabetes insipidus

      (2) Dipsogenic polydipsia: due to a structural brain lesion involving the hypothalamic thirst center; also known as dipsogenic diabetes insipidus

      (3) Beer potomania

      (4) Iatrogenic

         (a) Excessive hypotonic IV fluid administration

         (b) Excessive water administration by gastric or enteral tube

         (c) Excessive hypotonic irrigation fluid: e.g., during transurethral prostate resection surgery, endometrial ablation procedures, lithotripsy, enemas

   b. Renal failure

   c. Syndrome of inappropriate antidiuresis (see Chapter 54, Syndrome of Inappropriate Antidiuresis)

   d. Reset osmostat

      (1) Also known as *sick cell syndrome* or *essential hyponatremia*

      (2) Due to abnormal resetting of brain osmoreceptor

      (3) Renal concentrating and diluting functions are normal.

      (4) Normal response to salt loading, water loading, and water deprivation, except plasma sodium tends to be maintained at a lower than normal level

   e. Glucocorticoid deficiency

   f. Hypothyroidism

Clinical Findings

A. Patients with serum levels below 120 mmol/L or who develop hyponatremia within 24 hours are more likely to manifest CNS aberrations.

B. Symptoms

   1. Fatigue, malaise

   2. Apathy

   3. Headache

   4. Muscle cramps

   5. Anorexia, nausea, vomiting

   6. Hypogeusia

C. Physical findings

   1. Lethargy

   2. Agitation, irritability, personality changes, inappropriate or bizarre behavior

3. Disorientation, confusion, hallucinations

4. Abnormal sensorium, stupor, coma

5. Muscle weakness; bulbar or pseudobulbar palsy

6. Depressed deep tendon reflexes, pathologic reflexes, myoclonus, asterixis

7. Seizures

8. Other: ataxia, incontinence, hypo- or hyperthermia, Cheyne-Stokes respirations, signs of increased intracranial pressure, respiratory arrest

Key Clinical Findings

- Mild to moderate hyponatremia is usually asymptomatic.

- The most common manifestations of severe hyponatremia are altered mental status and seizures.

Treatment

A. Iso-osmolar hyponatremia

 1. Pseudohyponatremia: no treatment required, plasma sodium is actually normal

 2. Isotonic mannitol (or other osmotic agent) infusion: discontinue infusion

B. Hyperosmolar hyponatremia

 1. Hypertonic mannitol (or other osmotic agent) infusion: discontinue infusion

 2. Hyperglycemia

    a. Stop or decrease glucose administration.

    b. Administer insulin and IV fluids.

    c. Target a drop in glucose concentration of 75 to 100 mg/dL per hour.

C. Hypo-osmolar hyponatremia

 1. General measures

    a. Closely monitor vital signs.

    b. Monitor serum sodium concentration frequently (e.g., every 2 to 3 hours in severe cases) to monitor progress of therapy and periodically recalculate fluid requirements.

    c. Monitor fluid intake and output (Foley catheterization).

    d. Monitor output and (if volume is excessive) electrolyte composition of non-urinary body fluid losses; e.g., liquid diarrhea, nasogastric drainage.

    e. Obtain urine osmolality and urine electrolyte measurements.

    f. Order routine tests.

    g. Assure adequate IV access.

    h. Provide supplemental potassium if the patient is hypokalemic.

    i. Stop drugs that may be affecting ADH secretion or action.

    j. Calculate the patient's current total body water (TBW, L) from current weight (kg) and water fraction factor (f) by: TBW = $f \times$ weight:

       (1) Use 0.6 for f in nonelderly men.

       (2) Use 0.5 for f in nonelderly women and elderly men.

       (3) Use 0.4 for f in elderly women.

    k. If IV fluids are to be administered, anticipate the effect of each liter of IV fluid on the patient's serum sodium concentration.

       (1) Calculate the estimated change in serum sodium concentration (ΔNa_s, mmol/L) from the patient's current serum sodium concentration (Na_s, mmol/L), TBW (L), and the infusate sodium concentration (Na_{inf}, mmol/L) by

       $$\Delta Na_s = (Na_{inf} - Na_s) \div (TBW + 1)$$

       (2) Infusate sodium concentration (Na_{inf} in above equation)

          (a) 5% saline: 856 mmol/L

          (b) 3% saline: 513 mmol/L

          (c) Normal (0.9%) saline: 154 mmol/L

          (d) Ringer's lactate: 130 mmol/L

       (3) Assumes there are no gains of sodium or water other than the IV infusate, and no losses of body water or sodium during the infusion

    l. If IV saline solutions are to be used, estimate the volume (mL) of the selected infusate to achieve the targeted increment in serum sodium concentration (ΔNa_s, mmol/L) over the next 1 hour using:

       $$\text{Volume} = (1000 \times \Delta Na_s \times TBW) \div (Na_{inf})$$

       (1) For example, if TBW is 42 L, and 3% saline will be used as the infusate (513 mmol/L), and an increase in serum sodium concentration of 0.3 mmol/L is desired over the next 1 hour (extrapolates to ~7 mmol/L per 24 hours), then the resultant infusion rate is (1000 × 0.3 × 42) ÷ 513 ≈ 25 mL during the first 1 hour.

       (2) Recalculate at frequent intervals based on serial serum sodium levels.

       (3) Assumes there are no gains of sodium

or water other than the IV infusate, and no losses of body water or sodium

m. Recalculate applied formulas frequently during treatment, based on serial serum sodium determinations, to allow ongoing adjustments to IV composition and infusion rate.

n. Treat underlying cause.

o. Provide supportive care.

2. If ECF space is contracted:

a. If patient is hypotensive or shows other signs of perfusion failure, administer sufficient IV isotonic (0.9%) saline to correct hypovolemia and ensure adequate perfusion.

b. In the absence of hypovolemic shock (or after it is corrected), titrate the saline infusion (see above) to raise serum sodium no more than 8 mmol/L per day (0.3 mmol/L per hour).

3. If ECF space is expanded (edematous), hyponatremia is chronic (developed over >12 hours), and patient is asymptomatic

a. Calculate water excess (L) from current serum sodium concentration (Na_s, mmol/L) and current TBW (L) as:

$$\text{Water excess} = \text{TBW} \times [1 - (Na_s \div 140)]$$

b. For chronic (developing over >12 to 24 hours) asymptomatic hyponatremia, restrict water intake (generally 500 to 1000 mL/day) and sodium intake.

c. Target a rise in serum sodium of less than 8 mmol/L per day (0.3 mmol/L per hour).

d. Treat congestive heart failure, if present.

4. If ECF space is expanded or normal, hyponatremia is chronic (developed over >12 hours) and severe, and patient is symptomatic:

a. If symptoms are mild and urine osmolality is less than 200 mOsm/kg H_2O: institute fluid restriction.

b. If symptoms are severe or urine osmolality is greater than 200 mOsm/kg H_2O, administer IV hypertonic (3% or 5%) saline to raise serum sodium by ~0.3 mmol/L per hour, but no more than 8 mmol/L per 24 hours.

(1) Calculate hourly IV infusion rate (see above) needed to achieve targeted hourly change in serum sodium concentration.

(2) If seizures are present, treat with standard anticonvulsant therapy.

(3) Consider giving sufficient IV hypertonic (3% or 5%) saline to raise serum sodium by up to 3 mmol/L per hour for 1 to 2 hours if:

(a) Seizures are present, especially if they persist despite anticonvulsant therapy.

(b) Neurologic status deteriorates despite above measures.

(4) Consider use of loop diuretic to enhance free water excretion, especially if ECF space is expanded.

(5) Stop hypertonic saline administration when

(a) Life-threatening manifestations cease.

(b) Serum sodium concentration reaches 125 to 130 mmol/L (lower if initial sodium concentration was less than 100 mmol/L).

(6) Restrict free water.

5. To avoid osmotic demyelination syndrome

a. Do not exceed a rise in serum sodium of 8 mmol/L per 24 hours.

b. Do not allow overshoot hypernatremia.

6. Treat endocrine deficiency (hypothyroidism or adrenal insufficiency), if present.

Key Treatment Points

- Obtain frequent serum sodium measurements.

- Monitor intake and output closely.

- Discontinue drugs that stimulate antidiuretic hormone release or effect.

- Avoid an overly rapid (greater than 8 mmol/L per 24 hours) rise in serum sodium.

- Avoid rapid normalization of the serum sodium concentration.

- Avoid overcorrection of the serum sodium concentration (i.e., hypernatremia).

Complications

A. Of untreated or undertreated hyponatremia

1. Seizures (usually generalized)

2. Coma

3. Respiratory arrest

4. Permanent neurologic deficits

5. Persistent vegetative state

6. Death

B. Of overtreatment (i.e., overcorrection or overly

rapid correction of hyponatremia), resulting in osmotic demyelination syndrome

1. Spastic quadriparesis or quadriplegia
2. Pseudobulbar palsy, dysarthria, mutism
3. Pupillary or oculomotor abnormalities
4. Depression, psychosis
5. Stupor or coma
6. Ataxia, dystonia, parkinsonism
7. Death

Bibliography

Adrogué HJ, Madias NE. Aiding fluid prescription for the dysnatremias. Intensive Care Med 1997;23:309–316.

Fraser CL, Arieff AI. Epidemiology, pathophysiology, and management of hyponatremic encephalopathy. Am J Med 1997;102:67–77.

Oh MS, Kim H-J, Carroll HJ. Recommendations for treatment of symptomatic hyponatremia. Nephron 1995;70:143–150.

Verbalis JG. Adaptation to acute and chronic hyponatremia: implications for symptomatology, diagnosis, and therapy. Semin Nephrol 1998;18:3–19.

38 Hypernatremia

James A. Kruse

The most common cause of hypernatremia is simple dehydration. This develops when there is pure water loss or hypotonic fluid loss from the body, associated with inadequate water intake. Although much less common, excessive intake or administration of salt or hypertonic sodium solutions can lead to hypernatremia associated with extracellular fluid overload. In general, hypernatremia does not occur in subjects with a normal sensorium and an intact thirst mechanism who have access to and receive adequate water. When it occurs in the hospital setting it is iatrogenic; i.e., due to inadequate prescription of oral, enteral, or parenteral electrolyte-free water, or (less commonly) due to administration of hypertonic fluids. Although the extracellular fluid status is variable, there is associated intracellular dehydration in all cases. Assessment of the extracellular fluid status (e.g., by physical examination, central venous pressure measurement, etc.) serves to classify the underlying etiology or mechanism and facilitates the differential diagnosis. The associated mortality rate in hospitalized patients with severe hypernatremia is about 50%.

Etiology and Classification

A. Isovolemic hypernatremia (clinically normal extracellular fluid volume). Includes subclinical hypovolemic hypernatremia. Associated extracellular water loss is common, and clinically apparent hypovolemia can occur in severe cases (see later under B. Hypovolemic hypernatremia).
  1. Iatrogenic
    a. Free water deprivation
    b. Isotonic fluid replacement of hypotonic losses
  2. Cutaneous water loss
  3. Respiratory losses
    a. Tachypnea or Kussmaul respirations
    b. Nonhumidified supplemental oxygen use
  4. Diabetes insipidus
    a. Central diabetes insipidus
    b. Nephrogenic diabetes insipidus
  5. Rare brain lesions involved in thirst regulation (see later under b. Impaired thirst mechanism)
B. Hypovolemic hypernatremia (decreased extracellular fluid volume)
  1. Decreased water intake
    a. Impaired access to water

      (1) Lack of available water source
      (2) Debilitation or injury preventing water access
      (3) Marked iatrogenic water deprivation
    b. Impaired thirst mechanism
      (1) Generalized alteration in sensorium (common)
        (a) Cerebrovascular accident
        (b) Central nervous system (CNS) infection
        (c) Metabolic encephalopathy
        (d) Drugs causing CNS depression
        (e) Traumatic brain injury
        (f) Cerebral anoxia
        (g) Impaired consciousness from any other cause
      (2) Rare specific CNS lesions (e.g., involving hypothalamus)
        (a) Primary hypodipsia (osmoreceptor dysfunction)
        (b) Essential hypernatremia (also known as hypertonic reset osmostat syndrome)
  2. Increased renal water loss
    a. Diuretics (e.g., loop, thiazide, and potassium-sparing diuretics)
    b. Osmotic diuresis
      (1) Glycosuria (hyperglycemia)
      (2) Osmotic diuretics (e.g., mannitol, glycerol)
      (3) Post-obstructive diuresis
      (4) Diuretic phase of acute tubular necrosis
    c. Salt-wasting nephropathy
    d. Polyuric renal failure
    e. Diabetes insipidus
    f. Urinary concentrating defects of any cause
  3. Increased nonrenal water loss
    a. Gastrointestinal losses
      (1) Vomiting
      (2) Nasogastric suction
      (3) Diarrhea
      (4) Biliary drainage
      (5) Fistula fluid loss
    b. Cutaneous losses

(1) Insensible water loss

(2) Perspiration

(3) Burn injury

(4) Open wounds

   c. Respiratory losses

C. Hypervolemic hypernatremia (increased extracellular fluid volume)

   1. Iatrogenic

      a. Excessive $NaHCO_3$ therapy

      b. Excessive IV hypertonic saline

      c. Therapeutic abortion

      d. Peritoneal dialysis or hemodialysis

         (1) Incorrect dialysate prescription

         (2) Malfunction of proportioning system

      e. Complication of enteral or total parenteral nutrition (TPN)

   2. Mineralocorticoid excess

      a. Cushing's syndrome

      b. Conn's syndrome

      c. Therapeutic steroid administration

      d. Glycyrrhizic acid induced

         (1) Excessive licorice ingestion

         (2) Chewing tobacco

   3. Excessive sodium ingestion

      a. Salt tablet ingestion

      b. Sea water ingestion or near drowning

      c. Sodium hypochlorite (bleach) ingestion

Clinical Manifestations

A. Constitutional

   1. Malaise

   2. Thirst

   3. Fever

B. Neurologic

   1. Generalized weakness

   2. Lethargy

   3. Confusion, irritability, or delirium

   4. Obtundation, stupor, or coma

   5. Seizures

   6. Myoclonus, spasticity, or hyperreflexia

   7. Intracerebral or subarachnoid hemorrhage

C. Gastrointestinal

   1. Nausea

   2. Vomiting

D. Manifestations of altered extracellular fluid volume

   1. Findings in hypovolemic hypernatremia

      a. Weight loss

      b. Decreased skin turgor, sunken eye globes

      c. Dry mucous membranes, furrowed tongue

      d. Decreased axillary perspiration

      e. Flat neck veins, decreased central venous pressure

      f. Tachycardia

      g. Orthostatic or frank hypotension

      h. Cool extremities

      i. Slowed capillary refilling

   2. Findings in hypervolemic hypernatremia

      a. Weight gain

      b. Absence of signs of extracellular fluid deficit

      c. Distended neck veins

      d. Peripheral edema

      e. Pulmonary rales

      f. Increased central venous and pulmonary artery occlusion pressures

Laboratory Findings

A. Hypernatremia

B. Hyperosmolality (plasma)

C. Azotemia

D. Urine osmolality (Fig. 38–1)

   1. Highly concentrated urine (>700 mOsm/kg H_2O)

      a. Excessive free water loss

      b. Insufficient water intake

      c. Excessive sodium intake

      d. Osmoreceptor defect and marked volume depletion

   2. Moderately concentrated urine (300 to 700 mOsm/kg H_2O)

      a. Renal failure

      b. Osmotic diuresis

      c. Loop diuretic

      d. Partial central or nephrogenic diabetes insipidus

      e. Hyperaldosteronism

      f. Essential hypernatremia without severe volume depletion

   3. Dilute urine (urine osmolality less than plasma osmolality)

      a. Complete central diabetes insipidus

      b. Severe nephrogenic diabetes insipidus

      c. Gestational diabetes insipidus

E. Increased cerebrospinal fluid protein (without pleocytosis)

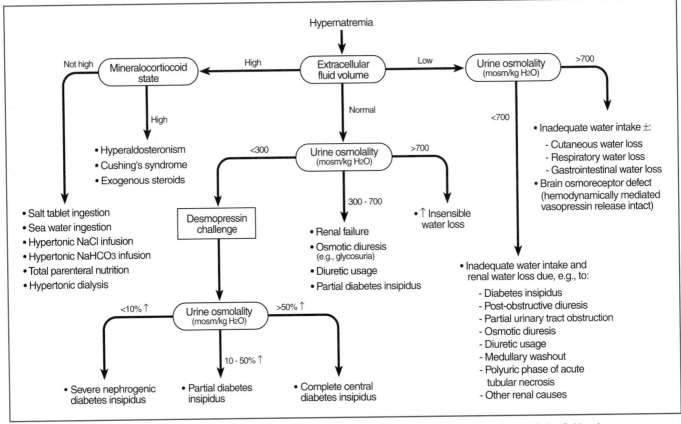

Figure 38–1 Simplified approach to the differential diagnosis of hypernatremia based on extracellular fluid volume, mineralocorticoid state, and urine osmolality. (From Kruse JA. Diagnosis and treatment of hyperosmolar emergencies. In: Vincent J-L (ed). Yearbook of Intensive Care and Emergency Medicine. New York: Springer-Verlag, 2000, pp 544–559, with permission.)

Key Preventive Measures

- Recognize that development of hypernatremia in hospitalized patients is iatrogenic.

- Ensure adequate frequency of serum sodium monitoring (at least daily in critically ill patients and those susceptible to dehydration and hypernatremia).

- Increase monitoring frequency in patients with serious alterations in consciousness, burn injuries, hyperglycemia, those recovering from renal failure, and those receiving diuretics, cathartics, or sodium bicarbonate.

- Anticipate insensible losses (typically 0.6 mL/kg per hour and increasing by 20%/°C increase in body temperature above normal).

- Increase administration of free water (e.g., IV hypotonic saline, IV 5% dextrose in water, enteral tap water) when serum sodium rises to or beyond upper normal limit.

Treatment

A. General measures

1. Closely monitor vital signs.

2. Monitor fluid intake and output; Foley catheterization.

3. Measure serum sodium concentration every 2 to 12 hours (depending on severity) to monitor progress of therapy and periodically recalculate fluid requirements.

4. Monitor serum electrolytes, glucose, urea nitrogen, creatinine, etc.

5. Obtain urine osmolality and urine electrolyte measurements.

6. Monitor output and (if volume is excessive) electrolyte composition of nonurinary body fluid losses.

7. Assure adequate IV access.

8. Consider hemodynamic monitoring to assess intravascular volume.

   a. Central venous pressure measurement may be helpful in severe cases.

b. Pulmonary artery catheterization is not required in most patients but may be useful in very unstable patients, those not responding to initial fluid resuscitation, elderly patients, and those with severe sepsis, underlying severe heart disease, or sustained circulatory shock.

9. Provide supportive therapy as needed.

B. Fluid therapy

1. Rapidly administer 500 mL to 2 L of normal saline or colloid intravenously in patients with evidence of hypovolemia and compromised perfusion.

2. Change IV fluid to hypotonic saline (1/3 or 1/2 normal saline) or 5% dextrose in water (if not hyperglycemic) once any intravascular volume deficit is corrected.

   a. May alternate between 5% dextrose and hypotonic saline (or use two IVs, one of each fluid type, and use different infusion rates as needed) to avoid excessively rapid drop in plasma sodium concentration

   b. Avoid IV dextrose solutions in patients with history of hyperglycemia or diabetes.

   c. Tap water via nasogastric or nasoenteric tube can also be utilized for fluid replacement.

      (1) Effect on water deficit is equivalent to 5% dextrose in water.

      (2) Particularly helpful in patients with glucose intolerance

3. Base free water replacement on calculated free water deficit.

   a. Deficit (L) = 0.6 × Wt × [(Na ÷ 140) − 1], where Wt is current body weight (kg), and Na is serum sodium concentration (mmol/L).

   b. The factor 0.6 represents the normal proportion of body weight that is water. Use slightly lower values in young women and elderly men (0.5), and in elderly women (0.4). Even lower values may be more representative in markedly obese subjects.

   c. Recognize that this formula estimates only the free water deficit; i.e., the volume of pure water required to normalize plasma sodium.

   d. Formula does not account for concomitant hypovolemia or other extracellular fluid deficits.

4. Select the targeted rate of sodium correction.

   a. For hyperacute hypernatremia, i.e., developing over less than 12 hours (rare): more rapid correction (e.g., 1 mmol/L per hour) is warranted.

   b. For the more typical, slowly developing hypernatremia, usually evolving over more than 2 days:

      (1) In asymptomatic patients, target a correction rate of 0.3 mmol/L per hour or less.

      (2) In symptomatic cases, consider using a rate of 0.4 to 0.6 mmol/L per hour initially.

      (3) To avoid causing cerebral edema

         (a) Avoid overly rapid correction.

         (b) Do not exceed a correction rate of 10 mmol/L per 24 hours.

         (c) Avoid complete normalization of sodium concentration within the first 48 hours.

         (d) Avoid over-treatment of the free water deficit (i.e., hyponatremia).

5. Recalculate the free water deficit frequently during treatment, based on serial serum sodium determinations, to provide ongoing adjustments to the rate of fluid replacement.

6. Anticipate the effect of each liter of infused intravenous fluid on the patient's plasma sodium concentration.

   a. Calculate the estimated change in plasma sodium (ΔNa, mmol/L) by:

   $$\Delta Na^+ = (\text{infusate Na concentration} - \text{current serum Na}) \div (0.6 \times Wt + 1)$$

   from the patient's current serum sodium concentration (mmol/L), body weight (Wt, kg), and the infusate sodium concentration (mmol/L).

   b. Infusate sodium concentration (for above equation)

      (1) Normal (0.9%) saline: 154 mmol/L

      (2) Ringer's lactate: 130 mmol/L

      (3) Half-normal (0.45%) saline: 77 mmol/L

      (4) 5% dextrose in 0.2% saline: 34 mmol/L

      (5) 5% dextrose in water: 0 mmol/L

   c. Recognize assumptions underlying the above calculation.

      (1) Total body water (L) equals six-tenths of body weight (kg); see earlier comment regarding female and elderly subjects.

(2) There are no other gains of sodium or water other than the IV infusate.

(3) There are no losses of body water or sodium during the infusion.

7. Replace no more than half the free water deficit in the first 24 hours; replace the remainder over the next 24 to 72 hours or more.

8. Titrate fluids (especially sodium-containing fluids) cautiously in elderly patients and those with underlying cardiac failure.

9. Monitor serum or blood glucose levels and avoid hyperglycemia.

10. After the water deficit is corrected, titrate the rate and composition of IV fluids and the rate of enteral water administration to provide maintenance requirements and replacement of ongoing losses.

C. Minimize unnecessary fluid losses

1. Discontinue diuretics (in isovolemic or hypovolemic hypernatremia).

2. Discontinue cathartics (e.g., lactulose, sorbitol, bowel preparations, laxatives).

3. Control hyperglycemia, if present.

4. Dress open wounds.

5. Minimize nasogastric suction and other gastrointestinal losses, if possible.

6. Avoid excessive amino acid (in TPN) or dietary protein administration.

7. Minimize insensible losses.

a. Treat fever, if present.

b. Use aerosolized supplemental oxygen.

D. Discontinue hypertonic saline or sodium bicarbonate solutions.

E. Enhance sodium and water elimination in patients with hypervolemic hypernatremia (i.e., due to sodium excess rather than water loss).

1. Consider loop diuretic if inadequate spontaneous diuresis.

2. Consider peritoneal dialysis or hemodialysis if renal function is markedly impaired.

F. Evaluate for possible underlying cause; depending on setting, this may include:

1. Computed tomography of brain

2. Cultures of blood, urine, and other body fluids as indicated by fever, leukocytosis, or other signs of possible infection

3. Other tests and evaluations as indicated by history, physical examination, screening laboratory tests, and imaging studies

G. Provide appropriate specific management of underlying cause (e.g., desmopressin administration for central diabetes insipidus).

Key Treatment

- Intravenous fluids: normal saline (if hypovolemic) followed by hypotonic saline

- Avoid overly rapid (>0.7 mmol/L per hour) decreases in serum sodium concentration.

- Frequent serum electrolyte testing: usually every 2 to 6 hours

- Monitor intake and output closely.

- Control associated hyperglycemia, if present.

- Discontinue cathartics and (in most cases) diuretics.

Bibliography

Adrogué HJ, Madias NE. Aiding fluid prescription for the dysnatremias. Intensive Care Med 1997;23:309–316.

Mandal AK, Saklayen MG, Hillman NM, et al. Predictive factors for high mortality in hypernatremic patients. Am J Emerg Med 1997;15:130–132.

Palevsky PM. Hypernatremia. Semin Nephrol 1998;18:20–30.

Polderman KH, Schreuder WO, Strack van Schijndel RJ, et al. Hypernatremia in the intensive care unit: An indicator of quality of care? Crit Care Med 1999;27:1041–1042.

Portel L, Hilbert G, Gruson D, et al. Survival with extreme hypernatremia at 209 mmol/L (letter). Intensive Care Med 1998;24:197–198.

39 Hypokalemia

James A. Kruse

Hypokalemia is a frequent problem encountered in the intensive care unit (ICU) setting. Plasma potassium concentration is normally a function of potassium intake and renal excretion. Small decreases in plasma potassium can signal large total body losses. Although total body potassium averages about 50 mmol/kg, only 2% of this is distributed in the extracellular fluid.

Etiology

A. Inadequate intake: starvation, anorexia nervosa, alcoholism, certain fad diets, inadequate potassium supplementation, parenteral nutrition formulas with insufficient potassium, geophagia

B. Drugs and toxins: thiazide and loop diuretics, mannitol, carbonic anhydrase inhibitors (e.g., acetazolamide), insulin, glucose, sodium bicarbonate, β-adrenergic agonists (including inhaled agents), corticosteroids, sodium penicillin, ampicillin, nafcillin, oxacillin, carbenicillin, ticarcillin, aminoglycosides, rifampicin, amphotericin B, outdated tetracycline, granulocyte–macrophage colony-stimulating factor, vitamin B_{12}, lithium, cation exchange resin, L-dopa, foscarnet, carbenoxolone, soluble barium salts, cisplatin, glycyrrhizic acid, gossypol, toluene, barium, thallium

C. Transcellular redistribution: insulin (including as treatment of diabetic ketoacidosis), alkalemia, refeeding syndrome, parenteral hyperalimentation, treatment of folate or vitamin B_{12} deficiency, barium poisoning, hypokalemic periodic paralysis

D. Gastrointestinal loss: vomiting, nasogastric suction, gastric lavage, biliary drainage, diarrhea, enterocutaneous fistula, ileostomy, villous adenoma, laxative abuse, non-insulin-secreting islet cell tumor, post–intestinal bypass surgery

E. Renal loss: uncontrolled diabetes, diuretic phase of acute tubular necrosis, post-obstructive diuresis, renal tubular acidosis types 1 and 2, Fanconi's syndrome, hypochloremia, hypomagnesemia, hypercalcemia, ketosis, ureterosigmoidostomy, renal artery stenosis, Barrter's syndrome, Liddle's syndrome, Gitelman's syndrome, polyuria of any cause

F. Mineralocorticoid excess: primary hyperaldosteronism (Conn's syndrome), secondary hyperaldosteronism, malignant or renovascular hypertension, Cushing's syndrome, ectopic ACTH syndrome, ad-

renogenital syndromes, hypernephroma, Wilms' tumor, juxtaglomerular cell tumor, excessive licorice ingestion

G. Miscellaneous: post-resuscitation, post–myocardial infarction, burn injury, hematologic malignancies, acute intermittent porphyria, pseudohypokalemia (due to leukocytosis with in vitro uptake of potassium by white blood cells)

Manifestations

A. Clinical manifestations are unreliable for assessment of hyperkalemia.

B. Symptoms: constipation, weakness, myalgias, muscle cramps, restless legs, fasciculations, respiratory distress, polyuria, polydipsia, nausea, vomiting

C. Physical findings: weakness, lethargy, gastroparesis, abdominal distention, paralytic ileus, paresthesias, hyporeflexia, paralysis, respiratory failure

D. Metabolic: metabolic alkalosis, rhabdomyolysis, nephrogenic diabetes insipidus, renal acidification defects, impaired glucose tolerance, negative nitrogen balance, renal phosphate wasting, exacerbation of hepatic encephalopathy (due to increased ammonium production), exacerbation of digoxin toxicity

E. Electrocardiogram (Fig. 39–1): tachydysrhythmias, flattened T waves, prominent U waves, ST segment depression, conduction abnormalities, enhanced digitalis effect

Key Preventive Measures

- Anticipate renal and gastrointestinal potassium losses.

- Provide adequate potassium in maintenance IV fluids.

- Ensure adequate potassium in total parenteral nutrition formulas.

- Monitor serum potassium at appropriate intervals.

Approach to Differential Diagnosis

A. Exclude transmembrane redistribution etiologies.

B. If leukocytosis (white blood cell count >50,000 cells/mm³), exclude pseudohypokalemia by rapid

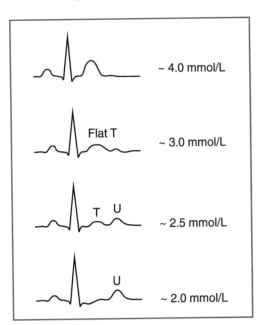

~ 4.0 mmol/L

Flat T   ~ 3.0 mmol/L

T U   ~ 2.5 mmol/L

U   ~ 2.0 mmol/L

Figure 39–1 Typical electrocardiographic (ECG) findings in hypokalemia. Correlation between actual potassium concentration and ECG findings is variable.

separation of plasma and measurement of plasma potassium.

C. Obtain history to exclude drug-induced etiologies and inadequate intake.

D. If urine potassium is less than 20 mmol/L (<30 mmol/day): consider inadequate intake, diarrhea, biliary loss, gastrointestinal fistula loss, prior diuretic use, cutaneous loss.

E. If urine potassium is greater than 20 mmol/L (>30 mmol/day), consider chronic blood pressure level:

1. Normotensive
   a. If normal anion gap metabolic acidosis: consider type I or II renal tubular acidosis or acetazolamide use.
   b. If elevated anion gap metabolic acidosis: consider diabetic ketoacidosis.
   c. If metabolic alkalosis: check urine chloride concentration.
      (1) Urine chloride less than 10 mmol/L: consider vomiting, nasogastric suctioning.
      (2) Urine chloride greater than 15 mmol/L: consider diuretic use, profound potassium depletion, Barrter's syndrome, magnesium deficiency.

2. Hypertensive
   a. If high plasma renin: consider malignant hypertension, renal artery stenosis, hypernephroma, Wilms' tumor, juxtaglomerular cell tumor.
   b. If low plasma renin, check plasma aldosterone.

(1) Plasma aldosterone less than 22 μg/dL: consider mineralocorticoid ingestion, Cushing's syndrome, adrenogenital syndrome.
(2) Plasma aldosterone greater than 22 μg/dL: consider primary hyperaldosteronism.

Treatment

A. Difficult to estimate total body potassium deficiency from serum levels: statistically, for every 100 mmol deficit in total body potassium, serum potassium decreases by approximately 0.3 mmol/L.

B. Amount of replacement depends on total body deficit, ongoing losses, and any factors affecting transcellular distribution.

C. Mild degrees may be treated with oral supplements, if patient can take solutions by mouth.
   1. Use potassium citrate formulations in patients with metabolic acidosis.
   2. Use potassium chloride formulations in patients with metabolic alkalosis.

D. Intravenous supplements are necessary if hypokalemia is severe or if patient cannot take potassium preparations orally or enterally.
   1. Infusate potassium concentration greater than 40 mmol/L may result in pain or phlebitis at the peripheral IV infusion site; central IV access preferred for higher concentrations.
   2. With continuous electrocardiographic (ECG) monitoring in an ICU setting, potassium can be safely given as a controlled IV infusion consisting of 20 mmol KCl in at least 100 mL saline infused over at least 1 hour ("IV piggy-back"), but generally for not more than 3 consecutive infusions without reevaluating serum potassium.
   3. The average increase in serum potassium using this protocol of replacement is 0.25 mmol/L per 20 mmol infusion (caution: considerable individual variation).
   4. Profound degrees of hypokalemia may rarely require infusion rates faster than 20 mmol/hour, but require cautious and more frequent monitoring.
   5. Potassium phosphate can be used in lieu of KCl in patients with concomitant severe hypophosphatemia: 15 mmol potassium phosphate (contains 22 mmol potassium) in at least 100 mL saline infused over at least 1 hour.
   6. Dangerous degrees of hyperkalemia are possible during IV potassium replacement, especially in patients with renal dysfunction, those receiving drugs that can cause hyperkalemia, and those receiving potassium supplementation by other routes (e.g., concomitant oral supplements or parenteral nutrition formulas).

Key Treatment Points

- Oral or enteral potassium preparations are adequate for mild hypokalemia in patients able to take by mouth.

- Exercise caution whenever prescribing parenteral potassium.

- In ICU patients unable to take oral or enteral supplements, or for marked hypokalemia, 20 mmol KCl in at least 100 mL saline given by IV infusion over at least 1 hour is generally safe.

- Avoid dextrose infusions, which stimulate insulin secretion and can exacerbate hypokalemia.

- Monitor serum potassium levels to avoid under treatment or overtreatment.

7. Never administer IV push because this can precipitate cardiac arrest.

8. Serial serum potassium assays are necessary to assess adequacy of supplementation and to protect against overshoot hyperkalemia; frequency depends on severity of hypokalemia, ongoing losses, and rate of replacement (e.g., every 2 hours in severe cases).

Bibliography

Gennari FJ. Hypokalemia. N Engl J Med 1998;339:451–458.

Halperin ML, Kamel KS. Potassium. Lancet 1998;352:135–140.

Kruse JA, Clark VL, Carlson RW, et al. Effects of concentrated potassium chloride infusions in critically ill patients with hypokalemia. J Clin Pharmacol 1994;34:1077–1082.

Kruse JA, Carlson RW. Rapid correction of hypokalemia using concentrated intravenous potassium chloride infusions. Arch Intern Med 1990;150:613–617.

40 Hyperkalemia

James A. Kruse

Severe hyperkalemia can be rapidly fatal. Milder degrees of hyperkalemia in the intensive care unit setting may progress to life-threatening hyperkalemia if vigilant potassium monitoring and early treatment measures are overlooked. Renal dysfunction is involved in the majority of cases.

Etiology

A. Excessive intake: oral or intravenous potassium supplements, salt substitutes, parenteral nutrition formulas, drugs formulated as potassium salts (e.g., potassium penicillin), blood transfusions, cardioplegic solutions, renal allograft preservatives

B. Primary renal causes: renal failure (acute or chronic), including acute tubular necrosis, any tubulointerstitial nephritis, sickle cell nephropathy, analgesic nephropathy, chronic pyelonephritis, lupus nephritis, amyloidosis, diabetic nephropathy, AIDS, obstructive uropathy, renal transplant

C. Transcellular redistribution: insulin deficiency, rhabdomyolysis, tumor lysis, massive hemolysis, extensive burns, severe exercise, reabsorption of hematoma, gastrointestinal hemorrhage, mesenteric infarction, marked catabolic states, inorganic (hyperchloremic) metabolic acidosis, respiratory acidosis, α-adrenergic stimulation, malignant hyperthermia, hyperkalemic periodic paralysis

D. Mineralocorticoid deficiency: Addison's disease, bilateral adrenalectomy, hypo- or hyperreninemic hypoaldosteronism, type 4 renal tubular acidosis, congenital adrenal hyperplasia, pseudohypoaldosteronism, 21 β-hydroxylase deficiency, angiotensin deficiency or insensitivity

E. Pharmacologic agents: amiloride, spironolactone, triamterene, angiotensin converting enzyme inhibitors, trimethoprim, nonsteroidal anti-inflammatory drugs, succinylcholine, β-adrenergic antagonists, α-adrenergic agonists, pentamidine, cyclosporin, somatostatin, digitalis intoxication, heparin, diazoxide, arginine HCl, lysine HCl

F. Pseudohyperkalemia: laboratory error, phlebotomy proximal to IV potassium infusion, prolonged tourniquet application, in vitro hemolysis, thrombocytosis ($>1,000,000$ platelets/mm³), leukocytosis ($>50,000$ cells/mm³)

Clinical Manifestations

A. Symptoms and physical findings are unreliable for assessment of hyperkalemia.

B. Manifestations often herald cardiac arrest.

C. Neuromuscular findings: weakness, dysarthria, dysphasia, paresthesias, paralysis, nausea, vomiting

D. Cardiovascular findings: tachydysrhythmias, cardiac arrest; more likely if hyperkalemia develops rapidly or is associated with hyponatremia, hypomagnesemia, or hypocalcemia

Electrocardiogram (see Fig. 40–1)

A. Early: tall, peaked T waves (especially in precordial leads)

B. Late

1. PR interval prolongation
2. QRS interval prolongation
3. Sinoventricular rhythm (absence of P waves despite underlying sinus rhythm)
4. Ventricular tachycardia, flutter, or fibrillation
5. Asystole

WARNING

The first electrocardiographic (ECG) manifestation of hyperkalemia may be ventricular tachycardia.

Treatment

A. All degrees of hyperkalemia

1. Discontinue potassium supplements by all routes (e.g., dietary, oral supplements, IV solutions, parenteral nutrition formulas).
2. Discontinue and avoid potassium-containing drugs (e.g., potassium penicillins).
3. Discontinue and avoid drugs favoring potassium retention (e.g., potassium-sparing diuretics, angiotensin converting enzyme inhibitors) or redistribution (e.g., succinylcholine).
4. Avoid or correct factors that may shift potassium out of cells (e.g., acidemia, insulin deficiency, hyperosmolality).

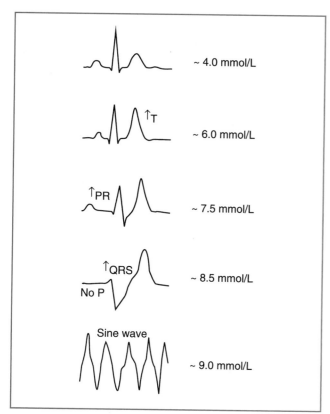

Figure 40–1 Typical ECG changes findings in hyperkalemia (correlation between actual potassium concentration and ECG findings is variable).

5. Order repeat serum potassium to confirm hyperkalemia (do not delay treatment while awaiting results if potassium higher than 6 mmol/L in credible setting).

6. Serially monitor serum potassium (e.g., every 2 hours in severe cases).

7. Investigate the underlying cause.

B. Severe hyperkalemia

1. Consider as an emergency.

2. Institute the measures outlined above.

3. Monitor ECG continuously.

4. Institute specific treatment measures immediately.

a. Provide pharmacologic cardioprotection with calcium.

(1) Mechanism of action: stabilizes cardiac membrane; does not lower plasma potassium

(2) Typical dosing: 10 to 20 mL of a 10% solution of calcium gluconate intravenously

(3) Kinetics: onset in seconds; duration only approximately 30 to 60 minutes

(4) Caution: calcium may precipitate or

worsen digoxin toxicity in patients receiving the drug

b. Redistribute potassium into cells

(1) Insulin and glucose

(a) Typical dosing: 10 U of regular insulin intravenously plus 25 g glucose intravenously

(b) Kinetics: onset is within minutes; duration of action is up to several hours

(c) Repeat every 2 to 5 hours, if necessary; monitor for hypo- or hyperglycemia.

(2) Albuterol

(a) Typical dosing: 10 to 20 mg by nebulized aerosol

(b) Kinetics: onset is within minutes; duration is up to several hours

(3) Sodium bicarbonate

(a) Mechanism of action: drives potassium into cells; may also act as membrane antagonist

(b) Typical dosing: 50 to 100 mmol IV

(c) Limited efficacy; may have some role if concomitant metabolic acidosis

(d) Caution: calcium carbonate precipitate will form if administered through the same IV as calcium chloride or gluconate without first thoroughly flushing the IV tubing

(e) Kinetics: onset within 15 minutes; duration of several hours

---

CAUTION

Insulin, bicarbonate, and albuterol do not remove potassium from the body; as their effects wane, plasma potassium will rise.

---

c. Promote elimination of potassium from the body.

(1) Sodium polystyrene sulfonate resin (Kayexalate)

(a) Mechanism of action: exchange of sodium and potassium within gastrointestinal tract; typically removes about 0.5 to 1.0 mmol of potassium per gram of administered resin

(b) Typical dosing: 25 to 50 g sodium polystyrene sulfonate, along with 20% sorbitol solution for cathartic effect; more effective orally or enterally than per rectum

    (c) Kinetics: onset is about 2 hours; duration of 4 to 6 hours; repeated dosing is usually necessary (e.g., every 3 to 6 hours)

(2) Loop diuretic: e.g., furosemide

    (a) Mechanism of action: increases renal potassium excretion

    (b) Typical dosing for furosemide is 40 mg intravenously, but depends on renal function

    (c) Kinetics: onset and duration parallel diuresis; efficacy parallels renal functional level

(3) Dialysis

    (a) Mechanism of action: removes potassium from body

    (b) Kinetics: onset is immediate upon initiation of hemodialysis (significantly slower for peritoneal dialysis)

    (c) Often necessary in renal failure

5. Hyperkalemia associated with digoxin toxicity

  a. Do not administer calcium.

  b. Give magnesium sulfate (e.g., 2 g intravenously) if no contraindication.

  c. Consider digoxin-specific antibody fragment treatment.

Key Treatment

- Levels higher than 6 mmol/L should be considered an emergency requiring immediate evaluation and treatment measures.
- Calcium offers immediate, but brief, cardioprotection.
- Insulin, bicarbonate, and albuterol shift potassium into cells.
- Cation exchange resin and dialysis remove potassium from the body.
- Dialysis is usually required to treat marked hyperkalemia in patients with end-stage renal disease.
- Frequent monitoring of serum or plasma potassium concentration is imperative.

Bibliography

Greenberg A. Hyperkalemia: treatment options. Semin Nephrol 1998;18:46–57.

Kemper MJ, Harps E, Müller-Wiefel DE. Hyperkalemia: therapeutic options in acute and chronic renal failure. Clin Nephrol 1996;46:67–69.

Marinella MA. Trimethoprim-induced hyperkalemia: an analysis of reported cases. Gerontology 1999;45:209–212.

Martinez-Vea A, Bardaji A, Garcia C, et al. Severe hyperkalemia with minimal electrocardiographic manifestations: a report of seven cases. J Electrocardiography 1999;32:45–49.

Wong SL, Maltz HC. Albuterol for the treatment of hyperkalemia. Ann Pharmacother 1999;33:103–106.

41 Hypocalcemia

Jorge A. Guzman
James A. Kruse

Definition

A. Hypocalcemia is present if serum total calcium concentration is less than 8.2 mg/dL, 4.1 mEq/L, or 2.1 mmol/L (Table 41–1).

1. Symptoms are unusual unless total calcium level is lower than 7.0 mg/dL.

2. The above threshold values assume a normal relationship between total and ionized calcium (i.e., they assume serum albumin concentration is normal).

3. If serum albumin concentration (g/dL) is abnormal, serum total calcium concentration (mg/dL) may be "corrected" by:

Corrected total Ca = measured total Ca + 0.8
× (4.0 − albumin)

B. Hypocalcemia is present if serum or plasma ionized calcium concentration is lower than 4.1 mg/dL, 2.1 mEq/L, or 1.1 mmol/L.

1. Ionized fraction normally accounts for about half of the total serum calcium concentration.

2. Ionized fraction is physiologically more relevant than total calcium concentration.

3. Measurement of ionized fraction is more accurate than estimating effect of abnormal albumin concentration by the above formula.

4. Ionized calcium assays are increasingly available in clinical chemistry and blood gas laboratories.

Etiologies

A. Decreased activity of parathormone (PTH)

1. Hypoparathyroidism

   a. Idiopathic (rare)

      (1) Inherited forms

      (2) Sporadic form

   b. Post-surgical hypothyroidism/hungry bone syndrome

      (1) Post-thyroidectomy

      (2) Post-parathyroidectomy

      (3) Post–carotid artery surgery

      (4) Following other operations involving neck dissection

   c. Metastasis to the parathyroid glands (rare)

   d. Iron deposition to the parathyroids due to hemochromatosis (rare)

   e. Copper deposition to the parathyroids due to Wilson's disease (rare)

2. Pseudohypoparathyroidism (target organ unresponsiveness to PTH)

   a. Type I (Albright's hereditary osteodystrophy): PTH levels normal or high, but PTH fails to raise nephrogenic cyclic adenosine monophosphate (cAMP)

   b. Type II: PTH raises nephrogenic cAMP but not plasma calcium

3. Hypomagnesemia (can lead to relative PTH deficiency and end-organ resistance to PTH action)

4. Gentamicin (induces magnesuria leading to hypomagnesemia)

B. Decreased vitamin D activity

1. Vitamin D deficiency

   a. Inadequate dietary intake (rare in the United States)

   b. Intestinal malabsorption

   c. Vitamin D dependent rickets

      (1) Type I: deficiency of enzyme that converts $25(OH)D_3$ to $1,25(OH)_2D_3$

      (2) Type II: target organ unresponsiveness to $1,25(OH)_2D_3$

   d. Altered vitamin D metabolism by drugs (phenytoin, phenobarbital, rifampin)

2. Hepatobiliary disease

3. Renal disease: kidney converts $25(OH)D_3$ to $1,25(OH)_2D_3$, needed for intestinal calcium absorption

4. Malabsorption syndromes

5. Acute and chronic alcoholism

C. Drugs

1. Antihypercalcemic agents: bisphosphonates, calcitonin, plicamycin, gallium nitrate

2. Phosphate salts

3. Furosemide

4. Phenytoin

5. Phenobarbital

6. Estrogens

7. Cimetidine

8. Ethylenediaminetetraacetate (EDTA): some radiocontrast agents, chelation therapy

9. Heparin

TABLE 41-1. CONVERSION FACTORS FOR MEASUREMENTS OF SERUM OR PLASMA CALCIUM CONCENTRATION

To Convert	To	Multiply By
mg/dL	mEq/L	0.50
mg/dL	mmol/L	0.25
mEq/L	mg/dL	2.00
mEq/L	mmol/L	0.50
mmol/L	mg/dL	4.00
mmol/L	mEq/L	2.00

Key Risk Factors in ICU Patients

- Renal failure
- Alkalemia
- Sepsis
- Citrate-buffered blood products
- Gastrointestinal tract bleeding

10. Foscarnet
11. Antimicrobials: rifampin, pentamidine, ketoconazole
12. Chemotherapeutic agents: cisplatin, doxorubicin, asparaginase
13. Theophylline
14. Glutethimide
15. Propylthiouracil

D. In vivo calcium chelation or precipitation
   1. Hyperphosphatemia
   2. Citrate administration (banked blood products)
   3. Pancreatitis (formation of calcium soaps from lipolytic products)
   4. Rhabdomyolysis
   5. Ethylene glycol ingestion (calcium oxalate precipitation)
   6. Parenteral nutrition with lipid emulsion
   7. Protamine sulfate administration

E. Renal disease or failure
   1. Due to renal tubular dysfunction
   2. Due to decreased renal $1,25(OH)_2D_3$ production
   3. Due to hyperphosphatemia

F. Decreased bone turnover

G. Hypothyroidism

H. Sepsis (multifactorial mechanisms)

I. Osteoblastic bone metastases (e.g., breast or prostate cancer)

J. Alkalemia (decreases ionized calcium fraction by increasing protein binding)

K. Hypermagnesemia

L. Spurious hypocalcemia
   1. Hypoalbuminemia (ionized fraction not affected)
   2. In vitro anticoagulant chelation
      a. Specimen (vacuum) tubes containing EDTA or citrate
      b. Specimens obtained from indwelling arterial catheters with citrate flush
      c. Chelation with heparin
   3. Sporadic laboratory or sampling error

Clinical Manifestations

A. Neuromuscular effects
   1. Tetany
      a. Overt tetany
      b. Latent tetany
         (1) By Chvostek's sign: elicited by tapping the facial nerve and producing involuntary contractions of the facial muscles
         (2) By Trousseau's sign: carpopedal spasm developing after inflation of a blood pressure cuff to 20 mm Hg above the systolic pressure for 3 min
   2. Seizures
   3. Extrapyramidal manifestations: parkinsonian tremors, dystonia, ataxia, or choreoathetosis
   4. Muscle cramps, proximal muscle weakness

B. Neuropsychiatric
   1. Psychiatric disturbances: anxiety, emotional instability, depression, frank psychosis
   2. Altered mentation: confusion, encephalopathy, dementia

C. Cardiovascular
   1. Impaired cardiac contractility
   2. Hypotension
   3. Catecholamine insensitivity
   4. Cardiac arrest
   5. Electrocardiographic Q-T interval prolongation
   6. Electrocardiographic ST segment changes
   7. Electrocardiographic T wave changes

D. Respiratory
   1. Laryngospasm
   2. Bronchospasm

E. Ocular
   1. Cataract (long-term hypocalcemia)
   2. Kayser-Fleischer ring (hypoparathyroidism due to Wilson's disease)
   3. Papilledema

> **WARNING**
>
> Calcium chloride is more irritating to tissue than other parenteral calcium formulations. If used, it should be administered by central vein. It can cause thrombophlebitis if given by peripheral vein and severe tissue necrosis if it extravasates. IM administration is contraindicated.

Treatment

A. Indications

1. Immediate parenteral treatment is indicated for acute symptomatic hypocalcemia; i.e., if attributed clinical manifestations are apparent.

2. Treatment may be indicated for asymptomatic patients with plasma ionized calcium concentration less than 3 mg/dL.

B. Calcium supplementation

1. Oral calcium administration

    a. Calcium carbonate: 1.25 g contains 500 mg elemental calcium.

    b. Also available as acetate, citrate, gluconate, and lactate salts

    c. Typical oral maintenance: 1 to 2 g/day of elemental calcium in the form of one of the above salts (in addition to dietary calcium) in divided doses, with meals

2. IV calcium administration

    a. Formulations (Table 41–2)

    (1) Calcium gluconate: 10 mL of 10% solution contains 1 g of the salt and 93 mg of elemental calcium.

    (2) Calcium chloride: 10 mL 10% solution contains 1 g of the salt and 273 mg of elemental calcium.

    (3) Calcium gluceptate: 10 mL of 22% solu-tion contains 180 mg (9 mEq) of elemental calcium.

    b. Initial dose: administer 10 mL of any of the above solutions, diluted in 100 mL of 5% dextrose in water, and given intravenously over 10 to 30 min as initial dose (effect may last only a few hours)

    c. Repeat initial dose as necessary or follow with a continuous IV infusion of calcium gluconate at 0.3 to 2 mg/kg per hour of elemental calcium (with frequent serum calcium determinations) until plasma ionized calcium concentration exceeds 4.0 mg/dL.

C. Magnesium supplementation

1. Hypocalcemia is refractory to calcium administration if there is concomitant hypomagnesemia.

2. Sustained effect of supplemental calcium will not be achieved until hypomagnesemia is corrected.

D. Vitamin D supplementation (rarely required during critical illness)

1. Consider if calcium supplementation alone does not maintain adequate serum calcium level.

2. Not effective unless there is adequate calcium and phosphate intake

3. Use with caution in patients with renal failure.

4. Oral dosing

    a. Ergocalciferol (vitamin D_2): 750 to 2500 μg/day

    b. Calcitriol ($1,25(OH)_2D_3$): 0.25 to 2.0 μg/day

    c. Calcifediol ($25\text{-}OHD_3$): 50 to 200 μg/day

    d. Dihydrotachysterol ($1\text{-}OHD_3$): 200 to 1000 μg/day

5. Monitor serum calcium periodically to avoid hypercalcemia due to vitamin D excess.

E. Renal failure patients

1. Oral calcium supplementation

2. Dietary phosphate restriction

3. Oral phosphate binding agents

TABLE 41–2. EQUIVALENCE FACTORS FOR PARENTERAL CALCIUM SALT FORMULATIONS

FORMULATION	GRAMS (OF THE SALT)	MILLIMOLES (OF CALCIUM OR THE SALT)	MILLIEQUIVALENTS (OF CALCIUM OR THE SALT)	MILLIGRAMS (OF ELEMENTAL CALCIUM)
Calcium chloride for injection ($CaCl_2 \cdot 2H_2O$)	1*	6.8	13.6	273
Calcium gluconate for injection ($CaC_{12}H_{22}O_{14}$)	1*	2.32	4.65	93
Calcium gluceptate for injection ($CaC_{14}H_{26}O_{16}$)	1	2.0	4.1	80
	2.2†	4.5	9.0	180

*Amount (mass) contained in 10 mL of a 10% solution of the salt.
†Amount (mass) contained in 10 mL of a 22% solution of the salt.

a. Calcium carbonate (see above)

b. Aluminum-containing phosphate binding antacids: chronic use may cause dementia and osteomalacia in patients receiving dialysis

4. Dialysis

WARNING

Intravenous calcium supplementation can provoke ventricular dysrhythmias in patients receiving digoxin. Employ continuous electrocardiographic monitoring if IV calcium supplementation must be given. Avoid in digoxin intoxication.

Bibliography

Geheb MA, Kruse JA, Haupt MT, et al. Fluid and electrolyte abnormalities in critically ill patients: fluid resuscitation, lactate metabolism, and calcium metabolism. In: Narins RG (ed). Maxwell and Kleeman's Clinical Disorders of Fluid and Electrolyte Metabolism. 5th ed. New York: McGraw-Hill, 1994, pp 1463–1489.

Lind L, Carlstedt F, Rastad J, et al. Hypocalcemia and parathyroid hormone secretion in critically ill patients. Crit Care Med 2000;28:266–268.

Toffaletti J. Physiology and regulation. Ionized calcium, magnesium and lactate measurements in critical care settings. Am J Clin Pathol 1995;104:S88–S94.

Vincent J-L, Bredas P, Jankowski S, et al. Correction of hypocalcemia in the critically ill: what is the haemodynamic benefit? Intensive Care Med 1995;21:838–841.

Zaloga G. Hypocalcemia in critically ill patients. Crit Care Med 1992;20:251–262.

42 Hypercalcemia

Jorge A. Guzman
James A. Kruse

Definition

A. Hypercalcemia is present if serum total calcium concentration is greater than 10.5 mg/dL, 5.2 mEq/L, or 2.6 mmol/L.

1. Immediate treatment is indicated if greater than 14 mg/dL (3.5 mmol/L), even if asymptomatic.

2. Immediate treatment may be indicated if greater than 12 mg/dL (3.0 mmol/L), depending on clinical manifestations.

3. Above threshold values assume a normal relationship between total and ionized calcium (i.e., they assume serum albumin concentration is normal).

4. If serum albumin concentration (alb, g/dL) is abnormal, serum total calcium concentration (total Ca, mg/dL) may be "corrected" by:

Corrected total Ca
$$= \text{measured total Ca} + 0.8 \times (4.0 - \text{albumin})$$

B. Hypercalcemia is present if serum or plasma ionized calcium concentration is greater than 5.2 mg/dL, 2.6 mEq/L, or 1.3 mmol/L.

1. Normally accounts for about half of the total serum calcium concentration

2. Physiologically more relevant than total calcium concentration

3. Measurement of ionized fraction is more accurate than estimating effect of abnormal albumin concentration by the above formula.

4. Ionized calcium assays are increasingly available in clinical chemistry and blood gas laboratories.

Etiologies

A. Endocrine disorders
1. Parathyroid-related
   a. Primary hyperparathyroidism
      (1) Solitary adenomas
      (2) Parathyroid hyperplasia
      (3) Multiple endocrine neoplasia (MEN) type I: hyperparathyroidism plus pituitary and pancreatic islet cell adenomas
      (4) Multiple endocrine neoplasia type IIa: parathyroid hyperplasia, pheochromocytoma, and medullary thyroid carcinoma
   b. Secondary or tertiary hyperparathyroidism

   c. Familial hypocalciuric hypercalcemia (generally benign, may have mild hypercalcemia)
2. Hyperthyroidism
3. Addison's disease
4. Pheochromocytoma
5. Vasoactive intestinal peptide hormone–producing tumor

B. Malignancy
1. Solid tumor with bone metastases (e.g., breast cancer)
2. Solid tumor with humoral mediation by parathormone (PTH) or PTH-like substances produced by the neoplasm (e.g., lung or kidney cancer)
3. Hematologic malignancies (multiple myeloma, lymphoma, leukemia)

C. Renal failure
1. Acute and chronic renal insufficiency
2. Recovery phase of rhabdomyolysis
3. Renal transplantation

D. Granulomatous disorders
1. Sarcoidosis
2. Tuberculosis
3. Histoplasmosis, coccidioidomycosis
4. Leprosy
5. Berylliosis

E. Drugs
1. Calcium preparations
2. Milk-alkali syndrome
3. Lithium therapy
4. Thiazide diuretics
5. Estrogens
6. Tamoxifen
7. Vitamin D intoxication
8. Vitamin A intoxication

F. Miscellaneous causes
1. Immobilization with high bone turnover
2. Paget's disease
3. Parenteral nutrition
4. Idiopathic hypercalcemia of infancy
5. Spurious hypercalcemia of multiple myeloma with calcium-binding immunoglobulin

PEARL

90% of cases of hypercalcemia are secondary to malignancy or hyperparathyroidism.

Clinical Findings

A. Neurologic
  1. Lethargy, fatigue, apathy, obtundation, stupor, coma
  2. Irritability, confusion, disorientation, memory loss, delirium
  3. Weakness
  4. Seizures (rare)
B. Musculoskeletal
  1. Reduced muscle tone and strength
  2. Myalgias, bone pain, arthralgia
  3. Osteitis fibrosa cystica, osteopenia, pathological fracture
C. Gastrointestinal
  1. Anorexia, nausea, vomiting
  2. Constipation, ileus
  3. Pancreatitis (acute or chronic)
  4. Abdominal pain (pancreatitis or peptic ulcer-related)
D. Cardiovascular
  1. Hypertension
  2. Hypovolemia
E. Renal
  1. Polyuria and polydipsia (nephrogenic diabetes insipidus, decreased renal concentrating ability)
  2. Nephrolithiasis, nephrocalcinosis, obstructive uropathy
  3. Decreased glomerular filtration (renal insufficiency)
  4. Interstitial nephritis
  5. Hyperchloremic acidosis (mild)

Key Clinical Findings

- "Bones, stones, belly groans, and mental status overtones"
- Mental status changes are more likely in elderly patients.
- May be asymptomatic, especially if mild or moderate hypercalcemia

Laboratory and Other Tests

A. Hypercalcemia (elevated total and ionized plasma or serum calcium concentration)
B. Abnormal intact PTH levels
C. Hypo- or hyperphosphatemia
D. Non-anion gap metabolic acidosis (mild)
E. Abnormal thyroid function tests (if hyperthyroidism is the cause)
F. Abnormal adrenal function tests (if adrenal insufficiency is the cause)
G. Electrocardiographic changes
  1. Q-T interval shortening
  2. T wave broadening
  3. Conduction disturbances
  4. Dysrhythmias (especially in conjunction with digoxin)

Treatment

A. Intravenous hydration
  1. Decreases circulating calcium concentration by dilution and by facilitating calciuresis
  2. Typically can decrease serum calcium concentration by 1.6 to 2.4 mg/dL by hydration alone
  3. Use IV isotonic saline at 100 to 200 mL/hr (or more) to achieve a like diuresis.
  4. Saline volumes as high as 10 L/day or more have been used.
B. Loop diuretic
  1. Further increases renal calcium excretion by inhibition of distal tubular calcium reabsorption (of marginal added value to hydration if cardiorenal function adequate)
  2. Helps prevent fluid overload from saline loading, particularly in patients with underlying cardiorenal dysfunction
  3. Typical dosing: IV furosemide 10 to 40 mg every 4 to 12 hours to maintain adequate diuresis
  4. Larger and more frequent dosing may be indicated in patients with underlying renal insufficiency or established fluid overload.
  5. Do not administer until patient is well hydrated.
  6. Do not allow hypovolemia to develop.
C. Calcitonin
  1. Inhibits osteoclastic activity; also has analgesic properties
  2. Dose: 4 U/kg subcutaneously or IM every 12 hours (after optional skin testing)

3. Onset within hours, peak effect within 12 to 24 hours, but effective for only 2 to 7 days because of tachyphylaxis

4. Typically lowers serum calcium by only 2 to 3 mg/dL

5. Adverse effects include flushing, mild nausea and abdominal cramps, allergic reactions.

D. Bisphosphonates

1. Pyrophosphate analogs that are resistant to phosphatase action and therefore inhibit osteoclastic bone resorption

2. Effective in rehydrated patients, particularly those with malignancy as the cause of hypercalcemia

3. Etidronate disodium

a. Dose: 7.5 mg/kg per day in 250 mL normal saline intravenously over 4 hours for 3 to 7 days

b. Onset within 2 days; peak effect within 7 days

c. Adverse effects include osteomalacia (with long-term use) and transient elevation of serum phosphorus and creatinine concentrations.

4. Pamidronate disodium

a. Dose: 60 to 90 mg in 250 mL by continuous IV infusion over 2 to 24 hours (avoid in renal insufficiency)

b. Typically given as a single dose, but may be given as often as daily for 2 to 7 days or more

c. Peak effect observed in approximately 4 days

d. Adverse effects include transient leukopenia, temperature increase (<2°C), and mild lowering of serum phosphorus concentration.

5. Combination treatment with pamidronate and calcitonin reported to produce rapid and sustained decrements in calcium levels

E. Gallium nitrate

1. Inhibits bone resorption by lowering hydroxyapatite solubility

2. Dose: 200 mg/m² per day by continuous IV infusion for 5 days

3. Adverse effects include nephrotoxicity and hypophosphatemia.

4. Contraindicated in renal insufficiency; avoid concomitant nephrotoxic agents (e.g., aminoglycosides)

F. Corticosteroids

1. Inhibit vitamin D–mediated calcium absorption in the intestine and neoplastic growth in lymphoid tissue

2. Effective in granulomatous disorders and hematologic neoplasms; not likely to be effective in solid neoplasms or hyperparathyroidism

3. May prolong the duration of effectiveness of calcitonin

4. Typical dosing: hydrocortisone 200 mg/day in divided doses, or prednisone 20 to 60 mg/day, for 2 or 5 days

G. Plicamycin (formerly mithramycin)

1. An antineoplastic agent that inhibits osteoclastic ribonucleic acid synthesis thereby decreasing bone resorption

2. Dose: 25 μg/kg per day given intravenously over 4 to 6 hours for 1 to 4 days (commonly a single dose)

3. Onset within 12 hours; peak effect in 2 to 3 days; effective for 5 days to several weeks

4. Has potential for causing skin necrosis and cellulitis (if extravasates into subcutaneous tissue), nausea, nephrotoxicity, hepatotoxicity (in ~20% of cases), and serious thrombocytopenia

5. Contraindicated in renal or hepatic dysfunction, thrombocytopenia or coagulopathy

6. Largely supplanted by bisphosphonates

H. Inorganic phosphate

1. Inhibits bone resorption and forms complexes with calcium

2. Intravenous administration is extremely hazardous in hypercalcemia and therefore is not recommended.

3. Oral administration (500 to 1500 mg elemental phosphorus daily) allowable in hypophosphatemic patients (<2 mg/dL)

I. Other medical therapies of limited efficacy

1. Chloroquine: may be effective in hypercalcemia due to sarcoidosis.

2. Indomethacin or aspirin: limited efficacy in malignancy-associated hypercalcemia

3. Estrogens: limited efficacy in postmenopausal women with primary hyperparathyroidism

J. Dialysis

1. Effectively removes calcium from the body

2. Both peritoneal dialysis and hemodialysis are effective.

K. Parathyroidectomy

1. Definitive treatment for moderate to severe, symptomatic primary hyperparathyroidism

2. Initial hydration and other medical treatment still necessary for acute hypercalcemic crisis

Key Treatment

- Main goal of treatment is to prevent or ameliorate the adverse central nervous system effects of hypercalcemia.

- Aggressive hydration and diuresis are the mainstays of treatment.

- Calcitonin has rapid onset of action but a small effect on lowering the calcium level.

- Bisphosphonates have a slower onset of action but a larger impact on serum calcium concentration.

Bibliography

Gucalp R, Theriault R, Gill I, et al. Treatment of cancer-associated hypercalcemia. Arch Intern Med 1994;154: 1935–1944.

Mundy GR, Guise TA. Hormonal control of calcium homeostasis. Clin Chem 1999;45(8 Pt 2):1347–1352.

Nussbaum SR. Pathophysiology and management of severe hypercalcemia. Endocrinol Metab Clin North Am 1993; 22:343–362.

Sekine M, Takami H. Combination of calcitonin and pamidronate for emergency treatment of malignant hypercalcemia. Oncol Rep 1998;5:197–198.

43 Hypomagnesemia

Jorge A. Guzman
James A. Kruse

Definitions

A. Hypomagnesemia is present if plasma or serum total magnesium concentration is lower than 1.7 mg/dL, 0.70 mmol/L, or 1.4 mEq/L.

B. Dimensional conversions
1. Magnesium concentration of 1 mg/dL = 0.41 mmol/L = 0.82 mEq/L
2. Magnesium concentration of 1 mmol/L = 2 mEq/L = 2.43 mg/dL
3. Magnesium concentration of 1 mEq/L = 0.5 mmol/L = 1.2 mg/dL

Etiologies

A. Decreased intake
1. Fasting or malnutrition
2. Alcoholism
3. Prolonged IV fluid therapy
4. Parenteral nutrition with inadequate magnesium

B. Decreased intestinal absorption
1. Malabsorption syndromes
2. Short bowel syndrome

C. Excessive urine loss
1. Drug effects
   a. Diuretics: thiazides, loop diuretics, osmotic agents
   b. Antimicrobials: aminoglycosides, amphotericin B, pentamidine, ticarcillin
   c. Ethanol
   d. Cisplatin
   e. Cyclosporin A
   f. Foscarnet
2. Renal or metabolic disorders
   a. Diabetic ketoacidosis
   b. Diuretic phase of acute renal failure
   c. Post-obstructive diuresis
   d. Interstitial nephropathy
   e. Renal tubular acidosis
   f. Primary aldosteronism
   g. Hypercalcemia
   h. Hypokalemia
   i. Hypophosphatemia
   j. Post–renal transplantation
   k. Hyperthyroidism
   l. Syndrome of inappropriate antidiuresis
   m. Bartter's syndrome
   n. Gitelman's syndrome
   o. Familial renal magnesium wasting
3. Intravascular volume expansion

D. Excessive non-urinary fluid loss
1. Nasogastric suction
2. Severe diarrhea, including excessive laxative use
3. Biliary or intestinal fistula

E. Transcellular redistribution
1. Refeeding after starvation
2. Adrenergic agonists
3. Digoxin
4. Insulin
5. Diabetic ketoacidosis (during treatment phase)
6. Cardiopulmonary bypass

F. Miscellaneous causes
1. Acute pancreatitis
2. Multiple transfusions
3. Dialysis with magnesium-free dialysate
4. Acute myocardial infarction
5. Idiopathic hypomagnesemia

PEARL

Hypomagnesemia is common in hospitalized patients; the most frequent mechanism is increased renal magnesium excretion.

Clinical Findings

A. Central nervous system manifestations
1. Vertigo
2. Ataxia
3. Nystagmus
4. Dysarthria
5. Psychosis
6. Altered mentation
7. Irritability
8. Obtundation
9. Paresthesias
10. Seizures

B. Neuromuscular manifestations

1. Hyperreflexia
2. Weakness
3. Tetany
4. Muscle spasms
5. Tremor

C. Cardiovascular manifestations
   1. Arterial hypertension
   2. Cardiac dysrhythmias
   3. Hypotension or cardiac arrest (from ventricular tachycardia or fibrillation)

D. Gastrointestinal symptoms
   1. Anorexia, nausea
   2. Dysphagia
   3. Constipation, adynamic ileus
   4. Abdominal cramps
   5. Hypersalivation

Laboratory Findings

A. Hypomagnesemia
B. Hypocalcemia
C. Hypokalemia
D. Hypophosphatemia
E. Hypocalciuria

Electrocardiographic Findings

A. T wave changes
B. Prolonged Q-T interval
C. Widened QRS complex
D. Atrial and ventricular extrasystoles
E. Tachydysrhythmias, including torsade de pointes
F. Potentiation of digoxin effects

Treatment

A. Parenteral magnesium supplementation is indicated in symptomatic patients or for those with serum levels less than 1 mEq/L.

B. Symptomatic patients generally have a deficit of 1 to 2 mEq/kg body weight.

C. As much as 2 to 4 mEq/kg body weight may be necessary in patients with increased renal excretion.

D. Up to 49 mEq of magnesium can be administered every 12 hours for a limited period.

E. Parenteral magnesium supplementation
   1. Magnesium sulfate for injection ($MgSO_4 \cdot 7H_2O$)
      a. Each 1 g of the hydrated salt contains 4.1 mmol of the salt and 4.1 mmol (99 mg) of elemental magnesium.

   b. Each 1 g of the hydrated salt contains 8.1 mEq of the salt and 8.1 mEq of magnesium.

   c. Available as 10%, 20%, and 50% solutions for injection; the concentrated solutions must be diluted due to their hyperosmolarity and irritating effects on vasculature (osmolarity of 50% solution is 4060 mOsm/L)

> **WARNING**
>
> Do not specify dosing of magnesium sulfate in "amps." $MgSO_4 \cdot 7H_2O$ is available in vials and ampules of various concentrations (e.g., 10%, 20%, and 50%) and volumes (e.g., 2 mL and 50 mL). Inadvertent substitution of one size unit for another has led to fatal overdoses.

2. Emergent treatment of life-threatening ventricular dysrhythmias associated with severe hypomagnesemia
   a. Initially give 2 g $MgSO_4 \cdot 7H_2O$ IV over 2 minutes.
   b. Follow with 5 g in 250 mL of saline over 6 hours.
   c. If necessary, follow with 10 g/day by continuous infusion until hypomagnesemia resolves.

3. Moderate magnesium depletion treated with magnesium sulfate
   a. Dose of 2 to 6 g is given over 2 to 6 hours and repeated every 6 to 12 hours.
   b. Titrate dosing by serial serum magnesium levels.

4. Mild
   a. Oral magnesium supplements may be employed.
   b. Typical dosing: 10 mmol PO every 6 to 12 hours (see later under Oral magnesium formulations)
   c. Alternatively, supplementation may be accomplished by IM (e.g., 2 to 4 mL 50% magnesium sulfate for injection at two sites) or IV administration of magnesium sulfate.

F. Oral magnesium formulations
   1. Magnesium chloride hexahydrate tablets: one 833 mg tablet contains 100 mg, 4.1 mmol, or 8.2 mEq of elemental magnesium.
   2. Magnesium oxide tablets: e.g., one 400 mg tablet contains 241 mg, 10 mmol, or 20 mEq of elemental magnesium.

3. Magnesium gluconate dihydrate tablets: e.g., one 500 mg tab contains 27 mg, 1.1 mmol, or 2.2 mEq of elemental magnesium.

4. Magnesium lactate: e.g., one 835 mg tablet contains 84 mg, 3.5 mmol, or 7.0 mEq of elemental magnesium

5. Other formulations include magaldrate and magnesium hydroxide, trisilicate, and citrate tablets or suspension.

G. Follow serum magnesium concentration, especially in patients with renal dysfunction.

H. Correct any coexisting electrolyte deficiencies.

B Bibliography

Agus ZS, Massry SG. Hypomagnesemia and hypermagnesemia. In: Narins RG (ed). Clinical Disorders of Fluid and Electrolyte Metabolism, 5th ed. New York: McGraw-Hill; 1994, pp 1099–1119.

Baran DT. Disorders of mineral metabolism. In: Irwin RS, Cerra FB, Rippe JM (eds). Intensive Care Medicine, 4th ed. Philadelphia: Lippincott-Raven; 1999, pp 1283–1289.

Fawcett WJ, Haxby EJ, Male DA. Magnesium: physiology and pharmacology. Br J Anaesth 1999;83:302–320.

Frakes MA, Richardson LE II. Magnesium sulfate therapy for certain emergency conditions. Am J Emerg Med 1997;15:182–187.

Kelepouris E, Agus ZS. Hypomagnesemia: renal magnesium handling. Semin Nephrol 1998;18:58–73.

44 Hypermagnesemia

Jorge A. Guzman
James A. Kruse

Definition

Hypermagnesmia is present when the plasma or serum magnesium concentration is greater than 2.3 mg/dL, 0.95 mmol/L, or 1.90 mEq/L.

Etiology

A. Acute or chronic renal insufficiency or failure

B. Magnesium therapy (excessive supplementation in hypomagnesemia or eclampsia)

C. Administration of magnesium-containing antacids, laxatives, and urologic irrigation solutions

D. Adrenal insufficiency

E. In vivo hemolysis

F. Hyperparathyroidism

G. Diabetic ketoacidosis (transient)

H. Lithium intoxication

I. Spurious hypermagnesemia
  1. Sporadic laboratory error
  2. In vitro hemolysis

Clinical Findings

A. Hyporeflexia, anticonvulsant effects (>4 mg/dL)

B. Loss of deep tendon reflexes, flushing, lethargy (>5 mg/dL)

C. Flushing, diaphoresis, drowsiness (>6 mg/dL)

D. Nausea, emesis, weakness, somnolence (>7 mg/dL)

E. Diplopia, prolonged electrocardiographic PR interval (>9 mg/dL)

F. Respiratory depression, hypotension (>10 mg/dL)

G. Complete heart block, paralysis, respiratory arrest, cardiac arrest (>13 mg/dL)

PEARLS

- The most common cause of hypermagnesemia in hospitalized patients is renal failure.

- The actions of magnesium on the central nervous system are antagonized by calcium.

- Definitive treatment of hypermagnesemia requires increasing magnesium excretion (via kidneys or dialysis).

Treatment

A. Institute continuous electrocardiographic monitoring to detect life-threatening dysrhythmias.

B. Discontinue all magnesium administration, including magnesium-containing antacids and parenteral nutrition formulas.

C. Calcium
  1. Calcium antagonizes the actions of magnesium on neuromuscular function.
  2. Emergent treatment should be instituted when magnesium-induced central nervous system depression is suspected.
  3. Administer 20 ml of 10% calcium gluconate (contains 2 g of the salt and 180 mg of elemental calcium) intravenously over 2 to 10 minutes.
  4. Repeat calcium dosing, if necessary, based on electrocardiographic findings.

D. Enhance magnesium excretion
  1. Intravenous fluid administration: e.g., 0.45% saline at 250 mL/hour
  2. Furosemide: e.g., 40 to 80 mg intravenously (if renal function is adequate for diuresis)

E. Intravenous glucose and insulin
  1. May promote movement of magnesium into cells
  2. Effect is temporary; probably lasts no more than 2 hours.

F. Hemodialysis
  1. Highly effective at removing magnesium from the body
  2. Provides definitive treatment for severe cases of hypermagnesemia
  3. Required in patients with marked hypermagnesemia and renal dysfunction

G. Follow serial serum magnesium levels.

B Bibliography

Cao Z, Bideau R, Valdes R Jr, et al. Acute hypermagnesemia and respiratory arrest following infusion of MgSO$_4$ for tocolysis. Clin Chim Acta 1999;285:191–193.

McLaughlin SA, McKinney PE. Antacid-induced hypermagnesemia in a patient with normal renal function and bowel obstruction. Ann Pharmacother 1998;32:312–315.

Navarro-Gonzalez JF. Magnesium in dialysis patients: serum levels and clinical implications. Clin Nephrol 1998; 49:373–378.

Schelling JR. Fatal hypermagnesemia. Clin Nephrol 2000; 53:61–65.

45 Hypophosphatemia

James A. Kruse

Key Physiology

- Phosphorus, as organic and inorganic phosphate, is the main intracellular anion.

- Total body content is about 700 g (23,000 mmol), with approximately 80% existing in bone.

- Normal dietary intake is approximately 1 g/day.

- Only about 1% is located in extracellular fluid.

- Phosphorus is filtered by the glomerulus and largely reabsorbed by the proximal renal tubules.

- Extracellular concentration is regulated by parathormone and 1,25-dihydroxy-vitamin D_3.

- Serum phosphorus normally ranges from 2.4 to 5.0 mg/dL (0.77 to 1.61 mmol/L).

Etiology and Classification

A. Nutritional
   1. Carbohydrate loading (glucose, fructose, glycerol, lactate)
   2. Total parenteral nutrition with inadequate phosphate
   3. Intravenous glucose infusion
   4. Low phosphate intake
   5. Alcoholism
   6. Malnutrition, cachexia
   7. Refeeding syndrome
   8. Vitamin D deficiency

B. Acid-base
   1. Respiratory or metabolic alkalosis
   2. Vomiting
   3. Post-hypercapnia
   4. Metabolic acidosis

C. Drugs
   1. Antacids and related compounds
      a. Aluminum-containing antacids (e.g., aluminum hydroxide, aluminum carbonate)
      b. Calcium-containing antacids or calcium supplements (e.g., calcium carbonate, calcium acetate)
      c. Sevelamer
      d. Sucralfate
   2. Diuretics: acetazolamide, loop diuretics, thiazide diuretics, metolazone, osmotic agents (e.g., mannitol, glycerol)
   3. Androgens
   4. Salicylate intoxication
   5. Sodium bicarbonate, sodium lactate
   6. Pamidronate, alendronate
   7. Gallium nitrate
   8. Steroids
   9. Ifosfamide
   10. Acute barium poisoning
   11. Acetaminophen (overdose)
   12. Aminoglycoside (toxicity)
   13. Cisplatin

D. Illnesses
   1. Alcohol withdrawal
   2. Gastrointestinal
      a. Malabsorption, steatorrhea
      b. Dietary deficiency
      c. Vomiting, nasogastric suction
      d. Diarrhea or gastrointestinal fistula loss
   3. Increased renal phosphate loss
      a. Diuretics (see 2. above)
      b. Renal tubular dysfunction: Fanconi's syndrome, multiple myeloma, lupus erythematosus
      c. Hyperparathyroidism
      d. Post−renal transplantation
      e. Diuretic phase of acute renal failure
      f. Familial X-linked (vitamin D-resistant) rickets
      g. Hereditary hypophosphatemic rickets with hypercalciuria
      h. Idiopathic hypercalciuria
      i. Gitelman's syndrome
      j. Volume expansion
      k. Sodium bicarbonate infusion
      l. Steroids
      m. Hypokalemia
      n. Hypomagnesemia
      o. Pregnancy

4. Periodic paralysis

5. Acute gout

6. Acute myocardial infarction

7. Sepsis

8. Exacerbation of chronic obstructive lung disease

9. Acute asthma

10. Acute respiratory failure

11. Pancreatitis

12. Hungry bone syndrome

13. Neuroleptic malignant syndrome

14. Oncogenic hypophosphatemia

15. Paraneoplastic hypophosphatemia

16. Hypophosphatemic bone disease

17. Acute malaria

18. Essential hypertension

E. Hormonal

1. Diabetes

a. Hyperglycemia

b. Treatment phase of diabetic ketoacidosis

c. Hyperosmolar nonketotic syndrome

2. Hyperinsulinemia

3. Hyperparathyroidism (primary and secondary)

4. Androgen use

5. Corticosteroids

6. Adrenergic agents: epinephrine, dopamine, terbutaline, albuterol

7. Erythropoietin

8. Other hormones: insulin, calcitonin, glucagon, gastrin

F. Other

1. Hemodialysis

2. Osteomalacia

3. Severe burn injury

4. Recovery from hypothermia

5. Rickets (vitamin D deficient, dependent, resistant

6. Postoperative state

7. Bone marrow transplantation

PEARL

In the intensive care unit setting, hypophosphatemia is common and the etiology is often multifactorial.

Clinical Manifestations

A. Musculoskeletal: muscle weakness (especially proximal muscles), myalgia, bone pain, rhabdomyolysis, myopathy, osteomalacia, osteopenia, rickets, fractures, pseudofractures

B. Respiratory: respiratory muscle weakness, respiratory failure, mechanical ventilator dependence

C. Cardiac: decreased myocardial contractility, impaired vasopressor response

D. Renal: rhabdomyolysis-related acute tubular necrosis

E. Hematologic: hemolytic anemia, impaired leukocyte function, platelet dysfunction

F. Neurologic: malaise, weakness, paresthesias, Guillain-Barré-like syndrome, altered mentation, irritability, dysarthria, ataxia, encephalopathy, tremor, seizures

Laboratory Findings

A. Hypophosphatemia

1. Mild hypophosphatemia: 2.0 to 2.3 mg/dL (0.65 to 0.74 mmol/L)

2. Moderate hypophosphatemia: 1.0 to 1.9 mg/dL (0.32 to 0.61 mmol/L)

3. Severe hypophosphatemia: lower than 1.0 mg/dL (<0.32 mmol/L)

B. Spurious hypophosphatemia

1. Described in multiple myeloma and polyclonal hyperglobulinemia, as being due to immunoglobulin interference with assay

2. Described after large doses of mannitol as being interference with some molybdate-based colorimetric assays

3. Leukemia with blast crisis, due to in vitro phosphate uptake by leukocytes

C. Other associated blood abnormalities

1. Hypermagnesemia

2. Hemolytic anemia

3. Hyperglycemia

D. Possible associated urine abnormalities

1. Hypercalciuria

2. Hypermagnesuria

3. Bicarbonaturia

Treatment

A. Stop phosphate-binding antacids or other causative agents

B. Phosphate supplementation

1. General

   a. Do not express therapeutic phosphate orders in milliequivalents (because the mass or molar amount of phosphate, or elemental phosphorus contained in the preparation, will vary with the pH of the preparation).

   b. Express therapeutic phosphate in mmol/L (conversion to mEq/L is a function of pH).

   c. Sometimes expressed as milligrams of elemental phosphorus (i.e., the phosphorus content of the phosphate preparation)

   d. 1 mmol of phosphate converts to 31 mg elemental phosphorus.

   e. 1 mmol/L solution of phosphate converts to 3.1 mg/dL of elemental phosphorus.

2. Oral supplementation

   a. Generally preferred over IV, unless hypophosphatemia is severe or patient is n.p.o.

   b. Recommended initial oral dose: 1 to 2 g/day (~30 to 60 mmol) in three or four divided doses

   c. Mild hypophosphatemia can be treated orally with milk (phosphorus content: approximately 1 mg/mL or 0.3 mmol/mL), neutral phosphate tablets or powders, or sodium phosphate laxatives

   d. Neutral phosphate

      (1) Contains a 4:1 ratio of $HPO_4^{2-}:H_2PO_4^-$, with a resulting pH of 7.4 at 37°C

      (2) Several sodium and potassium-containing preparations are commercially available.

      (3) Product formulations vary, but neutral phosphate tablets and unit-dose powdered concentrates typically provide the equivalent of approximately 250 mg (~8 mmol) elemental phosphorus per tablet or unit dose, with varying amounts of sodium and potassium depending on the preparation.

   e. Diarrhea is a common side effect of oral phosphates.

3. Intravenous supplementation

   a. For severe hypophosphatemia or if patient is n.p.o.

   b. Do not give IV phosphate in hypercalcemia.

   c. First select sodium or potassium phosphate.

      (1) Consider potassium phosphate if the patient is significantly hypokalemic.

      (2) Consider sodium phosphate if the patient is not significantly hypokalemic.

      (3) 15 mmol of potassium phosphate contains 22 mmol potassium.

   d. Conventional slow IV infusion method: 7 to 15 mmol sodium or potassium phosphate in at least 100 mL saline intravenously over 6 to 12 hours, depending on severity of hypophosphatemia

   e. Rapid infusion method: 15 mmol sodium or potassium phosphate in at least 100 mL saline IV over 1 to 3 hours; repeat up to a total of three successive infusions (depending on severity of hypophosphatemia)

   f. Reassess serum potassium (if given as potassium salt) and phosphorus after infusion prior to administering additional phosphate supplements.

   g. Stop parenteral administration when serum phosphorus reaches approximately 2.0 mg/dL.

4. Phosphate use in total parenteral nutrition (TPN)

   a. Typical TPN orders include 10 to 15 mmol/L phosphate in the TPN solution.

   b. Up to 20 mmol/L may be necessary initially if the patient is hypophosphatemic.

   c. Measure serum phosphorus daily and titrate the phosphate concentration of the TPN solution.

5. Reassess serum phosphorus levels during therapy.

6. Monitor serum calcium and magnesium levels.

C. Treat underlying cause.

D. Complications of parenteral phosphate

1. Hyperphosphatemia

2. Secondary effects

   a. Hypocalcemia

   b. Hypomagnesemia

   c. Hyperkalemia (with use of potassium phosphate salts)

   d. Metastatic calcinosis

   e. Hypotension

   f. Cardiac dysrhythmias

   g. Conduction disturbances, heart block

   h. Cardiac dysrhythmias, prolonged QT interval, cardiac arrest

   i. Acute renal failure

Key Treatment

- Express phosphate orders in millimoles phosphate, millimoles phosphorus, or milligrams elemental phosphorus.

- Do not express phosphate orders in milliequivalents.

- Typical oral supplement dose: 250 mg elemental phosphorus as neutral phosphate three times a day, initially

- Intravenous supplementation for severe hypophosphatemia in the ICU: 15 mmol or less sodium or potassium phosphate in at least 100 mL saline over at least 1 hour

- Recheck serum phosphorus level after supplementation.

Bibliography

Ambuhl PM, Meier D, Wolf B, et al. Metabolic aspects of phosphate replacement therapy for hypophosphatemia after renal transplantation: impact on muscular phosphate content, mineral metabolism, and acid/base homeostasis. Am J Kidney Dis 1999;34:875–883.

Bugg NC, Jones JA. Hypophosphatemia. Pathophysiology, effects and management on the intensive care unit. Anaesthesia 1998;3:895–902.

Kruse JA, Al-Douahji M, Carlson RW. Rapid intravenous phosphorus replacement in critically ill patients. Crit Care Med 1992;20:S104.

Perreault MM, Ostrop NJ, Tierney MG. Efficacy and safety of intravenous phosphate replacement in critically ill patients. Ann Pharmacother 1997;31:683–688.

Subramanian R, Khardori R. Severe hypophosphatemia. Pathophysiologic implications, clinical presentations, and treatment. Medicine 2000;79:1–8.

46 Hyperphosphatemia

James A. Kruse

Etiology

A. Increased exogenous phosphate load
1. Increased dietary phosphate intake
2. Oral or enteral phosphate supplementation
   a. Oral intake of phosphate supplements
   b. Oral intake of phosphate-containing laxatives
   c. Rectal administration of phosphate-containing enema products
3. Iatrogenic IV phosphate administration
   a. Phosphate-containing IV fluids used to treat hypophosphatemia
   b. Phosphate-containing total parenteral nutrition (TPN) formula
4. Vitamin D intoxication
5. Transfusion of stored blood
6. Acute white or yellow elemental phosphorus poisoning
7. Cutaneous injury from white phosphorus

B. Decreased renal phosphate excretion
1. Decreased glomerular filtration rate
   a. Chronic renal failure
   b. Acute renal failure
2. Increased tubular reabsorption
   a. Hypoparathyroidism
   b. Pseudohypoparathyroidism (type I or type II)
   c. Magnesium deficiency
   d. Etidronate disodium
   e. Furosemide
   f. Clonidine
   g. Acromegaly
   h. Hyperthyroidism
   i. Post-menopausal state or post-oophorectomy
   j. Estrogen therapy in women with osteoporosis
   k. Glucocorticoid withdrawal
   l. Post–unilateral adrenalectomy
   m. Tumoral calcinosis
   n. Juvenile hypogonadism
   o. Cortical hyperostosis
   p. Hypophosphatasia
   q. Insulin-like growth factor I
   r. Heparin

C. Transcellular shift
1. Respiratory acidosis
2. Untreated diabetic ketoacidosis
3. Lactic acidosis
4. Rhabdomyolysis
5. Tumor lysis syndrome (postcytolytic therapy)
   a. Burkitt's lymphoma
   b. Lymphoblastic leukemia
   c. Metastatic small-cell lung cancer
   d. Adenocarcinoma of the breast
6. In vivo hemolysis
7. Extensive intestinal infarction
8. Fulminant hepatic necrosis
9. Malignant hyperthermia
10. Severe hypothermia
11. Spontaneous hyperphosphatemia of leukemia

D. Spurious hyperphosphatemia
1. Prolonged delay in measurement
2. In vitro hemolysis
3. Hyperbilirubinemia
4. Hyperglobulinemia
5. Hyperlipidemia
6. Heparin sodium contamination

E. Other
1. Volume contraction, hemorrhagic shock
2. Familial hyperphosphatemia
3. Fluoride poisoning
4. β-Adrenergic blocking drugs
5. Verapamil
6. Sleep deprivation

Key Etiology and Epidemiology

- Most commonly seen in patients with chronic renal failure

- Otherwise an uncommon electrolyte disturbance

- Can be iatrogenic from excess phosphate administration from various sources

151

Clinical Manifestations

A. Usually asymptomatic
B. Metastatic tissue calcification
   1. Responsible for most manifestations
   2. More likely in alkaline tissues
   3. Occurs in heart, blood vessels, lungs, kidneys, gastric mucosa, cornea
C. Systemic findings
   1. Soft tissue
      a. Soft-tissue calcification
      b. Papular skin eruptions
      c. Osteodystrophy
      d. Necrosis of skin, fingers, toes from vascular calcinosis (calciphylaxis)
      e. Muscle tetany from associated hypocalcemia
   2. Ophthalmologic
      a. Corneal clouding
      b. Conjunctivitis
   3. Cardiac
      a. Conduction disturbances
      b. Dysrhythmias
      c. Heart failure
      d. Cardiac arrest
   4. Renal
      a. Underlying renal failure (commonly the cause of hyperphosphatemia)
      b. Acute renal dysfunction
         (1) Caused by nephrocalcinosis
         (2) Caused by myoglobinuria (in rhabdomyolysis)
         (3) Caused by urate nephropathy (in tumor lysis syndrome)
   5. Gastrointestinal
      a. Anorexia
      b. Nausea, emesis
      c. Ileus
      d. Hemorrhage

Laboratory Findings

A. By definition, serum phosphorus level higher than 5.0 mg/dL (1.61 mmol/L)
B. Calcium-phosphate product
   1. Multiply serum calcium by serum phosphate concentration.
   2. Normal is approximately 40 mg^2/dL^2.
   3. In vitro solubility product is 58 mg^2/dL^2.
   4. Metastatic calcification likely when product is more than 70 mg^2/dL^2.

C. Usually there is underlying renal insufficiency (i.e., increased serum creatinine concentration)
D. If caused by cell lysis (especially if concomitant renal dysfunction)
   1. Possible concomitant hyperkalemia
   2. Possible concomitant hyperuricemia
E. May be associated hypocalcemia, which can be symptomatic
F. Parathormone level may be increased or decreased.
G. Metabolic acidosis can occur with exogenous phosphate intoxication.

Treatment

A. Stop all forms of phosphate administration.
   1. Oral phosphate supplements
   2. Phosphate in IV solutions, including TPN solutions
   3. Phosphate-containing laxatives
   4. Phosphate-containing enema preparations
B. Restrict dietary phosphate intake (e.g., 600 to 900 mg/day).
C. Administer oral or enteral phosphate binders (best effect if taken with meals).
   1. Calcium salts (e.g., carbonate, acetate)
      a. Typical initial dosing in renal failure: 1 g with each meal
      b. Increase to 2 to 12 g/day.
      c. Contraindicated if patient is hypercalcemic
      d. May predispose to metastatic calcification in severe hyperphosphatemia
   2. Aluminum hydroxide or carbonate
      a. Can be used acutely if hyperphosphatemia is accompanied by hypercalcemia
      b. Associated morbidity from aluminum toxicity, especially with chronic use
   3. Sevelamer
      a. Nonabsorbable calcium- and aluminum-free phosphate binder
      b. Less increase in serum calcium and serum calcium-phosphate product compared to calcium salts
   4. Sucralfate
      a. Sucrose octasulfate and polyaluminum hydroxide complex
      b. Has phosphate-binding properties
D. Intravenous glucose and insulin: shifts a limited amount of phosphate into cells transiently
E. Improve underlying renal dysfunction, if possible.
F. Special circumstances
   1. Renal failure or intractable, severe hyperphosphatemia

a. Hemodialysis

b. Peritoneal dialysis

c. Hemodiafiltration

2. End-stage renal disease or hypoparathyroidism

a. Oral calcium supplementation

b. Vitamin D supplementation

c. Monitor serum calcium levels to avoid hypercalcemia

3. Tumor lysis syndrome or rhabdomyolysis

a. Saline diuresis (if adequate urine output)

b. Urinary alkalinization to promote phosphate excretion (if patient is not oliguric)

(1) Acetazolamide

(2) Intravenous sodium bicarbonate

c. Caution: in profound hyperphosphatemia alkalinization may aggravate renal dysfunction by causing renotubular calcium phosphate precipitation

G. Monitor serum phosphorus levels during therapy.

H. Monitor serum calcium and magnesium levels.

I. Treat underlying cause.

Key Treatment

- Stop phosphate administration.

- Main treatment is oral phosphate binders.

- Dialysis is also effective treatment.

Bibliography

Bleyer AJ, Burke SK, Dillon M, et al. A comparison of the calcium-free phosphate binder sevelamer hydrochloride with calcium acetate in the treatment of hyperphosphatemia in hemodialysis patients. Am J Kidney Dis 1999; 33:694–701.

Janigan DT, Perey B, Marrie TJ, et al. Skin necrosis: an unusual complication of hyperphosphatemia during total parenteral nutrition therapy. JPEN 1997;21:50–52.

Kirschbaum B. The acidosis of exogenous phosphate intoxication. Arch Intern Med 1998;158:405–408.

Llach F. Hyperphosphatemia in end-stage renal disease patients: pathophysiological consequences. Kidney Int 1999; 56:S31–S37.

Orias M, Mahnensmith RL, Perazella MA. Extreme hyperphosphatemia and acute renal failure after a phosphorus-containing bowel regimen. Am J Nephrol 1999;19:60–63.

47 Acid-Base Disturbances

James A. Kruse

Definitions

A. Acidemia: abnormally low arterial blood pH (<7.36)

B. Alkalemia: abnormally high arterial blood pH (>7.44)

C. Acidosis: a pathological process tending to acidify body fluids

D. Alkalosis: a pathological process tending to alkalinize body fluids

E. Respiratory disorder: an acid-base disturbance caused by pathological alteration involving the respiratory system or its central nervous system control

F. Metabolic disorder: an acid-base disturbance caused by pathological accumulation of organic or inorganic acids, other than H_2CO_3, or loss of HCO_3^- from the body

G. Acute disorder: a respiratory acid-base disturbance that is present for minutes to hours

H. Chronic disorder: a respiratory acid-base disturbance that is present for a matter of days or longer

I. Simple (or uncomplicated) disorder: an isolated cardinal acid-base disturbance, uncomplicated by another cardinal acid-base disturbance

J. Mixed (or complicated) disorder: an acid-base disturbance in which two or three simple acid-base disorders are simultaneously present

K. Serum total CO_2 content (tCO_2)
   1. Assay is commonly performed along with serum Na^+, K^+, and Cl^- concentrations.
   2. Related to bicarbonate (mmol/L) and P_{CO_2} (torr) by: $tCO_2 = HCO_3^- + 0.03 \times P_{CO_2}$

L. Serum anion gap
   1. Calculated as: $Na^+ - Cl^- - tCO_2$
   2. Conventional normal range is 8 to 16 mEq/L

M. Urine anion gap
   1. Calculated from urine electrolyte concentrations as: $Na^+ + K^+ - Cl^-$
   2. Normal is a positive value or approximately 0 mEq/L.

N. Serum osmole gap
   1. Calculated as:

$$Osm - (2 \times Na^+) + (BUN \div 2.8) + (glucose \div 18) + (ethanol \div 4.6)$$

   2. Where serum osmolality (Osm) is expressed as mOsm/kg H_2O; serum sodium is expressed as mmol/L; and serum urea nitrogen (BUN), glucose, and ethanol are expressed as mg/dL
   3. Normal is less than 10 mEq/L.

O. Delta gap ($\Delta gap/\Delta tCO_2$)
   1. The ratio of the change in serum anion gap (mEq/L) over the change in tCO_2 (mmol/L)
   2. Calculated as (serum anion gap $- 12) \div (24 - tCO_2)$
   3. Aids in the differential diagnosis of high anion gap metabolic acidosis and uncovers occult or mixed metabolic disorders

Etiology

A. Respiratory alkalosis
   1. Voluntary hyperventilation
   2. Central nervous system disorders: trauma, tumor, infection, vascular
   3. Psychiatric disorders: anxiety, hysteria, panic disorder
   4. Pulmonary disorders: pulmonary edema, pulmonary embolism, infection, early restrictive disease, pneumothorax
   5. Drug or toxin induced: salicylates, progesterone, methylxanthines, catecholamines, analeptics, dinitrophenol, nicotine
   6. Tissue hypoxia: circulatory shock, hypoxemia, severe anemia
   7. Altered metabolic rate: sepsis, fever, burn injury, thyrotoxicosis
   8. Other causes: post–metabolic acidosis, hepatic failure, mechanical ventilation

B. Respiratory acidosis
   1. Central nervous system disorders
      a. Drugs: sedative, hypnotic, narcotic, anesthetic
      b. Brainstem respiratory center lesions: trauma, tumor, vascular disorders
      c. Central nervous system infections
      d. Intracranial hypertension
      e. Central sleep apnea
   2. Neuromuscular and related disorders
      a. Primary neuromuscular diseases: muscular

dystrophy, myasthenia gravis, Guillain-Barré syndrome, polymyositis

b. Drug or toxin induced: organophosphates, botulism, neuromuscular blocking agents, aminoglycosides

c. Miscellaneous: hypokalemia, myxedema, periodic paralysis

3. Pulmonary disorders

a. Upper airway obstruction: foreign body aspiration, laryngospasm, obstructive sleep apnea

b. Lower airway obstruction: chronic obstructive pulmonary disease, status asthmaticus, foreign body aspiration

c. Severe pulmonary parenchymal disease: pneumonia, pneumonitis, smoke inhalation

d. Severe pulmonary edema

e. Restrictive disorders: kyphoscoliosis, spinal arthritis, fibrothorax, pulmonary fibrosis, flail chest, pneumoconiosis, progressive systemic sclerosis, obesity, ascites, pleural effusion, pneumothorax

f. Mechanical ventilation–induced

C. Metabolic acidosis

1. Normal serum anion gap

a. Diarrhea

b. Renal tubular acidosis

c. HCl or NH_4Cl administration

d. Parenteral nutrition: HCl salts of amino acids

e. Ureteral diversion surgery

f. Some villous adenomas

g. Dilutional acidosis (IV saline administration)

2. High serum anion gap

a. Diabetic or alcoholic ketoacidosis

b. Renal failure

c. Lactic acidosis

d. Methanol poisoning

e. Ethylene glycol poisoning

f. Salicylate overdose

g. Chronic paraldehyde intoxication

D. Metabolic alkalosis

1. Urine chloride concentration lower than 10 mmol/L

a. Vomiting

b. Nasogastric suction

c. Alkali administration

d. Contraction alkalosis

e. Post–diuretic use

f. Decreased chloride intake

g. Posthypercapnia

h. Some villous adenomas

2. Urine chloride concentration higher than 20 mmol/L

a. Ongoing diuretic use

b. Corticosteroid therapy

c. Cushing's syndrome

d. Hyperaldosteronism

e. Barrter's syndrome

f. Hypokalemia

Diagnosis

A. A nomogram (Fig. 47–1) can be used to determine whether arterial blood gas values are consistent with one of the six simple cardinal acid-base disturbances.

B. The following formulas can be used in lieu of the nomogram to determine the expected degree of compensatory change in $PaCO_2$ (torr) or HCO_3^- (mmol/L).

1. Metabolic acidosis:

$$\text{expected } PaCO_2 \approx 1.5 \times HCO_3^- + 8$$

2. Metabolic alkalosis:

$$\text{expected } PaCO_2 \approx 0.9 \times HCO_3^- + 15$$

3. Acute respiratory acidosis:

$$\text{expected } \Delta HCO_3^- \approx 0.1 \times \Delta PaCO_2$$

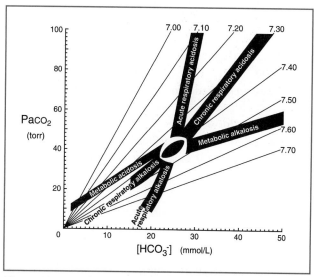

Figure 47–1 Acid-base nomogram. Diagonals represent lines of equal pH. Central ellipse defines normal values. Values lying within the black confidence bands are consistent with the indicated simple acid-base disorder; values elsewhere indicate the presence of a mixed disturbance. (From Kruse JA. Acid-base interpretations. In: Prough DS, Traytsman RJ (eds). Critical Care—State of the Art. Anaheim, CA: Society of Critical Care Medicine, 1993, pp 275–297, with permission.)

4. Chronic respiratory acidosis:

expected $\Delta\,HCO_3^- \approx 0.35 \times \Delta PaCO_2$

5. Acute respiratory alkalosis:

expected $\Delta\,HCO_3^- \approx 0.2 \times \Delta PaCO_2$

6. Chronic respiratory alkalosis:

expected $\Delta\,HCO_3^- \approx 0.4 \times \Delta PaCO_2$

C. If the expected value, calculated from the above formulas, differs substantially from the actual value, either a different isolated disturbance is present or there is a mixed acid-base disturbance.

D. Use of the serum anion gap in the differential diagnosis of metabolic acidosis can be misleading if factors that decrease the serum anion gap are present, e.g.,

1. Hypoalbuminemia
2. Multiple myeloma (with immunoglobulin G)
3. Profound increase in serum K^+, Ca^{2+}, Mg^{2+}
4. Li^+, Br^-, or I^- intoxication

E. Use of the urine anion gap in the differential diagnosis of metabolic acidosis

1. Negative values
   a. Proximal renal tubular acidosis
   b. Diarrhea
   c. Administration of acetazolamide or HCl
2. Positive
   a. Normal
   b. Distal renal tubular acidosis

F. Use of the serum osmole gap in the differential diagnosis of metabolic acidosis

1. High in methanol and ethylene glycol intoxication
2. Also elevated in the following conditions (which are not necessarily associated with metabolic acidosis or a high anion gap)
   a. Ethanol intoxication (will not increase osmole gap if ethanol term is included in equation)
   b. Isopropanol intoxication
   c. Hyperlipidemia or hyperproteinemia (spurious)
   d. Intravenous mannitol infusion
   e. Elevated in circulatory shock (due to largely unidentified endogenous circulating osmoles)

G. Use of the $\Delta gap/\Delta tCO_2$ in the differential diagnosis of metabolic acid-base disturbances

1. $\Delta Gap/\Delta tCO_2$ below 0.3 indicates the presence of a pure normal anion gap metabolic acidosis.

2. $\Delta Gap/\Delta tCO_2$ of approximately 0.8 to 1.2 indicates the presence of a pure high anion gap metabolic acidosis.

3. $\Delta Gap/\Delta tCO_2$ of approximately 0.3 to 0.7 indicates the presence of a normal anion gap metabolic acidosis plus a high anion gap metabolic acidosis.

4. $\Delta Gap/\Delta tCO_2$ exceeding 1.2 indicates the simultaneous presence of metabolic alkalosis plus a high anion gap form of metabolic acidosis.

Key Laboratory Tests

- All cases: arterial blood gases; serum electrolytes, glucose, urea nitrogen, creatinine

- Metabolic acidosis: serum anion gap (if elevated, consider blood lactate and serum ketones, osmole gap, salicylate level; if not elevated, consider urine anion gap)

- Metabolic alkalosis: spot urine chloride concentration

Treatment

A. General management

1. Appropriate treatment requires recognition and accurate characterization of the particular acid-base disturbance(s).
2. Specific treatment options depend on the underlying cause; e.g., dialysis for renal failure, insulin for diabetic ketoacidosis, improving tissue oxygenation and perfusion in hypoxic lactic acidosis, ethanol or 4-methylpyrazole for methanol or ethylene glycol poisoning.

B. Metabolic acidosis

1. Provide specific treatment directed against the underlying cause.
2. Severe acidemia (pH <7.10) may warrant treatment with IV $NaHCO_3$, particularly if due to renal failure, renal tubular acidosis, or intoxication with ethylene glycol, methanol, or salicylate.
3. The necessity and benefit of $NaHCO_3$ treatment in lactic acidosis and ketoacidosis is controversial, but it may be unnecessary even when the acidemia is severe.
4. If $NaHCO_3$ is used, generally do not correct plasma HCO_3^- completely; in severe metabolic acidosis initially aim at raising HCO_3^- to more than 10 mmol/L.
5. The HCO_3^- deficit (mmol) can be estimated

from the current plasma bicarbonate ($HCO_3^-{}_{pre}$) from body weight (in kg) using:

$$HCO_3^- \text{ deficit} = [(2.4/HCO_3^-{}_{pre}) + 0.4] \times \text{weight} \times (HCO_3^-{}_{post} - HCO_3^-{}_{pre})$$

6. Give no more than half of the calculated amount of $NaHCO_3$ initially; rapid IV infusion can have adverse hemodynamic effects.

7. Ongoing H^+ production and HCO_3^- losses are not accounted for in calculated HCO_3^- deficit; therefore, serially assay tCO_2 or arterial blood gases frequently to assess effects of $NaHCO_3$ therapy.

8. Complications of $NaHCO_3$ therapy include fluid overload, hypernatremia, hyperosmolality, over-shoot alkalemia, and hypokalemia.

C. Metabolic alkalosis

1. If possible, discontinue diuretics, nasogastric suction, and corticosteroids; treat underlying cause.

2. Correct any extracellular fluid volume deficit using IV normal saline; high urine Cl^- varieties of metabolic alkalosis are resistant to saline loading.

3. Replace potassium deficits.

4. In rare cases of profound alkalemia with acute potential for life-threatening end-organ consequences (e.g., seizures, ventricular tachydysrhythmias) consider brief HCl infusion.

5. The hydrogen ion deficit (in mmol) can be estimated from the current bicarbonate level (pre), the desired bicarbonate level (post), and body weight (in kg) using:

$$H^+ \text{ deficit} = K \times \text{weight} \times (HCO_3^-{}_{pre} - HCO_3^-{}_{post})$$

a. Value of K in the above formula is 0.2 (conservative) to 0.5.

b. Final HCl concentration is 100 to 200 mmol/L, always infused by central venous catheter.

c. Maximal infusion rate not to exceed approximately 0.2 mmol/kg per hour

d. Monitor arterial blood gases frequently.

D. Respiratory alkalosis

1. Treat underlying cause, if possible.

2. In mechanically ventilated patients, decrease ventilator rate, tidal volume, or mandatory minute ventilation settings (often not effective if patient is actively triggering mechanical ventilator).

3. If not due to inappropriate mechanical ventilator settings, mild to moderate respiratory alkalosis usually does not require treatment, per se.

4. Added dead space (between endotracheal tube and ventilator circuit) is employed by some practitioners; add in 50 mL increments and re-check blood gases.

5. High level sedation ± neuromuscular blockade is effective in mechanically ventilated patients but usually is not required.

6. Consider sedation ± paralysis if severe alkalemia is complicated by dysrhythmias or seizures.

E. Respiratory acidosis

1. Treat underlying cause (e.g., naloxone if opiate-induced, bronchodilators if bronchospasm-induced).

2. Spontaneously breathing patients may require mechanical ventilation.

3. In mechanically ventilated patients, increase minute ventilation, rate, or tidal volume settings.

 Key Treatment Points

- Appropriate treatment requires recognition and accurate characterization of the particular acid-base disturbance(s).

- Specific treatment options depend on the underlying cause; e.g., dialysis for renal failure, insulin for diabetic ketoacidosis, improving tissue oxygenation and perfusion in hypoxic lactic acidosis, 4-methylpyrazole for ethylene glycol poisoning, diuresis for pulmonary edema.

 Bibliography

Adrogué HJ, Madias NE. Management of life-threatening acid-base disorders. N Engl J Med 1998;338:26–34 and 107–111.

Arieff AI. Indications for use of bicarbonate in patients with metabolic acidosis. Br J Anaesth 1991;67:165–177.

Friedman BS, Lumb PD. Prevention and management of metabolic alkalosis. J Intensive Care Med 1990;5(Suppl): 522–527.

Kruse JA. Calculation of plasma bicarbonate concentration versus measurement of serum CO_2 content. pK' revisited. Clin Intensive Care 1995;6:15–20.

Kruse JA. Clinical utility and limitations of the anion gap. Int J Intensive Care 1997:51–66.

Shapiro BA, Peruzzi WT, Templin R. Clinical Application of Blood Gases. 5th ed. St. Louis: Mosby, 1994.

Urbina LR, Kruse JA. Blood gas monitoring. In: Carlson RW, Geheb MA (eds). Principles & Practice of Medical Intensive Care. Philadelphia: WB Saunders, 1993, pp 235–251.

48 Lactic Acidosis

James A. Kruse

Although hyperlactatemia is a physiologic response to strenuous exercise, elevated resting blood lactate levels are a serious finding in the intensive care unit (ICU) patient. The most common cause is hypoperfusion due to frank circulatory shock, which results in tissue hypoxia and partial reliance on anaerobic metabolism that generates lactate. Sepsis and seizures are also frequent causes. In severe sepsis and septic shock, the mechanism of the hyperlactatemia is an imbalance between tissue oxygen demand and availability. Seizures, while not uncommon in the ICU, are usually a relatively benign and transient cause. In the occasional patient with unexplained lactic acidosis there are many other potential causes to be considered. However, with some notable exceptions, most of these are either uncommon or are uncommonly associated with significant hyperlactatemia.

Etiologies

A. Secondary to tissue hypoxia (type A)

1. Cardiac arrest
2. Circulatory shock (cardiogenic, hypovolemia, septic, obstructive, etc.)
3. Severe hypoxemia
4. Profound anemia
5. Grand mal seizures
6. Carbon monoxide poisoning
7. Status asthmaticus (mainly due to decreased venous return from increased intrathoracic pressure)
8. Arterial thromboembolism

B. Secondary to other mechanisms (type B)

1. Associated with certain diseases or illnesses (type B_1)
   a. Thiamine deficiency (an enzyme cofactor necessary for lactate metabolism)
   b. Sepsis (mechanism not elucidated; may be tissue hypoxia in some cases)
   c. Certain neoplasms (e.g., lymphoma, leukemia, lung cancer, breast cancer)
   d. Liver disease (if associated tissue hypoxia)
   e. Short-bowel syndromes (D-lactic acidosis; see Laboratory Diagnosis, C 7, below)
   f. Pheochromocytoma (catecholamine-stimulated glycolysis)
   g. Respiratory alkalosis (may cause mild hyperlactatemia)

2. Secondary to drugs and toxins (type B_2)
   a. Biguanide hypoglycemic drugs (mainly occurs in patients with renal insufficiency)
      (1) Phenformin
      (2) Metformin
   b. Alcohols (uncommon as sole mechanism)
      (1) Ethanol (alcoholic beverages)
      (2) Methanol (wood alcohol)
      (3) Isopropanol (rubbing alcohol)
   c. Glycols
      (1) Ethylene glycol (found in most automotive antifreeze formulations)
      (2) Propylene glycol (diluent in some parenteral drugs: e.g., phenytoin, lorazepam, nitroglycerin)
   d. Sympathomimetic agents
      (1) Epinephrine (and certain other catecholamines)
      (2) Terbutaline
      (3) Ritodrine
   e. Acetaminophen overdose
   f. Salicylate overdose
   g. Antiretroviral nucleoside analogs
   h. Sorbitol and xylitol
   i. Cyanide (metabolite of sodium nitroprusside)
   j. Isoniazid
   k. Streptozotocin
   l. Fructose
   m. Sodium bicarbonate
   n. Strychnine

3. Congenital forms (type B_3)
   a. von Gierke's disease (type I glycogen storage disease)
   b. Hereditary fructose intolerance
   c. Pyruvate carboxylase deficiency
   d. Fructose 1,6-bisphosphatase deficiency
   e. Inborn defects of oxidative phosphorylation
   f. Pyruvate dehydrogenase deficiency
   g. Kearns-Sayre syndrome
   h. MELAS syndrome (mitochondrial encephalomyopathy with lactic acidosis and stroke)

PEARL

The most common cause of lactic acidosis is circulatory shock.

Clinical Manifestations

A. The signs and symptoms of lactic acidosis are non-specific.

B. Historical and physical findings reflect the underlying cause.

C. Kussmaul respirations may be present if there is significant associated acidemia.

D. Because shock is the most common cause, clinical signs of perfusion failure are common bedside findings.
   1. Hypotension
   2. Oliguria
   3. Altered sensorium
   4. Cool extremities

Laboratory Diagnosis

A. Arterial blood gas analysis
   1. Metabolic acidosis is classically present.
   2. Absence of metabolic acidosis by blood gas analysis does not exclude clinically significant hyperlactatemia.
      a. Discrepancy is due in part to relatively low levels of lactate that can be clinically significant (e.g., 2.5 to 4.0 mmol/L) but have little impact on acid-base balance.
      b. Also due to the frequency of concomitant respiratory or metabolic alkalosis in patients with hyperlactatemia

B. Serum anion gap determination
   1. Calculated from serum electrolyte panel as: $Na^+ - (Cl^- + total\ CO_2\ content)$
   2. Conventional normal range: 8 to 16 mEq/L
   3. Classically elevated in lactic acidosis and other organic acidoses
   4. The finding of an elevated serum anion gap, not explained by ketoacidosis, renal failure, or a toxic ingestion, strongly implicates lactic acidosis.
   5. Normal anion gap does not exclude hyperlactatemia.

C. Direct assay lactate
   1. More sensitive and specific than blood gas analysis or anion gap determination
   2. Should be obtained in all suspected cases

3. Obtaining and handling specimens
   a. Determined on arterial or mixed venous blood samples
   b. Transport heparinized blood sample on ice and assay immediately.
   c. Alternatively, place in grey-top vacuum tube and assay as soon as possible.

4. Upper limit of normal at rest: approximately 1.5 mmol/L

5. Concentrations up to 2.5 mmol/L are of questionable clinical significance.

6. Concentrations higher than 2.5 mmol/L should be considered clinically significant.

7. Commonly employed enzymatic assays detect only L-lactate, not D-lactate.
   a. D-lactate is produced by bowel flora of some patients after intestinal bypass surgery.
   b. Associated with otherwise unexplained metabolic acidosis
   c. Anion gap classically elevated
   d. Blood L-lactate levels normal
   e. Associated with encephalopathy and ataxia

Key Laboratory Findings

- Metabolic acidosis by arterial blood gas analysis

- Elevated anion gap may be present by serum electrolyte panel.

- Absence of laboratory findings suggesting alternative explanations for the above (e.g., serum ketones, hyperglycemia, severe azotemia)

- Elevated blood lactate concentration

Clinical Significance

A. There is a strong, direct correlation between blood lactate concentration and mortality.

B. Resting blood lactate levels higher than 8 mmol/L are associated with a mortality of over 90%.

C. Hyperlactatemia also correlates with the development of multiple organ system failure.

D. In hyperlactatemia due to hypoperfusion, serial blood lactate concentrations allow assessment of the effectiveness of therapeutic interventions and can be used as a physiologic end point for resuscitation.

E. Decreasing lactate signifies improvement in tissue oxygenation, whereas continual elevation is the characteristic pattern in nonsurvivors.

Treatment

A. Primary focus is treatment of the underlying cause.

B. Measures to augment systemic oxygen delivery (effective in hyperlactatemia due to tissue hypoxia or hypoperfusion)

 1. Ensure adequate airway control, ventilation, and arterial blood oxygenation ($SaO_2 > 90\%$).

 2. Administer packed red cells for significant anemia or blood loss.

 3. Employ measures to increase cardiac output, if inadequate.

    a. Control cardiac dysrhythmias.

    b. Intravascular fluid expansion with colloid or isotonic crystalloid if the patient is hypovolemic

    c. Afterload reduction for patients that are not hypotensive and are either hypertensive or have left ventricular dysfunction

    d. Inotropic agents

    e. Vasopressor-inotropic agents for refractory hypotension

    f. Intra-aortic balloon counterpulsation for appropriate cardiogenic causes

 4. Consider systemic and pulmonary artery catheterization for hemodynamic assessment and monitoring.

C. IV alkalinizing agents

 1. Sodium bicarbonate

    a. Traditionally given to reverse the adverse hemodynamic and metabolic consequences of severe acidemia

    b. Controlled trials have failed to show hemodynamic benefit.

    c. Raises blood pH, but may worsen acidosis at the cellular level by generating additional CO_2

    d. Other putative detrimental effects include hyperosmolality, hypervolemia, hypotension, decreased ionized calcium, decreased P_{50}, and increased lactate generation.

 2. Carbicarb

    a. A 1:1 mixture of sodium carbonate and sodium bicarbonate

    b. Generates less CO_2 than sodium bicarbonate

    c. Limited clinical experience; therapeutic role unclear

 3. Tromethamine

    a. Also known as tris(hydroxymethyl)aminomethane or THAM

    b. Does not generate CO_2 during buffering; therefore, should avoid worsening intracellular acidosis

    c. Limited clinical experience; therapeutic role unclear

D. Thiamine

 1. Indicated for lactic acidosis caused by thiamine deficiency

 2. Routinely administered prophylactically with total parenteral nutrition formulas to avoid inducing thiamine deficiency and empirically to patients with alcoholism

 3. Of unproven value for other forms of type B lactic acidosis

E. Dichloroacetate

 1. An investigational drug that indirectly stimulates pyruvate dehydrogenase activity

 2. Effective at lowering blood lactate levels in patients with lactic acidosis

 3. A large clinical trial has shown it to have no effect on survival compared to placebo.

F. Putative treatments of unproven efficacy

 1. Methylene blue

 2. Nitroprusside

 3. Glucose and insulin

 4. Hemodialysis

Key Treatment

- Therapy is directed at underlying etiology.

- Remember that shock is the most common cause.

- Always ensure adequate tissue oxygenation and perfusion.

- $NaHCO_3$ is probably not useful.

Bibliography

Forsythe SM, Schmidt GA. Sodium bicarbonate for the treatment of lactic acidosis. Chest 2000;117:260–267.

Kruse JA. Lactic acidosis: understanding pathogenesis and causes. J Crit Illness 1999;14:456–466.

Kruse JA. Lactic acidosis: clinical significance, diagnosis, and treatment. J Crit Illness 1999;14:514–521.

Stacpoole PW, Wright EC, Baumgartner TG, et al. Natural history and course of acquired lactic acidosis. Am J Med 1994;97:47–54.

49 Alcoholic Ketoacidosis

James A. Kruse

Alcoholic ketoacidosis (AKA) develops in a small minority of chronic alcohol users. Its pathophysiology is incompletely understood but probably involves the combined effects of recent ethanol metabolism, starvation, volume depletion, and abnormal insulin and counterregulatory hormone levels. Although the accompanying acidosis can be severe, it usually follows a transient and benign course if treated with IV fluids and dextrose. On the other hand, the disorder can be complicated by accompanying alcohol-related illnesses.

History

A. Chronic alcohol abuse
B. History of a recent alcoholic binge
C. Binge is followed by 1 to 3 days of little or no caloric intake and abstinence from alcohol.
D. Anorexia, nausea, and vomiting are prominent features.
E. Patient may also complain of malaise and abdominal pain.
F. No history of diabetes mellitus (some patients may have mild glucose intolerance)

Physical Findings

A. Abdomen: tenderness, especially in epigastrium
B. Respiratory: dyspnea, Kussmaul respirations, tachypnea, acetone breath odor
C. Neurologic: lucid sensorium (unless associated alcohol intoxication, withdrawal, or other process)
D. Signs of volume depletion, e.g., tachycardia, flat neck veins
E. Stigmata of chronic liver disease may be present.

Key Differential Diagnosis

- Diabetic ketoacidosis: blood glucose is markedly elevated in diabetic ketoacidosis.

- Starvation ketosis: degree of acidosis can be more severe in AKA than in starvation ketoacidosis.

- Exogenous acetone, methanol, isopropanol, ethylene glycol, or salicylate intoxication: exclude by toxicologic assays and osmole gap.

- Lactic acidosis: significant lactate elevation (>3 mmol/L) suggests underlying severe illness, frank or impending circulatory shock, sepsis, recent seizures, or other cause of lactic acidosis.

Associated Illnesses

A. Alcohol intoxication (in most cases resolved by the time of presentation)
B. Alcohol withdrawal (including seizures)
C. Alcoholic gastritis
D. Pancreatitis
E. Gastrointestinal hemorrhage (from Mallory-Weiss tear, gastritis, ulcers, esophageal varices, hemorrhoids)
F. Alcoholic hepatitis
G. Thiamine deficiency
H. Circulatory shock from volume depletion or hemorrhage
I. Aspiration pneumonitis
J. Rhabdomyolysis

Laboratory Findings

A. Acid-base disturbances
 1. Metabolic acidosis
    a. Always present; due to excessive production of ketoacids
    b. Usually manifests as low serum CO_2 content and low arterial blood pH and bicarbonate concentration and pH
    c. Acidemia may be mild to severe, or absent if concomitant alkalosis.
    d. Serum anion gap ($Na - Cl - CO_2$ content) is elevated (>16 mmol/L).
 2. Concomitant metabolic alkalosis is a possibility.
    a. Secondary to vomiting and volume contraction
    b. In some cases the metabolic alkalosis is severe enough to counter the acidemia and yield a normal or even elevated arterial blood pH (underlying acidosis remains detectable by high anion gap).
 3. Concomitant respiratory alkalosis may be present, secondary to sepsis, alcohol withdrawal, or underlying liver disease.
B. Ketosis
 1. Due to elevated plasma acetone, acetoacetate, and (particularly) β-hydroxybutyrate concentrations

2. Detectable levels of acetone and acetoacetate are usually present in serum or urine.

3. Serum β-hydroxybutyrate level is always elevated.

4. The β-hydroxybutyrate-to-acetoacetate ratio is higher (4 to 10:1) in AKA than in diabetic ketoacidosis (~3:1).

5. Because ketosis is usually assessed by the semiquantitative nitroprusside test, which reacts with acetone and acetoacetate but not with β-hydroxybutyrate, the degree of detectable ketosis may be disproportionately less than the degree of acidosis.

6. In some cases there may be no evidence of ketosis by the nitroprusside test.

C. Elevated blood lactate

1. Usually normal or slightly elevated

2. Higher levels suggest another explanation such as circulatory shock, sepsis, or recent seizures.

D. Blood glucose concentration

1. Hypoglycemia may occur.

2. Mild hyperglycemia may occur.

E. Serum osmole gap

1. Calculate as: measured serum osmolality [mOsm/kg H_2O] − (2 × serum sodium [mmol/L]) − (serum urea nitrogen [mg/dL] ÷ 2.8) − (serum glucose [mg/dL] ÷ 18) − (serum ethanol [mg/dL] ÷ 4.6).

2. Normal is usually defined as less than or equal to 10 mOsm/kg H_2O.

3. Slight elevations have been described in AKA.

4. Elevation also suggests methanol, isopropanol, or ethylene glycol poisoning, all of which must be considered and excluded.

F. Toxicology studies: negative for salicylates, toxic alcohols, and glycols

---

Key Laboratory Findings

- High anion gap metabolic acidosis

- Increased serum and urine ketones

- Acidosis out of proportion to ketosis by nitroprusside test

- Normal, low, or mildly elevated blood glucose

- Blood ethanol may be present or undetectable.

- Negative toxicologic studies for methanol and ethylene glycol

---

Treatment

A. General measures

1. Ensure all relevant diagnostic tests are ordered.

a. Serum sodium, potassium, chloride, CO_2 content, magnesium, calcium, phosphorus, glucose, urea nitrogen, creatinine, osmolality, creatine phosphokinase, semiquantitative ketone test, liver function tests, ethanol, methanol, ethylene glycol, isopropanol, and (if available) β-hydroxybutyrate and quantitative acetone levels

b. Complete blood cell count, prothrombin time and partial thromboplastin time

c. Urine semiquantitative ketone test

d. Arterial blood gases

e. Monitor glucose frequently to detect hypoglycemia or hyperglycemia.

f. Calculate serum anion and osmole gaps (see Chapter 47, Acid-Base Disturbances and Chapter 68, Alcohol and Glycol Intoxications).

g. Chest and abdominal x-ray films

h. Serial glucose, electrolytes, and arterial blood gases

2. Nothing by mouth, due to frequent occurrence of associated nausea, vomiting, and other gastrointestinal disturbances

3. Nasogastric intubation may be necessary in the presence of active vomiting, pancreatitis, or gastrointestinal bleeding.

4. Monitor fluid intake and output.

5. Establish IV access.

6. Consider central venous pressure monitoring, especially if there is bleeding, pancreatitis, or signs of instability.

7. Monitor for signs of alcohol withdrawal.

8. Institute seizure precautions.

B. Intravenous fluid

1. Administer 500 mL to 1 L of 5% dextrose in normal saline for at least 1 hour.

2. After correcting hypovolemia, use 5% dextrose in either normal or hypotonic saline.

3. Titrate further administration to provide maintenance fluid, cover for any ongoing losses, and correct any remaining fluid deficit.

C. Dextrose

1. Parenteral dextrose administration is central to rapid recovery.

2. Intravenous fluid solutions should contain 5% dextrose (with or without saline).

3. If hypoglycemia occurs

    a. Give 50 mL 50% dextrose.

    b. Increase rate or concentration of continuous dextrose infusion.

    c. Increase frequency of blood glucose monitoring.

D. Vitamins

    1. Give 100 mg IV thiamine daily.

    2. Give IV multivitamin supplement daily.

E. Insulin

    1. Not necessary in most cases

    2. Regular insulin may be utilized in unusual cases if marked hyperglycemia develops after IV dextrose is given.

F. Electrolyte monitoring and supplementation

    1. Monitor serial potassium, CO_2 content, magnesium, phosphorus, and anion gap levels.

    2. Provide potassium, magnesium, and phosphorus supplementation if necessary.

G. Sodium bicarbonate

    1. Generally unnecessary, even in severe AKA

    2. If administered, overshoot alkalemia may occur, especially if there is underlying concomitant metabolic alkalosis.

H. Evaluate for associated illnesses, as indicated:

    1. Cultures of blood, urine, and other body fluids as indicated by fever, leukocytosis, or other signs of infection

2. Serum amylase and lipase to evaluate for pancreatitis

3. Complete blood count to evaluate for anemia, thrombocytopenia, leukocytosis

4. Evaluation for gastrointestinal hemorrhage: stool guaiac testing, nasogastric intubation

5. Other blood tests, imaging studies, etc. as indicated by history, physical examination, screening laboratory tests

Key Treatment

- Intravenous fluids, dextrose, vitamins
- Insulin rarely necessary
- Sodium bicarbonate not indicated
- Serial blood tests (including glucose)
- Exclude alternative diagnoses.
- Assess for complicating illness.

Bibliography

Cuevas-Korensky CE, Kruse JA, Carlson RW. Characteristic findings in patients with alcoholic ketoacidosis. Chest 1991;100:81S.

Dillon ES, Dyer WW, Smelo LS. Ketone acidosis in nondiabetic adults. Med Clin North Am 1940;24:1813–1822.

Fulop M. Alcoholic ketoacidosis. Endocrinol Metab Clin North Am 1993;22:209–219.

Schelling JR, Howard RL, Winter SD, et al. Increased osmolal gap in alcoholic ketoacidosis and lactic acidosis. Ann Intern Med 1990;113:580–582.

50 Diabetic Ketoacidosis

James A. Kruse

Diabetic ketoacidosis (DKA) occurs when there is complete or near complete lack of insulin, resulting in decreased peripheral glucose utilization and increased gluconeogenesis, lipolysis, and ketogenesis. It can also occur when a severe physiologic stress markedly increases insulin requirements that cannot be met by the diabetic pancreas. It may occur in patients with a previous diagnosis of insulin-dependent or non-insulin-dependent diabetes, or as the first manifestation of diabetes mellitus.

Precipitating Factors

A. Noncompliance with diet or insulin therapy
B. Infection
C. Trauma
D. Acute myocardial infarction
E. Cerebrovascular accident
F. Pregnancy
G. Pancreatitis
H. Drug or alcohol use
I. Other intercurrent illness

Clinical Manifestations

A. Constitutional symptoms: malaise, generalized weakness, myalgias, thirst, polydipsia, polyuria
B. Gastrointestinal: nausea, vomiting, anorexia, abdominal pain, abdominal tenderness, gastroparesis, ileus
C. Neurologic: orthostatic lightheadedness, lethargy, headache, delirium, obtundation
D. Respiratory: dyspnea, Kussmaul respirations, tachypnea, pleurisy, acetone breath odor
E. Cardiovascular: tachycardia, flat neck veins, orthostatic or frank hypotension
F. Other: signs of volume depletion and hypoperfusion; e.g., slowed capillary refilling, decreased skin turgor, furrowed tongue, dry mucous membranes, sunken eye globes, decreased axillary perspiration, cool extremities

Laboratory Findings

A. Hyperglycemia
 1. Blood glucose typically elevated to 400 to 800 mg/dL, higher in some cases
 2. Secondary glycosuria and plasma hyperosmolality
B. Metabolic acidosis
 1. Low blood HCO_3^- and serum total CO_2 content (tCO_2): typically less than 15 mmol/L, but may be severely decreased (<5 mmol/L); rarely they can be normal or even elevated if there is concomitant metabolic alkalosis that is severe.
 2. Low blood pH: lower than 7.35, but may be severely decreased (<7.00); rarely may be normal or even elevated if there is concomitant metabolic or respiratory alkalosis of sufficient severity
 3. Acidosis is due to excessive production of ketoacids.
 4. See Chapter 47, Acid-Base Disturbances, for differential diagnosis of metabolic acidosis.
C. Serum anion gap ($Na^+ - Cl^- - tCO_2$)
 1. Serum anion gap is usually elevated (>16 mEq/L) due to increased circulating acetoacetate and β-hydroxybutyrate concentrations.
 2. The high anion gap metabolic acidosis present initially usually changes to a nonanion gap metabolic acidosis during the treatment phase.
 3. Rarely, the anion gap is within normal limits at presentation in spite of significant ketoacidosis. This occurs in patients who can maintain a near-normal hydration state that allows urinary ketoacid anion losses to parallel ketoacid production, thus preventing significant excess ketoacid anion accumulation.
D. Ketosis
 1. Detectable levels of acetone, acetoacetate, and β-hydroxybutyrate are usually present in serum and urine.
 2. The standard semiquantitative test for serum and urine "ketones" is the nitroprusside reaction, which detects acetone and acetoacetate but not β-hydroxybutyrate.
 3. β-Hydroxybutyrate and acetoacetate are interconvertible in vivo, typically present in a 3:1 ratio in DKA. This ratio increases in the presence of concomitant tissue hypoperfusion and hypoxia, which shifts acetoacetate to β-hydroxybutyrate and decreases the apparent ketone level as detected by the nitroprusside reaction,

even if the total ketone concentration has not changed.

4. Although acetoacetate and β-hydroxybutyrate are metabolized once adequate insulin is available during treatment, acetone is only slowly eliminated by the kidney and respiratory tract. Therefore, persistent acetonemia may not reflect ongoing ketoacid production during the recovery phase.

E. Azotemia

1. Serum urea nitrogen concentration and the serum urea to creatinine ratio are usually increased because of extracellular volume depletion.

2. Serum creatinine may be elevated for various reasons:

   a. Underlying chronic diabetic nephropathy

   b. Acute renal dysfunction related to intravascular volume depletion

   c. Interference with certain laboratory assays for creatinine (Jaffe reaction) by high levels of circulating acetoacetate

F. Hypokalemia or hyperkalemia

1. Hyperkalemia is typically present initially as a consequence of insulinopenia (not acidemia), in spite of a marked total body potassium deficit that averages 3 to 6 mmol/kg.

2. Hypokalemia usually manifests shortly after insulin therapy is initiated, which causes potassium to move from the extracellular space to the intracellular space.

G. Hyponatremia or hypernatremia

1. Sodium generally decreases in proportion to the degree of hyperglycemia.

2. This hyponatremia is real, not spurious. The mechanism is dilution secondary to a shift of water from the intracellular space to the extracellular space caused by the osmotic effect of hyperglycemia. This form of hyponatremia resolves in parallel with resolution of the DKA and requires no specific therapy.

3. The expected decrease in serum sodium concentration (mmol/L) can be estimated from the glucose concentration (mg/dL) by:

$$\Delta Na^+ = -0.016 \times (glucose - 100)$$

This is an average relationship and the actual deviation of serum sodium from normal can vary appreciably if there are concomitant independent derangements in total body water balance. Thus, the formula allows detection and quantification of concomitant free water deficits while the patient is hyperglycemic.

4. Excessive pure water losses will tend to counter the dilutional hyponatremia. In some cases this can result in sodium concentrations within normal limits, or hypernatremia.

5. Apart from the above effects, artifactual hyponatremia (i.e., pseudohyponatremia) can occur in patients with extreme hyperlipidemia.

H. Hypophosphatemia and hypomagnesemia

1. May be present initially or develop during treatment

2. Chiefly occur secondary to urinary losses during the glycosuria-induced osmotic diuresis

I. Miscellaneous

1. Elevated serum lipid concentrations

2. Elevated amylase levels: may be of pancreatic or salivary origin

3. Mild leukocytosis: may be seen in the absence of infection

4. Increased hematocrit: due to hemoconcentration

Key Laboratory Findings

- Hyperglycemia and glycosuria
- Increased serum and urine ketones
- Metabolic acidosis with high anion gap
- Hyperkalemia often present initially
- Hypokalemia develops soon after insulin therapy is initiated.

Treatment

A. General measures

1. Closely monitor vital signs.

2. Obtain routine laboratory studies: serum chemistry profile, complete blood count, urinalysis, etc.

3. Monitor serial laboratory tests frequently while the patient is receiving IV insulin.

   a. Measure serum or blood glucose every 1 to 2 hours to monitor progress of therapy and to avoid and detect hypoglycemia.

   b. Measure serum electrolytes every 2 to 6 hours; serial potassium monitoring is particularly important.

   c. Monitor serial arterial blood gas measurements at selected intervals in severe cases.

4. Employ continuous electrocardiographic (ECG) monitoring in severe cases and those with severe hypokalemia or hyperkalemia.

5. Nothing by mouth (due to frequent occurrence of associated nausea, vomiting, other gastrointestinal symptoms, gastric atony, ileus)

6. Nasogastric suction may be necessary in selected patients and those with vomiting.

7. Monitor fluid intake and output; consider need for Foley catheter in severe cases.

8. Hemodynamic monitoring

   a. Central venous pressure measurement helpful in guiding fluid requirements in severe cases

   b. Pulmonary artery catheterization is not required in most patients but may be useful in very unstable patients, those not responding to initial fluid resuscitation, elderly patients, and those with severe sepsis, underlying heart disease, or sustained circulatory shock.

   c. Systemic arterial catheterization may be useful in selected cases for facilitating frequent blood testing and, in unstable patients, for blood pressure monitoring.

9. Evaluate for a precipitating cause; depending on setting, this may include:

   a. Cultures of blood, urine, and other body fluids as indicated by fever, leukocytosis, or other signs of possible infection

   b. Urinalysis

   c. Chest x-ray

   d. Serial 12-lead ECGs and cardiac marker tests

   e. Computed tomography of brain

   f. Other tests and evaluations as indicated by history, physical examination, screening laboratory tests, and imaging studies.

B. Intravenous fluid

1. Rapidly administer 1 or 2 L of normal saline (average fluid deficit in DKA is 4 to 9 L).

2. Follow with 1 L/hour for 1 hour, 500 mL/hour for 1 to 2 hours, and then 200 to 300 mL/hour until the extracellular deficit is corrected; titrate fluids cautiously in elderly patients and those with underlying cardiac failure.

3. Once the intravascular volume deficit is corrected, change fluid to hypotonic saline during the above regimen; most patients can be changed to hypotonic fluid after the first 2 to 4 liters of normal saline.

4. Subsequently, titrate infusion rate to provide maintenance fluid, plus additional fluid to replace ongoing losses, until DKA resolves and patient is tolerating oral intake.

C. Insulin

1. Give 0.1 to 0.2 U/kg of regular human insulin by IV injection.

2. Start a continuous infusion at 0.1 U/kg per hour in normal saline solution.

   a. Double the insulin infusion rate if blood glucose does not respond within 2 or 3 hours.

   b. Titrate the infusion to target a fall in blood glucose of 75 to 100 mg/dL per hour.

   c. Slow the insulin infusion rate as the serum glucose level declines.

   d. Hyperglycemia is typically controlled within the first 8 to 12 hours; ketoacidosis usually persists for an additional 8 to 24 hours or longer.

   e. Continue insulin infusion until ketoacidosis resolves, as assessed by laboratory tests, using an IV dextrose infusion to avoid hypoglycemia (see later under D. Dextrose).

      (1) In most cases, resolution of ketoacidosis is best discerned by normalization of the serum anion gap.

      (2) Near-normalization of HCO_3^-, tCO_2, acetone, and/or arterial pH provide supplementary information on abatement of the ketoacidosis but these tests are usually less useful than the anion gap in judging resolution of ketoacidosis.

3. Once both hyperglycemia and ketoacidosis are controlled, IV regular insulin is replaced by subcutaneous insulin.

   a. Give subcutaneous dose of regular insulin 30 to 60 minutes before stopping IV insulin infusion.

   b. Begin sliding-scale regular insulin coverage doses every 4 to 6 hours according to serum or blood glucose levels.

   c. For patients able to tolerate dietary intake, start subcutaneous intermediate-acting insulin.

      (1) Begin with half the patient's usual dose, if known.

      (2) Sliding-scale coverage of regular insulin every 6 hours may be initiated simultaneously to cover for under-dosing of initial intermediate insulin regimen.

      (3) Titrate intermediate insulin dose to blood glucose levels.

D. Dextrose

1. Begin 5% dextrose (in normal saline, half-normal saline, or water, as appropriate for serum sodium and osmolality) infusion when blood glucose falls to approximately 250 mg/dL while on IV insulin infusion.

2. The purpose of the dextrose infusion is to prevent hypoglycemia while allowing additional IV insulin to be given to continue to treat the ketoacidosis.

3. Continue the titrated insulin infusion until ketoacidosis abates.

   a. Titrate the insulin infusion rate upward if ketoacidosis is not steadily improving.

   b. Titrate the dextrose infusion rate upward if necessary to avoid hypoglycemia.

   c. Titrate the dextrose infusion rate downward (or the insulin infusion rate upward) if glucose climbs above 300 mg/dL.

   d. Titrate the insulin infusion rate downward as long as the glucose level is controlled and ketoacidosis is abating.

4. Stop the dextrose infusion once IV insulin infusion is discontinued and the patient is taking oral calories.

E. Potassium

   1. Patients with hypokalemia at presentation are severely potassium depleted and require urgent initiation of potassium replacement.

   2. Withhold potassium if the patient is hyperkalemic at presentation, but once potassium falls to within normal limits, or if hypokalemia manifests, initiate IV potassium administration (typically at 5 to 20 mmol/hour).

   3. Titrate further potassium administration as guided by frequent serial potassium assays and the level of renal function.

F. Sodium bicarbonate

   1. Generally unnecessary, even in severe DKA; has not been shown to improve outcome.

   2. Some clinicians choose to administer $NaHCO_3$ (e.g., 50 mmol or more) if arterial blood pH is below 7.0, to target a pH between 7.0 and 7.2.

   3. $NaHCO_3$ administration can worsen hypokalemia by shifting potassium into cells, cause overshoot alkalemia, and precipitate or worsen hypernatremia.

G. Phosphorus

   1. Supplementation is not routinely necessary, but many patients with DKA develop hypophosphatemia.

   2. Supplementation is indicated in patients who present with or develop hypophosphatemia during the treatment phase.

   3. May be administered IV as phosphate salts: e.g., 15 mmol potassium or sodium phosphate in at least 100 mL saline over at least 1 hour (contains 22 mmol of potassium or sodium)

Key Treatment

- Intravenous fluids: normal saline followed by hypotonic saline

- Intravenous insulin infusion: titrated according to blood glucose and continued as long as there is significant ketoacidosis, usually judged by high anion gap

- Potassium supplementation: begin as soon as hyperkalemia resolves.

- Intravenous dextrose: begin when blood glucose reaches approximately 250 mg/dL while the patient is receiving IV insulin.

- Frequent laboratory testing: blood glucose every 1 to 2 hours; serum electrolytes every 2 to 4 hours

Bibliography

Laffel L. Ketone bodies: a review of physiology, pathophysiology and application of monitoring to diabetes. Diabetes Metab Res Rev 1999;15:412–426.

Oschatz E, Mullner M, Herkner H, Laggner AN. Multiple organ failure and prognosis in adult patients with diabetic ketoacidosis. Wien Klin Wochenschr 1999;111:590–595.

Silver SM, Clark EC, Schroeder BM, Sterns RH. Pathogenesis of cerebral edema after treatment of diabetic ketoacidosis. Kidney Int 1997;51:1237–1244.

Singh RK, Perros P, Frier BM. Hospital management of diabetic ketoacidosis: are clinical guidelines implemented effectively? Diabetic Med 1997;14:482–486.

Viallon A, Zeni F, Lafond P, Venet C. Does bicarbonate therapy improve the management of severe diabetic ketoacidosis? Crit Care Med 1999;27:2690–2693.

51 Hyperosmolar Nonketotic Coma

James A. Kruse

Hyperosmolar nonketotic dehydration syndrome (HONK) occurs when there is insufficient insulin to prevent hyperglycemia but enough to prevent significant ketoacidosis. It most often develops during a severe illness or physiologic stress in elderly patients either with no history of diabetes or with a history of non-insulin dependent diabetes.

Precipitating Factors

A. Noncompliance with diet or insulin therapy
B. Infection
C. Trauma
D. Acute myocardial infarction
E. Cerebrovascular accident
F. Pancreatitis
G. Other intercurrent illness
H. Parenteral glucose administration, total parenteral nutrition
I. Drugs: glucocorticoids, thiazides, phenytoin, β-adrenergic blockers, calcium channel blockers

Clinical Manifestations

A. Constitutional: malaise, thirst, polydipsia, polyuria, generalized weakness, somnolence
B. Gastrointestinal: nausea, vomiting, anorexia, abdominal pain, abdominal tenderness, gastroparesis, ileus
C. Neurological: lethargy, delirium, obtundation, stupor, coma (the syndrome is also known as hyperglycemic, nonketotic coma), focal or generalized seizures, focal neurologic findings
D. Cardiovascular: tachycardia, flat neck veins, orthostatic or frank hypotension
E. Other findings: signs of volume depletion and hypoperfusion; e.g., slowed capillary refilling, decreased skin turgor, furrowed tongue, dry mucous membranes, sunken eye globes, decreased axillary perspiration, cool extremities

Laboratory Findings

A. Hyperglycemia
   1. Blood glucose elevated above 800 mg/dL; usually higher than 1,000 mg/dL; much higher in some cases
   2. Secondary glycosuria

3. Secondary plasma hyperosmolality (>340 mOsm/kg H_2O), which in many cases can be severe and is the cause of the neurologic manifestations

B. Absence of significant ketoacidosis
   1. Metabolic acidosis is either absent or present to only a mild degree.
   2. Serum anion gap $(Na^+ - Cl^- - tCO_2)$ may be normal or mildly elevated.
   3. Ketosis is either absent or present to only a limited extent.

C. Azotemia: increased serum urea nitrogen concentration and serum urea-to-creatinine ratio

D. Hyponatremia or hypernatremia
   1. Plasma sodium generally decreases in proportion to the degree of hyperglycemia. The resulting hyponatremia is real, not spurious. The mechanism is dilution secondary to a shift of water from the intracellular space to the extracellular space caused by the osmotic effect of hyperglycemia. This form of hyponatremia resolves in parallel with resolution of the hyperglycemia and requires no other specific therapy. The expected decrease in serum sodium concentration (mmol/L) can be estimated from the glucose concentration (mg/dL) by: $\Delta Na^+ = -0.016 \times (glucose - 100)$. This is an average relationship, and the actual deviation of serum sodium from normal can vary appreciably if there are concomitant independent derangements in total body water balance.
   2. Marked free water deficits are common in HONK, and this tends to counter the effect of glucose to cause dilutional hyponatremia. Thus, in many cases the free water deficit results in hypernatremia despite the sodium-lowering effect of hyperglycemia.
   3. The above formula allows the effects of glucose on sodium to be determined apart from any other abnormality of water balance, allowing more accurate detection and quantification of concomitant free water deficits while the patient is hyperglycemic (apply above formula before inserting sodium concentration into free water deficit formula; see Chapter 38, on Hypernatremia).
   4. Apart from the above effects, artifactual hyponatremia (i.e., pseudohyponatremia) can occur

in patients with extreme hyperlipidemia, although this is uncommon.

E. Other electrolyte disturbances

1. Hypokalemia
2. Hypophosphatemia
3. Hypomagnesemia

Key Clinical and Laboratory Findings

- Typical patient is an elderly nursing home resident.
- Severe hyperglycemia
- Marked dehydration (typically 6 to 18 L)
- Hyperosmolality
- Stupor or coma
- Glycosuria
- Seizures or focal neurologic signs
- Hyponatremia or hypernatremia
- Some cases overlap with diabetic ketoacidosis.
- Absent or slight ketoacidosis

Treatment

A. General measures

1. Close monitoring of vital signs
2. Maintenance of patent airway: endotracheal intubation and mechanical ventilation, if necessary
3. Nothing by mouth; nasogastric suctioning
4. Strict monitoring of fluid intake and output; Foley catheterization
5. Continuous electrocardiographic (ECG) monitoring; serial 12-lead ECGs
6. Routine laboratory studies: serum chemistry profile, arterial blood gases, blood lactate, complete blood count, urinalysis, serial cardiac markers, etc.
7. Frequent serial laboratory tests while the patient is receiving IV insulin
   a. Serum or blood glucose every 1 to 2 hours to monitor progress of therapy and to avoid and detect hypoglycemia
   b. Serum electrolytes every 2 to 6 hours
8. Prophylaxis against venous thromboembolism: subcutaneous heparin (5,000 units every 12 hours) or lower extremity intermittent pneumatic compression devices
9. Hemodynamic monitoring
   a. Central venous pressure measurement helpful in guiding fluid requirements
   b. Pulmonary artery catheterization considered in very unstable patients, those not responding to initial fluid resuscitation, and those with severe sepsis, underlying heart disease, or sustained circulatory shock
   c. Systemic arterial catheterization may be useful in selected cases for facilitating frequent blood testing, and in unstable patients for blood pressure monitoring.
10. Evaluate for a precipitating cause
    a. Cultures of blood and urine; consider culture of other body fluids as indicated.
    b. Urinalysis
    c. Chest x-ray
    d. Serial 12-lead ECGs and cardiac marker tests
    e. Consider computed tomography of brain.
    f. Other tests and evaluations as indicated by history, physical examination, screening laboratory tests, and imaging studies

B. IV fluid

1. Rapidly administer 1 or 2 L of normal saline (typical fluid deficit is 6 to 18 L)
2. Follow with 1 L/hour for 1 hour, 500 mL/hour for 1 to 2 hours, and then 200 to 300 mL/hr until the intravascular volume deficit is corrected; titrate fluids cautiously in elderly patients and those with underlying cardiac failure.
3. Change fluid to hypotonic (e.g., 0.45%) saline during the above regimen once the intravascular volume deficit is corrected; most patients can be changed to hypotonic fluid after the first 2 to 4 liters of normal saline.
4. Subsequently, titrate the hypotonic fluid infusion rate to target a decrease in osmolality of approximately 1 to 2 mOsm/kg H_2O per hour initially, with normalization of plasma osmolality over 48 hours or more, taking into account any ongoing fluid losses.

C. Insulin

1. Give 0.1 to 0.2 U/kg of regular human insulin by IV injection.
2. Start a continuous infusion of regular insulin at 0.1 U/kg per hour in normal saline solution and titrate the infusion to target a fall in blood glucose of 75 to 100 mg/dL per hour.
3. Once the blood glucose reaches 250 to 300 mg/dL, stop the IV insulin infusion, administer a dose of subcutaneous regular insulin, and begin sliding-scale regular insulin coverage dosed every 4 to 6 hours according to serum or blood glucose levels.

Key Treatment

- Intravenous fluids: normal saline followed by hypotonic saline

- Intravenous insulin infusion: titrated to blood glucose

- Frequent laboratory testing: blood glucose every 1 to 2 hours, serum electrolytes every 2 to 6 hours

- Electrolyte supplementation (potassium, phosphorus, magnesium): guided by serial serum assays

- Supportive care: airway maintenance, mechanical ventilation, etc., as required

- Search for precipitating cause.

4. Once the patient recovers, regains consciousness, and is tolerating an oral diet, subcutaneous intermediate-acting insulin can be used in place of or in addition to the sliding-scale regular insulin coverage. Some patients may not require insulin therapy once they have recovered.

D. Electrolyte replacement

1. Patients are likely to be severely potassium depleted and require urgent initiation of potassium replacement.

2. Hypophosphatemia and hypomagnesemia are also common and likely to require supplementation.

3. Monitor electrolyte concentrations frequently and titrate electrolyte supplementation accordingly.

Bibliography

Genuth SM. Diabetic ketoacidosis and hyperglycemic hyperosmolar coma. Curr Ther Endocrinol Metab 1997;6: 438–447.

Gupta S, Prabhu MR, Gupta MS, et al. Severe non-ketotic hyperosmolar coma—intensive care management. Eur J Anaesthesiol 1998;15:603–606.

Kennedy DD, Fletcher SN, Ghosh IR, et al. Reversible tetraplegia due to polyneuropathy in a diabetic patient with hyperosmolar non-ketotic coma. Intensive Care Med 1999;25:1437–1439.

52 Hypoglycemia

James A. Kruse

Depending on its severity and duration, hypoglycemia spans a spectrum of seriousness and complications ranging from the asymptomatic patient to the patient in deep coma who develops irreversible neurologic damage with the sequela of persistent vegetative state. Although symptoms usually prompt otherwise healthy subjects with hypoglycemia to seek medical attention, the disorder can go unrecognized in the critically ill patient because of the effects of sedative drugs or underlying disease affecting the sensorium.

Etiologies

A. Fasting hypoglycemia
   1. Infections, sepsis
   2. Hepatic failure
   3. Renal failure
   4. Drugs
      a. Ethanol
      b. Sulfonylurea hypoglycemic agents
      c. Metformin
      d. Quinine, quinidine
      e. Pentamidine
      f. Disopyramide
      g. Ritodrine
      h. β-Adrenergic blockers
      i. Salicylates
      j. Phenylbutazone
      k. Haloperidol
      l. Trimethoprim-sulfamethoxazole
      m. Nonsteroidal anti-inflammatory drugs may prolong effects of sulfonylurea agents.
   5. Non-β-cell tumors (some are mediated by insulin-like growth factor II)
      a. Mesenchymal tumors (~50%): sarcoma, rhabdomyosarcoma, fibrosarcoma, leiomyosarcoma, mesothelioma, hemangiopericytoma
      b. Hepatomas, including hepatocellular cancer (20% to 25%)
      c. Other gastrointestinal tumors
      d. Lymphoma and leukemia
      e. Carcinoid and carcinoid-like tumors
      f. Adrenal carcinoma
   6. Most β-cell tumors (insulinomas)
   7. Adrenal insufficiency
   8. Thyroid dysfunction
   9. Pheochromocytoma
   10. Hypopituitarism, growth hormone deficiency
   11. Glycogen storage disease
   12. Autoimmune causes
      a. Insulinomimetic antibodies
      b. Insulin receptor antibodies
   13. Critical illness (substrate limitation, increased substrate demand, with or without any of the preceding)

B. Reactive (fed) hypoglycemia
   1. Abrupt discontinuation of total parenteral nutrition
   2. Gastrointestinal motility disorders (dumping syndrome, postgastrointestinal resection surgery)
   3. Fructose intolerance
   4. Some β-cell tumors
   5. Galactosemia
   6. Leucine-induced
   7. Akee fruit poisoning

Symptoms

A. Mediated by the autonomic nervous system
   1. Tremulousness
   2. Sweating
   3. Anxiety
   4. Palpitations
   5. Nausea, vomiting
   6. Weakness

B. Mediated by the central nervous system
   1. Hunger
   2. Headache
   3. Nervousness
   4. Blurred vision, diplopia
   5. Irritability, restlessness
   6. Impaired cognitive function
   7. Confusion, amnesia
   8. Paresthesia

171

Laboratory Findings

A. Hypoglycemia

  1. Defined as a serum, plasma, or whole blood glucose concentration lower than 45 mg/dL

  2. Values between 45 and approximately 60 mg/dL should prompt monitoring or therapy in critically ill patients.

B. Optional diagnostic tests

  1. Serum urea nitrogen, serum creatinine, urinalysis: to exclude renal disease

  2. Prothrombin time, serum transaminases, total and direct bilirubin, lactate dehydrogenase, and alkaline phosphatase: to exclude hepatic disease

  3. Drug screen (e.g., ethanol, sulfonylurea agents, metformin, salicylate)

  4. Insulin: to exclude hyperinsulinism or factitious use

  5. C-peptide or proinsulin: to confirm that hyperinsulinism is endogenous

  6. β-Hydroxybutyrate: to exclude hyperinsulinism

  7. Other hormone tests: e.g., cortisol to exclude adrenal insufficiency, thyroid function tests to exclude thyroid disease, etc

  8. Provocative testing (e.g., in conjunction with a 72-hour fast) is usually unnecessary and generally is not indicated in intensive care unit (ICU) patients (if necessary, can be pursued after condition stabilizes).

PEARL

Spurious hypoglycemia (pseudohypoglycemia) can be caused by delay in analysis (due to white and red cell glycolysis) or extreme leukocytosis (e.g., leukemia); it can be averted by prompt assaying or by use of a NaF-containing specimen tube to inhibit glycolysis.

Treatment

A. Monitoring

  1. Patients at risk for hypoglycemia

    a. Serial blood glucose determinations indicated

    b. Frequency determined by

      (1) Risk of developing hypoglycemia (e.g., patients receiving insulin infusions may require hourly glucose determinations)

      (2) Level of consciousness (more frequent if there is an underlying alteration in sensorium)

      (3) Recent level of glycemic stability

B. Dextrose supplementation

  1. Give dextrose-containing IV fluids to patients at risk for hypoglycemia, especially if not receiving nutritional support.

C. For hypoglycemic episode

  1. First, obtain blood for glucose determination.

    a. Bedside blood glucose assay

    b. Draw blood for serum glucose (do not await test results).

    c. Skip glucose testing if it will delay dextrose administration significantly.

  2. Second, administer bolus dose of glucose.

    a. May give fruit juice or other sweetened beverage to alert patients able to take food by mouth.

    b. All others and most ICU patients: 50 mL of 50% dextrose IV push

  3. Administer continuous dextrose infusion.

    a. If patient is not receiving dextrose intravenously, start with 5% dextrose-containing IV fluid.

    b. If patient is receiving 5% dextrose intravenously, increase infusion rate or change to 10% dextrose solution or both.

    c. If patient is receiving 10% dextrose, increase infusion rate or change to higher concentration (solutions containing more than 10% dextrose must be given by central venous catheter).

  4. For symptomatic or otherwise unconscious patients with hypoglycemia and no immediate IV access, give 0.5 to 1.0 mg glucagon intramuscularly or subcutaneously.

  5. For refractory hypoglycemia

    a. Inject additional 50% dextrose boluses intravenously + increase concentration or rate of continuous IV dextrose infusion or both.

    b. Inject 0.5 to 1.0 mg glucagon intramuscularly or subcutaneously.

Key Treatment

- Give 50% dextrose to all patients with unexplained alterations of their sensorium (may check blood glucose at bedside by reflectance meter first, if available).

- After administering 50% dextrose by IV injection, start IV dextrose infusion (or increase rate or concentration if patient is already receiving IV dextrose infusion).

c. Administer hydrocortisone for empiric coverage of possible adrenal insufficiency.

d. Consider IV diazoxide infusion (antihypertensive effect may limit use in patients who are hemodynamically unstable).

6. Institute frequent blood glucose monitoring; if hypoglycemia is detected by routine periodic glucose monitoring, increase the frequency of monitoring.

7. Pursue specific diagnosis if the underlying etiology is unclear (usually done after patient discharge from ICU).

8. Provide specific treatment for the underlying etiology.

Bibliography

Marks V, Teale JD. Drug-induced hypoglycemia. Endocrinol Metab Clin North Am 1999;28:555–577.

Marks V, Teale JD. Hypoglycemia: factitious and felonious. Endocrinol Metab Clin North Am 1999;28:579–601.

Roberge RJ, Martin TG, Delbridge TR. Intentional massive insulin overdose: recognition and management. Ann Emerg Med 1993;22:228–234.

Service FJ. Diagnostic approach to adults with hypoglycemic disorders. Endocrinol Metabol Clin North Am 1999;28:519–532.

Virally ML, Guillausseau PJ. Hypoglycemia in adults. Diabetes Metabol 1999;25:477–490.

53 Diabetes Insipidus

James A. Kruse

Diabetes insipidus (DI) is a polyuric disorder of water balance due to either diminished secretion of the antidiuretic hormone (ADH) arginine vasopressin (central or neurogenic DI) or specific resistance to its action at the level of the distal renal tubules and collecting ducts (nephrogenic DI).

Clinical Manifestations

A. Subjective and physical findings
1. Polyuria (>3 L/day), nocturia, and polydipsia
2. Findings attributable to the underlying etiology (e.g., visual field deficit when etiology is pituitary tumor)
3. Findings attributable to the resulting dehydration and hypernatremia (e.g., thirst, tachycardia, hypotension, hypertonic encephalopathy)
4. Fatigue, anorexia, constipation, or weight loss may occur.

B. Laboratory findings
1. Hypernatremia: does not occur in DI if the patient is conscious, has access to water, and has an intact thirst mechanism; however, it is common in seriously ill patients and intensive care unit (ICU) patients who lack at least one of these factors
2. Low urine osmolality
   a. Urine osmolality lower than 300 (often lower than 150) mOsm/kg H_2O (urine specific gravity <1.005) in complete DI; values up to approximately 750 mOsm/kg H_2O may be seen in partial DI
   b. Urine osmolality higher than 800 mOsm/kg H_2O excludes DI.
3. Laboratory findings related to underlying etiology or resulting dehydration (e.g., azotemia)

C. Clinical patterns of central DI that can occur after brain surgery or head trauma
1. Most common pattern is acute-onset polyuria, usually within 24 hours of event, that usually resolves in 3 to 5 days (occasionally longer).
2. Second most common is permanent central DI.
3. Least common (5% to 10% of cases after trauma) is the classic triphasic response, usually following resection of suprasellar tumors or stalk injury due to severe trauma.
   a. Phase 1: intense polyuria develops 2 to 48 hours after injury and lasts 2 to 4 (some-

times up to 8) days; caused by abrupt cessation of ADH secretion due to hypothalamic dysfunction
   b. Phase 2: antidiuresis phase lasting approximately 5 to 7 days, due to slow release of stored ADH from the degenerating posterior pituitary; hyponatremia may develop
   c. Phase 3: permanent central DI (in some cases this improves over time)

Differential Diagnosis of Polyuria

A. Water diuresis: caused by excess fluid intake or administration
1. Serum osmolality low to normal; urine osmolality usually <150 mOsm/kg H_2O
2. Primary polydipsia
   a. Psychogenic polydipsia
      (1) Due to psychiatric disturbances
      (2) Also known as *compulsive water drinking* or (in classification schemes that categorize it as a form of DI) *psychogenic DI*
   b. Dipsogenic polydipsia
      (1) Due to an abnormality in the central nervous system (CNS) thirst mechanism caused by a structural brain lesion, CNS infection, head injury, or certain drugs (lithium, carbamazepine)
      (2) Also known as *dipsogenic DI* in classification schemes that categorize it as a form of DI
3. Iatrogenic: excessive enteral or parenteral fluid administration

B. Solute diuresis
1. Suggested by urine osmolality lower than 400 mOsm/kg H_2O (in the absence of volume contraction) and higher than 250 mOsm/kg H_2O (specific gravity 1.008 to 1.012), and normal to high serum osmolality
2. Causes include hyperglycemia, the polyuric phase of acute renal failure, the postobstructive phase of urinary tract obstruction, and administration of radiocontrast agents, mannitol, glycerol, glucose, NaCl, or $NaHCO_3$.

C. Diabetes insipidus
1. Urine osmolality lower than 300 mOsm/kg H_2O, if complete; 300 to 800 mOsm/kg H_2O, if partial

2. Central diabetes insipidus (i.e., lack of ADH secretion)

3. True nephrogenic diabetes insipidus (specific lack of effect of ADH on renal collecting duct)

4. Other disorders sometimes classified as DI

   a. Generalized medullary or tubulointerstitial renal disease or loss of corticomedullary osmotic gradient (classified as nephrogenic DI in some categorization schemes)

   b. Psychogenic polydipsia (see A.2. above); classified as a form of DI by some investigators

   c. Increased peripheral breakdown of ADH due to circulating vasopressinase synthesized by placenta in pregnancy ("transient gestational DI")

Etiology

A. Central diabetes insipidus

1. Idiopathic: accounts for approximately one-third of cases

   a. Autoimmune

   b. Inherited: includes approximately one-third of cases of Wolfram's disease, also known as *DIDMOAD*, an acronym for DI, diabetes mellitus, optic atrophy, deafness

   c. Lymphocytic infundibuloneurohypophysitis

2. After brain surgery (especially hypophysectomy) or head trauma

3. Hypoxic encephalopathy: e.g., following cardiac arrest or carbon monoxide poisoning

4. Cerebrovascular: brain infarction, intraparenchymal brain hemorrhage, subarachnoid hemorrhage, internal carotid or circle of Willis aneurysm, pituitary apoplexy, sickle cell crisis, Sheehan's syndrome (postpartum pituitary hemorrhage), cavernous sinus thrombosis

5. Brain tumors affecting pituitary or hypothalamus: e.g., macroadenoma, craniopharyngioma, dysgerminoma, meningioma, glioma, pinealoma, choristoma, hamartoma, gangliocytoma, or metastatic lesions (e.g., from breast, lung, colon, lymphoma, or nasopharyngeal cancer); leukemia

6. Central nervous system infection: e.g., meningitis, encephalitis, lues, tuberculosis, fungal infection

7. Infiltrative CNS disease: e.g., neurosarcoidosis, Wegener's granulomatosis, histiocytosis X, Schüller-Christian disease, eosinophilic granuloma, xanthoma disseminatum

8. Other: cranial radiation therapy, post-aortocoronary bypass grafting, congenital brain malformations, certain snake envenomization, tetrodotoxin

B. Nephrogenic DI

1. Intrinsic abnormality of collecting duct resulting in insensitivity to ADH, in the presence of normal renal anatomy and corticomedullary solute gradient

   a. Congenital nephrogenic DI: vasopressin V_2-receptor (X-linked recessive) or aquaporin-2 mutations (autosomal recessive)

   b. Electrolyte abnormalities: hypercalcemia, severe hypokalemia

   c. Drugs: foscarnet, lithium, amphotericin B, demeclocycline, methoxyflurane, colchicine, vinblastine

   d. True nephrogenic DI associated with pregnancy (not due to circulating vasopressinase)

2. Any medullary or tubulointerstitial renal disorder (sometimes classified as *nephrogenic DI*); however, polyuria is absent in many cases and urine osmolality usually is not significantly lower than plasma osmolality

   a. Generalized acute or chronic renal failure of any etiology, including radiocontrast and aminoglycoside induced, and the diuretic phase of acute tubular necrosis

   b. Other medullary, papillary, or tubulointerstitial renal disease: e.g., obstructive nephropathy, pyelonephritis, post-renal transplant, polycystic kidney disease, sickle-cell nephropathy, medullary sponge kidney, analgesic abuse nephropathy, sarcoidosis, amyloidosis, multiple myeloma, Sjögren's syndrome

   c. Loss of corticomedullary osmotic gradient: e.g., due to loop diuretic use, osmotic diuresis, protein malnutrition, or after sustained polyuria of any etiology including prolonged water or solute diuresis

Key Etiologies

- Central DI: CNS surgery, radiation, tumor, infection, infarction, bleeding, or infiltrative disease

- Nephrogenic DI: drug-induced, obstructive uropathy, tubulointerstitial renal disease, recovery phase of acute tubular necrosis, hypercalcemia, severe hypokalemia, or sustained polyuria of any cause

Diagnostic Testing

A. Water-deprivation test

1. A provocative diagnostic test for DI in patients not already hypernatremic

   a. Withhold all fluids for up to 18 hours (6 to 12 hours typically required) during test.

b. Perform every 2 hours paired determinations of serum and urine osmolality, every 2 hours measurements of body weight, and strict collection of fluid output.

c. Monitor closely for clinical signs of excessive dehydration and ensure timely evaluation of serial laboratory tests and weight changes.

d. Stop test when two or three sequential urine osmolality measurements vary by less than 30 mOsm/kg H_2O, or when weight loss reaches 3% to 5% of body weight.

e. See B.1. below for interpretation and B.2. below for subsequent testing to differentiate central DI from nephrogenic DI.

2. This test is not safe to perform in critically ill subjects because of the risks from attendant dehydration.

3. Intensive care unit patients often are already hypernatremic, obviating the need for water deprivation.

B. Diagnostic testing in hypernatremic patients (most ICU patients in whom DI is a consideration)

1. For patients already hypernatremic, diagnosis of DI is made by finding an inappropriately low urine osmolality.

a. In otherwise normal individuals urine is hyperosmolar (>800 mOsm/kg H_2O) and plasma ADH levels are higher than 2 pg/mL.

b. Patients with complete central DI elaborate urine with an osmolality lower than 300 mOsm/kg H_2O, and have undetectable plasma ADH levels.

c. Patients with partial (also termed "incomplete") central DI elaborate urine with an osmolality between 300 and 700 mOsm/kg H_2O, and have ADH levels up to 1.5 pg/mL.

d. Patients with severe nephrogenic DI elaborate urine with an osmolality lower than 300 mOsm/kg H_2O, and have ADH levels higher than 5 pg/mL.

e. Patients with partial nephrogenic DI elaborate urine with an osmolality between 300 and 700 mOsm/kg H_2O, and have ADH levels greater than 5 pg/mL.

2. Distinguish central from nephrogenic DI by measuring urine osmolality before and 60 minutes after desmopressin challenge (1 to 2 mg subcutaneously).

a. Normal response (also seen in primary polydipsia): urine osmolality increases by less than 5%

b. Complete central DI: urine osmolality increases by more than 50%

c. Partial central DI: urine osmolality increases by 10% to 50%

d. Nephrogenic DI: urine osmolality shows essentially no change or concentrates only to level of serum osmolality

---

WARNING

The water-deprivation test is not safe to perform in intensive care unit patients because of the risks associated with inducing dehydration during critical illness.

Treatment

A. General measures

1. Some patients may have prodigious urine outputs (e.g., >20 L/day), sufficient to cause a severe hyperosmolar state or hypovolemic shock in a matter of hours.

2. Monitor intake and output closely.

3. Titrate fluid administration to avoid hyperosmolality and hypovolemia.

4. Assay serum sodium concentration frequently.

5. Administer IV normal saline to patients who are hypovolemic and hemodynamically unstable (even if they are hypernatremic).

6. Administer hypotonic IV fluids once intravascular volume is restored.

7. Target correction of half of the free-water deficit over the first 24 hours (see Chapter 38, Hypernatremia), and correct the remaining deficit over the next 48 hours or more.

8. Avoid overhydration, which can result in washout of renal medullary concentration gradient and exacerbate or perpetuate the polyuric state.

9. Consider central venous pressure or pulmonary artery occlusion pressure monitoring in selected cases.

10. Monitor for electrolyte losses (i.e., hypokalemia, hypomagnesemia, and hypophosphatemia), which may develop secondary to polyuria, and provide supplements as necessary.

B. Central DI

1. Exogenous antidiuretic hormone replacement therapy

a. Employed to limit polyuria (especially important in patients who are unstable or have urine outputs higher than 6 to 8 L/day)

(1) Aqueous vasopressin

(a) Typical dose: 1 to 10 U subcutaneously, intramuscularly, or intravenously; or by continuous IV infusion, typically starting at 2.5 U/hour

  (b) Onset of action: 30 minutes to 2 hours

  (c) Duration of action: 2 to 8 (typically 4 to 6) hours allows dosage titration (e.g., targeting a urine output of 100 mL/hour) and ease of recognition of recovery in patients with transient DI

(2) Desmopressin acetate: 1-desamino-8-D-arginine-vasopressin (dDAVP), a synthetic vasopressin analog selective for V_2 receptors

  (a) Injection formulation is given subcutaneously or intravenously, typically at 2 to 4 μg/day in two divided doses; intranasal formulation is typically dosed at 10 to 60 μg/day using two or three divided doses.

  (b) Onset of action: 30 to 60 minutes

  (c) Duration of action: 8 to 24 hours

(3) Vasopressin tannate in oil: used for chronic control of polyuria (generally not used in ICU setting)

  (a) Typical dosing: 1.5 to 5 U intramuscularly

  (b) Onset of action: 2 to 4 hours

  (c) Duration of action: 24 to 72 hours

b. Excessive vasopressin administration can cause hyponatremia, analogous to the syndrome of inappropriate antidiuresis (see Chapter 54).

c. Use vasopressin cautiously in patients with coronary artery disease because it is a potent vasoconstrictor. Topical nitrates may be given concurrently to selected patients; dDAVP is safer in this regard.

d. Other side effects: nausea, vomiting, abdominal cramps, and diarrhea

e. For new-onset central DI, particularly in response to trauma or surgery, hormone replacement can be withheld every 3 to 5 days to determine whether DI has resolved. Alternatively, the patient can be allowed to develop hypotonic polyuria between doses to assess the need for continuing replacement.

2. Chlorpropamide, clofibrate, carbamazepine, and thiazide diuretics have been used as alternative or adjunctive chronic pharmacotherapy in partial DI by increasing ADH release or augmenting its action on kidney.

C. Nephrogenic DI

1. Discontinue potentially causative drugs.

2. Exogenous ADH is generally ineffective; large doses of dDAVP may have some effect in partial nephrogenic DI.

3. Restrict solute (sodium, protein) intake.

4. Thiazide diuretics: cause mild volume contraction, stimulating sodium and water reabsorption in the proximal tubules and decreasing water delivery to the distal nephron

5. Other pharmacotherapy: indomethacin, amiloride (may be particularly useful in lithium-induced cases)

Key Treatment

- Careful monitoring of fluid balance and serum electrolyte levels

- Avoidance of hypovolemia or hypervolemia

- Vasopressin or desmopressin replacement for central DI

- Amiloride or thiazide diuretic for nephrogenic DI

- Treatment of underlying cause

Bibliography

Bendz H, Aurell M. Drug-induced diabetes insipidus: incidence, prevention and management. Drug Safety 1999; 21:449–456.

Bichet DG. Nephrogenic diabetes insipidus. Am J Med 1998;105:431–442.

Decaux G, Prospert F, Namias B, et al. Hyperuricemia as a clue for central diabetes insipidus (lack of V_1 effect) in the differential diagnosis of polydipsia. Am J Med 1997; 103:376–382.

Saito T, Ishikawa S, Ito T, et al. Urinary excretion of aquaporin-2 water channel differentiates psychogenic polydipsia from central diabetes insipidus. J Clin Endocrinol Metab 1999;84:2235–2237.

54 Syndrome of Inappropriate Antidiuresis

James A. Kruse

Key Etiologies

- Excessive production of the antidiuretic hormone (ADH) arginine vasopressin by the posterior pituitary

- Production of ADH or ADH-like substances from an ectopic site

- Therapeutic administration of ADH, ADH-like substances, or drugs that stimulate ADH production

- Therapeutic administration of drugs that potentiate the effects of ADH on the kidney

Differential Diagnosis

A. Exclude other forms of hyponatremia (see Chapter 37).

  1. Exclude iso- and hyperosmolar causes of hyponatremia.

  2. Exclude hypervolemic hyponatremia (i.e., edematous states).

  3. Exclude hypovolemic hyponatremia (i.e., clinical signs of volume depletion).

  4. Exclude alternative causes of isovolemic hyponatremia.

    a. Water intoxication (urine osmolality <100 mOsm/kg H_2O)

    b. Renal failure

    c. Reset osmostat

    d. Adrenal insufficiency

    e. Hypothyroidism

B. Syndrome of inappropriate antidiuresis (SIAD)

  1. Neoplasms (ectopic production of ADH or ADH-like factor)

    a. Lung cancer, especially small-cell lung cancer

    b. Mesothelioma

    c. Mediastinal tumors

    d. Pancreatic cancer

    e. Duodenal cancer

    f. Prostate cancer

    g. Sarcoma

    h. Thymoma

    i. Lymphoma

    j. Ureteral and bladder cancer

  2. Pulmonary causes (non-neoplastic)

    a. Pneumonia, including viral, bacterial, tubercular, and fungal etiologies

    b. Lung abscess, other intrathoracic abscess, empyema

    c. Positive pressure ventilation

    d. Chronic obstructive lung disease or acute bronchial asthma

    e. Miscellaneous: pulmonary embolism, rib fracture, Goodpasture's syndrome, pneumoconioses, pneumothorax, hemothorax, pulmonary fibrosis, bronchiectasis, cystic fibrosis

  3. Neurologic causes

    a. Meningitis, encephalitis, brain abscess

    b. Head trauma

    c. Brain tumor: primary or metastasic, benign or malignant

    d. Brain infarction, intraparenchymal brain hemorrhage, subdural hematoma, subarachnoid hemorrhage

    e. Psychosis

    f. Miscellaneous: Guillain-Barré syndrome, post-electroconvulsive therapy, lupus cerebritis or other central nervous system vasculitis, hydrocephalus, multiple sclerosis, cavernous sinus thrombosis, delirium tremens

  4. Cardiac causes

    a. Atrial tachydysrhythmias

    b. Post–mitral commissurotomy

  5. Metabolic and endocrine causes

    a. Acute intermittent porphyria

    b. Adrenal insufficiency (?)

    c. Hypothyroidism (?)

  6. Drugs

    a. Antidiuretic hormone and ADH analogs: e.g., vasopressin, oxytocin, desmopressin

    b. Drugs stimulating ADH release: e.g., opiates, opioids, barbiturates, nicotine, thiazides, isoproterenol, carbamazepine, cyclic antidepressants (e.g., amitriptyline, desipramine, protriptyline), fluphenazine, thioridazine, thiothixine, monoamine oxidase inhibitors, haloperidol, risperidone, vincristine, vinblastine, vinorelbine, clofibrate, acetylcholine, carbachol, bethanecol, bromocriptine, ifosfamide

   c. Drugs enhancing sensitivity of renal tubule to ADH: e.g., nonsteroidal anti-inflammatory drugs, acetaminophen

   d. Drugs stimulating ADH release and enhancing renal sensitivity: e.g., chlorpropamide, tolbutamide, cyclophosphamide, chlorambucil

   e. Phosphodiesterase inhibition: e.g., theophylline

   f. Other implicated agents: amiodarone, serotonin reuptake inhibitors (e.g., fluoxetine, paroxetine, sertraline, fluvoxamine), angiotensin-converting enzyme inhibitors (lisinopril), loop and thiazide diuretics, polymyxin B, thiotepa, general anesthesia

7. Acquired immunodeficiency syndrome (?)
8. Physiologic stress stimulating ADH release
   a. Trauma
   b. Surgery
   c. Anesthesia
   d. Pain
   e. Nausea
   f. Alcohol withdrawal
   g. Emotional factors

Key Clinical Manifestations

- Manifestations of hyponatremia (see Chapter 37)
- Manifestations related to the underlying cause

Diagnostic Findings

A. Clinical examination
   1. Extracellular fluid space appears clinically isovolemic (no edema or hypovolemia).
   2. No evidence of cardiac, hepatic, renal, adrenal, or thyroid disease

B. Laboratory tests
   1. Serum testing
     a. Hyponatremia (serum sodium <135 mmol/L)
     b. Hypo-osmolality (serum osmolality <280 mOsm/kg H_2O)
     c. Serum urate concentration is usually low.
     d. Renal, hepatic, thyroid, and adrenal function tests normal

   2. Urine testing
     a. Urine is not maximally (<100 mOsm/kg H_2O) dilute.
     b. Urine osmolality is usually greater than 300 mOsm/kg H_2O.
     c. Urine sodium concentration is usually greater than 30 mmol/L; may be lower if sodium intake is low or after marked fluid restriction.

C. Hyponatremia improves with fluid restriction.
D. Water loading test (usually unnecessary)
   1. Performed only on stable patients
     a. Performed after other causes of hyponatremia are excluded
     b. Serum sodium must first be corrected to a level greater than 125 mmol/L.
     c. Performed in the absence of pain, nausea, hypovolemia, or hypotension
     d. Carried out in morning hours
     e. Patient recumbent except to void
   2. Water load: e.g., 20 mL/kg up to 1.5 L over 10 to 20 minutes
   3. Collect hourly urine samples over 5 hours.
   4. Normal response
     a. At least 65% of load excreted by 4 hours
     b. At least 85% of load excreted by 5 hours
     c. Nadir of urine osmolality less than 100 mOsm/kg H_2O
   5. Restrict fluid after end of test to avoid further drop in plasma sodium.

Key Criteria for SIAD

- Hypo-osmolar hyponatremia
- Clinically isovolemic (no edema)
- No cardiac, hepatic, renal, adrenal, and thyroid dysfunction
- Urine is not maximally dilute.
- Urine sodium concentration is usually higher than 30 mmol/L.
- Hyponatremia improves with fluid restriction.

Treatment

A. See Chapter 37 under Treatment: C. Hypo-osmolar hyponatremia.
B. Assess serum sodium concentration frequently during treatment.
C. Monitor fluid intake and output closely.

D. Obtain urine osmolality and urine electrolyte measurements.

E. Stop drugs that may be affecting ADH secretion or action.

F. Stop all unnecessary hypotonic fluid administration.

G. Impose fluid restriction (typically 600 to 1,000 mL/day, depending on severity of hyponatremia).

H. If there is severe hyponatremia with severe associated neurologic symptoms, infuse a controlled amount of hypertonic saline (see Chapter 37).

I. Avoid osmotic demyelination syndrome secondary to overly rapid correction.

    a. Do not exceed a rise in serum sodium of 8 mmol/L per 24 hours.

    b. Do not allow overshoot hypernatremia to occur.

J. Once stabilized, consider adjunctive pharmacotherapy in the patient with chronic SIAD in whom the underlying cause cannot be completely corrected.

1. Demeclocycline

    a. Generally the preferred agent

    b. Attenuates the action of ADH on kidney

2. Other agents not commonly used

    a. Phenytoin: decreases ADH secretion; efficacy often negligible

    b. Lithium: attenuates ADH action on kidney, but high potential for significant side effects

    c. Urea: not commonly used

Bibliography

Chan TY. Drug-induced syndrome of inappropriate antidiuretic hormone secretion. Causes, diagnosis and management. Drugs Aging 1997;11:27–44.

Liu BA, Mittman N, Knowles SR, et al. Hyponatremia and the syndrome of inappropriate antidiuretic hormone associated with the use of selective serotonin reuptake inhibitors: a review of spontaneous reports. Can Med Assoc J 1996;155:519–527.

Musch W, Decaux G. Treating the syndrome of inappropriate ADH secretion with isotonic saline. Q J Med 1998;91:749–753.

55 Thyroid Storm

James A. Kruse

Thyroid storm is severe thyrotoxicosis that is accompanied by life-threatening manifestations, usually involving cardiovascular or neurologic abnormalities. It can occur as the culmination of insidiously worsening hyperthyroidism, but can also occur abruptly either in the case of massive thyroid hormone overdose or as a result of a precipitating physiologic stress. Any of the findings of hyperthyroidism may be present.

Etiologies

A. Primary hyperthyroidism
  1. Graves' disease
  2. Toxic multinodular goiter
  3. Toxic adenoma (Plummer's syndrome)
  4. Other etiologies of primary hyperthyroidism (e.g., thyroiditis, thyroid cancer) rarely if every lead to thyroid storm
B. Secondary hyperthyroidism
  1. Due to excessive pituitary production of thyroid stimulating hormone (TSH)
  2. Unlikely cause of thyroid storm
C. Tertiary hyperthyroidism
  1. Due to excessive hypothalamic production of thyrotropic releasing hormone (TRH)
  2. Unlikely cause of thyroid storm
D. Ectopic hormone production (e.g., struma ovarii) also an unlikely cause of thyroid storm
E. Drug-induced thyrotoxicosis
  1. Lithium carbonate
  2. Iodine-containing drugs: amiodarone, SSKI (saturated solution of potassium iodide)
  3. Excess dietary iodine: Jod-Basedow phenomenon
  4. Ingestion of excess thyroid hormone
    a. Iatrogenic overdose
    b. Intentional or accidental overdose
    c. Surreptitious use

PEARL

The most common cause of thyroid storm is Graves' disease.

Precipitating Events

A. Physical events
  1. Surgery
  2. Trauma
  3. Tooth extraction
B. Childbirth
C. Severe intercurrent illness
  1. Stroke
  2. Myocardial infarction
  3. Sepsis
  4. Diabetic ketoacidosis
  5. Pulmonary embolism
D. Following ablative therapy
  1. Radioactive iodine ablation
  2. Thyroidectomy
E. Overtreatment of hypothyroidism
F. Iodine-containing drugs or radiocontrast agents

Symptoms

A. Constitutional
  1. Fatigue
  2. Heat intolerance
  3. Weight loss
  4. Excessive sweating
B. Cardiovascular
  1. Symptoms of congestive heart failure
  2. Angina pectoris (if there is underlying coronary artery disease)
  3. Palpitations
C. Respiratory
  1. Dyspnea
  2. Symptoms of airway obstruction
D. Gastrointestinal
  1. Diarrhea
  2. Increased appetite
E. Central nervous system
  1. Tremor
  2. Insomnia
  3. Impaired cognitive function
  4. Nervousness, emotional lability, personality changes, psychosis

F. Miscellaneous
1. Dry eyes
2. Weakness (especially proximal muscle weakness)
3. Oligomenorrhea or amenorrhea
4. Onycholysis
5. Hair changes: thin or fine hair
6. Skin changes
   a. Warm, moist, smooth skin
   b. Hyperpigmentation
   c. Vitiligo

Physical Findings

A. Vital signs
1. Hyperthermia
2. Tachycardia
3. Tachypnea
4. Systolic hypertension with widened pulse pressure (hypotension can occur)
B. Eyes (infiltrative ophthalmopathy of Graves' disease leading to any of the following)
1. Thyroid stare
2. Palpebral edema
3. Conjunctival injection
4. Lid lag; unilateral lid retraction
5. Proptosis
6. Ophthalmoplegia
7. Corneal scarring
8. Decreased visual acuity
C. Neck
1. Thyromegaly, with or without tracheal deviation or airway compromise
2. Cervical bruit
D. Cardiovascular
1. Premature beats
2. Tachydysrhythmias, especially sinus tachycardia, atrial fibrillation, and atrial flutter
3. Signs of high-output heart failure
   a. Bounding pulses
   b. Widened pulse pressure
   c. Active precordium
   d. Gallop rhythm
   e. Flow murmur
   f. Rales
   g. Hepatomegaly
E. Dermopathy
1. Pretibial myxedema
   a. Nontender, nonpitting, brawny swelling of shins

   b. From soft tissue infiltration by mucopolysaccharides
   c. Seen in approximately 1% of patients with Graves' disease
2. Alopecia
3. Onycholysis
4. Jaundice
F. Central nervous system
1. Tremor
2. Hyperreflexia
3. Apathy
4. Agitation
5. Dementia
6. Delirium
7. Psychosis
8. Coma

Laboratory Findings

A. Thyroid function tests
1. General
   a. Use to confirm thyrotoxicosis.
   b. No thyroid hormone blood levels are diagnostic of thyroid storm.
2. Total thyroxine (T_4)
   a. More than 99% is bound to thyroxine-binding globulin, thyroxine-binding prealbumin, and albumin.
   b. Generally increased in thyrotoxicosis, but numerous factors affecting protein binding can confound interpretation.
3. Free T_4
   a. Increased in thyrotoxicosis
   b. Represents active fraction of circulating thyroxine (~0.02% of total T_4)
4. Free thyroxine index (FTI)
   a. Product of total T_4 and triiodothyronine (T_3) resin uptake test results
   b. Provides an estimate of free T_4
5. First-generation TSH: cannot distinguish thyrotoxicosis from euthyroid state
6. Sensitive thyrotropin (sTSH): decreased in primary hyperthyroidism
7. Triiodothyronine: detects T_3 thyrotoxicosis (rare)
B. Miscellaneous laboratory findings
1. Hypercalcemia
2. Hyperglycemia
3. Elevated liver function tests (including hyperbilirubinemia)
4. Low creatine phosphokinase activity
5. Decreased cholesterol and triglyceride levels

Key Laboratory Findings

- Free T$_4$: elevated (except in T$_3$ thyrotoxicosis)

- Free thyroxine index: usually elevated (used only if free T$_4$ unavailable)

- Sensitive TSH: low (first-generation tests not useful)

- Free T$_3$: assay needed only if T$_3$ thyrotoxicosis suspected

Treatment

A. Inhibit hormone synthesis
1. Ablative therapy (thyroidectomy or radioactive iodine therapy) definitively halts hormone production but has no role in the acute management of thyroid storm.
2. Thiourea drug therapy
   a. Propylthiouracil: 1 g load followed by 300 mg orally every 6 hours, or
   b. Methimazole: 20 mg every 4 hours initially for thyroid storm, then 20 to 40 mg/day orally or rectally
   c. Major side effect is agranulocytosis (<1% incidence)

B. Blunt end-organ effects
1. Propranolol
   a. Drug of choice
   b. Dose: 1 to 10 mg slow IV push then 20 to 120 mg orally every 6 hours
2. Esmolol infusion
   a. Useful if relative contraindication to β-blocker
   b. Dose: 250 μg/kg per minute loading dose followed by 50 μg/kg per minute infusion
3. Reserpine
   a. Consider if absolute contraindication to β-blocker
   b. Dose: 1 to 2.5 mg intramuscularly every 6 hours
4. Calcium channel blocker (for atrial fibrillation, if β-blocker contraindicated)

C. Stop hormone release
1. Iodide salts (withhold until 1 hour after thiourea drug therapy started, otherwise these measures could stimulate synthesis)
   a. Lugol's solution: 10 gtt orally every 8 hours
   b. SSKI: 1 to 5 gtt orally every 8 hours

   c. Sodium iodide 0.5 g intravenously every 8 hours
   d. Oral radiocontrast preparations: iopanoic acid (Telepaque) or ipodate (Oragrafin)
2. Corticosteroids (may inhibit hormone release)
3. Lithium (not usually recommended because of its low therapeutic index)

D. Block peripheral conversion of T$_4$ to T$_3$
1. Propranolol (see B. above)
2. Corticosteroids (also recommended to cover possibility of coexisting adrenal insufficiency)
3. Iopanoic acid (blocks conversion and inhibits release)

E. Supportive treatment
1. Intensive care unit monitoring
2. Identify and treat precipitating factors.
3. Treatment of congestive heart failure therapy
4. Treat hyperthermia.
   a. Cooling blanket
   b. Acetaminophen
   c. Avoid aspirin because it can theoretically worsen thyrotoxicosis by displacing hormone from circulating proteins
   d. Chlorpromazine + meperidine
5. Hemodialysis or plasmapheresis: treatment for massive thyroid hormone overdose

Key Treatment

- Propylthiouracil: 1000 mg loading dose + 300 mg orally every 6 hours

- Propanolol: 20 to 40 mg orally every 6 hours and titrate

- Sodium iodide: 500 mg orally or intravenously every 8 hours

- Hydrocortisone: 50 to 100 mg intravenously every 8 hours

- Specific treatment for underlying precipitating process

- Supportive measures

Bibliography

Brunette DD, Rothong C. Emergency department management of thyrotoxic crisis with esmolol. Am J Emerg Med 1991;9:232–234.

Choudhary AM, Roberts I. Thyroid storm presenting with liver failure. J Clin Gastroenterol 1999;29:318–321.

Dillmann WH. Thyroid storm. Curr Ther Endocrinol Metab 1997;6:81–85.

Feroze M, May H. Apathetic thyrotoxicosis. Int J Clin Pract 1997;51:332–333.

56 Myxedema Coma

James A. Kruse

Myxedema coma is severe hypothyroidism accompanied by life-threatening manifestations, usually involving cardiopulmonary and neurologic dysfunction. It can represent the culmination of insidiously worsening hypothyroidism, or it can occur suddenly, as a result of a precipitating physiologic stress. Any of the findings of hypothyroidism may be present.

Etiologies

A. Primary hypothyroidism
 1. Autoimmune: most commonly from prior Hashimoto's or other forms of thyroiditis
 2. Iatrogenic
    a. Prior radioactive iodine therapy or thyroidectomy for treatment of hyperthyroidism
    b. Radiation treatment for head and neck malignancy
 3. Drug-induced
    a. Propylthiouracil
    b. Methimazole
    c. Lithium carbonate
    d. Amiodarone
    e. Radioactive iodine
 4. Other, uncommon causes
    a. Infiltrative diseases
    b. Iodine deficiency
    c. Cystinosis
    d. Congenital causes
B. Secondary hypothyroidism
 1. Due to lack of anterior pituitary production of thyroid stimulating hormone (TSH)
 2. Unlikely cause of myxedema coma
C. Tertiary hypothyroidism
 1. Due to lack of hypothalamic production of thyrotropin releasing hormone (TRH)
 2. Unlikely cause of myxedema coma

Key Precipitating Factors

- Physical factors: surgery, trauma, cold exposure
- Intercurrent illness: e.g., infection, cerebrovascular accident, myocardial infarction, gastrointestinal hemorrhage
- Following ablative therapy: radioactive iodine ablation or thyroidectomy
- Drug-induced: sedative, hypnotic, narcotic drug therapy

Symptoms

A. Constitutional
 1. Fatigue
 2. Cold intolerance
 3. Weight gain (usually modest)
 4. Anorexia
 5. Myalgias
 6. Decreased sweating
B. Cardiopulmonary
 1. Symptoms of congestive heart failure
 2. Dyspnea
C. Neurologic
 1. Somnolence
 2. Weakness, lethargy
 3. Impaired memory and cognitive function
 4. Hearing impairment
D. Miscellaneous
 1. Facial and peripheral swelling
 2. Constipation
 3. Urinary retention
 4. Menorrhagia

Physical Examination

A. Vital signs
 1. Hypothermia
 2. Bradycardia
 3. Slow, shallow breathing
 4. Diastolic hypertension with narrowed pulse pressure (hypotension can occur)
B. Head and neck
 1. Puffy facies, periorbital edema
 2. Macroglossia (may cause airway obstruction)
 3. Hoarseness (vocal cord thickening)
 4. Cervical scar from previous thyroidectomy
 5. Goiter (with or without tracheal deviation or airway compromise)
C. Cardiovascular
 1. Sinus bradycardia
 2. Signs of congestive heart failure
    a. Neck vein distension
    b. S_3 gallop rhythm
    c. Pulmonary rales
    d. Ascites
    e. Peripheral edema

3. Signs of pericardial effusion
   a. Pericardial friction rub
   b. Distant heart sounds
   c. Quiet precordium
   d. Kussmaul's sign
   e. Pulsus paradoxus
D. Respiratory
   1. Rales
   2. Signs of pleural effusion
   3. Hypoventilation or respiratory failure (the respiratory response to hypoxemia and hypercapnia is blunted)
E. Abdomen and pelvis
   1. Absent or diminished bowel sounds
   2. Distended bladder (urinary retention)
F. Neurologic
   1. Hyporeflexia, especially: delayed relaxation phase to deep-tendon reflexes
   2. Decreased motor strength
   3. Apathy, lethargy, dulled sensorium
   4. Mental confusion, encephalopathy
   5. Psychotic behavior
   6. Stupor or coma
G. Dermopathy
   1. Myxedema (mucopolysaccharide infiltration)
   2. Dry, rough skin; hyperkeratosis involving extensor surfaces of elbows and knees
   3. Coarse, brittle, unruly hair
   4. Alopecia, especially lateral aspect of eyebrows
   5. Thick, brittle, ridged nails

Laboratory Findings

A. Thyroid function tests in hypothyroidism
   1. Thyrotropin: high, except in secondary and tertiary hypothyroidism, which are rare
      a. Best diagnostic test for primary hypothyroidism
      b. Marked elevation confirms primary hypothyroidism.
      c. There is no value that distinguishes myxedema coma from uncomplicated hypothyroidism.
   2. Free T_4: low
   3. Free thyroxine index (FTI): product of total T_4 and triiodothyronine (T_3) resin uptake test results; provides an estimate of free T_4: low
   4. Total thyroxine: usually low
   5. Triiodothyronine: variable
B. Thyroid function tests in nonthyroidal illness (euthyroid sick syndrome)

1. Mild alterations of TSH, T_4, or both can occur in either direction in the absence of thyroid dysfunction in the setting of critical illness.
2. T_3 is low in most intensive care unit (ICU) patients; decreases early in ICU course.
3. T_4 typically decreases later in course and only with more severe degrees of nonthyroidal illness.
4. Dopamine infusions can depress thyroid hormone levels in patients without thyroid disease.
5. Mild elevation of TSH in conjunction with elevated reverse T_3 (rT_3) level suggests nonthyroidal illness.
C. Miscellaneous laboratory findings in hypothyroidism
   1. Hypoxemia, hypercapnia
   2. Elevated creatine phosphokinase activity
   3. Elevated cholesterol and triglyceride levels
   4. Hyponatremia
   5. Hypoglycemia

Key Laboratory Tests

- Thyroid stimulating hormone is high (secondary and tertiary hypothyroidism are rare exceptions).
- Free T_4 (or free T_4 index) is low.
- Quick cosyntropin stimulation test can be performed to exclude concomitant adrenal insufficiency.
- Other diagnostic tests as appropriate to detect precipitating or concomitant diseases

Electrocardiogram

A. Sinus bradycardia
B. Low QRS complex voltage
C. Flat or inverted T waves
D. Prolonged PR, QRS, or QT intervals
E. Any degree of heart block

Treatment

A. Intensive care unit monitoring
   1. Continuous electrocardiographic monitoring for dysrhythmias and conduction disturbances; transcutaneous or transvenous cardiac pacing may be required
   2. Pulse oximetry monitoring of oxygenation (does not detect hypoventilation or hypercapnia)
   3. Frequent clinical assessments of airway control and level of sensorium

4. Serial arterial blood gas analysis to detect hypercapnia and acid-base disturbances

5. Temperature monitoring

6. Blood glucose monitoring to detect hypoglycemia

B. Thyroxine supplementation

1. Initial dose 300 to 500 μg intravenously (single dose)

2. Subsequent daily doses of 50 to 100 μg intravenously, or 100 to 200 μg orally each day

3. Consider somewhat lower dosing in patients at high risk for coronary events.

C. Corticosteroid supplementation

1. To cover for possible concomitant adrenal insufficiency

2. Hydrocortisone: 100 mg intravenously every 8 hours, or 12.5 mg/hour by continuous IV infusion

3. Consider rapid cosyntropin stimulation test prior to initiating hydrocortisone (see Chapter 58, Adrenal Insufficiency).

D. Supportive measures

1. Passive rewarming (active rewarming may precipitate hypotension)

2. Endotracheal intubation and mechanical ventilation are frequently required.

3. Dextrose containing IV solutions to avoid hypoglycemia

4. Culture relevant body fluids to exclude infection.

Key Treatment

- Thyroxine: 300 to 500 μg intravenously on day one, followed by 50 to 100 μg intravenously or 100 to 200 μg orally each day thereafter

- Hydrocortisone: 100 mg every 8 hours, or 12.5 mg/hour intravenously

- Temperature, electrocardiographic, and blood gas monitoring

- Close respiratory monitoring; mechanical ventilation is frequently required

- Supportive measures, including passive rewarming

- Specific treatment for underlying precipitating process

Bibliography

Camacho PM, Dwarkanathan AA. Sick euthyroid syndrome. What to do when thyroid function tests are abnormal in critically ill patients. Postgrad Med 1999;105: 215–219.

Girvent M, Maestro S, Hernández R, et al. Euthyroid sick syndrome, associated endocrine abnormalities, and outcome in elderly patients undergoing emergency operation. Surgery 1998;123:560–567.

Saadi H. Clinical implications of the interaction between hypothyroidism and the cardiovascular system. Cleveland Clin J Med 1997;64:93–98.

Yamamoto T, Fukuyama J, Fujiyoshi A. Factors associated with mortality of myxedema coma: report of eight cases and literature survey. Thyroid 1999;9:1167–1174.

57 Pheochromocytoma

James A. Kruse

Definition

A. An uncommon, catecholamine-producing chromaffin cell tumor causing hypertension and symptoms related to catecholamine excess

B. Can potentially lead to life-threatening hypertensive crisis

C. May produce only norepinephrine, a combination of norepinephrine and epinephrine, or, rarely, only epinephrine or predominantly dopamine

Pathology

A. Tumor is located in the adrenal medulla in most cases (~90%); more commonly in the right adrenal gland.

B. Bilateral adrenal tumors occur in approximately 10% of cases.

C. Most common extraadrenal location is the organs of Zuckerkandl.

D. Other extraadrenal locations are rare: neck, mediastinum, genitourinary system

E. Approximately 5% to 10% are malignant.

Epidemiology

A. Overall incidence of approximately 1 in 50,000 persons; accounts for approximately 1 of 1,000 cases of hypertension

B. Peak incidence is in fourth or fifth decade.

C. No gender predominance in benign variety in adults; female predominance in malignant variety (3:1); more common in male gender in children

D. Some cases are associated with von Recklinghausen's disease, von Hippel-Lindau disease, and multiple endocrine neoplasia syndrome types IIa and IIb.

Clinical Findings

A. Manifestations may be paroxysmal (due to episodic catecholamine secretion) and last for minutes to days (typically ~20 minutes), or continuous (due to sustained catecholamine secretion).

B. Paroxysmal manifestations may be precipitated by eating, activity, anxiety, postural changes, abdominal compression or palpation of the tumor, and certain drugs (e.g., phenothiazines, tricyclic antidepressants); however, usually no specific precipitating factor is identifiable.

C. Symptoms

1. Most common: headache, diaphoresis, and palpitations

2. Other potential symptoms: cutaneous flushing, anxiety attacks, feeling of impending doom, tremulousness, dizziness or lightheadedness, abdominal or chest pain, nausea or vomiting, dyspnea, constipation or diarrhea, weight loss, fatigue, visual disturbances, and paresthesias

D. Physical findings

1. Hypertension: the predominant physical finding; may be paroxysmal or sustained with superimposed paroxysms

2. Orthostatic hypotension or hypertension; rarely frank hypotension (seen with predominantly epinephrine-secreting pheochromocytoma)

3. Tachycardia, extrasystoles, other tachydysrhythmias; baroreceptor reflex–mediated bradycardia can occur

4. Other findings: tremors, pallor, palpable abdominal mass (uncommon), or pupillary dilation

E. Other manifestations

1. Direct consequences of hypertension: e.g., hypertensive encephalopathy, aortic dissection, intracerebral hemorrhage

2. Direct consequences of congestive heart failure (secondary to hypertension or catecholamine-induced myocarditis): e.g., pulmonary edema

3. Sudden death following minor trauma

Laboratory Findings

A. Possible nonspecific laboratory findings: hyperglycemia, increased hematocrit, hypercalcemia, increased plasma renin

B. Conventional biochemical confirmation is by assay of 24-hour urinary excretion of catecholamines (epinephrine, norepinephrine, and dopamine) and catecholamine metabolites (metanephrine, normetanephrine, and vanillylmandelic acid [VMA]).

1. Elevated in pheochromocytoma

2. Theoretically, compared to spot plasma assays,

24-hour urine measurements are less likely to miss intermittent catecholamine surges.

3. False negatives possible, especially for VMA; therefore, normal values do not exclude diagnosis.

4. May be elevated during stress states and in patients receiving certain drugs (see later under G).

C. Plasma catecholamine (epinephrine, norepinephrine, and dopamine) concentrations

1. Generally elevated in pheochromocytoma

2. Normal values do not exclude diagnosis, especially if sampling not performed during a paroxysm.

3. May be elevated during stress and in patients receiving interfering drugs

D. Plasma metanephrine concentrations

1. Elevated in pheochromocytoma

2. Normal plasma levels likely exclude the possibility of pheochromocytoma

3. Probably the best screening test

E. Provocative tests

1. Histamine, tyramine, or glucagon provocation provoke catecholamine release and increased blood pressure but are unreliable and hazardous; should not be employed.

2. Phentolamine provocation

   a. Phentolamine (5 mg by IV bolus) provokes a decrease in blood pressure, typically within 2 minutes or so of injection.

   b. Typical response in subjects without pheochromocytoma is a blood pressure drop of less than 35/25 mm Hg.

   c. Typical response in patients with pheochromocytoma is a blood pressure drop of more than 35/25 (typically 60/25) mm Hg.

   d. Contraindicated if normotensive

F. Clonidine suppression test

1. This centrally acting α_2-adrenergic receptor agonist decreases sympathetic neural activity, thereby suppressing catecholamine levels and exerting an antihypertensive effect in normal subjects or patients with essential hypertension.

2. Blood is sampled immediately before and at 30-minute intervals for 2 hours after clonidine (300 μg PO) is administered; blood pressure is monitored at frequent intervals.

3. Pheochromocytoma cells are not innervated by the central nervous system and therefore act autonomously; as a result, catecholamine levels and blood pressure are unchanged in patients with pheochromocytoma after clonidine administration, but they decrease in subjects with essential hypertension.

4. May be useful in patients with suspected pheochromocytoma who have only moderately abnormal biochemical tests

G. Factors that interfere with interpretation of biochemical assays for pheochromocytoma

1. Physical stress: due to acute or, in some cases, chronic illnesses (e.g., congestive heart failure, myocardial infarction, respiratory failure, renal failure, sepsis, anemia, hypoglycemia, hypothyroidism, peptic ulcer, dehydration, delirium tremens, coma), raised intracranial pressure, spinal cord or burn injury, or surgery

2. Drugs: catecholamines and related sympathomimetic agents, adrenergic receptor blocking agents, vasodilators, phenothiazines, most antihypertensive agents (except clonidine), monoamine oxidase inhibitors, most diuretics, tricyclic antidepressants, cocaine

3. Critical illness: since many intensive care unit patients have one or more of the above factors present, definitive biochemical confirmation of pheochromocytoma is deferred until a patient has been stabilized and no longer requires intensive care.

Anatomic Localization

A. Computed tomography (CT) scan

1. Particularly useful for localizing intraadrenal pheochromocytoma

2. Has greater than 95% sensitivity for localizing tumors larger than 1 cm within adrenal gland

3. Contrast agent administration may induce hypertensive crisis.

B. Magnetic resonance imaging (MRI) scan

1. T2-weighted spin resonance mode provides relatively specific enhancement of pheochromocytoma tissue.

2. Advantages over CT scanning: does not require radiocontrast administration; better for localizing extraadrenal pheochromocytoma

3. Sensitivity approaches 100% for adrenal tumors and is greater than 90% for extraadrenal tumors.

4. May aid in discriminating malignant from benign tumors

C. Radioiodinated meta-iodobenzylguanidine (MIBG) scintigraphy

1. MIBG is a guanethidine analogue structurally related to norepinephrine and is selectively taken up by catecholamine-producing cells.

2. Scans are repeated over several days.

3. Sensitivity 80% to 90%; specificity is greater than 95%.

4. Particularly useful for localizing extraadrenal, metastatic, or recurrent pheochromocytoma.

Key Diagnostic Points

- Diagnosis is based on clinical manifestations, clinical suspicion, and confirmation by specific laboratory tests.

- Most common manifestations are hypertension, headache, palpitations, and diaphoresis, commonly occurring in paroxysms.

- Elevated concentrations of circulating metanephrines may be the single best diagnostic biochemical test; normal levels exclude the diagnosis.

- Once confirmed biochemically, imaging studies are performed for anatomic localization.

Treatment

A. Pharmacologic treatment

1. Conventional antihypertensive agent of choice for acute emergencies: phentolamine mesylate, a short-acting α-adrenergic receptor blocking drug (typically starting with an IV bolus of 2 to 5 mg and repeating at intervals of at least 5 minutes until blood pressure is stabilized); a continuous infusion of sodium nitroprusside can also be used.

2. Standard antihypertensive agent of choice for chronic treatment: phenoxybenzamine hydrochloride (a long-acting α-adrenergic receptor blocking drug), starting at 10 mg every 12 hours and titrating dose to control of blood pressure and symptoms (typically to 20 to 40 mg 2 to 3 times a day)

3. β-Adrenergic receptor blocking drugs: e.g., propranolol, metoprolol, or esmolol

a. May be added, after α-adrenergic blockade is achieved, to control β-adrenergic manifestations such as tachycardia or cardiac dysrhythmias (e.g., propranolol, 1 to 2 mg intravenously every 5 to 10 minutes and then 30 to 60 mg/day initially, PO, in divided

doses; or esmolol, 0.5 mg/kg intravenously over 1 minute, followed by 0.1 to 0.3 mg/kg per minute intravenously)

b. Caution: do not administer β-adrenergic receptor blocking drugs unless patient is already receiving an α-adrenergic blocking drug, lest the unopposed α-adrenergic stimulation result in hypertensive crisis; this can lead to myocardial infarction, stroke, pulmonary edema, or death.

4. Other pharmacotherapy

a. α_1-Adrenergic receptor blocking drugs: prazosin, terazosin, or doxazosin

b. Metyrosine (α-methyl-L-tyrosine): decreases catecholamine synthesis by inhibiting tyrosine hydroxylase; used primarily in inoperable patients.

c. Labetolol: has combined α- and β-adrenergic receptor blocking action; rarely, can aggravate hypertension associated with pheochromocytoma.

B. Surgery

1. Surgical removal is the treatment of choice when feasible

2. Significant hazards associated with anesthesia and surgical manipulation; minimized by preoperative phenoxybenzamine administration for 1 to 2 weeks prior to surgery, with or without propranolol (80 to 360 mg/day) if significant tachydysrhythmias are present, and maintenance of optimal plasma volume intra- and perioperatively

3. Hypotension and hypoglycemia can occur once the tumor is removed.

4. Nonoperative candidates are treated pharmacologically.

C. Malignant pheochromocytoma is generally resistant to chemotherapy and radiation therapy; combination chemotherapy with vincristine, cyclophosphamide, and dacarbazine may be effective

D. Supportive measures for perioperative or crisis situations

1. Intensive care unit monitoring

2. Continuous electrocardiographic monitoring

3. Intraarterial pressure monitoring mandatory

4. Central venous or pulmonary artery pressure monitoring for optimization of intravascular volume

5. Use meperidine rather than morphine if narcotic analgesia required; histamine release caused by latter drug may provoke catecholamine surge.

6. Frequent blood glucose monitoring

Key Treatment Points

- Treatment of choice for pheochromocytoma-related hypertensive crisis is phentolamine mesylate.

- Use of a β-adrenergic receptor blocking agent alone is contraindicated.

- Definitive treatment is surgical removal, a potentially high-risk procedure requiring expert surgical, anesthesia, and perioperative management.

Prognosis

A. About 75% of patients are cured by surgery.

B. Lifelong follow-up is required because approximately 5% of patients thought to be cured develop early or late recurrence of hypertension.

C. Five-year survival for metastatic malignant pheochromocytoma is approximately 45%.

Bibliography

Frishman WH, Kotob F. Alpha-adrenergic blocking drugs in clinical medicine. J Clin Pharmacol 1999;39:7–16.

Goldstein RE, O'Neill JA Jr, Holcomb GW III, et al. Clinical experience over 48 years with pheochromocytoma. Ann Surg 1999;229:755–766.

Raber W, Raffesberg W, Bischof M, et al. Diagnostic efficacy of unconjugated plasma metanephrines for the detection of pheochromocytoma. Arch Intern Med 2000;160:2957–2963.

Shapiro B, Gross MD. Pheochromocytoma. Crit Care Clin 1991;7:1–21.

58 Adrenal Insufficiency

James A. Kruse

Adequate glucocorticoid secretion is necessary for normal carbohydrate and protein metabolism and immune function, especially during periods of stress or intercurrent illness. Primary adrenal insufficiency (Addison's disease) is due to destruction of the adrenal gland. This is most commonly caused by autoimmune disease (75% of cases) and tuberculosis (20% of cases). Secondary forms of the disease are due to failure of the hypothalamic–pituitary axis to produce corticotropin (adrenocorticotropic hormone, ACTH). Inadequate mineralocorticoid secretion occurs in primary adrenal failure and results in salt wasting, hyperkalemia, and hypovolemia. Mineralocorticoid secretion is regulated by changes in blood pressure, salt balance, and the renin–angiotensin system; thus, patients with secondary adrenal failure do not develop hypovolemia.

Etiologies

A. Primary adrenal insufficiency
  1. Autoimmune
  2. Autoimmune polyglandular syndromes
      a. Type I: autoimmune adrenalitis associated with panhypopituitarism, hypoparathyroidism, or mucocutaneous candidiasis
      b. Type II: autoimmune thyroid disease and diabetes
  3. Infections
      a. Meningococcemia
      b. Tuberculosis
      c. *Pseudomonas* sepsis
      d. Fungal infection
      e. Acquired immunodeficiency syndrome (AIDS)-related infections
      f. Cytomegalovirus
  4. Metastatic disease
      a. Lung
      b. Breast
      c. Colon
      d. Kidney
      e. Pancreas
  5. Granulomatous disease
      a. Tuberculosis
      b. Sarcoidosis
      c. Systemic fungal infections
  6. Infiltrative diseases
      a. Cancer
      b. Tuberculosis
      c. Sarcoidosis
      d. Histiocytosis X
      e. Hemochromatosis
      f. Amyloidosis
  7. Drugs
      a. Ketoconazole
      b. Etomidate
      c. Aminoglutethimide
  8. Adrenal hemorrhage
      a. Coagulopathy
      b. Therapeutic anticoagulation
      c. Trauma
  9. Adrenal infarction
      a. Thrombosis
      b. Arteritis
      c. Antiphospholipid syndrome
  10. Miscellaneous causes
      a. Adrenomyeloneuropathy
      b. Congenital causes
      c. AIDS (adrenal destruction by Kaposi's sarcoma or opportunistic pathogens)
B. Secondary adrenal insufficiency
  1. Pituitary or hypothalamic tumor (e.g., craniopharyngioma or adenoma) or infiltrative disease (e.g., sarcoidosis)
  2. Head trauma
  3. Pituitary surgery
  4. Cranial radiation
  5. Stroke
  6. Anoxic encephalopathy
  7. Withdrawal of chronic corticosteroid therapy

Symptoms

A. Constitutional
  1. Fatigue
  2. Malaise
  3. Lethargy
  4. Weakness
  5. Myalgia

191

6. Arthralgia

7. Weight loss

B. Gastrointestinal

1. Anorexia

2. Abdominal pain

3. Nausea and vomiting

4. Diarrhea

C. Central nervous system

1. Orthostatic lightheadedness

2. Confusion

3. Salt craving

Physical Examination

A. Vital signs

1. Fever

2. Tachycardia

3. Supine or orthostatic hypotension

B. Cardiovascular: flat neck veins

C. Abdomen

1. Tenderness

2. Rigidity

D. Neurological

1. Visual disturbances

2. Features of acromegaly

3. Amenorrhea

4. Galactorrhea

E. Skin

1. Hyperpigmentation (not seen in secondary forms), particularly involving the knuckles, palmar creases, other skinfolds, gingivae, mucosal surfaces, areolae, and scars

2. Vitiligo

F. Other: signs of hypothyroidism (secondary form only)

Laboratory Findings

A. Hyponatremia

B. Hyperkalemia

C. Prerenal azotemia

D. Hypoglycemia

E. Hypercalcemia (uncommon)

F. Non-anion gap metabolic acidosis (mild)

G. Anemia (normochromic and normocytic)

H. Neutropenia, eosinophilia, lymphocytosis

Key Findings

- Weakness
- Weight loss
- Vomiting
- Abdominal pain
- Hypotension
- Volume depletion
- Hyponatremia
- Hyperkalemia

Diagnosis

A. Rapid cosyntropin stimulation test is performed as follows:

1. Obtain blood sample for baseline cortisol assay.

2. Give 250 μg of cosyntropin (synthetic subunit of ACTH) IV.

3. Obtain blood samples 30 and 60 minutes later for cortisol assays.

B. Adrenal failure is likely present if the peak post-cosyntropin cortisol level is less than 15 μg/dL (400 nmol/L), or if a prestimulation (or random) cortisol level is less than 15 μg/dL in a critically ill patient.

C. Cortisol levels higher than 18 μg/dL are usually interpreted as excluding adrenal failure; however, cortisol levels lower than 25 mg/dL may be inadequate in some critically ill patients.

D. In patients with confirmed adrenal insufficiency, plasma ACTH assay distinguishes primary from secondary forms (levels >100 pg/mL [22 pmol/L] indicate primary adrenal failure); however, ACTH assay cannot be used to diagnose adrenal insufficiency.

Treatment

A. Hormone replacement

1. If the diagnosis is confirmed, the preferred treatment is hydrocortisone: 200 mg initially, followed by either 100 mg every 8 hours as IV boluses, or 300 mg/day as a continuous IV infusion.

2. In unstable patients with suspected adrenal failure, start empiric treatment before results of random cortisol assay and stimulation testing are available.

3. If necessary, begin emergency treatment prior to stimulation testing by using dexamethasone initially (10 mg stat and every 6 hours) because this steroid will not interfere with plasma cortisol measurements on subsequently obtained blood samples.

4. After blood samples are obtained and stimula-

tion testing is completed, substitute hydrocortisone for dexamethasone.

5. High doses of hydrocortisone contain sufficient mineralocorticoid activity so that fludrocortisone treatment is unnecessary (but fludrocortisone will be necessary if hydrocortisone dosing is later reduced to less than 100 mg/day).

6. During recovery, taper hydrocortisone dose and change to oral route; when hydrocortisone dose is less than 100 mg/day, add fludrocortisone (0.05 to 0.3 mg/day).

7. Target replacement dosing after complete recovery is 15 mg each morning and 10 mg each evening using hydrocortisone (for unstressed subjects).

B. Fluid therapy

1. Give 50 mL of 50% dextrose by IV injection initially if the patient has an altered sensorium and unknown blood glucose level.

2. Fluid resuscitate using IV 5% dextrose in normal saline to provide volume expansion and prevent or treat hypoglycemia (500 to 1,000 mL/hour is sometimes necessary initially).

3. Continue 5% dextrose and normal saline for maintenance IV fluid; potassium supplementation may be necessary after hyperkalemia resolves.

Key Management

- Perform rapid stimulation test to confirm diagnosis; if unstable, begin treatment before assay results are available.

- Intravenous hydrocortisone: 200 mg, then 100 mg every 8 hours

- Intravenous volume expansion using 5% dextrose in 0.9% saline

- Treat underlying cause.

Bibliography

Chin R. Adrenal crisis. Crit Care Clin 1991;7:23–42.

Henriques HF III, Lebovic D. Defining and focusing perioperative steroid supplementation. Am Surg 1995;61:809–813.

Lamberts SWJ, Bruining HA, de Jong FH. Corticosteroid therapy in severe illness. N Engl J Med 1997;337:1285–1292.

Oelkers W. Adrenal insufficiency. N Engl J Med 1996;335:1206–1212.

Rusnak RA. Adrenal and pituitary emergencies. Emerg Med Clin North Am 1998;7:903–925.

59 Approach to Poisoning and Drug Overdose

Suzanne R. White

Epidemiology

A. More than 2.17 million toxic exposures were reported to U.S. poison centers in 2000.

B. Most poisonings occur in children younger than 6 years old; however, most deaths from poisoning (>90%) occur in adults.

C. Substances most commonly related to fatality are carbon monoxide, analgesics, antidepressants, and cardiovascular drugs.

D. Approximately 10% of toxic exposures are intentional.

E. Only 1.2% of patients require the use of specific antidotes, and 0.3% require the use of specialized methods to enhance intoxicant elimination, underscoring the primary importance of monitoring and supportive care.

Diagnosis

A. The poisoned patient may present a diagnostic dilemma, but important clues may be obtained from a complete history and thorough physical examination.

B. History
   1. History provided by patient is often inaccurate and should be verified by friends, family, police, paramedics, or a search of the scene for the offending agent.
   2. Always attempt to retrieve the original container for exact ingredient determination.
   3. Poison centers may assist with ingredient identification.
   4. Important historical information includes route of exposure, time of ingestion, dose, prior vomiting, reason for exposure, whether others are ill, and whether the exposure is acute, chronic, or acute-on-chronic (e.g., was this the patient's own medication?).

C. Physical examination
   1. Focus on vital signs, pupils, mental status, skin, mucous membranes, peristalsis, and the presence of odors or end-organ toxicity.
   2. Certain toxins may characteristically alter vital signs (Table 59–1)

3. Certain substances may cause characteristic ophthalmologic findings.
   a. Miosis is most helpful and may be caused by cholinergic agents (organophosphates, carbamates, certain mushrooms, nerve agents) clonidine, opioids, phenothiazines, and phencyclidine.
   b. Mydriasis may be caused by anticholinergics, glutethimide, meperidine, lysergic acid diethylamide, certain mushrooms, sympathomimetic drugs, and withdrawal states.
   c. Nystagmus may be caused by alcohols (ethanol, ethylene glycol, isopropanol, methanol), barbiturates, carbamazepine, ketamine, lithium, phencyclidine, phenytoin, or thiamine depletion.

4. Certain substances render a characteristic odor to the patient, e.g.
   a. Garlic: arsenic, arsine gas, dimethyl sulfoxide (DMSO), mustard (vesicant), organophosphates, phosphorus, tellurium, thallium
   b. Bitter almonds or macaroons: cyanide
   c. Ketones: isopropanol, ethanol, lacquer, alcoholic ketoacidosis
   d. Peanuts: Vacor (N-3-pyridylmethyl-N′-p-nitrophenylurea)
   e. Gasoline or airplane glue: hydrocarbon inhalants
   f. Shoe polish: nitrobenzene
   g. Violets: turpentine
   h. Pears: chloral hydrate
   i. Geraniums: lewisite (2-chlorovinyldichloroarsine; vesicant)
   j. Freshly mown grass: phosgene

5. Skin findings may also provide useful clues.
   a. Bullae may be caused by barbiturates, caustics, carbon monoxide, other sedative hypnotics (e.g., glutethimide, methaqualone, meprobamate), snake or spider envenomation, or prolonged coma.
   b. Cyanosis unresponsive to oxygen suggests methemoglobinemia from nitrates or nitrites, "caine" anesthetics, aniline dyes, chlorates, dapsone, sulfonamides, or other substances.

TABLE 59–1. TOXINS THAT CHARACTERISTICALLY ALTER VITAL SIGNS

HYPOVENTILATION	HYPERVENTILATION
Anesthetics	Amphetamine
Carbon monoxide	Camphor
Clonidine	Central nervous system
Cyanide (late)	stimulants
Ethanol	Cocaine
γ-Hydroxybutyrate (GHB)	Cyanide (early)
Opiates and opioids	Ethylene glycol
Sedative-hypnotics	Hydrocarbons
	Metabolic acidosis (drug-induced)
	Methanol
	Salicylates
	Theophylline
	Withdrawal states

BRADYCARDIA	TACHYCARDIA
β-Adrenergic blockers	Amphetamines
Calcium channel blockers	Anticholinergic agents
Clonidine	Antihistamines
Digitalis	Arsenic
Membrane stabilizers	Atropine
Mushrooms	Caffeine
Opioids	Cocaine
Organophosphates	Cyanide
Quinidine	Ethanol
Sedative-hypnotics	Hypoglycemic agents
	Nicotine
	Salicylates
	Sympathomimetic drugs
	Theophylline
	Tricyclic antidepressants
	Withdrawal states

HYPOTENSION	HYPERTENSION
Antihypertensive drugs	Amphetamines
Antipsychotic drugs	Cocaine
β-Adrenergic blockers	Lead
Calcium channel blockers	Monoamine oxidase inhibitors
Diuretics	(early)
Ethanol	Nicotine
Monoamine oxidase inhibitors	Phencyclidine
(late)	Sympathomimetic agents
Nitrates	Tricyclic antidepressants
Meprobamate	
Opiates and opioids	
Sedatives-hypnotic agents	
Thiamine deficiency	
Tricyclic antidepressants	

HYPOTHERMIA	HYPERTHERMIA
Antipsychotics	Amphetamines
Carbon monoxide	Anticholinergic agents
Clonidine	Antihistamines
Cyanide	Cocaine
Ethanol	Dinitrophenol
Hydrogen sulfide	Ethanol withdrawal
Hypoglycemia	Lysergic acid diethylamide
Opiates and opioids	Sympathomimetics
Sedative-hypnotics	Tricyclic antidepressants
Thiamine depletion	

c. Alopecia is rare and points toward arsenic, colchicine, thallium, or antineoplastic exposure.

d. Flushing may be caused by the disulfiram- or metronidazole–ethanol interaction, niacin, anticholinergics, scombroid food poisoning, or ethanol.

e. Persistent erythema of the skin ("boiled lobster" appearance) may suggest boric acid exposure.

f. Stigmata of chronic drug abuse

   (1) Linear scars overlying blood vessels: heroin

   (2) Cheilosis: "huffing" inhalants

   (3) Perforation of the nasal septum: cocaine

6. Combining the above features will potentially allow the recognition of a toxidrome or characteristic constellation of physical findings resulting from exposure to a given intoxicant class (Table 59–2).

7. Unfortunately, toxidromes are not always obvious, since multiple drugs may be ingested, drugs may have multiple autonomic effects, and complications of drug overdose such as hypoxia or cardiovascular collapse alter the "classic" presentation.

Laboratory and Other Tests

A. High anion gap metabolic acidosis may result from metabolic products of paraldehyde, ethylene glycol, methanol, toluene, or salicylates. Additionally, lactate may accumulate as a result of intoxication with drugs that

1. Cause hypoxemia through pulmonary toxicity: opioids, salicylates, hydrocarbons, paraquat, sedative-hypnotics, toxic inhalants

2. Impair oxygen delivery: carbon monoxide, methemoglobin-inducing agents, sulfhemoglobin-inducing agents, drugs that cause hypotension

3. Impair mitochondrial function: carbon monoxide, cyanide, hydrogen sulfide, iron, formic acid

4. Increase oxygen demand through seizures or agitation: cocaine, cyclic antidepressants, isoniazid, theophylline, anticholinergic or sympathomimetic agents, lindane, strychnine, camphor, water hemlock

5. Alter lactate metabolism: isoniazid, metformin

B. A decreased anion gap may be attributed to lithium, bromide, or iodide intoxication.

C. An increased osmole gap may suggest the presence of certain substances.

1. Includes methanol, ethanol, isopropanol, ethyl-

TABLE 59–2. CLINICAL TOXIDROMES

PARAMETER	OPIATE, OPIOID	ANTICHOLINERGIC	CHOLINERGIC	SYMPATHOMIMETIC
Pulse	Decreased	Increased	Decreased	Increased
Blood pressure	Decreased	Variable	Variable	Increased
Respirations	Decreased	Variable	Variable	Increased
Temperature	Decreased	Increased	Decreased	Increased
Bowel sounds	Decreased	Decreased	Hyperactive	Normal
Skin	Sweaty	Dry, flushed	Sweaty	Sweaty
Mental status	Depressed	Agitation, delirium, seizures	Depressed	Agitation, delirium, seizure
Pupils	Miosis	Mydriasis	Miosis	Mydriasis
Other	Track marks, hyporeflexia	Urinary retention	Fasciculations, weakness, lacrimation defecation, urination, bronchospasm, bronchorrhea	

ene glycol, acetone, propylene glycol, acetonitrile, and osmotic diuretics (mannitol, glycerol)

   2. See Chapter 68, Alcohol and Glycol Intoxications.

D. Methods for toxin identification

   1. Most laboratories limit drug screens to those substances commonly ingested.

   2. Rapid drug screens are typically antibody-mediated tests (false positive results may occur).

   3. These commonly include

     a. Serum: salicylates, acetaminophen, ethanol, tricyclic antidepressants (qualitative)

     b. Urine (drugs of abuse): cocaine, amphetamines, opiates, cannabinoids, phencyclidine, methadone, propoxyphene, benzodiazepines, barbiturates

   4. More definitive analytical methods are available and may be accessed via close communication with the laboratory.

   5. Several intoxicants require immediate analysis because management decisions depend on the quantitative level.

     a. These assays are not typically reported on routine drug screens.

     b. Includes iron, methanol, ethylene glycol, carbon monoxide, digoxin, lithium, methemoglobin, theophylline, phenytoin, carbamazepine

Imaging Findings

A. The mnemonic *CHIPES* denotes those substances that are potentially radiopaque.

   1. C = chloral hydrate

   2. H = heavy metals

   3. I = iodine and iron

   4. P = phenothiazines and tricyclic antidepressants

   5. E = enteric coated formulations

   6. S = solvents

B. Bismuth preparations (Pepto-Bismol) and drug packets may also be visualized.

C. A negative radiograph does not rule out intoxication with the above substances.

Monitoring

A. Anticipate complications (e.g., seizures from cyclic antidepressants or cardiovascular collapse from sustained-release calcium channel blockers).

B. Frequent reassessment of airway status, oxygenation, vital signs, mental status, and cardiac rhythm are necessary.

C. Observation is one of the most important aspects of managing poisoned patients.

   1. Duration of the observation period will be dictated by the nature of the toxin, quantity ingested, route of exposure, and pharmaceutical formulation (enteric coated).

   2. Beware of substances with potential for delayed onset of toxicity (Tables 59–3 and 59–4).

Treatment

A. Stabilization

   1. Assure an adequate airway and ventilation.

   2. Hypotension should be treated with volume expansion, followed by vasopressors as needed (α-adrenergic agent for cyclic antidepressants, mixed α-β agent for β-blocker or calcium channel blocker).

   3. All patients with altered mental status should receive oxygen, naloxone, thiamine, glucose (or undergo rapid glucose determination).

   4. Flumazenil should be avoided in patients who may have ingested drugs that cause seizures, who have a history of seizures, or who may be chronically benzodiazepine-dependent.

B. Measures to reduce absorption

TABLE 59–3. TOXINS FOR WHICH 24-HOUR (PROLONGED) MONITORING IS RECOMMENDED AFTER EXPOSURE

AGENT	REASON FOR MONITORING
Acrylonitrile, acetonitrile, propionitrile	Cyanide toxicity
Aniline	Methemoglobinemia
Antidiarrheals (diphenoxylate, loperamide)	Central nervous system (CNS) and respiratory depression
Arsine	Hemolysis
Botulinum	Neuroparalysis, respiratory depression
Calcium channel blockers (sustained-release)	Cardiovascular collapse
Castor bean (ricin)	Gastrointestinal, multisystem organ failure
Chemotherapeutics	Bone marrow suppression, multisystem organ failure
Colchicine	Multisystem organ failure
Coral snake, Mojave rattlesnake	Neurologic toxicity
Cyanogenic plants	Cyanide toxicity
Dapsone	Methemoglobinemia, hemolysis
Hypoglycemic (sulfonylurea) drugs	Hypoglycemia
Methadone	CNS and respiratory depression
Methyl bromide	Pulmonary edema
Methylene chloride	Carbon monoxide toxicity, cardiac dysrhythmias
Monoamine oxidase inhibitors	Cardiovascular collapse, seizures, hyperadrenergic state
Mushrooms:	
Amanita phalloides	Hepatic necrosis
Gyromitra esculenta	Neurotoxicity, hepatotoxicity, methemoglobinemia
Nail primers with oxidants (nitroethane, paratoluidine)	Methemoglobinemia, skin and gastrointestinal burns
Nitrogen oxides	Pulmonary edema, methemoglobinemia
Organophosphates (highly lipid soluble, or dermal exposure to nerve agents)	Cholinergic toxicity
Ozone (rare)	Pulmonary edema
Paraquat, diquat	Pulmonary fibrosis
Pennyroyal oil	Hepatotoxicity
Phenylbutazone	Cardiopulmonary failure, aplastic anemia
Phosgene	Pulmonary edema
Podophyllin	Multisystem organ failure
Rodenticides:	
Bromethalin	Uncoupled oxidative phosphorylation, neurotoxicity
Sodium monofluoroacetate	Shock, hypocalcemia, multisystem organ failure
Vacor	Hyperglycemia, autonomic neuropathy
Rosary pea (abrin)	Multisystem organ failure
Thioridazine, mesoridazine	Cardiac dysrhythmias

TABLE 59–4. AGENTS THAT MAY CAUSE DELAYED TOXICITY*

AGENT	REASON
Benzene	Bone marrow suppression and leukemia
Chlorine	Pulmonary edema
Cadmium	Pneumonitis
Ethylene glycol	CNS, cardiopulmonary, renal toxicity, acid-base disturbance
Ethylene oxide	Pulmonary edema and neurotoxicity
Halogenated solvents (ingestion)	Hepatorenal toxicity
Hydrofluoric acid	Pulmonary edema, dermal burn, electrolyte disturbance
Hydrogen sulfide	Pulmonary edema
Methanol	Neurologic (CNS, blindness), acid-base disturbance
Phosphine	Pulmonary edema
Zinc phosphide	Pulmonary edema

*Prolonged observation should be considered unless significant exposures can be excluded (e.g., methanol level and acid-base picture exclude exposure).

1. Eye exposure requires immediate irrigation with copious volumes of normal saline or lactated Ringer's solution, followed by an assessment of corneal integrity.

2. Skin contamination requires repeated cleansing with soap and water; certain skin exposures may require specific topical therapy (e.g., calcium for hydrofluoric acid burns, polyethylene glycol for phenol burns).

3. Induced emesis: there is no role for the use of syrup of ipecac in the hospital setting

4. Gastric lavage is not employed routinely but may be considered for those patients arriving within 60 to 90 minutes after the ingestion of a potentially life-threatening substance.

   a. Contraindications to gastric lavage include the ingestion of corrosive or caustic agents.

   b. Complications from gastric lavage are not infrequent and include pulmonary aspiration of gastric contents or charcoal; epistaxis; pharyngeal, esophageal, or gastric perforation; hypothermia; or hyponatremia.

5. Activated charcoal is generally safe and effective.
   a. Dosed empirically at 0.5 to 1 g/kg of body weight
   b. Directly but reversibly adsorbs most substances except iron, lithium, hydrocarbons, corrosives, pesticides, and most alcohols
   c. May interrupt enterohepatic recirculation of some drugs and their metabolites (e.g., carbamazepine, dapsone)
   d. May create a concentration gradient that allows diffusible drugs already absorbed into the bloodstream to return to the intestinal lumen for elimination ("gastrointestinal dialysis")
   e. Multiple-dose charcoal
      (1) May be indicated for the treatment of phenobarbital, theophylline, carbamazepine, dapsone, and quinine intoxication
      (2) Commonly used for the treatment of salicylate and phenytoin toxicity, but its benefit in this setting is less clear
      (3) Dosing: 0.5 g/kg of body weight every 2 to 6 hours
      (4) Recommended that a cathartic be given only with the first dose of charcoal each day to avoid dehydration
      (5) Close attention must be given to the status of gut motility to avoid impaction of charcoal if ileus develops.
6. Cathartics
   a. Sorbitol
      (1) Demonstrated to be the most rapidly acting cathartic in terms of time to first stool
      (2) Improved outcome in poisoned patients with cathartic use has not been reported.
      (3) Repeated doses may be harmful.
   b. Whole bowel irrigation
      (1) Large volumes of polyethylene glycol solution are given to achieve mechanical cleansing of the gastrointestinal (GI) tract without fluid or electrolyte imbalance.
      (2) May be used to treat patients with certain ingestions, e.g. massive amounts of a toxic substance, metals (do not adsorb to charcoal) such as iron or lithium, sustained-release preparations, wrapped packages of cocaine or heroin, or foreign bodies
      (3) May also be used to remove drugs that have formed concretions in the GI tract such as barbiturates, iron, extended-release theophylline, salicylates, or sedative-hypnotics (e.g., glutethimide, meprobamate)
      (4) Concretions should be suspected in the setting of waxing and waning clinical status or drug levels.
      (5) The dose of polyethylene glycol solution is 2 L/hour until rectal effluent is clear.
C. Measures to enhance intoxicant elimination
   1. Urinary alkalinization (ion trapping) can enhance the elimination of certain drugs having a low pKa by preventing their tubular reabsorption.
      a. Effective for salicylates, phenobarbital, chlorpropamide, and 2,4-dichlorophenoxyacetic acid (2,4-D; herbicide)
      b. A distinction should be made between urinary and blood alkalinization; the latter is employed to decrease binding of drugs to cardiac sodium channels (tricyclic antidepressants, cocaine, others).
      c. Target urine pH is 7.5 (may be monitored every 1 to 2 hours).
      d. A plasma potassium level lower than 4 mmol/L will impair ability to alkalinize the urine.
      e. Monitor closely for fluid and electrolyte disturbances (e.g., hypocalcemia, hypokalemia, volume overload).
      f. The most important manipulation is that of urinary pH and not volume of output.
   2. Forced diuresis
      a. Entails administration of large volumes of fluid to maintain high urinary flow rate
      b. It is hazardous and no longer recommended for the treatment of poisoned patients.
   3. Urinary acidification
      a. Formerly used in cases of phencyclidine, amphetamine, or strychnine intoxication
      b. May predispose the patient to myoglobinuric renal failure and is no longer performed
   4. Hemodialysis
      a. May remove intoxicants that have low molecular weight, high water solubility, low protein binding and a small volume of distribution (<1 L/kg)
      b. May be indicated for treating intoxication from salicylates, phenobarbital, methanol, ethylene glycol, lithium, certain metals, and certain other toxins in patients with renal failure
   5. Hemoperfusion
      a. Passage of blood through an extracorporeal circuit containing a cartridge filled with charcoal or resin beads

b. Allows removal of certain higher molecular weight, nonpolar or highly protein bound substances

c. Has been used to treat theophylline, carbamazepine, colchicine, phenobarbital, and *Amanita* species (mushroom) intoxication

d. Potential complications related to hemoperfusion include thrombocytopenia, leukopenia, reduced glucose and calcium levels, and hemorrhage secondary to heparinization.

6. Hyperbaric oxygen

a. May enhance the elimination of carbon monoxide and may provide additional support to victims of cyanide or hydrogen sulfide poisoning or those with severe, refractory methemoglobinemia

b. Anecdotal improvement has been noted with carbon tetrachloride poisoning.

D. Specific antidotes (Table 59–5)

Key Treatment

- Stabilization
- Measures to reduce intoxicant absorption
- Measures to enhance intoxicant elimination
- Specific antidotes, if applicable
- Supportive care
- Recognition of co-morbidities and complications

Complications

A. Respiratory: aspiration, hypoxia, secondary pneumonia, pulmonary edema, respiratory depression, apnea

B. Cardiovascular: dysrhythmias, cardiovascular collapse, hypotension

TABLE 59–5. ANTIDOTES FOR THE TREATMENT OF POISONING

ANTIDOTE	TOXIN
Antivenom	Crotalids (rattlesnakes)
	North American coral snake
	Exotic snake species
	Black widow spider
	Scorpion
	Sea wasp or box jelly fish
Atropine	Organophosphates
	Carbamates
Physostigmine	*Clitocybe* or *Inocybe* species of mushrooms
Benztropine or diphenhydramine	Dystonic reaction from neuroleptic medication
Calcium	Hydrofluoric acid
	Calcium channel blocker
Chelators:	
Calcium disodium ethylenediaminetetraacetate	Lead, cadmium, copper, zinc
Deferoxamine	Iron, aluminum
Dimercaprol (BAL)	Arsenic, lead, gold, inorganic mercury
D-penicillamine	Investigational for copper, lead, mercury, arsenic, bismuth
Dimercaptosuccinic acid (succimer)	Lead, mercury
Cyanide antidote kit	Cyanide
	Hydrogen sulfide
Digoxin-specific antibodies	Digoxin, digitoxin, certain plants (e.g., oleander, foxglove, lily of the valley)
Ethanol	Methanol, ethylene glycol, glycol ethers
Fomepizole (4-methylpyrazole)	Ethylene glycol, methanol
Flumazenil	Benzodiazepines
Folic acid (leucovorin)	Methanol, methotrexate, trimethoprim
Glucagon	β-Adrenergic blockers, calcium channel blockers, insulin, oral hypoglycemic agents
Glucose	Insulin, oral hypoglycemic agents
Methylene blue	Drugs causing methemoglobinemia
N-acetylcysteine	Acetaminophen, pennyroyal oil, cyclopeptide mushrooms, carbon tetrachloride
Naloxone	Opiates, opioids, dextromethorphan, clonidine
Oxygen	Carbon monoxide
Pralidoxime (2-PAMCl)	Organophosphates, carbamates
Protamine	Heparin
Pyridoxine (vitamin B_6)	Isoniazid, *Gyromitra esculenta*, ethylene glycol, disulfiram, carbon disulfide
Thiamine	Ethanol (Wernicke-Korsakoff syndrome), ethylene glycol
Vitamin B_{12a}	Cyanide, nitroprusside
Vitamin K_1	Coumarin anticoagulants, long-acting anticoagulant rodenticides

C. Neurologic: central nervous system depression, hypoxic encephalopathy, cerebral edema, seizures, agitation

D. Renal: myoglobinuric renal failure, acute tubular necrosis

E. Gastrointestinal: ileus, bleeding, perforation, colonic ischemia, hepatic failure

F. Other: hyperthermia or hypothermia; acid-base, fluid, or electrolyte derangements

---

PEARL

Consider the possibility of suicidal intention and necessity for psychiatric evaluation.

Bibliography

American Academy of Clinical Toxicology/European Association of Poisons Centres and Clinical Toxicologists: Position statements: gut decontamination, single-dose activated charcoal, gastric lavage, cathartics, whole bowel irrigation, ipecac syrup. Clin Toxicol 1997;35:695–762.

American Academy of Clinical Toxicology/European Association of Poisons Centres and Clinical Toxicologists: Position statements and practice guidelines on the use of multi-dose activated charcoal in the treatment of acute poisoning. Clin Toxicol 1999;37:731–751.

Litovitz TL, Klein-Schwartz W, White SR, et al. 1999 Annual Report of the American Association of Poison Control Centers Toxic Exposure Surveillance System. Am J Emerg Med 2000;18:517–574.

60 Acetaminophen Overdose

James A. Kruse

Pharmacology

A. Acetaminophen is widely available in many over-the-counter analgesic formulations for its antipyretic and analgesic properties.

B. Absorption

1. Rapidly absorbed, typically reaching peak therapeutic levels in 30 minutes to 2 hours

2. Delayed absorption is possible if gastric emptying is delayed or if concretions form in the stomach (can occur in massive overdose).

C. Pharmacokinetics

1. Volume of distribution is approximately 0.9 L/kg.

2. Protein binding is approximately 10%.

3. At therapeutic dosing, plasma half-life is approximately 3 hours, but can increase to more than 10 hours in overdose.

D. Metabolism

1. Approximately 93% is conjugated to sulfate and glucuronide moieties forming nontoxic, water-soluble molecules that are excreted by kidneys.

2. Approximately 2% is excreted unchanged by kidneys.

3. Approximately 5% is metabolized by hepatic cytochrome P-450 cyp2E1 to *N*-acetyl-*p*-benzoquinoneimine (NAPQI).

Toxicology

A. The metabolite NAPQI is responsible for the toxicity of acetaminophen.

B. It is a highly reactive, toxic intermediate produced within the hepatocyte and is capable of irreversibly reacting with intracellular macromolecules, leading to hepatic necrosis.

C. Normally, NAPQI formed from therapeutic dosing of acetaminophen is inactivated by conjugation with hepatic glutathione.

D. In acetaminophen overdose the acetaminophen conjugation enzymes become saturated, the fraction metabolized to NAPQI increases, and glutathione stores become rapidly depleted, leading to hepatic necrosis.

E. Toxicity typically occurs with acute ingestions of at least 7.5 g.

F. Fatalities usually involve acute ingestions of more than 13 g.

G. Toxicity risk is higher in states of glutathione depletion.

1. Chronic alcoholism (serious toxicity can occur even at therapeutic doses)

2. Malnutrition

H. Toxicity risk is higher after induction of increased cytochrome P-450 activity by certain drugs.

1. Ethanol

2. Phenytoin

3. Phenobarbital

4. Carbamazepine

5. Omeprazole

6. Isoniazid

7. Rifampin

Key Prognosis

Without treatment, approximately two-thirds of patients with serum acetaminophen concentrations above the recommended treatment level by the Rumack-Matthew nomogram will develop evidence of significant hepatic necrosis (i.e., serum aspartate aminotransferase activity of more than 1,000 U/L), and approximately 5% will require liver transplantation or succumb to hepatic failure.

Clinical Manifestations

A. Phase 1 (from time of ingestion to approximately 24 hours postingestion)

1. Anorexia, nausea, vomiting

2. Malaise

3. Pallor

4. Diaphoresis

5. May be asymptomatic

6. Altered mental status at this stage suggests a concomitant overdose.

B. Phase 2 (24 to 48 hours postingestion)

1. May be asymptomatic

2. Right upper quadrant pain and tenderness may occur.

3. Biochemical evidence of developing hepatic necrosis

a. Serum alanine aminotransferase (ALT), aspartate aminotransferase (AST), and lactate dehydrogenase (LDH) activities increase.

b. Serum bilirubin concentration may increase.

4. Mild to moderate cases do not progress beyond phase 2 (typically <15 g).

C. Phase 3 (72 to 96 hours postingestion)

1. Occurs in severe toxicity

2. Characterized by the syndrome of fulminant hepatic failure

   a. Serum transaminase activities increase to high levels (in some cases to > 20,000 U/L).

   b. Serum lactate dehydrogenase activity increases.

   c. Serum total bilirubin concentration increases and jaundice occurs.

   d. Prothrombin time increases.

   e. Hepatic encephalopathy develops and may progress to coma.

   f. Centrilobular hepatic necrosis is apparent on liver biopsy.

   g. Hypoglycemia can occur.

   h. Gastrointestinal bleeding is common.

   i. Cerebral edema can occur.

   j. Renal dysfunction is common.

   k. Risk of sepsis is increased.

   l. May be fatal

D. Phase 4

1. Occurs in patients who survive phase 3 without liver transplantation

2. Hepatic damage normalizes over days to weeks depending on the extent of hepatic necrosis.

E. Other manifestations

1. Lactic acidosis has been reported in a minority of serious intoxications prior to the development of hepatic failure.

2. Rarely, coma has been reported prior to the development of hepatic failure and ostensibly unrelated to concomitant drug ingestions or other causes.

Treatment

A. Consider the possibility of a mixed overdose.

1. Mixed overdoses involving acetaminophen are common.

2. Obtain blood and urine for screening toxicologic analysis (e.g., opiates, salicylates), in addition to serum acetaminophen assay.

3. Other specific therapeutic measures may be indictated if there is a concomitant toxic ingestion.

B. Gastric lavage

1. May be considered if the patient presents soon after ingestion

2. Syrup of ipecac is not recommended (may result in prolonged vomiting and interfere with antidote administration).

C. Activated charcoal

1. Effectively binds acetaminophen in the gastrointestinal tract, thereby decreasing acetaminophen absorption

2. Use is controversial because charcoal also adsorbs the antidote.

3. Consider only if the patient presents less than 6 hours postingestion.

4. Do not give multiple doses.

D. *N*-acetylcysteine (NAC)

1. Acts as an effective antidote by directly inactivating NAPQI and generating glutathione

2. Efficacy of NAC decreases progressively if given 8 to 24 hours postingestion.

3. Indications for use

   a. Results of serum acetaminophen (≥4 hr postingestion) assay available

   (1) Treat if serum concentration exceeds critical value indicated by the Rumack-Matthew nomogram (see the package insert for NAC).

   (2) Critical serum acetaminophen value (μg/mL) can be calculated as: $10^{[2.477-(0.076 \times hr)]}$, where hr is hours postingestion (restricted to 4 to 24 hours).

   (3) Example critical values: higher than 150 μg/mL at 4 hours, higher than 30 μg/mL

Key Laboratory Tests

- Stat serum acetaminophen concentration

- Toxicologic screening tests, including quantitative salicylate assay

- Routine serum electrolytes, urea nitrogen, creatinine, and glucose assays

- Serum ALT, AST, LDH, and alkaline phosphatase activities

- Prothrombin time and serum total bilirubin concentration

- Arterial blood gases and lactate concentration

at 13 hours, or higher than 9 μg/mL at 20 hours postingestion

b. History of known or suspected ingestion of at least 7.5 g of acetaminophen in an adult

(1) If the patient presents less than 8 hours postingestion and a serum acetaminophen level is immediately obtainable: perform stat assay and begin treatment if level exceeds critical value

(2) If the patient presents at least 8 hours postingestion or the serum acetaminophen level is not immediately obtainable

(a) Begin NAC treatment immediately.

(b) Await serum acetaminophen level.

(c) Discontinue NAC if level is below critical value.

c. Begin NAC therapy immediately in pregnant women with suspected overdose; treatment can be discontinued if the serum acetaminophen level is below threshold for toxicity.

d. Instituting treatment more than 24 hours postingestion

(1) Based on original clinical studies, NAC has conventionally been accepted as having no utility if given more than 24 hours postingestion.

(2) Presentation more than 24 hours postingestion with measurable acetaminophen levels is a rational indication for NAC use.

(3) Newer information suggests that NAC may have therapeutic value in patients with biochemical evidence of acetaminophen-induced hepatic injury (i.e., elevated liver enzymes) or established hepatic failure.

e. Caveats to the Rumack-Matthew nomogram

(1) Serum levels obtained less than 4 hours postingestion are unreliable.

(2) Serum levels obtained at least 4 hours postingestion may be unreliable if overdose involves an extended-release preparation (repeat assay 4 to 6 hours later).

(3) Mixed overdoses may involve drugs that slow gastrointestinal absorption of acetaminophen (e.g., involving opioids or anticholinergic drugs).

(4) Precise timing of the ingestion is often inaccurate or not possible.

(5) Patients with low glutathione levels can develop significant degrees of toxicity at lower acetaminophen levels.

4. Dosing

a. Loading dose

(1) 140 mg/kg of the 10% (1.4 mL/kg) or 20% (0.7 mL/kg) solution diluted to approximately 5% in fruit juice or soda

(2) May be given while serum acetaminophen testing is awaited; if the serum level is found to be in the nontoxic range by the nomogram, further NAC administration is unnecessary.

b. Maintenance dosing

(1) Conventional recommendation: 17 doses of 70 mg/kg each given at 4-hour intervals, diluted in fruit juice or soda

(2) For patients who develop significant hepatic necrosis, consider continuing maintenance administration until recovery, transplantation, or death.

5. Vomiting can interfere with administration of the antidote.

a. Repeat dose if patient vomits within 1 hour of administration.

b. Pharmacologic agents to combat vomiting

(1) Prochlorperazine: 10 mg intravenously

(2) Metoclopramide: 25 mg (maximum of 1 mg/kg) intravenously or intramuscularly

(3) Diphenhydramine: 25 to 50 mg intravenously

(4) For refractory emesis: consider ondansetron (0.15 mg/kg intravenously) or droperidol (1.25 to 2.5 mg intravenously)

c. Delivery of NAC via nasogastric or nasoenteric feeding tube may circumvent regurgitation.

d. Endoscopic placement of a duodenal feeding tube assures postpyloric delivery of NAC.

e. Investigational pyrogen-free NAC preparations may be available through some poison control centers, but they have not been approved for general use in the United States as of this writing.

f. Preparation and off-label clinical use of NAC for slow IV administration by passage of the standard solution through a 0.2 μm filter has been described in the literature.

6. Adverse effects of NAC include nausea, emesis, diarrhea, and allergic reactions.

E. Administer IV dextrose and monitor blood glucose concentration to detect hypoglycemia.

F. Anticipate evolution of hepatic failure.

G. Consider hepatic transplantation for patients developing hepatic failure.

Key Treatment

- Single dose (1 g/kg) of activated charcoal if less than 6 hours postingestion

- NAC: 140 mg/kg followed by 17 doses of 70 mg/kg every 4 hours, if indicated

- Antiemetic pharmacotherapy (prochlorperazine, metoclopramide, diphenhydramine) for nausea or vomiting

- If serious hepatotoxicity becomes manifest or is anticipated, transfer to a facility with liver transplantation capabilities.

Bibliography

Bond GR, Hite LK. Population-based incidence and outcome of acetaminophen poisoning by type of ingestion. Acad Emerg Med 1999;6:1115–1120.

Johnston SC, Pelletier LL Jr. Enhanced hepatotoxicity of acetaminophen in the alcoholic patient. Medicine 1997; 76:185–191.

Woo OF, Mueller PD, Olson KR, et al. Shorter duration of oral N-acetylcysteine therapy for acute acetaminophen overdose. Ann Emerg Med 2000;35:363–368.

Wright RO, Anderson AC, Lesko SL, et al. Effect of metoclopramide dose on preventing emesis after oral administration of N-acetylcysteine for acetaminophen overdose. J Toxicol Clin Toxicol 1999;37:35–42.

Yip L, Dart RC, Hurlbut KM. Intravenous administration of oral N-acetylcysteine. Crit Care Med 1998;26: 40–43.

61 Salicylate Intoxication

James A. Kruse

Etiology

A. Classification
1. Intentional, self-induced overdose (usually a one-time, acute ingestion)
   a. Suicide attempt
   b. Suicidal gesture
2. Accidental overdose (more commonly due to chronic overdose)

B. Formulations and availability
1. Salicylates are widely available in many oral and topical over-the-counter analgesic remedies.
2. Aspirin (acetylsalicylic acid)
   a. The most commonly available form of salicylate
   b. Also available as enteric-coated preparations
3. Nonacetylated salicylic acid derivatives
   a. Bismuth subsalicylate: active ingredient in Pepto-Bismol (salicylate content approximately 9 mg/mL)
   b. Methyl salicylate
      (1) Active ingredient in oil of wintergreen, the most potent form of salicylate (salicylate content approximately 1.4 g/mL)
      (2) Contained in some over-the-counter topical liniments (e.g., Ben-Gay)
   c. Extensive use of topical preparations (e.g., liniments containing methyl salicylate or keratolytic agents containing salicylic acid) can potentially result in toxicity.

C. Aspirin toxicity
1. Acute intoxication
   a. Mild salicylate toxicity typically occurs with acute aspirin ingestions of 150 mg/kg.
   b. Moderate toxicity occurs with ingestions of 150 to 300 mg/kg.
   c. Serious toxicity typically occurs with ingestions of more than 300 mg/kg.
2. Chronic intoxications
   a. Often more serious than acute intoxication
   b. More difficult to assess degree of intoxication

Pharmacology

A. Absorption
1. Orally ingested salicylates are absorbed chiefly in the small bowel.
2. Enteric coated salicylate products can take 12 to 24 hours for complete absorption.

B. Metabolism
1. Aspirin (acetylsalicylic acid) is rapidly de-acetylated to salicylic acid.
2. Salicylate is the active form that has both therapeutic and toxic properties.
3. Salicylate is metabolized chiefly to water-soluble conjugates that are eliminated by the kidney.

C. Pharmacokinetics
1. Volume of distribution is approximately 0.2 L/kg.
2. Protein binding
   a. Salicylate has a high binding affinity for albumin.
   b. Free plasma salicylate concentration is increased in hypoalbuminemia and in the presence of drugs that compete for albumin binding (e.g., warfarin), thus increasing toxicity.
3. Elimination
   a. Follows Michaelis-Menten kinetics, changing from first-order to zero-order within the therapeutic range
   b. Thus, small changes in dosage can result in large changes in plasma concentration.
   c. Toxic elimination half-life is approximately 24 hours.

D. Renal handling
1. Both salicylate ions and uncharged salicylic acid molecules are filtered by the glomerulus.
2. Acid urine results in protonation of filtered salicylate ions, converting them to uncharged salicylic acid molecules that can be reabsorbed from the renal tubules, perpetuating the toxicity.
3. Alkaline urine maintains salicylate anions in the charged state within the renal tubule, preventing their reabsorption and hastening excretion.

Pathophysiology

A. General cytotoxic effects of salicylates
1. Uncoupling of oxidative phosphorylation
2. Inhibition of tricarboxylic acid cycle

3. Stimulation of glycolysis

4. Mechanism of metabolic acidosis is multifactorial and poorly defined.

B. Central nervous system effects

1. Lowered seizure threshold

2. Cerebral edema

C. Gastrointestinal effects

1. Gastric and intestinal erosions and ulcers

2. Gastrointestinal hemorrhage

D. Hepatic effects

1. Hepatocellular necrosis

2. Inhibition of vitamin K–dependent clotting factor synthesis

E. Renal effects

1. Decreased glomerular filtration rate

2. Interstitial nephritis

3. Acute tubular necrosis

F. Hematologic effects

1. Impaired platelet function

2. Hypoprothrombinemia

3. Disseminated intravascular coagulation

G. Cardiovascular effects

1. Increased cardiac output

2. Hypotension

3. Low systemic vascular resistance

4. Cardiac dysrhythmias

5. Cardiac arrest

H. Pulmonary effects

1. Hyperpnea

2. Pulmonary edema

a. Probably caused by increased permeability of pulmonary capillary endothelium

b. Risk factors

(1) Smoking history

(2) Chronic intoxication

(3) Metabolic acidosis

(4) Serum salicylate level higher than 40 mg/dL

Key Risk Factors for Poor Prognosis	
• Delayed presentation	• Hyperpyrexia
• Unrecognized intoxication	• Older age
• Pulmonary edema	• Acidemia
• Serum salicylate level higher than 70 mg/dL	• Coma

Clinical Manifestations

A. General

1. Diaphoresis

2. Tachypnea

3. Paradoxical hyperpyrexia

4. Bounding pulses

B. Central nervous system

1. Decreased auditory acuity

2. Tinnitus

3. Irritability

4. Delirium

5. Lethargy, stupor, coma

6. Seizures

C. Gastrointestinal

1. Nausea and vomiting

2. Epigastric pain

3. Gastrointestinal bleeding

4. Peritoneal signs from perforated hollow viscus

D. Pulmonary

1. Kussmaul breathing pattern

2. Signs of pulmonary edema

3. Respiratory failure

E. Renal

1. Oliguria

2. Renal failure

F. Hematologic

1. General bleeding diathesis

2. Purpura

G. "Pseudo-sepsis syndrome"

1. Fever

2. Tachycardia

3. Tachypnea

4. Hypotension

5. Leukocytosis

6. Multiple organ system dysfunction

a. Noncardiogenic pulmonary edema

b. Renal failure

c. Encephalopathy

d. Disseminated intravascular coagulation

Laboratory Findings

A. Serum salicylate concentration higher than 30 mg/dL

B. Acid-base derangements

1. Respiratory alkalosis

a. Develops at low toxic levels

b. Develops early in course in severe intoxication, prior to metabolic acidosis

2. Metabolic acidosis

   a. Uncommon at low toxic levels; present in severe intoxications

   b. Develops soon after respiratory alkalosis manifests

   c. May be associated with an increased serum anion gap

C. Electrolyte disturbances

  1. Hypokalemia

  2. Hypocalcemia

D. Glycemic disturbances

  1. Hypoglycemia

  2. Hyperglycemia

E. Miscellaneous

  1. Increased prothrombin time

  2. Increased bleeding time

  3. Low serum urate

  4. Ketosis

  5. Mild blood lactate elevation

  6. Abnormal liver function tests

  7. Azotemia

  8. Proteinuria

Key Findings

- History of acute drug overdose or chronic salicylate ingestion
- Tinnitus or decreased auditory acuity
- Kussmaul breathing pattern
- Mental status abnormalities
- Respiratory alkalosis
- Metabolic acidosis with increased anion gap

Treatment

A. General measures

  1. Ensure adequate airway, breathing, and circulation.

  2. Monitor vital signs and neurologic status frequently.

  3. Consider continuous cardiac monitoring.

  4. Consider possibility of concomitant drug ingestions.

  5. Obtain quantitative serum salicylate and acetaminophen measurements in all cases of suspected community-acquired drug overdose; repeat salicylate assay until the level is shown to be decreasing.

  6. Respiratory care

   a. Monitor for development of hypoxemia and pulmonary edema.

    (1) Pulse oximetry

    (2) Serial physical examinations

    (3) Serial chest x-rays

   b. Provide supplemental oxygen.

   c. Endotracheal intubation and mechanical ventilation may be necessary.

  7. Seizure precautions

   a. Correct hypoglycemia and electrolyte and acid-base derangements.

   b. Correct hyperthermia, if present.

   c. Anticonvulsant therapy (e.g., benzodiazepines, phenytoin, barbiturates) may be necessary.

B. Dextrose

  1. Give concentrated IV dextrose solution if sensorium is abnormal.

  2. Cerebral glucose may be low despite normal blood concentration.

C. Gastric emptying

  1. Syrup of ipecac is not recommended.

  2. Gastric lavage

   a. May be considered for patients arriving at least 1 hour after an acute, life-threatening overdose

   b. Endotracheal intubation is required for patients lacking protective airway reflexes.

D. Activated charcoal

  1. Standard dose is 1 g/kg

  2. Multiple dose administration

   a. Use is controversial, as benefit has not been proven.

   b. If used, dose is 0.5 g/kg every 6 hours.

E. Intravenous fluid

  1. Restore any concomitant fluid deficits.

  2. If fluid status is normal, typical starting rate is 200 mL/hour.

  3. Target a urine output of approximately 2 mL/kg per hour, but vigorous diuresis is unnecessary.

  4. Temper fluid administration if pulmonary edema develops and the patient is hemodynamically stable.

F. Sodium bicarbonate

  1. Given to alkalinize the urine and hasten renal elimination

  2. Suggested dosing routine

   a. 50 to 100 mmol $NaHCO_3$ intravenously over 30 minutes

   b. Followed by 100 mmol in 1 L of 5% dextrose in water at at least 100 mL per hour intravenously

  c. Titrate rate to achieve urine pH of at least 7.5, if possible.

  d. If fluid overload becomes a concern, provide $NaHCO_3$ as an isotonic solution (150 mmol/L in sterile water or 5% dextrose) at a lower infusion rate.

  e. Monitor arterial blood gases and avoid arterial pH higher than 7.5.

  f. Discontinue $NaHCO_3$ when serum salicylate level is lower than 35 mg/dL.

  3. Monitor serum potassium level closely and provide potassium supplementation as needed to avoid bicarbonate-induced hypokalemia.

G. Pulmonary artery catheterization

  1. Not routinely necessary

  2. May be helpful in selected cases to guide fluid management in the face of hypotension, oliguria, or pulmonary edema

H. Calcium

  1. Monitor plasma ionized calcium concentration.

  2. Give IV calcium gluconate if symptomatic hypocalcemia develops.

I. Monitoring and prophylaxis for bleeding

  1. Give H_2-receptor blocker or proton pump inhibitor for gastrointestinal prophylaxis.

  2. Correct coagulopathy with vitamin K or, if necessary, fresh frozen plasma.

  3. Order serial hemoglobin assays.

  4. Monitor for clinical signs of bleeding.

J. Extracorporeal therapy

  1. Salicylate is effectively removed from the body by dialysis (peritoneal or hemodialysis) or hemoperfusion.

  2. Hemodialysis is preferred because it allows concomitant treatment of fluid and electrolyte derangements.

  3. Indications for dialysis

    a. Hemodynamic instability

    b. Pulmonary edema

    c. Acidosis refractory to alkali therapy

    d. Seizures

    e. Fluid and electrolyte derangements refractory to conventional treatment

    f. Marked elevation of serum salicylate concentration

      (1) More than 90 mg/dL in single-dose acute ingestions

      (2) Severity of chronic intoxication is difficult to judge by serum levels, and dialysis may be indicated at much lower levels (e.g., >60 mg/dL).

  4. Continue hemodialysis until the serum salicylate level is lower than 10 mg/dL.

K. Obtain psychiatric evaluation if suicide attempt is suspected.

Key Treatment

- Activated charcoal (? multiple dose)
- Intravenous $NaHCO_3$ to alkalinize urine
- Repeat serum salicylate level
- Hemodialysis for severe cases
- Monitoring for complications
- Psychiatric evaluation and follow-up

Bibliography

Higgins RM, Connolly JO, Hendry BM. Alkalinization and hemodialysis in severe salicylate poisoning: comparison of elimination techniques in the same patient. Clin Nephrol 1998;50:178–183.

Juurlink DN, McGuigan MA. Gastrointestinal decontamination for enteric-coated aspirin: what to do depends on who you ask. J Toxicol Clin Toxicol 2000;38:465–470.

Leatherman JW, Schmitz PG. Fever, hyperdynamic shock, and multiple-system organ failure. A pseudo-sepsis syndrome associated with chronic salicylate intoxication. Chest 1991;100:1391–1396.

Raschke R, Arnold-Capell PA, Richeson R, et al. Refractory hypoglycemia secondary to topical salicylate intoxication. Arch Intern Med 1991;151:591–593.

Yip L, Dart RC, Gabow PA. Concepts and controversies in salicylate toxicity. Emerg Med Clin North Am 1994;12:351–364.

62 Sedative-Hypnotic and Narcotic Drug Overdose

James A. Kruse

Definition

A. Overdose involving drugs capable of depressing the sensorium and causing sedation, induced sleep (hypnosis, narcosis), or coma

  1. Some agents also possess anxiolytic properties at low doses.

  2. The opiate and opioid narcotics also possess analgesic properties.

B. General anesthetic agents (e.g., halothane, nitrous oxide) are commonly excluded from this category in a toxicologic context.

C. Although overdoses of many other classes of drugs can depress the sensorium (e.g., antidepressants, lithium, salicylate), they are not considered pure sedative-hypnotic agents and are not covered in this chapter (see specific chapters).

Classification

A. Benzodiazepines: e.g., alprazolam, chlordiazepoxide, clonazepam, clorazepate, diazepam, estazolam, flunitrazepam, flurazepam, halazepam, lorazepam, midazolam, oxazepam, prazepam, temazepam, triazolam

B. Barbiturates: e.g., amobarbital, barbital, butabarbital, pentobarbital, phenobarbital, secobarbital

C. Opiate and opioid narcotics: e.g., buprenorphine, butorphanol, codeine, dextromethorphan, diphenoxylate, fentanyl, heroin, hydrocodone, hydromorphone, levorphanol, loperamide, meperidine, methadone, morphine, nalbuphine, opium, oxycodone, oxymorphone, paregoric, pentazocine, propoxyphene, sufentanil, tramadol

D. Alcohols

  1. Ethanol

  2. Toxic alcohols: e.g., isopropanol, methanol (commonly not considered in the category of sedative-hypnotic agents because of the cytotoxic properties of their metabolites; see Chapter 68, Alcohol and Glycol Intoxications)

  3. Chloral hydrate

  4. Ethchlorvynol

E. Miscellaneous sedative-hypnotic agents: e.g., buspirone, etomidate, γ-hydroxybutyric acid, glutethimide, meprobamate, methaqualone, methyprylon, paraldehyde, propofol, zolpidem

Clinical Findings

A. Central nervous system (CNS)

  1. Sedation, narcosis, coma

  2. Seizures (particularly meperidine, propoxyphene, tramadol)

  3. Delirium

  4. Muscle rigidity (IV fentanyl)

  5. Myoclonus

B. Ocular

  1. Miosis (opiate narcotics)

  2. Blurred vision

  3. Retinal hemorrhage (methaqualone)

C. Respiratory

  1. Bradypnea, shallow breathing

  2. Signs of aspiration

  3. Signs of pulmonary edema (opioids, opiates, ethchlorvynol, meprobamate)

  4. Chest wall rigidity (IV fentanyl)

D. Cardiovascular

  1. Hypotension

  2. Cardiac dysrhythmias (particularly chloral hydrate, meprobamate, propoxyphene)

E. Gastrointestinal

  1. Nausea, emesis, ileus (particularly opioid narcotics)

  2. Hemorrhagic gastritis (particularly ethanol, chloral hydrate, methaqualone)

F. Miscellaneous

  1. Hypothermia or hyperthermia

  2. Cutaneous bullae

Treatment

A. Resuscitation

  1. Ensure patent airway.

    a. Clear oral cavity and pharynx; remove dentures.

    b. Chin-lift, head-tilt maneuvers

    c. Insertion of nasal airway or endotracheal tube may be necessary.

2. Ensure adequate ventilation and gas exchange.
   a. Provide supplemental oxygen.
   b. Provide artificial ventilation using bag-valve mask or mechanical ventilation, as necessary.
   c. Close observation may suffice for stable patients with altered sensorium but adequate spontaneous ventilation.
3. Secure IV access.
4. Infuse isotonic crystalloid fluids for hypotension.
5. Infuse vasopressor agent for refractory hypotension.
6. Obtain laboratory tests.
   a. Blood test for routine biochemical, hematologic, and coagulation assays
   b. Screen for sedative-hypnotic and narcotic drugs; except for ethanol, quantitative analysis is not generally useful.
   c. Screen for other toxic ingestions (e.g., tricyclic antidepressants, salicylate, acetaminophen).
B. Monitoring
   1. Frequent assessment of vital signs
   2. Continuous electrocardiographic monitoring
   3. Continuous pulse oximetry
   4. Arterial blood gas analysis
   5. Consider Foley catheterization in unconscious or unstable patients.
   6. Consider systemic and pulmonary artery catheterization in patients with refractory hypotension or signs of pulmonary edema.
C. Naloxone use for possible or known opiate or opioid overdose
   1. Assurance of an adequate airway, ventilation, and perfusion takes precedence over naloxone administration.
   2. Dose
      a. 2 mg by IV bolus
      b. 0.4 mg can be given initially if sensorium is depressed but respiration is not impaired; if partial or no response, administer an additional 0.8 mg.
      c. If no IV access, intramuscular, subcutaneous, sublingual, or endotracheal route may be used.
      d. Lack of response after 10 mg makes opioid overdose unlikely as sole cause of depressed sensorium.
      e. Repeated doses may be necessary because the half-life of naloxone is 20 to 60 minutes.
   3. Positive response indicated by improvement in sensorium, increased respiratory rate and tidal volume, increased heart rate and blood pressure, or pupillary dilation.
   4. Can precipitate acute withdrawal reaction in chronic opiate users (e.g., agitation, diaphoresis, nausea, vomiting, abdominal pain, diarrhea, body aches, lacrimation, piloerection)
   5. Continuous IV infusion
      a. Especially useful for longer-acting opioids (e.g., methadone, propoxyphene)
      b. Prepared as 10 mg of naloxone in 250 mL normal saline
      c. Initiate infusion at an hourly dose 2/3 that initially required to reverse respiratory depression, or 0.4 mg/hour.
      d. Infusion can be maintained for 12 hours or more.
D. Flumazenil use for benzodiazepine overdose (see Chapter 170, Benzodiazepines and Flumazenil)
   1. Competitively antagonizes the actions of benzodiazepines at CNS receptors
   2. Indicated for overdose known to be due solely to acute benzodiazepine use
   3. Assurance of an adequate airway, ventilation, and perfusion takes precedence over flumazenil administration.
   4. Not indicated for routine use in patients with mixed or unknown drug overdose
   5. Can precipitate seizures and other withdrawal manifestations in patients with recent benzodiazepine use
   6. Because of the potential to precipitate seizures, contraindicated in patients with concurrent cyclic antidepressant overdose
   7. Dose
      a. Initial dose is 0.1 to 0.3 mg by IV injection over 15 seconds.
      b. If no response after 30 seconds to 1 minute, an additional 0.3 mg can be given.
      c. Additional doses of 0.5 mg can be given over 30 seconds at 1-minute intervals, to a total of 3 mg.
      d. An IV infusion of 0.25 to 1.0 mg/hour can be used in responders to prevent relapse into coma.
E. Gastrointestinal decontamination
   1. Gastric lavage using a large-bore orogastric tube may be considered for life-threatening overdoses.
   2. Insertion of a cuffed endotracheal tube precedes lavage.
   3. Syrup of ipecac is contraindicated.
   4. Whole-bowel irrigation has been employed, but its therapeutic value is uncertain.

F. Activated charcoal

1. Should be administered to all patients, at a dose of 1 g/kg, along with a cathartic (e.g., sorbitol or magnesium citrate)

2. Multiple-dose activated charcoal (0.5 g/kg every 4 hours for at least three doses)

   a. Recommended for life-threatening overdoses involving phenobarbital

   b. Value uncertain in other sedative–hypnotic overdoses

G. Forced diuresis: not recommended

H. Alkalinization with IV NaHCO₃

1. Recommended in phenobarbital overdose

   a. Promotes urinary excretion of the drug

   b. Target a urine pH of 7.5 to 8.0; avoid blood pH higher than 7.55.

2. Not useful for other sedative–hypnotic or narcotic overdoses

3. Useful for certain mixed overdoses (see Chapter 61, Salicylate Intoxication, and Chapter 74, Cyclic Antidepressant Drug Overdose)

I. Analeptic or respiratory stimulant drugs are not recommended.

J. Consider other etiologies of sensorial depression.

1. Exclude glycemic disturbances.

   a. Give concentrated dextrose intravenously or perform bedside blood glucose assay to exclude hypoglycemia.

   b. Exclude hyperglycemia; diabetic ketoacidosis; hyperglycemic, hyperosmolar coma.

2. Give IV thiamine in case there is a deficiency.

3. Consider mixed or alternative drug overdose with agents that can cause CNS depression but are not pure sedative–hypnotic or narcotic agents.

   a. Examples: tricyclic antidepressants, salicylate, lithium

   b. Some of these alternative toxic ingestions require specific therapy (see chapters on specific agents).

4. Screen for metabolic causes (e.g., hypercalcemia, uremia, hepatic encephalopathy).

5. Consider computed tomography of the brain to exclude structural causes of coma.

6. Perform lumbar puncture if meningitis is a consideration.

K. Extracorporeal elimination (hemodialysis, hemoperfusion)

1. No role for most pure sedative–hypnotic or narcotic agents

2. Hemoperfusion is effective at removing phenobarbital; however, supportive care alone is suf-

ficient in most cases and avoids complications associated with extracorporeal treatment.

3. Hemoperfusion may have efficacy in hastening elimination of meprobamate.

4. Definite role for some agents that have intrinsic toxicity beyond CNS depression effects (e.g., hemodialysis for methanol or lithium intoxication); however, these agents should not be considered pure sedative–hypnotic drugs)

L. Special considerations for "body-packers" (individuals smuggling heroin by intentional ingestion of condoms or other packets containing the drug)

1. Confirm by plain abdominal or contrast x-ray.

2. Administer multiple doses of activated charcoal.

3. Administer a cathartic.

4. The use of whole-bowel irrigation with polyethylene glycol solutions has been recommended but also criticized on the basis that it may dissolve drug-containing packets and interfere with adsorptive properties of activated charcoal.

5. Monitor until drug packets have passed through gastrointestinal tract.

6. Package rupture can be managed with continuous infusion of naloxone and supportive care.

M. Supportive measures

1. Titration of mechanical ventilation

2. Correction of fluid and electrolyte abnormalities

3. Cooling or warming blanket for hyperthermia or hypothermia

4. Frequent repositioning to avoid soft tissue pressure injury

5. Ocular lubrication to prevent corneal drying in patients with prolonged coma

6. Prophylaxis for deep venous thrombosis

Key Treatment

- Maintenance of a patent airway

- Artificial ventilation with bag-valve mask or mechanical ventilator

- Intravenous volume expansion for hypotension; vasopressors for refractory cases

- Activated charcoal administration

- Exclusion of alternative or mixed overdoses, or other causes of sensorial depression

- Monitoring and supportive care in an intensive care unit

Complications

A. Respiratory
1. Upper airway obstruction
2. Atelectasis
3. Hypoxemia
4. Respiratory acidosis
5. Aspiration pneumonitis
6. Noncardiogenic pulmonary edema (opiates, opioids, ethchlorvynol, meprobamate)
7. Respiratory failure or arrest

B. Cardiac
1. Circulatory shock
2. Cardiac dysrhythmias
3. Cardiac arrest

C. Neurologic
1. Anoxic encephalopathy
2. Prolonged coma
   a. Secondary to anoxia
   b. Secondary to specific agents (e.g., ethchlorvynol, glutethimide, meprobamate, methaqualone)
3. Compression neuropathy

D. Renal and metabolic
1. Rhabdomyolysis
2. Myoglobinuric renal failure
3. Acute tubular necrosis from hypotension, hypoxia
4. Electrolyte disturbances

E. Infectious and inflammatory complications
1. Nosocomial infection or sepsis
2. Complications of IV drug abuse
   a. Bacteremia
   b. Endocarditis
   c. Pneumonia
   d. Soft-tissue infection at injection site
   e. Phlebitis
   f. Mycotic aneurysm
3. Cutaneous pressure sores

F. Miscellaneous
1. Hyperthermia (e.g., methyprylon)
2. Hypothermia (e.g., ethchlorvynol)
3. Drug withdrawal syndrome
4. Deep vein thrombosis

CAUTION

Flumazenil may precipitate seizures in patients with chronic benzodiazepine dependence, concurrent cyclic antidepressant overdose, or underlying seizure disorder.

Bibliography

Gaudreault P, Guay J, Thivierge RL, et al. Benzodiazepine poisoning. Clinical and pharmacological considerations and treatment. Drug Saf 1991;6:247–265.

Lin J-L, Jeng L-B. Critical, acutely poisoned patients treated with continuous arteriovenous hemoperfusion in the emergency department. Ann Emerg Med 1995;25:75–80.

Manoguerra AS. Gastrointestinal decontamination after poisoning. Where is the science? Crit Care Clin 1997;13:709–725.

Sporer KA. Acute heroin overdose. Ann Intern Med 1999;130:584–590.

Weinbroum AA, Flaishon R, Sorkine P, et al. A risk-benefit assessment of flumazenil in the management of benzodiazepine overdose. Drug Saf 1997;17:181–196.

Yell RP. Ethchlorvynol overdose. Am J Emerg Med 1990;8:246–250.

63 Theophylline Overdose

James A. Kruse

Pharmacology

A. Action
1. Inhibits phosphodiesterase
2. Results in increased intracellular cyclic adenosine and guanosine monophosphate
3. Decreases smooth muscle calcium levels and causes smooth muscle dilation
4. Myocardial and central nervous system stimulation at toxic doses

B. Absorption
1. Peak plasma levels achieved within 90 to 120 minutes
2. Delayed with sustained-release and enteric-coated formulations

C. Protein binding: approximately 60%

D. Elimination
1. Hepatic metabolism by cytochrome P-450 system (~90%)
2. Renal excretion (~10%)

E. Pharmacokinetics
1. Volume of distribution: approximately 0.5 L/kg
2. Half-life: 4 to 10 hours
3. Nonlinear kinetics can occur at toxic levels (and at therapeutic levels in some patients).
4. Factors that decrease theophylline clearance
   a. Drugs: e.g., cimetidine, ciprofloxacin, erythromycin, propranolol
   b. Heart failure
   c. Liver disease
   d. Severe, acute illness
5. Factors that increase theophylline clearance
   a. Drugs: e.g., barbiturates, carbamazepine, isoniazid, rifampin
   b. Cigarette smoking
   c. Hyperthyroidism

Key Risk Factors for Major Toxicity

- Chronic theophylline intoxication
- Peak serum concentration higher than 100 μg/mL (acute overdose)
- Age greater than 60 years (chronic intoxication)

Clinical Findings

A. General
1. Tachycardia
2. Tachypnea
3. Flushing

B. Gastrointestinal
1. Nausea, vomiting
2. Abdominal pain (may be crampy)
3. Diarrhea
4. Gastrointestinal hemorrhage
5. Dysphagia

C. Cardiovascular
1. Tachydysrhythmias
   a. Sinus tachycardia
   b. Atrial fibrillation or flutter
   c. Other supraventricular tachydysrhythmias
   d. Ventricular tachycardia or fibrillation
2. Hypotension
3. Chest pain
4. Cardiac arrest

D. Neurologic
1. Anxiety
2. Tremors
3. Confusion
4. Irritability, restlessness
5. Headache
6. Hallucinations, acute psychosis
7. Seizures
8. Lethargy, stupor, coma

E. Renal
1. Diuresis
2. Urinary retention
3. Acute renal failure

Key Clinical Findings

- History of acute drug overdose or chronic theophylline usage
- Nausea, vomiting
- Cardiac tachydysrhythmias
- Agitation, confusion
- Seizures

Laboratory Findings

A. Increased serum theophylline concentration

1. Interpretation

   a. Upper therapeutic limit: 15 to 20 μg/L

   b. Mild toxic range: 20 to 35 μg/mL

   c. Serious toxicity: more than 35 μg/mL

   d. High risk of death: more than 90 μg/mL in acute overdose; more than 50 μg/mL (but more variable) in chronic intoxication

2. Serial assays are indicated to determine peak level and to use as end point for active treatment measures.

B. Hyperglycemia

C. Hypokalemia

D. Hypercalcemia

E. Hypophosphatemia

F. Hypobicarbonatemia

1. Metabolic (lactic) acidosis

2. Respiratory alkalosis

G. Leukocytosis

PEARL

There is poor correlation between the serum theophylline level and clinical manifestations in patients with chronic intoxication.

Treatment

A. General measures

1. Assure adequate airway and ventilation; endotracheal intubation.

2. Assure adequate perfusion; cardiopulmonary resuscitation may be necessary.

3. Monitor vital signs frequently.

4. Obtain 12-lead electrocardiogram.

5. Continuous electrocardiographic monitoring

6. Seizure precautions

7. Consider evaluation for other etiologies; e.g.,

   a. Give concentrated dextrose, thiamine, and naloxone intravenously if altered sensorium.

   b. Computed tomography indicated if seizures occur

   c. Consider concomitant drug intoxication.

B. Blood tests

1. Obtain serum glucose, electrolytes, other routine biochemical tests, and complete blood cell and platelet counts.

2. Obtain serum theophylline level initially and repeat every 2 to 4 hours until peak established.

3. Obtain serum and urine for toxicologic screening tests to exclude mixed overdose.

C. Use of gastric lavage may be considered in the following circumstances.

1. Presentation within 1 hour of ingestion

2. Overdose involving sustained-release theophylline products

3. Massive overdose

D. Activated charcoal

1. Adsorbs theophylline remaining within the gastrointestinal tract

2. Also removes systemically absorbed theophylline by establishing a concentration gradient across the bowel wall favoring back-diffusion into the gut lumen

3. Give 1 g/kg orally or by nasogastric tube initially, then 0.5 g/kg every 2 to 4 hours until the serum theophylline level is less than 25 mg/L.

4. Give 0.5 mL/kg sorbitol or 4 mL/kg magnesium citrate orally or by nasogastric tube with the first dose of charcoal to promote elimination.

5. Antiemetic drug therapy (e.g., metoclopramide) may be necessary to suppress vomiting.

E. Charcoal hemoperfusion

1. Rapidly lowers serum theophylline levels, but requires specialized equipment and personnel

2. Complications

   a. Complications of central venous access

   b. Hypotension

   c. Thrombocytopenia

   d. Leukopenia

   e. Hemolysis

   f. Anemia

   g. Hypocalcemia

   h. Hypophosphatemia

   i. Hypoglycemia

3. Indications

   a. Life-threatening theophylline intoxication

   b. Deterioration despite conventional treatment

   c. Intolerance of oral or enteral activated charcoal (e.g., intractable vomiting, ileus, bowel obstruction)

   d. Serum theophylline concentration of at least 100 mg/L in patients with acute intoxication

   e. Serum theophylline concentration of at least 60 mg/L in patients with chronic intoxication

   f. Serum theophylline concentration of at least 40 mg/L in patients with chronic intoxication and coexisting respiratory failure, serious liver disease, or congestive heart failure

4. Alternatives
   a. Resin hemoperfusion
   b. Hemodialysis (less effective than hemoperfusion, but can be used if hemoperfusion is unavailable)

F. Treat seizures
   1. Benzodiazepine (e.g., IV diazepam or lorazepam) for active seizures
   2. Phenobarbital may be administered after benzodiazepine.
   3. Anticonvulsant prophylaxis with phenobarbital may be considered in high-risk patients.
      a. Serum theophylline level higher than 80 μg/mL (acute ingestion)
      b. Serum theophylline level higher than 40 μg/mL (chronic ingestion)
      c. Age greater than 60 years
   4. Perform electroencephalogram in patients in coma to exclude nonconvulsive status epilepticus.

G. Treat cardiac dysrhythmias.
   1. Supplement potassium if hypokalemic.
   2. β-Adrenergic antagonists may be considered for supraventricular tachydysrhythmias.
      a. Often contraindicated because of underlying bronchospastic disease
      b. Potential for causing hypotension by negative inotropic effect, but propranolol has been used
      c. Esmolol advantageous because any adverse effects are reversed rapidly after discontinuation of infusion
   3. Lidocaine or phenytoin for ventricular tachycardia or fibrillation

H. Treat hypotension
   1. Consider intravascular volume expansion before vasopressor agents.
   2. If vasopressor necessary, choose agent with minimal β-adrenergic agonist action (e.g., phenylephrine, norepinephrine, dopamine)
   3. Address severe tachydysrhythmias.

Bibliography

Kempf J, Rusterholtz T, Ber C, et al. Haemodynamic study as guideline for the use of beta blockers in acute theophylline poisoning. Intensive Care Med 1996;22:585–587.

Shannon M. Life-threatening events after theophylline overdose: a 10-year prospective analysis. Arch Intern Med 1999;159:989–994.

Shannon MW. Comparative efficacy of hemodialysis and hemoperfusion in severe theophylline intoxication. Acad Emerg Med 1997;4:674–678.

Tsai J, Chern TL, Hu SC, et al. The clinical implication of theophylline intoxication in the emergency department. Hum Exp Toxicol 1994;13:651–657.

Vassallo R, Lipsky JJ. Theophylline: recent advances in the understanding of its mode of action and uses in clinical practice. Mayo Clin Proc 1998;73:346–354.

64 Lithium Overdose

James A. Kruse

Pharmacology

A. Action

1. Stabilizes serotoninergic neurotransmission
2. Inhibits release and reuptake of norepinephrine at synapses
3. Interferes with the action of arginine vasopressin at the renal tubule and collecting duct

B. Absorption

1. Gastrointestinal tract absorption results in peak blood concentration in 0.5 to 4 hours (except for sustained-release formulations).
2. Because of slow tissue absorption and renal excretion, 5 to 6 days are normally required to reach steady-state levels with therapeutic dosing.

C. Elimination

1. Entirely renal, except for trace amounts excreted in feces and sweat
2. Filtered at the glomerulus and reabsorbed (~80%) at the proximal tubule
3. Excretion decreased by sodium depletion, renal insufficiency, and thiazide diuretic use (risk factors for toxicity)

D. Pharmacokinetics

1. Volume of distribution: 0.7 L/kg
2. No protein binding
3. Half-life is approximately 6 hours (early) and 18 to 60 hours (late), with normal renal function.
4. Equilibrates slowly into and out of the central nervous system; thus, clinical improvement can be slow even if serum levels are lowered by dialysis

Clinical Findings

A. Central nervous system

1. Fatigue, lethargy, weakness
2. Confusion, irritability
3. Inability to concentrate, impaired memory
4. Lethargy, stupor, coma
5. Hyperreflexia
6. Tremors, including intention tremor
7. Myoclonus, fasciculations
8. Increased muscle tone
9. Ataxia, dysarthria
10. Seizures
11. Visual disturbances
12. Choreoathetosis
13. Malignant neuroleptic syndrome
14. Transient neurologic asymmetries

B. Cardiovascular

1. Sinus bradycardia
2. Sinus node dysfunction
3. U waves
4. T wave inversions
5. ST segment depression
6. Intraventricular conduction defects
7. Ventricular dysrhythmias
8. Hypotension

C. Gastrointestinal

1. Anorexia
2. Nausea, vomiting
3. Abdominal cramps or pain
4. Diarrhea
5. Excessive salivation

D. Renal

1. Polyuria and polydipsia (nephrogenic diabetes insipidus)
2. Nephrosis
3. Partial distal renal tubular acidosis
4. Renal failure

E. Miscellaneous

1. Dehydration
2. Hypothyroidism
3. Skin reactions (e.g., psoriatic, acneiform, folliculitis)
4. Acute respiratory distress syndrome

Key Clinical Findings

- Mental status abnormalities
- Myoclonus, ataxia, hyperreflexia
- Electrocardiographic changes
- Nausea, vomiting

Laboratory Findings

A. Increased serum lithium concentration
1. Therapeutic range: 0.6 to 1.4 mmol/L
2. Mild to moderate toxicity: 1.5 to 2.5 mmol/L
3. Serious toxicity: 2.5 to 3.5 mmol/L
4. Life-threatening toxicity: greater than 3.5 mmol/L
5. Spuriously elevated levels can occur if vacuum tubes or blood gas sampling devices containing lithium heparin are used for specimen collection.

B. Hyperglycemia with or without ketoacidosis
C. Hypercalcemia
D. Hypermagnesemia
E. Decreased serum anion gap
F. Hypernatremia
G. Azotemia
H. Neutrophilia
I. Lymphocytopenia
J. Thrombocytosis
K. Proteinuria

PEARL

Response to treatment is slower in chronic intoxication than in an acute overdose.

Treatment

A. General
1. Continuous electrocardiographic monitoring
2. Consider early endotracheal intubation.
3. Obtain routine serum biochemical tests: electrolytes, glucose, urea nitrogen, creatinine, etc.
4. Obtain serial serum lithium concentrations.
   a. Needed to determine peak level
   b. Multiple delayed peaking may occur in intoxication involving extended-release products.
   c. Allows evaluation of need for repeated dialysis
5. Obtain toxicologic screening tests if there is a possibility of a mixed overdose.
6. Monitor for clinical deterioration, which typically can evolve over 48 hours.
7. Careful monitoring of fluid intake and output

B. Discontinue offending and potentiating drugs.
1. Discontinue lithium carbonate.
2. Discontinue diuretics.
3. Discontinue drugs with potentially overlapping effects, e.g.: phenothiazines, haloperidol, cyclic antidepressants.

C. Gastric lavage may be considered if patient presents within 1 hour of acute overdose.

D. Perform whole-bowel irrigation.
1. Polyethylene glycol solution (GoLYTELY) at 2 L/hr for 5 hours
2. Contraindicated if bowel sounds are absent
3. Activated charcoal does not adsorb lithium, although it can be of value in cases of mixed overdose.

E. Intravenous fluids
1. Replace any existing fluid and sodium deficit.
2. Use normal saline or half-normal saline to provide maintenance fluids.
3. Urine output of at least 1 mL/kg per hour is generally adequate.
4. Beyond replacing deficits, forced diuresis is not recommended.

F. Hemodialysis
1. Indications
   a. Recommended for moderate to severe intoxication (serum lithium concentration higher than 3.5 or 4 mmol/L), even if asymptomatic
   b. Consider when serum concentration is in 2.0 to 4.0 mmol/L range if there is underlying renal insufficiency.
   c. Obtain at least 2 serum lithium concentrations, at least 3 hours apart, and plot the logarithm of drug concentration versus time; consider dialysis if linear extrapolation to 0.6 mmol/L reveals a corresponding elimination time longer than 36 hours.
   d. Hemodynamic instability
2. Continue dialysis until serum lithium concentration is below 1 mmol/L.
3. Monitor serum lithium level postdialysis; concentration may rebound 6 to 12 hours later.
4. Repeat dialysis if necessary.
5. Continuous venovenous hemodiafiltration has been used successfully and may obviate rebound.
6. Peritoneal dialysis has only approximately one-third the clearance of hemodialysis, but may be used initially if hemodialysis or continuous renal replacement modalities are not immediately available.

G. Multiple-dose sodium polystyrene sulfonate
1. Cation exchange resin has been used as adjunctive therapy for hastening lithium elimination.
2. No recommendation for routine use because available data are limited
3. Not a substitute for dialysis

H. Recognize and treat nephrogenic diabetes insipidus, if present.

   1. See Chapter 53, Diabetes Insipidus.

   2. Amiloride may be useful for treating persistent diabetes insipidus caused by lithium.

I. Consultation and follow-up

   1. Nephrologic follow-up (irreversible renal dysfunction can occur from lithium intoxication)

     a. Nephrogenic diabetes insipidus

     b. Tubulointerstitial nephropathy

     c. Nephrotic syndrome

   2. Psychiatric evaluation

     a. If overdose was intentional

     b. For management of underlying psychiatric disorder, if present

   3. Neurologic follow-up

     a. Persistent cerebellar dysfunction, nystagmus, tremor, rigidity, and memory deficits can occur.

     b. Neurologic sequelae can last for days or weeks, or be permanent.

Key Treatment

- Close monitoring and supportive care
- Whole-bowel irrigation
- Hemodialysis
- Serial serum lithium level assessments

Bibliography

Dupuis RE, Cooper AA, Rosamond LJ, et al. Multiple delayed peak lithium concentrations following acute intoxication with an extended-release product. Ann Pharmacother 1996;30:356–360.

Gallinat J, Boetsch T, Padberg F, et al. Is the EEG helpful in diagnosing and monitoring lithium intoxication? A case report and review of the literature. Pharmacopsychiatry 2000;33:169–173.

Groleau G. Lithium toxicity. Emerg Med Clin North Am 1994;12:511–531.

Timmer RT, Sands JM. Lithium intoxication. J Am Soc Nephrol 1999;10:666–674.

Van Bommel EF, Kalmeijer MD, Ponssen HH. Treatment of life-threatening lithium toxicity with high-volume continuous venovenous hemofiltration. Am J Nephrol 2000; 20:408–411.

65 Cocaine Intoxication

James A. Kruse

Pharmacology

A. Formulations

  1. Cocaine hydrochloride

    a. Crystalline form of cocaine (benzoylmethy-lecgonine)

    b. Commonly abused by nasal insufflation (snorting), oral ingestion, or IV injection

    c. Cannot be smoked because its chemical structure breaks down at high temperature

  2. Solid alkaloid form

    a. Commonly known as *free base* or *crack* cocaine

    b. Can be smoked because heat vaporizes the compound without breaking down its chemical structure

  3. Cocaine sulfate

  4. Adulterants (common in illicit formulations or ersatz cocaine)

    a. Inert substances that simulate appearance of cocaine: e.g., talc, cornstarch, flour, plaster of Paris, lactose, mannitol

    b. Local anesthetics, added to impart topical anesthetic properties: e.g., procaine, lidocaine, tetracaine, benzocaine

    c. Stimulants, added to impart sympathomimetic properties: e.g., phenylpropanolamine, caffeine, amphetamine, ephedrine

    d. Toxins, added to impart bitter taste similar to cocaine: e.g., strychnine, quinine

    e. Other illicit or over-the-counter drugs: e.g., heroin, phencyclidine, aspirin, acetaminophen

B. Absorption: rapidly and highly absorbed from the nasal mucosa, gastrointestinal tract, and (when smoked) the lungs

C. Actions

  1. Central nervous system (CNS) stimulant

    a. Inhibits presynaptic reuptake of dopamine and norepinephrine

    b. Increase in excitatory neurotransmitter levels

  2. Sympathomimetic vasoconstrictor properties

    a. Centrally mediated α and β-adrenergic stimulation

    b. Blockade of catecholamine reuptake

  3. Blockade of fast sodium channels

    a. Local anesthetic effects

    b. Type I antidysrhythmic effects on myocardium

D. Metabolism

  1. Approximately 40% hydrolyzed by plasma cholinesterase and hepatic esterases to ecgonine methyl ester

  2. Approximately 40% hydrolyzed nonenzymatically to benzoylecgonine

  3. Approximately 20% metabolized by hepatic demethylation to norcocaine

E. Pharmacokinetics

  1. Onset of action

    a. By insufflation: less than 3 minutes

    b. By smoking or IV injection: less than 15 seconds

    c. By ingestion: approximately 10 minutes

  2. Peak effect

    a. By insufflation: 20 to 30 minutes

    b. By smoking or IV injection: 3 to 5 minutes

    c. By ingestion: approximately 60 minutes

  3. Elimination

    a. Duration of effect: 20 to 90 minutes

    b. Half-life of cocaine: 30 to 90 minutes

    c. Half-life of metabolites: 4 to 8 hours (allows detection by urine testing for 2 days or more after cocaine use)

Clinical Findings

A. Central nervous system

  1. Anxiety, restlessness

  2. Euphoria, hyperactivity, psychosis

  3. Delirium, stupor, coma

  4. Hallucinations (uncommon)

  5. Syncope

  6. Seizures (typically brief and self-limited, or absent)

  7. Headache

B. Cardiovascular

  1. Hypertension

  2. Dysrhythmias

    a. Sinus tachycardia

    b. Supraventricular tachydysrhythmias

c. Ventricular tachycardia or fibrillation

d. Bradydysrhythmias

3. Ischemic chest pain

4. Signs of congestive heart failure

5. Delayed conduction (prolonged QRS and QT intervals)

C. Miscellaneous

1. Increased body temperature

2. Mydriasis

3. Abdominal pain (see complications)

4. Constipation, bowel obstruction from "body packing" (e.g., condoms, latex gloves, or balloons filled with cocaine and swallowed for purposes of smuggling; see Treatment, G., below)

5. Increased muscle tone

WARNING

β-Adrenergic blocking drugs are contraindicated in cocaine intoxication.

Complications

A. Central nervous system

1. Status epilepticus

2. Transient ischemic attack

3. Cerebral infarction

4. Subarachnoid hemorrhage

5. Intracerebral hemorrhage

6. Central nervous system vasculitis

7. Dystonic reactions

8. Cerebral atrophy

B. Ocular

1. Blindness

a. Retinal artery vasospasm

b. Optic tract or occipital cortex infarction or vasculitis

c. Optic neuropathy

2. Corneal defects (crack eye syndrome)

C. Cardiovascular

1. Myocardial ischemia and infarction, mediated by several potential mechanisms:

a. Coronary vasospasm

b. Increased myocardial oxygen demand

c. Intimal smooth muscle proliferation

d. Premature coronary atherosclerosis

e. Coronary thrombosis

2. Congestive heart failure, which may be due to:

a. Myocarditis

b. Cardiomyopathy

c. Contraction band necrosis

d. Endocarditis-mediated valvular disease (from IV use)

3. Aortic dissection

4. Aortic rupture

5. Cardiac arrest

D. Pulmonary

1. Asthma exacerbation

2. Noncardiogenic pulmonary edema

3. Pulmonary hemorrhage

4. Thermal airway injury

5. Diffuse pulmonary infiltrates, hypersensitivity pneumonitis (crack lung)

6. Bronchiolitis obliterans and organizing pneumonia

7. Barotrauma

a. Pneumothorax

b. Pneumomediastinum

c. Pneumopericardium

E. Gastrointestinal

1. Mesenteric ischemia, infarction, perforation

2. Bowel obstruction from "body packing" (see Treatment, G., below)

3. Hepatotoxicity

F. Obstetric

1. Preterm labor and delivery

2. Abruptio placentae

3. Chorioamnionitis

4. Spontaneous abortion or stillbirth

5. Adverse prenatal effects

a. Teratogenesis

b. Growth retardation

c. Other congenital anomalies (e.g., microcephaly, myelomeningocele, agenesis of corpus callosum)

G. Miscellaneous

1. Rhabdomyolysis

2. Hyperthermia

3. Disseminated intravascular coagulation

4. Metabolic acidosis

5. Respiratory distress, failure

6. Acute renal failure

7. Priapism

8. Sudden massive overdose from "body packing" (see Treatment, G., below)

a. Due to rupture of swallowed cocaine-filled packets

b. Can result in severe complications (e.g., hyperthermia, myocardial infarction, brain hemorrhage, status epilepticus, respiratory arrest and ventricular arrhythmias) or death

Key Complications

- Hypertension
- Seizures
- Rhabdomyolysis
- Tachydysrhythmias
- Acute myocardial infarction
- Cerebral hemorrhage or infarction

Treatment

A. General
  1. Ensure adequate airway and ventilation.
  2. Monitor vital signs frequently.
  3. Secure IV access.
  4. Monitor electrocardiogram continuously.
  5. Assess oxygenation using pulse oximetry.
  6. Provide supportive measures.

B. Obtain laboratory and other tests.
  1. Urine toxicologic assay to confirm presence of cocaine metabolites
  2. Urine and serum toxicologic screening to exclude mixed intoxication
  3. Routine hematologic, coagulation, and serum biochemical tests
  4. Blood glucose monitoring to detect hypoglycemia or hyperglycemia
  5. Serum total creatine phosphokinase activity to exclude rhabdomyolysis
  6. Serum creatine phosphokinase MB isoenzyme and cardiac troponin levels to exclude myocardial infarction
  7. 12-lead electrocardiogram
  8. Arterial blood gas analysis (selected cases)
  9. Imaging studies
     a. Chest x-ray to detect pulmonary complications
     b. Computed tomography of the brain if CNS abnormalities present
     c. Abdominal x-ray if body packing is suspected

C. Gastric evacuation
  1. May be considered if there is a history of oral consumption
  2. Syrup of ipecac not recommended

D. Activated charcoal: 1 g/kg

E. Sedation
  1. Benzodiazepines (e.g., lorazepam, diazepam) are first-line agents; administer intravenously initially.
  2. Neuroleptic agents have been used, but they may lower the seizure threshold and impair heat dissipation.

F. Tachydysrhythmias
  1. Supraventricular tachydysrhythmias
     a. Benzodiazepines are first-line agents.
     b. Sodium bicarbonate, adenosine, calcium channel blockers, and possibly labetolol have a role.
  2. Ventricular tachycardia
     a. Lidocaine
     b. Magnesium sulfate
     c. Overdrive pacing
     d. Sodium bicarbonate
     e. Labetolol (?)

G. Treatment for body packing
  1. Confirm by plain abdominal or contrast x-ray.
  2. Administer multiple doses of activated charcoal.
  3. Administer laxatives or perform whole-bowel irrigation (the use of whole-bowel irrigation with polyethylene glycol solutions has been recommended but also criticized on the basis that it may dissolve drug-containing packets and interfere with adsorptive properties of activated charcoal).
  4. Monitor until drug has passed through gastrointestinal tract.
  5. Consider endoscopic or surgical removal if clinical signs of toxicity manifest or there is bowel obstruction (role is controversial).

H. Hypertension
  1. Benzodiazepines may be sufficient for mild cases.
  2. β-Adrenergic blockers are contraindicated.
     a. May exacerbate hypertension by blocking basal opposing vasodilatory effect mediated by endogenous peripheral β-adrenergic receptors
     b. Can cause coronary artery vasoconstriction and precipitate cardiac ischemia
     c. Labetolol, which has combined α and β-adrenergic blocking effects, has been advocated, but its role is not well established.
  3. Other conventional antihypertensive agents can be used (e.g., nitroglycerin, phentolamine, nitroprusside).

Key Treatment

- Activated charcoal
- Benzodiazepines
- Electrocardiographic monitoring
- Monitor for and treat hypertension.
- Monitor for and treat hyperthermia.
- Seizure precautions

I. Treat myocardial ischemia and infarction.
   1. Provide standard treatment.
   2. Exceptions to standard management
      a. Thrombolytic therapy may be contraindicated by hypertension.
      b. β-Adrenergic blocking agents are contraindicated.

J. Treat hypotension.
   1. Give isotonic crystalloids intravenously.
   2. Norepinephrine is useful for hypotension refractory to volume loading.

K. Treat seizures.
   a. Give IV benzodiazepines initially.
   b. Follow with barbiturate (or phenytoin).

L. Treat hyperthermia: may require external cooling measures or other methods of lowering body temperature

M. Treat rhabdomyolysis (see Chapter 153, Rhabdomyolysis).

Bibliography

Boghdadi MS, Henning RJ. Cocaine: pathophysiology and clinical toxicology. Heart Lung 1997;26:466–485.

Haim DY, Lippmann ML, Goldberg SK, et al. The pulmonary complications of crack cocaine. A comprehensive review. Chest 1995;107:233–240.

Kleerup EC, Wong M, Marques-Magallanes JA, et al. Acute effects of intravenous cocaine on pulmonary artery pressure and cardiac index in habitual crack smokers. Chest 1997;111:30–35.

Mittleman MA, Mintzer D, Maclure M, et al. Triggering of myocardial infarction by cocaine. Circulation 1999;99: 2737–2741.

Pitts WR, Lange RA, Cigarroa JE, et al. Cocaine-induced myocardial ischemia and infarction: pathophysiology, recognition, and management. Prog Cardiovasc Dis 1997;40:65–76.

Winbery S, Blaho K, Logan B, et al. Multiple cocaine-induced seizures and corresponding cocaine and metabolite concentrations. Am J Emerg Med 1998;16:529–533.

66 Calcium Channel and β-Blocker Drug Overdoses

Adriana H. Wechsler
Richard W. Carlson

Classification

A. Calcium channel antagonists

   1. Dihydropyridine derivatives (e.g., nifedipine)

      a. Predominant effect is reduction of systemic vascular resistance.

      b. Can cause hypotension

      c. May cause reflex tachycardia

      d. Nifedipine is the most potent vasodilator.

   2. Phenylalkylamine (verapamil) and benzothiazepine (diltiazem) derivatives

      a. Delay sinus node activity

      b. Slow atrioventricular (A-V) conduction and significantly decrease myocardial contractility

      c. Cardiac effects predominate.

   3. Diarylaminopropylamine ether derivative (bepridil)

      a. Acts as a class I antidysrhythmic agent

      b. The only calcium channel blocker to cause QT interval prolongation; may induce ventricular tachycardia and torsade de pointes

   4. T-channel blockers, such as mibefradil (Posicor), are not currently available.

B. β-Adrenergic receptor antagonists

   1. Cardioselectivity

      a. Nonselective and selective β-adrenergic blockers have differing effects at therapeutic doses.

      b. β-Adrenergic selectivity is reduced at toxic doses.

   2. Membrane stabilizing effects: may occur with various agents at toxic doses

   3. Lipid solubility

      a. Varies substantially among agents

      b. Correlates with extent of liver metabolism and penetration across the blood–brain barrier

   4. Sotalol

      a. A nonselective β-adrenergic receptor antagonist with unique antidysrhythmic activity

      b. Can produce torsade de pointes

> **PEARL**
>
> There are many similarities in the clinical features of overdoses with β-adrenergic receptor antagonists and calcium channel antagonists. Adverse effects are intensified with co-ingestion of both drugs or other agents that affect cardiac conduction or cause hypotension.

Pharmacology

A. Calcium channel antagonists (Table 66–1)

   1. Effects and mechanisms of action

      a. Block the slow (L-type) calcium channels in myocardium and vascular smooth muscle

      b. Inhibit sinoatrial (SA) and A-V nodal conduction

      c. Decrease heart rate, cardiac output, and arterial blood pressure

      d. Bepridil is the only agent to also block fast sodium and potassium channels, prolonging A-V nodal refractory period, action potential, and myocardial repolarization.

   2. Metabolism and pharmacokinetics

      a. Rapid oral absorption

      b. Predominate liver metabolism

      c. First-pass hepatic metabolism reduces bioavailability.

      d. Substantial protein binding

      e. Large volume of distribution

      f. Standard formulations have rapid onset of action; toxicity appears typically within 30 to 60 minutes of ingestion, rarely beyond 3 hours.

      g. Sustained-release formulations manifest symptoms within 6 to 8 hours, but may be delayed up to 24 hours.

   3. Therapeutic indications

      a. Hypertension

      b. Angina pectoris

      c. Supraventricular dysrhythmias

      d. Left ventricular diastolic dysfunction

      e. Other indications include migraine headache,

TABLE 66-1. CLASSIFICATION, REPRESENTATIVE AGENTS, PHARMACOLOGY AND METABOLISM OF CALCIUM CHANNEL RECEPTOR BLOCKING DRUGS*

CLASS	GENERIC NAME	BRAND NAME	CARDIOVASCULAR EFFECTS	PEAK LEVEL (HR)[†]	HALF-LIFE (HR)
Phenylalkylamine	Verapamil	Calan, Isoptin, Verelan	↓ SVR, ↓ HR, ↓ ↓ CC, ↑ ↑ ↑ AVC	1 to 2	4.5 to 12
	Verapamil[‡]	Calan SR	(Same as above)	1 to 2	4.5 to 12
Benzothiazepine	Diltiazem	Cardizem, Dilacor, Tiazac	↓ SVR, ↓ HR, ↑ AVC, 0 to ↓ CC	0.5 to 1	3 to 4.5
	Diltiazem[‡]	Cardizem CD	(Same as above)	10 to 14	5 to 8
Diarylaminopropylamine ether	Bepridil	Vascor	↓ SVR, ↑ HR, ↓ CC, ↑ ↑ AVC	2 to 3	26 to 64
Dihydropyridine	Nifedipine	Procardia, Adalat	↓ ↓ SVR, ↑ HR, ↓ CC, ↑ AVC (overdose)	0.5	2
	Nifedipine[‡]	Procardia XL, Adalat CC	(Same as above)	6	2
	Nicardipine	Cardene	↓ SVR, ↑ HR	0.5 to 2	2 to 10
	Nicardipine[‡]	Cardene SR	0 to ↓ CC, 0 AVC	1 to 2	9
	Felodipine	Plendil	↓ SVR, ↑ HR, 0 to ↓ CC, 0 AVC	2.5 to 5	11 to 16
	Amlodipine	Norvasc	↓ SVR, ↑ HR, 0 to ↓ CC, 0 AVC	6 to 12	30 to 50
	Nisoldipine[‡]	Sular	↓ SVR, 0 to ↑ HR, 0 to ↓ CC, 0 AVC	6 to 12	7 to 12

* ↓ to ↓ ↓ ↓ = expected degree of decrease; ↑ = expected to increase; 0 = no effect; SVR = systemic vascular resistance; HR = heart rate; CC = cardiac contractility; AVC = atrioventricular conduction time.
[†] After oral dosing.
[‡] Sustained-release or extended-release formulation.

subarachnoid hemorrhage (nimodipine), Raynaud's phenomenon, preterm labor, esophageal spasm, and bipolar disorders.

B. β-Adrenergic receptor antagonists (Table 66-2)
  1. Effects and mechanism of action
    a. Molecular structures are similar to isoproterenol.
    b. Exhibit competitive antagonism of catecholamines at β-adrenergic receptors with reduction of adenyl cyclase activity
    c. Decrease inotropism, chronotropism, and dromotropism (conduction)
    d. Can impair glycogenolysis and gluconeogenesis; can augment free fatty acid release
    e. Increase bronchial tone and alter smooth muscle tone
    f. Agents such as propranolol also have "membrane stabilizing effects," which block fast sodium channels.
  2. Metabolism and pharmacokinetics
    a. Rapid absorption with peak effects of standard formulations in 1 to 4 hours
    b. Half-lives vary from 10 minutes (esmolol) to more than 24 hours (nadolol); extended-re-

TABLE 66-2. FEATURES OF REPRESENTATIVE β-ADRENERGIC RECEPTOR BLOCKING DRUGS

NAME	CARDIO-SELECTIVE	ADRENERGIC RECEPTOR ANTAGONIST ACTIVITY	MEMBRANE STABILIZATION (NA CHANNEL BLOCKADE)	VOLUME OF DISTRIBUTION (L)	PROTEIN BINDING	HALF-LIFE (HR)	LIPID SOLUBILITY	METABOLISM AND ELIMINATION
Atenolol	Yes	β_1	No	1	Low	5+	Low	Renal (dialyzable)
Esmolol	Yes	β_1		2+	Moderate	Minutes	Low	Esterase
Labetalol	No	$\alpha_1, \beta_1, \beta_2$	No	9+	Moderate	4 to 6	Moderate	Hepatic
Metoprolol	Yes	β_1	Low	5+	Low	3 to 4	Moderate	Hepatic
Nadolol	No	β_1, β_2	No	2	Low	<24	Low	Dialyzable
Pindolol	No	β_1, β_2*	Low	2	Moderate	<12	Moderate	Renal and hepatic
Propranolol[†]	No	β_1, β_2	Moderate to high	3 to 4	High	3 to 6	High	Hepatic
Sotalol	No	β_1, β_2	No	2	Very low	12	Low	Renal

* Also possesses intrinsic sympathomimetic activity.
[†] Associated with the most fatalities from overdose.

lease preparations increase duration of action.

   c. Volume of distribution greater than 1 L/kg

   d. Water-soluble agents are associated with reduced hepatic metabolism and greater excretion in unchanged form.

   e. Protein binding varies from approximately 0% (sotalol) to more than 90% (propranolol).

3. Therapeutic indications

   a. Hypertension

   b. Angina

   c. Tachydysrhythmias

   d. Other indications include migraine, panic attack, hyperthyroidism, aortic dissection, idiopathic hypertrophic subaortic stenosis, glaucoma, withdrawal states, pheochromocytoma, congestive heart failure (carvedilol), and mitral valve prolapse.

Key History

- History of β-adrenergic receptor antagonist or calcium channel antagonist use

- History of previous overdose or suicide attempts with any drug

- Symptoms from β-adrenergic blocker overdose usually develop within 2 to 6 hours after ingestion; calcium channel blocker toxicity can manifest within 30 minutes of ingestion.

Clinical Findings

A. Findings common to overdoses with either calcium channel antagonists or β-adrenergic receptor antagonists

1. Constitutional: fatigue, generalized weakness

2. Cardiovascular: hypotension, bradycardia (dihydropyridine derivatives can cause reflex tachycardia), conduction disturbances (heart block, wide QRS interval, prolonged QT interval), orthostasis, torsade de pointes (sotalol and bepridil), congestive heart failure, pulmonary edema

3. Pulmonary: pulmonary edema, aspiration pneumonitis, respiratory depression, apnea

4. Gastrointestinal: nausea, vomiting, mesenteric ischemia or bowel infarction (rare)

5. Central nervous system: lethargy, dizziness, obtundation, delirium, coma, seizures (rare), anoxic encephalopathy (after prolonged hypotension)

B. Additional findings that may be seen in calcium channel antagonist overdose

1. Cardiovascular: reflex tachycardia (dihydropyridines), ventricular dysrhythmias (ventricular tachycardia, torsade de pointes; uncommon except with bepridil)

2. Metabolic: hyperglycemia (secondary to inhibition of insulin release), lactic acidosis

C. Additional findings that may be seen in β-adrenergic receptor antagonist overdose

1. Cardiovascular: hypertension (rarely, with pindolol)

2. Pulmonary: bronchospasm

3. Metabolic: hypoglycemia, hyperkalemia, metabolic acidosis

4. Renal: acute renal failure

Key Laboratory and Other Tests

- Drug levels: generally not available or not helpful; diltiazem and verapamil levels available on some urine toxicology surveys

- Electrocardiogram: may show bradydysrhythmias, conduction disturbances, prolonged QRS interval, QT interval prolongation, torsade de pointes

- Chest x-ray: pulmonary edema, aspiration pneumonia

- Blood tests: routinely assess serum electrolytes, urea nitrogen, creatinine, glucose, and calcium concentrations; liver function tests; arterial blood gases

Differential Diagnosis

A. Toxic overdoses

1. β-Adrenergic antagonist overdose vs. calcium channel antagonist overdose

2. Digoxin toxicity

3. Clonidine and other α-adrenergic agonist toxicity

4. Antidysrhythmic agents

5. Other agents: organophosphates, cyclic antidepressants, opioids, sedative-hypnotics, cyanide, hydrogen sulfide, cardioactive steroids, carbamates

B. Other disorders

1. Cardiac: coronary artery disease, rhythm disturbances, pulmonary edema, cardiogenic shock

2. Cerebrovascular accident

3. Anaphylactic, hypovolemic, or septic shock

4. Adrenal insufficiency, myxedema coma

Treatment

A. Resuscitation

1. Ensure adequate airway and ventilation.

   a. Intubate trachea, if indicated.

   b. Consider atropine (0.5 mg intravenously) prior to intubation, to prevent aggravating bradycardia.

   c. Provide assisted ventilation as needed.

2. Maintain large-bore peripheral or central intravenous access.

3. Treat hypotension: crystalloid fluid resuscitation is first priority.

4. Treat symptomatic bradycardia.

   a. First priority is atropine (0.5 to 1.0 mg intravenously every 2 to 3 minutes up to 3 mg maximum), but effects are typically modest and there may be little or no effect on arterial blood pressure.

   b. Temporary transvenous or transcutaneous pacing may be required in severe bradycardia.

5. Consider overdrive pacing to treat torsade de pointes caused by sotalol intoxication.

6. Intra-aortic balloon counterpulsation (as an adjuvant to pacing) and cardiopulmonary bypass may be considered in cases of extreme circulatory failure.

7. Treat seizures.

   a. Lorazepam loading with up to 0.1 mg/kg intravenously

   b. Correct hypoglycemia.

   c. See Chapter 79, Status Epilepticus.

B. Decontamination

1. Induction of emesis (syrup of ipecac)

   a. Contraindicated in both calcium channel antagonist and β-adrenergic receptor antagonist overdoses, because resulting vagal stimulation can aggravate bradycardia.

   b. Generally contraindicated for drug overdoses in the hospital setting.

2. Gastric lavage: consider for ingestions occurring within 1 hour (calcium channel blocker) or 2 hours (β-adrenergic blocker) of presentation

3. Activated charcoal

   a. 1 g/kg by mouth or by nasogastric or orogastric tube

   b. Consider additional doses 0.5 g/kg every 1 to 2 hours for up to 72 hours for massive ingestions, for ingestions of sustained release preparations, and (in β-adrenergic blocker overdose) to reduce enterohepatic recirculation.

4. Whole bowel irrigation

   a. Consider for ingestions of large amounts of sustained-release preparations.

   b. Accomplished using polyethylene glycol (GoLytely, CoLyte) by nasogastric tube at 1 to 2 L/hour until clear rectal drainage is obtained

   c. Consider concomitant antiemetic treatment during whole bowel irrigation (e.g., ondansetron or chlorpromazine).

5. Dialysis and hemoperfusion

   a. Of little benefit in most of these overdoses because of high protein binding, high volume of distribution, or lipid solubility of the drugs

   b. Consider for propranolol, atenolol, or sotalol overdose.

C. Monitoring

1. Airway, vital signs, and continuous electrocardiographic monitoring for at least 6 hours for suspected ingestion

2. Intensive care unit monitoring for at least 24 hours for symptomatic patients

3. Serial neurologic examinations for level of consciousness

4. Seizure precautions

5. Routine laboratory testing: serum electrolytes, glucose, renal and hepatic function tests

6. Serial arterial blood gases, pH, and lactate concentration

7. Urine output

8. Consider invasive hemodynamic monitoring (systemic and pulmonary artery catheterization) in patients with hypotension, bradycardia, or conduction disturbances.

9. Chest x-ray

D. Glucagon

1. Bypasses β_1-adrenergic receptors to directly activate adenylate cyclase and cyclic adenosine monophosphate, increasing heart rate and arterial blood pressure; particularly helpful for refractory hypotension

2. Consider use early in severe overdoses; effects usually evident within 1 to 3 minutes and peak in 5 to 7 minutes.

3. Initial dose is 2 to 5 mg (up to 10 mg in β-adrenergic antagonist overdose) by IV bolus, followed by 4 to 10 mg over 5 minutes if no response.

4. Consider maintenance infusion at "response

dose" (1 to 5 mg/hour); mix in 5% dextrose-water or normal saline.

5. Caution: may induce nausea and vomiting; protect airway

6. May cause hyperglycemia, hypokalemia, and rarely Stevens-Johnson syndrome or allergic reactions

E. Calcium salts

1. Have a clear role as first-line treatment of calcium channel antagonist overdoses, but are less helpful in β-adrenergic receptor antagonist overdoses and may inhibit the actions of glucagon

2. Improve cardiac contractility; less effective for bradycardia and conduction disturbances

3. Initial dose is 10 to 20 mL of 10% calcium chloride intravenously; repeat boluses every 15 to 20 minutes up to 3 to 4 doses, or give an infusion of 0.5 mEq/kg per hour (0.2 to 0.4 mL/kg per hour of 10% calcium chloride).

4. Calcium gluconate is an alternative to calcium chloride (see Chapter 41, Hypocalcemia, for dose conversions and precautions).

5. Monitor serum calcium concentration and discontinue IV calcium if concentration exceeds 14 mg/dL or signs of hypercalcemia develop.

WARNING

Avoid calcium salts if suspicion of co-ingestion of digoxin; or give calcium after digoxin-specific Fab therapy.

F. Catecholamines

1. β-Adrenergic agonists stimulate receptors on myocardium and peripheral vasculature to ameliorate bradycardia, impaired contractility, and vasodilation.

2. For β-adrenergic receptor antagonist overdose:

   a. Isoproterenol may be the optimal agent for β-blocker–induced bradycardia.

   b. High infusion rates may be required; start at 2 to 10 μg/minute and titrate to response.

   c. Consider norepinephrine or epinephrine for β-blocker–induced hypotension; may be used in conjunction with isoproterenol.

3. For calcium channel antagonist overdose:

   a. Isoproterenol (2 to 10 μg/minute) or dobutamine (2 to 30 μg/kg per minute) may be used for chronotropic and inotropic effects.

   b. For significant calcium channel antagonist overdoses addition of a catecholamine with

α-adrenergic activity is often necessary to offset the β2-activated peripheral vasodilation. Typically dopamine (at adrenergic doses, i.e., ≥10 μg/kg per minute) and isoproterenol can be used; epinephrine, norepinephrine, or phenylephrine can also be considered.

G. Phosphodiesterase inhibitors

1. Amrinone and milrinone are second-line agents for improving inotropic state.

2. See Chapter 160, Amrinone and Milrinone.

CAUTION

The use of vasodilating inotropic agents (i.e., milrinone, amrinone, dobutamine, isoproterenol) can lead to peripheral vasodilation and hypotension; always use in conjunction with a vasopressor to counteract hypotension.

H. Insulin + glucose

1. Anecdotal reports suggest efficacy in calcium channel blocker overdose; consider in severe toxicity.

2. Insulin 0.5 U/kg per hour plus dextrose infusion by central access at approximately 20 g/hour and titrated to maintain blood glucose concentration above 100 mg/dL but without marked hyperglycemia

I. Hypertonic sodium chloride and bicarbonate (investigational)

1. Hypertonic sodium chloride may improve cardiac contractility, increase vascular smooth muscle contraction, and overcome inhibition of sodium channel blockade, thereby offsetting effects on potassium.

2. Hypertonic bicarbonate therapy has been shown to be effective in an experimental model of verapamil intoxication.

3. Bicarbonate not demonstrated to help in experimental β-adrenergic receptor antagonist intoxication

J. 4-Aminopyridine (investigational treatment for calcium channel blocker overdose): facilitates synaptic transmission by calcium-dependent transmitter release

Prognosis

A. Factors affecting severity of toxicity in calcium channel antagonist overdose

1. Dose ingested

a. Toxicity reported with <1.5 g of diltiazem

b. Survival reported after ingestion of more than 16 g of verapamil

2. Comorbid conditions

a. Patients with underlying cardiovascular disease: greater morbidity and mortality

b. Elderly patients and those with cardiovascular disease: symptomatic at lower, and even therapeutic doses

c. Liver disease exacerbates toxicity.

3. Co-ingestions

a. β-Adrenergic receptor antagonists, calcium channel antagonists, and digoxin will potentiate conduction abnormalities caused by one another, and co-ingestion leads to more severe bradydysrhythmias.

b. Calcium channel antagonists decrease clearance of digoxin, with concomitant digoxin toxicity.

4. Formulation and pharmacologic class

a. Verapamil causes the greatest impairment of cardiac conduction and contractility, most often leads to toxicity that is resistant to pharmacotherapy (often requiring pacing), and is associated with the greatest number of fatalities.

b. Dihydropyridines (e.g., nifedipine) have limited myocardial binding, and bradycardia is therefore uncommon, except with massive ingestions (fatalities are rare).

c. Phenylalkamine (e.g., verapamil) and benzothiazepine (e.g., diltiazem) classes exert significant negative inotropic and chronotropic effects; atrioventricular blockade is more common.

d. Sustained-release drugs induce more severe and prolonged toxicity.

B. Clinical course in β-adrenergic receptor antagonist overdose

1. If asymptomatic for 6 hours, serious toxicity is unlikely, although observation for up to 24 hours is suggested for ingestion of extended-release preparations.

2. Toxicity with critical hemodynamic and metabolic disturbances may persist for 48 to 72 hours.

3. Mortality rate is up to 25%; greater risk is associated with co-ingestions.

4. The prognosis for full recovery is good if the patient survives the acute period of toxicity.

Bibliography

Abernathy DR, Schwartz JB. Calcium-antagonist drugs. N Engl J Med 1999;341:1447–1457.

Boyer EW, Shannon M. Treatment of calcium-channel-blocker intoxication with insulin infusion. N Engl J Med 2001;344:1721–1722.

Kerns W II, Schroeder D, Williams C, et al. Insulin improves survival in a canine model of acute β-blocker toxicity. Ann Emerg Med 1997;29:748–757.

Love JN, Howell JM, Litovitz TL, et al. Acute β-blocker overdose: factors associated with the development of cardiovascular morbidity. J Toxicol-Clin Toxicol 2000;38:275–281.

Reith DM, Dawson AH, Epid D, et al. Relative toxicity of β-blockers in overdose. J Toxicol-Clin Toxicol 1996;34:273–278.

Snook CP, Sigvaldason K, Kristinsson J. Severe atenolol and diltiazem overdose. J Toxicol-Clin Toxicol 2000;38:661–665.

Tanen DA, Rula AM, Curry SC, et al. Hypertonic sodium bicarbonate is effective in the management of verapamil toxicity in a swine model. Ann Emerg Med 2000;36:547–553.

67 Digoxin Overdose

Salmaan Kanji
John W. Devlin

Etiology

A. Mechanism of toxicity

1. Cardiac glycosides inhibit the function of the sodium–potassium–adenosine triphosphatase (Na-K-ATPase) pump.

   a. Transient late depolarizations may be seen at toxic concentrations.

   b. Hyperkalemia

      (1) Frequently results from acute ingestion

      (2) May cause further depolarization of myocardial conduction tissue, especially in the atrioventricular (AV) node

   c. Hypokalemia

      (1) Often seen with chronic toxicity

      (2) May be related to concomitant diuretic use

      (3) By causing receptor down regulation, may exacerbate Na-K-ATPase pump inhibition and decrease the volume of distribution of the drug

2. Directly prolongs the AV nodal refractory period, thus decreasing conduction velocity in the atria, ventricles and AV node

   a. Prolongs electrocardrographic (ECG) PR interval, decreases QT interval

   b. If increased vagal tone is present, digoxin may result in varying degrees of AV block along with accelerated junctional rhythms.

   c. ST-segment depression and inverted T waves

      (1) Usually seen soon after an acute intoxication

      (2) Caused by increased vagal tone

3. Enhanced atrial and ventricular excitability and automaticity may result in extrasystoles and tachydysrhythmias.

B. Risk factors contributing to digoxin toxicity

1. Hyperkalemia

2. Hypokalemia

3. Hypomagnesemia

4. Hypercalcemia

5. Renal or hepatic insufficiency

6. Advanced age

7. Alkalemia

8. Cor pulmonale

9. Drug interactions (e.g., loop and thiazide diuretics, quinidine, verapamil, diltiazem, amiodarone, propafenone, spironolactone, cyclosporin A)

Clinical Findings

A. Cardiovascular

1. AV block (varying degrees)

2. Ectopic rhythms

   a. Atrial tachycardia

   b. Non-paroxysmal junctional tachycardia

   c. Ventricular premature extrasystoles (PVCs)

   d. Bidirectional ventricular tachycardia

   e. Ventricular flutter

   f. Ventricular fibrillation

3. Sinoatrial block

4. Sinus bradycardia

5. Hypotension and circulatory shock can occur with significant dysrhythmias.

6. Electrocardiographic changes

   a. ST-segment depression

   b. T wave inversion

   c. Increased PR interval

   d. AV block

   e. Decreased QT_c interval

B. Gastrointestinal

1. Nausea

2. Vomiting

3. Anorexia

4. Abdominal pain

C. Visual disturbances

1. Photophobia

2. Blurred vision

3. Scotoma

4. Aberrations of color vision (usually limited to chronic toxicity)

5. Amblyopia

D. Central nervous system

1. Confusion

2. Disorientation

3. Drowsiness

4. Hallucinations

5. Convulsions (rare)

229

Laboratory Findings

A. Measure serum electrolyte concentrations, including K, Mg, and Ca.

   1. Hyperkalemia: serum potassium concentrations greater than 5.5 mEq/L are associated with severe toxicity

   2. Hypokalemia and hypomagnesemia (usually seen in chronic overdose situations, often due to concomitant diuretic use)

B. Measure serum urea nitrogen and creatinine concentration to assess renal function.

C. Measure serum digoxin concentration.

   1. Therapeutic range for digoxin is 0.8 to 2.0 ng/mL.

   2. Relationship of clinical signs of digoxin toxicity to serum digoxin concentration

      a. Signs and symptoms of acute digoxin toxicity are usually seen at concentrations greater than 10 ng/mL but may occur with lower concentrations (especially in the elderly).

      b. Serum digoxin concentrations may be misleading if obtained during the post-ingestion distribution phase, thus serum digoxin concentrations should not be drawn less than 6 hours after the last ingestion.

Key Findings

- Virtually any dysrhythmia can occur with digitalis toxicity, although AV block and increased ventricular automaticity are the most common, occurring in 30% to 40% of patients.

- Severity of hyperkalemia is a better prognostic indicator of mortality related to digoxin toxicity than serum drug concentrations or ECG changes.

- Visual disturbances generally are manifestations of chronic toxicity.

- Serum digoxin concentrations obtained within 6 hours of ingestion will likely overestimate the degree of intoxication.

Treatment

A. Supportive care

   1. Maintain airway and provide assisted ventilation, if necessary.

   2. Secure IV access.

   3. Support cardiovascular function, if necessary.

   4. Provide continuous ECG monitoring for patients who are symptomatic, have ECG changes, or have hyperkalemia.

   5. Any patient with suspected digoxin overdose should be monitored for at least 12 to 24 hours because of the possibility of delayed tissue distribution.

B. Prevention of further gastrointestinal absorption

   1. Induction of emesis: use of ipecac syrup is controversial because it is ineffective if given more than 30 minutes after an acute ingestion, and the vagal stimulation induced by emesis may exacerbate bradycardia and heart block

   2. Activated charcoal

      a. Most effective if administered within 1 hour of ingestion

      b. Multiple doses of activated charcoal may enhance digoxin elimination by reducing enterohepatic and enteroenteric recirculation.

      c. Dose: 25 to 100 g PO or via nasogastric tube in a slurry every 2 to 4 hours

      d. Sorbitol may be added to the first one or two doses.

      e. Several doses may be required for large ingestions or for patients with renal failure.

   3. Gastric lavage

      a. Should only be considered within 60 minutes of acute ingestion.

      b. Caution: gastric lavage may enhance vagal stimulation and exacerbate digoxin-induced bradycardia and heart block

   4. Whole bowel irrigation

      a. May be considered for large ingestions

      b. Contraindicated in patients with bowel obstruction, perforation, toxic megacolon, or toxic colitis

      c. Dose: polyethylene glycol (GoLYTELY) PO or via nasogastric tube at 2 L/hour until rectal effluent is clear

C. Enhancing elimination

   1. Forced diuresis, hemodialysis, and hemoperfusion are not effective in removing digoxin or digitoxin from the serum because only 1% of the total body digoxin stores are found in the serum at any one time, and of this amount approximately 25% is protein bound.

   2. Multiple dose charcoal may be effective in enhancing elimination as digoxin undergoes both enterohepatic and enteroenteric recirculation.

   3. Cholestyramine and colestipol have been used to bind digitoxin, and to a lesser extent digoxin, in the gastrointestinal tract in patients with renal failure.

D. Digoxin-specific antibody fragments (Fab)

   1. Mechanism of action

a. Fab binds both intravascular free digoxin (immediately after IV administration) as well as digoxin that has diffused into the interstitial space.

b. Digoxin has a greater affinity for Fab than for the Na-K-ATPase pump.

c. The Fab–digoxin complex is renally eliminated.

d. Fab promotes the dissociation of digoxin from cardiac Na-K-ATPase by decreasing the serum free digoxin concentration.

2. Efficacy and safety

a. Mean time to initial response is 19 minutes after the end of infusion.

b. Mean time to complete response is 88 minutes.

c. Reported adverse effects include hypokalemia (4%), allergic reactions (<1%), and exacerbations of congestive heart failure (3%).

3. Indications for use

a. Ventricular dysrhythmias

b. Progressive bradydysrhythmias

c. Second- or third-degree heart block not responsive to atropine

d. Serum potassium level greater than 5.0 mEq/L in the setting of suspected digitalis toxicity

e. Post-distribution serum digoxin concentrations of at least 10 ng/mL (more than 6 hours after ingestion)

f. Known ingestion of at least 10 mg digoxin

4. Dosing

a. Each vial of Digibind contains 38 mg of digoxin-specific Fab fragments, which will bind approximately 0.5 mg digoxin or digitoxin.

b. Dosing based on amount ingested (body load): Digibind dose = body load/0.5, where body load (mg) = dose (mg) × 0.8, and dose is in number of vials

c. Dosing based on a 6-hour post-ingestion serum concentration:

$$\text{Digibind dose} = \text{digoxin level} \times \text{Wt} / 100$$

where digoxin level is the serum digoxin concentration (ng/mL), Wt is the patient's weight (kg), and dose is in number of vials

d. Each vial is reconstituted with 4 mL of sterile water and administered IV over 30 minutes through a 0.22 μm membrane filter (it may be given as an IV bolus to highly unstable patients).

5. Renal failure

a. In patients with renal failure the half-life of Fab is substantially prolonged (~10-fold).

b. Fab is not appreciably removed by dialysis because of its large molecular weight, extensive tissue binding, and large volume of distribution.

c. A rebound phenomenon has been described up to 3 to 11 days after the initial Fab dose.

(1) Serum digoxin concentrations begin to rise as the digoxin begins to dissociate from the Fab that was initially administered.

(2) This may indicate the need for another dose.

6. Serum digoxin levels

a. Serum digoxin concentrations usually peak 3 to 24 hours after Fab administration before slowly declining.

b. This phenomenon is observed because most assays cannot differentiate free digoxin and digoxin bound to Fab.

c. After Fab administration, total serum digoxin levels are no longer clinically useful and should not be used to guide therapy.

E. Managing complications

1. Hyperkalemia

a. Treatment is recommended if serum potassium concentration is greater than 5.0 mEq/L.

b. Fab should be administered as quickly as possible because it will restore Na-K-ATPase pump function and rapidly reverse hyperkalemia.

c. Glucose and insulin: 100 mL of 50% dextrose IV push plus 5 to 10 units of regular insulin IV push (recommended for life-threatening hyperkalemia >6.5 mEq/L or when Fab is not available)

d. Sodium bicarbonate: 88 mEq intravenously (recommended for life-threatening hyperkalemia >6.5 mEq/L or when Fab is not available)

e. Calcium should not be administered as it may precipitate cardiac dysrhythmias.

f. Sodium polystyrene sulfonate (Kayexalate)

(1) Not recommended because it lowers total body potassium and may not benefit the patient.

(2) The hyperkalemia associated with digoxin toxicity is related to a shift of potassium from the intracellular space to the extracellular space.

g. Continuous ECG monitoring

2. Severe hypokalemia (<3.0 mEq/L)

   a. Provide cautious potassium replacement.

   b. Monitor serial serum potassium levels.

3. Hypomagnesemia: provide supplemental magnesium (e.g., 2 to 4 g MgSO$_4$ intravenously over 20 minutes)

4. Severe supraventricular bradydysrhythmia or AV block

   a. Atropine 0.5 to 1.0 mg intravenously or endotracheally (if IV access is unavailable) every 5 minutes to a maximum dose of 0.04 mg/kg

   b. While atropine is used to block the vagotonic effects of digoxin, it may be only partially effective at restoring a normal heart rate because the depressant effects of digoxin are only partly mediated by the vagus nerve.

   c. The use of isoproterenol is contraindicated as it may increase the incidence of ventricular ectopic activity.

   d. Transvenous or external cardiac pacing should be considered in patients who have severe bradycardia or severe AV block that is unresponsive to phenytoin, atropine, or both, and where Fab therapy is not available.

5. Ventricular dysrhythmias (PVCs, ventricular tachycardia, bigeminy)

   a. Fab is first-line therapy.

   b. Phenytoin or lidocaine

      (1) Both depress ventricular automaticity without significantly slowing AV node conduction (phenytoin may improve conduction through the AV node).

      (2) Either agent is indicated for termination of ventricular dysrhythmias when Fab is not available.

      (3) Phenytoin dose: 15 mg/kg loading dose intravenously at 50 mg/minute; with IV or PO maintenance doses of 300 to 400 mg/day, targeting a therapeutic level between 10 and 20 μg/mL

      (4) Lidocaine dose: 1.0 to 1.5 mg/kg loading dose IV push (a 0.5 to 1.0 mg/kg dose may be given 10 to 15 minutes after the loading dose), followed by continuous maintenance infusion of 1.0 to 4.0 mg/minute

      (5) The maintenance dose of lidocaine should be reduced by 50% in patients with impaired hepatic blood flow (e.g., congestive heart failure, cardiogenic shock, acute myocardial infarction).

   c. All Vaughn-Williams class 1A antidysrhythmic agents are contraindicated as they may worsen both AV nodal blockade and have additional proarrhythmogenic effects.

   d. Magnesium sulfate

      (1) Has been used successfully in the management of ventricular dysrhythmias due to its ability to suppress early afterdepolarizations and antagonize digoxin at the Na-K-ATPase pump

      (2) Typical dose: 2 to 4 g intravenously over 20 minutes, followed by a continuous infusion of 1 to 2 g/hour, with serial serum assays

      (3) Contraindicated in bradycardia or AV block

      (4) Monitor for ECG changes, bradypnea, hyporeflexia, and hypotension.

Key Treatment (Indications for Digoxin-Specific Antibody Fragments)

- Ventricular dysrhythmias
- Second- or third-degree heart block, not responsive to atropine
- Serum potassium level greater than 5.0 mEq/L in the setting of suspected digitalis toxicity
- Progressive bradydysrhythmias
- Known ingestion of at least 10 mg digoxin
- Serum digoxin concentration of at least 10 ng/mL more than 6 hours post-ingestion

 Bibliography

Lip GYH, Metcalfe MJ, Dunn FG. Diagnosis and treatment of digoxin toxicity. Postgrad Med J 1993;69:337–339.

Martiny SS, Phelps SJ, Massey KL. Treatment of severe digitalis intoxication with digoxin-specific antibody fragments: a clinical review. Crit Care Med 1988;16:629–635.

Williamson KM, Thrasher KA, Fulton KB, et al. Digoxin toxicity: an evaluation in current clinical practice. Arch Intern Med 1998;158:2444–2449.

68 Alcohol and Glycol Intoxications

James A. Kruse

Etiology

Alcohol and glycol ingestions can be accidental or intentional, sporadic or epidemic. A common scenario for consumption of non-ethanol toxins is the desperate alcoholic without access to ethanol-containing beverages that resorts to intentional ingestion of these agents as an alcohol substitute. The following are common sources and uses of these intoxicants.

A. Ethanol intoxication
   1. Alcoholic beverages
   2. Pharmaceuticals containing ethanol as vehicle (e.g., some cough syrups, parenteral nitroglycerin, paclitaxel)
   3. Various toiletries, cosmetics, colognes, mouthwashes
   4. Food extracts
   5. Cleaners, detergents, cements, paint removers
   6. Gasohol

B. Methanol (wood alcohol)
   1. Denaturing agent
   2. Industrial solvent and synthetic precursor
   3. Automotive products (e.g., windshield washer fluids)
   4. Paint products (e.g., paints, stains, varnishes, lacquer thinner)
   5. Other commercially available solvents and cleaners
   6. Sterno and other brands of "canned heat"
   7. Gasohol, dry gas

C. Isopropanol
   1. Rubbing alcohol
   2. Alcohol sponges
   3. Antiseptics and disinfectants
   4. Cosmetics, lotions, liniments, hair products
   5. Commercially available cleaning, automotive, and other products

D. Ethylene glycol
   1. Commercially available automotive ("permanent") antifreezes and coolants
   2. Industrial solvent, antifreeze, plasticizer, humectant, and synthetic precursor
   3. Automotive products (e.g., hydraulic brake fluid, car wash fluids)
   4. Paint products (e.g., paints, lacquers) and inks

E. Propylene glycol
   1. Automotive antifreeze and coolant
   2. Cosmetics and toiletries
   3. Pharmaceutical vehicle (e.g., parenteral preparations of diazepam, lorazepam, digoxin, phenytoin, etomidate, esmolol, hydralazine, nitroglycerin, trimethoprim-sulfamethoxazole; topical silver sulfadiazine)
   4. Use in food industry (food additive, emulsifier, humectant, dairy and brewery antifreeze)
   5. Industrial solvent

F. Diethylene glycol
   1. Industrial solvent, humectant, plasticizer, antifreeze, and synthetic precursor
   2. Has been mistakenly and fraudulently substituted as vehicle in pharmaceutical formulations (e.g., in place of glycerin or propylene glycol), resulting in epidemic fatalities

---

PEARL

A common scenario for consumption of toxic alcohols (other than ethanol) or glycols is the desperate alcoholic without access to ethanol-containing beverages who resorts to intentional ingestion of one of these agents as an alcohol substitute.

Toxicology

A. Ethanol
   1. A clear, colorless, volatile liquid with a characteristic, pleasant odor and a burning taste
   2. Ingestion of approximately 4 ounces of liquor or 48 ounces of beer by a 70 kg person typically results in a blood ethanol concentration of approximately 100 mg/dL.
   3. Fatalities have occurred at serum levels of approximately 400 mg/dL; however, survival has occurred at levels as high as 700 mg/dL.
   4. Main physiologic effects are inebriation and central nervous system (CNS) depression.
   5. Metabolized by hepatic alcohol dehydrogenase to acetaldehyde, and then to acetate by hepatic acetaldehyde dehydrogenase; also metabolized by a microsomal enzyme pathway

6. Rate of metabolism can vary widely, but typically decreases at a rate of 10 to 30 mg/dL per hour depending on prior exposure history; chronic use of ethanol, benzodiazepines, barbiturates, and certain other drugs induces high-level activity of microsomal enzymes and leads to more rapid metabolism.

B. Methanol (wood alcohol)

1. A clear, colorless, volatile liquid with a mildly alcoholic odor

2. The lethal dose is highly variable (<10 to >500 mL).

3. Methanol itself has inebriating and sedating properties, but it is otherwise relatively innocuous.

4. Its metabolic by-products are formaldehyde and formic acid, which are highly toxic agents responsible for ocular and CNS toxicity.

C. Isopropanol (isopropyl alcohol)

1. A clear, colorless, volatile liquid with a distinctive odor and a burning, bitter taste

2. The lethal dose is estimated to be approximately 200 mL; mild symptoms have occurred after ingestion of 20 mL and at serum concentrations of approximately 50 mg/dL.

3. Metabolized directly to acetone

D. Ethylene glycol

1. Clear, colorless, practically odorless, slightly viscous liquid with a sweet taste

2. The lethal dose is typically 1 to 2 mL/kg, but substantial variability has been reported.

3. The only toxic effects of the parent compound are neurologic; however, it is metabolized to several highly toxic by-products (notably glycolic, glyoxylic, and oxalic acids) that can cause acidosis and renal dysfunction.

E. Propylene glycol

1. Clear, colorless, viscous liquid with a slightly acrid taste

2. Very low toxicity compared to other glycols; approved by World Health Organization for use as food additive at less than 25 mg/kg per day

3. Metabolized directly to lactic acid

F. Diethylene glycol

1. Clear, colorless, practically odorless liquid with a sharply sweetish taste

2. Mean lethal dose in one epidemic poisoning was 38 g in children and 71 g in adults.

3. Only documented metabolite is 2-(hydroxy)-ethoxyacetic acid, but its role in pathogenesis is unclear; not metabolized to glycolic, glyoxylic, or oxalic acids.

Clinical Manifestations

A. Ethanol

1. Central nervous system

a. Sensorial depression (although low concentrations can initially result in exuberant behavior due to loss of high-level CNS inhibition)

b. Chronic use leads to some degree of tolerance because of CNS adaption.

c. Dose response is therefore variable, but typified by the following:

(1) 50 to 150 mg/dL: exuberant verbal and motor activity, impaired judgment and concentration, mild ataxia, slowed reaction time, blurred vision

(2) 150 to 250 mg/dL: ataxia, dysarthria, impaired visual pursuit, nystagmus, diplopia, lethargy interrupted by brief periods of exuberant activity

(3) 250 to 400 mg/dL: stupor, intermittently interrupted by brief periods of hostile verbal and physical behavior; incoherent speech; hypoglycemia; hypothermia; seizures

(4) More than 400 mg/dL: coma, respiratory arrest, death

2. Gastrointestinal (GI): epigastric pain, nausea, emesis, hemorrhage, gastritis, pancreatitis

3. Cardiorespiratory: characteristic breath odor; pulmonary aspiration caused by impaired airway reflexes and obtundation; respiratory failure or arrest; tachycardia; vasodilation; hypotension

4. Miscellaneous: flushed facies, hypothermia

B. Methanol

1. Central nervous system: drunkenness, stupor, coma, meningeal signs, cerebral edema, cerebral infarction (involving basal ganglia), seizures

a. As with ethanol, inebriation occurs shortly after ingestion.

b. Conversion to toxic metabolites takes hours, so there is typically a delay of 12 to 24 hours before other manifestations (other than inebriation and GI effects) occur.

2. Gastrointestinal: epigastric pain, nausea, emesis, hemorrhage, gastritis, pancreatitis

3. Ocular: decreased visual acuity, scotomata, scintillations, blurred vision, unreactive pupils, papilledema, partial or complete blindness

4. Cardiorespiratory: faint odor of methanol or formaldehyde may be detectable on patient's

breath, dyspnea, Kussmaul respirations, respiratory failure, circulatory shock

C. Isopropanol

1. Central nervous system: headache, confusion, dizziness, slurred speech, ataxia, miosis, lethargy, obtundation, coma; isopropanol is roughly twice as potent as ethanol with respect to CNS effects (coma reported with isopropanol serum concentrations of approximately 120 mg/dL)

2. Gastrointestinal: nausea, vomiting, abdominal pain, hemorrhagic gastritis, diarrhea, hepatic dysfunction

3. Cardiorespiratory: characteristic odor of isopropanol or acetone may be detectable on the patient's breath; dyspnea; hypoxemia; pulmonary edema; respiratory failure; bradycardia; circulatory shock

4. Miscellaneous: flushing, renal dysfunction, myopathy, rhabdomyolysis, hemolysis, hypothermia

D. Ethylene glycol

1. Central nervous system (effects can manifest within minutes of ingestion): initial excitement, confusion, lethargy, ataxia, stupor, coma, seizures

2. Cardiorespiratory (effects typically occur 12 to 24 hours after ingestion): dyspnea, Kussmaul respirations, pulmonary edema, respiratory failure, circulatory shock

3. Renal (effects manifest 24 to 72 hours after ingestion): acute tubular necrosis, oliguric or nonoliguric renal failure; may require dialysis

E. Propylene glycol

1. Central nervous system: inebriation, sensorial depression, coma, seizures

2. Cardiorespiratory: tachycardia, tachypnea, cardiac dysrhythmias, hypotension

F. Diethylene glycol

1. Central nervous system: coma, clonus, facial palsy, fever, dilated pupils, seizures

2. Gastrointestinal: nausea, emesis, diarrhea, hepatomegaly, hepatic injury with central degeneration

3. Cardiorespiratory: shock, respiratory failure

4. Renal: acute tubular necrosis with vacuolar nephropathy (but no calcium oxalate deposition), renal failure, oligoanuria

Laboratory Findings

A. Ethanol

1. Slight increase in blood lactate concentration can occur; significant elevation should prompt consideration of another cause (e.g., circulatory shock, alternative intoxication).

2. Confirmed by positive serum ethanol assay

3. Increase in serum osmolality

4. Hypoglycemia can occur.

5. Alcoholic ketoacidosis is uncommon; occurs during resolution phase of a recent binge.

B. Methanol

1. Metabolic acidosis

a. Resulting from metabolism to formic acid

b. Lactic acidosis can also occur.

(1) Especially likely if there is secondary circulatory shock

(2) Can also occur due to high redox state produced by metabolism of methanol, leading to an increased lactate : pyruvate ratio.

c. Acidosis can be profound in severe poisoning.

2. Increased serum anion gap caused by the accumulation of formate (and possibly lactate)

3. Increased serum osmole gap caused by high circulating concentrations of methanol and formate

a. Calculated as the difference (in mOsm/kg H_2O) between measured (Osm_m) and estimated (Osm_c) serum osmolality using:

$$\text{Osmole gap} = Osm_m - Osm_c$$

b. Estimated serum osmolality is calculated from simultaneously obtained measurements of serum glucose, urea nitrogen, and ethanol (in mg/dL) and sodium concentration (in mmol/L) using:

$$Osm_c = 2 \times \text{sodium} + (\text{glucose}/18) \\ + (\text{urea nitrogen}/2.8) + (\text{ethanol}/4.6)$$

c. Normal osmole gap is less than 10 mOsm/kg H_2O.

d. Significant elevations suggest an excessive circulating concentration of an osmotically active solute, such as methanol.

4. Positive serum methanol assay confirms diagnosis.

C. Isopropanol

1. Does not cause metabolic acidosis, per se

a. Neither isopropanol nor its metabolite, acetone, is an acid.

b. Severe cases can have associated lactic acidosis by the same mechanisms described for methanol.

2. No associated increased serum anion gap (unless significant lactic acidosis)

3. Increased serum osmole gap from high concentrations of circulating isopropanol and acetone

4. Positive serum isopropanol assay confirms diagnosis.

5. May be associated with hypoglycemia

6. Spuriously increased serum creatinine concentration can occur.

D. Ethylene glycol

1. Metabolic acidosis

a. Mainly from metabolism to glycolic and glyoxylic acids

b. Severe cases can have associated lactic acidosis by the same mechanism as described for methanol.

c. Can be extremely severe

2. Increased serum anion gap: mainly from accumulation of glycolate and glyoxylate

3. Increased serum osmole gap from high circulating concentrations of ethylene glycol and its metabolites

4. Crystalluria

a. Caused by formation calcium oxalate, a terminal metabolite of ethylene glycol

(1) Calcium oxalate monohydrate (whewellite): hempseed-shaped, prismatic, or needle-like crystals

(2) Calcium oxalate dihydrate (weddellite): octahedral crystals

b. Presence of oxalate crystalluria corroborates the diagnosis, but its absence does not exclude the diagnosis.

5. Fluorescent urine

a. Yellow-green fluorescence of urine upon exposure to ultraviolet light has been reported after ingestion of certain commercial antifreeze preparations.

b. These antifreeze preparations include fluorescein dye to facilitate identification of automotive cooling system leaks.

c. False positive fluorescence can occur.

(1) Presence of other fluorescent substances in urine (e.g., carbamazepine, benzodiazepine metabolites, carotene, niacin)

(2) Use of plastic specimen containers with high native fluorescence

d. False negative fluorescence can occur

(1) Ingestion of antifreeze (or other ethylene glycol containing solution) formulated without fluorescein

(2) Urine collected more than 4 hours after ingestion

(3) Urine pH lower than 4.5, which prevents fluorescence (can obviate by pH testing and, if necessary, in vitro adjustment of pH)

6. Hypocalcemia may occur as a result of calcium oxalate precipitation.

7. Positive serum ethylene glycol assay confirms diagnosis.

E. Propylene glycol

1. Hyperlactatemia, a result of direct conversion of propylene glycol to lactic acid

2. Metabolic acidosis from lactic acidosis

3. Increased serum anion gap from accumulation of lactate

4. Increased serum osmole gap from high circulating concentrations of propylene glycol and lactate

5. Hemolysis can occur.

6. Positive serum propylene glycol assay confirms diagnosis.

Key Laboratory Findings*

Intoxicant	Metabolic Acidosis	↑ Serum Osmole Gap	↑ Serum Anion Gap	↑ Serum Acetone	Oxalate Crystalluria	Specific Assay
Ethanol	−	+†	−	−	−	+
Methanol	+	+	+	−	−	+
Isopropanol	−	+	−	+	−	+
Ethylene glycol	+	+	+	−	+	+
Propylene glycol	+	+	+	−	−	+
Diethylene glycol	+	±	+	−	−	+

*plus sign = characteristic finding; minus sign = not a characteristic finding.
†Serum osmole gap is elevated only if ethanol term is excluded from formula for estimating serum osmolality.

F. Diethylene glycol

1. Metabolic acidosis due to metabolism to 2-(hydroxy)-ethoxyacetic acid and resultant renal failure

2. Increased serum anion gap may occur as a result of accumulation of 2-(hydroxy)-ethoxyacetate.

3. Increased serum osmole gap possible (but not as sensitive for detecting diethylene glycol as for identifying compounds with lower molecular weight or lower toxicity)

4. Crystalluria not expected (not metabolized to oxalate)

5. Positive serum diethylene glycol assay confirms diagnosis

Treatment

A. General measures

1. Ensure adequate oxygenation, ventilation, and perfusion.

   a. Respiratory support: endotracheal intubation and mechanical ventilation may be required in patients with severe sensorial depression, impending or frank respiratory failure, and in patients undergoing gastric lavage

   b. Treatment of shock: which may include fluid therapy, inotropic drugs, and vasopressor agents; pulmonary artery catheterization may be helpful for titrating therapy

2. Monitor vital signs and neurologic status, institute seizure precautions.

3. Ensure all relevant diagnostic tests are obtained; initiation of specific therapy should not be delayed if a presumptive diagnosis can be made before specific toxicologic identification is available.

4. Gastric lavage should be performed in patients presenting soon after ingestion (emesis should not be induced, even in awake patients, because sensorial depression may develop and place patient at risk for aspiration).

5. Activated charcoal may be administered but is unlikely to be of benefit unless there is another toxin present.

6. Consider evaluation for and treatment of conditions commonly associated with intoxication by alcohol and alcohol substitutes.

   a. Other forms of intoxication or drug overdose (administer naloxone routinely to patients with unexplained alterations in consciousness; perform drug screening assays)

   b. Subdural hematoma or other serious head injuries (consider computed tomography of brain)

   c. Infections (e.g., pneumonia, meningitis, spontaneous bacterial peritonitis)

   d. Hypoglycemia (check blood glucose and administer dextrose routinely to patients with unexplained alterations in consciousness)

   e. Fluid and electrolyte disturbances

   f. Hepatitis, cirrhosis, hepatic encephalopathy

   g. Pancreatitis (check serum amylase and lipase activities)

   h. Gastrointestinal hemorrhage

   i. Rhabdomyolysis (check serum creatine phosphokinase activity)

B. Ethanol intoxication

1. Provide reassurance and a calm environment with close observation.

2. Administer thiamine (e.g., 50 to 100 mg intravenously) to cover possibility of Wernicke's encephalopathy.

3. Administer multivitamin.

4. Administer dextrose-containing IV fluid.

5. Avoid sedative agents during acute intoxication.

6. Institute withdrawal precautions and routine supportive measures.

7. Hemodialysis has been used in cases of profound intoxication to remove ethanol, but it is rarely necessary unless intoxication is extreme or there is an additional indication for dialysis (e.g., established renal failure or concomitant methanol poisoning).

C. Methanol intoxication

1. Ethanol (therapeutic administration)

   a. Slows conversion of methanol to formaldehyde and formate by competitive inhibition of alcohol and aldehyde dehydrogenase

   b. Routes of administration

      (1) Intravenous: given as a 5% or 10% (volume/volume) ethanol solution in 5% (weight/volume) dextrose; must be given by central vein because of hyperosmolality

      (2) Enteral: oral dosing can be used in mild cases if the patient is sufficiently alert, or by nasogastric tube if sufficiently diluted (<20%); may produce emesis and abdominal pain

   c. Loading dose

      (1) In terms of absolute ethanol: 600 mg/kg or 0.76 mL/kg (based on V_d of 0.6 L/kg, specific gravity of absolute ethanol of

0.79, and targeted serum level of 100 mg/dL)

  (2) Oral loading dose using 100 proof liquor (i.e., 50% ethanol, v/v; or 40 g/dL): 1.52 mL/kg

  (3) Intravenous loading dose using 5% (v/v, i.e., 4 g/dL) ethanol solution: 15.2 mL/kg

  d. Maintenance dose

    (1) In terms of absolute ethanol: 66 mg/kg per hour

    (2) Intravenous dosing using 5% ethanol solution: 1.66 mL/kg per hour

    (3) Oral dosing using 100 proof liquor: 0.17 mL/kg per hour (must be diluted)

    (4) Increase dose (typically by a factor of 2 to 3) if the patient uses ethanol chronically.

    (5) Increase the dose (typically by a factor of 2 to 3) during hemodialysis.

  e. Serial serum ethanol levels should be obtained every 1 to 2 hours to allow frequent titration of ethanol administration to maintain a serum ethanol level of 100 to 150 mg/dL.

2. Fomepizole

  a. Potent inhibitor of alcohol dehydrogenase

  b. May be considered for use in place of ethanol.

3. NaHCO$_3$

  a. Titrate to arterial blood gas findings to treat metabolic acidosis.

  b. Anecdotal reports suggest NaHCO$_3$ ameliorates toxic manifestations and may improve survival.

  c. Avoid complete correction of acidemia or overshoot alkalosis.

4. Folic (e.g., 50 to 100 mg every 4 hours intravenously) or folinic acid is given to augment metabolic conversion of formate to CO$_2$.

5. Hemodialysis is performed in patients with the following findings to remove methanol and toxic metabolites from the body.

  a. Ocular findings

  b. Renal impairment

  c. Serum methanol levels above 50 mg/dL

  d. Metabolic acidosis

  e. Severe poisoning

6. Attention to fluid balance is important, particularly in patients given ethanol therapeutically because of the large fluid volumes involved.

D. Isopropanol

1. Hemodialysis should be considered in patients with high serum isopropanol levels ($\geq$ 400 mg/dL), coma, or hypotension.

2. Peritoneal dialysis is less effective than hemodialysis, but it can be used if hemodialysis is unavailable.

3. Continuous nasogastric suction may be of benefit based on the possibility of enterosalivary or enterogastric recirculation of absorbed isopropanol.

E. Ethylene glycol

1. Treatment is similar to that of methanol poisoning.

  a. NaHCO$_3$ (limited experimental evidence suggests survival benefit)

  b. Ethanol

    (1) Administer if there is presumptive evidence of ethylene glycol intoxication or a serum level greater than 20 mg/dL.

    (2) Use at the same dosage as for methanol (see above).

  c. Fomepizole

    (1) May be used in lieu of ethanol

    (2) Possesses the same mechanism of action as ethanol, but with the following advantages

      (a) Easier to dose and titrate

      (b) No sedating effects

      (c) Less chance of volume overload compared to IV ethanol

      (d) No nausea, emesis, abdominal pain compared to oral ethanol

  d. Hemodialysis removes ethylene glycol and its toxic metabolites from the body; used in all patients with toxic symptoms, acidosis, evidence of renal dysfunction, or serum ethylene glycol levels higher than 50 mg/dL.

2. Vitamin therapy: value in ethylene glycol poisoning is speculative, but it is not harmful

  a. Pyridoxine (vitamin B$_6$) supplementation: some evidence suggests that pyridoxine deficiency impairs glyoxylate metabolism

  b. Thiamine supplementation: may promote degradation of glyoxylate

  c. Folic acid supplementation: folate promotes conversion of formate to CO$_2$, and there is limited evidence that formate may be a minor product of ethylene glycol metabolism

3. Calcium chloride or gluconate was previously recommended to prevent hypocalcemia and intentionally precipitate oxalate in vivo, but this may have adverse consequences; not recommended except to treat symptomatic hypocalcemia.

Key Dosing for Fomepizole

- Load with 15 mg/kg, followed by 10 mg/kg every 12 hours for 4 doses, followed by 15 mg/kg every 12 hours until serum ethylene glycol level is lower than 20 mg/dL (all doses given intravenously over 30 minutes).

- At beginning of hemodialysis:
  If less than 6 hours since last dose, do not administer dose.
  If at least 6 hours since last dose, administer next scheduled dose.

- During hemodialysis: dose every 4 hours

- At completion of hemodialysis:
  If less than 1 hour between last dose and end of hemodialysis, do not administer dose at end of hemodialysis.
  If 1 to 3 hours between last dose and end of hemodialysis, administer half of the next scheduled dose at end of hemodialysis.
  If more than 3 hours between last dose and end of hemodialysis, administer next scheduled dose at end of hemodialysis.

- Maintenance dosing off hemodialysis: every 12 hours

F. Propylene glycol

1. Usually responds to removal of offending agent and supportive care alone

2. Hemodialysis can be considered in severe cases.

G. Diethylene glycol

1. Hemodialysis

2. Although not well studied for this agent, other treatment as for ethylene glycol is recommended, including either ethanol or fomepizole.

Bibliography

Kruse JA. Methanol poisoning. Intensive Care Med 1992; 18:391–397.

Kruse JA. Ethylene glycol intoxication. J Intensive Care Med 1992;7:234–243.

Kruse JA. Methanol, ethylene glycol, and related intoxications. In: Carlson RW, Geheb MA (eds). Principles & Practice of Medical Intensive Care. Philadelphia: WB Saunders, 1993, pp. 1714–1723.

Kruse JA, Cadnapaphornchai P. The serum osmole gap. J Crit Care 1994;9:185–197.

Winter ML, Ellis MD, Snodgrass WR. Urine fluorescence using a Wood's lamp to detect the antifreeze additive sodium fluorescein: a qualitative adjunctive test in suspected ethylene glycol ingestions. Ann Emerg Med 1990; 19:663–667.

69 Alcohol Withdrawal Syndrome

Richard W. Carlson
Jaya M. Raj

Acute alcohol intoxication and effects of chronic use, as well as the alcohol withdrawal syndrome (AWS) lead to considerable morbidity and mortality. The AWS includes multiple systemic manifestations that affect the severity of the syndrome.

Key Epidemiology

- Up to 40% of patients in emergency departments have consumed ethanol.

- More than 15 million Americans have alcohol dependence or heavy use.

- More than 200,000 alcohol-related deaths occur each year in the United States.

- In the United States, there are 1.2 million yearly hospital admissions for alcohol-related problems.

- 6% develop delirium tremens, with a mortality rate of up to 20%.

- 13% to 71% of patients seen for alcohol detoxification will develop the AWS.

Pathophysiology

A. Repeated ethanol use induces tolerance and dependence.

B. The AWS follows cessation or reduction of intake after prolonged use.

C. Chronic alcohol use has many effects on neurotransmission within the central nervous system (CNS), including alterations in

1. Adrenergic receptors
2. Dopamine turnover
3. γ-Aminobutyric acid (GABA) release
4. GABA receptor function
5. Excitatory N-methyl-D-aspartate receptor function

D. Circulating catecholamine levels correlate with the severity of the AWS.

PEARLS

(Features Distinguishing Ethanol Intoxication from AWS)

Intoxication	Withdrawal
• Relaxation	• Hypervigilant
• Sedation	• Easily startled
• Euphoria	• Hyperadrenergic
• Ataxia	• Falling blood ethanol levels
• Reduced inhibitions	• High catecholamine levels
• Memory loss	• Hyperventilation
• Poor judgment	• Seizure potential
• Obtundation or coma at higher ethanol levels	

Key Differential Diagnosis

(Caution: many conditions may co-exist with AWS)

- Heat stroke or hypothermia
- Drug ingestion
- Sepsis
- Trauma
- CNS bleeding
- Thyroid storm
- Wernicke's encephalopathy
- Epilepsy
- Hypoglycemia
- Subdural hematoma
- Acute myocardial infarction
- Respiratory failure
- Aspiration or bacterial pneumonia
- Dementia
- Parkinsonism
- Meningitis
- Pancreatitis
- Pneumonia
- Alcoholic ketoacidosis
- Vitamin deficiency states

TABLE 69–1. STAGES OF ALCOHOL WITHDRAWAL SYNDROME

STAGE	APPROXIMATE ONSET	SIGNS AND SYMPTOMS
1	6 to 8 hours after last drink or decreased consumption	Tremulousness, anxiety tachycardia, hypertension, diaphoresis
2	24 hours	Hallucinations (visual, tactile, or auditory); may be lucid
3	7 to 48 hours	Grand mal seizures
4	3 to 5 days or more	Autonomic hyperactivity, global confusional state (delirium tremens)

Clinical Findings

A. Stages of AWS (see Table 69–1)
  1. Do not occur sequentially in all patients
  2. Correlate with catecholamine levels

Laboratory Findings

A. General
  1. Laboratory abnormalities are nonspecific.
  2. Abnormal findings are related to acute medical problems, trauma, or chronic effects of ethanol on the liver and other organs.
B. Hematologic abnormalities
  1. Hemoglobin or hematocrit increase (because of third spacing) or decrease (because of bleeding)
  2. Leukocytosis or leukopenia
  3. Thrombocytopenia
C. Coagulation abnormalities
  1. Elevated prothrombin time
  2. Elevated partial thromboplastin time
D. Serum biochemical abnormalities
  1. Electrolyte disturbances (e.g., alterations of potassium, magnesium, phosphorus, and calcium concentrations)
  2. Hyperglycemia or hypoglycemia
  3. Elevated urea nitrogen and creatinine concentrations
  4. Elevated enzyme activities
    a. Elevated serum amylase and lipase
    b. Elevated creatine phosphokinase (CK) activity
  5. Abnormal toxic drug assays or screening tests (including the serum osmole gap)
  6. Hyperuricemia
  7. Abnormal liver function tests
    a. Increased serum aspartate aminotransferase activity
    b. Increased serum alanine aminotransferase activity
    c. Increased serum bilirubin concentration
  8. Thyroid function disturbances
E. Arterial blood gas and acid-base derangements
  1. Hypoxemia
  2. Hypocapnia or hypercapnia
  3. Ketosis or ketoacidosis
  4. Elevated blood lactate concentration
F. Positive blood, sputum, or urine microbiologic cultures
G. Positive occult blood detected in gastric aspirate or stool
H. Electrocardiographic abnormalities
I. Electroencephalographic abnormalities

Special Considerations: Indications for Intensive Care Unit Admission

A. Age more than 40 years
B. Cardiac disease, dysrhythmias, congestive heart failure, coronary artery disease, recent (past 6 months) myocardial infarction
C. Hemodynamic or respiratory instability
D. Marked acid-base disturbances
  1. Severe derangements
  2. "Double" or "triple" acid-base disorders
E. Fluid and electrolyte derangements
  1. Hyponatremia or hypernatremia
  2. Hypokalemia or hyperkalemia
  3. Hypomagnesemia
  4. Hypophosphatemia
  5. Hypocalcemia
  6. Volume depletion
F. Hypoglycemia or marked hyperglycemia
G. Sepsis
H. Acute gastrointestinal disorders
  1. Bleeding
  2. Pancreatitis
  3. Hepatic insufficiency
  4. Spontaneous bacterial peritonitis
I. Hypothermia or hyperthermia
J. Trauma or burn injury
K. Rhabdomyolysis

TABLE 69-2. ALCOHOL WITHDRAWAL SYNDROME SEDATON THERAPY

Agent	Dose	Interval	Half-life	Comments
Lorazepam	1 to 2 mg orally, intravenously, or intramuscularly (may give as continuous IV infusion at 1+ mg/hour after front-loading with 1+ mg intravenously)	Every 2 to 4 hours	10 to 20 hours	Helpful in liver disease and in old age
Midazolam	2 to 4 mg intravenously 2 to 6+ mg/hour by continuous IV infusion	—	1 to 12 hours	—
Diazepam	5 to 20 mg orally or intravenously	Every 6 hours	>40 hours	Reduce dose in liver disease; has long half-life and long-acting metabolites
Chlordiazepoxide	25 to 100 mg orally	Every 6 hours	5 to 15 hours	Useful in unmonitored settings (mild-moderate AWS)
Oxazepam	15 to 20 mg orally	Every 4 hours	5 to 10 hours	As above
Propofol	0.05 to 0.4 mg/kg intravenously initially, then 0.01 to 0.2 mg/kg per minute IV infusion	—	10+ minutes	Respiratory depression (must secure airway and provide mechanical ventilation)

L. Renal insufficiency or failure

M. Prior history of delirium tremens, alcohol-withdrawal seizures, complicated AWS

N. Poor score on sedation-anxiety evaluation

PEARL

Survival is linked to management of intercurrent medical or surgical problems, as well as to treatment of AWS.

Treatment

A. Treatment goals
  1. Allay symptoms of anxiety, agitation.
  2. Ensure protective environment.
  3. Manage delirium.
  4. Provide treatment or prophylaxis for hyperadrenergic state.
  5. Observe for progression of syndrome.
  6. Correct nutritional, fluid, and electrolyte defects.
  7. Provide psychiatric evaluation, if necessary.

B. Sedation
  1. Sedate with cross-tolerant agents to achieve a light sleep.
    a. Benzodiazepines are first-line agents (see Table 69-2).
    b. Barbiturates have also been used for sedation.
    c. Propofol can be used in patients with a cannulating airway who are receiving mechanical ventilation.
  2. Titrate sedative dosing as needed.

  a. Use somatic complaints and symptoms score or Ramsay score (Table 69-3).
  b. Aim for a Ramsay score of 2 to 3.

C. Adjunctive pharmacotherapy for controlling hyperadrenergic manifestations (may be helpful)
  1. β-Adrenergic antagonists
  2. Central-acting adrenergic agonists

D. Manage seizures.
  1. Treat AWS seizures with benzodiazepines.
  2. Use phenytoin for underlying seizure disorder, head trauma, or primary central nervous system pathology.

E. Give vitamins prophylactically.
  1. Thiamine: 100 mg daily for 5 days
  2. Folate: 1 mg daily
  3. Multivitamin formulation

F. Prophylaxis against deep vein thrombosis

G. After recovery, refer for counseling and rehabilitation.

TABLE 69-3. RAMSAY SEDATION SCALE*

Score	Level of Consciousness
1	Awake, anxious, agitated, restless
2	Awake, cooperative, oriented, tranquil
3	Awake; responds only to commands
4	Asleep; brisk response to tactile or load auditory stimulation
5	Asleep; sluggish response to tactile or load auditory stimulation
6	Unresponsive

*From Ramsay MAE, Savage TM, Simpson BRJ, Goodwin R. Controlled sedation with alphaxolone-alphadolone. Br Med J 1974;2: 656–659.

Key Treatment

- Benzodiazepines are the agent of choice.

- Barbiturates, β-blockers, central-acting adrenergic agonists may be helpful.

- Frequently reassess sedation level and titrate benzodiazepine dosing.

- Treat AWS seizures with benzodiazepines.

Bibliography

American Psychiatric Association. Practice guideline for the treatment of patients with delirium. Am J Psychiatry 1999:156(Suppl 5):1–20.

Barr J, Donner A. Optimal intravenous dosing strategies for sedatives and analgesics in the intensive care unit. Crit Care Clin 1995;11:827–847.

Carlson RW, Keske B, Cortez A. Alcohol withdrawal syndrome: alleviating symptoms, preventing progression. J Crit Illness 1998;13:311–317.

D'Onofrio G, Rathlev NK, Ulrich AS, et al. Lorazepam for the prevention of recurrent seizures related to alcohol. N Engl J Med 1999;340:915–919.

Mayo-Smith MF. Pharmacological management of alcohol withdrawal: a meta-analysis and evidence-based practice guideline. American Society of Addiction Medicine Working Group on Pharmacological Management of Alcohol Withdrawal. JAMA 1997;278:144–151.

McMicken DB. Alcohol withdrawal syndromes. Emerg Med Clin North Am 1990;8:805–819.

Saitz R, Friedman LS, Mayo-Smith MF. Alcohol withdrawal: a nationwide survey of inpatient treatment practices. J Gen Intern Med 1995;10:479–487.

Saitz R, O'Malley SS. Pharmacotherapies for alcohol abuse: withdrawal and treatment. Med Clin North Am 1997; 81:881–907.

Zacharias S, Rodriguez-Garcia A, Honz N, et al. Development of an alcohol withdrawal clinical pathway: an interdisciplinary process. J Nurs Care Qual 1998;12:9–18.

70 Cyanide Poisoning

James A. Kruse

Pathophysiology

A. The cyanide ion (C≡N⁻) is a potent histotoxic agent.

1. Inhibits mitochondrial cytochrome oxidase, stopping the electron transport chain and oxidative phosphorylation

2. Although commonly said to cause cellular hypoxia, by stopping intracellular oxidative metabolism, cyanide raises rather than lowers tissue oxygen content.

3. In severe poisoning, marked lactic acidosis and death can ensue within minutes.

B. Forms and sources

1. Hydrogen cyanide (H—C≡N)

   a. A colorless gas or liquid, also known as *hydrocyanic acid* or *prussic acid*

   b. Produced by pyrolysis of various combustibles, including paper; nylon, polyurethane, melamine, nitrocellulose, and polyacrylonitrile plastics; photographic film; wool; silk; and tobacco

2. Inorganic cyanide salts

   a. Examples: KCN, $NaCN$, $Ca(CN)_2$, $Hg(CN)_2$, $CNCl$, $CNBr$

   b. Used, e.g., as fumigants and rodenticides, as industrial and laboratory synthetic precursors, in electroplating and metallurgical processing

   c. Lethal dose for KCN is approximately 250 mg

3. Cyanogenic organic chemicals

   a. Examples: acetonitrile (CH_3CN), acrylonitrile (CH_2CHCN), proprionitrile (CH_3CH_2CN), aliphatic thiocyanates

   b. Used as industrial and laboratory solvents and synthetic precursors, particularly in the production of plastics

4. As a metabolite of nitroprusside

5. Cyanogenic plants and extracts

   a. Bitter almonds and almond extracts

   b. Apple, apricot, choke cherry, crab apple, peach, pear, plum seeds

   c. Certain other plants: e.g., bamboo, sorghum, elderberry, hydrangea, cassava

   d. Amygdalin (D-mandelonitrile-β-D-glucoside-6-β-D-glucoside)

(1) Active ingredient in or synonym for most forms of Laetrile, a putative antineoplastic extract from apricot pits or peach pits

(2) Metabolized to cyanide when ingested, but not if given intravenously

C. Metabolism

1. Cyanide is chiefly metabolized by conversion to thiocyanate (SCN^-), catalyzed by rhodanese, a transsulfurase enzyme that is overwhelmed by the presence of significant cyanide exposure.

2. Cyanide can also combine with methemoglobin to form cyanmethemoglobin, a reversible reaction.

3. Thiocyanate

   a. Has mild intrinsic neurotoxicity, but is much less toxic than cyanide

   b. It is excreted by the kidney with a half-life of 3 to 4 days in the presence of normal renal function (can accumulate to toxic levels in patients with renal insufficiency).

Clinical Findings

A. Exposure history (typical examples)

1. Sudden collapse of industrial, commercial, or laboratory personnel with access or exposure to cyanide or cyanide-containing compounds

2. Ingestion of cyanogenic plants or extracts

3. Ingestion of rodenticide or other cyanide formulations or precursors

4. Exposure to fire or smoke inhalation

5. Therapeutic use of nitroprusside, with unexplained coma and lactic acidosis

6. Suicide attempts with unexplained coma and lactic acidosis

B. Symptoms

1. Bitter or almond-like taste

2. Headache, dizziness

3. Apprehension

4. Dyspnea

5. Palpitations or chest pain

6. Nausea, vomiting, abdominal pain

C. Physical findings

1. General

a. Odor of bitter almonds on breath or gastric aspirate

b. Flushing

c. Cyanosis may be absent or present (lack of cyanosis in patients that otherwise clinically appear hypoxic is the classic description of cyanide intoxication).

2. Central nervous system (CNS)

a. Giddiness, agitation, restlessness

b. Mental status changes

c. Lethargy, stupor, coma

d. Ataxia, opisthotonos, trismus, paralysis

e. Seizures

3. Ocular

a. Equalization or near-equalization of red coloration of retinal arteries and veins

b. Mydriasis (miosis can be seen with thiocyanate toxicity)

4. Respiratory

a. Hyperpnea, tachypnea (early)

b. Pulmonary edema (cardiogenic or noncardiogenic)

c. Bradypnea, respiratory failure or arrest (late)

5. Cardiovascular

a. Hypertension (early) or hypotension (late)

b. Tachydysrhythmias or bradydysrhythmias

PEARL

The ability to detect the characteristic odor of bitter almonds associated with cyanide and found on the breath of cyanide-poisoned patients is genetically determined (X-linked) and cannot be appreciated by approximately 30% of the population.

Laboratory Findings

A. Cyanide concentration

1. Stat cyanide levels are not commonly available and are not useful for deciding on necessity for acute treatment.

2. Average normal whole blood cyanide concentration is typically much less than 0.2 μg/mL, but varies with assay and laboratory.

a. Can be twice as high in smokers

b. Serum and plasma levels are considerably lower because cyanide is concentrated in erythrocytes.

3. Typical clinical correlates at various concentrations

a. 0.5 μg/mL or less: may be asymptomatic

b. 0.5 to 1.0 μg/mL: tachycardia, flushing

c. 1.0 to 2.5 μg/mL: agitation or sensorial depression

d. 2.5 to 3.0 μg/mL: coma

e. More than 3.0 μg/mL: potentially fatal

B. Thiocyanate concentration

1. Not useful for diagnosis or treatment of cyanide poisoning

2. May have utility for monitoring patients receiving prolonged nitroprusside therapy (to detect thiocyanate toxicity)

3. Normal plasma concentration is typically 3 to 15 μg/mL (50 to 250 μmol/L).

4. Levels of approximately 60 μg/mL are associated with mild neurotoxic effects; e.g., diaphoresis, meiosis, dizziness, tinnitus, confusion, hyperreflexia, muscle twitching, seizures, nausea, vomiting.

5. Levels higher than 200 μg/mL are life-threatening.

C. Arterial blood gases

1. Metabolic (lactic) acidosis

2. Respiratory acidosis can occur from respiratory arrest or failure.

3. PaO_2 is expected to be normal (high if supplemental oxygen is given), unless there is a concomitant reason for hypoxemia or marked hypercapnia.

4. Methemoglobin saturation (see Chapter 72, Methemoglobinemia)

a. May be normal or elevated from smoke inhalation or therapeutic nitrite administration

b. Monitor serial methemoglobin levels once $NaNO_2$ administered and avoid raising to higher than 25%.

5. Arterial oxyhemoglobin saturation (SaO_2) calculated from measured PaO_2 and assumed normal P_{50} may yield spurious results, especially after therapeutic nitrites have been administered, unless measured by CO-oximetry.

D. Mixed venous blood gases

1. Unexplained mixed venous hyperoxemia

a. Increased mixed venous oxygen content, tension, and oxyhemoglobin saturation

b. Decreased a$\bar{v}$DO$_2$ and oxygen extraction ratio (see Chapter 216, Monitoring Oxygen Transport)

c. Mixed venous hyperoxemia also occurs with carbon monoxide and hydrogen sulfide poisoning.

2. As with arterial oxyhemoglobin saturation, spu-

rious values can occur if specimens are not assayed by CO-oximetry.

E. Serum anion gap elevated because of lactate accumulation

F. Blood lactate concentration elevated

G. Cardiac markers (creatine phosphokinase MB isoenzyme activity and cardiac troponin levels) may be elevated.

Electrocardiographic Findings

A. Classic progression of heart rate: initial bradycardia, followed by transient tachycardia, followed by terminal bradycardia, followed by asystole

B. Other bradydysrhythmias or tachydysrhythmias

C. Conduction disturbances

D. Nonspecific ST segment changes

E. Changes consistent with ischemia or infarction

Treatment

A. Resuscitation
   1. Ensure adequate airway, ventilation, and circulation.
   2. Administer supplemental oxygen at F_{IO_2} of 1.00.

B. Remove source of exposure.
   1. Remove from contaminated atmosphere if source is cyanide gas.
   2. Provide cutaneous decontamination if applicable.
   3. Syrup of ipecac is contraindicated.
   4. Perform gastric lavage if source was ingestion; however, do not delay institution of antidotal therapy.
   5. Activated charcoal (1 g/kg) should be administered.
   6. Discontinue nitroprusside if that is the suspected source; discontinuation and empiric treatment cannot be delayed while awaiting blood cyanide assay.

C. Specific measures
   1. Indicated for cyanide-exposed patients with serious signs and symptoms
   2. Patients whose only manifestations are restlessness, hyperventilation, or anxiety may not require antidotal treatment.
   3. Do not delay antidotal therapy; if it is indicated, it should be started while the initial resuscitation is underway.
   4. First administer amyl nitrite.
      a. Rapidly induces methemoglobinemia (typi-

cally to a methemoglobin saturation of approximately 3%), which has higher affinity for cyanide than cytochrome oxidase
      b. If patient has IV access and sodium nitrite is available, proceed directly to $NaNO_2$ injection and do not administer amyl nitrite.
      c. If patient lacks IV access or sodium nitrite is not immediately available, crack one pearl of amyl nitrite wrapped in gauze or cloth and administer by inhalation.
      d. Allow patient to inhale the drug for 30 seconds of each minute; use a fresh pearl every 3 to 4 minutes.
      e. Stop amyl nitrite administration once IV access is available and IV sodium nitrite is being injected.
   5. Second, give sodium nitrite by IV injection.
      a. Results in formation of methemoglobin, which binds cyanide
      b. Dose is 300 mg or 4 to 6 mg/kg of 3% (10 mL of 30 mg/mL) solution of $NaNO_2$ over 5 min; typically results in methemoglobin level of approximately 10%.
      c. Monitor blood pressure closely; $NaNO_2$ is a vasodilator and can cause marked hypotension, especially if rapidly injected.
      d. The conventional goal for patients not responding to therapy is a methemoglobin saturation level of 25%; lower levels (e.g., 10%) are acceptable in responders.
      e. Methemoglobin saturation levels >30% can result in life-threatening hypoxemia and should be avoided if at all possible (see Chapter 72, Methemoglobinemia).
      f. If there is concomitant significant carbon monoxide intoxication, proceed to sodium thiosulfate injection and withhold $NaNO_2$ until hyperbaric oxygen therapy can be initiated.
      g. For cases in which the diagnosis is not certain, consider foregoing $NaNO_2$ and using sodium thiosulfate alone.
   6. Third, inject sodium thiosulfate intravenously.
      a. Facilitates rhodanese-mediated conversion of cyanide to thiocyanate by acting as a sulfur source
      b. Dose is 12.5 g or 150 to 200 mg/kg of 25% (50 mL of 250 mg/mL) solution of $Na_2S_2O_3$ over 15 minutes.
      c. Has no significant adverse effects
   7. May repeat $NaNO_2$ and $Na_2S_2O_3$ once, at half-dose, 30 minutes after first doses

a. Limit to those with inadequate response to initial dosing.

b. If possible, check stat methemoglobin level before repeating $NaNO_2$ administration.

D. Sodium bicarbonate

1. Conventional recommendation is to administer intravenously for treatment of severe metabolic acidosis.

2. Guide dosing by serial arterial blood gases.

E. Hemodialysis

1. Not standard therapy for cyanide poisoning in patients with adequate renal function

2. Efficacy is unclear for removing cyanide.

3. Efficacious at removing thiocyanate (applicable to patients with renal dysfunction; see below under Special Consideration, B. Nitroprusside-induced cyanide intoxication)

F. Supportive care

1. Intensive care unit monitoring

2. Treat circulatory shock.

a. Intravascular volume expansion with isotonic crystalloid or colloid-containing fluids

b. Vasopressor infusion for refractory hypotension

3. Treat serious cardiac dysrhythmias: use conventional antidysrhythmic agents

4. Treat seizures: use conventional anticonvulsant agents

G. Investigational therapies

1. Cyanide binding agents

a. Hydroxocobalamin: not available as a practicable formulation in the United States

b. α-Ketoglutaric acid (a normal intermediate metabolite of the Krebs' cycle)

c. Stroma-free methemoglobin: improves survival in animal models

d. Dicobalt ethylenediaminetetraacetate

2. 4-Dimethylaminophenol: induces methemoglobinemia more rapidly than $NaNO_2$

3. Encapsulated rhodanese and thiosulfonates: hastens conversion of cyanide to thiocyanate; improves survival in animal models

4. Hyperbaric oxygen therapy

a. Efficacy for cyanide intoxication unconfirmed and contradictory

b. Useful for combined cyanide and carbon monoxide poisoning (i.e., from smoke inhalation)

Key Treatment

- Perform cardiopulmonary resuscitation if necessary.

- Administer 100% O_2 and (until IV access obtained) amyl nitrite by inhalation.

- Administer IV sodium nitrite to induce controlled methemoglobinemia.

- Administer IV sodium thiosulfate to convert cyanide to thiocyanate.

Special Considerations

A. Smoke inhalation

1. Consider cyanide intoxication (from HCN gas exposure) and co-intoxication with carbon monoxide.

2. Important clues are evidence of decreased arteriovenous oxygen difference, severe metabolic acidosis, and hyperlactatemia despite treatment with 100% oxygen and declining carboxyhemoglobin levels.

3. Induction of methemoglobinemia with sodium nitrite may be dangerous if there is significant carboxyhemoglobinemia.

4. Empiric treatment with oxygen and sodium thiosulfate is safe.

B. Nitroprusside-induced cyanide intoxication

1. Sodium nitroprusside ($Na_2[Fe(CN)_5NO]\cdot 2H_2O$) is metabolized by reaction with hemoglobin to form cyanmethemoglobin, cyanide, and then thiocyanate.

2. Minimize risk of toxicity by avoiding unnecessary, high-dose, or prolonged use of sodium nitroprusside.

3. Addition of 1 g sodium thiosulfate per 100 mg of sodium nitroprusside in the IV solution decreases the risk of cyanide (but not thiocyanate) toxicity.

4. Suspect nitroprusside-induced cyanide intoxication if there are suggestive clinical findings in a patient receiving the drug, particularly the constellation of unexplained CNS abnormalities, hemodynamic instability, and lactic acidosis.

5. Extra caution for thiocyanate intoxication is warranted for patients with renal insufficiency; the treatment for thiocyanate toxicity is hemodialysis.

C. Acetonitrile (methyl cyanide) ingestion

1. A common industrial solvent that has been

used in some sculpted, artificial fingernail removal products

2. Manifestations of cyanide poisoning are delayed by 3 to 24 hours by the slow conversion of acetonitrile via the cytochrome P-450 system to cyanide and formaldehyde.

3. Increases in the serum anion gap and the osmole gap may occur.

Key Complications (in survivors)

- May completely recover or sustain residual or delayed-onset neuropsychiatric deficits

- Neurologic sequelae may include encephalopathy, memory disturbances, intellectual deficits, personality change, or Parkinsonism-like syndrome.

Bibliography

Barillo DJ, Goode R, Esch V. Cyanide poisoning in victims of fire: analysis of 364 cases and review of the literature. J Burn Care Rehabil 1994;15:46–57.

Beasley DM, Glass WI. Cyanide poisoning: pathophysiology and treatment recommendations. Occup Med 1998;48:427–431.

Mueller M, Borland C. Delayed cyanide poisoning following acetonitrile ingestion. Postgrad Med J 1997;73:299–300.

Salkowski AA, Penney DG. Cyanide poisoning in animals and humans: a review. Vet Human Toxicol 1994;36:455–466.

Yen D, Tsai J, Wang LM, et al. The clinical experience of acute cyanide poisoning. Am J Emerg Med 1995;13:524–528.

71 Carbon Monoxide Poisoning

Suzanne R. White

Carbon monoxide (CO) is a colorless, odorless, and nonirritating gas formed by the incomplete combustion of carbonaceous material. Common sources include fires, cigarette smoke, defective heating systems, automobile exhaust, and in vivo formation following dermal, gastrointestinal (GI) or respiratory exposure to dihalogenated solvents such as methylene chloride, bromide, or iodide. Carbon monoxide is an insidious and highly lethal toxin that represents the leading cause of fatality from poisoning. Symptoms resulting from exposure are notoriously vague, especially with low-level or chronic exposures, and the diagnosis may be easily overlooked. Long-term neurologic sequelae are common.

Pathophysiology

A. Carbon monoxide binds to hemoglobin with high affinity, forming carboxyhemoglobin (COHb), which
   1. Decreases oxygen carrying capacity of blood
   2. Impairs normal oxygen unloading
B. Carbon monoxide induces hypotension through cyclic guanosine monophosphate–mediated vasodilatation.
C. At high COHb levels (>50%), CO binds to cytochrome *c* oxidase and inhibits subcellular respiration.
D. Other proposed histotoxic mechanisms include the induction of perivascular oxidative stress, release of excitotoxic neurotransmitters or catecholamines, and modulation of nitric oxide production.

Key Epidemiology

- Causes approximately 5,600 deaths/year in the United States
- Causes 40,000 significant, nonfatal exposures annually
- Fifty percent of fatalities are unintentional.

Symptoms

A. Constitutional
   1. Fatigue
   2. Weakness
B. Neurologic
   1. Headache (especially in fall or winter)
   2. Syncope
   3. Dizziness or vertigo
   4. Confusion, lethargy, coma
   5. Seizures
C. Gastrointestinal
   1. Nausea
   2. Vomiting
D. Cardiovascular
   1. Syncope
   2. Dyspnea on exertion
   3. Angina

PEARL

Have a high index of suspicion for CO intoxication when evaluating patients with altered mental status.

Physical Findings

A. Vital signs: tachycardia, bradycardia, hypotension, cardiovascular collapse (with severe exposures)
B. Neurologic
   1. Altered mental status, ataxia, nystagmus, hyperreflexia, compression-related peripheral neuropathy, decreased visual acuity
   2. Abnormal Carbon Monoxide Neuropsychiatric Screening Battery (CONSB) psychometric test
      a. Assesses performance on tasks such as digit span, short-term memory, trail-making, aphasia screening
      b. Sensitive marker of subtle CO-related neuropsychiatric deficit
      c. Predictive of persistent or delayed neurologic sequelae from CO poisoning (see below)
   3. A lucid interval following acute exposure with delayed deterioration in neurologic status is seen in 10% to 43% of patients and has been termed the "delayed neuropsychiatric syndrome," which is associated with
      a. Memory deficits
      b. Personality changes
      c. Speech impairment

d. Parietal lobe dysfunction (apraxia, agnosia, dysgraphia)

e. Motor dysfunction (parkinsonism, gait disturbance, tremor, hemiparesis)

f. Incontinence

C. Pulmonary: pulmonary edema (rare, unless following smoke inhalation)

D. Ophthalmologic: retinal hemorrhage (generally with exposures of >12 hours)

E. Dermatologic: bullae (rare) secondary to sweat gland necrosis

Laboratory Findings

A. Arterial blood gases

1. Severe hypoxemia (decreased blood oxygen content) can occur despite normal or high PaO_2.

2. Blood gas panels that report oxyhemoglobin saturations based on calculation from PO_2 can substantially overestimate true oxyhemoglobin saturation.

3. Accurate oxyhemoglobin saturation can only be obtained by CO-oximetry.

4. Metabolic (lactic) acidosis can occur.

B. Blood COHb level

1. The best indicator of exposure; does not, however, correlate well with toxicity.

2. Does not reflect the severity of poisoning or the potential for delayed sequelae.

3. May be low with chronic exposures, delayed presentation, or prior oxygen therapy

4. May be elevated in disease states associated with hemolysis (e.g., sickle cell anemia, thalassemia, or preeclampsia)

5. Venous COHb levels correlate well with arterial levels.

6. Some CO-oximeters report fetal hemoglobin as COHb.

C. Arterial blood lactate elevation is common.

D. Hyperglycemia is common.

E. Plasma cardiac markers: creatine phosphokinase (CK), CK-MB isoenzymes troponin T or I levels

1. Elevations are noted in 10% to 18% of cases, often without electrocardiographic (ECG) changes.

2. Reflective of global cardiac ischemia

F. Abnormal renal function tests from hypoxic injury to the kidneys

G. Elevated CK-MM activity

1. Due to rhabdomyolysis

2. Related to immobility and hypoxic injury to skeletal muscle

H. Other abnormalities: leukocytosis, hemoconcentration, elevated serum transaminase activity, proteinuria

I. Consider pregnancy test in women of child-bearing potential.

Imaging Findings

A. Chest x-ray may show pulmonary edema with smoke inhalation.

B. Computed tomography (CT) and magnetic resonance imaging (MRI)

1. Bilateral, symmetric hypodensities in the basal ganglia, characteristically the globus pallidi

2. Cerebral edema

3. Diffuse white matter changes

C. Positron emission tomography abnormalities

D. Single photon emission computed tomography abnormalities

Other Tests

A. Pulse oximetry: overestimates oxyhemoglobin saturation by the amount of COHb present and is therefore unreliable

B. 12-lead ECG: useful screen for subclinical ischemia in patients with altered mental status along with plasma cardiac marker studies

---

Key Findings

- Constitutional and GI symptoms: fatigue, weakness, nausea, vomiting

- Neurologic symptoms: headache, syncope, dizziness, vertigo, confusion, lethargy, coma, seizures

- Cardiovascular findings: dyspnea on exertion, angina, tachycardia, bradycardia, hypotension

- Laboratory findings: elevated blood lactate level, hyperglycemia, metabolic acidosis, cardiac enzyme elevations. Normal pulse oximetry and oxygen saturation by blood gas analysis if co-oximeter not used

- Imaging studies: CT or MRI findings of cerebral edema, diffuse white matter changes, or bilateral basal ganglia lucencies

- Other: abnormal CO Neuropsychiatric Screening Battery

C. Electroencephalography: findings usually nonspecific

D. Neuropsychiatric testing is warranted prior to discharge to assess for persistent neuropsychiatric injury and to establish baseline for follow-up.

Differential Diagnosis

A. Metabolic causes of altered mental status

B. Other intoxicants that cause mental status changes or metabolic acidosis: e.g., sedative hypnotics, opioids, ethanol, cyanide, salicylates, toxic alcohols, iron, γ-hydroxybutyrate, clonidine, antidepressants, antipsychotics

C. Infectious illness

D. Endocrinopathy

E. Traumatic or other neurosurgical emergencies

F. Differential for bilateral basal ganglia abnormalities

1. Other intoxicants: methanol, cyanide, hydrogen sulfide, pesticides, manganese, carbon disulfide, disulfiram

2. Hypoxia, hypoglycemia, hemolytic-uremic syndrome, osmotic demyelination syndrome, encephalitis, Huntington's chorea

Treatment

A. Normobaric 100% oxygen by tight-fitting nonrebreather or continuous positive airway pressure mask should be started as soon as the diagnosis is suspected.

1. Intubation may be necessary to deliver adequate dosage of oxygen to patients with chronic obstructive lung disease and hypercapnia.

2. The half-life of COHb is 4.5 hours while breathing ambient air, 1.5 hours while breathing normobaric 100% oxygen, and 20 minutes during hyperbaric oxygen therapy.

3. Duration of treatment with normobaric oxygen will be approximately 4 half-lives (4 to 6 hours if COHb level is <20%).

B. Hyperbaric oxygen (HBO) therapy

1. Indications and potential benefit in terms of preventing delayed neuropsychiatric sequelae are controversial.

2. Proposed indications include

a. COHb level greater than 25%

b. Abnormal CONSB (see above)

c. Neurologic findings

d. Ongoing myocardial ischemia

Key Treatment

- Initiate treatment with 100% oxygen once diagnosis is suspected.

- Exclude other causes of altered mental status.

- Monitor for subclinical myocardial ischemia.

- Careful patient selection for hyperbaric oxygen therapy (role unproven)

- Consider empiric treatment for cyanide toxicity if smoke inhalation.

- Consider pre-discharge neuropsychiatric testing and arrange for follow-up within 3 weeks.

e. Metabolic acidosis

f. History of syncope

g. Refractory or worsening symptoms despite treatment with normobaric oxygen

h. Pregnancy with COHb level higher than 10% to 15%

3. If used, HBO is ideally administered within 6 hours of exposure.

4. Role for sequential HBO treatments or for its use if given late or after chronic exposure is unproven.

5. Putative neuroprotective mechanisms of HBO include inhibition of polymorphonuclear-endothelial cell adhesion molecule elaboration, prevention of xanthine dehydrogenase to oxidase conversion, shortened half-life of COHb, hyperoxygenation of bloodstream improving oxygen delivery and restoring mitochondrial respiration, and protection against cerebral edema.

6. HBO is considered safe in pregnancy.

a. Carbon monoxide is a potent fetotoxin and teratogen.

b. Carbon monoxide-fetal hemoglobin has a considerably longer half-life (7 hours) than COHb A.

c. The pregnant patient will generally require oxygen therapy 5 times longer than needed to clear maternal COHb.

C. Treat rapidly reversible causes of coma.

D. Continuous ECG monitoring is indicated.

E. Avoid sodium bicarbonate administration (further impairs unloading of oxygen based on leftward shift of hemoglobin-oxygen dissociation curve).

F. Consider co-intoxication with cyanide in victims of smoke inhalation (see Chapter 70, Cyanide Poisoning, and Chapter 145, Thermal Burn Injury).

Prognosis

A. While mortality is low (1.8%), persistent or delayed neuropsychiatric sequelae develop in 10% to 43% of adults.

B. Follow-up with a neurologist at 3 weeks after exposure for assessment for delayed neuropsychiatric changes is recommended.

Bibliography

Ernst A, Zibrak JD. Carbon monoxide poisoning. N Engl J Med 1998;339:1603–1608.

Scheinkestel CD, Bailey M, Myles PS, et al. Hyperbaric or normobaric oxygen for acute carbon monoxide poisoning: a randomised controlled clinical trial. Med J Aust 1999;170:203–210.

Thom SR. Options for treatment of carbon monoxide poisoning, including hyperbaric oxygen therapy. In: Penney DG (ed). Carbon Monoxide. Boca Raton, FL: CRC Press, 1996, pp 271–283.

Weaver LK. Carbon monoxide poisoning. Crit Care Clin 1999;15:297–317.

White SR. Update on the clinical treatment of carbon monoxide poisoning. In: Penney DG (ed). *Carbon Monoxide Toxicity*. Boca Raton, FL: CRC Press, 2000, pp 261–289.

72 Methemoglobinemia

James A. Kruse

Pathophysiology

A. Methemoglobin (metHb) is formed when the iron in hemoglobin molecules is oxidized from the normal ferrous (Fe^{2+}) to the ferric (Fe^{3+}) state.

B. Can occur when hemoglobin is exposed to relatively high levels of certain oxidizing agents, either by ingestion or in some cases topical use

C. Enzymes normally present in the body are capable of reducing excess metHb to its normal form, thereby maintaining metHb levels at 1% or less of total hemoglobin.

D. Acquired forms of the illness occur when the rate of formation of metHb exceeds the rate of its reduction.

E. MetHb is incapable of binding oxygen, and high metHb levels can cause life-threatening tissue hypoxia.

F. The presence of metHb also shifts the oxyhemoglobin dissociation curve to the left, which decreases oxygen unloading in peripheral tissues.

Etiology

A. Congenital methemoglobinemia

1. Deficiency of erythrocyte cytochrome-b_5 nicotinamide adenine dinucleotide metHb reductase

   a. This enzyme, also known as metHb reductase I or diaphorase I, is normally responsible for approximately 95% of metHb reduction.

   b. Deficiency inherited as an autosomal recessive trait

   c. Increased risk in Inuit and Alaskan Native Americans

   d. Homozygotes have chronic cyanosis with metHb levels of 15% to 30%, but are usually asymptomatic except for cyanosis.

   e. Heterozygotes are asymptomatic and do not normally have cyanosis but are predisposed to develop methemoglobinemia after exposure to oxidizing agents.

2. Hemoglobin M

   a. Rare autosomal dominant trait causing a dyshemoglobinemia

   b. Caused by any of a variety of amino acid substitutions in α or β chains of hemoglobin

   c. Homozygous forms are incompatible with life.

   d. Heterozygotes typically have metHb levels of 25% to 30%.

B. Acquired methemoglobinemia (see Precipitating Agents below)

1. Exposure to certain pharmaceutical agents

   a. Therapeutic use, especially in patients with metHb reductase I deficiency

   b. Overdose

2. Exposure to certain toxins

Precipitating Agents

A. Analgesic, antipyretic drugs: acetaminophen (theoretical only), phenacetin, phenazopyridine

B. Aniline dyes and dye-manufacturing reagents

1. Reagents: acetanilid, aminobenzene, nitrobenzene, *p*-toluidine, phenylhydrazine

2. Consumer products: dyed blankets, diaper marking pens, laundry markers, hair dyes, inks, paint products, shoe polishes, red or orange wax crayons, shoe and leather dyes

C. Antibiotics

1. Antimalarials: chloroquine, pamaquine, primaquine, quinine

2. Sulfa drugs: sulfamethoxazole, sulfisoxazole, sulfonamide, sulfoxone

3. Others: dapsone, nitrofurantoin, *p*-aminosalicylic acid

D. Antiseptics, disinfectants: resorcinol (also an antipruritic and keratolytic agent), cresol

E. Arsine

F. Chlorates: explosives, match heads, pyrotechnics, herbicides

G. Copper sulfate

H. Kerosine

I. Local anesthetics (including topical use): ethyl aminobenzoate (benzocaine), lidocaine, prilocaine, procaine

J. Monuron (herbicide)

K. Methylene blue (in high doses)

L. Naphthalene (moth repellant)

M. Nitrates and nitrites: amyl nitrite, butyl nitrite, isobutyl nitrite, methyl nitrite, silver nitrate, sodium nitrite, meat preservatives, well water high in nitrates

N. Nitrobenzene: gun-cleaning products, industrial solvents

O. Nitroethane and *N,N*-dimethyl-*p*-toluidine (in artificial fingernail solutions)

P. Other drugs: flutamide, ifosfamide, inhaled nitric oxide, menadione, metoclopramide, nitroglycerin, nitroprusside (rare), phenelzine

Clinical Manifestations

A. MetHb levels 3% to 15%
   1. Asymptomatic
   2. Skin may appear pale or have a slate-gray color.

B. MetHb levels 15% to 20% (>1.5 g/dL)
   1. Cyanosis, brown or blue coloration of mucous membranes
   2. Blood is chocolate-brown in color.

C. MetHb levels 20% to 45%
   1. Headache, lethargy, generalized weakness, dizziness, altered mental status, syncope
   2. Tachycardia, myocardial ischemia

D. MetHb levels greater than 45%
   1. Dyspnea, cardiac dysrhythmias, heart failure
   2. Seizures, coma
   3. Lactic acidosis

E. MetHb levels greater than 70% are associated with a high fatality rate.

Key Manifestations

- Cyanosis
- Dyspnea
- Altered mental status
- Chocolate-brown-colored blood

Diagnosis

A. Blood metHb level measurement
   1. Readily determined from arterial blood gas analysis on modern CO-oximeters
   2. MetHb values can be expressed in absolute concentration units: normal is less than 0.15 g/dL
   3. More commonly expressed as the fraction or percentage of total hemoglobin that is metHb
      a. Levels at least 2% of total hemoglobin considered abnormal
      b. For a given degree of absolute methemoglobinemia, the fractional metHb value will vary in proportion to the degree of anemia, if present.

B. Blood with high metHb levels has a characteristic chocolate-brown color, and does not turn red upon exposure to air.

C. Hemoglobin M can be identified by hemoglobin electrophoresis.

D. Urine may be brown or black because of the presence of metHb in urine.

E. In the presence of metHb, oxygenation must be assessed using a CO-oximeter.
   1. Non-CO-oximeters cannot differentiate oxyhemoglobin from metHb and can yield a falsely high fractional arterial oxyhemoglobin saturation (SaO_2).
   2. Oxyhemoglobin saturation determined by an algorithm based on measured PaO_2 and the oxyhemoglobin dissociation function will yield a falsely high value.
   3. Methylene blue administration can interfere with in vitro CO-oximetry, causing falsely lowered SaO_2 values.

F. MetHb interferes with pulse oximetry (SpO_2).
   1. SpO_2 values tend toward a value of approximately 85% if there is significant methemoglobinemia, regardless of the true SaO_2.
   2. If the true SaO_2 is normal or near normal, the presence of elevated metHb will result in underestimation of the true SaO_2.
   3. If the true SaO_2 is markedly low, the presence of elevated metHb will tend to overestimate the true SaO_2.

G. Arterial oxygen tension (PaO_2)
   1. PaO_2 values remain accurate regardless of metHb or methylene blue levels.
   2. Nevertheless, PaO_2 can be misleading because in the presence of high levels of metHb the arterial oxygen content can be severely decreased even when PaO_2 is normal or high.

Key Diagnostic Points

- Measure metHb levels by CO-oximetry.
- Pulse oximetry is unreliable with high metHb levels.
- Monitor SaO_2 by CO-oximetry; do not use values calculated from PaO_2.

Treatment

A. General measures
   1. Closely monitor vital signs.
   2. Give supplemental oxygen (FIO_2 1.00, if possible).
   3. Provide cardiorespiratory support, if necessary.

B. Remove offending oxidant.

1. Discontinue any possible precipitating drugs.

2. If due to oral ingestion of a precipitating drug:

    a. Consider gastric lavage.

    b. Administer activated charcoal.

3. If due to topical drug or toxin, provide cutaneous decontamination.

4. Hemodialysis has been used in unusual cases to remove precipitating drugs or toxins that are dialyzable and have a long half-life.

C. Consider methylene blue treatment.

1. Acts as a co-factor to accelerate metHb reduction by the alternate erythrocyte enzyme, nicotinamide adenine dinucleotide phosphate (NADPH) metHb reductase (also known as metHb reductase II or diaphorase II)

2. Contraindicated in patients with known glucose-6-phosphate dehydrogenase (G6PD) deficiency; however, small initial doses (0.3 to 0.5 mg/kg) titrated upward with careful monitoring have been advocated by some investigators in severe cases

3. Methylene blue therapy may be unnecessary in stable patients without serious cardiopulmonary disease or anemia if the metHb level is lower than 30%.

4. Dose is 1 to 2 mg/kg intravenously given over at least 5 min; may repeat in 1 hour and every 4 hours thereafter.

5. Maximum total dose is 7 mg/kg; high doses (especially if greater than 15 mg/kg) may increase the level of metHb.

6. Potential side effects: dyspnea, diaphoresis, apprehension, restlessness, confusion, nausea, vomiting, diarrhea, dysuria, increased urinary frequency, chest pain, tremor, burning sensation in mouth or abdomen, hemolytic anemia, blue discoloration of skin and urine

7. Some patients are refractory to methylene blue therapy.

    a. Caused by low levels of NADPH secondary to reduced activity of G6PD, in patients with G6PD deficiency

    b. Caused by erythrocyte NADPH metHb reductase deficiency

    c. Caused by overwhelming oxidant stress secondary to high doses or high oxidant potency of the precipitating agent

    d. Patients with hemoglobin M

    e. Patients with sulfhemoglobinemia misdiagnosed as methemoglobinemia

8. Can precipitate severe hemolysis in patients with underlying G6PD deficiency, which is more common in Native Americans, African Americans, and Asians

9. Monitor closely for signs of hemolytic anemia if methylene blue given: blood for erythrocyte count, hemoglobin, hematocrit, reticulocyte count; plasma hemoglobin; serum unconjugated bilirubin, lactate dehydrogenase, etc.

D. Ascorbic acid

1. Limited efficacy for lowering metHb levels in chronic methemoglobinemia

2. Used mainly for cosmetic therapy in chronic setting

3. Effect is too weak and too slow to be of clinical use in acute methemoglobinemia.

E. Other possible treatments (? efficacy)

1. Packed red cell transfusion or exchange transfusion

2. Hyperbaric oxygen treatment

3. N-acetylcysteine has not been shown to be effective in lowering metHb levels in healthy volunteers in whom mild methemoglobinemia was induced with IV $NaNO_2$

4. Cimetidine has been advocated for methemoglobinemia specifically caused by dapsone, to inhibit, cytochrome P-450 conversion of dapsone to its oxidant metabolite.

Key Management

- Administer supplemental oxygen.
- Stop the offending drug(s).
- Obtain blood for stat erythrocyte G6PD level, if possible.
- Consider giving 1 to 2 mg/kg methylene blue in severe cases.

B Bibliography

Dötsch J, Demirakça S, Hahn D, et al. Accuracy of methemoglobin measurements: comparison of six different commercial devices and one manual method. Crit Care Med 1999;27:1191–1194.

Khan NA, Kruse JA. Methemoglobinemia induced by topical anesthesia: a case report and review. Am J Med Sci 1999;318:415–418.

Lu HC, Shih RD, Marcus S, et al. Pseudomethemoglobinemia: a case report and review of sulfhemoglobinemia. Arch Pediatr Adolesc Med 1998;152:803–805.

73 Neuroleptic Drug Overdose

Ho-Yin Adrian Li

Classification of Neuroleptic Drugs

A. Typical agents (predominantly D_2-receptor antagonists)

  1. Representative structural classes

    a. Phenothiazine: chlorpromazine, promethazine, thioridazine, mesoridazine, prochlorperazine, fluphenazine

    b. Butyrophenone: haloperidol, droperidol

    c. Thioxanthene: thiothixene

    d. Dibenzoxazepine: loxapine

    e. Indole: molindone

  2. Potency

    a. Low: chlorpromazine, thioridazine, mesoridazine

    b. Medium: droperidol, perphenazine, loxapine, molindone

    c. High: haloperidol, fluphenazine, thiothixene

B. Atypical agents (predominantly 5-hydroxytryptamine$_2$-receptor antagonists, except for risperidone, also a potent D_2-antagonist)

  1. Representative structures

    a. Benzisoxazole: risperidone

    b. Dibenzodiazepine: clozapine, olanzapine

    c. Dibenzothiazepine: quetiapine

Key Epidemiology

- About 11,000 cases of neuroleptic drug overdose occur every year in the United States.

- Most cases (~75%) involve ingestion of multiple agents.

Pharmacology

A. Pharmacokinetics (similar among various classes)

  1. Volume of distribution: 15 to 30 L/kg

  2. Highly protein bound (~92% to 95%)

  3. Half-life: 20 to 40 hours (oral formulation) and 2 to 10 days (depot formulation)

  4. Highly lipophilic (clinical observation suggests that they cross the placenta)

  5. Some have active (hepatic) metabolites that may contribute to dissociation between the blood level of the parent drug and the observed clinical effects.

B. Pharmacodynamics and toxic effects

  1. D_2-receptor antagonism

    a. Mesolimbic system effects: improvement of positive symptoms of schizophrenia

    b. Mesocortical and nigrostriatal tract effects: involved in causing extrapyramidal symptoms and worsening of negative symptoms

  2. 5-Hydroxytryptamine$_2$ antagonism

    a. Affects dorsolateral prefrontal cortex

    b. Improves negative symptoms

  3. α_1-Adrenergic receptor blockade

    a. Can cause hypotension, priapism, miosis

    b. More likely with low-potency D_2-receptor antagonists

  4. Anticholinergic (muscarinic) effects

    a. Tachycardia, dry mouth, constipation, urinary retention, hyperthermia

    b. Occur more often with low-potency D_2-receptor antagonists

  5. Antihistaminic effects

    a. Sedation

    b. Weight gain

  6. Antagonism on other subtypes of dopamine receptors: hyperprolactinemia

C. Toxicology

  1. Clinical toxicity is more likely with low-potency phenothiazines; thioridazine and mesoridazine are more cardiotoxic.

  2. Acute toxicity may be superimposed on chronic side effects.

  3. Lethal doses are not well defined, but fatalities have occurred with ingestions of individual drugs, such as more than 1.5 g of thioridazine and 2.5 g of clozapine, loxapine, and mesoridazine.

Symptoms and Physical Findings

A. Neurologic

  1. Slurred speech

  2. Confusion, lethargy, obtundation

  3. Loss of brain-stem and deep-tendon reflexes (dose-dependent)

  4. Miosis

5. Seizures (clozapine, loxapine, and the low-potency phenothiazines)

6. Sialorrhea (clozapine)

7. Extrapyramidal manifestations (increased incidence with high-potency D_2-receptor antagonists and in the elderly)

   a. Acute: dystonia, akathisia (hours or days after starting treatment or increasing dosage)

   b. Subacute: Parkinsonism (after weeks to months; may coexist with acute symptoms)

   c. Chronic: tardive dyskinesia (typically after more than 1 year of therapy; not readily reversible in 50%); may mimic inadequate treatment for Parkinsonism

8. Acute visual loss (after thioridazine overdose)

B. Pulmonary

1. Respiratory depression: usually from co-ingestion of neurodepressant drug

2. Respiratory distress: usually secondary to aspiration pneumonitis

C. Cardiovascular

1. QTc interval prolongation: related to sodium or potassium channel blockade; predisposes to torsade de pointes

2. QRS widening

3. T wave inversion

4. Supraventricular and ventricular dysrhythmias

5. Hypotension

6. Hypertension (with risperidone)

7. Myocardial infarction or myocarditis

D. Fever or hypothermia

1. Severe hyperthermia may lead to thrombocytopenia, hemolysis, bleeding diathesis, and hepatic injury.

2. Hypothermia can occur from hypothalamic effects or environmental exposure during periods of unconsciousness.

3. Neuroleptic malignant syndrome

   a. Rare: 0.07% to 0.9% of patients treated with neuroleptic drugs

   b. Has not been reported in acute neuroleptic overdose

   c. See Chapter 86, Neuroleptic Malignant Syndrome and Malignant Hyperthermia.

E. Hematologic: agranulocytosis

1. Occurs in 1% to 2% of patients treated with clozapine; may involve N-desmethylclozapine

2. Also reported with haloperidol

F. Acute pancreatitis, possibly after olanzapine overdose

Key Findings

- Altered mental status
- Orthostatic hypotension
- Temperature dysregulation
- Extrapyramidal symptoms
- Anticholinergic effects
- Cardiac dysrhythmias

Laboratory and Other Tests

A. Electrocardiogram

B. Imaging studies

1. Chest x-ray

2. Computed tomography of brain

C. Electroencephalography (EEG), in selected cases

D. Routine blood tests

1. Serum electrolyte, glucose, urea nitrogen, and creatinine concentrations; liver and thyroid function tests

2. Serial serum creatinine phosphokinase activity

3. Coagulation screen

4. Complete blood cell count

5. Arterial blood gases

E. Toxicologic tests

1. Routine toxicologic screening

2. Serum lithium level, if indicated

F. Urine myoglobin

Treatment

A. Resuscitation

1. Ensure adequate airway control and ventilation (laryngeal dystonia may be present).

2. Treat ventricular tachydysrhythmias.

   a. Amiodarone: 2 to 4 mg/kg (up to 300 mg) intravenously followed by maintenance infusion of 0.015 mg/kg per minute for 6 hours, then 0.0075 mg/kg per minute for 18 hours

   b. Lidocaine: 1 to 1.5 mg/kg intravenously, then 1 to 4 mg/minute for 24 to 30 hours; may be tried if the above fails

   c. If there is no response, consider early direct-current cardioversion or defibrillation.

   d. Magnesium sulfate: 1 to 2 g bolus intravenously

   e. Overdrive pacing or IV isoproterenol infusion has been used to maintain heart rate above 90 beats/minute as a treatment for torsade de pointes.

f. Avoid class Ia, Ic, II, and III antidysrhythmic drugs.

g. Consider alkalinization using an infusion of NaHCO₃ in dextrose in water to maintain pH at 7.45 to 7.55 for 12 hours, then taper gradually.

(1) If QRS interval widening does not normalize at targeted pH, NaHCO₃ may be discontinued.

(2) Concomitant serum potassium monitoring is required.

3. Hypotension

a. The α_1-adrenergic receptor agonists norepinephrine or phenylephrine are recommended for hypotension refractory to IV fluids.

b. Epinephrine may result in further lowering of blood pressure in phenothiazine-induced hypotension.

c. Dopamine has been reported to be ineffective in the treatment of some patients overdosed with phenothiazines.

B. Decontamination

1. Should not be initiated until immediately life-threatening derangements have been controlled

2. Orogastric lavage using a 36 to 40 Fr tube (in airway protected patients) may be useful, particularly if there is known recent ingestion of a large quantity of thioridazine or mesoridazine, or if the patient had ventricular dysrhythmias.

3. Activated charcoal: 1 g/kg, up to 100 g, orally or by nasogastric or orogastric tube

C. Stop neuroleptic agents and drugs that may exacerbate their effects (e.g., lithium).

D. Provide continuous neurologic, cardiovascular, respiratory, renal, and temperature monitoring.

E. Control seizures (IV drug formulations should be used).

1. Lorazepam: 0.05 mg/kg up to 2 mg intravenously every 10 to 15 minutes

2. Or, phenobarbital 10 to 20 mg/kg, given in normal saline at 25 to 50 mg/minute, followed by 120 to 240 mg every 20 minutes as needed

3. Or, propofol infusion (requires mechanical ventilation)

4. Consider continuous EEG monitoring in refractory cases, if available.

F. Antiparkinsonian treatment options

1. Sinemet: one 25/100 tablet every 8 hours; may increase by one tablet per day to a maximum of 8 tablets per day

2. Amantadine: 50 to 100 mg every 12 hours

3. Diphenhydramine: 10 to 50 mg intravenously

4. Benztropine: 1 to 2 mg intravenously (should be stopped if temperature is at or rises above 38°C, which also suggests that it is ineffective)

G. Dystonia treatment options (treatment should be continued for 2 to 3 days after resolution of symptoms)

1. Benztropine: 0.02 to 0.05 mg/kg intravenously, up to 1 to 2 mg, followed by 1 to 2 mg every 12 hours

2. Diphenhydramine: 1 to 2 mg/kg intravenously, up to 50 mg at a time; max 300 mg/day

3. Benzodiazepine: e.g., lorazepam 0.05 mg/kg intravenously, up to 2 mg

H. Akathisia treatment options

1. Propranolol: incremental IV doses of 1 mg, with continuous electrocardiographic and blood pressure monitoring

2. Antiparkinsonian drugs

3. Benzodiazepine

I. Hemodialysis is ineffective.

J. Psychiatric reassessment

Key Treatment

- Airway and ventilation control
- Seizure control
- Gut decontamination
- Circulation control
- Treatment of extrapyramidal symptoms
- Observation for recurrence
- Dysrhythmia control

Bibliography

Acri AA, Henretig FM. Effects of risperidone in overdose. Am J Emerg Med 1998;16:498–501.

Buckley NA, Sanders P. Cardiovascular adverse effects of antipsychotic drugs. Drug Safety 2000;23:215–228.

Buckley NA, Whyte IM, Dawson AH. Cardiotoxicity more common in thioridazine overdose than with other neuroleptics. J Toxicol Clin Toxicol 1995;33:199–204.

Gerber JE, Cawthon B. Overdose and death with olanzapine: two case reports. Am J Forensic Med Pathol 2000; 21:249–251.

Hustey FM. Acute quetiapine poisoning. J Emerg Med 1999;17:995–997.

Li C, Gefter WB. Acute pulmonary edema induced by overdosage of phenothiazines. Chest 1992;101:102–104.

74 Cyclic Antidepressant Drug Overdose

James A. Kruse

Classification of Antidepressant Drugs

A. First-generation cyclic antidepressants
1. Tricyclic antidepressants
   a. Tertiary amines: amitriptyline (Elavil, Endep, Enovil), doxepin (Sinequan, Adapin), imipramine (Tofranil, Janimine), trimipramine (Surmontil), clomipramine (Anafranil)
   b. Secondary amines: desipramine (Norpramin, Pertofrane), nortriptyline (Pamelor, Aventyl), protriptyline (Vivactil)
   c. Dibenzoxazepine derivative: amoxapine (Asendin)
2. Tetracyclic antidepressants: maprotiline (Ludiomil), mirtazapine (Remeron)
B. Other antidepressants (not covered further in this chapter; some have substantially lower overdose morbidity and mortality)
1. Serotonin-modulating drugs: trazodone (Desyrel), nefazodone (Serzone)
2. Selective serotonin reuptake inhibitors (SSRI): paroxetine (Paxil), sertraline (Zoloft), fluoxetine (Prozac), fluvoxamine (Luvox), citalopram (Celexa)
3. Serotonin-norepinephrine reuptake inhibitor: venlafaxine (Effexor)
4. Dopamine-norepinephrine reuptake inhibiting unicyclic aminoketone derivative: bupropion (Wellbutrin, Zyban)
5. Monoamine oxidase inhibitors: phenelzine (Nardil), tranylcypromine (Parnate), moclobemide (Aurorix, Manerix)
6. Lithium (see Chapter 64, Lithium Overdose)

Pharmacology

A. Actions
1. Presynaptic reuptake inhibition of norepinephrine, dopamine, and serotonin, affecting responsiveness of neurotransmitter receptors
2. Acetylcholine, histamine, serotonin, and α-adrenergic receptor blockade
3. Quinidine-like cardiac effects by inhibition of voltage-gated sodium channels
4. Hypotension by myocardial depression and α-adrenergic antagonism–induced vasodilation
5. Large variability in response to given quantity of overdose and plasma concentration
B. Absorption
1. Rapidly and completely absorbed from gastrointestinal tract
2. Blood levels normally peak in 2 to 8 hours but may be delayed up to 12 hours or more in overdose.
C. Metabolism
1. Hepatic metabolism, with first-pass effect, by demethylation, hydroxylation, and glucuronide conjugation
2. Urinary excretion of conjugates
3. Small proportion of the drug undergoes enterohepatic recirculation.
D. Pharmacokinetics
1. Volume of distribution: 9 to 60 L/kg
2. Protein binding
   a. Normally approximately 90% bound to plasma proteins
   b. Bound fraction (physiologically inactive) increases with increasing pH
3. Half-life: 8 to over 100 hours (in overdose)

Clinical Findings

A. General
1. Dry mucous membranes
2. Warm, dry skin
3. Hyperthermia
B. Ophthalmologic
1. Blurred vision
2. Mydriasis
C. Cardiovascular
1. Tachycardia (early sign)
2. Cutaneous flushing
3. Hypotension
4. Hypertension (early sign, usually mild)
5. Cardiac arrest
D. Central nervous system
1. Confusion, agitation, delirium
2. Hallucinations
3. Dizziness

4. Hyperreflexia

5. Dystonia

6. Myoclonic, ataxic, or choreoathetoid movements

7. Seizures (especially with amoxapine, maprotiline)

8. Sedation, stupor, coma

E. Gastrointestinal

1. Constipation, ileus

2. Intestinal pseudo-obstruction

3. Toxic megacolon

4. Cecal perforation

5. Pancreatitis

F. Pulmonary

1. Acute respiratory distress syndrome

2. Aspiration pneumonitis

G. Uroexcretory

1. Urinary retention

2. Hydronephrosis

Key Findings

- History of depression, access to offending drug

- Peripheral anticholinergic findings: tachycardia, mydriasis, hyperthermia, dry flushed skin, urinary retention, ileus

- Central nervous system derangements: sedation, agitation, coma, seizures

- Cardiac dysrhythmias: sinus tachycardia is most common

- QRS interval duration greater than 100 msec (signifies high risk of serious overdose)

Electrocardiographic Findings

A. Cardiac dysrhythmias

1. Sinus tachycardia

2. Supraventricular tachydysrhythmias

3. Ventricular tachycardia, including torsade de pointes

4. Idioventricular rhythm

B. Other electrocardiographic changes

1. Intraventricular conduction defects, especially right bundle branch block

2. Atrioventricular block

3. Quinidine-like effects

a. ST segment changes

b. T wave changes

c. PR, QRS, and QT interval prolongation

d. Rightward deviation of the terminal 40 msec of the frontal plane QRS axis to greater than 120°

C. Cardiac arrest

1. Ventricular tachycardia or fibrillation

2. Pulseless electrical activity

3. Asystole

Treatment

A. General

1. Ensure adequate airway and ventilation.

2. Obtain IV access.

3. If sensorium is depressed, consider other etiologies and give naloxone, thiamine, and dextrose intravenously (do not administer flumazenil).

4. Continuous electrocardiographic monitoring

5. Obtain 12-lead electrocardiogram.

6. Obtain chest x-ray.

7. Obtain blood for laboratory tests.

a. Serum for electrolytes, urea nitrogen, creatinine, glucose

b. Complete blood cell count

c. Arterial blood gases

d. Serum cyclic antidepressant levels do not correlate well with toxicity and are generally unnecessary.

B. Gastric evacuation

1. Consider endotracheal intubation and orogastric lavage for serious cases.

2. Syrup of ipecac is not recommended.

C. Activated charcoal

1. Give 50 to 100 g (1 g/kg) activated charcoal, along with a cathartic (sorbitol, magnesium sulfate, or magnesium citrate).

2. Multidose charcoal administration

a. Rationale for use is enterohepatic recirculation of drug; however, this treatment is probably ineffective and is not necessary.

b. If used, give half the initial dose, without cathartic, every 2 to 4 hours for one or more additional doses.

c. Not recommended if bowel sounds are absent

D. Alkalinization

1. Indications

a. QRS interval prolongation to more than 100 msec

b. Rightward terminal QRS axis deviation greater than 120°

c. Clinical signs of serious toxicity (e.g., seizures, hypotension, ventricular dysrhythmias)

2. Decreases the circulating fraction of free (not protein-bound) drug and decreases cardiovascular toxicity

3. Usually accomplished using IV NaHCO$_3$; e.g., 1 to 2 mmol/kg initially, followed by a continuous IV infusion of 0.10 to 0.15 M NaHCO$_3$ started at 5 to 40 mmol/hour

4. Target arterial blood pH between 7.45 and 7.55; higher pH levels may precipitate seizures or cardiac dysrhythmias.

5. In mechanically ventilated patients, hyperventilation may also be employed as an adjunct to effect alkalemia.

6. NaHCO$_3$ can induce hypokalemia; monitor serum potassium closely and provide supplemental potassium as necessary.

E. Forced diuresis is not recommended.

F. Cardiac tachydysrhythmias

1. Sinus tachycardia requires no treatment unless there is a cause other than drug effect (e.g., hypovolemia, hypoxemia).

2. Supraventricular tachycardia

a. First-line treatment is alkalinization.

b. Vagal maneuvers may be attempted.

c. If necessary, β-adrenergic or calcium channel blockers may be considered, with due caution for negative inotropic and vasodilator properties.

3. Ventricular tachydysrhythmias

a. Lidocaine and cardioversion are first-line treatments.

b. Alkalinize blood, as for supraventricular tachycardia.

c. Overdrive pacing may be considered.

d. Phenytoin has been used, but it has the potential for provoking dysrhythmias, conduction disturbances, and hypotension.

e. Class Ia, Ic, and III antiarrhythmic drugs are contraindicated.

4. Second- and third-degree heart block

a. Alkalinize blood as described.

b. Correct hyperkalemia and hyponatremia, if present.

c. Atropine is often ineffective.

d. Temporary cardiac pacing may be necessary.

5. Cardiac arrest: prolonged cardiopulmonary resuscitation (e.g., >1 hour) has been effective

G. Hypotension

1. Expand intravascular volume with isotonic crystalloids.

2. Alkalinize blood.

3. For hypotension refractory to fluid therapy, norepinephrine is the vasopressor of choice; phenylephrine is an alternative.

4. Dobutamine may worsen hypotension, tachycardia, and dysrhythmias.

5. Glucagon (10 mg bolus and 1.7 mg/hour intravenously) has been anecdotally associated with reversal of hypotension.

H. Seizures

1. Treat with benzodiazepine followed by phenobarbital.

2. Phenytoin may not be effective and has the potential for provoking dysrhythmias, conduction disturbances, and hypotension.

3. Propofol may be effective in refractory cases.

I. Physostigmine

1. Inhibits acetylcholinesterase and increases acetylcholine levels

2. Has been used to treat the anticholinergic effects of cyclic antidepressants, including coma and supraventricular dysrhythmias

3. However, its use in the treatment of cyclic antidepressant overdose is not recommended because of the potential for serious side effects (cholinergic crisis).

a. Bradycardia

b. Seizures

c. Nausea, emesis

d. Salivation, lacrimation, bronchorrhea

e. Urination, defecation

J. Extracorporeal removal

1. Hemodialysis: not effective

2. Resin hemoperfusion: low efficacy and generally not recommended

K. Triage considerations

1. Lack of the following findings at 6 hours after ingestion signify low likelihood for developing serious toxicity; these patients generally do not require admission to the intensive care unit (ICU).

a. Altered sensorium

b. Hypotension

c. Absent bowel sounds

d. Seizures

e. Cardiac dysrhythmias

f. QRS interval prolongation

g. Right axis deviation

2. Sinus tachycardia, prolonged QRS interval or right axis deviation may be harbingers of serious complications (e.g., cardiac dysrhythmias, seizures, hypotension) and necessitate ICU monitoring.

3. Psychiatric follow-up necessary if intentional overdose with suicidal ideation

Key Treatment

- Ensure airway, ventilation, and perfusion.
- Continuous cardiac monitoring
- Activated charcoal administration
- Systemic alkalinization with IV sodium bicarbonate
- Isotonic IV fluids and, if necessary, norepinephrine for hypotension

Bibliography

Foulke GE. Identifying toxicity risk early after antidepressant overdose. Am J Emerg Med 1995;13:123–126.

Glauser J. Tricyclic antidepressant poisoning. Cleve Clin J Med 2000;67:709–713, 717–719.

Harrigan RA, Brady WJ. ECG abnormalities in tricyclic antidepressant ingestion. Am J Emerg Med 1999;17:387–393.

Liebelt EL, Ulrich A, Francis PD, et al. Serial electrocardiographic changes in acute tricyclic antidepressant overdoses. Crit Care Med 1997;25:1721–1726.

Ross JP, Small TR, Lepage PA. Imipramine overdose complicated by toxic megacolon. Am Surg 1998;64:242–244.

75 Anticholinergic Poisonings

Suzanne R. White

Etiology

A. The 1998 report of the American Association of Poison Control Centers listed more than 194,000 toxic exposures to anticholinergic substances.

B. Anticholinergic (antimuscarinic) toxicity is prototypically caused by the belladonna alkaloids (atropine, scopolamine, hyoscyamine, and hyoscine) found naturally in plants such as deadly nightshade, mandrake, Jimson weed, and black henbane.

C. Toxicity can also occur following drug overdose or as a side effect of pharmaceuticals used to treat a wide variety of symptoms.

1. Motion sickness: scopolamine, meclizine
2. Gastrointestinal (GI) spasm: dicyclomine, propantheline
3. Diarrhea: diphenoxylate, atropine
4. Bladder instability: oxybutyrin
5. Skeletal muscle spasm: cyclobenzaprine, orphenadrine
6. Asthma: ipratropium
7. Parkinsonism: benztropine, trihexyphenidyl, amantadine
8. Coryza and allergies: diphenhydramine, chlorpheniramine, hydroxyzine, cyproheptadine, astemizole, terfenadine, loratadine, fexofenadine, cetirizine
9. Seizures: carbamazepine
10. Cardiac dysrhythmias: procainamide, quinidine
11. Psychiatric illness: cyclic antidepressants (TCAs), phenothiazines, atypical antipsychotics

D. Even patients taking the above drugs therapeutically may become ill under conditions of heat stress.

E. Anticholinergic toxicity outbreaks have occurred in certain settings.

1. Intentional abuse: jimsonweed, scopolamine-adulterated heroin
2. Malicious administration: scopolamine-tainted alcoholic beverages

Pathophysiology

A. Muscarinic receptors
1. Affect smooth muscles in the eye, bronchi, GI tract, and bladder
2. Regulate heart rate, sweat, salivary and mucous gland activity
3. Central nervous system (CNS) muscarinic receptor activation facilitates new memory formation, motor coordination, perception, and cognition.

B. All of the agents listed above have the ability to competitively block muscarinic receptors within peripheral and central cholinergic neurons, potentially causing the "anticholinergic toxidrome" (see later under Key Physical Findings).

C. In addition to the antimuscarinic effects, some of these agents have other more serious neurologic and cardiovascular effects with overdose, including

1. α-Adrenergic blockade resulting in hypotension (TCAs, phenothiazines)
2. Cardiac sodium channel blockade resulting in seizures, myocardial depression, and widened QRS complex on the electrocardiogram (ECG) (TCAs, carbamazepine, procainamide)
3. Cardiac potassium channel blockade resulting in QT prolongation and torsade de pointes (diphenhydramine, terfenadine, astemizole, mesoridazine, thioridazine, quinidine, procainamide, diisopyramide)
4. Interference with neurotransmitters such as γ-hydroxybutyrate, adenosine, serotonin, or dopamine resulting in seizures, movement disorders, or rigidity (TCAs, phenothiazines, carbamazepine)

D. The major morbidity and mortality associated with anticholinergic drug toxicity stems from hyperthermia and rhabdomyolysis, resulting from agitation and ineffective heat dissipation.

Key Risk Factors

- Heat stress
- Dehydration
- Use of multiple anticholinergic agents
- Extremes of age

Clinical Findings

A. The diagnosis hinges on recognition of the clinical anticholinergic toxidrome and elicitation of a care-

263

ful medication history, including herbal tea remedy exposure.

B. The onset of symptoms is usually rapid except following the ingestion of jimsonweed seeds, diphenoxylate/atropine, cyclobenzaprine, and thioridazine.

C. Physical findings

1. Vital signs: tachycardia, hyperthermia; hypotension and bradycardia are rare and typically occur with massive ingestion

2. Cardiac: sinus tachycardia or other tachydysrhythmias

3. Respiratory: delayed fatal respiratory depression has occurred following diphenoxylate/atropine ingestion

4. Neurologic: agitation, delirium, hallucinations, amnesia, cognitive dysfunction, "babbling" speech, picking movements, choreoathetosis, extrapyramidal reactions, seizures, coma

5. Eyes:

a. Mydriasis is expected unless the drug has other significant actions.

(1) TCAs and phenothiazines also cause α_1-adrenergic receptor blockade; therefore, pupils are midrange or miotic.

(2) Combination opioid-containing products (diphenoxylate/atropine) may cause miosis.

b. Loss of accommodation

6. Skin: dry axillae, flushing

7. Gastrointestinal: dry mucous membranes, decreased bowel sounds, ileus

8. Genitourinary: palpable bladder, urinary retention

D. Typically, acutely poisoned patients exhibit both peripheral and central anticholinergic toxicity, yet some patients with chronic use may display only central anticholinergic toxicity (perceptual and cognitive dysfunction, dementia, psychosis), especially the elderly.

E. Adults are less susceptible to the CNS stimulant effects and less commonly develop seizures than children.

Differential Diagnosis

A. Hypoxia

B. Metabolic disturbances (e.g., hypoglycemia)

C. Salicylism

D. Lithium intoxication

E. Sympathomimetic toxidrome due to cocaine, phencyclidine, amphetamines, or monoamine oxidase inhibitors (differentiate by presence of bowel sounds and sweating)

F. Central nervous system infection or trauma

G. Endocrine crisis

H. Withdrawal from ethanol or other sedative-hypnotic drug

I. Neuroleptic malignant syndrome

J. Serotonin syndrome

Laboratory Findings

A. Elevated serum creatine phosphokinase activity secondary to rhabdomyolysis (especially doxylamine)

B. Hyperkalemia, hyperphosphatemia, hypocalcemia related to rhabdomyolysis

C. Lactic acidosis secondary to seizures or agitation

D. Disseminated intravascular coagulation related to hyperthermia

E. Drug screening

1. Rapid antibody-based drug screens generally do not detect these agents, other than TCAs.

2. Based on structural similarity, a positive TCA screen may be seen with high serum levels of cyclobenzaprine, diphenhydramine, carbamazepine, and some phenothiazines.

F. Plasma acetaminophen level

1. Should be checked in the setting of any intentional drug ingestion

2. Many over-the-counter sleep and cough-and-cold preparations contain acetaminophen in

---

Key Physical Findings

Peripheral	Central
• Tachycardia	• Amnesia, cognitive dysfunction
• Hyperthermia	• Delirium, babbling speech
• Mydriasis	• Hallucinations
• Dry mucous membranes and axillae	• Agitation, picking movements
• Flushing	• Extrapyramidal reactions
• Decreased bowel sounds	• Seizures, coma
• Palpably distended bladder	• Circulatory collapse

combination with anticholinergic substances (sleep aids and cough-and-cold preparations).

3. A single 4-hour acetaminophen level may not be adequate after ingestion of such mixed products.

4. A delayed peak is often noted secondary to decreased gut motility; therefore, serial acetaminophen levels are indicated.

Other Tests

A. Electrocardiogram: any finding other than sinus tachycardia should suggest a massive exposure to anticholinergic toxins or the presence of a more cardiotoxic substance

B. Computed tomography of the brain: may be indicated to exclude other neurologic or neurosurgical emergencies

C. Lumbar puncture: may be necessary to exclude other causes of altered mental status

Key Complications

- Rhabdomyolysis (especially with doxylamine overdose)

- Myoglobinuric renal failure

- Trauma related to behavioral disturbance

- Hepatic necrosis

- Disseminated intravascular coagulation

- Cerebral edema

- Ileus

- Glaucoma

Treatment

A. Provide supplemental oxygen and assess oxygenation.

B. Administer thiamine.

C. Perform rapid dextrose determination to exclude hypoglycemia.

D. Naloxone is not indicated in the agitated or seizing patient.

E. Flumazenil is contraindicated in the setting of anticholinergic toxicity (may predispose to seizures).

F. Consider GI decontamination.

1. Ipecac is contraindicated.

2. Gastric lavage may be considered only if within 60 to 90 minutes of ingestion (risks of large-bore lavage tube outweigh benefits in an agitated patient).

3. Whole bowel irrigation with polyethylene glycol solution at 2 L/hour may be considered for seed ingestion if ileus is not present.

4. Multiple-dose charcoal may be considered for patients with prolonged symptoms, if gut motility is present.

G. Treat hyperthermia.

1. Employ continuous rectal or bladder (core) temperature monitoring.

2. Antipyretics are generally not effective.

3. Evaporative cooling most effective

4. No role for dantrolene

H. Provide adequate sedation with IV benzodiazepines.

1. Titrated to effect

2. Avoid phenothiazines and butyrophenones (they have synergistic neurologic and cardiac effects and may further inhibit heat dissipation).

3. Physical restraint alone may be detrimental.

I. Provide adequate IV hydration.

J. Treat seizures aggressively.

1. Use benzodiazepines and barbiturates.

2. Phenytoin is not effective for drug-induced seizures.

3. Status epilepticus is rare.

K. Monitor and treat cardiac dysrhythmias.

1. Continuous ECG monitoring is indicated.

2. Wide complex cardiac dysrhythmias are treated with IV sodium bicarbonate (bolus or continuous infusion) to a targeted arterial blood pH of 7.45 to 7.50.

3. Lidocaine is a second-line agent for ventricular dysrhythmias.

4. Quinidine, diisopyramide, procainamide are contraindicated.

L. Physostigmine use

1. Physostigmine is a carbamate acetylcholinesterase inhibitor that crosses the blood–brain barrier and potentially reverses both peripheral and central antimuscarinic blockade by increasing acetylcholine levels at cholinergic synapses.

2. Its role as an antidote is controversial.

3. Potential adverse effects

a. Asystole in the setting of conduction disturbance or TCA toxicity

b. Seizures

c. Muscle weakness

d. Cholinergic crisis: bradycardia, salivation, lacrimation, bronchospasm, bronchorrhea, diarrhea

4. Indications

a. Only when first-line therapies (sedation and cooling) have failed

b. Intractable seizures

c. Hemodynamically significant supraventricular tachydysrhythmias

d. Diagnostic use is controversial (never use routinely in unknown drug overdose setting as a "coma cocktail").

5. Dose: 1 to 2 mg in 10 mL normal saline over 5 minutes by IV injection (repeat doses are rarely needed and continuous infusions should not be given)

6. Careful patient selection is critical.

a. Must have baseline ECG showing no conduction disturbances, QRS of less than 100 msec duration, and no axis deviation of the terminal portion of the QRS complex

b. No history of exposure to other toxins with potential cardiac effect

c. Patient must have peripheral and central signs of antimuscarinic toxicity.

d. Absence of the following

(1) Bronchospastic disease

(2) Vagotonic symptoms, especially bradycardia

(3) Intestinal or bladder obstruction

(4) Severe peripheral vascular disease (gangrene)

(5) Diabetes mellitus

(6) Cardiovascular disease

(7) Recent co-administration of succinylcholine

7. Have atropine available at the bedside as a precaution.

Key Treatment

- Most complications result from agitation and hyperthermia.

- Aggressive cooling measures

- Adequate sedation using benzodiazepines

- Adequate hydration

- Physostigmine is rarely needed.

Bibliography

Bowden CA, Krenzelok EP. Clinical applications of commonly used contemporary antidotes: a US perspective. Drug Safety 1997;16:9–47.

Chan TC, Evans SD, Clark RF. Drug-induced hyperthermia. Crit Care Clin 1997;13:785–808.

Delaney KA. Anticholinergics. In: Rosen P, Barkin R (eds). Emergency Medicine: Concepts and Clinical Practice. St. Louis: Mosby, 1998, pp 1300–1306.

Feinberg M. The problems of anticholinergic adverse effects in older patients. Drugs Aging 1993;3:335–348.

Kirk MA. Anticholinergics and antihistamines. In: Haddad LM, Shannon MW, Winchester JF (eds). Clinical Management of Poisoning and Drug Overdose. Philadelphia: WB Saunders, 1998, pp 641–649.

76 Serotonin Syndrome

Jane E. Sundberg

The serotonin syndrome (SS) is a complication of serotonergic drug toxicity. It is chiefly caused by antidepressive drugs, often in combination with monoamine oxidase (MAO) inhibitors, leading to excess of intrasynaptic 5-hydroxytryptamine with stimulation of postsynaptic serotonin receptors. Diagnosis of SS is by clinical presentation and exclusion of other conditions. The serotonin syndrome may be acutely life-threatening, but it typically resolves within hours.

Key Pathophysiology

- Hyperstimulation of brain stem and spinal cord postsynaptic 5-hydroxytryptamine$_{1A}$ receptors

- Typically precipitated by a change in dose of selective serotonin reuptake inhibitor medication or addition of an MAO inhibitor, cyclic antidepressive, or other agent that inhibits serotonin reuptake, or another serotonergic drug

Etiology (Often in Combination)

A. Selective serotonin reuptake inhibitors
   1. Paroxetine
   2. Sertraline
   3. Fluoxetine
   4. Fluvoxamine
   5. Citalopram
B. Serotonin modulating drugs
   1. Nefazodone
   2. Trazodone
C. Serotonin-norepinephrine reuptake inhibitor: Venlafaxine
D. Dopamine-norepinephrine reuptake inhibiting unicyclic aminoketone derivative: Bupropion
E. Other psychotropic drugs
   1. Tricyclic antidepressants and mirtazapine
   2. Monoamine oxidase inhibitors
      a. Phenelzine
      b. Tranylcypromine
      c. Moclobemide
      d. Isocarboxazid
      e. Selegiline
   3. Lithium
   4. Buspirone
   5. St. John's wort

F. Cocaine
G. Bromocriptine
H. Amantadine
I. Sympathomimetic drugs
   1. Pseudoephedrine
   2. Amphetamines
   3. Methylenedioxymethamphetamine (ecstasy)
J. Dihydroergotamine
K. Serotonin 5-HT, receptor agonists (sumatriptan, rizatripan, etc.)
L. Opioids
   1. Meperidine
   2. Fentanyl
   3. Dextromethorphan
   4. Tramadol
   5. Pentazocine
M. Carbamazepine
N. Levodopa
O. Hallucinogens
   1. Lysergic acid diethylamide
   2. Morning glory seeds

Clinical Findings

A. Diagnostic criteria of Sternbach (see Key Diagnosis box)
B. Manifestations
   1. Usually develop within minutes to hours after initiating or changing the dose of serotonergic agent or adding another agent
   2. 70% of cases resolve within 24 hours.
C. Signs and symptoms
   1. Mental status: agitation, coma, confusion, delirium, disorientation, hallucinations, insomnia, mania, mutism
   2. Neuromuscular alterations: akathesia, clonus, hyperactivity, nystagmus, ocular oscillation, oculogyric crisis, opisthotonos, rhabdomyolysis, rigidity (may be more pronounced in lower extremities), seizures, tremor, trismus, stiff neck, Babinski sign
   3. Autonomic dysfunction: abdominal cramping, vomiting, blood pressure increases/decreases, diaphoresis, flushing, headache, hyperthermia, lacrimation, mydriasis, salivation, tachycardia,

teeth chattering, dilated pupils, decreased sexual function, salivation

4. Pulmonary: respiratory distress

D. Complications may persist beyond resolution of primary signs and symptoms.

Key Diagnosis (More than Three Features Required)

- Agitation
- Hyperreflexia
- Fever
- Myoclonus
- Diaphoresis
- Tremor
- Shivering
- Incoordination
- Diarrhea
- Mental status change: confusion, hypomania

Differential Diagnosis

A. Disorders requiring exclusion
   1. Infectious disorders
      a. Intracranial infection
      b. Sepsis
   2. Metabolic disturbances
   3. Substance abuse or withdrawal
   4. Intracranial catastrophe
   5. Neuroleptic drug effect

B. Conditions often confused with SS
   1. Delirium tremens
   2. Neuroleptic malignant syndrome
   3. Malignant hyperthermia (Table 76–1)
   4. Lethal catatonia
   5. Anticholinergic toxicity
   6. Tyramine-cheese reaction

TABLE 76–1. DIFFERENTIATING FEATURES OF SEROTONIN SYNDROME VERSUS NEUROLEPTIC MALIGNANT SYNDROME

FEATURE	SEROTONIN SYNDROME	NEUROLEPTIC MALIGNANT SYNDROME
Putative agonist/antagonist	Serotonin	Dopamine
Onset after drug administration or dose adjustment	Minutes to hours	Days
Course	<24 hours	Days
Fever	+	+++
Autonomic changes	++	+++
Altered consciousness	++	+++
Rigidity	++	+++
Rhabdomyolysis	+	+++
Myoclonus, hyperreflexia	+++	±
Leukocytosis	+	+++

Key Monitoring

- Autonomic parameters
- Cardiac rhythm
- Coagulation
- Acid-base balance
- Serum muscle enzymes

Treatment

A. Discontinue all serotonergic drugs.

B. Administer IV hydration.

C. Provide supportive care.

D. Treat muscle rigidity and myoclonus.
   1. Benzodiazepines, such as clonazepam, are the treatment of first choice.
   2. Treatment with dantrolene has been reported.

E. Control seizures.
   1. Benzodiazepines
   2. Barbiturates

F. Consider use of a serotonin antagonist, such as cyproheptadine or methysergide; chlorpromazine has also been used.

G. Use cooling measures as indicated (antipyretics are usually ineffective).

Key Complications

- Rhabdomyolysis
- Renal failure
- Respiratory failure
- Disseminated intravascular coagulation

Bibliography

Bodner RA, Lynch T, Lewis L, Kahn D. Serotonin syndrome. Neurology 1995;45:219–223.

Carbone JR. The neuroleptic malignant and serotonin syndromes. Emerg Med Clin North Am 2000;18:317–325.

Gillman PK. The serotonin syndrome and its treatment. J Psychopharmacol 1999;13:100–109.

Lejoyeux M, Ades J, Rouillon F. Serotonin syndrome: incidence, symptoms and treatment. CNS Drugs 1994;2:132–143.

Martin TG. Serotonin syndrome. Ann Emerg Med 1996;28:520–526.

Mason PJ, Morris VA, Balcezak TJ. Serotonin syndrome. Medicine 2000;79:201–209.

Mills KC. Serotonin syndrome: a clinical update. Crit Care Clin 1997;13:763–783.

Nierenberg DW, Semprebon M. The central nervous system serotonin syndrome. Clin Pharmacol Ther 1993;53:84–88.

Sternbach H. The serotonin syndrome Am J Psychiatry 1993;148:705–713.

77 Organophosphate Poisoning

Ali A. Hamdan

Organophosphates (OPs) are the most widely used insecticides. They can cause serious or fatal poisoning if accidentally or deliberately ingested. Symptoms are caused by their inhibitory effect on cholinesterase enzymes, which leads to accumulation of acetylcholine (Ach) at cholinergic receptors. The diagnosis is based on a history of exposure, symptoms of cholinergic overactivity, and a decrease in erythrocyte (RBC) or plasma cholinesterase activity. Early recognition is essential to avoid lethal complications, particularly ventricular dysrhythmias, respiratory failure, central nervous system (CNS) depression, and seizures. Treatment is aimed at decontamination, administration of anticholinergic drugs, and general supportive care. Relapse may occur after seemingly successful treatment.

Key Pharmacology

- Common insecticide OPs include malathion, parathion, dichlorvos, and diazinon.

- Neostigmine and physostigmine are pharmacologic OP agents.

- Organophosphates are highly lipid-soluble agents, well absorbed from skin, oral mucosa, conjunctivae, and gastroenteric and respiratory routes.

- Organophosphates widely distribute in tissues and are slowly eliminated by hepatic metabolism.

Pathophysiology

A. Cholinergic processes
1. Acetylcholine is a neurotransmitter released at the terminal nerve endings of all postganglionic parasympathetic nerves, and at both sympathetic and parasympathetic ganglia.
   a. Acetylcholine is also a CNS neurotransmitter.
   b. It is released at skeletal muscle myoneural junctions.
   c. Acetylcholine is normally inactivated by cholinesterases in RBCs (true cholinesterase) and plasma (pseudocholinesterase).
2. Organophosphates bind and inactivate both types of cholinesterase.

   a. Binding is irreversible unless early pharmacologic intervention is instituted.
   b. The result is an accumulation of Ach at synapses, leading to a hypercholinergic state.

B. Severity
1. Determined by the route of exposure and the degree and duration of the poisoning
2. Varies with the specific OP agent according to its lipid solubility, rate of metabolism, and other factors

Clinical Findings

A. Acute exposure (cholinergic crisis): onset of signs and symptoms is within minutes to 12 hours
1. Peripheral muscarinic effects
   a. Cardiac: bradycardia, hypotension
   b. Gastrointestinal (GI): salivation, vomiting, diarrhea, abdominal pain, fecal incontinence
   c. Pulmonary: bronchorrhea, bronchospasm, cough
   d. Ocular: miosis, lacrimation
   e. Genitourinary: frequency, incontinence
2. Peripheral nicotinic effects
   a. Cardiac: tachycardia, hypertension
   b. Neuromuscular: fasciculations, weakness, paralysis, cramps
3. Central nervous system effects
   a. Altered mental status, ranging from agitation to coma
   b. Seizures
   c. Respiratory depression
   d. Ataxia, dysarthria
   e. Tremor

B. Intermediate syndrome
1. Occurs 1 to 4 days after apparent recovery from cholinergic crisis
2. Characterized by paralysis of respiratory, cranial motor, neck flexor, and proximal limb muscles

C. Delayed polyneuropathy
1. Occurs 6 to 21 days after exposure
2. Manifests as a sensorimotor polyneuropathy

Key Diagnostic Points

- History of exposure
- "Sludge": salivation, lacrimation, urination, defecation, GI distress, emesis
- Neuromuscular effects
- Decreased plasma or RBC cholinesterase activity
- Positive response to treatment

Diagnosis

A. Diagnostic criteria
   1. Presence of the aforementioned signs and symptoms
   2. 50% depression of plasma or RBC cholinesterase activity
   3. Positive response to treatment
B. Other considerations to be included in differential diagnosis
   1. Infection
   2. Metabolic disturbances (e.g., hypoglycemia, thyrotoxicosis)
   3. Other acute neurologic disorders
   4. Other poisonings

Key Treatment

- Decontamination
- Airway protection
- Respiratory and hemodynamic support
- Avoidance of succinylcholine
- Atropinization and oxime therapy
- Monitoring for complications
- Adequate observation prior to discharge

Treatment

A. Decontamination
   1. For oral ingestions
      a. Consider induction of vomiting using oral syrup of ipecac (10 to 30 mL) if patient is fully awake; contraindicated if altered mental status.
      b. Perform gastric lavage if patient presents soon after ingestion.
      c. For patients in coma or at risk for seizures, perform endotracheal intubation prior to lavage.
      d. Do not lavage if there is co-ingestion of a corrosive substance.
      e. Administer activated charcoal: 25 to 200 g.
   2. For inhalation exposure
      a. Move patient to fresh air.
      b. Administer humidified supplemental oxygen at an FIO_2 of 1.00.
      c. Monitor for respiratory and systemic symptoms.
   3. For ocular exposure
      a. Perform copious irrigation for 10 to 15 minutes.
      b. Observe closely for local or systemic symptoms development and treat accordingly.
   4. Cutaneous exposure
      a. Remove contaminated clothing.
      b. Vigorously wash skin, hair, and nails.
      c. Systemic effects can occur.
B. Maintain airway and oxygenation.
   1. Frequent suctioning of oral secretions is often required.
   2. If sensorium is affected, consider early endotracheal intubation to protect airway and prevent aspiration.
   3. Because of the potential for prolonged paralysis, avoid succinylcholine if a paralytic agent is needed for intubation.
C. Treat hypotension with IV fluids; add a vasopressor (e.g., dopamine) if necessary.
D. Control seizures.
   1. Use IV benzodiazepines (diazepam or lorazepam) as first-line drugs.
   2. Consider phenytoin, fosphenytoin, or phenobarbital, if seizures are otherwise refractory.
E. Health care personnel should protect themselves from exposure by avoiding contact with contaminated patient's skin, clothing, secretions, etc.
F. Atropine
   1. Indicated to control muscarinic symptoms
   2. Has no effect on nicotinic or CNS symptoms
   3. Dosing methods
      a. Repeated IV bolus dosing: 2 to 5 mg IV every 5 to 10 minutes to effect; additional IV boluses can be used as needed to quickly control breakthrough cholinergic symptoms
      b. Continuous IV infusion: 30 mg in 200 mL of normal saline, titrated to effect
   4. Assess for signs of atropine effects, e.g., dry mucous membrane, tachycardia, and mydriasis.

5. Adequacy of atropine dosing is assessed by ability to control secretions and bradycardia.

6. Maintain atropine therapy for at least 2 days, or up to several weeks, depending on the severity of poisoning.

7. Be aware of atropine CNS toxicity that may mimic OP poisoning, relapse after treatment, or sepsis.

G. Pralidoxime

1. Reactivates cholinesterase

2. Use is controversial, but generally employed for severe nicotinic and CNS poisoning; e.g., profound skeletal muscle or diaphragmatic weakness, respiratory depression, coma, seizures.

3. Most effective if given shortly after exposure

4. Administer 1 to 2 g IV at 0.25 to 0.5 g/minute, as early as possible and within the first 24 hours after exposure.

5. May repeat dose in 2 hours and every 6 to 12 hours for up to 48 hours (several days may be necessary in some cases)

6. Use by continuous infusion (at 0.5 mg/hour) has been suggested.

H. Treatment of intermediate syndrome

1. Respiratory support is a key measure.

2. Atropine and pralidoxime are not effective.

3. Recovery is expected 5 to 15 days after onset.

I. Supportive measures

J. Observation

1. Relapse can occur after treatment.

2. May be due to inadequate decontamination of skin or gastrointestinal tract, premature discontinuation of atropine, or redistribution of OP from subcutaneous fat stores

Key Complications

- Respiratory failure
- Ventricular dysrhythmias
- Liver function abnormalities
- Coagulopathy
- Ulcerative stomatitis
- Relapse after treatment
- Delayed peripheral neuropathy
- Pancreatitis
- Blood dyscrasias
- Delayed CNS toxicity (impaired memory, psychosis)

Bibliography

Bardin PG, van Eeden SF, Moolman JA, et al. Organophosphate and carbamate poisoning. Arch Intern Med 1994; 154:1433–1441.

Clegg DJ, van Gemert M. Expert panel report of human studies on chlorpyrifos and/or other organophosphate exposures. J Toxicol Environ Health B Crit Rev 1999;2: 257–279.

Geller RJ, Singleton KL, Tarantino ML, et al. Nosocomial poisoning associated with emergency department treatment of organophosphate toxicity—Georgia 2000. J Toxicol Clin Toxicol 2001;39:109–111.

Gude W, Shepherd S. Pesticides. In: Howell JM (ed). Emergency Medicine. Philadelphia: WB Saunders, 1998, pp 1499–1506.

Marcello I. Treatment of acute organophosphate poisoning. Med J Aust 1991;154:51–55.

Marrs TC. Organophosphate poisoning. Pharmacol Ther 1993;58:51–66.

78 Venom Injuries: Snake and Arthropod

Syed K. Shahryar
Richard W. Carlson

Snakes and arthropods cause thousands of injuries each year. Most bites and stings are caused by nonvenomous animals or less dangerous species. However, contact with nonvenomous forms or those with less toxic venom may lead to life-threatening allergic reactions to the venom or therapy (antivenin). The intensivist should have a basic knowledge of venomous organisms and their toxins, priorities of management, and measures to assess severity. Poison control centers, zoos, and universities and colleges may provide additional information and tips on management of specific injuries.

Definitions

A. *Poison:* a toxic substance that is typically delivered orally and has specific (and often limited) deleterious effects

B. *Venom:* an animal poison delivered parenterally via a venom apparatus (fang, stinger, or venom gland) and containing several toxins that may affect multiple organ systems as well as produce local effects

Epidemiology (U.S.)

A. Snakes: 45,000 snakebites occur annually, more than 8,000 of them by venomous animals (<10 deaths/year)
  1. Family Crotalidae (pit vipers): rattlesnakes, copperheads, cottonmouths, and massasaugas
  2. Family Elapidae (coral snakes): Eastern coral snake, *Micrurus fulvius fulvius:* Texas coral snake *M. f. tenere*; and Western, Sonoran, or Arizona coral snake, *Micruroides euryxanthus*
  3. Occasionally, non-indigenous "exotic" snakes

B. Arthropods: there are more than 1 million species, but few are dangerous to humans; only those with very toxic venom (independent of anaphylaxis) are presented here
  1. Spiders
    a. Black and brown widow spiders (family Theridiidae, genus *Latrodectus*)
    b. Violin or brown "recluse" (family Loxoscelidae)
  2. Scorpions (class Arachnida, family Buthidae): Southwest United States and Mexico

  3. Bees, wasps, hornets (class Insecta, order Hymenoptera): painful and occasionally dangerous stings; potentially fatal anaphylactic reactions
  4. Ants: multiple species, including fire ants

Key Epidemiology

- Snakebites usually follow attempts to catch or handle; random wilderness bites are uncommon.
- Undisturbed snakes can usually be avoided.
- Arthropod injuries are typically random and occur in urban and rural settings.

Diagnosis

A. Crotalid snake envenomation
  1. Clinical findings
    a. History usually reliable, except for children or if animal not seen
    b. Fang marks, local edema, blebs, bullae, ecchymoses
    c. Pain, paresthesias, fasciculations
    d. Nausea, vomiting, weakness
    e. Local or systemic bleeding; petechiae
    f. Circulatory shock, cardiac dysrhythmias
    g. Central nervous system (CNS) alterations
  2. Assessing severity of crotalid envenomation
    a. Confirm bite: history, fang marks.
    b. Consider both local and systemic findings.
      (1) Score (mild, moderate, severe) local finding: pain, edema, ecchymoses, blebs or bullae (often hemorrhagic), nerve or muscle compression, myonecrosis.
      (2) Evaluate systemic findings: cardiovascular (hypotension, dysrhythmias), pulmonary (pulmonary edema, hemorrhage), gastrointestinal (nausea, vomiting, bleeding), hematologic (thrombocytopenia, coagulopathy), neurologic (fasciculations, pain, taste in mouth, paresthesias, rarely seizures or coma, CNS bleeding), renal failure (myoglobinuria, hypovolemia).
    c. Patient factors that influence risk of injury:

272

extremes of age; allergies; underlying cardio-pulmonary, neurologic, or hematologic conditions

d. There are multiple species of pit vipers with significant differences in toxicity and composition of venoms.

3. Early laboratory findings

    a. Complete blood cell count: fall in hemoglobin (bleeding) may be obscured by plasma loss with hemoconcentration

    b. Thrombocytopenia: may correlate with severity

    c. Coagulation changes: prolonged prothrombin or partial thromboplastin times, hypofibrinogenemia

    d. Creatine phosphokinase activity: reflects muscle damage and potential for development of compartment syndrome

---

PEARLS (Coral Snake Envenomations)

• Eastern species are the most dangerous, Texas species may be dangerous, Western, Arizona, and Sonoran species usually cause less serious envenomations.

• Venoms contain neurotropic factors; cranial nerve and other CNS changes may occur, as may local neurotropic findings (occasionally respiratory failure).

• Cause less local tissue damage than crotalid bites

• Symptoms and signs may be delayed up to 12 hours.

B. Spiders

1. *Latrodectus* (black widow)

    a. Description

      (1) Large-bodied black or brown spider with an "hourglass" shape on the abdomen

      (2) May be aggressive

    b. Location

      (1) Indigenous in most states

      (2) Often found in garages, on woodpiles, or under stones

    c. Clinical features

      (1) Moderate local pain, typically with minimal local swelling or erythema

      (2) Local or regional muscle irritation and

increased tone; possible fasciculations or spasms

      (3) Risk of hypertensive crisis, especially in elderly, children, or those with underlying hypertension

      (4) Hemolysis and CNS changes, including seizures, may occur.

      (5) Nausea, vomiting, diaphoresis, fever, and other nonspecific signs and symptoms can occur.

2. *Loxosceles* (recluse, violin, or fiddle-back spiders)

    a. Description

      (1) Several species

      (2) Tan-to-brown spider with long, spindly legs and a "violin" shape on the dorsal surface of the cephalothorax

    b. Location and behavior

      (1) Common in South and South-Central United States, as well as West and Midwest

      (2) Found in woodpiles, garages, privys, storage sites

      (3) Usually not aggressive

    c. Clinical features

      (1) Local

        (a) Swelling and pain

        (b) Within 12 to 24 hours: erythema, often with vesicle and expanding central cutaneous necrosis, which may persist for weeks (necrotic arachnidism)

      (2) Systemic (uncommon): hemolysis, thrombocytopenia, coagulopathy, disseminated intravascular coagulation, circulatory shock

      (3) No distinctive or specific laboratory features

C. Scorpion envenomation (family Buthidae)

1. Description

    a. There are several species.

    b. The most dangerous species is *Centruroides exilicauda* (previously known as *C. sculpturatus*)

2. Location

    a. Found in Southwest United States, especially Arizona and New Mexico

    b. Nocturnal, desert habitat

    c. May enter homes or buildings

3. Clinical features (see Table 78–1)

    a. Most stings are on feet or hands.

    b. Symptoms appear within an hour: local

CAUTION

Arachnid bites are commonly mistaken for multiple other conditions. To confirm *Loxosceles* envenomation, the animal should be obtained and identified, together with a typical clinical presentation and course.

Conditions That May Be Mistaken for Loxoscelism

- Other arthropod bites or stings
- Foreign body
- Purpura fulminans
- Local embolic events
- Rocky Mountain spotted fever
- Vasculitis: leukocytoclastic, drug-induced, collagen vascular disease associated

- Pyoderma gangrenosum
- Ecthyma gangrenosum
- Cellulitis, necrotizing fasciitis
- Bacterial infection
- Fungal infection
- Raynaud's phenomenon, ergotism

---

    pain, pain on movement, or "tapping" lesion.

    c. *C. exilicauda* may produce a hyperadrenergic state with irritability, hypertension, salivation, tachycardia, dysrhythmias, cardiac damage, and CNS disturbances (including altered mentation, cranial nerve defects and seizures).

Treatment

A. Snake
  1. General measures
    a. Immobilize and keep patient quiet.
    b. Transport to hospital.

    c. Obtain assistance from local poison control center.
  2. Local measures
    a. Cleanse wound, immobilize, avoid excessive debridement.
    b. Surgical evaluation for local care or possible compartment syndrome; fasciotomy only for confirmed compartment syndrome (elevated compartmental pressures)
    c. Treat secondary infection.
    d. Avoid local injections, electroshock, or cooling.
  3. Systemic measures
    a. Intravenous fluids (for hypotension)
    b. Antivenin (for hypotension)
      (1) The only specific therapy (not to be used for trivial bites or envenomations)
      (2) Obtain informed consent prior to use, if possible.
      (3) Crotalid Polyvalent Antivenin (Wyeth) is available for crotalid envenomations (see Table 78–2).
        (a) Use only for moderate to serious envenomations; more than 20% of crotalid bites are not associated with envenomation ("dry bite").
        (b) Test skin first; give intravenously in monitored setting.
        (c) Risk of anaphylaxis: if skin test is positive or the patient is sensitive to horse serum, weigh the risk–benefit ratio
        (d) Use progression of signs and symptoms to quantify envenomation severity, and titrate therapy accordingly.
      (4) Antivenin is available for Eastern and Texas coral snake envenomations.
        (a) Dose of antivenin is not standardized; often, 4 to 10 or more vials are used for serious envenomations.

TABLE 78–1. GRADING SEVERITY OF *C. exilicauda* ENVENOMATIONS

Grade I	Pain and swelling, ± local paresthesias
Grade II	Pain and paresthesias locally and at other site(s)
Grade III	Grade II findings plus cranial nerve or somatic neuromuscular dysfunction, including blurred vision, salivation, difficulty swallowing, fasciculations, airway problems, slurred speech, or muscle spasms
Grade IV	Local plus cranial and somatic findings

TABLE 78–2. CROTALID ENVENOMATION: ANTIVENIN TREATMENT

SEVERITY	POTENTIAL ANTIVENIN DOSE (NUMBER OF VIALS)
No envenomation	None
Local (mild to moderate)	0 to 10
Local (severe)	10+
Systemic (moderate to severe)	20+

  (b) Not effective for Western, Arizona, and Sonoran species

  (5) Ovine-derived fragment antibody to crotalid venoms (recently available)

  (a) Monovalent immunoglobulin Fab fragments from sheep immunized with venoms of *C. adamanteus, C. scutulatus, C. atrox,* and *Agkistrodon piscivorus*

  (b) Preliminary data suggest efficacy in patients with minimal to moderate envenomation.

  (c) Dosage is 4 to 6 vials initially, plus subsequent dosing.

  (d) Should not be administered to patients with hypersensitivity to papaya or papain

  c. Avoid heparin and corticosteroids.

Key Treatment: Crotalid Polyvalent Antivenin (Wyeth)

- Use only for moderate to serious envenomations; more than 20% of crotalid bites are not associated with envenomation ("dry bite").

- Obtain informed consent prior to use, if possible.

- Test skin first; give intravenously in monitored setting.

- Risk of anaphylaxis: if skin test is positive or the patient is sensitive to horse serum, weigh the risk–benefit ratio.

- Use progression of signs and symptoms to quantify envenomation severity, and titrate therapy accordingly.

B. Spiders

  1. *Latrodectus* (black widow)

  a. Monitor for cardiopulmonary instability, muscle rigidity.

  b. Apply cooling pack locally.

  c. Possibly effective: muscle relaxants, calcium channel blockers, analgesia

  d. Control hypertension as needed.

  e. For severe reactions, administer *Latrodectus* antivenin (Merck) intravenously or intramuscularly.

  (1) Follow package insert.

  (2) Skin testing should be performed.

  (3) Risk of serum sickness or anaphylaxis (derived from horse serum)

Key Treatment: *Latrodectus* envenomation

Consider antivenin therapy in the very young or old, in pregnant patients, and in those with severe injuries or underlying medical problems, especially cardiopulmonary disorders.

  2. *Loxosceles*

  a. Monitor for cardiopulmonary or neurologic instability.

  b. Supportive care: rest, ice compresses, elevation (RICE), salicylates; consider antibiotics in ulcerating lesions

  c. Possibly effective therapies

  (1) Debridement (avoid early debridement)

  (2) Hyperbaric oxygen

  (3) Dapsone (4,4-diamonodiphenylsulfone)

  (a) Dose is 50 to 200 mg/day orally in divided doses; monitor for side effects.

  (b) Use remains controversial; no controlled clinical trials.

  (4) Steroids have been used by some authors for systemic reactions (hemolysis).

  d. No antivenin is currently available.

  e. Secondary infection is common.

CAUTION

Current management of necrotic arachnidism is controversial and often unsatisfactory.

C. Scorpion envenomation (family Buthidae)

  1. Local: rest, ice compress, elevation (RICE), analgesia

  2. Systemic

  a. Observe patient in the intensive care unit if hypertensive, CNS changes, extremes of age.

  b. Monitor arterial pressure and ensure adequate airway.

  c. Benzodiazepines for sedation

  d. Vasodilators for hypertension (nitroprusside, prazosin, hydralazine, calcium channel blockers)

  e. For severe reactions to *C. exilicauda*: goat serum antivenin is available in Arizona (Samaritan Regional Poison Control Center, Phoenix).

Bibliography

Anderson PC. Spider bites in the United States. Dermatol Clin 1997;15:307–311.

Bond GR. Antivenin administration for *Centruroides* scorpion sting: risks and benefits. Ann Emerg Med 1992;21: 788–791.

Boyer LV, Seifert SA, Clark RF, et al. Recurrent and persistent coagulopathy following pit viper envenomation. Arch Intern Med 1999;159:706–710.

Carlson RW, Pineda-Roman M, Ramamrutham R. Injuries by venomous and poisonous animals. *In:* Shoemaker W, Ayres SM, Grenvik A, et al (eds). Textbook of Critical Care Med, 4th ed. Philadelphia: WB Saunders, 2000, pp 223–246.

Holstege CP, Miller MB, Wermuth M, et al. Crotalid snake envenomation. Crit Care Clin 1997;13:889–921.

Kitchens CS, Van Mierop LH. Envenomation by the Eastern coral snake (*Micrurus fulvius fulvius*): a study of 39 victims. JAMA 1987;258:1615–1618.

Sams HH, Dunnick CA, Smith ML, et al. Necrotic arachnidism. J Am Acad Dermatol 2001;44:561–573.

Walter FG, Bilden EF, Gibly RL. Envenomations. Crit Care Clin 1999;15:353–386.

79 Status Epilepticus

James A. Kruse

Definition and Classification

A. Seizures
1. Defined as excessive hypersynchronous neuronal activity in the cerebral cortex
2. Descriptive categories
    a. Partial (focal) vs. generalized
    b. Simple vs. complex
    c. Convulsive vs. nonconvulsive
    d. Tonic, clonic, tonic-clonic, or myoclonic
    e. New onset vs. recurrent

B. Status epilepticus (SE)
1. Conventional definitions
    a. At least 30 minutes of continuous seizure activity, or
    b. At least 2 sequential seizures without recovery of consciousness in the interictal period
2. Operant definition
    a. Seizure activity lasting at least 10 minutes
    b. Basis is that, in practice, treatment is initiated within 10 minutes, thus not allowing 30 minutes of seizure activity to elapse (except in cases refractory to treatment).
3. Most cases manifest as generalized tonic-clonic activity (grand mal), but focal (epilepsia partialis continua), absence, complex partial, and other forms can occur.

Etiology

A. Preexisting seizure disorder of any cause
1. Noncompliance with anticonvulsant pharmacotherapy
2. Refractory underlying epilepsy
3. Alcohol or drug (e.g., barbiturate) withdrawal
4. Hysterical or feigned (pseudoseizures)
5. Superimposed acute process resulting in lowered seizure threshold (see B. new-onset seizure)

B. New-onset seizure
1. Head trauma (acute or prior)
2. Brain infarction (acute or prior)
3. Intracranial bleeding: e.g., intracerebral or subarachnoid hemorrhage, subdural hematoma
4. Brain tumors
5. Central nervous system (CNS) infection: meningitis, encephalitis, brain abscess
6. Anoxic encephalopathy: e.g., post-cardiac arrest
7. Hypertensive encephalopathy
8. Metabolic causes
    a. Drug or alcohol withdrawal
    b. Hypoglycemia
    c. Hyponatremia
    d. Hypocalcemia
    e. Hypomagnesemia
    f. Hyperosmolality
    g. Uremia
    h. Hepatic encephalopathy
    i. Sepsis
9. Toxic causes
    a. Poisoning or drug intoxication: e.g., salicylate, theophylline, lidocaine, meperidine, penicillin, cyclic antidepressants, cocaine
    b. Alcohol or drug withdrawal
10. Idiopathic epilepsy
11. Miscellaneous: lupus cerebritis, human immunodeficiency virus-related, degenerative CNS diseases

Key Tests

- Serum biochemical tests: glucose, electrolyte profile, urea nitrogen, creatinine, hepatic function tests, creatine phosphokinase activity

- Complete and differential blood cell and platelet counts

- Coagulation tests: prothrombin and partial thromboplastin times

- Arterial blood gases and lactate concentration

- Anticonvulsant drug levels

- Ethanol and toxicologic analysis, as indicated

- Brain computed tomography or magnetic resonance imaging

- Electroencephalography

Treatment (also see Chapter 172, Anticonvulsants)

A. Maintain ventilation and perfusion.
1. Establish airway and ventilate with bag-valve mask; this will usually be followed by endotracheal intubation.
2. Provide supplemental oxygen.
3. Monitor vital signs, continuous electrocardiogram and pulse oximetry.
4. Secure IV access.
5. Obtain blood samples for routine tests (see box, Key Tests).

B. Consider hypoglycemia as a cause for seizure.
1. Inject 50 mL of 50% dextrose (after or with 100 mg thiamine) intravenously, or
2. Test blood using rapid beside glucose assay, if readily available, and forego dextrose if patient is not hypoglycemic.

C. Terminate active ictus.
1. Lorazepam
   a. First-line anticonvulsant
   b. Dose: 0.1 mg/kg no faster than 2 mg/minute
   c. Duration of anticonvulsant effect: more than 4 hours
   d. Success rate: 65%
2. Diazepam
   a. Second-line alternative agent to lorazepam
   b. Dose: 0.15 to 0.3 mg/kg no faster than 5 mg/min intravenously; has also been effective per rectum at 0.2 to 0.5 mg/kg
   c. Duration of anticonvulsant effect: approximately 20 minutes
   d. Success rate (when followed by phenytoin): 56%
   e. May have greater respiratory depressant effect than lorazepam
3. May give additional benzodiazepine dosing if seizures continue after recommended initial dose.
   a. The aim of this approach is to titrate dose to control seizure activity as long as side effects (hypotension) can be controlled.
   b. Current data suggest that this approach has limited efficacy.
4. Monitor for drug-induced hypotension.
   a. Usually responds to IV fluid loading
   b. In some cases, hypotension may limit the infusion rate or total dose of drug.
5. Respiratory depression is treated by bag-valve ventilation using a face mask or endotracheal intubation.

6. Always immediately follow benzodiazepine administration with a loading dose of phenytoin, fosphenytoin, or phenobarbital.

D. Prevent seizure recurrence
1. Phenytoin
   a. Phenytoin administration should be preceded by one of the above agents in treating SE.
      (1) At maximum recommended infusion rate, phenytoin typically requires approximately 25 minutes to administer a loading dose.
      (2) The efficacy of phenytoin as a sole agent for terminating ictus is only 44%, significantly less than lorazepam.
   b. Phenytoin is the agent of choice to prevent recurrence.
   c. Give full loading dose (20 mg/kg) to patients who have not received the drug.
   d. Precautions
      (1) Infuse no faster than 50 mg/minute, and do not infuse through glucose-containing IV fluids.
      (2) Monitor blood pressure and electrocardiogram during loading infusion.
      (3) Rapid infusion can induce hypotension, dysrhythmias, or conduction disturbances induced by phenytoin or its propylene glycol-based diluent.
      (4) These complications usually respond to slowing the infusion rate.
   e. An additional 5 mg/kg may be considered in patients who continue to seize despite standard benzodiazepine and phenytoin loading doses.
   f. Follow loading dose with intermittent maintenance doses (typically started at 100 mg every 8 hours and guided by serial serum phenytoin levels)
   g. Aim for serum levels at or somewhat above the upper therapeutic limit (20 μg/mL).
2. Fosphenytoin
   a. A water-soluble prodrug alternative to phenytoin; converted to phenytoin in vivo with a 7 to 15 minute half-time conversion
   b. Can achieve therapeutic level in approximately 15 minutes (~10 min faster than phenytoin)
   c. Dosing is expressed as "milligrams phenytoin equivalents" and is the same as for phenytoin.
   d. Less risk of inducing hypotension than with phenytoin; can be administered faster than

phenytoin IV (150 mg/minute vs. 50 mg/minute)

    e. Has special utility for patients lacking IV access (can be given intravenously, whereas phenytoin cannot)

  3. Phenobarbital

    a. Second-line agent, in place of phenytoin or fosphenytoin

    b. Also conventionally used as an adjunctive anticonvulsant for patients with seizures refractory to phenytoin

    c. Loading dose is 20 mg/kg intravenously, infused no faster than 100 mg/minute (50 mg/minute if not actively seizing); 10 mg/kg may be sufficient for some patients.

    d. Typical maintenance dosing is 60 to 300 mg/day.

    e. Aim for serum levels at or above the upper therapeutic limit (40 μg/mL).

E. For SE refractory to the above measures, one or more of the following agents should be used.

  1. Pentobarbital

    a. Start with 5 mg/kg intravenously and infuse up to 20 mg/kg (typically 12 mg/kg), until seizure activity stops.

    b. Then give 0.5 to 5 (typically 1 to 3) mg/kg per hour.

    c. For additional seizures, give a bolus dose of 3 to 5 mg/kg and increase the maintenance infusion; infusions as high as 10 mg/kg per hour or more may be considered if hemodynamic status can be controlled.

    d. This technique can be used to induce barbiturate coma.

  2. Midazolam infusion

    a. Dose: 0.1 to 0.3 mg/kg intravenously loading, followed by continuous infusion at 0.05 to 2.0 mg/kg per hour and titrated to suppress seizure activity

    b. Major complications are tachyphylaxis and hypotension.

  3. Propofol infusion

    a. Dose: 1 to 5 mg/kg intravenously, followed by continuous infusion at 1 to 15 mg/kg per hour and titrated to suppress seizure activity

    b. Rapid discontinuation may precipitate withdrawal seizures.

  4. Other drugs that have been used as adjuvants in refractory cases include thiopental, methohexital, valproic acid, etomidate, paraldehyde, lidocaine, chloral hydrate, and inhalational anesthetic agents such as halothane, isoflurane, and nitrous oxide.

  5. The major complication of these forms of pharmacotherapy is hypotension (especially with pentobarbital).

    a. Hypotension may result from myocardial depression or vasodilation.

    b. It may limit the dose.

    c. Consider use of hemodynamic monitoring.

    d. It may require fluid loading, vasopressor, or inotropic drug therapy.

  6. Procedure for stopping continuous infusion anticonvulsant therapy

    a. First achieve seizure control.

      (1) No clinical evidence of seizures

      (2) Electroencephalogram (EEG) with either burst-suppression pattern or absence of seizure activity

    b. After at least 12 hours without seizures, decrease the infusion rate by half or titrate downward.

    c. If seizures recur, give a bolus dose of the drug and increase the infusion rate.

    d. Try again to titrate the infusion after an additional 12 hours or more without seizures.

  7. Continuous or serial EEG studies

    a. Allows titration of anticonvulsant therapy

    b. Electroencephalographic testing should be performed for patients remaining unresponsive, but without clinically apparent seizure activity, to exclude subclinical nonconvulsive SE.

    c. Evidence of subclinical SE warrants additional pharmacological treatment.

F. Establish cause.

  1. Review history, physical examination, and laboratory studies to establish reason for seizures.

  2. If cause is unclear, consider a brain imaging study followed by lumbar puncture, if not contraindicated.

G. Correct factors that can lower seizure threshold.

  1. Correct hypoxemia.

  2. Correct severe alkalemia or acidemia.

  3. Correct severe electrolyte disturbances (e.g., hyponatremia, hypocalcemia).

  4. Lower body temperature if the patient is hyperthermic.

H. Monitor blood anticonvulsant concentrations and adjust maintenance drug doses if levels are suboptimal.

I. Treat underlying conditions (e.g., meningitis, uremia, cardiac dysrhythmias, stroke).

J. Recognize, prevent, and treat complications.

1. Institute seizure precautions and prophylaxis against deep venous thrombosis.
2. Monitor serum creatine phosphokinase activity to detect rhabdomyolysis.
3. Treat hyperthermia (body temperature ≥40°C).

Key Treatment

- Ensure adequate airway, ventilation, and circulation.

- Give IV lorazepam or diazepam.

- Next, administer IV phenytoin or (if patient is intolerant to IV phenytoin or has no IV access) fosphenytoin.

- Consider phenobarbital if seizures recur while receiving adequate phenytoin.

- For refractory cases, induce anesthesia using continuous IV infusion of propofol, benzodiazepine, or pentobarbital.

Complications

A. Neurologic
1. Neuronal injury
2. Unrecognized (subclinical, nonconvulsive) SE
3. Autonomic system involvement
   a. Upper and lower airway hypersecretion
   b. Bronchoconstriction
B. Respiratory
1. Hypoxemia
2. Hypercapnia
3. Aspiration pneumonitis
4. Noncardiogenic pulmonary edema
5. Respiratory failure
   a. Airway obstruction
   b. Ictal interference with ventilation
   c. Respiratory depression secondary to anticonvulsant therapy

   d. Pulmonary complications (e.g., from aspiration)
C. Cardiovascular
1. Cardiac dysrhythmias from hypoxemia, anticonvulsant therapy, or other mechanisms
2. Hypotension resulting from impaired venous return or anticonvulsant therapy
D. Renal and metabolic
1. Rhabdomyolysis
2. Myoglobinuric renal failure
3. Electrolyte disturbances, particularly hyperkalemia
4. Lactic acidosis
   a. Production by skeletal muscles during seizures
   b. Circulatory shock
   c. Propylene glycol intoxication (diluent of some anticonvulsant formulations; metabolized to lactic acid)
5. Hypoglycemia or hyperglycemia
6. Hyperthermia
E. Miscellaneous
1. Disseminated intravascular coagulation
2. Orthopedic injury

PEARL

Myoclonic seizures post-cardiac arrest are often refractory to treatment but may sometimes respond to clonazepam or sodium valproate.

 ## Bibliography

Bleck TP. Management approaches to prolonged seizures and status epilepticus. Epilepsia 1999;40(Suppl. 1):S59–S63.

Jordan KG. Nonconvulsive status epilepticus in acute brain injury. J Clin Neurophysiol 1999;16:332–340.

Towne AR, Waterhouse EJ, Boggs JG, et al. Prevalence of nonconvulsive status epilepticus in comatose patients. Neurology 2000;54:340–345.

Treiman DM, Meyers PD, Walton NY, et al. A comparison of four treatments for generalized convulsive status epilepticus. N Engl J Med 1998;339:792–798.

Willmore LJ. Epilepsy emergencies. The first seizure and status epilepticus. Neurology 1998;51(Suppl. 4):S34–S38.

80 Cerebral Infarction

Seemant Chaturvedi

Stroke is one of the most important public health problems. It is the third leading cause of death and the leading cause of disability among adults. In recent years there have been significant advances in both prevention and acute treatment. This chapter focuses on cerebral infarction, as opposed to cerebral hemorrhage. Cerebral infarction is the more common cause of stroke, accounting for 80% to 85% of neurovascular events.

Etiology

A. Large-vessel atherosclerosis (20%)
   1. Carotid artery stenosis
   2. Vertebral artery stenosis
   3. Basilar artery stenosis
B. Small-vessel, lacunar infarction (25%)
C. Cardioembolism (20%)
D. Cryptogenic (undetermined) etiology (30%)
E. Miscellaneous causes (5%)
   1. Hypercoagulable states
   2. Arterial dissection
   3. Migraine
   4. Sympathomimetic drugs
   5. Vasculitis

Clinical Findings

A. Carotid distribution ischemia
   1. Retinal ischemia
      a. Amaurosis fugax
      b. Retinal artery occlusion
   2. Hemispheric ischemia
      a. Contralateral weakness
      b. Contralateral numbness
      c. Dysphasia (dominant hemisphere infarction)
      d. Neglect, acute confusion (nondominant hemisphere infarction)
B. Vertebrobasilar ischemia
   1. Vertigo
   2. Diplopia
   3. Facial or perioral numbness

4. Dysarthria
5. Dysphagia
6. Ataxia
7. Limb dysmetria
8. Unilateral or bilateral weakness
9. Crossed sensory loss

Key Symptoms

- Unilateral weakness
- Unilateral numbness
- Dysphasia
- Vertigo
- Dysarthria
- Diplopia

Differential Diagnosis

A. Cerebral hemorrhage
B. Mass lesions (brain tumors)
C. Demyelinating disease
D. Migraine
E. Focal seizures with postictal paralysis
F. Hypoglycemia
G. Toxic and metabolic states
H. Sepsis
I. Encephalitis
J. Conversion reaction

Imaging Studies

A. Brain computed tomography
   1. Infarcted tissue is hypodense compared to normal brain.
   2. Hypodensity may take 12 to 24 hours to become apparent.
   3. As the infarct becomes more chronic, hypodensity increases.
B. Magnetic resonance imaging
   1. Increased signal intensity on T2-weighted images

2. May take 6 to 24 hours to become apparent

3. Chronic lesions have low signal intensity on T1-weighted images.

4. Diffusion-weighted imaging can reveal acute infarction, even within first hour.

Treatment

A. Acute intervention

1. Intravenous thrombolytic therapy

a. Useful if treatment can be started within 3 hours of symptom onset

b. Blood pressure should be below 185/110 pretreatment and for the first 24 hours.

c. Tissue plasminogen activator dose: 0.9 mg/kg (90 mg maximum) IV, 10% as bolus and remainder over 1 hour

d. No aspirin or heparin given for 24 hours post-treatment

e. Intensive care unit monitoring recommended for 24 hours

f. Multiple exclusionary criteria

2. Intra-arterial (IA) thrombolysis

a. Not approved by Food and Drug Administration

b. One phase III study showed IA prourokinase to be useful up to 6 hours after middle cerebral artery occlusion.

c. Requires immediate access to angiography

d. Low-dose heparin conventionally given after IA thrombolysis

3. Heparin

a. Commonly administered

b. Remains controversial

c. Two recent studies showed no net benefit for heparin in an unselected stroke population.

d. One study showed that patients with large-vessel atherosclerosis benefit.

e. No bolus administered

f. Partial thromboplastin time maintained at 1.5 to 2.0 times control

4. Aspirin

a. Modest benefit when used in first 48 hours

b. Preferred dose is 325 mg/day

5. Neuroprotective agents

a. Remain investigational

b. None proven useful thus far

Key Treatment

- Intravenous thrombolysis
- Intra-arterial thrombolytic therapy
- Antiplatelet therapy
- Intravenous heparin

Complications

A. Cerebral edema

B. Seizures

C. Deep-vein thrombosis

D. Pneumonia

E. Urinary tract infection

F. Decubitus ulcers

G. Hemorrhagic transformation

1. Incidence with IV thrombolytic therapy is approximately 6%.

2. Incidence with IV heparin use is approximately 2%.

Prevention

A. Antiplatelet agents

1. Aspirin: recommended dose is 50 to 325 mg/day

2. Ticlopidine

a. Dose: 250 mg every 12 hours

b. Risk of thrombotic thrombocytopenic purpura

c. Complete blood cell and platelet count monitoring required

3. Clopidogrel

a. Dose: 75 mg/day

b. Increased risk of rash, diarrhea

c. Rare cases of thrombotic thrombocytopenic purpura

4. Aspirin/extended release dipyridamole

a. Dose: 25 mg/200 mg every 12 hours

b. Shown to be more effective than aspirin alone (23% risk reduction)

c. Increased risk of headache, gastrointestinal distress

B. Anticoagulation (warfarin)

1. Most useful for cardioembolic stroke prevention

a. Atrial fibrillation

b. Cardiomyopathy

c. Prosthetic heart valves

2. Investigational use for intracranial atherosclerosis

C. Carotid endarterectomy

1. Beneficial for carotid distribution minor stroke or transient ischemic attack if there is greater than 70% angiographic stenosis

2. Surgical morbidity and mortality should be less than 6%.

3. Not very effective for asymptomatic stenosis

a. Low risk of stroke with asymptomatic narrowing (2% per year)

b. Risk–benefit ratio less attractive

D. Angioplasty/stenting

1. May be useful in selected cases

a. Refractory intracranial stenosis

b. Poor surgical candidates

c. Investigational use as an alternative to endarterectomy

Bibliography

Brott TG, Hacke W. Thrombolytic and defibrinogenating agents for ischemic and hemorrhagic stroke. In: Barnett HJM, Mohr JP, Stein BM, Yatsu FM (eds). Stroke, 3rd edition. New York: Churchill Livingstone, 1998; pp 1155–1176.

International Stroke Trial Collaborative Group. The International Stroke Trial (IST): a randomized trial of aspirin, subcutaneous heparin, both, or neither among 19,435 patients with acute ischaemic stroke. Lancet 1997;349: 1569–1581.

The National Institutes of Neurological Disorders and Stroke rt-PA Stroke Study Group. Tissue plasminogen activator for acute ischemic stroke. N Engl J Med 1995; 333:1581–1587.

The Publications Committee for the Trial of ORG 10172 in Acute Stroke Treatment (TOAST) investigators. Low molecular weight heparinoid, ORG 10172 (danaparoid), and outcome after acute ischemic stroke. JAMA 1998; 279:1265–1272.

81 Intracerebral Hemorrhage

Lakshmipathi Chelluri

Epidemiology

A. Each year there are 40 to 70,000 cases of intracerebral hemorrhage (ICH) in the United States.
B. Accounts for 10% of all strokes
C. Responsible for 50% of all stroke-related deaths
D. Anatomic location
   1. Supratentorial: 85%
      a. Lobar: 25%
      b. Caudate nucleus: 5%
      c. Thalamus: 20%
      d. Putamen: 35%
   2. Infratentorial: 15%
      a. Pons: 7%
      b. Cerebellum: 8%

Etiology

A. Hypertension is the most common risk factor.
B. Risk factors other than hypertension include
   1. Amyloid angiopathy
      a. Older patients
      b. Associated with lobar ICH
   2. Anticoagulation
   3. Fibrinolytic agents
   4. Hemorrhagic transformation after ischemic stroke
   5. Vascular malformations
   6. Tumors
   7. Trauma
   8. Vasculitis
   9. Drug abuse

Symptoms and Signs

A. Severity depends on location and size of ICH.
B. Symptoms
   1. Headache
   2. Decreased level of consciousness
   3. Vomiting
   4. Seizures (common with lobar hemorrhage)
C. Signs
   1. Hemiplegia
   2. Hemisensory syndrome
   3. Aphasia is absent with cerebellar hemorrhage.
   4. Brain stem signs
      a. Unilateral after thalamic or cerebellar hemorrhage
      b. Pontine hemorrhage causes pinpoint pupils, respiratory rhythm abnormalities, and decerebrate rigidity.
   5. Clinical features are not sufficient to distinguish ischemic from hemorrhagic stroke.

Imaging Studies

A. Computed tomography provides information about
   1. Location of lesion
   2. Size of lesion
   3. Presence of structural abnormalities
      a. Aneurysms
      b. Vascular malformations
      c. Tumors
   4. Complications
      a. Herniation
      b. Intraventricular hemorrhage
      c. Hydrocephalus
B. Magnetic resonance imaging and magnetic resonance angiography provide better visualization of some structural abnormalities, such as cavernous malformations.
C. Cerebral angiography
   1. Useful for delineating arteriovenous malformations and aneurysms
   2. Should be considered for all patients without a clear cause for hemorrhage
   3. Indicated for patients being considered for surgical intervention
   4. Part of the evaluation of younger patients without hypertension

Key Tests

- Computed tomography
- Magnetic resonance imaging (selected patients)
- Cerebral angiography (selected patients)
- Coagulation studies and platelet count
- Assessment of renal function
- Chest radiograph

Treatment

A. Assess and ensure adequacy of airway, breathing, and circulation.

B. Assess neurologic function.

C. Intubation and mechanical ventilation are indicated for patients with
   1. Decreased level of consciousness and increased risk of aspiration
   2. Inadequate oxygenation or ventilation

D. Adequate sedation should be provided prior to intubation to avoid increases in systemic blood pressure or intracranial pressure (ICP).

E. Position
   1. Avoid compression of jugular veins.
   2. Elevate head of bed 15 to 30 degrees.

F. Control blood pressure.
   1. Optimal pressure depends on prior history of hypertension, ICP, and time elapsed since onset of symptoms.
      a. Rebleeding during the first 24 hours is common; therefore, control of hypertension during this period is especially important.
      b. If ICP is high, lowering systemic blood pressure too much will compromise cerebral perfusion pressure.
      c. Usual goal is to maintain systolic blood pressure between 140 to 180 mm Hg.
      d. If ICP is monitored, keep cerebral perfusion pressure (i.e., mean arterial pressure minus ICP) higher than 70 mm Hg.
   2. Anti-hypertensive agents
      a. Sodium nitroprusside, although easy to titrate, may promote dilatation of cerebral vessels, leading to increased cerebral blood flow and worsening of intracranial hypertension.
      b. β-Adrenergic blockers are the preferred agents for controlling blood pressure in ICH.
         (1) Labetalol
         (2) Esmolol
      c. Other agents
         (1) Hydralazine
         (2) Angiotensin converting enzyme inhibitors
   3. Guidelines
      a. If systolic blood pressure is higher than 230 mm Hg or diastolic blood pressure is higher than 140 mm Hg on two measurements 5 minutes apart, then use sodium nitroprusside.
      b. If systolic blood pressure is between 180

and 230 mm Hg or diastolic blood pressure is between 105 and 140 mm Hg on two measurements 5 minutes apart, then use labetalol.
      c. If systolic blood pressure is lower than 180 mm Hg or diastolic blood pressure is lower than 105 mm Hg, then administer an oral β-adrenergic blocker, hydralazine, or angiotensin converting enzyme inhibitor.

G. Seizure prophylaxis
   1. Use phenytoin to achieve a plasma level between 15 and 20 μg/mL.
   2. Use additional anticonvulsants as needed.

H. Intracranial pressure monitoring
   1. May be appropriate for patients with a Glasgow coma score lower than 9 or continued neurological deterioration
   2. Aim to keep ICP lower than 20 mm Hg.

I. Treatment of intracranial hypertension
   1. Sedation
   2. Therapeutic paralysis
   3. Osmotherapy
      a. Mannitol (0.25 to 0.5 g/kg intravenously every 4 to 6 hours)
      b. Monitor serum osmolality and seek to maintain less than 310 mOsm/kg H_2O.
   4. Cerebrospinal fluid drainage using an intraventricular catheter
   5. Mild hyperventilation ($PaCO_2$ between 30 and 35 torr)
   6. Barbiturate coma

J. Other medical considerations
   1. Fever
      a. Increases cerebral metabolism and oxygen consumption
      b. Treat with acetaminophen or ibuprofen to keep temperature below 38°C.
   2. Monitor and maintain normal fluid, acid-base, and electrolyte status.
   3. Provide prophylaxis against deep venous thrombosis using pneumatic compression devices.
   4. Provide prophylaxis against stress ulceration.
      a. H_2-receptor antagonist
      b. Sucralfate
      c. Proton pump inhibitor
   5. Provide rehabilitation services.
      a. Physical therapy
      b. Occupational therapy
      c. Speech therapy

K. Surgical intervention

1. The role of surgical therapy is controversial.
2. Indications
   a. Massive hematoma (>3 cm diameter) with brain stem compression or intracranial hypertension
   b. Hydrocephalus
   c. Surgically accessible structural lesions
   d. Aneurysm
   e. Arteriovenous malformation

Key Treatment

- Ensure adequacy of airway, breathing, and circulation.
- Assess and monitor neurologic function.
- Provide adequate sedation prior to intubation.
- Ensure proper positioning of patient to minimize risk of increasing ICP.
- Control blood pressure.
- Provide seizure prophylaxis.
- Monitor ICP (selected patients).
- Treat intracranial hypertension (using osmotherapy, cerebrospinal fluid drainage, mild hyperventilation, and, possibly, administration of barbiturates).

Prognosis

A. Predictors of poor prognosis
   1. Intraventricular hemorrhage
   2. Older age
   3. Need for surgical treatment
   4. Basal ganglion hemorrhage
   5. Hypertension as the only etiologic factor
B. Mortality at 30 days is 35% to 52%.
C. Only 10% and 20% patients are living independently at 30 days and 6 months, respectively.

Bibliography

Broderick JP, Adams HP Jr, Barsan W, et al. Guidelines for the management of spontaneous intracerebral hemorrhage: A statement for healthcare professionals from a special writing group of the Stroke Council, American Heart Association. Stroke 1999;30:905–915.

Massaro AR, Sacco RL, Mohr JP, et al. Clinical discriminators of lobar and deep hemorrhages. The Stroke Data Bank. Neurology 1991;41:1881–1885.

Rosenow F, Hojer C, Meyer-Lohmann C, et al. Spontaneous intracerebral hemorrhage. Acta Neurol Scand 1997; 96:174–182.

Shah MV, Biller J. Medical and surgical management of intracerebral hemorrhage. Semin Neurol 1998;18:513–519.

Taylor CL, Selman WR, Ratcheson RA. Brain attack: the emergent management of hypertensive hemorrhage. Neurosurg Clin North Am 1997;8(2):237–244.

82 Subarachnoid Hemorrhage

Marie R. Baldisseri

Pathogenesis

A. Subarachnoid hemorrhage (SAH) results from the sudden rupture of a cerebral artery with hemorrhage into the subarachnoid space.

B. Vasospasm
1. Most commonly occurs 4 to 14 days after the initial bleed
2. There is angiographic evidence of vasospasm in up to 75% of patients.
3. Clinical evidence of vasospasm is present in 30% to 40% of patients.
4. Despite therapy, vasospasm-induced delayed cerebral ischemia is associated with significant mortality and morbidity (neurologic disability).

Etiology

A. Cerebral aneurysms
1. Saccular ("berry")
2. Mycotic
3. Fusiform
4. Diffuse
5. Globular

B. Perimesencephalic, nonaneurysmal SAH

C. Subarachnoid hemorrhage (SAH) secondary to trauma, coagulopathy, vasculitis, and idiopathic causes

Risk Factors for Aneurysmal SAH

A. Preexisting hypertension (20% of patients with SAH)

B. Cigarette smoking

C. Alcohol consumption

D. Personal or family history of SAH

E. Polycystic kidney disease

F. Hereditary connective tissue diseases
1. Ehlers-Danlos syndrome (type IV)
2. Pseudoxanthoma elasticum
3. Fibromuscular dysplasia

G. Sickle cell anemia

H. α_1-Antitrypsin deficiency

Clinical Findings

A. "Thunderclap" headache

B. Loss of consciousness

C. Emesis

D. Nuchal rigidity

E. Localized neurologic deficits

F. Seizures

G. Inappropriate behavior and agitation

H. Lethargy, stupor, and coma

I. Retinal subhyaloid hemorrhages

Classification

A. Rationale
1. Severity of SAH is classified on the basis of clinical presentation and computed tomography (CT) findings.
2. Clinical and radiographic grading of SAH is important because there is a significant correlation between outcome and the initial grading level.
3. Grade also guides the timing of surgery.

B. Clinical classification by World Federation of Neurological Surgeons
   1. Grade I: Glasgow coma scale 15, motor deficit absent
   2. Grade II: Glasgow coma scale 14 to 13, motor deficit absent
   3. Grade III: Glasgow coma scale 14 to 13, motor deficit present
   4. Grade IV: Glasgow coma scale 12 to 7, motor deficit present or absent
   5. Grade V: Glasgow coma scale 6 to 3, motor deficit present or absent
C. Clinical classification by Hunt-Hess scale
   1. Grade I: asymptomatic or mild headache
   2. Grade II: moderate to severe headache, nuchal rigidity with or without cranial nerve deficits
   3. Grade III: confusion, lethargy, or mild focal symptoms
   4. Grade IV: stupor, hemiparesis, or both
   5. Grade V: coma or extensor posturing

Diagnosis

A. High index of clinical suspicion required.
B. Emergent noncontrast head CT scan is 95% sensitive if performed within 24 hours.
C. Lumbar puncture
   1. Performed if CT scan is unavailable, negative, equivocal, or technically inadequate
   2. The presence of xanthochromia is the primary criterion for a diagnosis of SAH with a negative CT scan.
D. Four-vessel angiography
E. Diagnosis of vasospasm
   1. Clinical examination
   2. Cerebral angiogram
   3. Transcranial Doppler ultrasonography
   4. Xenon-enhanced CT scan
   5. Positron emission tomography
F. Cardiac findings
   1. Electrocardiographic changes
      a. Prolongation of the QT interval
      b. Inverted T waves
      c. Prominent U waves
      d. Elevation or depression of ST segments
   2. Ventricular and supraventricular dysrhythmias in up to 90% of patients
   3. Myocardial ischemia or infarction
   4. Transient left ventricular dysfunction ("catecholamine-induced cardiomyopathy")

G. Pulmonary complications
   1. Aspiration pneumonitis or pneumonia
   2. Cardiogenic pulmonary edema
   3. Neurogenic pulmonary edema
H. Laboratory findings
   1. Cerebrospinal fluid xanthochromia
   2. Hyponatremia secondary to syndrome of inappropriate antidiuresis or cerebral salt-wasting syndrome
I. Radiographic (CT) diagnostic categories according to the Fisher scale
   1. No SAH on CT scan
   2. Broad diffusion of subarachnoid blood, no clots, and no layers of blood greater than 1 mm deep
   3. Either localized blood clots in the subarachnoid space or layers of blood greater than 1 mm deep
   4. Intraventricular and intracerebral blood present, in the absence of significant subarachnoid blood

Treatment

A. Initial management
   1. Intensive care unit admission
   2. Neurologic clinical evaluations every 1 to 2 hours
   3. Blood pressure monitoring (intra-arterial catheter)
   4. Central venous pressure monitoring or pulmonary artery pressure monitoring if cardiac disease is present
   5. Intracranial pressure (ICP) monitoring with external ventricular drain
   6. Electrocardiogram and chest x-ray on admission to the intensive care unit
   7. Baseline serum electrolyte concentrations, hematologic and coagulation profiles, type and crossmatch, and arterial blood gas analysis
   8. Frequent monitoring of serum sodium concentration
B. Preoperative management
   1. Assess level of consciousness and ensure adequacy of airway and breathing.
      a. Endotracheal intubation and mechanical ventilation, if required
      b. Premedicate (sedate) prior to intubation to avoid hypertension.
   2. Maintain arterial blood pressure within 5% to 10% of premorbid values using

a. β-Adrenergic blocker

(1) Labetalol: 10 to 20 mg intravenously every 10 to 15 minutes, as needed

(2) Esmolol: 500 mg/kg IV loading dose, then 25 to 200 mg/kg per minute infusion

b. Hydralazine: 10 to 20 mg intravenously every 10 to 15 minutes as needed

3. Treat increased ICP

a. Drainage of cerebrospinal fluid via ventriculostomy

b. Premedicate (sedate) prior to ventricular drain placement to avoid hypertension.

4. Vasospasm prophylaxis

a. Nimodipine: 60 mg orally every 4 hours, or 30 mg every 2 hours if the larger dose causes hypotension

b. "HH" therapy using infusion of colloid solution (e.g., 6% hetastarch) to induce mild hypervolemia and hemodilution (target hematocrit is 30% to 35%)

5. Seizure prophylaxis

a. Phenytoin: 15 mg/kg IV loading dose, then approximately 300 mg/day

b. Avoid phenobarbital.

6. Pain control with short-acting agents

a. Narcotics (e.g., morphine, fentanyl, codeine)

b. Avoid benzodiazepines.

7. Treat fever with acetaminophen.

8. Deep-vein thrombosis prophylaxis using pneumatic compression devices

9. Stress ulcer prophylaxis using H_2-receptor antagonist, sucralfate, or proton pump inhibitor

10. Early enteral nutrition or oral diet

11. Stool softener

12. Bed rest

C. Timing of surgical intervention

1. Early aneurysm clipping for Hunt-Hess grades I to III improves outcome.

2. Surgery should be delayed for Hunt-Hess grades IV to V, unless there is spontaneous clinical improvement or the patient improves after placement of an external ventricular drain.

D. Endovascular (nonsurgical) treatment

1. Obliteration of aneurysm with platinum coils (particularly useful for basilar artery aneurysms)

2. Balloon occlusion

E. Postoperative management

1. Blood pressure control

a. Aggressive blood pressure control for the first 24 hours postoperatively using β-adrenergic blocker (labetalol or esmolol) or hydralazine

b. Allow blood pressure to rise to premorbid values (keeping systolic pressure lower than 200 mm Hg) after the first postoperative day.

2. Vasospasm prophylaxis

a. Nimodipine

b. Expand intravascular volume using crystalloid solution (normal saline), colloid solution (6% hetastarch or 5% human serum albumin), or packed red blood cells (if hemodilution concentration <8 g/dL) with normal saline.

c. Hemodilution

3. Vasospasm treatment

a. "HHH" therapy: hypervolemia, hemodilution, and induced-hypertension using dopamine or phenylephrine to increase cerebral perfusion pressure (mean arterial pressure minus ICP) to greater than 70 mm Hg

b. Percutaneous transluminal angioplasty with or without intra-arterial papaverine

4. Correct hyponatremia.

a. Oral NaCl for cerebral salt wasting

b. IV 0.9% or 3% (in selected cases) saline

c. Fludrocortisone acetate (0.2 mg intravenously every 12 hours)

Key Treatment

- Good outcome with appropriate preoperative medical treatment and early surgical treatment requires prompt recognition using clinical and radiographic evidence of SAH.

- Institute "HHH" therapy for prophylaxis and treatment of vasospasm-induced delayed cerebral ischemia.

- Consider emergent angioplasty for patients refractory to "HHH" therapy.

Prognosis

A. The primary cause of mortality after SAH is acute brain injury caused by the initial bleed.

B. In those patients who survive the initial insult, the

major causes of increased morbidity and mortality are recurrent bleeding and cerebral vasospasm.

C. The incidence of rebleeding within the first three months is 30%.

D. Rebleeding is associated with a 50% mortality rate.

B Bibliography

Edlow JA, Caplan LR. Avoiding pitfalls in the diagnosis of subarachnoid hemorrhage. N Engl J Med 2000;342:29–36.

Miller J, Diringer M. Management of aneurysmal subarachnoid hemorrhage. Neurol Clin 1995;13(3):451–478.

Oropello JM, Weiner L, Benjamin E. Hypertensive, hypervolemic, hemodilutional therapy for aneurysmal subarachnoid hemorrhage. Is it efficacious? No. Crit Care Clin 1996;12(3):709–730.

Ullman JS, Bederson JB. Hypertensive, hypervolemic hemodilutional therapy for aneurysmal subarachnoid hemorrhage. Is it efficacious? Yes. Crit Care Clin 1996;12(3):697–707.

Wijdicks EFM. Aneurysmal subarachnoid hemorrhage. In: Wijdicks EFM. The Clinical Practice of Critical Care Neurology. Philadelphia: Lippincott-Raven, 1997, pp 132–157.

83 Subdural Hematoma

Marie R. Baldisseri

Key Pathogenesis

- Subdural hematomas result from tearing of cerebral bridging veins located between the inner surface of the dura mater and the arachnoid layers of the meninges.

- Usually results from violent movement of the brain within the skull

- Venous bleeding is usually slowed or stopped by rising intracranial pressure.

Classification

A. Acute
   1. Trauma is the most common etiologic event.
   2. Infrequent causes
      a. Bleeding from a cortical artery
      b. Ruptured aneurysm
      c. Superficial arteriovenous malformation
B. Subacute
C. Chronic
   1. The etiology can be less dramatic compared to acute subdural hematoma.
   2. History may consist of remote minor head trauma, especially in high-risk patients, such as the elderly and those on oral anticoagulant drugs.

Key Epidemiology

- Subdural hematomas are most frequently caused by acute trauma.

- One-fourth of all trauma deaths result from head injury.

Clinical Findings

A. Acute subdural hematoma
   1. Symptoms result from compression of the brain by the rapidly evolving and expanding fresh clot.
   2. Symptoms occur within 48 hours after injury.
   3. Typically there is brief lucid period prior to coma.
   4. Patient can be stuporous at the onset, with deepening coma over time.
   5. Patients can present with signs of rapidly increasing intracranial pressure (headache and decreased level of consciousness) and then worsening symptoms with cerebral edema and herniation (pupillary dilatation and contralateral hemiparesis).
   6. It is sometimes difficult to determine the contribution of subdural hematoma to the overall clinical picture because subdural hematomas often present with epidural hematomas, cerebral contusion, or lacerations.
   7. Posterior fossa subdural hematomas present with headache, vomiting, pupillary dilatation, dysphagia, cranial nerve palsies, and rarely, neck stiffness and ataxia of the trunk and gait disturbance.
B. Subacute subdural hematoma
   1. Symptoms occur within 48 hours to 2 weeks after the initial injury.
   2. There can be gradual improvement after head injury but then deterioration with signs of an acute subdural hematoma.
C. Chronic subdural hematoma
   1. Symptoms can occur after a relatively long interval (weeks to months) after the initial trauma.
   2. Mental status changes include drowsiness, inattentiveness, giddiness or depression, or confusion.
   3. Headaches
   4. Seizures
   5. Choreiform movements
   6. Transient ischemic attacks
   7. Rarely, focal or lateralizing signs (e.g., contralateral or ipsilateral hemiparesis, aphasia, homonymous hemianopia) are present.

Key Findings

- Acute bleeds are almost always associated with coma, which may deepen over time.

- Chronic bleeds are associated more frequently with mental status changes and occasional focal or lateralizing signs.

Diagnosis

A. Computed tomography (CT) of the head without contrast

   1. 90% accurate for acute subdural hematoma

   2. The classic appearance is a concave or half-moon shaped, hyperdense lesion that is denser than the adjacent cortex.

   3. For less acute hematomas, the fluid may be isodense with the cortex and the CT scan may reveal only ventricular shift.

B. Magnetic resonance imaging is useful for less acute hematomas, and shows a widened space between the skull and the brain.

C. Computed tomography with contrast and magnetic resonance imaging are the best ways to visualize less acute subdural hematomas.

D. Cerebral arteriogram

E. Electroencephalography often shows reduced voltage or electrical silence over the area of the hematoma.

F. Skull films can reveal areas of calcification surrounding a chronic subdural hematoma.

G. Examination of cerebrospinal fluid is not diagnostic, although the presence of xanthochromic fluid with a relatively low protein count should raise the suspicion of a chronic subdural hematoma.

Treatment

A. Emergency placement of burr holes for evacuation of clot can be life-saving for patients at risk for impending herniation.

B. Surgery

   1. Acute subdural hematomas require large wide craniotomy for control of bleeding and evacuation of clot.

   2. 10% to 15% of acute subdural hematomas require reoperation for evacuation.

   3. Chronic hematomas require craniotomy to allow stripping away the pseudomembranes that surround the clot.

C. Corticosteroid treatment is an alternative to surgery for chronic subdural hematomas with minor symptoms or when there are contraindications to surgery.

Key Treatment

- Surgery with wide craniotomy is usually needed for larger bleeds with more extensive brain compression and for chronic subdural hematomas for removal and stripping of pseudomembranes.

- Small clots can resolve spontaneously; accordingly, surgical intervention is not indicated if no or only minor symptoms are present.

Prognosis

A. The size of the initial bleed is important, because larger bleeds will continue to enlarge rather than remain solid or resorb spontaneously.

B. Acute subdural hematoma is associated with high mortality, in part because of concomitant brain injury, which occurs in more than half of cases.

C. If brain injury is absent, then baseline medical condition is a key determinant of outcome after acute subdural hematoma.

D. Negative prognostic factors include advanced age, poor neurologic status, and prolonged delay from the time of injury to surgical intervention.

E. Patients with a Glasgow coma scale score lower than 6 have a mortality rate as high as 76%; mortality usually results from severe cerebral compression and herniation.

F. Early surgical evaluation of acute subdural hematomas is associated with the best outcome.

G. Prognosis is less predictable for surgical evacuation of chronic subdural hematomas; these lesions tend to recur frequently, particularly in the elderly, because cerebral atrophy increases the available space within the cranium.

 Bibliography

Dent DL, Croco MA, Menke PG, et al. Prognostic factors after acute subdural hematoma. J Trauma 1995;39:36–43.

Friedman AH (ed). Craniocerebral injuries. In: Sabiston's Textbook of Surgery (15th ed). Philadelphia: WB Saunders, 1997; pp 1355–1360.

Raimond J, Taylor JW. Neurological Trauma. In: Neurological Emergencies: Effective Nursing Care. Baltimore: Aspen Systems, 1986; pp 189–242.

Victor M, Ropper AH (eds). Craniocerebral trauma. In: Adams and Victor's Principles of Neurology. New York: McGraw-Hill, 2001; pp 925–953.

84 Intracranial Hypertension

Daniel B. Michael

Definitions

A. Intracranial pressure (ICP)
   1. Force per unit area, relative to atmospheric pressure, within the skull
   2. Measured in millimeters of mercury (mm Hg = cm $H_2O \div 1.36$)
   3. Normal ICP is 0 to 10 mm Hg.

B. Intracranial hypertension
   1. Elevated ICP
   2. Complicates many brain diseases; e.g., traumatic brain injury, stroke, and meningitis
   3. Compromises cerebral blood flow and can lead to brain herniation
   4. Treatment indicated if ICP is greater than 20 mm Hg

C. Monro-Kellie doctrine
   1. Changes in ICP are related to changes in intracranial volume.
   2. Average normal adult intracranial volume is approximately 1500 mL and consists of 80% brain, 10% blood, and 10% cerebrospinal fluid (CSF).
   3. In the face of an increase in volume of one compartment, ICP homeostasis is maintained by an equal decrease involving one or both of the other compartments.

D. Langfitt curve (Fig. 84–1)
   1. Describes the relationship between ICP and intracranial volume
   2. Intracranial elasticity
      a. The first derivative (i.e., dP/dV) of the Langfitt pressure–volume curve
      b. Corresponds to the slope of the Langfitt curve at any given point on the curve
   3. Intracranial compliance
      a. The reciprocal of intracranial elastance
      b. Decreases as intracranial volume and ICP increase.

E. Pressure–volume index
   1. The volume of fluid required to increase ICP by a factor of 10
   2. Normal is 25 mL.
   3. Assessed by injection of 1 mL sterile saline into ventricle
   4. Low values indicate low compliance.

   5. Not a routine assessment due to risk of herniation or infection

F. Cerebral perfusion pressure (CPP)
   1. Calculated as CPP = MAP − ICP
   2. MAP = mean arterial blood pressure
   3. Normal CPP is greater than 60 mm Hg.
   4. Low values compromise cerebral blood flow (CBF).

G. Cerebral vascular resistance (CVR)
   1. CVR = CPP/CBF, or
   2. CVR = $k \times l \times v/d^4$
   3. Where k = a constant; l = blood vessel length; v = blood viscosity; d = blood vessel diameter
   4. Influenced by $PaCO_2$ and pH (e.g., increased $PaCO_2$ and decreased pH cause cerebral vasodilation and increase regional CBF by decreasing local CVR)

H. Cerebral blood flow
   1. CBF = CPP/CVR
   2. Normal is greater than 40 to 50 mL/min per 100 g brain tissue.
   3. Threshold for irreversible ischemic brain damage: 18 to 20 mL/min per 100 g

I. Cerebral autoregulation
   1. The physiologic process that maintains CBF constant and normal over a wide range of CPP
   2. Autoregulation may be lost in certain disease states and when CPP falls outside the physiologic limits (generally between ~50 to ~150 mm Hg).

J. Jugular venous oxyhemoglobin saturation (SjO_2)
   1. Measurement requires an indwelling vascular catheter lying within the jugular bulb.
   2. May be obtained intermittently by in vitro CO-oximetry or continuously with a fiberoptic monitoring catheter
   3. Normal range: 0.55 to 0.71
   4. Decreased values imply decreased CBF.

K. Cerebral arterial-venous oxygen content difference (cerebral $avDO_2$)
   1. The arterial-venous difference in oxygen content of blood entering and leaving the brain
   2. Calculated from jugular bulb oxygen tension (PjO_2, torr), SjO_2, hemoglobin concentration (Hb, g/dL), and systemic arterial oxygen tension (torr) and saturation: cerebral $avDO_2$ =

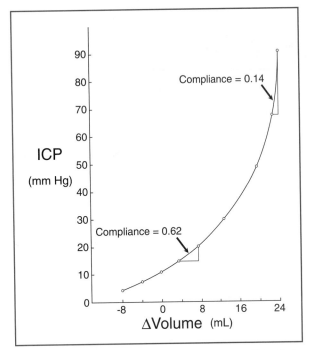

Figure 84–1 Intracranial pressure–volume curve. Note that as ICP rises, smaller increases in intracranial volume produce large increases in pressure. (Adapted from Michael DB. Intracranial Hypertension. Grosse Pointe Shores, MI: Daniel B. Michael, 2000, with permission.)

$$[1.39 \times Hb \times (SaO_2 - SjO_2)] + [0.0031 \times (PaO_2 - PjO_2)]$$

3. Normal avDO$_2$ range is 4.8 to 8.5 mL/dL.
4. Increased values imply decreased CBF.

L. Cerebral metabolic rate of oxygen utilization (CMRO$_2$)
   1. CMRO$_2$ = CBF × cerebral avDO$_2$
   2. Normal CMRO$_2$ range is 2.9 to 3.7 mL/100 g brain per minute.
   3. Decreased values occur with decreased cerebral blood flow.

Etiology

A. Traumatic brain injury (TBI)
B. Cerebrovascular disease
   1. Ischemic infarction
   2. Hemorrhage
      a. Intracerebral
      b. Intraventricular
      c. Subarachnoid: ruptured aneurysm or arteriovenous malformation
C. Intracranial neoplasm
D. Inflammatory disease
   1. Meningitis
   2. Cerebritis

3. Brain abscess
E. Benign intracranial hypertension (pseudotumor cerebri)
F. Systemic diseases
   1. Global cerebral ischemia following circulatory arrest
   2. Hepatic liver failure (e.g., Reye's syndrome)
G. Congenital or acquired hydrocephalus
H. Potential causes of elevated ICP in the ICU
   1. Expanding mass lesions (e.g., hematoma, hydrocephalus)
   2. Hypercapnia
   3. Hypoxia
   4. Respiratory procedures (e.g., suctioning airway, positive end-expiratory pressure)
   5. Isometric muscle contraction (e.g., posturing)
   6. Valsalva maneuver (e.g., cough, emesis)
   7. Emotional upset, noxious stimuli
   8. Awakening, rapid eye movement (REM) sleep
   9. Seizures
   10. Hyperthermia
   11. Hyponatremia
   12. Secondary injury mechanisms (e.g., free radical production)

Pathophysiology

A. Elevated ICP caused by uncompensated increase in intracranial volume
   1. Extravasated blood (e.g., TBI)
   2. Cerebrospinal fluid (e.g., hydrocephalus)
   3. Intracellular (i.e., cytotoxic) edema
   4. Extracellular (i.e., vasogenic) edema
B. Pressure–volume curve demonstrates logarithmic nature of compensation.
   1. Early mechanisms
      a. Cerebrospinal fluid displacement
      b. Intravascular blood exclusion (arteriolar vasoconstriction)
   2. Late mechanisms (if elevated ICP not treated)
      a. Brain displacement (herniation)
      b. Ischemia (stroke)
   3. Compensation is more effective with slower volume increase.
      a. Acute: less than 150 mL (e.g., acute epidural hematoma)
      b. Chronic: greater than 150 mL (e.g., brain neoplasm)
   4. Uncompensated or untreated mechanisms lead to further ICP elevation; positive feedback

mechanism or vicious cycle can thus occur and lead to death.

C. Elevated ICP may cause and be caused by ischemia.

1. If autoregulation is impaired, increased ICP decreases CPP and therefore CBF.

   a. Cerebral ischemia severely increases morbidity of elevated ICP (causes cytotoxic edema and cell death).

   b. Systemic hypertension may result from brainstem ischemia due to elevated ICP (can increase vasogenic edema).

   c. Hyperventilation is used to treat elevated ICP (>20 to 25 mm Hg); causes vasoconstriction and ischemia, especially in areas of injured brain.

   d. Hypoxia and increased regional lactate may increase ischemia.

2. If $CMRO_2$ is increased (e.g., due to fever or convulsions), associated increases in $PaCO_2$ and decreases in pH cause cerebral vasodilation (decreased CVR).

D. Decreased local CVR and increased regional CBF ("cerebral hyperemia") may be observed transiently in 30% of patients with severe TBI.

Key Epidemiology

- Incidence of intracranial hypertension is related to the incidence of the underlying injury or disease.

- Severe TBI cases: approximately 200 per 100,000 population per year in the United States, with elevated ICP in approximately 70%

- 150 new ischemic and 36 new hemorrhagic (including subarachnoid hemorrhage) strokes per 100,000 population per year in the United States, with 10 to 50% complicated by elevated ICP requiring monitoring

Clinical Findings

A. Clinical significance of elevated ICP is not completely understood.

B. Clinical manifestations are produced by brain herniation or ischemia, which may have caused the intracranial hypertension in the first place.

C. Degree or severity of ICP elevation cannot be inferred from clinical findings.

1. Fatal herniation may occur at ICP as low as 20 to 25 mm Hg in TBI or stroke.

2. Pseudotumor cerebri may be associated with relatively mild symptoms such as headache,

vomiting, and drowsiness at ICP levels as high as 90 mm Hg.

D. Early findings

1. Headache

2. Drowsiness

3. Confusion

4. Yawning

5. Vomiting without nausea

6. Cushing's triad

   a. Hypertension with widened pulse pressure

   b. Bradycardia

   c. Respiratory irregularity

7. Retinal hemorrhages (with abrupt, severe ICP elevation)

8. Papilledema (may take several hours to develop)

9. Neurogenic pulmonary edema with acute respiratory failure (with abrupt, severe ICP elevation)

E. Late findings (herniation syndromes)

1. Sub-falcine herniation

   a. Often accompanies or precedes lateral downward transtentorial herniation

   b. Cingulate gyrus herniates under the falx cerebri.

      (1) Compresses anterior cerebral artery

      (2) Produces weakness of the contralateral lower extremity

2. Downward transtentorial herniation (central or lateral)

   a. Central form causes rostral-to-caudal progression of brainstem dysfunction.

      (1) Midbrain dysfunction (coma, dilated pupils due to bilateral third cranial nerve palsy, extensor posturing and central neurogenic hyperventilation; compression of the posterior cerebral arteries may occur, leading to cortical visual loss if the patient regains consciousness)

      (2) Pontine dysfunction (includes the midbrain findings, the loss of the corneal reflex and ataxic breathing)

      (3) Medullary dysfunction (includes midbrain and pontine findings, loss of gag and vestibular reflexes, apnea, hypotension, and death)

   b. Lateral form causes medial portion of the temporal lobe (uncus) to herniate through the tentorial hiatus, initially causing unilateral midbrain compression.

      (1) Dilation of the ipsilateral pupil, which may occur before coma

(2) Contralateral hemiparesis typically occurs.

(3) Ipsilateral hemiparesis (Kernohan-Woltman notch phenomenon) occurs in 15% of cases.

(4) Progression as in central herniation

3. Upward transtentorial herniation

a. Can complicate ventriculostomy placement for posterior fossa mass

b. Associated with rapid loss of consciousness due to upward displacement of the brainstem

4. Trans–foramen magnum herniation (coning)

a. Caused by expanding infratentorial mass

(1) Caudal brainstem and cerebellar tonsils forced through the foramen magnum

(2) Reduces arterial blood flow to the central medulla

(3) Cushing's triad occurs.

(4) Rapid progression to apnea, hypotension and death

5. Fungoides cerebri

a. Herniation through a skull defect after (open craniocerebral injury of craniotomy)

b. Gives a mushroom appearance of brain prolapsing through the skull defect

---

PEARL

Intracranial hypertension may be inferred from clinical findings, but placement of an ICP monitor is required for diagnosis (see Chapter 220, Intracranial Pressure Monitoring).

Treatment

A. Treatment threshold depends on clinical context; generally treat ICP higher than 20 to 25 mm Hg.

B. Goal: control ICP without decreasing CBF

1. Often must achieve a compromise

2. Use clinical examination to individualize treatment.

C. Treat in stepwise fashion, beginning with simple measures (with low potential for complications) and proceeding to more complex and risky measures (Fig. 84–2).

D. Secure airway, establish normal ventilation, and maintain systolic blood pressure greater than 90 mm Hg.

E. Evacuate surgically accessible lesions.

F. Stepwise ICU management

1. Positioning

a. Remove constricting cervical devices.

b. Elevate the head (30 degrees).

2. Sedation (see Table 84–1)

a. Use short-acting, reversible agents.

b. Continue neurologic examinations every 1 to 2 hours.

3. Cerebrospinal fluid drainage

a. Use external ventricular drainage device (ventriculostomy).

b. Open drain at 15 mm Hg above the external auditory meatus.

c. Avoid excessive drainage.

4. Mannitol

a. Dose: 0.25 to 1.00 g/kg IV bolus every 6 hours until ICP controlled or serum osmolality greater than 315 to 330 mOsm/kg H_2O

b. May give 10 to 20 mg furosemide with each mannitol bolus

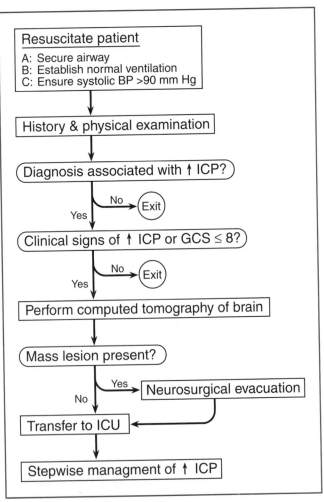

Figure 84–2 Treatment algorithm for intracranial hypertension. (Adapted from Michael DB. Intracranial Hypertension. Grosse Pointe Shores, MI: Daniel B. Michael, 2000, with permission.)

TABLE 84–1. SEDATIVES USEFUL IN LOWERING ICP

SEDATIVE	REVERSING AGENT
Morphine sulfate (0.05 to 0.1 mg/kg IV every 1 to 2 hours)	Naloxone (0.1 to 0.2 mg IV every 2 to 3 minutes)
Lorazepam (1 to 2 mg IV every 1 to 2 hours)	Flumazenil (0.2 mg IV every 30 to 60 seconds to maximum of 3 mg)
Propofol (5 to 50 μg/kg per minute IV, titrated in 5 μg/kg per minute increments every 5 to 10 minutes)	Time (allow 30 to 60 minutes after infusion is stopped)

From Michael DB. Intracranial Hypertension. Grosse Pointe Shores, MI: Daniel B. Michael, 2000, with permission.

5. Hyperventilation to maintain $PaCO_2$ at 30 to 35 torr
   a. Prolonged or profound hypocapnia may cause ischemia.
   b. Consider SjO_2 monitoring to maintain a level of 0.70.
6. Barbiturate coma
   a. Pentobarbital: 5 to 10 mg/kg per hour by continuous IV infusion
   b. May lead to hypotension or decreased cardiac output
   c. Consider pulmonary artery catheterization for hemodynamic monitoring.
7. Investigational therapy
   a. Corticosteroids
      (1) No class I evidence of efficacy

Key Stepwise Treatment

- Resuscitate and evacuate surgically accessible mass lesions.
- Elevate head and remove constricting neck devices.
- Sedate patient.
- Drain CSF via ventriculostomy.
- Give mannitol 0.25 to 1.00 g/kg IV bolus every 6 hours.
- Hyperventilate to maintain $PaCO_2$ at 30 to 35 torr.
- Consider barbiturate or investigational treatment if patient is salvageable.

   (2) New prospective trial for use in head injury currently under way
   b. Free-radical scavengers (e.g., vitamins C and E; polyethylene glycol conjugated supra oxide dismutase)
   c. N-methyl-D-aspartate receptor antagonists (e.g., Selfotel; MK 801); currently not available in the United States
   d. Selective cerebral calcium channel blockers (e.g., C-1009); currently not available in the United States
   e. Therapeutic hypothermia (36.5° to 32.5°C)
   f. Craniectomy or cerebral lobectomy

Outcome

A. No class I (prospective, randomized controlled) trials which may demonstrate improved outcome by monitoring or treating elevated ICP have been conducted.
B. Prolonged ICP elevations are associated with poor outcome.
C. Traumatic Coma Data Bank has demonstrated a strong association between the duration of intracranial hypertension and outcome.
D. Guidelines for management of severe head injury cite potential benefits from ICP monitoring.
   1. Helps in the earlier detection of mass lesions
   2. Can limit the indiscriminate use of therapies to control ICP that can be potentially harmful
   3. Can reduce ICP by CSF drainage and thus improve cerebral perfusion
   4. Helps in determining prognosis

Bibliography

Bullock R, Chesnut RM, Clifton G, et al. Part 1: guidelines for the management of severe head injury. J Neurotrauma 2000;17:451–553.
Cushing H. Some experimental and clinical observations concerning state of increased intracranial tension. Am J Med Sci 1902;124:375–400.
Lee KR, Hoff JT. Intracranial pressure. In: Youmans JR (ed). Neurological Surgery. Philadelphia: WB Saunders, 1996; pp 491–518.
Marmarou A, Anderson RL, Ward JD, et al. Impact of ICP instability and hypotension on outcome in patients with severe head trauma. J Neurosurg 1991;75:S59–S66.
Michael DB. Intracranial Hypertension. Grosse Pointe Shores, MI: Daniel B. Michael, 2000.
Narayan RK, Wilberger Jr JE, Povlishock JT (eds). Neurotrauma. New York: McGraw-Hill, 1996.
Plum F, Posner JB. Diagnosis of Stupor and Coma, 3rd ed. Philadelphia: F.A. Davis, 1980.
Troncale JA, Michael DB. Headache. In: Kozel RA, From D, Konen J (eds). When to Call a Surgeon. Philadelphia: F.A. Davis, 1996.

85 Spinal Cord Compression

Perry A. Ball

Etiology

A. Metastatic disease
   1. Compression may be due to direct invasion of epidural space or due to spread to vertebral bodies, with subsequent collapse.
   2. Common primary sites
      a. Lung
      b. Breast
      c. Prostate
      d. Kidney
      e. Thyroid
      f. Lymphoma
B. Epidural abscess
   1. Location
      a. Cervical (15%)
      b. Thoracic (50%)
      c. Lumbar (15%)
   2. Causative organisms
      a. *Staphylococcus aureus* (50% of cases)
      b. Aerobic and anaerobic streptococci
      c. Enteric Gram-negative bacilli
      d. *Mycobacterium tuberculosis*
C. Trauma
   1. Fracture
      a. Burst fracture
      b. Fracture dislocation
      c. No x-ray abnormality (more common in children and the elderly)
   2. Penetrating injuries
      a. Gunshot wound
      b. Stab injury
   3. Location
      a. Cervical (55%)
      b. Thoracic (15%)
      c. Thoracolumbar junction (15%)
      d. Lumbar (15%)
   4. Neurologic injury
      a. Complete injury (45%)
      b. Incomplete injury (55%)
   5. Associated injury
      a. Head trauma (25%)
      b. Chest and abdominal injury (25% to 50%)

Key Etiologies

- Fractures
- Penetrating injuries
- Metastatic tumors
- Epidural abscess

Clinical Findings

A. Complete injuries (no motor or sensory function below the level of the lesion)
   1. Initial flaccid paralysis below the level of the lesion, followed by the development of spasticity
   2. Cervical root levels
      a. C3 to C5: diaphragm is paralyzed by loss of phrenic nerve function
      b. C5: deltoid and biceps are paralyzed
      c. C6: wrist extensors are paralyzed
      d. C7: triceps are paralyzed
      e. C8: finger extensors and flexors are paralyzed
B. Incomplete injuries (some preservation of motor or sensory function below the lesion)
   1. Central cord syndrome
      a. Seen in cervical lesions
      b. Weakness of hands > arms > legs
   2. Anterior cord syndrome: loss of motor function with preservation of sensory function
   3. Brown-Sequard syndrome
      a. Compromise of half of cord
      b. Weakness and loss of proprioception on same side as the lesion and loss of light touch on the opposite side
   4. Cauda equina syndrome
      a. Seen in lumbar lesions
      b. Variable degree of leg weakness and loss of sphincter control
C. Spinal epidural abscess
   1. Presentation
      a. Back pain, fever, neurologic deficit
      b. Elevated erythrocyte sedimentation rate, leukocytosis

2. Risk factors
  a. Diabetes mellitus
  b. Intravenous drug abuse
  c. Alcoholism
  d. Renal failure
  e. Skin infection
  f. Invasive procedure, such as epidural injection and epidural catheterization
  g. Penetrating injury
  h. In a significant number of cases no clear etiology can be identified.

D. Pulmonary findings
  1. Lesions above C3 frequently result in apnea from loss of phrenic nerve function.
  2. Some 30% of mid and lower cervical spine injuries (C3 to C7) will lead to the need for mechanical ventilation at some point during the acute phase, but most patients can ultimately be weaned from ventilatory support.
    a. Early ventilatory failure is due in large part to initially flaccid chest wall muscles resulting in a progressive decline in forced vital capacity, manifested by increasing respiratory rate with falling tidal volume.
    b. Improvement in ventilatory mechanics occurs over weeks as chest wall muscles become spastic.
  3. Quadriplegic patients have better ventilatory mechanics supine rather than upright.
    a. The mechanism underlying this paradoxical relationship is overdistention of the diaphragm in the upright position.
    b. The use of an abdominal binder improves ventilatory mechanics in the upright position.

E. Hemodynamic findings
  1. Spinal cord compression above the cervicothoracic junction is associated with arterial hypotension.
  2. Sympathetic outflow to peripheral vasoconstriction arises from C8 to T1.
  3. Cardiac accelerator fibers arise from T1 to T4
  4. Thus, cord compression above C8 leads to peripheral vasodilation and bradycardia from unopposed vagal outflow.

Key Findings

- Neurologic deficit
- Respiratory embarrassment
- Hypotension
- Bradycardia

Imaging Studies

A. Plain x-rays
  1. Look for loss of vertebral alignment.
  2. May show bone destruction from tumor or end-plate erosion from infection
B. Computed tomography (CT)
  1. Sensitive for the detection of acute hemorrhage
  2. Delineates acute fractures
  3. Addition of myelography demonstrates degree of cord compression well.
C. Magnetic resonance imaging
  1. Demonstrates degree of cord compression well
  2. Addition of contrast helpful in identification of area of infection or tumor
  3. It is the most sensitive imaging methodology for detection and localization of spinal epidural abscess.
  4. Can be technically challenging in mechanically ventilated patients; images are degraded by patient motion

---

PEARL

For metastatic disease to spine where the primary site is unknown, consider a metastatic imaging survey (CT of chest, abdomen, pelvis, bone scan, mammograms) or needle biopsy of spinal lesion.

Treatment

A. Airway management
  1. Oral intubation with manual in-line traction is a safe means of obtaining control of the airway in the patient with spinal cord injury.
    a. Alternatives (blind nasal intubation, fiberoptic intubation or surgical airway) should be considered and planned for.
    b. Succinylcholine should be avoided in spinal cord injuries of longer than 24 hours duration because of the risk of inducing severe hyperkalemia.
  2. Tracheostomy should be performed if anticipated ventilatory dependence exceeds 2 weeks.
    a. Reduces dead space
    b. Facilitates weaning trials without the need for repeated airway manipulation
B. Hemodynamic
  1. Substantial volume resuscitation is often required in light of peripheral vasodilation.
    a. Invasive monitoring (central venous or pul-

monary artery catheterization) can be helpful in guiding fluid resuscitation.

   b. Foley catheterization should be performed to monitor urine output, because bladder emptying is usually compromised.

  2. Pharmacological support of the circulation may be necessary.

   a. Agents with both α- and β-adrenergic effects, such as dopamine and norepinephrine, are useful to counteract low peripheral resistance and bradycardia.

   b. Agents with purely α-adrenergic effects, such as phenylephrine, may be associated with persistent bradycardia.

C. Trauma

  1. Methylprednisolone

   a. Dose: 30 mg/kg IV bolus followed 1 hour later by 5.4 mg/kg per hour by continuous IV infusion for 23 hours

   b. Should be started within 8 hours of injury

   c. Corticosteroids offer no demonstrated benefit for patients with penetrating injuries.

  2. Immobilization

   a. Tong traction

   b. Cervical collar

   c. Rotating bed

   d. Halo vest

  3. Surgery: timing and indications for surgery remain controversial

D. Neoplasm

  1. High-dose dexamethasone: 12 mg intravenously, followed by 4 mg intravenously every 6 hours

  2. Decisions regarding radiation therapy alone versus surgical decompression followed by radiation therapy should be individualized based on

   a. Neurologic function

   b. Radiosensitivity of tumor

   c. Previous radiation treatment

   d. Extent of disease and spinal stability

   e. Life expectancy

  3. Radiation generally consists of 3000 cGy in fractionated doses.

  4. Surgery

   a. Laminectomy in cases of epidural mass

   b. Reconstruction and stabilization in cases of vertebral collapse

E. Spinal epidural abscess

  1. Surgical debridement is usually required.

  2. Selected cases without neurologic deficit or with severe concurrent illness can be managed cautiously by antibiotics alone.

  3. Antibiotic treatment

   a. Empiric coverage should include a third-generation cephalosporin and vancomycin.

   b. The antibiotic regimen should be tailored once an organism is identified.

   c. Typical duration of therapy is 6 to 8 weeks.

Key Treatment

- Delineate neurologic deficit.

- Identify etiology.

- Localize lesion using imaging studies.

- Give methylprednisolone for non-penetrating traumatic injuries within 8 hours.

- Support ventilation and hemodynamics.

- Avoid succinylcholine in injuries more than 24 hours old.

Bibliography

Bracken MB, Shepard MJ, Collins WF, et al. A randomized, controlled trial of methylprednisolone or naloxone in the treatment of acute spinal cord injury. Results of the second National Spinal Cord Injury Study. N Engl J Med 1990;322:1405–1411.

Cooper PR, Errico TJ, Martin R, et al. A systematic approach to spinal reconstruction after anterior reconstruction for neoplastic disease of the thoracic and lumbar spine. Neurosurgery 1993;32:1–8.

Curling OD, Gower DJ, McWhorter JM. Changing concepts in spinal epidural abscess: A report of 29 cases. Neurosurgery 1990;185–192.

86 Neuroleptic Malignant Syndrome and Malignant Hyperthermia

Vivek Padegal
Venkata Bandi
Peter J. Papadakos

Key Epidemiology

- Neuroleptic malignant syndrome is seen primarily in young and middle-aged adults.

- Malignant hyperthermia tends to occur in younger individuals. Most cases occur before the age of 15 years and the risk declines further beyond age 30 years.

Etiology and Risk Factors

A. Neuroleptic malignant syndrome
   1. Idiosyncratic drug reaction, mainly precipitated by neuroleptic drug use
      a. High doses, rapid dose escalation, and intramuscular injection increase risk.
      b. Longer-acting agents do not increase risk, but may prolong duration of syndrome if it develops.
      c. Specific drugs
         (1) Phenothiazines: chlorpromazine, thioridazine, fluphenazine, trifluoperazine
         (2) Butyrophenones: haloperidol
         (3) Thioxanthenes: thiothixene
         (4) Others: resperidone, clozapine, promethazine, loxapine
   2. Other precipitating drugs include dopamine antagonists and depleters (e.g., metoclopramide, tetrabenazine, reserpine, sulpiride, sultopride) and cyclic antidepressants.
   3. Can occur after withdrawal of anti-Parkinsonism drugs (e.g., levodopa)
   4. Potential adjuctive factors include dehydration and organic brain disease.

B. Malignant hyperthermia
   1. Idiosyncratic reaction precipitated by exposure to certain anesthetics and muscle relaxants
      a. Inhalational anesthetics: halothane, methoxyflurane, enflurane, isoflurane, cyclopropane, diethyl ether
      b. Depolarizing neuromuscular blocking agents: succinyl choline, decamethonium, gallamine
      c. Controversial inciting agents: ketamine, lidocaine, anticholinergics, theophylline

   2. Past history
      a. History of prior anesthetic procedure without incident does not negate risk.
      b. 24% to 50% of patients have had prior anesthetic procedures without incident.
   3. Other risk factors
      a. Family history (inherited risk)
      b. Emotional or heat stress
      c. Vigorous exercise
      d. Certain operative procedures are associated with higher risk: e.g., ocular, head, neck, and musculoskeletal surgery
      e. Musculoskeletal abnormalities (controversial): e.g., kyphoscoliosis, strabismus, myotonic or Duchenne muscular dystrophy, osteogenesis imperfecta, central core disease

Key Pathogenesis

- Neuroleptic malignant syndrome may be due to dopaminergic blockade at the level of the basal ganglia and hypothalamic thermoregulatory center.

- Malignant hyperthermia occurs secondary to abnormal efflux of calcium from the sarcoplasmic reticulum into the myoplasma, resulting in sarcomeric contraction.

- Both disorders are associated with excessive muscle contraction and resultant heat production.

Clinical Findings

A. Neuroleptic malignant syndrome
   1. Onset is from hours to months after initial exposure.
   2. Clinical features typically evolve over 24 to 72 hours.
   3. Mandatory findings
      a. High fever (>40°C)
      b. Marked muscle rigidity ("lead pipe" or "cogwheeling")
   4. Frequent accompanying features
      a. Autonomic dysfunction: tachycardia, diaphoresis, incontinence, labile blood pressure

b. Extrapyramidal dysfunction: tremulousness, involuntary movements, or catatonic akinesia

c. Alterations in mental status: mutism, agitation, stupor, or coma

d. Other: dysphagia, dysarthria, sialorrhea

B. Malignant hyperthermia

1. Onset is from minutes to hours after exposure to inciting agent; rarely seen in less than 15 minutes.

2. Classic findings

a. Hyperthermia (may be seen later in course)

b. Muscle rigidity

3. Other manifestations

a. Neuromuscular: early jaw spasm, trismus (intubation may be difficult with succinyl choline), or increased motor tone in jaw

b. Increased muscle tone in extremities or chest

c. Tachypnea, tachycardia

d. Hypertension, increased cardiac output

e. Diaphoresis, cyanosis

Key Clinical Findings

- Hyperthermia
- Muscle rigidity
- Exposure to inciting agent

Differential Diagnosis

A. Malignant hyperthermia

B. Infection

1. Sepsis

2. Encephalomyelitis

3. Tetanus (see Chapter 90)

C. Other causes of rhabdomyolysis (see Chapter 153, Rhabdomyolysis)

D. Seizures

E. Major psychoses, including lethal catatonia

F. Endocrinopathy (thyroid storm, pheochromocytoma)

G. Systemic lupus erythematosus

H. Heat stroke (see Chapter 149)

I. Toxic exposure

1. Strychnine

2. Carbon monoxide

3. Drug overdose (e.g., salicylates, dopamine antagonists, stimulants, anticholinergic drugs, monoamine oxidase inhibitors, serotonin reuptake inhibitors)

Key Laboratory Findings

- Marked increases in serum creatine phosphokinase activity
- Laboratory signs of dehydration (e.g., hypernatremia)
- Laboratory signs of renal dysfunction (e.g., azotemia)
- Increased end-tidal P_{CO_2}
- Hypercalcemia (malignant hyperthermia)
- Leukocytosis
- Lactic acidosis
- Hypoxemia
- Myoglobinuria
- Hyperkalemia

Treatment

A. Discontinue suspected offending drug or anesthetic (if intraoperative, stop procedure as soon as possible).

B. Avoid other dopamine agonists (e.g., metoclopramide) or agents known to be associated with these syndromes.

C. Institute aggressive cooling measures (see Chapter 149, Heat Stroke).

1. Evaporative water spray or misting, plus circulating fan

2. Ice packs or cooling blanket

3. Antipyretics

D. Increase FIO_2 to 1.00 and begin hyperventilation to avoid hypercapnia (malignant hyperthermia).

E. Begin specific pharmacotherapy.

1. Dantrolene

a. See Chapter 178, Dantrolene.

b. Delay in initiation worsens outcome in malignant hyperthermia.

2. Bromocriptine

a. Promotes release of endogenous dopamine within central nervous system

b. Dose: 10 to 25 mg every 6 to 8 hours orally or via nasogastric tube

c. May need 1 week of treatment

3. Benzodiazepine for muscular relaxation

4. Rigidity rarely may necessitate nondepolarizing neuromuscular blocking agents, such as cis-atracurium, if the above measures are insufficient.

F. Supportive measures

1. Intravenous hydration

2. Correction of electrolyte disturbances

3. Mechanical ventilation, if indicated

a. Monitor respiratory status.

b. Severe muscle rigidity involving diaphragm

or accessory respiratory muscles can lead to respiratory failure.

    c. Do not administer succinyl choline (e.g., during endotracheal intubation) because it may precipitate hyperkalemia if there is rhabdomyolysis or renal dysfunction.

4. Prophylaxis against deep-vein thrombosis (see Chapter 118, Deep Venous Thrombosis)

PEARL

More cases of neuroleptic malignant syndrome have been reported with the use of haloperidol than any other drug, but this may simply reflect the fact that haloperidol has been the most widely used neuroleptic.

Complications

A. Rhabdomyolysis
B. Acute myoglobinuric renal failure
C. Metabolic
    1. Hyperkalemia
    2. Lactic acidosis
D. Pulmonary
    1. Aspiration pneumonitis
    2. Acute respiratory distress syndrome
    3. Respiratory acidosis
    4. Respiratory failure
    5. Pulmonary embolism

E. Cardiac dysrhythmias (avoid digoxin because it affects intracellular calcium)
F. Deep venous thrombosis
G. Sepsis
H. Disseminated intravascular coagulation
I. Cerebral edema

Key Prognosis

- Recurrence of neuroleptic malignant syndrome is unusual.

- Mortality in both syndromes is approximately 7%.

Bibliography

Caroff SN, Mann SC. Neuroleptic malignant syndrome. Contemp Clin Neurol 1993;77:185–202.

Chan T, Evans S, Clark C. Drug-induced hyperthermia. Crit Care Clin 1997;13:785–808.

Granner MA, Wooten GF. Neuroleptic malignant syndrome or Parksonism hyperpyrexia syndrome. Semin Neurol 1991;11:228–235.

Hopkins PM. Malignant hyperthermia: advances in clinical management and diagnosis. Br J Anaesth 2000;85:118–128.

Larach MG, Localio A, Allen G, et al. A clinical grading scale to predict malignant hyperthermia susceptibility. Anesthesiology 1994;80:771–779.

Montgomery JN, Ironside JW. Neuroleptic malignant syndrome in the intensive therapy unit. Anaesthesia 1990; 45:311–313.

Rosenberg MR, Green M. Neuroleptic malignant syndrome: review of response to therapy. Arch Intern Med 1989;149:1927–1931.

87 Myasthenia Gravis

Robert P. Lisak

Myasthenia gravis (MG) is an autoimmune disease that results in muscle weakness. Normal amounts of acetylcholine (ACh) are released at the neuromuscular junction in this disorder. However, availability of postsynaptic nicotinic acetylcholine receptors (AChR) on skeletal muscle is reduced by the presence of antibodies to the receptor (anti-AChR). In a small number of patients the autoantibodies may be directed against other as yet unidentified postsynaptic components.

Etiology

In patients with MG anything that affects pre- or postsynaptic events may lead to further deterioration in neuromuscular transmission and increase weakness in bulbar and respiratory muscles, resulting in marked worsening including myasthenic crisis. In addition to autoimmune acquired MG there are other disorders of the neuromuscular junction that affect presynaptic, synaptic, and postsynaptic structures. These include toxins, drugs, other autoimmune diseases (Lambert-Eaton myasthenic syndrome caused by antibodies to presynaptic voltage-gated calcium channels) and a group of inherited disorders affecting several different presynaptic, synaptic, and postsynaptic proteins important to neuromuscular junctions (myasthenic syndromes), including defects in AChR itself. These are important to identify because therapy directed at the immune system is ineffective in congenital/inherited myasthenic syndromes and in neuromuscular junction disorders caused by drugs or toxins. Thus, there is essentially only one source of acquired myasthenia gravis (autoantibodies) but there are many disorders of neuromuscular transmission.

Symptoms

A. Primary symptoms (i.e., those directly related to weakness)
  1. Weakness is frequently variable in different muscle groups.
  2. Patients may complain of fatigue or variable weakness with effort and sometimes of general fatigue in response to motor activity.
  3. Subjective fatigue without motor symptoms is not a presentation of myasthenia gravis.
  4. Specific involvement
    a. Diplopia, ptosis
    b. Poor facial movement, including poor eye closure
    c. Dysphagia, dysarthria, difficulty chewing
    d. Weakness of neck muscles
    e. Dyspnea
    f. Weakness of upper and lower limbs (proximal more than distal)
    g. Fatigue of motor activity (but not subjective fatigue)
B. Secondary symptoms (may or may not be present depending on multiple factors including type, severity, and duration of primary symptoms)
  1. Symptoms of hypercarbia
  2. Symptoms of hypoxia
  3. Symptoms of respiratory infection (aspiration pneumonia)
  4. Weight loss (decreased caloric intake from dysphagia and decreased chewing)

Physical Findings

A. Respiratory: tachypnea or decreased respirations, poor air movement, use of accessory muscles of respiration
B. Cardiac: tachycardia may be present
C. Skin: cyanosis may be present
D. Neurologic
  1. Mental status is normal unless hypercarbia or hypoxia is present.
  2. Cranial nerve dysfunction
    a. Ptosis
    b. Restricted extraocular movement, with normal pupillary response to light
    c. Weakness of jaw and facial muscles, with normal facial sensation
    d. Weakness of palatal and pharyngeal muscles, with dysphagia and dysarthria
    e. Weakness of neck muscles and tongue
  3. Motor examination may show variable degrees of weakness, proximal often greater than distal; may have truncal, intercostal, and abdominal muscle weakness.
  4. Sensory examination is normal in the absence of other confounding diseases.
  5. Deep-tendon reflexes are normal to slightly brisk, with normal plantar response unless there are secondary central nervous system complica-

tions (hypoxia); hyporeflexia may be present secondary to concomitant diseases (e.g., diabetic neuropathy, vitamin B$_{12}$ deficiency).

E. Other: patients with MG may have other autoimmune diseases, and signs of those diseases might also be present (e.g., hyper- or hypothyroidism, lupus, rheumatoid arthritis)

Laboratory and Other Tests

A. Arterial blood gases may show hypercarbia and hypoxia (hypercarbia is more commonly seen early in respiratory failure that is due to neuromuscular disease).

B. Electromyography (EMG) and nerve-conduction studies

1. Show reduction of compound motor action potential at slow rates of stimulation (2 to 5 Hz) with no evidence of disease of the peripheral nerves (in the absence of a confounding disorder such as diabetes) or anterior horn cells

2. May show mild evidence of myopathy

3. Useful in detecting other causes of neuromuscular and peripheral nerve disease

4. Single-fiber EMG is positive in more than 90% of patients with MG.

C. Elevated titers of anti-AChR antibodies occur in 85% to 90% of patients with generalized MG.

Imaging Studies

A. Chest x-ray evidence of atelectasis or pneumonia may be present.

B. Mediastinal mass on chest x-ray (~50%) or computed tomography (>95%) of patients with MG and thymoma (10% to 15% of patients)

C. Enlarged thymus seen on chest computerized tomography in many of the 65% to 75% of MG patients with thymic hyperplasia

D. Elevated hemidiaphragm is seen in some patients with thymoma or status postthymectomy for thymoma (phrenic nerve involvement).

Diagnosis

A. Edrophonium test

1. Prepare syringes.

a. Fill one insulin syringe with 10 mg (1 mL) edrophonium and another with saline.

b. Label the syringes so that the examining physician is blinded as to which syringe contains drug.

2. Perform baseline muscle testing of 7 to 12 weak muscles (includes cranial nerves) and check vital capacity and negative inspiratory force (NIF).

3. Inject 0.2 mL intravenously and flush line.

4. Examine at 1½ to 3 min; if patient is stronger in several muscles, stop and see if worsens within 5 min.

a. If worsens, repeat test with the other solution.

b. If not, retest muscles and give an additional 0.6 to 0.8 mL, repeating testing as before.

c. If still no response, give remaining 0.2 mL and repeat procedure.

d. Always test with both solutions and then have the person who prepared the syringes break the blind.

5. Prophylactic atropine given subcutaneously or intravenously is not necessary unless the patient has bradycardia, but a prefilled syringe containing atropine should be readily available.

B. Electromyographic and nerve conduction studies should be performed by an experienced electromyographer.

C. Blood should be sampled for anti-AChR antibody testing before commencing immunotherapy.

Key Findings

- Ptosis
- External ophthalmoparesis
- Buccal, facial, oral, bulbar weakness
- Extremity and truncal weakness
- Abnormal repetitive stimulation on EMG
- Normal mental status
- Normal sensory exam
- Normal reflexes and tone
- Response to edrophonium
- Respiratory distress or insufficiency

Monitoring

A. Close clinical assessment of respiratory status and vital signs

B. Close monitoring for signs of hypercarbia or hypoxia

C. Frequent assessment of bulbar function (e.g., swallowing, gag, need for suctioning)

D. Frequent (every 4 to 6 hours) vital capacity and NIF testing, if not intubated

E. Arterial blood gases

1. Can be helpful as adjunctive measures, but clinical assessment of progression of respiratory and bulbar muscles is more important for de-

terminating the need for endotracheal intubation and mechanical ventilation

2. PaCO₂ changes first.

3. PaO₂ and oxyhemoglobin saturation are last to change and are far less useful for monitoring.

F. Endotracheal intubation and mechanical ventilation should be rapidly instituted if deterioration of respiratory or bulbar function occurs, rather than waiting for abnormal blood gases or fall of vital capacity to a specific level (1.0 L is commonly cited for the average-sized adult patient).

Treatment

A. Provide airway management, pulmonary toilet, ventilatory support.

B. Identify and treat any infection.

C. Avoid concomitant administration of drugs with neuromuscular blocking or membrane stabilizing properties (e.g., aminoglycosides, neuromuscular blocking agents), if possible.

D. If patient needs respiratory support, it is not necessary to try to distinguish myasthenic worsening from cholinergic crisis.

E. Plasma exchange: one plasma volume exchange every other day for 5 to 6 treatments; consider additional exchanges depending on patient's response

F. If cause for MG deterioration (e.g., infection or rapid reduction or discontinuation of previous MG drugs) is not obvious and there are no absolute contraindications, give prednisone or equivalent at 0.5 to 1.0 mg/kg per day.

1. Worsening due to steroids may occur before improvement.

2. In patients who are less weak and not monitored in an ICU, a low dose of prednisone is used and the dose is slowly increased to avoid temporary worsening.

G. Pyridostigmine

1. May be begun or reinstituted at low dose (30 to 60 mg every 4 hours)

2. Gradually increase, judging dose and frequency by clinical status.

3. Use of the edrophonium test for pyridostigmine

dosing, or to differentiate myasthenic vs cholinergic crisis, can be misleading.

4. Side effects include increased secretions, abdominal cramps (sometimes with diarrhea), diaphoresis, bradycardia; can be treated with atropine or atropine-like agents.

H. If prolonged mechanical ventilation seems likely, provide nutritional support and pyridostigmine via nasogastric route.

I. Intravenous immunoglobulin G therapy is slower in action than plasma exchange in MG and may not be as effective.

J. Thymectomy and immunosuppressive agents (e.g., azathioprine, cyclosporine, mycophenolate mofetil, cyclophosphamide) are useful in patients with MG but seldom need to be part of the care of crisis because their effects are frequently delayed.

Key Treatment

- Closely monitor respiratory and bulbar function.

- Endotracheal intubation and mechanical ventilation may be necessary.

- Rapidly establish diagnosis.

- Identify and treat precipitating factors.

- Plasma exchange

- Corticosteroids, as needed

- Pyridostigmine, as needed

Bibliography

Agrov Z, Wirgun I. Drugs and the neuromuscular junction: pharmacotherapy of transmission disorders and drug-induced myasthenic syndromes. In: Lisak RP (ed). Handbook of Myasthenia Gravis and Myasthenic Syndromes. New York: Marcel Dekker, 1994; pp 295–320.

Chaudrhy V, Cornblath DR. Immunosuppressive therapy for myasthenia gravis. In: Lisak RP (ed). Handbook of Myasthenia Gravis and Myasthenic Syndromes. New York: Marcel Dekker, 1994; pp 341–374.

Lewis RA, Selwa JF, Lisak RP. Myasthenia gravis: immunological mechanisms and immunotherapy. Ann Neurol 1995;37(Suppl 1):S51–S62.

Lisak RP. Myasthenia gravis. Current Treatment Options in Neurology 1999;1:239–249.

Watson DF, Lisak RP. Myasthenia gravis: an overview. In: Lisak RP (ed). Handbook of Myasthenia Gravis and Myasthenic Syndromes. New York: Marcel Dekker, 1994; pp 1–20.

88 Guillain-Barré Syndrome

Richard A. Lewis

Guillain-Barré syndrome (GBS) is a subacutely evolving autoimmune paralytic disorder. Formerly GBS was considered synonymous with acute inflammatory demyelinating polyradiculoneuropathy (AIDP), but more recently it has become clear that GBS is a true syndrome comprised of a number of similar but distinct disorders. These disorders include acute motor axonal neuropathy (AMAN), acute sensory axonal neuropathy (ASAN), acute motor sensory axonal neuropathy (AMSAN), acute autonomic neuropathy, and Miller-Fisher syndrome (MFS), although AIDP remains the most common form.

Guillain-Barré syndrome describes subacute disorders that progress over 2 to 4 weeks. Chronic inflammatory demyelinating polyneuropathy (CIDP) is a disorder similar to AIDP, but it is either chronically progressive or relapsing. It is considered to be a separate condition from GBS. The clinical symptoms and examination described below are based on those found in AIDP, although AMAN and AMSAN have similar findings.

Etiology

A. Infection
   1. Viral (definite or probable associations)
      a. Cytomegalovirus
      b. Epstein-Barr virus
      c. Human immunodeficiency virus
      d. Hepatitis B and C
      e. Varicella zoster
      f. Vaccinia, smallpox
   2. Bacterial
      a. *Campylobacter jejuni*
      b. *Mycoplasma pneumoniae*
B. Vaccination
   1. Rabies vaccines
   2. Swine flu (1979)
   3. Associations with other vaccines are less clear.
C. Surgery
   1. From 5% to 10% of GBS cases develop 1 to 4 weeks after a surgical procedure.
   2. No specific correlation has been shown with the type of surgery or anesthesia or with any complications.
D. Pregnancy and postpartum state

E. Autoimmune
   1. Systemic lupus erythematosus
   2. Thyroiditis
F. Malignancy
   1. Hodgkin's disease
   2. Non-Hodgkin's lymphoma
G. Drugs that can cause a GBS-like neuropathy
   1. Gold therapy
   2. Vincristine (high risk in patients with Charcot-Marie-Tooth disease)
   3. Other reported drugs: captopril, streptokinase, danazol, disulfiram

> ### PEARL
>
> Over 70% of patients with GBS have had a prior event that occurred between 1 and 4 weeks before the onset of neurologic symptoms.

Clinical Findings

A. Symptoms
   1. Initial symptoms
      a. Paresthesias of hands or feet
      b. Weakness
      c. Neck or back pain
      d. Occasionally begins with diplopia, facial weakness
   2. Progression (usually progresses over 3 weeks, but occasional patients develop complete paralysis within 72 hours)
      a. Symmetric weakness
      b. Can be ascending, descending, or global
      c. Dysphagia
      d. Respiratory embarrassment
   3. Symptoms that are not typical of uncomplicated GBS
      a. Urinary incontinence
      b. Fever
B. Physical examination
   1. General systemic findings that may be seen in GBS
      a. Tachycardia is common (the most common autonomic sign).

307

b. Bradycardia (irregular pulse and dysrhythmias)

c. Blood pressure can be elevated or reduced.

d. Tachypnea with use of accessory muscles of respiration

e. Abdominal distension and reduced bowel sounds if associated ileus

2. Neurologic findings

  a. Findings typical of GBS

    (1) Normal mental status

    (2) Pupils can be poorly reactive to light and occasionally are fully dilated.

    (3) Extraocular motor paresis or paralysis

    (4) Facial diplegia (the most common cranial nerve abnormality)

    (5) Absent gag reflex

    (6) Reduced muscle tone

    (7) Relatively symmetric weakness (some asymmetry is not unusual)

    (8) Areflexia or marked hyporeflexia

    (9) Minor sensory deficits

  b. Autonomically mediated findings that can occur

    (1) Flushing

    (2) Reduced sweating

    (3) Bronchoconstriction

    (4) Increased bronchial secretions

    (5) Syndrome of inappropriate antidiuresis

    (6) Diabetes insipidus

    (7) Paralytic ileus

    (8) Horner's syndrome

  c. Findings that are not typical of GBS and cast doubt on the diagnosis

    (1) Hyperreflexia

    (2) Spasticity

    (3) Babinski sign

    (4) Prominent bowel or bladder symptoms at onset

3. Cardiovascular findings (autonomic dysfunction occurs in the majority of cases and is a serious and potentially fatal aspect of the disorder)

  a. Cardiac dysrhythmias

    (1) Sinus tachycardia is frequent and an early sign but is usually benign.

    (2) Poor response to carotid sinus stimulation suggests reduced vagally mediated efferent response.

    (3) Bradycardia is more serious and may be followed by sinus arrest and asystole.

b. Blood pressure changes

  (1) Hypertension is frequent and may be an early sign.

  (2) Orthostatic hypotension is common; it results from a reduction in peripheral vascular tone.

C. Findings observed in variants of GBS

1. Miller-Fisher syndrome

  a. Diplopia and eye movement abnormalities

  b. Ataxia

  c. Areflexia

  d. Little or no weakness

  e. Anti-GQ1b antibodies

2. Sensory predominant GBS

  a. Ataxia

  b. Prominent paresthesias

  c. Marked vibration and proprioception abnormalities

3. Acute dysautonomia

  a. Orthostatic hypotension

  b. Pupillary abnormalities

  c. Cardiac dysrhythmias

  d. Urinary and bowel retention

D. Electrocardiographic findings

1. Dysrhythmias

2. Flattened T waves

3. T wave inversion

4. Reduced RR intervals

Diagnostic Studies

A. Cerebrospinal fluid (CSF)

1. Elevated protein

  a. Can be normal in first week

  b. If normal early, may need to repeat lumbar puncture

2. Mononuclear white blood cells

  a. Fewer than 10 cells/mm^3

  b. More than 50 mononuclear cells or presence of polymorphonuclear cells cast doubt on diagnosis.

B. Electromyography (EMG) and nerve-conduction studies

1. Conduction slowing and conduction block are hallmarks of AIDP.

2. Reduced amplitudes, prolonged distal motor latencies, and late responses (F waves) may be early findings consistent with early involvement of distal nerve fibers and proximal ventral roots.

3. Denervation on needle EMG suggests axonal degeneration and is associated with a worse prognosis.

Key Findings

- Symmetric weakness
- Facial weakness
- Respiratory insufficiency
- Dysphagia
- Areflexia
- Increased CSF protein and no cells
- Slow nerve conductions

Differential Diagnosis

A. Neuromuscular junction disorders
  1. Myasthenia gravis
  2. Botulism
B. Acute motor neuron disorders
  1. Poliomyelitis
  2. Other viral disorders
C. Acute intoxications
  1. Tick paralysis
  2. Diphtheria
  3. Ciguatoxin, tetrodotoxin, and saxitoxin (due to ingestion of certain marine animals)
  4. Organophosphate poisoning
D. Central nervous system disorders
  1. Locked-in syndrome
  2. Acute encephalomyelitis
  3. Acute transverse myelitis

Treatment

A. Treatments directed at the autoimmune process
  1. Plasmapheresis
  2. Intravenous immunoglobulin (IVIG)
  3. The above treatments are equally effective in shortening the course of the illness, reducing the time on mechanical ventilation, and improving overall recovery.
B. Prevention of complications (severely affected patients can be bedridden for weeks or months)
  1. Deep venous thrombosis prophylaxis
  2. Gastrostomy for dysphagia
  3. Prevention of pressure sores by frequent turning or use of specialized beds
  4. Prevention of joint contractures by passive range of movement and bracing
C. Symptomatic treatments (if quadriplegic and receiving mechanical ventilation, these patients are unable to communicate; the medical team needs to be aware of the patient's physical and psychological discomfort)
  1. Analgesics for pain
  2. Anxiolytics
D. Respiratory therapy
  1. Respiratory failure can occur rapidly.
  2. Careful and frequent monitoring of respiratory function is needed.
  3. Patients should be in an intensive care setting during the progressive stage of the illness.
  4. Respiratory monitoring
    a. Hypoxemia is a late sign of respiratory failure in GBS.
    b. Forced vital capacity (FVC) of less than 15 mL/kg or less than 1 L necessitates respiratory support in most patients
    c. Rapid decline of FVC requires special attention.
    d. Negative inspiratory force (NIF), tidal volume, and respiratory rate complement FVC monitoring.
    e. Air leaks in patients with facial diparesis may falsely lower FVC.
    f. Use of accessory muscles of respiration point to impending respiratory failure.
    g. Weak cough and inability to handle secretions may warrant intubation irrespective of other respiratory parameters.
  5. Other respiratory considerations
    a. Consider early tracheostomy in patients with severe disease.
    b. Continuous positive airway pressure by mask may be used in certain situations.
    c. Up to 25% of patients will require mechanical ventilation.
E. Cardiovascular therapy
  1. Pacemaker may be indicated if significant bradycardia develops.
  2. Drug therapy may be required for hypertension.
    a. α-Adrenergic inhibitors have been suggested along with β-blockers because the latter may increase the vasopressor response to increased levels of circulating catecholamines in GBS.
    b. Exaggerated hypotensive responses to nitroglycerin, morphine, furosemide, and other drugs can occur.

Key Treatment

- Plasmapheresis or IVIG
- Monitor FVC and NIF to determine need for mechanical ventilation.
- Monitor and treat blood pressure and cardiac rhythm abnormalities.
- Prevent complications of long-term paralysis.
- Gastrostomy

Prognosis

A. More than 70% of patients have excellent recovery, even those who are quadriplegic and require mechanical ventilation.

B. Indicators of poor prognosis
1. Older age
2. Quadriplegia and mechanical ventilation
3. Denervation on EMG

C. Most common causes of death
1. Autonomic dysfunction and fatal hypotension or dysrhythmia
2. Pulmonary embolism
3. Pulmonary edema
4. Sepsis

D. Relapses and recurrences
1. 5% to 10% of patients treated with IVIG or plasmapheresis will relapse within the first month; further treatment may be indicated.
2. 5% incidence of recurrence years later

 Bibliography

Arnason BG, Soliven B. Acute inflammatory demyelinating polyneuropathy. In: Dyck PJ, Thomas PK, Griffin JW, et al (eds). Peripheral Neuropathy, 3rd ed. Philadelphia: WB Saunders, 1993; pp 1437–1497.

Asbury AK. New concepts of Guillain-Barré syndrome. J Child Neurol 2000;15:183–191.

Ho T, Griffin J. Guillain-Barré syndrome. Curr Opin Neurol 1999;12:389–394.

Ropper AH, Wildreks EF, Traux BT. Guillain Barré Syndrome. Philadelphia: F.A. Davis, 1991.

89 Botulism

Anh Tu Duy Nguyen
Kalpalatha K. Guntupalli

Botulism is a neuroparalytic syndrome characterized by symmetrical descending paralysis caused by a toxin produced by *Clostridium botulinum*. Initially described in 1820 by Kerner in association with ingestion of sausage, the term is derived from the Latin word for sausage, *botulus*. Botulism is a rare but treatable condition in which prompt recognition coupled with intensive care unit (ICU) management and antitoxin therapy can be life-saving.

Etiology

A. Manifestations are due to a neurotoxin produced by *C. botulinum*, a spore-forming anaerobic Gram-positive bacterium.
   1. *C. botulinum* is present in soil and marine sediments.
   2. Heat-resistant spores enable the organism to survive food preparation conditions that kill most other organisms.
B. A given strain of *C. botulinum* usually produces a single neurotoxin.
   1. Eight different neurotoxins have been described: types A, B, C1, C2, D, E, F, and G.
   2. Neurotoxins A, B, E, F, and G cause human disease.
   3. The overwhelming majority of cases are due to type A, B, and E neurotoxins.

Pathophysiology

A. The toxins are odorless and tasteless polypeptides.
   1. They bind irreversibly to presynaptic junctions and prevent acetylcholine release.
   2. They are among the most potent toxins known.
   3. Can be absorbed via the lungs if aerosolized; there are concerns regarding potential use as a biological weapon.
B. Symptoms are caused by inhibition of acetylcholine release from the neuromuscular junctions and peripheral autonomic synapses.
   1. The toxin does not cross the blood–brain barrier; therefore, central nervous system symptoms are typically absent.
   2. Recovery involves sprouting new presynaptic junctions (takes up to 6 months).
C. Neurotoxin A has medicinal uses.
   1. Examples are treatment of torticollis and achalasia.

2. Therapy with neurotoxin A may cause inadvertent botulism.

Epidemiology (4 Major Forms)

A. Food-borne botulism: a form of food poisoning
   1. From ingestion of pre-formed toxin in contaminated foods (e.g., home-canned fruits and vegetables, salted and fermented fish, seal and whale meat)
   2. Recent cases have been due to contaminated salsa, baked potatoes in aluminum foil, cheese sauce, and garlic in oil.
B. Wound botulism
   1. *C. botulinum* wound infection with production of neurotoxin
   2. Can occur with any wound
   3. Described with intramuscular or subcutaneous injection of "black tar" (unpurified) heroin
C. Infantile botulism (the most common form)
   1. Acquired by ingestion of spores of *C. botulinum* (e.g., in dust, honey, or corn syrup)
   2. Honey is the most widely recognized source, but it accounts for a minority of cases.
   3. Results in colonization of the gastrointestinal (GI) tract, with production and absorption of the neurotoxin
D. Adult infectious botulism
   1. A rare, adult variant of infantile botulism, also characterized by intestinal colonization
   2. Risk factors include antibiotic use, abdominal surgery, and GI disorders with altered bacterial flora.

Clinical Findings

A. Food-borne botulism
   1. Incubation period is 18 to 36 hours (range 6 hours to 8 days).
   2. Prodromal GI symptoms: vomiting, abdominal pain, constipation, diarrhea (occasionally), and urinary retention prior to muscle weakness
   3. Progressive descending flaccid weakness; typically symmetrical
   4. Weakness begins with cranial nerve involvement, presenting as the "5 D's of botulism:" diplopia, dilated pupils, dysphagia, dysarthria, and dry mouth.

311

5. Descending paralysis with dyspnea and respiratory failure, which may develop suddenly

6. Typically there are no sensory (other than blurred vision) or cognitive abnormalities, or fever.

B. Wound botulism

1. Incubation period is 4 to 14 days from injury.

2. Presentation is similar to food-borne botulism.

3. The GI prodrome is usually absent, and fever (by non-clostridial wound bacteria) may be present.

4. Increasing incidence in "black tar" heroin use

C. Infantile botulism

1. Presents with GI symptoms (e.g., constipation, difficulty feeding), progressive weakness, hypotonia, and weak cry

2. Symptoms progress over 2 to 3 weeks, plateau for 2 to 3 weeks, and then improve slowly over several months.

Key Physical Findings

- Acute, bilateral cranial neuropathies

- Pupillary involvement (mydriasis, blurred vision)

- Descending symmetric weakness

- Normal or slow heart rate with normal blood pressure

- No fever, altered mental status, or sensory deficits

Diagnostic Tests

A. Neurotoxin detection

1. A mouse inoculation test can be performed at the U.S. Centers for Disease Control and Prevention (CDC) or designated state public health laboratories.

2. May be performed on serum, stool, remaining food, or gastric contents

B. Identification of *C. botulinum* in stool and food cultures

1. *C. botulinum* is not part of normal gut flora.

2. Presence of the organism in the setting of compatible clinical symptoms and signs suggests the diagnosis.

C. Electrophysiologic studies

1. Decreased action potential amplitude with characteristic marked incremental response to repetitive, high-frequency (20 Hz) stimuli

2. Nerve conduction is normal.

D. Other tests

1. Cerebrospinal fluid (CSF) is normal.

2. Erythrocyte sedimentation rate and complete blood cell counts are normal.

3. Brain computed tomography (CT) and magnetic resonance imaging are normal.

4. Edrophonium test is negative (may be falsely positive).

Differential Diagnosis

A. Guillain-Barré syndrome: ascending paralysis

1. Miller-Fischer variant may start with bulbar muscles similar to botulism.

2. CSF: elevated protein concentration

3. Electromyography distinguishes Guillain-Barré from botulism.

B. Myasthenia gravis: characteristic findings on electrophysiologic testing

C. Lambert-Eaton syndrome: no autonomic features of botulism

D. Cerebrovascular accident: CT of brain is usually abnormal in stroke.

E. Tick paralysis: skin examination is essential to reveal attached tick.

F. Drugs or poisons: e.g., organophosphates, atropine, carbon monoxide, aminoglycosides

G. Paralytic shellfish poisoning

H. Puffer fish poisoning ("fugu")

I. Hypermagnesemia

PEARL

Clinical suspicion should be high in patients presenting with key features of the syndrome, especially if a cluster of similar cases develop or if there are risk factors such as eating home-made canned foods, eating salted and fermented fish, or using injection drugs. Diagnosis is made in this clinical context by demonstrating the presence of either neurotoxin or *C. botulinum*.

Treatment

A. Initial management is empiric, based on clinical findings and a presumptive diagnosis. Awaiting results of confirmatory tests will delay treatment.

B. ICU monitoring is crucial because of the potential for rapid development of respiratory failure, a major cause of mortality.

C. Elective intubation is recommended when vital capacity decreases below 30% of predicted, or when there is concern over upper airway competency.

D. Remove unabsorbed toxin

1. Nasogastric aspiration

2. Administration of charcoal and cathartics

3. Enema may be helpful if no diarrhea.

E. Antitoxin: ABE trivalent equine serum for food-borne and wound botulism

1. There is retrospective evidence that antitoxin therapy shortens the course of illness and decreases mortality.

2. Side effects: 9% to 20% develop hypersensitivity reaction.

3. Skin sensitivity test required prior to therapy

4. One vial of antitoxin (7500 IU of type A, 5500 IU type B, 8500 IU of type E antitoxin) is recommended.

a. Based on the antitoxin half-life of 5 to 8 days and achieving serum antitoxin levels 100-fold greater than the neurotoxin

b. Antitoxin is available from CDC (daytime telephone: 404-639-2206; 404-639-2888 other times).

PEARL

Antitoxin can only neutralize neurotoxin that is not bound to nerve endings; has greatest efficacy when given early.

F. Wound botulism

1. High-dose penicillin (3 million units intravenously every 4 hours)

2. Metronidazole 500 mg intravenously every 8 hours, if penicillin allergic

3. Debridement is usually required.

4. Give tetanus booster as needed.

G. Notify public health department.

H. Investigational therapy

1. Plasmapheresis to remove neurotoxin

2. Human botulinum immunoglobulin trial: Treatment Investigational New Drug Protocol; California Department of Health Services (telephone 510-540-2646)

Key Treatment

- Provide supportive ICU care with monitoring for upper airway dysfunction and decrease in vital capacity.

- Give antitoxin for wound botulism and food-borne botulism; early treatment shortens disease course and may prevent death.

- Prevent further absorption of neurotoxin from the gut or wound.

- After recovery, educate patient to prevent recurrence.

Prevention

A. No person-to-person spread; isolation is not required.

B. Do not taste or eat food that appears spoiled or from bulging food containers.

C. No immunity develops to botulinum neurotoxin; patients remain susceptible.

1. Education is key to prevent recurrence.

2. Proper food handling and preparation are crucial.

D. Botulinum toxoid (pentavalent vaccine A, B, C, D, E) is recommended only for laboratory workers exposed to neurotoxin.

Key Prognosis

- Rapid diagnosis and management yield full recovery to baseline level of function for most patients.

- Hospital course is often prolonged (1 to 3 months).

- Most muscle strength is recovered in the first 3 months, with continued improvement over the next 12 months.

- Mortality is 5% to 7.5% with prompt treatment; can be up to 60% outside the critical care setting.

Bibliography

Bakheit AMO, Ward CD, McLellan DL. Generalized botulism-like syndrome after intramuscular injections of botulinum toxin type A: a report of two cases. J Neurol Neurosurg Psychiatry 1997;62:198.

Bleck TP. *Clostridium botulinum*. In: Mandell GL, Bennett JE, Dolin R (eds). Mandell, Douglas, and Bennett's Principles and Practice of Infectious Diseases, 5th edition. Philadelphia: Churchill Livingstone, 2000; pp 2543–2548.

Martin C, Schaller MD, Lepori M, Liaudet L. Cranial nerve palsies and descending paralysis in a drug abuser resulting from wound botulism. Intensive Care Med 1999;25:765–769.

McCroskey LM, Hatheway CL. Laboratory findings in four cases of adult botulism suggest colonization of the intestinal tract. J Clin Microbiol 1988;26:1052–1054.

Passaro DJ, Werner SB, McGee J, et al. Wound botulism associated with black tar heroin among injecting drug users. JAMA 1998;279:859–863.

Scully RE, Mark EJ, McNeely WF, et al. Case records of the Massachusetts General Hospital. N Engl J Med 1997;337:184–190.

Shapiro RL, Hatheway C, Swerdlow DL. Botulism in the United States: a clinical and epidemiologic review. Ann Intern Med 1998;129:221–228.

Werner SB, Passaro D, McGee J, et al. Wound botulism in California, 1951–1998: recent epidemic in heroin injectors. Clin Infect Dis 2000;31:1018–1024.

90 Tetanus

Adel Ghuloom
Venkata Bandi

Tetanus is a life-threatening bacterial infection. The organism *Clostridium tetani* releases a highly potent neurotoxin (tetanospasmin) resulting in muscle spasm. *C. tetani* is a motile, anaerobic Gram-positive rod found in soil and animal feces. It exists in a sporulated form in unfavorable environments and can survive for many months. Spores resist boiling and disinfectants. In tissues with low oxidative-reduction potential, such as necrotic wounds, the spores convert to germinative forms and produce toxin.

Key Epidemiology

- A disease of nonimmunized or partially immunized patients

- Completely immunized patients without adequate booster doses are also susceptible.

- Drug abusers are at increased risk of infection.

- Tetanus is uncommon in the United States; sporadic in underdeveloped countries with inadequate immunization.

Pathogenesis

A. Contamination of wounds with spores does not always lead to disease.
B. In a low oxidation-reduction potential environment spores convert to germinative cells and produce tetanospasmin.
C. Intraneuronal transport of toxin to the anterior horn of the spinal cord and cranial nerve nuclei
D. Toxin prevents release of inhibitory neurotransmitters at presynaptic terminals.
E. Unopposed excitatory neurotransmitters lead to muscle spasm.

Classification

A. Localized tetanus
  1. Muscle groups affected in proximity to portal of entry
  2. May progress to generalized form
  3. Prognosis good
B. Cephalic tetanus
  1. Cranial nerve involvement
  2. May progress to generalized form

  3. May result from ear infection or head injury
  4. High mortality
C. Generalized tetanus
  1. Most common form
  2. High mortality in elderly patients and heroin addicts

Clinical Findings

A. Trismus
B. Opisthotonos
C. Risus sardonicus
D. Nuchal rigidity
E. Dysphagia
F. Autonomic nervous system dysfunction
  1. Hypertension or hypotension
  2. Hyperpyrexia
  3. Bradycardia or tachycardia
  4. Diaphoresis
  5. Peripheral vasoconstriction
G. Abdominal muscle rigidity
H. Cranial nerve palsies
I. Respiratory failure secondary to spasm of the respiratory muscles
J. Touch, noise, or light can precipitate symptoms.
K. Mental status is normal.
L. Hands and feet can be spared.

Key Findings

- Trismus

- Opisthotonos

- Risus sardonicus

- Nuchal rigidity

- Dysphagia

Differential Diagnosis

A. Meningitis
B. Stiff-man syndrome
C. Rabies
D. Peritonitis
E. Strychnine poisoning

314

F. Neuroleptic malignant syndrome

G. Hypocalcemic tetany

H. Diseases of temporomandibular joints

Diagnosis

A. Tetanus is a clinical diagnosis; high index of suspicion is required.

B. Blood cultures are not helpful.

C. Wound culture may be positive in less than 50% of cases.

D. Leukocytosis

E. Normal cerebrospinal fluid

F. Increased serum creatine phosphokinase activity

PEARL

Think of tetanus if the patient's hands and feet are spared and mentation is normal.

Treatment

A. Supportive care

1. Intensive care unit admission is required.

2. Intubate trachea if there is generalized tetanus or severe dysphagia.

3. Correct hypovolemia and electrolyte deficits.

4. Provide prophylaxis for deep venous thrombosis.

5. Provide prophylaxis against gastrointestinal stress ulceration.

6. Provide nutritional support.

B. Toxin neutralization and infection management

1. Neutralize toxin with human tetanus immunoglobulin (hTIG).

   a. Generalized tetanus: 3000 U to 6000 U intramuscularly

   b. Intrathecal hTIG may prevent progression to generalized form in cephalic or localized forms.

   c. Give antitoxin before wound debridement.

2. Adequate wound debridement is crucial to prevent further toxin release.

3. Antibiotic therapy may help eradicate infection at entry site.

   a. Penicillin G is the drug of choice: one million units intravenously every 6 hours

   b. Tetracycline, clindamycin, erythromycin and metronidazole can be used in cases of penicillin allergy.

C. Treatment of muscle spasm

1. Diazepam 2.5 to 20 mg intravenously every 2 to 6 hours

2. Morphine sulfate 2 to 10 mg every 1 to 3 hours to reduce muscle spasm

3. Neuromuscular blocking agents, such as vecuronium

   a. For severe muscle spasms

   b. Give only to patients who are sedated, endotracheally intubated, and mechanically ventilated.

   c. Avoid depolarizing neuromuscular blockers (succinylcholine) because of the risk of hyperkalemia.

4. Dantrolene may reduce muscle spasm.

D. Autonomic instability

1. Consider continuous IV magnesium sulfate, if the patient is unresponsive to diazepam and morphine.

   a. Monitor serum magnesium concentration every 4 to 6 hours.

   b. Maintain serum magnesium level at 2.5 to 4 mmol/L.

2. Clonidine, 300 μg enterally every 8 hours, if the patient is unresponsive to magnesium

3. Epidural anesthesia may help control autonomic instability.

4. Warning: β-adrenergic blocking agents may result in sudden cardiac arrest

---

Key Treatment

- Protect airway.
- Neutralize toxin.
- Treat infection.
- Debride wound.
- Treat muscle spasm.
- Treat autonomic instability.
- Watch for complications.
- Immunize patient before discharge.

Prevention

A. If patient completes primary series: give 0.5 mL of tetanus/diphtheria (Td) vaccine intramuscularly every 10 years

B. Give Td vaccine for all patients, with a clean minor wound and a contaminated wound with unknown immunization history.

C. No immunization is required for patients with a clean minor wound or a contaminated wound with known immunization history in the last 10 and 5 years, respectively.

D. All contaminated wounds with unknown immunization history requires hTIG in addition to the Td vaccine. Administer in separate syringes at separate sites.

Key Prognosis

- Mortality is less than 10% with appropriate supportive care.

- Recovery is complete; muscle spasm may persist for 4 to 6 weeks.

- Infection does not confer immunity; immunization should be started before the patient leaves the hospital.

Bibliography

Abrahamian FM, Pollack CV Jr, Lo Vecchio F, et al. Fatal tetanus in a drug abuser with "protective" antitetanus antibodies. J Emerg Med 2000;18:189–193.

Abrutyn E, Berlin JA. Intrathecal therapy in tetanus. A meta-analysis. JAMA 1991;226:2262–2267.

Bardenheier B, Prevots DR, Khetsuriani N, et al. Tetanus surveillance—United States, 1995–1997. MMWR CDC Surveill Summ 1998;47(2):1–13.

Bhagwarjee S, Bosenberg AT, Muckaret DJ. Management of sympathetic overactivity in tetanus with epidural bupivacaine and sufentanil. Crit Care Med 1999;27:172–175.

Jolliet P, Magnenat JL, Kobel T, et al. Aggressive intensive care treatment of very elderly patients with tetanus if justified. Chest 1990;97:702–705.

Lee HC, Ko WC, Chuang YC. Tetanus of the elderly. J Microbiol Immunol Infect 2000;33:191–196.

Lipman J, James MF, Erskine J, et al. Autonomic dysfunction in severe tetanus: magnesium sulfate as an adjunct to deep sedation. Crit Care Med 1987;15:987–988.

Talan DA, Moran GJ. Tetanus among injecting-drug users—California, 1997. Ann Emerg Med 1998;32:385–386.

91 Sepsis and SIRS

Dane J. Nichols

The systemic inflammatory response syndrome (SIRS) encompasses a constellation of features that commonly develop in the wake of local or generalized tissue injury. The grading of the response is based on common findings readily available to the clinician. In the current schema, SIRS is further categorized according to whether the initiating event for the inflammatory response is an infectious agent or not.

Definitions

A. SIRS
   1. Body temperature lower than 36°C or higher than 38°C
   2. Pulse higher than 90 beats/minute
   3. Respirations more than 20 breaths/min or $PaCO_2$ lower than 32 torr
   4. White blood cell count <4,000 or >12,000 cells/mm^3, or ≥10% immature forms
B. Sepsis: SIRS resulting from an infectious process
C. Severe sepsis: sepsis associated with evidence of hypoperfusion or end-organ dysfunction
D. Hypotension: commonly defined in clinical trials as systolic pressure lower than 90 mm Hg or a fall in baseline pressure by more than 40% without other obvious cause
E. Septic shock: sepsis-associated hypotension after adequate fluid resuscitation and evidence of associated end-organ malperfusion, including but not restricted to oliguria, lactic acidosis, or altered mental status

Epidemiology

A. The systemic inflammatory response syndrome is present in 40% to 80% of ICU patients.
B. Approximately 25% will go on to develop sepsis.
C. Approximately 15% to 20% will develop severe sepsis.
D. Approximately 5% will progress to shock.

Etiology

Diverse processes may be involved in the generation and maintenance of the host inflammatory response; those most often identified include:

A. Infectious
   1. Bacterial
      a. Gram-negative bacilli
      b. Gram-positive cocci
      c. Anaerobic organisms
      d. Mycobacterial species
      e. *Legionella*
   2. Viral
      a. Cytomegalovirus
      b. Other herpes viruses
      c. Hepatitis A, B, or C
      d. Influenza virus
      e. Epstein-Barr virus
      f. Dengue
   3. Fungal
      a. Disseminated *Candida*
      b. *Blastomyces*
      c. *Coccidioides*
      d. *Histoplasma*
      e. *Aspergillus*
      f. *Pneumocystis carinii*
   4. Parasitic
      a. Toxoplasmosis
      b. Malaria
      c. *Babesia*
B. Noninfectious
   1. Pancreatitis
   2. Fulminant hepatic failure
   3. Severe trauma
   4. Severe thermal burn injury
   5. Severe gastrointestinal bleeding
   6. Subarachnoid hemorrhage
   7. Coronary artery bypass grafting

Physical Findings

A. Vital signs
   1. Tachycardia
   2. Tachypnea
   3. Fever or hypothermia
   4. Hypotension may be present

B. Cardiovascular: signs of hypovolemia and impaired perfusion are common
  1. Flat neck veins or low central venous pressure (prior to resuscitation)
  2. Widened pulse pressure
  3. Poor capillary refill (prior to resuscitation)
C. Neurologic: alterations in sensorium or mentation can occur
D. Other: findings specific to an underlying disorder (e.g., rebound abdominal tenderness from sepsis due to peritonitis, purulent sputum or signs of consolidation in sepsis due to pneumonia, fractures in SIRS due to multiple trauma, etc.)

Key Clinical and Laboratory Findings

- Fever or hypothermia

- Tachycardia

- Tachypnea or respiratory alkalosis

- Leukocytosis or leukopenia

Laboratory Findings

A. Microbiological
  1. Blood culture
    a. Unrevealing in about half of cases
    b. Specimens should be obtained no more frequently than every 24 hours
  2. Sputum Gram stain and culture
  3. Urine Gram stain and culture (should be obtained if pyuria present)
  4. Gram stains and culture of pleural, peritoneal, soft tissue, or abscess fluid (performed as indicated)
B. Hematologic
  1. Leukocyte abnormalities
    a. Leukocytosis or leukopenia
    b. Shift in leukocyte distribution toward immature forms
    c. Leukocyte inclusions (Döhle bodies)
  2. Thrombocytopenia
  3. Prolonged prothrombin or partial thromboplastin time
  4. Elevated fibrin monomer and D-dimer levels
  5. Elevated or decreased fibrinogen level
C. Arterial blood gases
  1. Respiratory alkalosis

  2. Metabolic (lactic) acidosis
  3. Widened alveolar–arterial PO_2 gradient
D. Metabolic and endocrine
  1. Hyperlactatemia
  2. Azotemia
  3. Hypo- or hyperglycemia
  4. Elevated plasma cortisol levels
  5. Ionized hypocalcemia
  6. Hypomagnesemia
  7. Abnormal thyroid function test results
E. Hepatic
  1. Elevated serum transaminase activity
  2. Conjugated hyperbilirubinemia
  3. Hypoalbuminemia
  4. Low serum prealbumin levels
F. Renal
  1. Proteinuria
  2. Azotemia
  3. Elevated serum creatinine level
G. Miscellaneous
  1. Increased C-reactive protein level
  2. Elevated procalcitonin level
  3. Elevated troponin I or troponin T level
  4. Hypocholesterolemia
  5. Abnormal cytokine levels

Testing

A. In the critically ill patient, determining the cause of the inflammatory response remains a challenge.
B. Evaluation should proceed in a logical fashion based on clinical clues and applied epidemiology.
C. Serial laboratory testing
  1. Routine serum biochemistry tests
  2. Complete blood count, including differential white blood cell and platelet counts
  3. Coagulation tests
  4. Arterial blood gases
  5. Arterial blood lactate concentration
D. Appropriate microbiological testing may include:
  1. Blood, urine, and sputum cultures
  2. Vascular catheter tip cultures
  3. Stool cultures
  4. Wound cultures (surgically obtained)
  5. Pleural or peritoneal fluid studies
  6. Cerebrospinal fluid analysis

E. Imaging studies

1. Chest x-ray

2. Consider sinus imaging.

3. Consider contrast-enhanced abdominal computed tomography.

Key Complications

- Acute respiratory distress syndrome (acute respiratory failure)

- Acute renal failure (acute tubular necrosis)

- Thrombocytopenia or disseminated intravascular coagulation

- Progression to multiple organ system failure or septic shock

Treatment

A. Intravascular volume expansion

1. Isotonic crystalloids remain the initial choice of fluids during the early phases of volume repletion for most patients with sepsis.

2. Also see Chapter 92, Septic Shock and Chapter 159, Intravenous Fluids.

3. Packed red blood cell transfusion may be appropriate in certain situations where oxygen carrying capacity is inadequate; e.g., patients with the following

   a. Concomitant coronary artery disease

   b. Refractory hypoxemia

   c. Persistent lactic acidosis

B. Control of inflammatory focus

1. Infectious

   a. Drainage of closed-space infections

   b. Removal of infected catheters or other devices

   c. Appropriate antibiotic therapy

2. Noninfectious

   a. Appropriate resuscitation

   b. Removal of devitalized tissue and necrotic debris

C. Innovative pharmacotherapies for sepsis

1. Agents that have been studied in large-scale clinical trials but that have not been shown to have benefit

   a. Monoclonal antibody against endotoxin (e.g., E5, HA1A)

   b. Interleukin-1 receptor antagonist

2. Drotrecogin alfa activated (human recombinant activated protein C)

   a. Has antithrombotic, profibrinolytic, and anti-inflammatory effects

   b. Shown in the Protein C Worldwide Evaluation in Severe Sepsis (PROWESS) trial to reduce 28-day mortality from 30.8% in controls to 24.7% in patients receiving drotrecogin

   c. Approved by the U.S. Food and Drug Administration for treatment of severe sepsis

   d. Contraindicated in patients with active hemorrhage or at risk for serious bleeding (see package insert)

   e. Serious bleeding events occurred in 3.5% of patients receiving drotrecogin compared to 2% of controls in the PROWESS trial.

   f. Administered by continuous intravenous infusion at 24 μg/kg per hour for 96 hours.

3. Other investigational agents

   a. Tissue factor pathway inhibitor

   b. Exogenous antithrombin III

   c. Platelet activating factor antagonists

   d. Monoclonal antibodies against tumor necrosis factor-α

Key Treatment

- Identification of inciting event

- Aggressive restoration of intravascular volume deficits

- Appropriate antibiotic therapy if SIRS is attributed to infection

- Removal of necrotic tissue or drainage of closed-space infection

- Monitoring and supportive care

Prognosis

A. The mortality rate associated with the development of sepsis or SIRS is strongly associated with the underlying illness.

B. Mortality is also associated with the duration and severity of the inflammatory response and the presence of sepsis or septic shock.

1. SIRS

   a. Meeting 2 SIRS criteria: 6%

   b. Meeting 3 SIRS criteria: 9%

   c. Meeting 4 SIRS criteria: 18%

2. Sepsis

    a. Culture positive: 16%

    b. Culture negative: 10%

3. Severe sepsis

    a. Culture positive: 20%

    b. Culture negative: 16%

4. Septic shock: approximately 50%, regardless of culture status

Bibliography

Bernard GR, Vincent J-L, Laterre P-F, et al. Efficacy and safety of recombinant human activated protein C for severe sepsis. N Engl J Med 2001;344:699–709.

Bone RC, Balk RA, Cerra FB, et al. Definitions for sepsis and organ failure and guidelines for the use of innovative therapies in sepsis. Chest 1992;101:1644–1655.

Brun-Buisson C, Doyon F, Carlet J, et al. Bacteremia and severe sepsis in adults: a multicenter prospective survey in ICUs and wards of 24 hospitals. Am J Respir Crit Care Med 1996;154:617–624.

Muckart DJJ, Bhagwanjee S. American College of Chest Physicians/Society of Critical Care Medicine Consensus Conference definitions on the systemic inflammatory response syndrome and allied disorders in relation to critically injured patients. Crit Care Med 1997;25:1789–1795.

Oberhoffer M, Karzai W, Meier-Hellmann A, et al. Sensitivity and specificity of various markers of inflammation for the prediction of tumor necrosis factor-α and interleukin-6 in patients with sepsis. Crit Care Med 1999;27:1814–1818.

O'Grady NP, Barie PS, Bartlett J, et al. Practice parameters for evaluating new fever in critically ill adult patients. Crit Care Med 1998;26:392–408.

Pittet D, Thiévent B, Wenzel RP, et al. Importance of pre-existing co-morbidities for prognosis of septicemia in critically ill patients. Intensive Care Med 1993;19:265–272.

Rangel-Frausto MS, Pittet D, Costigan M, et al. The natural history of the systemic inflammatory response syndrome (SIRS): a prospective study. JAMA 1995;273:117–123.

92 Septic Shock

Dane J. Nichols

Pathophysiology

A. Circulatory shock represents an imbalance between the body's metabolic demands for substrate and oxygen and its ability to meet those requirements.

B. In septic shock this imbalance may result from any of the following.

1. Global hypoperfusion
   a. Myocardial dysfunction
   b. Decreased perfusion pressure due to excessive vasodilation
   c. Concomitant hypovolemia
   d. Microcirculatory thrombosis

2. Regional maldistribution of nutrient blood flow or tissue oxygen delivery
   a. Microcirculatory shunting of blood flow from tissues with high metabolic demand to tissues with lower metabolic demand
      (1) Excessive nitric oxide production
      (2) Microcirculatory thrombosis
   b. Transluminal oxygen diffusion from arterioles to adjacent venules, augmented by increased countercurrent blood flow

3. Intracellular metabolic derangements
   a. Augmented glycolysis
   b. Mitochondrial dysfunction

4. Hypermetabolism
   a. Fever
   b. Systemic inflammation

C. Organ system dysfunction or failure

1. From perfusion failure, tissue dysoxia, or other mechanisms affecting one or more organ systems

2. Potentially involved organ systems and key manifestations:
   a. Lungs: acute respiratory distress syndrome and acute respiratory failure
   b. Kidneys: acute tubular necrosis and acute renal failure
   c. Central nervous system (CNS): altered sensorium, delirium, encephalopathy, coma
   d. Cardiovascular: heart failure (including high-output failure), hypotension, elevated filling pressures

   e. Liver: abnormal hepatic function tests, cholestasis, shock liver
   f. Hematologic: thrombocytopenia, coagulopathy
   g. Gastrointestinal (GI) tract: diarrhea, ileus, ischemic bowel

3. Factors that may contribute to the development of multiple organ system failure
   a. Lack of aggressive, early resuscitation
   b. Inappropriate antibiotic selection
   c. Failure to achieve local control of infection
   d. Exaggerated host responses to inflammatory stimuli

Key Definition

Septic shock: sepsis-associated hypotension, despite adequate fluid resuscitation, associated with evidence of end-organ malperfusion including but not restricted to oliguria, lactic acidosis, or altered mental status

Etiology

A. Site of infection

1. A presumptive focus of sepsis is identified in more than 95% of cases.

2. Common primary sites
   a. Pleuropulmonary
   b. Primary bacteremia
   c. Urinary tract
   d. Intra-abdominal source

3. A primary source cannot be identified in 3% to 4% of patients with septic shock.

B. Infectious agents

1. Microbiological confirmation occurs approximately 70% of the time.

2. Commonly involved organisms
   a. Gram-negative bacteria: approximately 30% to 40% of cases
      (1) *Escherichia coli*
      (2) *Klebsiella* species
      (3) *Pseudomonas aeruginosa*
   b. Gram-positive bacteria: approximately 30% to 50% of cases
      (1) *Staphylococcus aureus*

321

(2) *Streptococcus pneumoniae*

(3) *Enterococcus* species

  c. Polymicrobial: approximately 13% to 20%

  d. Anaerobic bacteria: approximately 2% to 5%

  e. Fungi: approximately 2 to 3%

Epidemiology

A. Approximately 1% of hospitalized patients develop bacteremia.

B. Approximately 0.3% of hospitalized patients develop severe sepsis from bacteremia.

C. Nosocomial bacteremia accounts for 45% of cases.

D. 40% to 70% of patients develop severe sepsis or septic shock 24 to 72 hours after recognition of the systemic inflammatory response syndrome (SIRS); see Chapter 91, Sepsis and SIRS.

E. Approximately 50 to 60% of patients will develop 2 or more organ system failures.

F. Mortality from septic shock ranges from 30% to 70%.

Risk Factors

A. Immunosuppression

B. Malignancy

C. Organ transplantation

D. Indwelling catheters or other implanted devices

E. Genetically determined cytokine expression (?)

Physical Findings

A. Vital signs
1. Hypotension
2. Tachycardia
3. Tachypnea
4. Fever or hypothermia

B. Cardiovascular
1. Flat neck veins or low central venous pressure (before resuscitation)
2. Widened pulse pressure (after resuscitation), unless hypotension is severe
3. Cool, mottled extremities

C. Pulmonary
1. Focal signs of consolidation
2. Rales secondary to permeability pulmonary edema

D. Gastrointestinal
1. Signs of regional inflammation: e.g., ileus, vomiting, rebound tenderness
2. Absent bowel sounds
3. Evidence of GI hemorrhage

E. Neurologic
1. Alterations in sensorium or mentation: e.g., confusion, somnolence, agitation
2. Signs of CNS infection: e.g., meningismus, seizures, focal weakness

F. Hematologic
1. Overt bleeding; e.g., epistaxis, GI hemorrhage, oozing from puncture sites
2. Petechiae or purpuric cutaneous lesions
3. Digital ischemia

G. Renal
1. Oliguria
2. Gross pyuria

Differential Diagnosis

A. Cardiogenic shock: e.g, myocardial infarction, valvular heart disease, cardiomyopathy (viral, ischemic, infiltrative, peripartum, or idiopathic)

B. Obstructive shock: e.g., aortic dissection, critical valvular stenosis, pulmonary embolism, cardiac tamponade, constrictive pericarditis

C. Hypovolemic shock: e.g., traumatic or nontraumatic hemorrhage, environmental exposure, severe gastroenteritis, pancreatitis

D. Distributive shock: e.g., salicylate intoxication, Addisonian crisis, fulminant hepatic failure, neurogenic causes

Key Complications

Organ System Dysfunction or Failure	Other Complications
• Catecholamine-refractory hypotension	• Fluid, electrolyte, and acid-base disturbances
• Acute tubular necrosis	• Critical illness polyneuropathy
• Acute respiratory distress syndrome	• Antibiotic-associated diarrhea
• Thrombocytopenia and coagulopathy	• Nosocomial superinfection
• Encephalopathy	

Treatment

A. General principles
1. Maintenance of adequate tissue perfusion and oxygenation

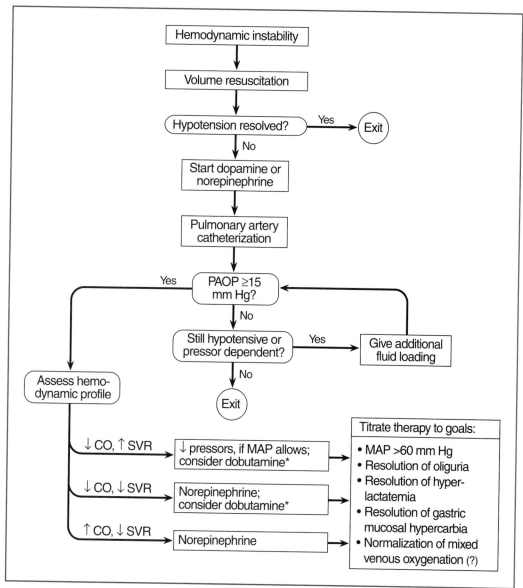

Figure 92-1 Suggested algorithm for management of hemodynamic instability in septic shock. PAOP = pulmonary artery occlusion pressure; MAP = mean arterial blood pressure; CO = cardiac output; SVR = systemic vascular resistance; * = blood pressure should be controlled with vasopressor prior to initiating dobutamine to minimize risk of precipitating severe hypotension.

2. Identification and control of the source of infection

3. Blunting the inflammatory cascade

B. General measures

  1. Intensive care unit admission

  2. Continuous electrocardiographic monitoring

  3. Continuous pulse oximetry

  4. Continuous intra-arterial blood pressure monitoring

  5. Serial laboratory testing (arterial blood gases and lactate, routine serum biochemistry tests, complete blood count, coagulation tests, etc.)

  6. Assure adequate airway and ventilation

C. Hemodynamic support (Fig. 92-1)

  1. Intravascular volume expansion

    a. Initial fluid requirements may be quite large, exceeding 6 to 10 L of crystalloid or 2 to 4 L of colloid in the first 24 hours in some cases.

    b. Continue until hemodynamic goals are met.

    c. Crystalloids

      (1) Recommended as initial choice for fluid resuscitation in most situations

      (2) Large volumes of normal saline are associated with the development of hyperchloremic metabolic acidosis.

(3) To achieve similar degrees of volume expansion, 2 to 5 times as much crystalloid as colloid is required.

(4) Result in decreased plasma colloid oncotic pressure and are less effective than colloids in achieving rapid intravascular volume expansion

d. Colloids

(1) Acceptable for use after administration of more than 2 L of crystalloids if hemodynamic end points are not achieved

(2) Vary in their ability to be retained in the vascular space

(3) Carry a small risk of anaphylaxis and are costly

(4) Hetastarch has been associated with alterations in coagulation profiles, but this appears to be of little consequence when administered volumes are less than 1.5 L/day.

e. Packed red blood cells

(1) Alter viscosity and rheologic properties of the blood

(2) Stored blood has impaired ability to unload oxygen to tissues.

(3) Alter immune response secondary to co-infused leukocytes

(4) In general, should be reserved for patients with hemoglobin concentrations lower than 8 g/dL, those demonstrating persistent lactic acidosis, low SvO_2, evidence of coronary ischemia, or bleeding

2. Vasoactive and inotropic support (see Chapter 161, Vasoactive Catecholamines)

a. Dopamine

(1) Initial drug of choice in septic shock

(2) Has been associated with lower gastric intramucosal pH, diminished thyrotropin and prolactin release, and blunted ventilatory response to hypercarbia

b. Norepinephrine

(1) More likely to achieve hemodynamic targets than dopamine

(2) Exhibits less chronotropic effect than dopamine

c. Epinephrine

(1) A potent α- and β-adrenergic agonist

(2) Combination therapy using dobutamine and norepinephrine is more effective in experimental settings.

d. Dobutamine

(1) Potent inotrope

(2) Has vasodilator properties that can precipitate or worsen hypotension

(3) Can have substantial chronotropic and dysrhythmogenic effects

e. Phenylephrine

(1) A pure α-adrenergic agonist having vasoconstrictive but no inotropic action

(2) Limited experience for use in treating septic shock

f. Vasopressin

(1) A potent, non-catecholamine vasoconstrictor

(2) May have a role for catecholamine-refractory hypotension

g. L-N^G-methylarginine

(1) An investigational inhibitor of nitric oxide synthesis with effective vasoconstrictive action

(2) Clinical trials involving this agent in the treatment of patients with septic shock showed a negative effect on outcome.

3. End points of hemodynamic therapy

a. Mean arterial blood pressure

(1) Should be maintained higher than 60 mm Hg

(2) Perfusion may be inadequate in chronically hypertensive patients maintained at this level.

(3) Central MAP may be underestimated by short radial artery catheters.

b. Pulmonary artery occlusion pressure

(1) Initial target is 12 to 15 mm Hg

(2) Further fluid loading should be guided by serial assessments of cardiac performance.

c. Cardiac index and systemic oxygen delivery

(1) Augmentation of subnormal levels is part of conventional therapy.

(2) Efforts to routinely drive patients to supranormal oxygen delivery (cardiac index higher than 4.5 L/min per m^2; oxygen delivery greater than 600 mL/min per m^2) have not been associated with improved survival in most randomized trials.

d. Arterial blood lactate: declining or normal concentration

e. Blood oxygenation: SpO_2 >92%

f. Urine output

(1) Oliguria can be secondary to inadequate systemic or regional (renal) perfusion.

(2) May also be due to intrinsic renal dysfunction; e.g., acute tubular necrosis

D. Anti-infective therapy

1. Use broad-spectrum agents directed at the most likely organisms.

2. Use appropriate loading regimens and dosing intervals.

3. Consider special coverage requirements for neutropenic hosts, transplant recipients, and HIV positive patients.

E. Adjunctive therapy

1. Mechanical ventilation

a. Improves short-term survival in animal models.

b. Up to 30% of cardiac output is directed to muscles of respiration during acute respiratory failure.

2. Antipyretic therapy

a. Lowers oxygen demand and consumption

b. May interfere with normal immune response

c. Consider in patients with marginal oxygenation.

d. Ibuprofen more effective antipyretic than acetaminophen

3. Sedation with or without therapeutic paralysis

a. Reduces oxygen demand and consumption

b. Consider for intubated patients.

4. Corticosteroids

a. Short-term high doses have been shown in randomized controlled clinical trials to be ineffective.

b. Physiologic doses may improve α- and β-adrenergic receptor function and decrease duration of vasopressor therapy.

5. Drotrecogin alfa activated and various novel, investigational pharmacotherapies (see Chapter 91, Sepsis and SIRS)

Prognosis

A. Outcome from septic shock is closely tied to several factors:

1. The host's hemodynamic response to sepsis

2. Development and extent of multiple organ dysfunction

3. Site of infectious focus and virulence of the involved organism

4. Underlying and co-morbid diseases

B. Mortality ranges from 30% to 80%.

1. 70% to 80% of the mortality is expressed within the first 7 to 14 days.

2. Mortality is higher in euthermic or hypothermic patients than in febrile patients.

C. Metabolic markers

1. Arterial blood lactate: marked and sustained elevations predict poor outcome

2. C-reactive protein

a. Reflects interleukin-6 activity

b. Sustained or increasing levels beyond day 3 are associated with higher mortality.

3. Low serum albumin or prealbumin: reflects ongoing reprioritization of hepatic protein synthesis and capillary leak

D. Hemodynamic markers

1. Prognosis is better in those patients capable of achieving supranormal perfusion and oxygen transport during the early phases of resuscitation.

a. Oxygen delivery >600 mL/min per m²

b. Oxygen consumption >170 mL/min per m²

c. Cardiac index > 4.5 L/min per m²

2. Prognosis is better in those patients capable of increasing oxygen consumption by more than 15% during infusion of dobutamine at 10 μg/kg per min (dobutamine flux test).

E. Organ dysfunction

1. Tenfold increase in mortality when any organ dysfunction complicates bacteremic sepsis

2. Survivors of bacteremic sepsis average one organ dysfunction, whereas nonsurvivors average three to four dysfunctions.

Key End Points of Resuscitation

- Mean arterial pressure greater than 60 mm Hg

- Pulmonary artery occlusion pressure 12 to 15 mm Hg

- Normal or elevated cardiac index

- Hemoglobin concentration greater than 8 g/dL

- Arterial oxyhemoglobin saturation greater than 92%

- Normal or declining arterial blood lactate concentration

Bibliography

Brun-Buisson C, Doyon F, Carlet J, et al. Incidence, risk factors, and outcome of severe sepsis and septic shock in adults. A multicenter, prospective study in intensive care units. JAMA 1995:274:968–974.

Carlet J, Artigas A, Bihari D, et al. Tissue hypoxia. How to detect, how to correct, how to prevent. Am J Respir Crit Care Med 1996;154:1573–1578.

Choi PTL, Yip G, Quinonez LG, et al. Crystalloids vs. colloids in fluid resuscitation: a systematic review. Crit Care Med 1999;27:200–210.

Dorman T, Breslow MJ, Lipsett PA, et al. Radial pressure monitoring underestimates central arterial pressure during vasopressor therapy in critically ill surgical patients. Crit Care Med 1998;26:1646–1649.

Hébert PC, Wells G, Blajchman MA, et al. A multicenter, randomized, controlled clinical trial of transfusion requirements in critical care. N Engl J Med 1999;340:409–417.

Heyland DK, Cook DJ, King D, et al. Maximizing oxygen delivery in critically ill patients: a methodologic appraisal of the evidence. Crit Care Med 1996;24:517–524.

Malay MB, Ashton RC Jr, Landry DW, et al. Low-dose vasopressin in the treatment of vasodilatory septic shock. J Trauma Infection Crit Care 1999;47:699–705.

Pittet D, Thiévent B, Wenzel RP, et al. Bedside prediction of mortality from bacteremic sepsis. A dynamic analysis of ICU patients. Am J Respir Crit Care Med 1996:153:684–693.

Task force of the American College of Critical Care Medicine, Society of Critical Care Medicine. Practice parameters for hemodynamic support of sepsis in adult patients in sepsis. Crit Care Med 1999;27:639–660.

93 Gram-Positive Infections

Donald P. Levine

Compared with their Gram-negative counterparts, far fewer Gram-positive pathogens are likely to be encountered by the critical care specialist. Nevertheless, they are just as likely to be associated with serious disease. Unlike Gram-negative bacteria, they are more capable of producing life-threatening or fatal infection in patients without an underlying immunologic abnormality or indwelling invasive device. Many species of Gram-positive organisms produce disease in humans. Those presented here are the ones most likely to cause infection serious enough to require management in an intensive care setting.

Epidemiology

A. *Staphylococcus aureus*
1. Represents 15% to 20% of all bacteremias; 10% of nosocomial infection
2. Intravenous catheter-related sepsis common; also cellulitis, other skin and soft tissue infections, pneumonia, endocarditis, bone, central nervous system (CNS) catheters
3. Anterior nasal (~20%) and vaginal carriage (~10%) common
4. High risk for colonization
   a. Injection drug use
   b. Insulin-dependent diabetes mellitus
   c. Hemodialysis and peritoneal dialysis
   d. Chronic skin lesions
   e. Burn injury
5. High risk of nosocomial transmission
   a. High carriage rate among physicians and nurses
   b. Airborne transmission from respiratory infection, shedders
   c. Lack of handwashing

B. Coagulase-negative staphylococci
1. Indwelling vascular catheters
2. Prosthetic devices
3. Cardiac pacemakers
4. Hemodialysis shunts
5. Neutropenia

C. Group A streptococci
1. Carriage is infrequent in adults
2. Carriage sites: pharyngeal (most common), skin, rectum, vagina

D. Group B streptococci
1. Elderly and debilitated hosts
2. Underlying conditions: diabetes mellitus, malignancy, chronic renal failure, liver disease, cerebrovascular disease, dementia, colonized urogenital tract, post-partum infection (especially post–cesarean section)

E. *Streptococcus pneumoniae*
1. Oropharyngeal colonization, highest in closed populations
2. Serious sepsis in splenectomized patients
3. Multiple myeloma
4. Congenital agammaglobulinemia
5. Chronic and acute myelogenous leukemia
6. Human immunodeficiency virus (HIV) infection

F. *Streptococcus viridans*
1. Hepatic disease
2. Diabetes mellitus
3. Cardiac valve defects, congenital or acquired

G. *Enterococcus*
1. Normal flora of gastrointestinal tract, vagina
2. Transmission via hand-to-hand contact in hospitals
3. Nosocomial acquisition
4. Urogenital tract instrumentation
5. Postoperative and postpartum infections
6. Burn injury
7. Prolonged intensive care unit stay

H. *Corynebacterium*
1. *C. jeikeium:* neutropenia, prolonged antibiotic use, prolonged hospitalization
2. *C. striatum:* normal flora of anterior nares and skin (face and upper trunk)
3. *C. pseudodiphtheriticum:* immunosuppression, cardiopulmonary abnormalities

I. *Listeria monocytogenes*
1. Age 60 years or older
2. Pregnant women
3. Immunosuppression: hematologic malignancy, HIV, organ transplantation, corticosteroid therapy
4. Foodborne illness: ready-to-eat (delicatessen) meats, soft cheeses

J. *Rhodococcus equi:* defective cell-mediated immunity, respiratory infection with dissemination

K. *Bacillus cereus:* device-related nosocomial infection, injection drug users

L. *Clostridium perfringens*

1. Ubiquitous in intestinal tract and soil

2. From traumatic wounds (e.g., motor vehicle, agricultural; most often with open fractures), surgical wounds (especially colon and biliary tract), abortion, and underlying vascular insufficiency

Diagnosis and Treatment of Staphylococcal Infections

A. *Staphylococcus aureus*

1. Bacteremia

a. Clinical findings: obtundation, fever, chills, tachycardia, pleuritic chest pain, joint pain or swelling, purulent discharge (e.g., from IV site), skin lesions (e.g., cellulitis, Osler nodes, Janeway lesions, petechiae, necrosis), meningeal signs, focal neurologic signs (from brain embolus or mycotic aneurysm), conjunctival hemorrhages, Roth spots, rales, pleural or pericardial friction rub, murmur, splenomegaly, back pain

b. Differential diagnosis: clinically indistinguishable from streptococcal infection

c. Tests: culture of blood and other suspected body fluids; imaging studies (e.g., echocardiogram if endocarditis suspected; x-rays of spine or joint, when involved; magnetic resonance imaging [MRI] for suspected intracranial lesions, Doppler-ultrasound of suspected involved vessels)

d. Treatment: remove all suspected infected vascular devices, drain all infected fluid collections if possible, administer antistaphylococcal antibiotic for 2 weeks (4 to 6 weeks if cardiac source)

2. Toxic shock syndrome (see Chapter 110, Toxic Shock Syndrome)

3. Pneumonia

a. Clinical findings: dyspnea, productive cough, chest pain, systemic toxicity, obtundation; clinically indistinguishable from other serious pneumonias

b. Tests

(1) Chest x-ray: infiltrates, typically multiple, bilateral, predominantly in lower lobes; cavitation and abscess common; pneumatoceles; pleural effusion

(2) Sputum Gram stain, sputum and blood cultures

c. Treatment: antistaphylococcal antibiotic

4. Empyema

a. Clinical findings: dyspnea, chest pain, tachycardia; loculation common

b. Tests

(1) Imaging studies: chest x-ray, with decubitus view; ultrasonography

(2) Thoracentesis: Gram stain, cell count, culture, biochemical tests on fluid

(3) Blood culture

c. Treatment: drainage of empyema, usually requiring tube thoracostomy; surgical repair of bronchopleural fistula, if present; antistaphylococcal antibiotic

5. Brain abscess (most often secondary to embolization from infected mitral or aortic valve)

a. Clinical findings: fever, meningism, focal neurologic findings; patients more often present with signs of sepsis than anaerobic or polymicrobial brain abscess, per se

b. Tests

(1) Blood cultures; aspirate abscess fluid for Gram stain and culture

(2) Imaging studies: MRI or computed tomography (CT) with contrast, often showing multiple, scattered abscesses throughout brain but favoring middle cerebral artery distribution; echocardiogram, if endocarditis suspected

c. Treatment: drainage may be required for large or encapsulated abscesses, significant effacement of ventricles, raised intracranial pressure; smaller abscesses may respond to antibiotic therapy alone

6. Spinal epidural abscess

a. Source: complication of spinal osteomyelitis or hematogenous dissemination

b. Clinical findings: fever, spinal ache, radiculitis, paralysis, other focal neurologic deficit; subtle presentation

c. Tests

(1) Imaging studies: x-ray, MRI, or CT of spine; echocardiogram, if findings suggestive of underlying endocarditis

(2) Aspiration or biopsy for Gram stain and culture

(3) Blood cultures

d. Treatment: urgent surgical drainage required if focal deficits, paresis, or paralysis; antibiotic therapy alone may be adequate if only pain or radiculitis

7. Subdural empyema

   a. Source: complication of sinusitis, surgery, or trauma

   b. Clinical findings: fever, headache, vomiting, meningism, altered mental status, seizures, focal neurologic signs

   c. Imaging: MRI with contrast

   d. Treatment: surgical drainage and antistaphylococcal antibiotic coverage

8. Intracranial septic thrombophlebitis

   a. Source: complication of sinusitis, orbital cellulitis, soft-tissue infection

   b. Clinical findings: depend on anatomic location

     (1) Cavernous sinus: ptosis, other cranial nerve deficits, proptosis

     (2) Sagittal sinus: altered mental state, upper and lower extremity weakness

   c. Imaging: MRI with contrast

   d. Treatment: antistaphylococcal antibiotic

B. Coagulase-negative staphylococci

1. Infective endocarditis (also see Chapter 105, Endocarditis)

   a. Sources: prosthetic valve involvement (40% *S. epidermidis*); native valve uncommon (requires prior valve damage)

   b. Clinical findings: prolonged fever common; prosthetic valve dysfunction common (defect of sewing ring); cardiac dysrhythmia (see Chapter 105)

   c. Tests: blood cultures, echocardiogram

   d. Treatment: antibiotics; valve replacement for valve dysfunction or hemodynamic instability

Key Antibiotic Treatment for Serious Staphylococcal Infections

- For *S. aureus* bacteremia: nafcillin or oxacillin 2 g every 4 hours; cefazolin 2 g every 8 hours, if non-life-threatening penicillin allergy; vancomycin 1 g every 12 hours, if life-threatening penicillin allergy or methicillin-resistant strain suspected; penicillin G 2 g every 4 hours, if susceptible

- For *S. aureus* pneumonia or empyema: same

- For *S. aureus* CNS infections: same except increase nafcillin or oxacillin to 2 to 3 g every 4 hours, vancomycin to 2 g every 12 hours

- Coagulase-negative endocarditis: use vancomycin 1 g every 12 hours (unless methicillin-sensitive), plus gentamicin and rifampin

Diagnosis and Treatment of Streptococcal Infections

A. Group A streptococci

1. Necrotizing fasciitis

   a. Clinical findings

     (1) Rapid evolution from unapparent skin lesion, superficial lesion, surgical or traumatic wound to extensive, inflammatory process

     (2) Fever; exquisite pain and tenderness, disproportionate to visible disease; swelling; erythema; dusky to ecchymotic skin; yellow or hemorrhagic bullae; skin necrosis; rapid development of septic shock

     (3) Resembles necrotizing fasciitis caused by other organisms or mixed infection

     (4) Rhabdomyolysis, may be delayed 2 to 3 days

   b. Differential diagnosis: deep vein thrombophlebitis, muscle strain, cellulitis, other causes of rhabdomyolysis

   c. Diagnosis

     (1) Requires high level of suspicion when patient has fever, severe pain, signs of sepsis, and elevated serum creatine phosphokinase (CK) activity

     (2) Immediate surgical exploration of lesion: assess muscle viability; biopsy or frozen section may help; blunt probe of fascia to determine if intact

   d. Tests: Gram stain and culture; x-ray, CT or MRI may reveal lesion or demonstrate soft tissue swelling, but these delay diagnosis and are unnecessary

   e. Treatment: extensive debridement, which should be repeated to assure removal of all non-viable tissue; antibiotic treatment; avoid nonsteroidal anti-inflammatory drugs as they are associated with worse prognosis

2. Streptococcal toxic shock syndrome (see Chapter 110, Toxic Shock Syndrome)

3. Pneumonia

   a. Clinical findings: abrupt onset, fever, chills, productive cough (frequently with blood streaking), pleuritic chest pain, signs of consolidation (uncommon), percussion dullness (up to 40% develop empyema), rales

   b. Tests: sputum Gram stain (indistinguishable from *S. pneumoniae*) and culture; blood cultures (bacteremia in up to 15%)

c. Treatment: penicillin, cefazolin, or clindamycin 900 mg every 8 hours (if life-threatening penicillin allergy)

B. Group B streptococci

1. Several typical clinical presentations

a. Primary bacteremia

b. Pregnancy-related infections: wound infection or endometritis after cesarean section; urinary tract infection; meningitis after epidural anesthesia

c. Endocarditis

d. Meningitis: malignancy; after neurosurgery or epidural catheterization

e. Recurrent infection common: associated with inadequate dose or duration of antibiotic therapy for initial infection

f. Almost always a serious underlying disease

2. Clinical findings

a. Fever, chills, malaise, local signs consistent with site of infection, meningeal irritation, uterine tenderness, signs of systemic embolization

b. Indistinguishable from symptoms associated with other organisms

3. Tests

a. Gram stain and cultures (as appropriate) of blood, cerebrospinal fluid (CSF), lochia, urine

4. Treatment

a. Penicillin, cefazolin, or vancomycin

b. Duration of antibiotic therapy

(1) Bacteremia: 10 days

(2) Meningitis: 14 to 21 days

(3) Endocarditis: 4 to 6 weeks

(4) Soft tissue infection: 10 days

C. *Streptococcus pneumoniae*

1. Pneumonia

a. Clinical findings: fever, chills, cough (usually productive), dyspnea, pleuritic pain, malaise, tachycardia, tachypnea, splinting on involved side, increased tactile fremitus (if consolidation; now uncommon), percussion dullness or flatness in patients with effusion, bronchial breath sounds (if consolidation), rales

b. Tests: chest x-ray; sputum Gram stain and culture; blood cultures

c. Empiric treatment: see Key Antibiotic Treatment box

2. Meningitis: there are no clinical features to distinguish pneumococcal meningitis from infection caused by any other organism (see Chapter 108, Meningitis)

3. Primary (spontaneous) bacterial peritonitis: indistinguishable from disease due to other organisms (see Chapter 94, Gram-Negative Infections)

D. *Streptococcus viridans*

1. Endocarditis

a. Clinical findings

(1) Insidious onset with progressive disease

(2) Fever; malaise; anorexia; weight loss; neurologic deficit (often secondary to embolus or ruptured mycotic aneurysm); murmur (~90%); splenomegaly (~50%); immunologic findings (~30%)—i.e., Osler nodes, Janeway lesions, Roth spots, splinter hemorrhages

b. Diagnosis and treatment (see Chapter 105, Endocarditis)

Key Antibiotic Treatment for Serious Streptococcal Infections

- For necrotizing fasciitis: penicillin G 1 to 2 million units intravenously every 4 hours, plus clindamycin (900 mg every 8 hours) for first several days to inhibit toxin production

- For pneumonia caused by group A streptococci: penicillin G 1 million units every 4 hours; or cefazolin 1 to 2 g every 8 hours, if non-life-threatening penicillin allergy; or clindamycin 900 mg every 8 hours, if life-threatening penicillin allergy

- For group B streptococci: penicillin G 2 million units every 4 hours; or cefazolin 2 g every 8 hours, if non-life-threatening penicillin allergy; or vancomycin 1 g every 12 hours, if life-threatening penicillin allergy

- For *S. pneumoniae* pneumonia: levofloxacin, ± vancomycin if penicillin resistance is suspected; or penicillin G 1 million units every 4 hours; or cefazolin 1 to 2 g every 8 hours, if non-life-threatening penicillin allergy; or clindamycin 900 mg every 8 hours, if life-threatening penicillin allergy

- For *S. pneumoniae* meningitis: see Chapter 108, Meningitis

- For *S. viridans* endocarditis: see Chapter 105, Endocarditis

Diagnosis and Treatment of Enterococcal Infections

A. *Enterococcus* (*E. faecalis* and *E. faecium*)

1. Bacteremia

a. Source

(1) Invariably occurs in patients with serious underlying disease; high mortality rate; septic shock can occur, usually as part of polymicrobial infection that includes Gram-negative organisms

(2) Nosocomial (e.g., urinary tract, IV catheter, burn wound; intra-abdominal abscess or peritonitis less common; frequently polymicrobial) or primary (usually in immunocompromised or otherwise severely ill patients; most often monomicrobial)

b. Tests: blood cultures; catheter tip cultures (vascular catheters only) to verify source

c. Treatment: Key Antibiotic Treatment box

2. Urinary tract infection

a. Source: cystitis, pyelonephritis, perinephric abscess, prostatitis; most often nosocomial, associated with urinary tract instrumentation

b. Diagnosis and treatment: see the Key Antibiotic Treatment box and Chapter 106, Urosepsis

3. Endocarditis

a. Source: frequently associated with prosthetic valve infection, especially left-sided infection; resembles sub-acute infection seen with *S. viridans*; more common in elderly men

b. Diagnosis and treatment: see Chapter 105, Endocarditis

Key Antibiotic Treatment for Enterococcal Infections

- Bacteremia: penicillin or ampicillin usually sufficient for uncomplicated cases; vancomycin for penicillin-allergic patients; gentamicin (if susceptible) may be added for acutely ill patients

- Urinary tract infection: ampicillin or penicillin adequate; vancomycin for penicillin-allergic patients; synergistic therapy rarely necessary

- Vancomycin-resistant strains: require alternative therapy, e.g., tetracycline, ampicillin, or penicillin (if susceptible); quinupristin-dalfopristin (vancomycin-resistant *E. faecium* only); linezolid (vancomycin-resistant *E. faecium* and *E. faecalis*)

- Endocarditis: see Chapter 105, Endocarditis

Diagnosis and Treatment of Other Gram-Positive Infections

A. *Corynebacterium jeikeium*

1. Source

a. Sepsis in immunocompromised patients, especially those with lymphoreticular neo-

plasms; rarely infect nonimmunosuppressed individuals

b. Prosthetic valve (and rarely native valve) endocarditis

c. Pneumonia (with cavitation), meningitis, CNS shunt infections

d. Risk factors: prolonged neutropenia and hospitalization, prior broad-spectrum antibiotics, vascular catheters or other invasive devices that break skin barrier, cardiac surgery

2. Treatment: vancomycin (virtually all strains are multiply resistant to all other antibiotics); removal of prosthetic material, unless infection rapidly controlled

B. *Corynebacterium striatum* and *pseudodiphtheriticum*

1. Clinical findings

a. Endocarditis, necrotizing pleuropulmonary disease, sepsis in neutropenic patients, catheter-related infections

b. Increasing reports of infection due to non-diphtheria strains with similar clinical profiles

2. Treatment: most isolates are vancomycin or penicillin susceptible; susceptibility testing advised because there is occasional broad resistance

C. *Listeria monocytogenes*

1. Meningitis

a. Clinical findings: may have subacute presentation; seizures more likely than with other pathogens; nuchal rigidity often absent

b. Differential diagnosis: tuberculous meningitis, aseptic meningitis, encephalitis

c. Tests

(1) Cerebrospinal fluid Gram stain positive in less than 50% of cases

(2) Cerebrospinal fluid glucose normal in most cases

(3) Approximately 1/3 of cases have mononuclear pleocytosis.

(4) Blood culture more often positive than with other pathogens (~75%)

d. Treatment

(1) Repeat lumbar puncture in 12 to 24 hours if initial tap is nondiagnostic.

(2) Ampicillin plus aminoglycoside is treatment of choice.

2. Sepsis in pregnancy

a. Source: late pregnancy (usually third trimester)

b. Clinical findings: acute-onset fever, arthralgia, myalgia, backache, headache; premature labor or stillbirth

   c. Tests: blood cultures

   d. Treatment: ampicillin or penicillin (equally effective); trimethoprim-sulfamethoxazole

D. *Rhodococcus equi*

  1. Clinical findings

   a. Most infections occur in patients with altered cellular immunity—most commonly patients with acquired immunodeficiency syndrome (AIDS).

   b. Pleuropulmonary infections predominate, frequently with cavitation.

   c. Disseminated disease uncommon (abscesses, endophthalmitis)

  2. Differential diagnosis: tuberculosis, nocardiosis, anaerobic lung abscess

  3. Tests

   a. Chest x-ray (cavitation common)

   b. Gram and acid-fast stain (frequently acid-fast) and culture of sputum or suspected body fluid

   c. Invasive procedure to obtain specimen often required

  4. Treatment

   a. Vancomycin is drug of choice; erythromycin plus rifampin is second choice.

   b. Treat for 2 to 3 months in most non-AIDS patients; continuous suppression may be necessary in AIDS patients.

E. *Bacillus* spp. *(B. cereus)* ophthalmic infection

  1. Source: post-traumatic, frequently with intraocular foreign body; injection drug use

  2. Clinical findings: periorbital edema, proptosis, corneal edema, panophthalmitis, ring abscess formation, destruction of vitreous and retina with rapid deterioration of vision (within 12 to 48 hours of inoculation)

  3. Diagnosis

   a. Requires a high index of suspicion in drug user or post-traumatic patient with rapid destructive process in the eye

   b. Immediate aspirate of ocular fluid for Gram stain and culture

  4. Treatment

   a. Immediate vitrectomy and intravitreous instillation of clindamycin plus gentamicin, and corticosteroids

F. *Clostridium perfringens* (clostridial gas gangrene)

  1. Source: after trauma, surgery (especially abdominal), abortion, burn injury

  2. Clinical findings

   a. Local: sudden-onset severe pain; swelling; pallor, edema; followed by bronze discoloration; crepitance, a late sign that may be absent; bullae; serosanguineous discharge with a sweet odor

   b. Systemic: extreme anxiety; diaphoresis; tachycardia, hypotension, coma; edema; discoloration of lesion site; exquisite tenderness disproportionate to lesion appearance; hemorrhagic bullae; crepitance; hemorrhage secondary to disseminated intravascular coagulation

  3. Differential diagnosis: crepitant cellulitis, necrotizing fasciitis, streptococcal myonecrosis; requires immediate exploration of wound to assess for viability of tissue

  4. Tests: Gram stain of discharge (but do not delay surgical exploration) shows large Gram-positive bacilli and few to absent polymorphonuclear cells; radiograph shows gas in soft tissue (do not delay surgical exploration awaiting tests)

  5. Treatment

   a. Extensive debridement, usually requiring amputation

   b. Hyperbaric oxygen may be useful, provided patient can be treated within 1 hour.

   c. Penicillin G 2 million units every 2 hours, plus clindamycin 900 mg every 8 hours (beneficial to suppress toxin production)

   d. Alternative antibiotics should be considered only when penicillin is absolutely contraindicated; e.g., chloramphenicol, metronidazole, imipenem, tetracycline (cephalosporins should be avoided).

Bibliography

Lorber B. Listeriosis. Clin Infect Dis 1997;24:1–11.

Maki DG, Agger WA. Enterococcal bacteremia: clinical features, the risk of endocarditis, and management. Medicine 1988;67:248–269.

Stevens DL. Invasive group A *Streptococcus* infections. Clin Infect Dis 1992;14:2–13.

94 Gram-Negative Infections

Donald P. Levine

Gram-negative infections, like any other, may range from mild to life-threatening. Those encountered in the intensive care unit (ICU) are among the most serious of all infections and may lead to death despite rapid and appropriate management. Patients may develop Gram-negative infection outside the hospital, but more commonly these are nosocomial infections that occur in compromised hosts with multiple comorbid conditions. Such infections are often a complication of an underlying condition, making management even more difficult. A favorable outcome is seldom assured, and even optimal management may not result in cure.

Etiology

A. Gram-negative bacilli that ferment lactose: *Escherichia coli, Klebsiella pneumoniae, Enterobacter* spp., *Serratia marcescens, Proteus mirabilis, Proteus* spp., *Shigella* spp., *Salmonella* spp., *Citrobacter* spp., other Enterobacteriaciae

B. Gram-negative bacilli that do not ferment lactose: *Pseudomonas aeruginosa, Acinetobacter baumanii, Stenotrophomonas maltophilia,* others

C. Gram-negative cocci: *Neisseria meningitidis, Haemophilus influenzae, Moraxella catarrhalis*

D. Origin of infection most often seen in ICU setting

1. Central nervous system: meningitis, brain abscess

2. Respiratory tract: pneumonia, sinusitis, tracheobronchitis

3. Cardiovascular system: endocarditis, suppurative thrombophlebitis

4. Gastrointestinal system: (often mixed, including anaerobes) cholecystitis, acalculous cholecystitis, ascending cholangitis, hepatic abscess, pancreatic abscess, splenic abscess, spontaneous peritonitis, secondary peritonitis, typhlitis

5. Urinary tract: pyelonephritis, prostatitis

6. Skin and skin structures: (often mixed, including anaerobes) necrotizing fasciitis with or without myositis

Clinical Findings

A. Meningitis

1. Settings for Gram-negative meningitis

a. Community-acquired, non-traumatic, normal host: *Neisseria meningitidis, Haemophilus influenzae*

b. Nosocomial or post-traumatic: enteric Gram-negative bacilli, including *Pseudomonas aeruginosa, Acinetobacter baumanii*

c. Other predisposing conditions: Gram-negative sepsis, old age, immunosuppression

2. Common manifestations: headache, fever, meningism, altered mentation, fulminant course, skin lesions, septic shock

B. Brain abscess

1. Usually no signs of sepsis

2. Often findings related to mass lesion or raised intracranial pressure: altered sensorium, headache, focal neurologic signs, seizures

C. Pneumonia

1. Risk factors

a. Nursing home residence

b. Immunosuppression

c. Prior use of antibiotics

d. Use of mechanical ventilation

e. Other: old age, diabetes mellitus, alcoholism, chronic obstructive lung disease, acute renal failure

2. Signs and symptoms indistinguishable from pneumonia of other etiologies

a. Cough, dyspnea, and fever (may be absent in the elderly)

b. Hemoptysis (in severe necrotizing infection)

c. Pleuritic pain

d. Pulmonary infiltrates (frequently multilobar,

PEARLS

- Gram-negative infections are frequently polymicrobial, including anaerobic bacteria.

- No clinical features differentiate from Gram-positive infection.

- Anaerobic bacteria should be covered in intra-abdominal infection other than primary peritonitis, even if not isolated.

- *Pseudomonas* is cultured frequently, but is often only colonizing the site.

may be superimposed on acute respiratory distress syndrome)

    e. Leukocytosis or leukopenia

    f. Hypoxemia

D. Sinusitis

  1. Risk factors

    a. Nasogastric or nasotracheal intubation

    b. Facial fractures

    c. Nasal packing

    d. Nasal colonization with enteric Gram-negative flora

    e. Sedation

    f. Depressed sensorium

    g. Supine position

    h. Poor pulmonary toilet

    i. Increased gastric pH

  2. Findings: frequently concurrent pneumonia or unidentified source of fever in intubated patient; also, concurrent otitis media

E. Tracheobronchitis

  1. Risk factors

    a. Endotracheal intubation and mechanical ventilation

    b. Corticosteroid or prior antibiotic therapy

  2. Suspect in febrile patients without pulmonary infiltrate

F. Infective endocarditis

  1. Major risk factors

    a. Injection drug use, especially *Pseudomonas aeruginosa* and *Serratia marcescens*

    b. Early prosthetic valve infection

    c. Cirrhosis

    d. Bacteremic urinary tract infection (rarely)

  2. Signs and symptoms

    a. Fever

    b. Unexplained anemia

    c. Heart murmur

    d. Sustained bacteremia, often in spite of effective antimicrobial therapy

    e. Systemic or pulmonary embolism with infected thrombus

    f. Valve destruction or dehiscence

G. Suppurative thrombophlebitis

  1. Risk factors

    a. Intravenous catheter insertion, especially in lower limbs for longer than 5 days; frequently with antibiotic administration

    b. Elderly or debilitated

    c. Burn injury

    d. Injection drug use

    e. Total parenteral nutrition (TPN)

    f. Post-partum (pelvic thrombophlebitis)

  2. Signs and symptoms

    a. Fever common

    b. Sepsis

    c. Septic pulmonary embolism and secondary pneumonia common

    d. Local signs (erythema, tenderness, swelling) frequently absent

H. Cholecystitis

  1. Major risk factor is obstruction of cystic or common bile duct (gallstones >90%; tumor rarely).

  2. Signs and symptoms

    a. Fever and slight icterus common

    b. Initially epigastric pain with nausea and vomiting

    c. Later shift of pain to right upper quadrant, occasionally with radiation to right shoulder

    d. If severe enough, or if extension beyond gallbladder, peritoneal signs may occur.

    e. Right upper quadrant mass (palpable gallbladder)

I. Acalculous cholecystitis

  1. Major risk factors

    a. Post trauma

    b. Perfusion failure

    c. Mechanical ventilation with positive end-expiratory pressure

    d. Biliary stasis, especially due to narcotics or TPN

  2. Signs and symptoms are nonspecific; requires high index of suspicion.

J. Ascending cholangitis

  1. Common pathway of risk factors is biliary obstruction.

    a. Gallstones

    b. Tumor

    c. Duct constriction secondary to previous surgery

    d. Chronic pancreatitis

    e. Occasionally after endoscopic retrograde cholangiopancreatography (ERCP)

  2. Signs and symptoms

    a. Charcot's triad: fever, chills, jaundice (85%)

    b. Acute onset of diffuse pain, fever, tenderness over liver

    c. Bacteremia with septic shock

K. Hepatic abscess

  1. Risk factors

    a. Underlying biliary sepsis

b. Infected gallbladder

c. Intra-abdominal focus of infection with spread via portal vein (appendicitis, diverticulitis)

d. Penetrating trauma to the liver

e. Distant infection with hematogenous spread via the hepatic artery

2. Signs and symptoms

a. Prolonged fever and chills

b. Right upper quadrant pain, often dull in character

c. Tender hepatomegaly

d. Occasionally respiratory symptoms if abscess located high in liver

e. May present as fever of unknown origin

f. Jaundice infrequent

L. Pancreatic abscess

1. Risk factors

a. Pancreatitis, usually severe

b. Complication of ERCP

c. Rarely a complication of penetrating ulcer or infected pseudocyst

2. Signs and symptoms

a. Sudden deterioration during treatment for acute pancreatitis

b. Failure to respond to treatment of acute pancreatitis

c. Nausea and vomiting are prominent features.

d. Fever is typical, but may be absent.

e. Abdominal pain radiating to back

f. Jaundice and signs of peritonitis are less common.

M. Splenic abscess

1. Risk factors

a. Infective endocarditis, especially in injection drug users

b. Splenic infarction secondary to trauma or sickle hemoglobinopathies

c. HIV infection with Salmonella bacteremia

2. Signs and symptoms

a. Left upper quadrant pain referred to left shoulder

b. Tender splenomegaly

c. Splenic rub

d. High fevers

N. Peritonitis (primary or spontaneous)

1. The major risk factor is ascites, most often associated with underlying alcoholic cirrhosis.

2. Additional risk factors

a. Postnecrotic cirrhosis

b. Acute viral hepatitis

c. Chronic active hepatitis

d. Malignancy (with ascites)

e. Congestive heart failure

3. Signs and symptoms

a. Presentation may be insidious or acute in onset.

b. In almost all cases, ascites is present prior to the onset of peritonitis.

c. Patients with cirrhosis have accompanying signs of end-stage hepatic failure.

d. Fever (up to 80%), diffuse abdominal pain and tenderness (often with rebound), nausea, vomiting, diarrhea

e. Diminished to absent bowel sounds

f. Absence of evidence of primary intra-abdominal cause for peritonitis (e.g., ruptured hollow viscus)

O. Secondary peritonitis

1. Invariably a mixed infection requiring synergistic activity of anaerobic organisms and facultative bacteria that are predominantly, but not exclusively, Gram-negative

2. Risk factors

a. Disruption of hollow abdominal viscus (solid organs such as liver and spleen are usually sterile) with spillage of contents into peritoneal cavity, due either to injury or to disease

b. Chronic ambulatory dialysis

c. Ascent from infection in pelvic organs

d. Extension of infection from shunts (ventriculoperitoneal or peritoneovenous)

3. Signs and symptoms

a. Initial symptoms usually reflect the underlying pathological process.

b. Abdominal pain and tenderness (eventually with rebound), which may localize over involved organ unless infection spreads to generalized peritonitis

c. Fever, nausea, vomiting, abdominal distention, decreased appetite, and inability to pass flatus or stool

d. Initial tachycardia and diminished pulses, progressing to shock

e. Guarding with rigid abdominal muscle wall is common, but may be absent.

f. Diminished to absent bowel sounds

P. Intraperitoneal abscess

1. Risk factors

a. May result from primary peritonitis

b. May be secondary to another intra-abdominal process, most often ruptured hollow abdominal viscus, e.g., appendicitis, diverticulitis, pancreatitis, cholecystitis, abdominal surgery or trauma, perforated ulcer

2. Signs and symptoms may be nonspecific, but usually localize to site of abscess.

   a. Acute onset of fever, chills, abdominal pain, and tenderness over involved area

   b. Illness may present with subacute, indolent course in the case of subphrenic abscess.

   c. Pleural effusions and chest pain associated with subphrenic abscess

Q. Typhlitis (inflammation of the cecum)

1. Risk factors

   a. Severe neutropenia

   b. Immunosuppression

2. Signs and symptoms

   a. Fever, right lower quadrant abdominal pain

   b. Diarrhea

   c. Rebound tenderness

   d. May progress rapidly to acute abdomen

R. Urinary tract infection

1. The commonest source of Gram-negative bacteremia; yet, unless complicated by bacteremia or sepsis syndrome, it seldom necessitates ICU admission.

2. Risk factors

   a. Urinary catheterization or surgical manipulation of urinary tract

   b. Obstruction by stricture, stone, or tumor

   c. Severe reflux

3. Signs and symptoms

   a. Urinary frequency, urgency, and dysuria are most typical of lower tract disease.

   b. Fever, flank pain with or without characteristic symptoms of lower tract infection most often reflect upper tract disease (pyelonephritis).

   c. Hematuria most often reflects lower tract disease.

   d. Sepsis and shock are seen exclusively in upper tract disease.

S. Necrotizing fasciitis with or without myositis

1. Primarily a disease caused by Gram-positive organisms; however, mixed Gram-negative (anaerobic and facultative anaerobic) infection occurs and may be extremely serious.

2. Risk factors

   a. Injection drug use

   b. Diabetes mellitus

   c. Alcoholism

   d. Abdominal trauma or surgery

   e. Perirectal infection

3. Signs and symptoms

   a. Exquisite pain and tenderness most important findings

   b. Erythema and edema with indistinct borders

   c. Rapid progression of skin changes from erythema to bullae with necrosis

   d. Tissue gas may be found in some cases.

   e. Skin anesthesia may occur as a late sign.

Diagnosis

A. Meningitis

1. Cerebrospinal fluid analysis

   a. Gram stain and culture

   b. White blood cell (WBC) count usually 1,000 to 5,000 cells/mm^3, predominantly neutrophils

   c. Serum glucose usually lower than 40 mg/dL

   d. Bacterial antigen detection (by latex agglutination if possible) may detect *Neisseria* and *Haemophilus*, some enteric Gram-negative bacilli.

   e. Limulus lysate assay may identify cause as Gram-negative meningitis in cases with negative Gram-stain and culture.

2. Computed tomography (CT) or magnetic resonance imaging (MRI)

   a. Assess for concomitant sinusitis.

   b. Assess for CSF leak.

   c. Assess for complications in nonresponding cases.

B. Brain abscess

1. Magnetic resonance imaging (preferably) or CT with contrast enhancement to determine location, size and configuration of abscess

2. Stereotactic aspiration for Gram stain, aerobic and anaerobic cultures

C. Sinusitis

1. Computed tomography of sinuses

2. Aspirate for culture

D. Tracheobronchitis and pneumonia

1. Chest x-ray

2. Computed tomography may help define pathology in difficult cases.

3. Sputum Gram-stain is highly specific.

4. Sputum culture

5. Fiberoptic bronchoscopy and bronchoalveolar lavage may be useful in ventilator-associated pneumonia.

6. Lung biopsy if etiology undiagnosed in immunocompromised patient

E. Infective endocarditis and suppurative thrombophlebitis

1. Blood cultures three times at 1-hour intervals

2. Chest x-ray

3. Echocardiogram

   a. Transthoracic most useful for right-sided infection and valve complications

   b. Transesophageal most useful for mitral valve infection, particularly helpful in prosthetic valve infection

F. Intra-abdominal infection

1. Cholecystitis and cholangitis

   a. Ultrasonography especially useful for right upper quadrant pathology

   b. Hepatobiliary iminodiacetic acid cholesintigraphy scan

   c. Computed tomography or MRI

   d. Endoscopic retrograde cholangiopancreatography may define obstruction but may not be feasible in critically ill patient.

2. Hepatic, pancreatic, or splenic abscess

   a. Plain x-ray films of abdomen and chest

   b. Ultrasonography

   c. Computed tomography or MRI

   d. Needle aspirate for cell count, culture

3. Peritonitis

   a. Supine and upright x-ray of abdomen and chest

   b. Computed tomography with oral and IV contrast to evaluate for secondary cause

   c. Needle aspiration for cell count, Gram stain, and culture

   d. Paracentesis to obtain fluid for cell count, Gram stain, and culture

4. Intra-abdominal abscess

   a. Plain x-ray films of chest and abdomen

   b. Ultrasonography

   c. Computed tomography with oral and IV contrast

   d. Indium 111-tagged WBC scan may identify location

G. Urinary tract infection

1. Urinalysis

2. Urine Gram stain and culture (may represent colonization rather than infection in absence of pyuria)

H. Necrotizing fasciitis

1. X-ray, CT, or MRI

2. Surgical exploration is critical for both diagnosis and management.

   a. Evaluate integrity of facial planes.

   b. Obtain material for Gram stain and culture.

Key Laboratory Tests

- Obtain Gram stain and culture of all clinical material and any purulent body fluids.

- Aspirate closed space infection to obtain diagnostic material.

- Obtain blood cultures, even in the absence of fever, at least 30 min apart.

- Culture specimens for aerobic and anaerobic organisms.

- Culture vascular catheter tips if infection suspected.

- Primary diagnostic goal is identification of the infecting pathogen(s); other tests may contribute to impression of infection, but not etiologic diagnosis.

- Obtain susceptibility testing of all isolates.

Treatment (empiric, i.e., for cases with unidentified pathogens)

A. Meningitis

1. Third-generation cephalosporin (cefotaxime or ceftriaxone)

2. Ceftazadime or cefepime if patient had surgery or trauma

3. Ampicillin added for patients with possible *Listeria* infection

4. Vancomycin if possible shunt-related infection or resistant *Streptococcus pneumoniae* infection

B. Brain abscess (empiric regimen depends on source of abscess, if known)

1. Sinus or mastoid: third-generation cephalosporin plus metronidazole

2. Trauma or neurosurgery: third-generation cephalosporin (ceftazadime or cefepime if *Pseudomonas* suspected), plus vancomycin

3. Abdominal site: third-generation cephalosporin plus metronidazole

C. Sinusitis: ampicillin/sulbactam; piperacillin/tazobactam if *Pseudomonas* suspected

D. Tracheobronchitis or pneumonia (in ICU patient)

1. Third-generation cephalosporin (cefotaxime, ceftriaxone; consider ceftazadime or cefepime if *Pseudomonas* likely), plus

2. Gentamicin (tobramycin if *Pseudomonas* likely)

E. Infective endocarditis or suppurative thrombophlebitis

1. Empiric therapy targeting Gram-negative organisms is frequently not recommended unless a specific pathogen is suspected, then

2. Third-generation cephalosporin (cefotaxime, ceftriaxone, ceftizoxime; ceftazadime or cefepime if *Pseudomonas* suspected), plus

3. Gentamicin: 8 mg/kg per day in divided doses every 8 hours (tobramycin if *Pseudomonas* suspected)

F. Intra-abdominal infection

1. Must cover for polymicrobial infection, including anaerobes.

2. Cannot rely on β-lactam alone for treatment of *Enterobacter, Pseudomonas, Serratia, Citrobacter,* or *Morganella,* because of development of resistance.

3. Efficacy of aminoglycosides questioned in this setting

4. Recommended combinations

   a. β-Lactam/β-lactamase inhibitor (ampicillin/sulbactam, ticarcillin/clavulanate, or piperacillin/tazobactam) ± aminoglycoside; or

   b. Third-generation cephalosporin (cefotaxime, ceftizoxime, or ceftriaxone; ceftazadime or cefepime, if *Pseudomonas* suspected) plus metronidazole; or

   c. Carbapenem: imipenem or meropenem, or

   d. Aztreonam plus clindamycin

G. Urinary tract infection (for Gram-negative bacilli in ICU patient)

1. Initial therapy based on Gram stain of urine

2. Community acquired

   a. Aminoglycoside (gentamicin or tobramycin), or

   b. β-Lactam: third-generation cephalosporin or aztreonam, or

   c. β-Lactam/β-lactamase inhibitor, or

   d. Quinolone

3. Nosocomial

   a. Anti-pseudomonal β-lactam (ceftazadime, cefepime, or aztreonam) ± aminoglycoside, or

   b. Antipseudomonas β-lactamase inhibitor combination: ticarcillin/clavulanate or piperacillin/tazobactam, or

   c. Carbapenem: imipenem or meropenem, or

   d. Quinolone

Key Treatment Points

- Invasive devices and vascular catheters should be removed as soon as possible, both as treatment of established infection and to prevent infection.

- Obtain material for culture before beginning antibiotic therapy.

- Consider parenteral therapy as initial approach for all critically ill patients.

- Cover for polymicrobial infection until etiology confirmed.

Bibliography

Bartlett JG. Intra-abdominal sepsis. Med Clin North Am 1995;79:599–617.

Bergeron MG. Treatment of pyelonephritis in adults. Med Clin North Am 1995;79:619–649.

Cohen PS, Maguire JH, Weinstein L. Infective endocarditis caused by Gram-negative bacteria: a review of the literature, 1945–1977. Prog Cardiovasc Dis 1980;22:205–242.

Green RJ, Dafoe DC, Raffin TA. Necrotizing fasciitis. Chest 1996;110:219–229.

Talmor M, Li P, Barie PS. Acute paranasal sinusitis in critically ill patients: guidelines for prevention, diagnosis, and treatment. Clin Infect Dis 1997;25:1441–1446.

Torres A, El-Ebiary M, Riquelme R, et al. Community-acquired pneumonia in the elderly. Semin Respir Infect 1999;14:173–183.

Unhanand M, Mustafa MM, McCracken GH Jr, et al. Gram-negative enteric bacillary meningitis: a 21 year experience. J Pediatr 1993;122:15–21.

95 Candidal Infections

Peter K. Linden

Yeasts belonging to the genus *Candida* are the most common fungal organisms causing infections in critically ill hospitalized patients. Common risk factors for these infections include breeches in anatomic host defenses, use of broad-spectrum antibiotics, and immunosuppression due to medical therapies or intrinsic diseases. Candidal infections are best categorized as superficial (e.g., stomatitis, esophagitis, cystitis) or tissue-invasive (e.g., candidemia, peritonitis, tissue abscess, osteomyelitis, endocarditis, or disseminated disease). Deep-seated candidal infections are associated with very high rates of morbidity and mortality. Unfortunately, the likelihood of complications or death is only partially modified by aggressive diagnosis and early treatment.

Classification

A. Morphology
1. Unicellular yeast (4 to 6 μm)
2. Budding yeast
3. Other morphologies
   a. Pseudohyphae (*C. albicans*)
   b. Hyphae
B. Ten species of *Candida* are capable of causing human infection.
1. *C. albicans* (50% to 70% of infection)
2. *C. tropicalis* (second most common)
3. *C. krusei*
4. *C. guillermondi*
5. *C. parapsilosis*
6. *C. pseudotropicalis*
7. *C. stellatoidea*
8. *C. lusitaniae*
9. *C. rugosa*
10. *C. glabrata* (formerly *Torulopsis glabrata*)

Pathogenesis

A. Superficial infection (overgrowth of *Candida* and inadequate host response)
1. Dermatitis: macerated, damaged skin
2. Cystitis: ascending route of infection from the peri-urethral area
3. Stomatitis (thrush)
4. Esophagitis: contiguous spread from the oropharynx

5. Tracheobronchitis: contiguous spread from oropharynx
6. Vaginitis: overgrowth of commensal *Candida* spp.
B. Systemic infection
1. Major portals of entry for *Candida*
   a. Transcutaneous invasion (including along the tracks of IV catheters)
   b. Transurethral invasion
   c. Gastrointestinal tract
   d. Operative contamination
2. Pathways of spread
   a. Hematogenous spread from the primary portal of entry
   b. Major targets are highly perfused organs (e.g., kidneys, vertebra, retinas, liver, spleen, and eyes).
   c. Dissemination is more prevalent in neutropenic patients, solid organ recipients, and other immunocompromised hosts.

Risk Factors and Predisposing Conditions

A. Immunosuppression
1. Oncologic conditions
2. Neutropenia
3. Acquired immunodeficiency syndrome (AIDS)
4. Organ transplant
5. Corticosteroid therapy
6. Diabetes mellitus
B. Anatomic factors
1. Indwelling bladder catheterization
2. Intravascular devices
3. Surgical wounds
4. Permanently implanted devices (cardiac valves, vascular grafts)
5. Burns
C. Broad-spectrum antibiotic therapy
D. Miscellaneous conditions
1. Pregnancy
2. Total parenteral nutrition
3. Intravenous drug abuse
4. Intrinsic defects in neutrophil-mediated killing of bacteria and fungi
5. Chronic mucocutaneous candidiasis

Clinical Findings

A. Superficial infection

1. Oropharyngeal candidiasis (thrush)

   a. Creamy white patches on the tongue, gingiva, buccal mucosa

   b. Raw bleeding surfaces after scraping

   c. No systemic signs

2. Esophagitis

   a. Painful swallowing (odynophagia)

   b. Difficulty swallowing (dysphagia)

   c. Substernal chest pain

   d. Endoscopic appearance is white patches on the mucosa.

   e. Concomitant thrush may or may not be present.

3. Cystitis

   a. Presence of a bladder catheter can obscure symptoms.

   b. Increased frequency of micturition may occur if bladder catheter is not in place.

   c. Dysuria (variable).

   d. Systemic symptoms are absent without upper tract involvement.

4. Vaginitis

   a. Vaginal discharge (thick or serous)

   b. Vulva pruritus

   c. Erythema of vulva

5. Tracheobronchitis

   a. Bronchoscopy reveals white plaques on large airway mucosal surfaces.

   b. Symptoms can include hemoptysis, bronchospasm, or cough.

   c. Isolation of *Candida* in respiratory specimens usually represents colonization rather than infection.

B. Invasive infection

1. Candidemia

   a. *Candida* grows in routine blood cultures.

   b. *Candida* should never be interpreted as a contaminant.

   c. Persistent candidemia on therapy suggests endovascular infection (e.g., endocarditis, septic phlebitis, infected vascular graft).

2. Peritonitis

   a. Associated with peritoneal dialysis, hollow viscus perforation, and bowel surgery

   b. Peritoneal signs (rebound tenderness, guarding) are variable.

   c. Findings at laparotomy can include (localized or diffuse) fibrinous peritonitis.

3. Hepatosplenic candidiasis

   a. This diagnosis should suspected in patients with resolving neutropenia but persistent fever, abdominal pain, and hepatosplenomegaly.

   b. Laboratory evaluations shows increased serum alkaline phosphatase concentration.

   c. Abdominal computed tomography shows hypodense, ring-enhancing hepatosplenic lesions.

4. Disseminated candidiasis

   a. Major target organs include the heart, brain, kidneys, bone, liver, spleen, and eyes.

   b. Physical findings include micronodular skin lesions; white, cotton-wool retinal exudates; and hepatosplenomegaly.

   c. Blood cultures are negative in more than 50% of cases.

   d. Biopsy shows micro- or macro-abscesses with yeast and hypheal forms.

Key Diagnostic Points

- Detection of *Candida* at non-sterile sites has poor positive predictive value for deep-seated infection but good negative predictive value.

- Growth of *Candida* in any number of blood culture sets is almost always significant.

- Absence of candidemia does not rule out deep-seated candidal infection.

- Serologic methods for diagnosing candidal infections have mediocre sensitivity and specificity.

Laboratory Findings

A. Oropharyngeal infection (thrush or esophagitis)

1. Potassium hydroxide (KOH) or Gram stain preparation from tongue scraping or esophageal mucosal brushing

   a. Pseudohyphae

   b. Hyphae

   c. Budding yeast forms

2. Esophageal biopsy (mucosal invasion)

3. Growth of *Candida* in culture is not sufficient evidence to make the diagnosis.

B. Tracheobronchitis

1. Bronchoscopy demonstrates white plaques on the mucosa of large airways.

2. Potassium hydroxide or Gram stain preparation (as above)

3. Transbronchial biopsy is usually not indicated.

C. Cystitis

1. Growth of *Candida* in urine (no quantitative threshold has been established)

2. Pyuria (>10 leukocytes/high-power field)

3. Yeast, hyphae, or leukocyte casts consistent with upper tract infection

4. Persistence of *Candida* despite bladder catheter removal or antifungal treatment may indicate presence of an upper tract infection (renal candidiasis, fungus ball).

D. Dermatitis

1. Potassium hydroxide preparation of scrapings of skin rash shows yeast, pseudohyphae, hyphae forms.

2. Presence of "satellite" lesions at periphery of confluent maculopapular rash

E. Tissue-invasive candidiasis

1. Diagnosis requires a high index of clinical suspicion based upon presence of risk factors and a clinical syndrome affecting one or more organ systems compatible with candidal infection.

2. Detection of candidemia

a. Routine aerated blood culture without special methods should be sufficient.

b. The diagnostic yield may be slightly higher with lysis-centrifugation tube (Isolator, Du-Pont) detection systems.

3. For detection of organ invasion, ideal specimens are aseptic percutaneous or operative fluid or tissue specimens.

a. *Candida* are best visualized in tissue using methenamine silver or periodic acid–Schiff stains.

b. Routine hematoxylin-eosin stains are less sensitive.

4. Serologic testing

a. Candida-antibody detection: rising titers may indicate disease, but this finding lacks both sensitivity and specificity

b. Candida-mannan detection by latex agglutination: variable sensitivity and specificity versus criterion standard diagnostic methods

Treatment

A. Superficial candidal infection

1. Oropharyngeal infection

a. Nystatin "swish and swallow": 100,000 units every 6 hours

b. Clotrimazole lozenges

c. Fluconazole: 400 mg/day

d. Amphotericin B oral suspension: 100 mg every 6 hours

2. Candidal cystitis

a. Oral fluconazole: 200 mg/day for 7 days

b. Continuous bladder irrigation with amphotericin B, 50 to 100 mg in 1 L 5% dextrose in water, daily for 5 days

3. Candidal dermatitis

a. Topical mycostatin powder

b. Topical miconazole cream

c. Consider systemic therapy for severe, refractory cases.

d. Correct conditions leading to macerated, damaged skin.

4. Tissue-invasive candidiasis

a. Amphotericin B and fluconazole have been shown to yield comparable rates of eradication for serious candidal infections, including candidemia in non-neutropenic patients, candidal infections in patients with post-chemotherapy neutropenia, and bone marrow transplant recipients.

b. Amphotericin B: 0.6 mg/kg per day

(1) Optimal total dose has not been established (500 to 2,000 mg).

(2) Consider adding 5-flucytosine (150 mg/kg per day) for infections caused by strains other than *C. albicans*.

(3) Consider saline loading (500 to 1,000 mL) prior to infusion to reduce nephrotoxicity.

(4) *C. lusitaniae* is resistant to amphotericin B.

c. Fluconazole: 400 to 800 mg/day

(1) *C. krusei* is always resistant to fluconazole.

(2) *C. glabrata* is often resistant to fluconazole.

(3) Fluconazole-resistant strains of *C. albicans* have been reported in AIDS patients and less commonly in other immunosuppressed hosts after long durations of prior exposure to fluconazole.

d. Lipid formulations of amphotericin B

(1) Improved outcomes for candidal infection have not been demonstrated; however, the lipid formulations are less nephrotoxic than conventional amphotericin B.

(2) These formulations are significantly more expensive than amphotericin.

(3) Specific formulations

(a) Amphotericin B lipid complex (Abelcet): 3 to 5 mg/kg per day

(b) Liposome encapsulated amphotericin B (Ambisome): most expensive agent

(c) Amphotericin B cholesteryl sulfate complex (Amphotec): high rates of infusion-related toxicity

Key Pharmacologic Treatment of Serious Candida Infection

- Amphotericin B and fluconazole have comparable efficacy in published randomized trials.

- Therapy should be initiated with the maximum daily target dose.

- High dose fluconazole (800 mg/day) should be considered for life-threatening *Candida* infection.

- Lipid amphotericin B formulations show comparable efficacy in Candida infection but are renal-sparing.

- Duration of therapy not firmly established. Consider patient severity, site of infection, rapidity of the clinical and mycologic response.

5. Special circumstances
   a. Central nervous system infection
      (1) Amphotericin B (1.0 mg/kg per day) + 5-flucytosine
      (2) Consider intrathecal amphotericin B (1 to 2 mg/day).
   b. Endocarditis
      (1) Amphotericin B: 0.6 to 0.8 mg/kg per day
      (2) Immediate valve replacement
      (3) Post-valve surgery administer amphotericin B for 6 to 8 weeks.
   c. Neutropenia
      (1) Amphotericin B (0.6 mg/kg per day) for persistent fever at 7 days
      (2) Continue until absolute neutrophil count is greater than 1,000 cell/mm^3.
      (3) In cases of disseminated disease, the total dose of amphotericin B should be at least 2 g.
6. Other considerations
   a. Reduce iatrogenic immunosuppression.
   b. Carry out surgical drainage and debridement or repair as indicated.
   c. Remove infected hardware.
   d. Give granulocyte colony stimulating factor

to maintain a neutrophil count greater than 1,000 cells/mm^3.

Key Indications for Anti-fungal Therapy

- A single positive blood culture from an "at risk" patient

- Isolation of *Candida* from any sterile body site

- Positive microscopic stain for yeast from a sterile body specimen

- Histopathologic evidence of yeast or hyphae forms in tissue

Prevention (Antifungal Prophylaxis)

A. Target populations
   1. Solid organ transplant recipients
   2. Bone marrow transplant recipients
   3. Patients with post-chemotherapy neutropenia
   4. Patients with AIDS
   5. Patients undergoing complicated abdominal surgery
B. Preventative approaches
   1. Fluconazole for high-risk period (most common)
      a. AIDS patients: lifelong
      b. Post-liver transplant: 4 to 8 weeks
      c. Neutropenic period (usually 2 to 3 weeks)
      d. Bone marrow engraftment period
   2. Other anti-fungal agents for prophylaxis against candidal infection
      a. Low dose amphotericin B (10 to 20 mg/day) for 7 to 14 days
      b. Lipid formulations of amphotericin B
   3. Other general measures
      a. Limit the spectrum and duration of therapy with antibiotics.
      b. Avoid unnecessary, prolonged intravascular catheter placement.
      c. Reduce iatrogenic immunosuppression when possible.
      d. Use granulocyte or granulocyte-monocyte colony stimulating factors to reduce the duration and severity of neutropenia after cytotoxic chemotherapy.

Bibliography

Anaissie EJ, Darouiche RO, Abi-Said D, et al. Management of invasive candidal infections: results of a prospective, randomized, multicenter study of fluconazole versus amphotericin B and review of the literature. Clin Infect Dis 1996;23:964–972.

Edwards JE Jr, Bodey GP, Bowden RA, et al. International Conference for the Development of a Consensus on the Management and Prevention of Severe Candidal Infections. Clin Infect Dis 1997;25:43–59.

Nguyen MH, Peacock JE Jr, Tanner DC, et al. Therapeutic approaches in patients with candidemia. Evaluation in a multicenter, prospective, observational study. Arch Intern Med 1995;155:2429–2435.

Reents S, Goodwin SD, Singh V. Antifungal prophylaxis in immunocompromised hosts. Ann Pharmacother 1993;27:53–60.

Rex JH, Bennett JE, Sugar AM, et al. A randomized trial comparing fluconazole with amphotericin B for the treatment of candidemia in patients without neutropenia N Engl J Med 1994;331:1325–1330.

Winston DJ, Pakrasi A, Busuttil RW. Prophylactic fluconazole in liver transplant recipients. A randomized, double-blind, placebo-controlled trial. Ann Intern Med 1999;131:729–739.

Candida species account for more than 90% of all fungal infections (superficial and invasive) in critically ill patients. However, a small but important segment of fungal infections are caused by yeasts other than *Candida* (e.g., *Cryptococcus neoformans, Malassezia furfur, Saccharomyces* spp., and *Pneumocystis carinii*), dimorphic fungi (*Histoplasma capsulatum, Coccidioides immitis, Blastomyces dermatidis*) and the molds (*Aspergillus* and other filamentous fungi, *Mucor*). Most patients who develop serious infection caused by these fungi are immunosuppressed, whether intrinsically or iatrogenically. The critical care clinician needs to have a keen appreciation for these sporadic but serious infections to facilitate early detection and prompt appropriate management.

Etiology and Pathogenesis

A. Non-candidal yeast infections
   1. *Cryptococcus neoformans*
      a. Encapsulated yeast which causes disease in patients with impaired T lymphocyte function due to HIV-1 related disease, organ recipients, steroid recipients, patients with Hodgkin's disease
      b. The lung is the portal of entry and the organism has a "tropism" for the central nervous system.
   2. *Malassezia furfur*
      a. Lipophilic yeast, which can colonize normal skin and cause superficial dermatophyte infections
      b. Rarely, this organism can cause systemic infection with fungemia (neonates receiving lipid parenteral formula).
   3. *Saccharomyces species:* outbreaks of bloodstream infection related to intravascular catheters have been reported
   4. *Rhodotorula rubra:* associated with primary fungemia in neutropenic patients and other immuncompromised hosts
   5. *Trichosporon beigelii*
      a. Usually observed in patients with neutropenia secondary to chemotherapy for leukemia
      b. Can cause fungemia, pneumonia, and disseminated disease

      c. May respond to azole therapy if neutropenia resolves
B. Dimorphic fungi (exist both as yeast and mold forms)
   1. *Histoplasma capsulatum*
      a. Causes histoplasmosis, the most common mycosis in the United States
      b. Most cases occur in the Ohio and Mississippi river valleys.
      c. Acquisition of infection is via inhalation of organisms that become airborne from contaminated soil.
   2. *Coccidioides immitis*
      a. Infection is acquired via inhalation of airborne arthroconidia, which develop from soil contaminated with mycelia forms.
      b. Most cases of coccidioidomycosis occur in the southwestern United States.
   3. *Blastomyces dermatitidis*
      a. Inhalation of spores of *B. dermatitidis* usually leads to pulmonary clearance without clinical signs of infection.
      b. Symptomatic pulmonary or extra-pulmonary blastomycosis is seen most often in the Ohio and Mississippi river valleys and the southeastern United States.
C. *Aspergillus* species
   1. Most infections are caused by *A. fumigatus* or *A. flavus.*
   2. Invasive disease is seen in patients with compromised neutrophil- or cell-mediated immunological defenses.
   3. Hematogenous dissemination is a hallmark of invasive disease.
D. Non-aspergillus molds
   1. Less common than *Aspergillus*, but clinical presentation, diagnosis, and management are generally similar
   2. Examples include *Pseudallescheria boydii, Fusarium,* and *Dactylaria.*
E. Mucormycosis
   1. Caused by a broad category of pathogens
   2. *Rhizopus* and *Rhizomucor species* cause most infections.
   3. Infection follows inhalation of airborne spores with primary sinus or pulmonary involvement.

4. Infection can disseminate to other viscera.

5. Poorly controlled diabetes, steroid therapy, neutropenia, and desferoxamine therapy are risk factors.

Key Risk Factors

- Diabetes mellitus
- Neutropenia
- Organ transplantation
- Acquired immunodeficiency syndrome
- Corticosteroid therapy

Clinical Findings

A. Cryptococcosis
   1. Meningitis
      a. Usually subacute onset (1 to 2 weeks)
      b. Symptoms include fever, headache, and lethargy.
      c. Frank meningismus is usually absent.
      d. Focal signs (including seizures) may be present.
   2. Non-meningeal syndromes
      a. Pneumonitis
      b. Skin lesions (cellulitis or discrete nodules)
      c. Bone and joint infection
      d. Ocular infection
      e. Prostatitis
      f. Dissemination to multiple visceral organs

B. Histoplasmosis (there are four distinct clinical presentations)
   1. Acute pulmonary infection
      a. If the size of the inoculum is low, exposure results in no detectable disease.
      b. If the size of the inoculum is high, exposure causes disease in at least 50%.
      c. Symptoms include nonproductive cough, pleuritic chest pain, fever, myalgias, headache, chills, and anorexia.
      d. Physical findings include rales and cervical or supraclavicular lymphadenopathy.
      e. Chest radiograph shows hilar or mediastinal adenopathy, patchy infiltrates, and pleural effusions (rare).
   2. Chronic pulmonary disease
      a. Symptoms include chronic cough, dyspnea, fatigue, fever, weight loss.
      b. Physical findings include abnormal chest sounds on auscultation, cachexia.
      c. Chest x-ray shows fibrotic/cavitary lesions with apical predominance.
   3. Disseminated histoplasmosis
      a. Seen almost exclusively in patients with defects in cell-mediated immunity (steroid therapy, AIDS)
      b. Pulmonary and extra-pulmonary disease is observed.
      c. Systemic symptoms include fever, weight loss, anorexia.
      d. Local symptoms and signs are referable to the involved organ system(s) and can include findings due to bone marrow infection (anemia, leukopenia, thrombocytopenia), and cutaneous and mucosal ulcers.
      e. Physical findings can include ulcerative lesions on skin or oral mucosa, lymphadenopathy, hepatosplenomegaly, or findings consistent with adrenal insufficiency
   4. Mediastinal granuloma or fibrosing mediastinitis: principal clinical symptoms are due to compression of a mediastinal structure (superior vena cava, esophagus, trachea, bronchi) by enlarged lymph nodes

C. Coccidioidomycosis
   1. Primary pulmonary infection
      a. Only 40% of patients are symptomatic.
      b. Can progress to pneumonia, chronic cavitary pulmonary disease, or disseminated disease especially in immunocompromised hosts
      c. Symptoms include productive cough, fever, pleuritic chest pain, malaise, arthralgia.
      d. Physical findings include erythema nodosum or erythema multiforme.
      e. Chest x-ray reveals minimal changes to frank pneumonia (thin-walled cavities or nodules may be seen in chronic phase).
   2. Disseminated disease
      a. 0.5% to 1% of cases
      b. Patients at higher risk include the very young or elderly, immunosuppressed patients, patients in late pregnancy.
      c. Most severe cases are now seen in AIDS patients.
      d. Extrameningeal disease most commonly involves skin, bones, and joints.
      e. Meningitis may have an acute or subacute onset.

D. Blastomycosis
   1. Acute pneumonia
      a. Symptoms include fever, chills, productive cough, hemoptysis.
      b. Physical findings are nonspecific.

c. Chest x-ray shows alveolar or mass-like lesions; cavities are rare; reticulonodular patterns are uncommon.

2. Chronic pneumonia is characterized by pneumonic symptoms and findings along with a "wasting illness" (anorexia, night sweats, weight loss).

3. Extra-pulmonary infection

a. Cutaneous lesions, the most common finding, can appear ulcerative or verrucous.

b. Osteomyelitis usually involves the vertebrae, ribs, or pelvic bones.

c. Genitourinary infection is more common in men and often presents as prostatitis or epididymo-orchitis.

4. Disseminated disease

E. Aspergillosis

1. Pulmonary

a. Chronic necrotizing aspergillosis

b. Indolent low-grade disease

c. Often seen in patients with underlying chronic lung disease

d. Can result in aspergilloma formation requiring surgical resection and amphotericin

2. Bronchopulmonary aspergillosis

a. Allergic manifestation is characterized by wheezing, infiltrates, and eosinophilia.

b. Managed with steroids

3. Tracheobronchitis: noninvasive involvement of the large airways

4. Invasive pulmonary aspergillosis

a. This form of the disease carries a high mortality rate and occurs exclusively in patients with compromised neutrophil-mediated or cell-mediated immunity.

b. Symptoms include fever, cough, pleuritic chest pain, and hemoptysis.

c. Physical findings are nonspecific.

d. Chest x-ray shows single or multiple nodular lesions (most common) or cavitary lesions, wedge-shaped peripheral densities, lobar or non-lobar alveolar infiltrates.

5. Extrapulmonary aspergillosis

a. Clinically inapparent hematogenous spread to almost any organ (kidneys, spleen, liver, thyroid, heart, and gastrointestinal tract) can occur.

b. Clinically apparent dissemination can present in these ways:

(1) Cutaneous involvement: nodular purple or red lesions

(2) Central nervous system involvement: single or multiple brain abscesses causing focal neurologic changes and seizures

(3) Bone involvement: localized bone pain, spinal cord compression

(4) Refractory sepsis

PEARL

The clinical significance of any *Aspergillus* isolate depends most on the presence and severity of underlying immune deficits. It is highest in neutropenia and in bone marrow or solid organ transplant recipients.

F. Mucormycosis

1. Sino-orbital infection is associated with retro-orbital pain, headache, peri-orbital cellulitis, proptosis, and visual loss.

2. Pulmonary infection presents in a manner similar to *Aspergillus*.

3. Gastrointestinal infection causes nonspecific gastrointestinal symptoms; findings can include ulceration, infarction, and bleeding due to angio-invasion.

4. Cutaneous infection can occur at wound or catheter sites due to primary cutaneous invasion or as a late sign of disseminated visceral infection.

PEARL

Infections involving the dimorphic fungi may present as acute fulminant illnesses in immunocompetent or immunocompromised individuals, or as reactivated dormant infections in immunosuppressed hosts.

Diagnosis

A. Cryptococcosis

1. Demonstration of *Cryptococcus* at any site should prompt a search for concomitant disease at sites.

2. Meningitis

a. Cerebrospinal fluid (CSF) sampling is essential.

b. Before performing lumbar puncture, perform computed tomography of the head to exclude contraindications (mass effect, midline shift).

c. Cerebrospinal fluid cryptococcal antigen (latex agglutination assay) has 95% to 100% sensitivity.

d. India ink assay: 50% sensitivity

e. Fungal culture: sensitivity is close to 100%, but results are unavailable for 24 to 72 hours

f. Nonspecific CSF findings include increased protein concentration, decreased glucose concentration, and moderately elevated leukocyte count with a predominance of lymphocytes on the differential count.

3. Non-meningeal infection

a. Serum cryptococcal antigen assay is 50% to 70% sensitive for meningeal or nonmeningeal disease.

b. Culture (blood, body fluid, or tissue)

(1) *C. neoformans* will grow in conventional or fungal blood culture systems (usually in 24 to 78 hours).

(2) Isolator (lysis-centrifugation) tubes appear to be more sensitive than radiometric systems.

(3) The organism also can be grown from respiratory specimens, pleural and peritoneal fluid, urine, and tissue biopsies.

c. Tissue stains

(1) Preliminary identification is best done with methenamine silver or periodic acid–Schiff stains.

(2) Distinction from other yeast types is done with Mayer's mucicarmine stain, which stains cryptococci (and only cryptococci) red.

B. Histoplasmosis

1. Fungal culture of appropriate specimen(s)

a. Blood cultures using lysis-centrifugation (isolator) methods are positive in up to 70% of disseminated cases.

b. Urine or sputum cultures are positive in 40% to 70% of disseminated cases.

c. Multiple cultures of the same site may increase diagnostic yield.

d. Bone marrow cultures have the highest diagnostic yield (about 80%).

e. Cultures take 2 to 3 weeks to grow.

2. Tissue stains

a. Demonstration of the organism in tissue is advantageous since it achieves a rapid diagnosis.

b. Wright's stain is used for blood or bone marrow.

c. Grocott-Gomori methenamine silver stain

can be used for any visceral tissue biopsy specimen.

3. *H. capsulatum* polysaccharide antigen detection

a. Antigen is detectable in urine of 90% of patients with disseminated disease.

b. Antigen is detectable in blood of 50% of patients with disseminated disease.

c. Serial assays are useful to confirm titer reduction as measure of response to antifungal therapy.

C. Coccidioidomycosis

1. Index of suspicion should be higher if the patient has been a resident of or traveled to an endemic area.

2. Definitive diagnosis requires obtaining appropriate specimens for culture and tissue stains or serologic confirmation.

a. Culture: *C. immitis* grows readily on routine fungal media in 7 to 10 days

b. Stain: visualization of characteristic "spherules" by hematoxylin-eosin or Grocott-Gomori methenamine silver stains

c. Serology: complement fixation antibody titer is sensitive for both diagnosis and monitoring response to therapy

D. Blastomycosis

1. Diagnosis must rely upon tissue or fluid specimens for special stains or culture; no reliable serological tests are available.

2. Culture: *B. dermatidis* grows on routine fungal media

3. Stain: *B. dermatidis* can be visualized with silver stains

E. Aspergillosis

1. Specimen stain

a. *Aspergillus* spp. are best seen by silver staining methods as dichotomous, 45-degree angle branching forms.

b. However, other mycelia (e.g., *Fusaria, Pseudallescheria boydii*) also have this appearance.

2. Culture

a. *Aspergillus* spp. grow on routine fungal media.

b. Growth of *Aspergillus* in respiratory specimens does not establish the diagnosis of invasive disease; however, in neutropenic patients and immunosuppressed transplant recipients, this finding strongly suggests invasive aspergillosis.

3. Serologic assays for *Aspergillus*-associated antigen(s) have shown variable sensitivity.

F. Mucormycosis

1. Tissue or body fluid stain: silver staining shows broad hyphae with 90-degree angle branching forms
2. Fungal culture
   a. These pathogens grow well on routine fungal media.
   b. Speciation is possible by microscopic examination of growth.

Treatment

A. *Cryptococcus neoformans* (meningitis or non-meningeal infection)
   1. Amphotericin B (0.4 to 0.6 mg/kg per day) plus 5-fluorocytosine (5-FC; 150 mg/kg per day in 4 divided doses)
      a. Total dose and duration are not established, but a minimum of 4 weeks of therapy is usually required.
      b. Longer therapy is needed for AIDS patients, slow responders, and patients with a burden of disease.
   2. Fluconazole (400 to 600 mg/day) is an alternative to amphotericin B; however, a high early mortality has been observed with this treatment regimen in AIDS patients with unfavorable prognostic variables.
   3. Combination therapy using fluconazole with 5-FC appears promising.
   4. Complicating hydrocephalus
      a. Therapeutic CSF drainage with a lumbar or ventricular drain may be required.
      b. Intrathecal amphotericin B (1 to 3 mg/day) can also be administered.
   5. Isolated pulmonary lesions: consider surgical excision
   6. AIDS patients: lifelong suppressive therapy with either fluconazole or itraconazole is warranted due to high relapse rate without such treatment

Key Treatment of Cryptococcosis

- Amphotericin B is preferred for severe cases.
- Combination with 5-FC enhances response in meningitis.
- Duration of treatment depends on severity of underlying immune deficits.

B. *Malassezia furfur*: treat systemic infection with amphotericin B
C. *Trichosporon beigelii*: may respond to azole therapy if neutropenia resolves

D. Histoplasmosis
   1. Acute pulmonary infection
      a. Mild cases: no therapy needed
      b. Severe cases: ketoconazole (400 mg/day) or itraconazole (200 mg/day) or 2 to 3 weeks of amphotericin B (0.7 to 1.0 mg/kg per day)
      c. Hypersensitivity reactions are managed with prednisone (80 mg/day with 2 to 3 week taper).
   2. Chronic pulmonary infection
      a. Symptomatic patients are treated with amphotericin B (35 mg/kg cumulative dose).
      b. Consider surgical resection of large, thick-walled cavities if the condition is refractory to medical therapy or the patient relapses after treatment.
   3. Disseminated disease
      a. Amphotericin B (0.7 to 1.0 mg/kg per day) to a minimum dose of 2.5 g followed by consolidation therapy with every-other-day amphotericin B or itraconazole (400 mg/day)
      b. Post-treatment suppression therapy with weekly amphotericin B or daily itraconazole (200 to 400 mg/day) is needed for patients with a high risk of relapse (e.g., patients with AIDS).
E. Coccidioidomycosis
   1. Symptomatic primary pneumonia may resolve without treatment but should be treated with itraconazole (400 mg/day) or fluconazole (400 mg/day) if the patient has any of the following conditions: AIDS, other immunosuppression, third trimester pregnancy, diabetes
   2. Non-meningeal, non-life-threatening disease should be treated with itraconazole (400 mg/day) or fluconazole (400 mg/day).
   3. Life-threatening or azole-refractory disease should be treated with amphotericin B.
   4. Meningeal disease should be treated with fluconazole (400 to 800 mg/day) indefinitely or amphotericin B (0.6 to 1.0 mg/kg per day) for a minimum total dose of 2.5 g, plus intrathecal (or intraventricular) amphotericin B (0.1 to 0.3 mg/day).
F. Blastomycosis
   1. Non-life-threatening disease
      a. Itraconazole (200 to 400 mg/day) for 6 to 12 months
      b. Fluconazole (400 to 800 mg/day)
   2. Life-threatening disease (including meningitis): amphotericin B (0.5 mg/kg per day) to a total

dose of at least 1.5 g, followed by itraconazole (200 mg/day)

G. Aspergillosis

1. High-dose amphotericin B (1 to 1.5 mg/kg per day): no prospective studies addressed duration or cumulative dose needed

2. Lipid formulations of amphotericin B (5 to 6 mg/kg per day) have been approved as second-line therapy for amphotericin-intolerant or refractory cases.

3. Itraconazole

   a. Mild-to-moderate infections have shown favorable responses to itraconazole (400 to 600 mg/day).

   b. The parenteral formulation is recommended for critically ill patients.

4. Investigational agents include voriconazole and pneumocandins.

5. Surgical resection of isolated pulmonary or central nervous system lesions or debridement of sinus infection should be considered.

H. Mucormycosis

1. Amphotericin B: these organisms are only partially responsive and thus require high doses (1.0 to 1.5 mg/kg per day)

2. Lipid formulations of amphotericin B

3. Early surgical debridement of necrotic sino-orbital tissue or excision of pulmonary lesions is essential for cure.

4. Promote recovery of underlying condition by using filgrastim for neutropenia, or insulin therapy for diabetic ketoacidosis.

Bibliography

Bradsher RW. Histoplasmosis and blastomycosis. Clin Infect Dis 1996;22(suppl. 2):S102–S111.

Denning DW. Therapeutic outcome in invasive aspergillosis. Clin Infect Dis 1996;23:608–615.

Lee FY, Mossad SB, Adal KA. Pulmonary mucormycosis: the last 30 years. Arch Intern Med 1999;159:1301–1309.

Robinson LA. *Aspergillus* and other fungi. Chest Surg Clin North Am 1999;9:193–225.

Stevens DA, Kan VL, Judson MA, et al. Practice guidelines for diseases caused by *Aspergillus:* Infectious Diseases Society of America. Clin Infect Dis 2000;30:696–709.

White MH, Armstrong D. Cryptococcosis. Infect Dis Clin North Am 1994;8:383–398.

97 Herpes Infections

Pranatharthi H. Chandrasekar

Herpes Simplex Virus

Clinical Findings (Table 97-1)

A. Oral-facial herpes simplex virus (HSV) infection (HSV 1 ≫ HSV 2)
   1. Gingivostomatitis (primary infection)
      a. Painful vesicles or shallow ulcers inside oral cavity and lower face
      b. Malaise
      c. Fever
      d. Difficulty eating
      e. Regional adenopathy
   2. Pharyngitis (primary infection): difficulty eating
   3. Herpes labialis (recurrent infection)
      a. Vesicles or ulcers on vermilion border of lips or intra-oral site
      b. Shorter duration with fewer symptoms than primary infection
B. Genital infection (HSV 2 ≫ HSV 1)
   1. Primary (first episode) infection
      a. Pain
      b. Dysuria
      c. Vaginal and urethral discharge
      d. Vesicles, pustules, ulcers over external genitalia
      e. Tender inguinal adenopathy
      f. Fever
      g. Malaise
      h. Headache
      i. Extragenital infection by autoinoculation (site: buttocks, groin, thigh, fingers, eyes)
      j. Aseptic meningitis
      k. Autonomic dysfunction
      l. Transverse myelitis
   2. Recurrent infection
      a. Typical: clusters of painful vesicles
      b. Atypical: linear fissures, painless lesions
   3. Perianal infection
   4. Proctitis (rectal infection): associated with rectal intercourse in homosexual men
      a. Anorectal pain
      b. Anorectal discharge
      c. Tenesmus
      d. Constipation
C. Herpes simplex encephalitis (>95% caused by HSV 1)
   1. Fever
   2. Altered sensorium
   3. Bizarre behavior
   4. Focal (temporal lobe) neurologic findings
D. Herpetic keratoconjunctivitis
   1. Acute pain
   2. Blurred vision, chemosis, conjunctivitis
   3. Dendritic lesions in cornea
E. Herpetic whitlow (infection of finger): occupational risks (e.g., respiratory therapy, dentistry)
   1. Fever
   2. Edema
   3. Erythema
   4. Vesicles or pustules
   5. Regional adenitis
F. Immunocompromised hosts
   1. Tracheobronchitis
   2. Pneumonia
   3. Esophagitis
   4. Hepatitis
   5. Extensive mucocutaneous disease
   6. Disseminated disease
G. Erythema multiforme
H. Bell's palsy (? HSV 1)

Laboratory

A. Tzanck preparation of infected material
B. Antibody detection: type-specific (HSV 1 or HSV 2) antibodies
C. Antigen detection: direct fluorescent antibody test
D. DNA detection: polymerase chain reaction; e.g., cerebrospinal fluid analysis in patients with encephalitis
E. Culture

Key Test for HSV Encephalitis

- HSV DNA in cerebrospinal fluid by polymerase chain reaction

TABLE 97–1. HERPESVIRUSES AND ASSOCIATED DISEASES

Herpes simplex virus 1	Gingivostomatitis, herpes labialis, keratoconjunctivitis, encephalitis, genital herpes, herpetic whitlow, esophagitis, hepatitis
Herpes simplex virus 2	Genital herpes, proctitis, cutaneous herpes, disseminated herpes, aseptic meningitis, meningoencephalitis, neonatal herpes
Varicella-zoster virus	Varicella (chickenpox), dermatomal (shingles) zoster, disseminated zoster
Cytomegalovirus	Congenital disease, mononucleosis, retinitis, pneumonitis, encephalitis, colitis, esophagitis (see Chapter 98, Cytomegalovirus Infections)
Epstein-Barr virus	Mononucleosis, hepatitis, oral hairy leukoplakia, post-transplant lymphoproliferative syndromes, African Burkitt's lymphoma, CNS lymphoma, nasopharyngeal carcinoma, leiomyosarcoma
Human herpes virus 6	Roseola infantum, febrile seizures (infants), pneumonitis, encephalitis
Human herpes virus 7	Roseola infantum
Human herpes virus 8	Kaposi's sarcoma, Castleman's disease, primary effusion lymphoma

Treatment

A. Mucocutaneous infections
  1. Orolabial or genital herpes (first episode): acyclovir 400 mg orally every 8 hours × 10 to 14 days
  2. Genital herpes (recurrent)
    a. Acyclovir 400 mg orally every 8 hours for 5 days
    b. Alternate: valacyclovir, famciclovir
  3. Orolabial herpes: recurrent
    a. Acyclovir 400 mg PO orally every 8 hours for 5 days
    b. Penciclovir cream (for 5 days)
  4. Suppressive therapy for recurrent HSV
    a. Acyclovir 400 mg orally every 12 hours
    b. Alternate: valacyclovir, famciclovir
  5. Prophylaxis in immunocompromised patients: acyclovir 400 mg orally every 12 hours
B. Herpetic whitlow: acyclovir 400 mg orally every 8 hours for 7 days
C. Herpes simplex virus esophagitis, pneumonia, or disseminated infection: acyclovir 5 mg/kg intravenously every 8 hours
D. Erythema multiforme with HSV: acyclovir 400 mg orally every 8 hours
E. Aseptic meningitis: acyclovir 5 mg/kg intravenously every 8 hours
F. HSV encephalitis: acyclovir 10 mg/kg intravenously every 8 hours for 14 to 21 days
G. Genital HSV at term: cesarean section
H. Acyclovir-resistant HSV: foscarnet 40 mg/kg intravenously every 8 hours

Varicella-Zoster Virus

Clinical Findings (and see Table 97–1)

A. Chickenpox (varicella)
  1. Truncal or facial rash
  2. Macules, papules, vesicles ("dew-drop" appearance)
  3. Pustules
  4. Mucosal involvement
  5. Fever
  6. Pneumonia (common in adults)
  7. Cerebellar ataxia
  8. Encephalitis
  9. Meningitis
  10. Transverse myelitis
  11. Reye's syndrome
  12. Bacterial superinfection
B. Herpes zoster
  1. Pain
  2. Vesicles, pustules
  3. Unilateral rash (shingles)
  4. Dermatomal distribution
  5. Zoster ophthalmicus
  6. Ramsay-Hunt syndrome
  7. Dissemination
  8. Meningoencephalitis
  9. Transverse myelitis
  10. Guillain-Barré syndrome
  11. Retinitis
  12. Acute retinal necrosis
  13. Pneumonitis
  14. Hepatitis

Differential Diagnosis

A. Impetigo
B. Herpes simplex rash
C. Enteroviral rash

Laboratory Tests

A. Tzanck smear
B. Direct fluorescent antibody test

C. Polymerase chain reaction for viral DNA

D. Culture

Prevention

A. High-risk individuals: varicella zoster immunoglobulin

B. Vaccine to prevent varicella

Treatment

A. Chickenpox
1. Hygiene
2. Antipruritic drugs
3. Acetaminophen (no aspirin)
4. Specific therapy
   a. Not for otherwise healthy children
   b. Acyclovir 800 mg orally 5 times each day for 5 days
   c. Acyclovir 5 to 10 mg/kg intravenously every 8 hours for 5 to 7 days (if seriously ill or there is intolerance to oral acyclovir)
5. Foscarnet 40 mg/kg intravenously every 8 hours (acyclovir-resistant varicella)

B. Herpes zoster
1. Valacyclovir 1 g orally every 8 hours for 7 days
2. Famciclovir 500 mg orally every 8 hours for 7 days
3. Acyclovir 800 mg orally 5 times each day for 7 days
4. Seriously ill, disseminated infection
   a. Acyclovir 10 mg/kg intravenously every 8 hours for 7 days
   b. Foscarnet 40 mg/kg intravenously every 8 hours for 7 days (acyclovir-resistant varicella-zoster)

Key Treatment for Herpes Simplex and Varicella-Zoster

- Oral treatment: acyclovir, valacyclovir, famciclovir
- Seriously ill patients: acyclovir intravenously
- Acyclovir-resistant: foscarnet intravenously

Infectious Mononucleosis (Epstein-Barr Virus)

Epidemiology

A. Epstein-Barr virus (EBV) resides in the upper respiratory tract.

B. Transmission via

1. Intimate contact between susceptible persons and asymptomatic shedders
2. Transfusion
3. Transplantation

Clinical Findings (Table 97–1)

A. Symptoms
1. Fever
2. Sore throat
3. Malaise

B. Physical findings
1. Lymphadenopathy
2. Exudate, pharyngitis
3. Splenomegaly

Differential Diagnosis

A. Cytomegalovirus mononucleosis
B. Primary human immunodeficiency virus (HIV-1) infection
C. Viral hepatitis
D. Acute toxoplasmosis
E. Group A streptococcal pharyngitis

Laboratory Findings

A. Lymphocytosis
B. Atypical lymphocytes
C. Neutropenia
D. Thrombocytopenia
E. Liver function abnormalities
F. Heterophile antibodies (Monospot test)
G. Epstein-Barr virus–specific antibodies (if heterophile antibody negative)
1. Viral capsid antigens
2. Early antigens
3. Nuclear antigens

Key Tests for EBV (infectious mononucleosis)

- Relative lymphocytosis in peripheral blood
- Monospot for heterophile antibodies

Treatment

A. Supportive care
B. Corticosteroids: indications

1. Impending airway obstruction (tonsillar enlargement)
2. Severe thrombocytopenia
3. Hemolytic anemia
4. Central nervous system involvement

Complications

A. Autoimmune hemolytic anemia
B. Splenic rupture
C. Encephalitis
D. Aseptic meningitis
E. Transverse myelitis

Key Treatment for Epstein-Barr Virus

• Corticosteroids for specific indications

Bibliography

Cohen JI, Brunell PA, Stratus SE, et al. Recent advances in varicella-zoster virus infection. NIH Conference. Ann Intern Med 1999;130:922–932.

Levy JA. Three new human Herpes viruses (HHV 6, 7, and 8). Lancet 1997;349:558–562.

Schooley RT. Epstein-Barr virus (infectious mononucleosis). In: Mandell GL, Bennett JG, Dolin R (eds). Principles and Practice of Infectious Diseases. Philadelphia: Churchill Livingstone, 2000; pp 1599–1613.

Whitley RJ, Kimberlin DW, Roizman B. Herpes simplex viruses. Clin Infect Dis 1998;26:541–553.

98 Cytomegalovirus Infections

Lawrence R. Crane

Cytomegalovirus (CMV) *infection* is widespread, asymptomatically infecting 60% to 70% of adult North Americans. At the same time, serious CMV *disease* requiring treatment in the intensive care unit (ICU) is mostly limited to the profoundly immunocompromised patient. It is responsible for a substantial fraction of morbidity and mortality in bone marrow and solid organ transplant recipients and in persons with human immunodeficiency virus type 1 (HIV-1) infection. Common to all human herpesviruses, CMV establishes a latent infection after recovery from an acute infection. Acute infection occurs either from maternal–infant transmission or as a sexually transmitted infection. Activation from the latent state occurs after immunosuppression. Acute infection may also occur after transfusion of infected blood products or by transplantation of infected organs.

Clinical Findings

A. In patients with acquired immunodeficiency syndrome
  1. Retinitis
  2. Central nervous system
    a. Encephalitis
      (1) Diffuse encephalitis
      (2) Ventriculitis
    b. Myelitis
    c. Polyradiculopathy
  3. Gastrointestinal tract
    a. Esophagitis
    b. Colitis
    c. Pancreatitis
    d. Biliary tract, including gallbladder (HIV-associated cholangiopathy)
  4. Pneumonitis
B. In post-transplantation patients
  1. Pneumonitis (bone marrow transplantation)
  2. Hepatitis (liver transplantation)
  3. Other end-organ disease (e.g., enteritis)

Diagnosis

A. Cultivation of CMV virus in tissue culture
B. Identification of CMV in tissue by histologic and histochemical means

PEARLS

- Cytomegalovirus disease occurs during the advanced stages of HIV-infection; the CD4 lymphocyte count is typically lower than 50 cells/mm^3.
- Major consequences of CMV disease in organ transplantation include superinfection and damage to organ transplant.
- Cytomegalovirus disease typically occurs 1 to 4 months after transplantation.
- Incidence is lowered with screening of donors, blood products, antiviral prophylaxis; most problems occur as result of reactivation of CMV in recipient or graft.

C. Identification of CMV-specific antigens or CMV-specific DNA
  1. CMV pp65 antigen detection (monoclonal antibody)
  2. Perform polymerase chain reaction (PCR).
D. Fourfold rise in CMV antibody titer
E. Typical appearance of retinal exudates by experienced examiner (in the case of CMV retinitis)

 Key Tests—HIV

- Demonstration of CMV antibodies or growth of CMV in respiratory tract, urine, blood, and other specimens (except cerebrospinal fluid [CSF]) in advanced stages of HIV is of little utility in establishing a diagnosis of CMV disease.
- The only reliable way to establish a diagnosis of CMV end-organ disease during advanced HIV is by (1) retinal examination in the event of retinitis, (2) demonstration of typical histological features of biopsied tissue, or (3) growth of CMV or demonstration of CMV DNA by PCR in CSF in the event of encephalitis or polyradiculitis.
- When CMV end-organ disease is suspected in an HIV-infected patient in the ICU, perform a retinal examination; the presence of CMV retinitis should raise the index of suspicion for CMV end-organ disease elsewhere.

Key Tests—Transplantation

- In contrast to HIV-infected patients, a diagnosis of CMV disease can be made with greater certainty in transplant recipients.

- Cytomegalovirus pneumonia: x-ray evidence of a progressive interstitial pulmonary process, with evidence of CMV infection by culture, antibody rise, CMV antigen detection, or histologic demonstration with no evidence of other causes of pneumonia

- Other end-organ disease generally requires histologic confirmation.

Treatment

A. Ganciclovir
1. Dosing: 5 mg/kg intravenously every 12 hours
2. Considered to be therapy of choice
3. Bone marrow toxicity is the major limiting side effect.

B. Foscarnet
1. Alternative to ganciclovir
2. Dosing: 60 mg/kg intravenously every 8 hours or 90 mg/kg every 12 hours
3. Used when ganciclovir resistance is suspected
4. Major toxicities include renal failure and electrolyte abnormalities.

C. Combination therapy with ganciclovir and foscarnet
1. Combination therapy is superior to monotherapy for CMV retinitis, but at a high toxicity and quality-of-life cost.
2. There are some favorable anecdotal data on combination therapy using ganciclovir and foscarnet in HIV patients with CMV encephalitis.

D. Intravenous immune globulin (IVIG)
1. Dosing: 500 mg/kg intravenously four times daily
2. Has been employed in several small, uncontrolled series along with ganciclovir for CMV pneumonitis in bone marrow transplant patients

 Bibliography

Crumpacker CS. Cytomegalovirus. In: Mandell GL, Bennett JE, Dolin R (eds). Principles and Practice of Infectious Diseases, 5th ed. Philadelphia: Churchill Livingstone, 2000, pp 1586–1599.

Drew WL, Lalezari JP. Cytomegalovirus. In: Cohen PT, Sande MA, Volberding P (eds). The AIDS Knowledge Base, 3rd ed. Philadelphia: Lippincott Williams & Wilkins, 1999, pp 713–719.

Hibberd PL, Snydman DR. Cytomegalovirus infection in organ transplant recipients. Infect Dis Clin North Am 1995;9:863–877.

Zaia JA, Forman SJ. Cytomegalovirus infection in the bone marrow transplant recipient. Infect Dis Clin North Am 1995;9:879–900.

99 Acquired Immune Deficiency Syndrome

Lawrence R. Crane

As human immunodeficiency virus (HIV) infection has moved from a palliative to a chronic disease model of care, more HIV-infected persons are cared for in intensive care units (ICUs). Additionally, the ICU setting may be where the diagnosis of HIV infection is first made. While HIV-infected patients may require intensive care for any number of reasons, acute respiratory failure caused by *Pneumocystis carinii* pneumonia (PCP) is the most common reason (~45%) for ICU admission. A basic principle in the management of HIV patients in the ICU is an appreciation of the appearance of certain opportunistic infections or malignancies in a hierarchic fashion associated with declining CD4+ T-lymphocyte counts (Table 99–1). Clearly, knowledge of the HIV-infected patient's absolute CD4+ count is key—not only in differential diagnosis, but also in prediction of outcome of an ICU admission. Another key principle is that most reasons for ICU admissions of HIV patients are infections. More than one infection may be present. Finally, the best outcomes occur when clinicians make a microbiological diagnosis—and avoid the "empiric downward spiral."

Key Management Points

- High index of suspicion for HIV disease in acute respiratory failure in otherwise healthy patients

- Immunologic status (CD4+ count) is key to differential diagnosis.

- Most common reason for ICU admission is infection.

- The best outcomes occur when a microbiological diagnosis is made.

- Initiating or maintaining antiretroviral therapy in ICU patients is rarely done and only after expert consultation.

Precipitating Factors for ICU Admission

A. Acute respiratory failure (50% to 75%)
  1. *Pneumocystis carinii* pneumonia
  2. Bacterial pneumonias
    a. *Streptococcus pneumoniae*
    b. *Haemophilus pneumoniae*
    c. *Pseudomonas aeruginosa*
    d. Other Gram-negative bacteria
    e. *Mycobacterium tuberculosis*
    f. Nontuberculous mycobacteria, particularly *M. kansasii*
    g. *Rhodococcus equi*
    h. Nocardial infections
  3. Fungal pneumonias
    a. *Cryptococcus neoformans*
    b. *Histoplasma capsulatum*
    c. *Coccidioides immitis*
    d. Aspergillosis
  4. Viral pneumonias
    a. Herpes simplex viruses
    b. Cytomegalovirus
    c. Varicella zoster virus
    d. Influenza virus
  5. Parasitic infections
    a. *Toxoplasma gondii*
  6. Noninfectious
    a. Neoplasia (Kaposi's sarcoma, lymphoma, lung cancer)
    b. Exacerbation of chronic lung disease
    c. Drug overdose
    d. Congestive heart failure
    e. Pulmonary embolism or infarction
B. Neurologic complications (10% to 15%)
  1. Mass lesions
    a. Toxoplasmic encephalitis
    b. Primary central nervous system lymphoma
    c. Tuberculoma
    d. Cryptococcoma
  2. Meningitis
    a. *Cryptococcus neoformans*
    b. *Mycobacterium tuberculosis*
    c. *Listeria monocytogenes*
    d. *Streptococcus pneumoniae*
    e. *Haemophilus influenzae*
    f. *Nocardia* sp.
    g. *Treponema pallidum*
  3. Other
    a. Myelopathy with respiratory failure (cyto-

TABLE 99–1. LIKELIHOOD OF OPPORTUNISTIC EVENTS IN HIV-INFECTED PATIENTS

IMMUNE FUNCTION LEVEL	LIKELIHOOD OF OPPORTUNISTIC EVENT	COMMENTS
Normal or near-normal (CD4+ count >400 cells/mm³)	Very low	Kaposi's sarcoma, bacterial pneumonias, mucosal candida and oral hairy leukoplakia
Moderately low (CD4+ count 200 to 400 cells/mm³)	Low	Kaposi's sarcoma; lymphomas; higher rates of bacterial pneumonias; nonspecific pneumonitis; HIV cardiomyopathy; HIV nephropathy; pulmonary tuberculosis, histoplasmosis and coccidioidomycosis in certain geographical areas; *Candida* esophagitis; *P. carinii* may be seen in pediatric patients
Low (CD4+ count 50 to 200 cells/mm³)	High	All opportunistic events possible
Very low (CD4+ count <50 cells/mm³)	Very high	Fatal opportunistic events possible

megalovirus, varicella-zoster virus, HIV-associated, *Toxoplasma*)

    b. Status epilepticus (HIV-associated, mass lesion)

C. Sepsis (10%)

    1. *Streptococcus pneumoniae*

    2. *Haemophilus pneumoniae*

    3. *Pseudomonas aeruginosa*

    4. Other Gram-negative bacteria

    5. *Mycobacterium tuberculosis*

    6. Nontuberculous mycobacteria, particularly *M. avium*

    7. *Staphylococcus aureus*

    8. Coagulase-negative staphylococci (device-related)

D. Other (10% to 20%)

    1. Gastrointestinal (bleed, perforation, obstruction, dehydration)

    2. Adrenal crisis

    3. Acid-base disturbance

    4. Post-procedure observation

Clinical Findings

A. Initial medical history

    1. Travel, residence since 1978

    2. Blood, transplant recipient (particularly before May 1985)

    3. Illicit drug use

    4. Sexual history

    5. Tuberculosis exposure and risk (homeless, unemployed, inner city, prison, group or nursing home, recreational drugs)

    6. Prior infections (mononucleosis syndrome, sexually transmitted diseases, hepatitis)

    7. Immunization record

B. Review of systems

    1. General: weight loss, anorexia, fever, sweats

    2. Skin: rash, pigmented lesions, pruritis, dryness

    3. Lymphatics: generalized adenopathy

    4. HEENT: headache, visual acuity, nasal discharge, sore throat, thrush

    5. Cardiopulmonary: cough, dyspnea

    6. Gastrointestinal: dsyphagia, odynophagia, diarrhea, abdominal pain

    7. Musculoskeletal: arthralgias, arthritis

    8. Gynecologic: persistent vaginitis, warts, menstrual difficulties, infertility

    9. Neurologic: depression, personality change, cognitive, bowel or bladder problems, peripheral weakness or paraesthesias

C. Physical findings

    1. Findings unique to HIV (or nearly so)

        a. Disseminated Kaposi's sarcoma

        b. Oral hairy leukoplakia

    2. Findings suggestive of HIV (other causes of immune suppression excluded)

        a. Oral thrush

        b. Cytomegalovirus retinitis

    3. Findings frequently seen, but not specific to HIV

        a. Integument: xerosis, tineas, folliculitis, molluscum, seborrhea, psoriasis

        b. Ocular fundi: cotton-wool spots

        c. Aphthous ulcers, herpes

        d. Generalized extrainguinal adenopathy

        e. Splenomegaly, hepatomegaly

        f. Genital or anal warts

        g. Neuropsychiatric

Key History in Known HIV-Infected Patients

- Date HIV diagnosed

- Transmission category

- Last CD4+ count and viral load

- Current antiretroviral therapy

- Current prophylaxis for opportunistic infection

- Event profile (prior opportunistic infections, malignancies)

- Advance directives and durable power of attorney

Laboratory Tests

A. Human immunodeficiency virus antibody test (if HIV infection not clearly documented)

B. CD4+ count

C. Serum HIV RNA (viral load); generally not necessary in the ICU setting

D. Complete blood count, differential, platelets

E. Routine serum biochemical assays

F. Tuberculosis cultures, gastrointestinal pathogens when appropriate

G. Serologic tests: syphilis; *Toxoplasma* IgG; hepatitis A, B, C; (cytomegalovirus serologies generally not useful)

Key Factors Adversely Affecting Survival

- Hospitals inexperienced in HIV care

- Empirical therapy for PCP

- High APACHE II score (mortality underestimated if CD4+ count less than 200 cells/mm^3)

- Glasgow Coma Scale score less than 7

- CD4+ lymphocyte count less than 50 cells/mm^3

- Baseline (pre-ICU admission) Karnofsky performance status less than 80%

- Previous opportunistic events, particularly PCP, disseminated *Mycobacterium avium* complex, cytomegalovirus disease, lymphoma, progressive multifocal leukoencephalopathy

Bibliography

Brown MC, Crede WB. Predictive ability of acute physiology and chronic health evaluation II scoring applied to human immunodeficiency virus-positive patients. Crit Care Med 1995;23:848–853.

Cohen PT, Katz MH. Long-term primary care management of HIV disease. In: Cohen PT, Sande MA, Volberding P (eds). The AIDS Knowledge Base, 3rd ed. Philadelphia: Lippincott Williams & Wilkins, 1999, pp 203–234.

Crane LR, Schuman P. Human immunodeficiency virus infection and the acquired immunodeficiency syndrome. In: Carlson RW, Geheb MA (eds). Principles and Practice of Medical Intensive Care. Philadelphia: WB Saunders, 1993, pp 589–601.

Zimmerman L, Huang L. Critical care of HIV-infected patients. In: Cohen PT, Sande MA, Volberding P (eds). The AIDS Knowledge Base, 3rd ed. Philadelphia: Lippincott Williams & Wilkins, 1999, pp 369–376.

100 *Pneumocystis carinii* Pneumonia

Lawrence R. Crane

During the pre-AIDS era, intensive care unit (ICU) admission rates for *Pneumocystis carinii* pneumonia (PCP) in the United States were less than 100 immunocompromised hosts/year. It was considered a eukaryotic protozoan. Diagnosis was made by open lung biopsy and treatment options were limited. Today, thousands of cases of PCP, mostly human immunodeficiency virus (HIV)-associated, are admitted to U.S. ICUs each year. It is the most common reason for ICU admission of an HIV-infected patient. *Pneumocystis* is now classified as a fungus, phylogenetically related to *Ascomycetes*. Diagnosis of PCP is much improved and there are better therapeutic approaches (Table 100–1).

Epidemiology (in HIV infection)

A. 53%: not on prophylaxis, not in care
B. 32%: on prophylaxis, immunologic breakthrough (CD4+ count <50 cells/mm^3)
C. 11%: not on prophylaxis, provider omission
D. 4%: outliers (CD4+ count >200 cells/mm^3)

Risk Factors

A. Human immunodeficiency virus infection (85% of cases)
  1. Adults: absolute CD4+ count less than 200 cells/mm^3 (or %CD4+ less than 20%)
  2. Infants and children younger than 6 years: absolute CD4+ count less than 500 cells/mm^3 (or %CD4+ less than 15%)
  3. History of previous PCP
  4. Thrush, B symptoms
B. Immunosuppressive therapy (corticosteroids, cytotoxic drugs)
  1. Organ transplantation
  2. Collagen vascular disease
  3. Malignancy (solid tumor more frequent than leukemia, lymphoma)
C. Other immunosuppression
  1. Protein-calorie malnutrition
  2. Idiopathic CD4+ lymphocytopenia

Clinical Findings

A. Symptoms: "classic" triad of dyspnea, fever, cough of gradual onset
B. Physical findings: minimal to marked dyspnea; lungs often clear

Differential Diagnosis

A. Bacterial pneumonias
  1. *Streptococcus pneumoniae*
  2. *Haemophilus pneumoniae*
  3. *Mycobacterium tuberculosis*
  4. Nontuberculous mycobacteria, particularly *M. kansasii, M. avium* complex
B. Fungal pneumonias
  1. *Cryptococcus neoformans*
  2. *Histoplasma capsulatum*
  3. *Coccidioides immitis*
C. Viral pneumonia: cytomegalovirus
D. Parasitic infections: *Toxoplasma gondii*
E. Noninfectious
  1. Neoplasia (Kaposi's sarcoma, lymphoma)
  2. Congestive heart failure
  3. Lymphoid interstitial pneumonitis

Diagnosis

A. Serum lactate dehydrogenase (LDH) activity
  1. Elevation can occur, but is nonspecific
  2. Is a predictor of outcome
B. Arterial blood gas
  1. PaO$_2$ ≤70 torr defines severe PCP.
  2. Alveolar–arterial oxygen tension difference ≥30 torr defines severe PCP.
C. Pulmonary function: decreased CO diffusion capacity is the most common abnormal finding
D. Chest x-ray
  1. "Classic" appearance: bilateral diffuse interstitial infiltrate
  2. May progress to alveolar consolidation as infection advances
  3. "Atypical" chest x-ray appearances
    a. Lung abscess
    b. Cavitary lung disease

TABLE 100–1. THERAPEUTIC OPTIONS FOR CRITICALLY ILL PATIENTS WITH *PNEUMOCYSTIS CARINII* PNEUMONIA

CRITICALLY ILL PATIENT, INITIAL THERAPY
- Trimethoprim (TMP)-sulfamethoxazole (SMX): 15–20 mg/kg per day (as TMP) intravenously in divided doses every 6 to 8 hours; *or*
- Pentamidine: 3 to 4 mg/kg per day, intravenously once daily

IF PaO$_2$ ≤70 TORR, OR ALVEOLAR–ARTERIAL OXYGEN TENSION DIFFERENCE >35 TORR
- Add prednisone: 40 mg PO every 12 hours, days 1 to 5; 40 mg once daily, days 6 to 10; 20 mg once daily, days 11 to 21
- May substitute methylprednisolone intravenously at 75% of prednisone doses

CRITICALLY ILL PATIENT, UNRESPONSIVE TO INITIAL THERAPY
- Switch to opposite first-line drug, consider desensitization if patient is on pentamidine and TMP-SMX allergic
- Primaquine: 30 mg/day PO once daily and clindamycin 900 mg intravenously every 8 hours; screen for glucose-6-phosphate dehydrogenase before starting primaquine
- Trimetrexate: 30 mg/m^2 per day intravenously in divided doses every 6 hours and leucovorin 20 mg/m^2 per day intravenously
- Other regimens: include aerosolized pentamidine, oral atovaquone, and dapsone/trimethoprim (have been evaluated only in patients who are mildly to moderately ill)

c. Lobar consolidation

d. Nodular densities

e. Pleural effusions

4. Upper lobe infiltrates, resembling tuberculosis

5. Normal chest x-ray

E. Nuclear medicine: gallium scan, indium scan (usually not practical in ICU setting)

F. Diagnostic microbiological procedures

1. Induced sputa collections

2. Deep tracheal suction specimens

3. Bronchoscopy with bronchoalveolar lavage (BAL) with or without transbronchial lung biopsy (TBBx)

4. Open lung biopsy

Key Diagnostic Considerations

- Establish a microbiological diagnosis: the differential diagnosis is broad, second pathogens can occur, and outcome will be better

- Microbiological diagnostic procedures for PCP dictated by the tempo of the disease: in the ICU setting generally do BAL with or without TBBx

- The gold standard for diagnosis is BAL with TBBx.

- In addition to stains and histologic examination for *Pneumocystis,* specimens should be stained and cultured for acid-fast organisms and fungi, and cultured for viruses.

- Repeat BAL, TBBx, and even open lung biopsy should be considered when a diagnosis is not made or for the patient with definite PCP failing first-line therapy.

Treatment (see Table 100–1)

Key Management Considerations

- For HIV patients with pulmonary infiltrates, tuberculosis must be considered in the differential diagnosis (in respiratory isolation until tuberculosis excluded).

- Clinical response is usually seen only after 3 to 5 days of effective therapy; maintain first round of therapy for 5 to 7 days before determining a clinical failure.

- Chest x-ray commonly shows worsening early during therapy; deterioration beyond 7 to 10 days signals therapeutic failure.

- *Pneumocystis* organisms will typically persist in BAL or induced sputum samples for at least 3 weeks in patients who have responded to therapy.

- There are no convincing data supporting combination therapy for PCP.

- When establishing prognosis, remember that most of the studies of predictors of outcome of PCP in HIV-infected patients were done before effective antiretroviral therapy was available.

Complications

A. Spontaneous pneumothorax

B. Extrapulmonary *Pneumocystis*

1. Usually occurs in patients receiving aerosol pentamidine

2. Retina, orbit, ear, heart, liver, spleen, small intestine, marrow, lymph nodes, kidneys, adrenals, pituitary, thyroid involvement can occur.

Prognosis

A. Predictors of poor outcome in mechanically ventilated patients

1. Empiric therapy for PCP

2. Spontaneous pneumothorax

3. High levels positive end-expiratory pressure (>10 mm Hg)

4. Previous PCP and other previous opportunistic events, particularly disseminated *Mycobacterium avium* complex, cytomegalovirus disease, lymphoma, progressive multifocal leukoencephalopathy

5. In ICU longer than 2 weeks

6. High APACHE II score underestimates mortality.

7. CD4+ lymphocyte count lower than 50 cells/mm³

8. Baseline (pre-ICU admission) Karnofsky performance status <80%

B. Predictors of survival in mechanically ventilated patients

1. Falling serum LDH; LDH less than 350 U/L

2. Higher serum albumin concentration

3. Mechanical ventilation for up to 96 hours

4. Adjunctive corticosteroid use

5. Treating center's familiarity with the disease (hospital has >30 HIV discharges per 10,000 discharges)

B Bibliography

Crane LR, Schuman P. Human immunodeficiency virus infection and the acquired immunodeficiency syndrome. In: Carlson RW, Geheb MA (eds). Principles and Practice of Medical Intensive Care. Philadelphia: WB Saunders, 1993, pp 589–601.

Horner RD, Bennett CL, Rodriguez D, et al. Relationship between procedures and health insurance for critically ill patients with *Pneumocystis carinii* pneumonia. Am J Respir Crit Care Med 1995;152:1435–1442.

Kazanjian P, Armstrong W, Hossler PA, et al. *Pneumocystis carinii* mutations are associated with duration of sulfa prophylaxis and with sulfa treatment failure and in AIDS patients. J Infect Dis 2000;182:551–557.

Leoung GS. *Pneumocystis carinii* pneumonia. In: Cohen PT, Sande MA, Volberding P (eds). The AIDS Knowledge Base, 3rd ed. Philadelphia: Lippincott Williams & Wilkins, 1999, pp 721–760.

101 Infections in Neutropenic Cancer Patients

George J. Alangaden

Patients with cancer, especially those with hematologic malignancies, who develop chemotherapy-induced neutropenia are at high risk for infection. The degree and duration of neutropenia determines the risk for infection and bacteremia. Most early infections are caused by Gram-positive cocci and Gram-negative bacilli. Fungal infections occur later in the course of neutropenia. Mucositis induced by chemotherapy and vascular access catheters facilitates entry of pathogens from the gastrointestinal (GI) tract and skin. These infections are difficult to evaluate because of the diminished inflammatory response associated with the lack of neutrophils. Fever is often the only clinical feature and may represent an occult infection in 50% to 60% of cases. Clinical evaluation of a febrile neutropenic patient requires particular attention to the mouth, pharynx, perirectal area, lungs, sinuses, skin, and vascular access sites. Signs of infection are often muted. Blood cultures, cultures from sites of identified or suspected infection, and chest x-rays should be performed. Infections can be rapidly progressive, and hence antimicrobial therapy is necessarily empiric prior to the identification of an infection. Selection of an initial antimicrobial regimen is guided by the potential sites of infection, pathogens likely present at these sites, antimicrobial susceptibilities of these pathogens at the local institution, and the severity of infection. In the absence of an identified infection or positive culture, a broad-spectrum antibiotic with activity against Gram-negative bacilli, including *Pseudomonas aeruginosa*, should be initiated. Therapy is modified to cover Gram-positive pathogens and fungi based on identification or increased likelihood of infection due to these pathogens, lack of response to initial antibiotics, or clinical worsening. Duration of antimicrobial therapy depends on the resolution of fever, neutropenia, or documented infection.

Key Definitions

- Fever: oral temperature higher than 38°C (100°F)
- Neutropenia: absolute neutrophil count less than 500 cells/mm³

Etiology

A. Fever
  1. Bacterial infections, including bacteremia
    a. Gram-positive cocci
    b. Gram-negative bacilli
  2. Fungal infections, including fungemia
    a. *Candida* spp.
    b. Molds (e.g., *Aspergillus* spp.)
  3. Chemotherapy-related
  4. Transfusions of blood products
  5. Underlying malignancy
B. Oral mucosal lesions
  1. Chemotherapy-related mucositis
  2. Herpes simplex virus (HSV)
  3. Anaerobic bacteria
  4. *Candida* spp.
C. Dysphagia
  1. Chemotherapy or radiation-related mucositis
  2. *Candida* spp.
  3. Herpes simplex virus
D. Diarrhea or abdominal pain
  1. *Clostridium difficile*
  2. Polymicrobial intra-abdominal infections
  3. Neutropenic enterocolitis or typhlitis (anaerobes)
  4. Chemotherapy-related
E. Perirectal pain: polymicrobial infections
F. Pneumonia
  1. Bacterial infection (Gram-negative bacilli)
  2. Mold infection (occurs after prolonged neutropenia)
  3. Other: pulmonary edema, drug or radiation toxicity
G. Sinusitis
  1. Bacterial infection
  2. Mold infection
  3. Respiratory viruses (particularly with rhinitis)
H. Rashes
  1. Chemotherapy or radiation-related toxicity
  2. Transfusion-related
  3. Bacteremia (ecthyma gangrenosum)
  4. Fungemia (*Candida* or molds such as *Fusarium* spp.)
I. Vascular access device infections
  1. Coagulase-negative staphylococci
  2. *Staphylococcus aureus*
  3. *Corynebacterium* spp.
  4. Gram-negative bacilli
  5. *Candida* spp.

J. Liver disease
1. Chemotherapy-related toxicity
2. *Candida* spp. (often manifests at resolution of neutropenia)

Key Etiology Points

- Bacterial pathogens and HSV account for most early infections.

- Fungal infections with *Candida* spp. are next in frequency.

- Molds (e.g., *Aspergillus* spp.) cause invasive disease when neutropenia is prolonged.

- Most infections result from endogenous GI tract or skin-associated microbial flora.

- Consider noninfectious causes such as chemotherapy or radiation-related toxicity, transfusion reactions, and underlying disease in the differential diagnoses.

Laboratory Tests

A. Routine
1. Complete blood cell count and differential
2. Routine serum biochemical tests
3. Serum liver function tests
4. Urinalysis
5. Chest x-ray
B. Specific:
1. Blood cultures for bacteria and fungi
2. Gram stains and cultures of specimens from any site of suspected infection
3. Oral mucosal, genital, or perianal lesions
   a. Direct fluorescent antibody, culture for HSV
   b. KOH smear and culture for *Candida* spp.
4. Diarrhea: *C. difficile* toxin assays of stool
5. Pneumonia
   a. Chest x-ray
   b. Computed tomography (CT) scans, if fungal infection suspected
   c. Sputum
   d. Bronchoalveolar lavage
   e. Lung biopsy
   f. Tests on clinical respiratory specimens
      (1) Gram stain, fungal stain, acid-fast stain
      (2) Cultures for bacteria, fungi, mycobacteria
      (3) Direct fluorescent antibody tests (dFA) and cultures for respiratory viruses

(4) *Legionella* dFA and culture
(5) Histopathology
6. Sinusitis
   a. Computed tomography scan
   b. Sinus aspirate: test for bacteria and fungi
   c. Nasopharyngeal wash (if rhinitis) test for respiratory viruses
7. Rash
   a. Viral dFA and cultures (vesicular lesions)
   b. Gram stain and culture (bacterial and fungal) of aspirate or biopsy
8. Vascular access device site inflammation: perform Gram stain and cultures from exit site, blood cultures
9. Liver disease
   a. Serum transaminase, alkaline phosphatase, amylase, and lipase activities and bilirubin concentration
   b. Serology for hepatitis viruses B and C, cytomegalovirus
   c. Ultrasonography, CT scan of abdomen
   d. Biopsy: tests for fungi, bacteria, viruses, and histopathology

Key Diagnostic Points

- Estimate duration of neutropenia.

- Determine relationship of fevers to transfusions and drug administration.

- Consider symptoms and signs of infection at sites commonly affected; i.e., GI tract, lungs, sinuses, skin, vascular access devices.

- Symptoms and signs of infection are often subtle in the absence of neutrophils.

- Reevaluate patient daily with attention to common sites of infection.

- Absence of neutrophils in appropriate clinical specimens does not invalidate microbiology results.

Treatment

A. Initial empiric therapy for fever in the absence of identified site or pathogen
1. Extended-spectrum antipseudomonal cephalosporins: cefepime or ceftazidime
2. Carbapenems: imipenem, meropenem
3. Combination therapy: e.g., antipseudomonal penicillin + aminoglycoside

4. Consider addition of empiric vancomycin to initial empiric therapy only if
   a. Vascular access device infection
   b. High likelihood of penicillin-resistant viridans streptococci
   c. Septic shock
5. Consider addition of anti-anaerobic agent, e.g., metronidazole or clindamycin, if
   a. Intra-abdominal infection
   b. Perirectal infection
   c. Severe mucositis

B. Follow-up evaluation and modification of initial empiric therapy if no identified site or pathogen
1. Afebrile within 4 days of initial antibiotic therapy: continue same therapy
2. Persistent fevers after 3 to 4 days of initial therapy
   a. Clinically stable
      (1) Continue same therapy.
      (2) Discontinue empiric vancomycin if no Gram-positive pathogen identified.
      (3) Consider consultation with infectious disease specialist.
   b. Clinically unstable
      (1) Broaden antibiotic coverage (e.g., add anti-anaerobic agent).
      (2) Add vancomycin, if indicated (see A.4. above).
      (3) Consider addition of amphotericin B.
   c. Persistent fevers after 5 to 7 days of initial therapy: add amphotericin B

C. Pathogen-specific directed therapy
1. Treat with optimal doses of standard antimicrobial agents directed against the pathogen(s) identified and based on results of susceptibility tests.
2. Intravenous administration is generally preferred.

D. Duration of therapy
1. Factors determining duration of therapy
   a. Resolution of neutropenia
   b. Resolution of fever
   c. Resolution of signs of infection
   d. Eradication of infecting pathogen
   e. Eradication of source: e.g., removal of infected catheter
2. Site and pathogen identified
   a. Duration of therapy is generally similar to that of non-neutropenic patients.
   b. Invasive fungal infections: treat until resolution of all clinical and radiological features of infection
3. Fever but no identified site or pathogen
   a. Afebrile and neutropenia resolved: total of approximately 7 days
   b. Afebrile, but persistently neutropenic: additional 7 to 14 days
   c. Febrile, but neutropenia resolved: 7 days postresolution of neutropenia
   d. Febrile and persistently neutropenic: 14 days, then reevaluate; if stable consider stopping antibiotics

Key Treatment Points

- Treat all neutropenic patients with fever or signs of infection promptly using empiric high-dose, IV, broad-spectrum antibiotics.

- Select initial antibiotics based on potential sites of infection, likely pathogens at those sites, and antimicrobial susceptibilities of the pathogens locally.

- Modify management based on daily evaluation, cultures, and response to therapy.

- Treat until resolution of neutropenia and signs of infection.

Prevention of Infection

A. Controversial issue
B. However, antimicrobial prophylaxis may be considered if expected duration of chemotherapy-induced profound neutropenia (<100 cells/mm^3) is longer than 7 days.
1. Bacterial: quinolones or trimethoprim/sulfamethoxazole
2. Fungal: fluconazole
3. HSV: acyclovir (if HSV-seropositive)
C. Once started, continue until resolution of neutropenia.

Bibliography

Hughes WT, Armstrong D, Bodey GP, et al. Guidelines for the use of antimicrobial agents in neutropenic patients with unexplained fever. Clin Infect Dis 1997;25:551–573.

Pizzo PA. Empirical therapy and prevention of infection in the immunocompromised host. In: Mandell GL, Bennett JE, Dolin R (eds). Principles and Practice of Infectious Diseases. Philadelphia: Churchill Livingstone, 2000, pp 3102–3112.

Rubenstein E, Wade JC, et al. NCCN practice guidelines for fever and neutropenia. Oncology 1999;13:197–257.

102 Infections in Bone Marrow Transplant Patients

Pranatharthi H. Chandrasekar

Blood and marrow transplantation (BMT) is performed worldwide for hematologic and oncologic diseases including aplastic anemia, leukemia, lymphoma, and solid tumors. The procedure consists of ablation of bone marrow and tumor followed by infusion of hemopoietic progenitor cells in order to restore the immunohemopoietic system. Profound immunodeficiency results from BMT; complete immune reconstitution requires 1 to 2 years after transplantation. Hence, BMT recipients are at high risk for common and opportunistic infections.

Definitions

A. Based on the source of graft (stem cells), the transplant is termed
   1. Autologous: stem cells are derived from recipient's own blood and marrow
   2. Allogeneic: stem cells are derived from another individual
   3. Umbilical cord: stem cells are derived from umbilical cord blood
   4. Marrow: stem cells are derived from bone marrow
   5. Peripheral blood: stem cells are derived from peripheral blood

B. Allogeneic transplantation is further classified as
   1. Matched-related: donor and recipient are related and have similar human leukocyte antigen (HLA) types
   2. Mismatched-related: donor and recipient are related and have dissimilar HLA types
   3. Matched-unrelated: donor and recipient are unrelated and have similar HLA types
   4. Minitransplantation
      a. A procedure combining the use of a nonmyeloablative conditioning regimen along with infusion of high numbers of donor CD 34 antigen-expressing cells
      b. Reserved for older and less medically fit patients
      c. Shorter duration of neutropenia is the anticipated goal.

C. Graft-versus-host disease (GVHD)
   1. A condition that occurs in allogeneic recipients as a consequence of donor lymphocytes attacking tissue sites (usually skin, gut, and liver) of the genetically different immunodeficient recipient
   2. Frequency of GVHD is highest among those receiving stem cells from mismatched or unrelated donors.

D. CD 34 antigen-positive stem cell transplant
   1. Infusion of blood rich in CD 34 antigen expressing stem cells
   2. The product is "devoid" of tumor cells and mature T and B lymphocytes; consequently, tumor relapse and GVHD are less frequent, but immune reconstitution is delayed.

Risk Factors

A. Allogeneic transplant
   1. Phase I: day of transplant to day 30 posttransplant
      a. Risk for infection
         (1) Neutropenia
         (2) Mucositis
         (3) Diarrhea
         (4) Acute GVHD
         (5) Vascular devices
      b. Common microorganisms
         (1) Bacteria: Gram-positive cocci, Gram-negative rods, *Clostridium difficile*
         (2) Viruses: herpes simplex virus (HSV), rotavirus
         (3) Fungus: *Candida*
   2. Phase II: 30 to 100 days posttransplant
      a. Risk for infection
         (1) Acute GVHD
         (2) Chronic GVHD
         (3) Immunosuppressive drugs
         (4) Corticosteroids
         (5) Impaired cellular immunity
         (6) Vascular devices

b. Common microorganisms
  (1) Viruses: cytomegalovirus, HSV, Epstein-Barr virus
  (2) Fungi: *Aspergillus, Candida, Pneumocystis carinii*
3. Phase III: >100 days posttransplant
  a. Risk for infection
    (1) Chronic GVHD
    (2) Immunosuppressive drugs
    (3) Corticosteroids
    (4) Impaired humoral and cellular immunity
  b. Common microorganisms
    (1) Bacteria: *Streptococcus pneumoniae, Haemophilus influenzae, Staphylococcus aureus,* Gram-negative bacteria
    (2) Fungi: *Aspergillus, Pneumocystis*
    (3) Viruses: varicella-zoster, cytomegalovirus, Epstein-Barr virus
    (4) Parasite: *Toxoplasma*
B. Autologous transplant
  1. Phase I: same risk factors as in allogeneic transplant
  2. Phases II and III: risk for infection is low since GVHD is not seen and no GVHD prophylaxis (e.g., cyclosporin A) is employed

Etiology

A. Fever
  1. Bacteremia: Gram-positive cocci, Gram-negative rods
  2. Fungemia: *Candida*
  3. Conditioning regimen
  4. Transfusions
  5. GVHD
B. Mucositis (oral)
  1. Herpes simplex virus
  2. *Candida*
  3. Anaerobic bacteria
C. Diarrhea
  1. Bacterial: *Clostridium difficile*
  2. Viral: rotavirus, adenovirus, cytomegalovirus
  3. GVHD
D. Rashes
  1. Conditioning regimen
  2. Drug allergies
  3. Transfusion-associated
  4. Virus-related: herpes simplex, varicella-zoster
  5. Fungi: *Candida, Aspergillus,* other fungi
  6. GVHD

E. Vascular device-associated infection
  1. Coagulase-negative staphylococci
  2. *Staphylococcus aureus*
  3. *Corynebacterium*
  4. Gram-negative bacilli
  5. *Candida*
F. Nasal drainage
  1. Respiratory syncytial virus
  2. Influenza virus
  3. Parainfluenza virus
  4. Adenovirus
G. Pneumonia
  1. Phase I
    a. Gram-negative bacilli
    b. Pulmonary edema
    c. Alveolar hemorrhage
    d. Drug-associated
    e. Engraftment syndrome
  2. Phase II and III
    a. Bacterial: *Streptococcus pneumoniae, Legionella, Nocardia*
    b. Viral: cytomegalovirus, human herpesvirus 6
    c. Fungal: *Aspergillus, Pneumocystis carinii*
    d. Drug-associated
    e. Radiation-associated
    f. Idiopathic pneumonia
    g. Bronchiolitis obliterans
H. Encephalitis
  1. Viral: cytomegalovirus, HSV, human herpesvirus 6
  2. Fungal: *Aspergillus*
  3. Protozoan: *Toxoplasma*
  4. Drug-associated (e.g., cyclosporin A)
I. Hepatitis
  1. Conditioning regimen (e.g., veno-occlusive disease)
  2. GVHD
  3. Drug-associated
  4. Fungal: *Candida, Aspergillus*
  5. Viral: HSV, varicella-zoster, adenovirus, hepatitis B, hepatitis C
J. Hemorrhagic cystitis
  1. Cyclophosphamide
  2. GVHD
  3. Viral: adenovirus, BK/JC virus

PEARLS

- Risks for infection vary according to the time from transplantation.

- Types and rates of infections are similar during phase I in allogeneic and autologous recipients; thereafter, infections are less frequent in autologous recipients.

- Commonly encountered organisms are skin and gut-associated bacteria, herpes simplex virus and *Candida* during phase I, cytomegalovirus and *Aspergillus* during phase II, and *Streptococcus pneumoniae*, varicella-zoster, and *Aspergillus* during phase III.

- Mimickers of infection include effects of underlying disease, conditioning-regimen effects, GVHD and immunosuppressive therapy.

Laboratory and Other Tests

A. Blood cultures
   1. Bacteria
   2. Virus: cytomegalovirus
   3. Fungi: *Candida, Fusarium*
B. Stool studies
   1. *Clostridium difficile* toxin
   2. Rotavirus
C. Oral ulcers
   1. Herpes simplex virus: direct fluorescent antibody test (DFA), culture
   2. *Candida*: KOH smear, culture
D. Skin rashes
   1. Herpes simplex virus: DFA, culture
   2. Varicella-zoster virus: DFA, culture
   3. Biopsy
      a. Gram stain
      b. Fungal stain
      c. Acid-fast bacilli stain
      d. Histology
      e. Bacterial, fungal, viral cultures
E. Pulmonary findings
   1. Radiographs
      a. Chest x-ray
      b. Computed tomography (CT) scan of chest
   2. Specimens
      a. Sputum
      b. Bronchoalveolar lavage
      c. Lung biopsy

   3. Tests
      a. Gram stain
      b. Fungal stain
      c. Acid-fast bacilli stain
      d. *Legionella*: DFA
      e. Respiratory viruses (respiratory syncytial virus, influenza and parainfluenza viruses, adenovirus, cytomegalovirus): DFA
      f. Staining for *Pneumocystis carinii*
      g. Cultures for bacteria, fungi, viruses, mycobacteria
F. Upper respiratory tract symptoms: nasal wash for respiratory viruses by DFA
G. Cerebrospinal fluid: polymerase chain reaction (PCR) and culture for viruses
   1. Cytomegalovirus
   2. Human herpesvirus 6
   3. Varicella-zoster
   4. Herpes simplex virus
H. Liver function abnormalities
   1. Serologies for hepatitis B and C viruses, cytomegalovirus
   2. Cytomegalovirus antigen in blood, DNA in blood by PCR
   3. Computed tomography scan of abdomen
   4. Biopsy

Treatment

A. Empiric therapy for fever during neutropenia (phase I): antibiotics active against Gram-negative bacilli, particularly against *Pseudomonas* (e.g., cefepime, ceftazidime, imipenem)
B. Therapy for specific pathogens
   1. Gram-negative bacilli
      a. Cefepime
      b. Ceftazidime
      c. Ciprofloxacin
   2. Gram-positive cocci
      a. Vancomycin
      b. Nafcillin
      c. Penicillin
   3. Anaerobic bacteria
      a. Clindamycin
      b. Metronidazole
      c. Imipenem
   4. Herpes simplex virus and varicella-zoster virus
      a. Acyclovir
      b. Valacyclovir
      c. Famciclovir
      d. Foscarnet (if acyclovir-resistant)

5. Cytomegalovirus
   a. Ganciclovir
   b. Foscarnet (if ganciclovir-resistant)
6. Repiratory syncytial virus: aerosol ribavirin
7. *Candida (C. albicans, C. tropicalis):* fluconazole
8. *Candida (C. krusei* and other fluconazole-resistant species)
   a. Amphotericin B
   b. Lipid formulations of amphotericin B
9. *Aspergillus*
   a. Amphotericin B
   b. Lipid formulations of amphotericin B
   c. Itraconazole
   d. Caspofungin
10. *Pneumocystis carinii*
    a. Trimethoprim-sulfamethoxazole
    b. Pentamidine
11. *Toxoplasma:* pyrimethamine plus sulfadiazine

C. Prophylaxis
   1. From transplantation to 30 days post-transplant
      a. Gram-negative bacilli: norfloxacin, ciprofloxacin
      b. *Candida:* fluconazole
      c. Herpes simplex: acyclovir
   2. From 30 to 100 days posttransplant
      a. Cytomegalovirus: ganciclovir
      b. *Streptococcus pneumoniae:* penicillin

   c. *Pneumocystis carinii:* trimethoprim-sulfamethoxazole
3. More than 100 days posttransplant: same as phase II in patients with ongoing GVHD and immunosuppressive therapy

Key Treatment

- Correction of immune deficiencies is as important as antimicrobial therapy during infection management.

- Antimicrobial agents are employed in empiric, therapeutic, and prophylactic settings; side effects and antimicrobial resistance are common.

- Prompt diagnostic tests and early empiric therapy are critical for successful management.

Bibliography

Hughes WT, Armstrong D, Bodey GP, et al. 1997 Guidelines for the use of antimicrobial agents in neutropenic patients with unexplained fever. Clin Infect Dis 1997;25: 551–573.

Momin F, Chandrasekar PH. Antimicrobial prophylaxis in bone marrow transplantation. Ann Intern Med 1995; 123:205–215.

Van Burik JA, Weisdorf D. Infections in recipients of blood and marrow transplantation. In: Mandell GL, Bennett JE, Dolin T (eds). Principles and Practice of Infectious Diseases. Philadelphia: Churchill Livingstone, 2000, pp 3136–3147.

Walter EA, Bowden RA. Infection in the bone marrow transplant recipient. Infect Dis Clin North Am 1995;9: 823–847.

103 Infections in Solid Organ Transplant Patients

Peter K. Linden

Solid organ recipients are susceptible to a diverse spectrum of infectious pathogens from the combined effects of the transplant surgery, iatrogenic immunosuppression to prevent and treat allograft rejection, underlying comorbid conditions (cirrhosis, diabetes) and exposure to pathogens derived from either the donor organ or the microflora in the hospital and community. The incidence of specific infections varies according to which solid organ has been transplanted, the dosage and type of immunosuppression, and the exposure history of the transplant recipient to pathogens. Early diagnosis and aggressive treatment are essential to reducing infection-related morbidity and mortality. Numerous preventive and preemptive strategies have evolved which can significantly reduce the impact of certain post-transplant infections.

Epidemiology

A. Early period (0 to 4 weeks)

1. Early infections are associated with complications related to the transplant surgery itself, incubating or undetected infections that were present prior to transplantation, allograft dysfunction, and iatrogenic immunosuppression.

2. Multi-resistant nosocomial pathogens: methicillin-resistant *Staphylococcus aureus,* vancomycin-resistant *Enterococcus* spp, *Pseudomonas aeruginosa* and *Candida* are common, probably because of heavy prior antimicrobial exposure during the pre- and peri-transplant period

   a. Technical complications of transplant surgery

      (1) Kidney: perinephric abscess, ureteral or vascular anastomotic leaks

      (2) Liver: peritonitis, infected intra-abdominal collection, bile leak, cholangitis, liver abscess from hepatic artery insufficiency

      (3) Heart: sternal wound infection, mediastinitis

      (4) Lung: bronchial anastomosis infection, empyema

      (5) Pancreas: enteric anastomotic leaks, intrapancreatic abscess

   b. Hospital-acquired infections: pneumonia, intravascular device infection, urinary tract infection, wound infection, *Clostridium difficile* colitis

   c. Herpes simplex virus (HSV) infection from reactivation of dormant preexisting infection: orolabial, genital, disseminated cutaneous, or visceral infection (rare)

B. Middle period (2 to 6 months)

1. The dominant pathogen(s) include cytomegalovirus (CMV), reactivated dormant agents (*Mycobacterium tuberculosis,* endemic mycoses, viral hepatitides), and exogenous pathogens (*Listeria monocytogenes, Aspergillus, Cryptococcus neoformans, Nocardia*).

2. Risk factors for infection during this interval include

   a. High doses of immunosuppressive agents during the early post-transplant period

   b. Necessity for repeat transplantation

   c. Prolonged hospitalization after the transplantation

   d. Lack of pair immunity

   e. Unusual epidemiologic exposure

3. Cytomegalovirus

   a. Patients with primary CMV infection (i.e., seropositive donor, seronegative recipient) have the highest rate (70%) and severity of invasive disease.

   b. Transplant recipients who are CMV seropositive have less severe disease.

   c. Cytomegalovirus disease is also likely to be severe in lung transplant recipients and patients receiving anti-lymphocyte therapy (OKT3 or anti-thymocyte globulin).

   d. The CMV syndrome is characterized by fever and constitutional symptoms.

   e. Cytomegalovirus pneumonitis is characterized by fever, symmetrical interstitial infiltrates, and hypoxemia.

   f. Cytomegalovirus hepatitis is associated with elevated liver enzyme levels.

   g. Cytomegalovirus enteritis is associated with esophagitis (odynophagia), gastroduodenitis (bleeding), and/or colitis (diarrhea).

   h. Disseminated CMV disease is present when there is invasive disease involving two or

369

more noncontiguous sites (e.g., lung and liver).

    i. Secondary effects of CMV: superinfection with other opportunistic pathogens, allograft rejection caused by up-regulation of class II HLA antigens, or late allograft dysfunction

4. Other viruses

    a. Epstein-Barr virus (EBV): responsible for the development of post-transplant lymphoproliferative disease with visceral B lymphocyte tumors of variable severity; EBV-seronegative recipients and patients treated with anti-lymphocyte agents are at highest risk for this infection

    b. Human herpesvirus (6, 7, or 8) infection may manifest in several ways.

        (1) Asymptomatic shedding

        (2) Viral syndrome

        (3) Invasive disease (encephalitis, hepatitis, or pneumonia)

    c. Viral hepatitides (hepatitis B, hepatitis C)

    d. Polyomavirus (JC, BK)

        (1) Progressive multifocal encephalopathy causes white matter lesions and multiple neurologic deficits; there is no proven effective therapy.

        (2) JCV or BKV viruria in renal transplant recipients may be asymptomatic or lead to ureteral ulcers or stenosis.

    e. Adenovirus

5. Bacteria

    a. *M. tuberculosis*: may be primary or reactivated infection; disseminated disease is more common than in the general population

    b. *Nocardia asteroides*: causes pulmonary lesions that can spread to soft tissue or the central nervous system

    c. *L. monocytogenes*: the most common cause of bacterial meningitis in organ recipients; can cause meningoencephalitis, focal central nervous system lesions, or bacteremia with sepsis

    d. *Legionella* infection causes pneumonia; extrapulmonary disease is rare.

6. Fungi

    a. *Candida* spp (responsible for most fungal infections in transplant recipients)

    b. *Aspergillus* and other filamentous fungi

    c. *Cryptococcus neoformans*

    d. *Pneumocystis carinii* (in absence of prophylaxis)

C. Late period (>6 months)

1. Most transplant recipients have good allograft function with low-dose maintenance immunosuppression and have infectious disease(s) similar to the general community in the absence of unusual exposures.

2. Chronic progressive infection(s) and sporadic opportunistic infections can occur in the late period.

3. Recipients with chronic rejection or receiving higher doses of immunosuppressive agents remain at higher risk.

4. Community-acquired infections

    a. Varicella zoster: primary infection (chickenpox) or reactivated (shingles)

    b. *Streptococcus pneumoniae*

    c. Influenza A or B

5. Chronic or progressive infections: viral hepatitides, CMV retinitis

6. Sporadic reactivation or primary infection with pathogens listed above

Key Risk Factors

- Prior infection with the pathogen

- High immunosuppressive burden (e.g., use of antilymphocyte agents or high-dose corticosteroid therapy)

- Lack of compliance with prophylactic drug regimen (trimethoprim-sulfamethoxazole)

Diagnosis

A. Pulmonary system

1. The time of post-transplant exposure, known or suspected environmental exposures, radiographic pattern, and compliance with chemoprophylaxis are key data elements that are required to construct a differential diagnosis.

2. Diagnostic evaluation

    a. Chest x-ray

        (1) Essential first study, but it may not be adequate for visualization of small lesions or those located in posterior-inferior areas

        (2) The radiographic pattern may narrow the differential diagnosis.

            (a) Discrete nodular or cavitary lesions: fungi (e.g., *Aspergillus*, *Mucor*, endemic mycoses), *M. tuberculosis*, pyogenic abscess (primary or metastatic), or other agents (e.g., *C. neoformans*, *Nocardia*)

            (b) Diffuse interstitial or alveolar pattern: CMV pneumonia, *P. carinii* (if not receiving prophylaxis), *Strongyloides stercoralis* (if prior inhabitant of tropical zones), adenovirus, or primary varicella infection

b. Computed tomography (CT) of the chest is the technique of choice to examine for a discrete nodule or cavity, mediastinal or hilar adenopathy, and pleural processes.

c. Sputum analysis for Gram, acid-fast, and silver stains

d. Bronchoscopy with lavage or transbronchial biopsy provides a better yield than sputum for acid-fast bacilli, *Aspergillus*, *P. carinii*, and other opportunistic pathogens.

e. Open lung biopsy should be reserved only for enigmatic cases or those not responding to well-chosen empiric therapy, or when it is not possible to establish the etiology with bronchoscopy.

B. Central nervous system

1. Altered mental status with or without subtle meningeal signs

a. Consider bacterial, viral, and fungal etiologies including *L. monocytogenes*, *S. pneumoniae*, *C. neoformans*, and Gram-negative bacilli.

b. Diagnostic evaluation

(1) Head CT or magnetic resonance imaging (MRI) should be obtained first to rule out mass effects and/or midline shift.

(2) Lumbar puncture should be performed and cerebrospinal fluid submitted for cell count, glucose and protein concentration, Gram and India ink stains, routine and fungal cultures, and polymerase chain reaction assay for HSV.

2. Focal neurologic signs including seizure, myoclonus, paresis, or sensory loss

a. Differential diagnosis includes abscess secondary to *Aspergillus* or other mycelial fungi, *Toxoplasma gondii*, *C. neoformans*, HSV encephalitis, *L. monocytogenes*, disseminated bacterial infection, progressive multifocal leukoencephalopathy, or demyelinating syndrome from cyclosporine or tacrolimus.

b. Diagnostic evaluation

(1) Head CT or MRI should be obtained; MRI is more sensitive for small lesions and brain-stem lesions and does not require injection of a nephrotoxic contrast agent.

(2) Lumbar puncture: see above

(3) Electroencephalogram to exclude seizure activity; temporal lobe localization may indicate HSV encephalitis

C. Skin

1. Discrete or confluent lesions may represent primary cutaneous inoculation or evidence of hematogenous dissemination.

2. Noninfectious etiologies including allergic reactions, tumor, and graft-versus-host disease need to be considered.

3. Diagnostic evaluation

a. Skin biopsy should be submitted for special stains, cultures, and histopathologic examination.

b. Examine other organ systems for evidence of dissemination and obtain routine and fungal blood cultures if dissemination is suspected.

D. Gastrointestinal system

1. Infection can present as localized pain (odynophagia due to esophageal candidiasis), diarrhea (CMV enterocolitis), hemorrhage (EBV-related lymphoma, *Mucor* enteritis, CMV enteritis).

2. Diagnostic evaluation

a. X-ray imaging (e.g., barium swallow, small bowel follow-through study) is of limited benefit but may localize an abnormality that can direct subsequent endoscopic examinations.

b. Diarrhea samples should be submitted to the laboratory and analyzed for presence of *Clostridium difficile* toxin, ova and parasites, and enteric pathogens.

c. Endoscopic studies (i.e., esophagogastroduodenoscopy or colonoscopy) are indicated to visualize the mucosa and to obtain mucosal biopsies where appropriate.

Special Considerations

A. Kidney transplantation

1. Lowest rates of post-transplant infection

2. Removal of the allograft (and resumption of hemodialysis) is a potential strategy for stopping immunosuppression in patients with life-threatening infections.

B. Liver transplantation

1. Major risk factors for early infection are large transfusion requirement, long operative time, and choledochojejunostomy biliary anastomosis.

2. The most common manifestation of CMV infection is CMV hepatitis.

3. Common post-transplant problems include

a. Recurrent hepatitis C: 100% rate of viremia with variable graft dysfunction

b. Candidal peritonitis

C. Heart transplantation

1. Highest risk for toxoplasmosis due to transmission from heart donor to a seronegative recipient

2. Highest rates of nocardial infection

3. Patients with implanted artificial heart devices can have residual infection after transplantation.

D. Lung transplantation

1. Several factors contribute to very high rates of lung infection.

a. Impaired cellular host defenses in the graft

b. Impaired lymphatic drainage

c. Airway denervation

d. Obliterative bronchiolitis

2. Cytomegalovirus pneumonitis is the most frequent manifestation of CMV infection.

3. Organisms in the donor lung can contribute to the development of early pneumonia.

4. Pulmonary colonization with *Aspergillus* is common during the pre-transplant period and may require post-transplant prophylaxis.

5. Because of retention of a diseased native lung in the recipient, pulmonary infections are more common in single-lung recipients than double-lung recipients.

6. The "at-risk" period for opportunistic respiratory infection (CMV, *P. carinii*) is prolonged beyond the first year and may require extended chemoprophylaxis.

E. Pancreas transplantation

1. Exocrine drainage of the pancreas by anastomosis to the bladder is associated with a higher incidence of urinary tract infection.

2. Exocrine drainage of the pancreas by enteric anastomosis has a higher rate of intra-abdominal infection.

3. Recipients of combined kidney and pancreas organs have higher rates of wound infection and CMV disease.

Prevention

A. Bacterial prophylaxis (regimens shown are those in use at the University of Pittsburgh Medical Center)

1. Surgical wound prophylaxis

a. Kidney: ampicillin-sulbactam

b. Liver: ampicillin-sulbactam or ampicillin + cefotaxime

c. Heart: cefazolin

d. Lung: cefipime plus clindamycin (modification may be needed based on results of donor lung cultures)

2. Urinary tract prophylaxis in kidney transplant recipients: 3 to 6 months of therapy with trimethoprim-sulfamethoxazole (TMP-SMX) or a fluoroquinolone reduces the incidence of urinary tract infection

3. If the organ donor is suspected to have bloodstream or other serious unsuspected infection at the time of organ procurement, then the prophylactic regimen for the recipient should be tailored to ensure coverage against the specific pathogen(s) and consideration given to using a longer course of therapy.

B. Fungal prophylaxis

1. Prevention of candidal infection

a. Low-dose amphotericin B: 10 to 20 mg/day for 7 to 14 days

b. Fluconazole: 400 mg/day for first month

c. Mycostatin: 2 to 8 million U/day

2. Prevention of *Aspergillus* infection

a. Itraconazole: 200 to 400 mg/day

b. Aerosolized amphotericin B

3. *Pneumocystis carinii* prophylaxis

a. All organ transplant recipients should receive 6 to 12 months of post-transplant prophylaxis.

b. Lung transplant recipients and patients with a chronically high immunosuppressive burden should receive prolonged *P. carinii* prophylaxis as their risk extends beyond 12 months.

c. Agents

(1) TMP-SMX: 1 single-strength daily for 12 months

(2) TMP-SMX: 1 double-strength every other day for 12 months

(3) Aerosolized pentamidine: 300 mg every 4 weeks

(4) Dapsone: 50 to 100 mg/day

Key Points to Guide Prevention

- Assessment of risk e.g., organ type, type and quantity of immunosuppression, exposure

- Target specific pathogens (e.g., CMV, *P. carinii*).

- Major approaches
  - Boost host immunity (vaccine).
  - Avoid exposure (donor screening).
  - Chemoprophylaxis (ganciclovir, TMP/SMX, INH)
  - Passive immunity (VZIG, HBIG)

C. Viral prophylaxis or preemptive strategies
  1. Herpes simplex virus: acyclovir, 800 mg twice a day
  2. Cytomegalovirus
     a. High-dose acyclovir: 3200 mg/day (effective in kidney transplantation)
     b. Parenteral ganciclovir: 5 mg/kg every 12 hours
        (1) Use for the first 14 to 28 post-transplant days.
        (2) Use for 14 days after evidence of CMV shedding by positive leukocyte CMV antigenemia or polymerase chain reaction testing.
        (3) Use for 14 days after antilymphocyte therapy.
     c. Oral ganciclovir is an option for long-term (6 to 12 months) prophylaxis in high-risk patients.
     d. Hyperimmune anti-CMV globulin
     e. Other approaches
        (1) Use only CMV seronegative blood products in CMV-negative recipients of CMV-negative organs.
        (2) Cytomegalovirus vaccination pre-transplant

Key Points in CMV Prevention

- Highest risk categories are CMV seronegative recipients of CMV positive donors, lung recipients and those receiving anti-lymphocyte therapy.

- Parenteral or oral ganciclovir is the most common antiviral agent.

- Prophylactic or preemptive approaches are both effective.

  3. Hepatitis B prophylaxis is usually indicated for liver transplant recipients with chronic HBV infection, because they are at high risk for recurrent infection.
     a. Hepatitis B immunoglobulin: 10,000 units intravenously (see Caution box) daily for 14 days, followed by 10,000 units every 2 to 4 weeks to maintain anti-HBs antibody titer greater than 500 IU/L and lamivudine (100 mg/day)
     b. Hepatitis B vaccination: seroconversion pretransplant is less than 50% because of poor immune response
D. Other pathogens
  1. *Toxoplasma gondii*
     a. Heart transplant recipients, who are seronegative for *T. gondii,* are at risk for primary toxoplasmosis.
     b. Prevention strategies: TMP-SMX (as used for prophylaxis against *P. carinii*) or pyrimethamine (25 mg/day for 6 weeks)
  2. *M. tuberculosis*: tuberculin skin test converters can be treated for 12 to 18 months with isoniazid (300 mg/day)
  3. Varicella zoster: seronegative recipients exposed to an incubating case of chickenpox should receive varicella zoster immune globulin (5 mL intramuscularly) within 24 to 72 hours of exposure
  4. *S. pneumoniae*: polyvalent pneumococcal vaccination
  5. Influenza: annual influenza vaccination

CAUTION

Caution is advised when using antihepatitis B immunoglobulin by the IV route because of the risk of anaphylactoid reactions. Premedication with diphenhydramine (25 to 50 mg IV), oral acetaminophen (650 mg), and meperidine (25 to 50 mg IV) may reduce the severity of infusion reactions (fever, chills, rigors). More severe reactions (bronchospasm, hypotension) may necessitate termination or slowing of the infusion and hydrocortisone or epinephrine administration.

Bibliography

Couchoud C, Cucherat M, Haugh M, et al. Cytomegalovirus prophylaxis with antiviral agents in solid organ transplantation: a meta-analysis. Transplantation 1998; 65:641–647.

Fishman JA, Rubin RH. Infection in organ-transplant recipients. N Engl J Med 1998;338:1741–1751.

Hadley S, Karchmer AW. Fungal infections in solid organ transplant recipients. Infect Dis Clin North Am 1995; 9(4):1045–1074.

Patel R, Paya C. Infections in solid-organ recipients. Clin Microbiol Rev 1997;10:86–124.

104 Tuberculosis

Dana G. Kissner

Etiology

A. *Mycobacterium tuberculosis* (TB), a non-motile, non-sporulating, 0.3 to 0.6 by 1 to 4 μm obligatory aerobic rod that is strongly acid-fast, weakly Gram positive, and slow growing

B. *M. tuberculosis* complex also includes *M. bovis*, Bacillus of Calmette and Guérin [BCG] *M. africanum*, and *M. microti*.

Clinical Findings

A. Nonspecific, constitutional manifestations
   1. Malaise
   2. Fever (including fever of unknown origin), chills, sweats
   3. Anorexia, weight loss, cachexia ("consumption")
   4. Clubbing
   5. Erythema nodosum or induratum
   6. Poncet's syndrome (non-infectious polyarthritis)
B. Pulmonary TB
   1. Constitutional signs and symptoms
   2. Cough, sputum (copious amounts are rare), hemoptysis
   3. Chest pain
   4. Dyspnea (rare unless extensive pulmonary involvement, large pleural or pericardial effusion, or miliary TB); respiratory failure can occur.
   5. Physical examination of the lungs is frequently normal.
C. Laryngeal TB (highly contagious)
   1. Constitutional signs and symptoms
   2. Cough, hoarseness
D. Central nervous system (CNS) TB: meningitis, brain abscess, tuberculoma
   1. Headache, papilledema, meningismus
   2. Confusion, delirium, altered level of consciousness
   3. Nausea, vomiting
   4. Focal neurologic signs, seizures
E. Miliary (disseminated) TB
   1. Weakness, anorexia, weight loss
   2. Fever
   3. Pain: headache, pleuritic, abdominal, back
   4. Dyspnea (respiratory failure can occur)
   5. Diarrhea
   6. Lymphadenopathy, hepatomegaly, splenomegaly
   7. Tubercles on funduscopic examination
   8. Evidence of adrenal insufficiency
F. Bone and joint TB
   1. Arthritis: monoarticular pain and swelling, most commonly in a weight-bearing joint, and often preceded by local trauma
   2. Spondylitis (Pott's disease)
      a. Back pain: low thoracic and lumbar most common locations
      b. Constitutional signs and symptoms
      c. Paraplegia, paresthesia
      d. Paravertebral abscess (posterior triangle of the neck; retropharyngeal; psoas muscle, which can extend into thigh, iliac fossa, above inguinal ligament, in gluteal folds): may fluctuate, drain, form sinus tracts
      e. Kyphosis, gibbous deformity
   3. Rib lesions at costochondral junctions produce cold abscesses that appear as chest wall masses.
G. Gastrointestinal (GI) and peritoneal TB
   1. Peritonitis
      a. Constitutional signs and symptoms
      b. Abdominal pain
      c. Ascites
      d. "Doughy" abdomen or mass
      e. Signs or symptoms of bowel obstruction
   2. Enteritis: ileal and ileocecal regions most common locations
      a. Constitutional signs and symptoms
      b. Abdominal pain
      c. Abdominal mass
      d. Signs or symptoms of bowel perforation, obstruction, or fistula
      e. Diarrhea (not common), hematochezia
H. Genitourinary (GU)
   1. Constitutional signs and symptoms not common
   2. May be asymptomatic
   3. Dysuria, frequency, urgency, flank pain
   4. Gross hematuria or pyuria
   5. Tender or nontender epididymal, testicular, or prostatic mass or induration

374

6. Draining scrotal sinus

7. Pelvic pain, menstrual disturbances, cervical erosions, adnexal masses, female infertility

I. Lymphatic

1. Lymphadenopathy: matting of lymph nodes, fluctuation, and sinus tract formation are common; sites include axilla, mediastinum, hilum, abdomen, groin, and especially cervical and supraclavicular regions

2. Cough, sputum, and hemoptysis from mediastinal lymph node erosion through bronchi

3. Sternal pain and abscess from erosion of mediastinal lymph nodes

4. Dysphagia, cough, dyspnea from esophageal displacement or tracheal–esophageal fistula formation

J. Pleural TB

1. Constitutional signs and symptoms; may be asymptomatic

2. Thoracic symptoms: cough, dyspnea, chest pain

3. Decreased breath sounds and dullness to percussion

K. Pericardial TB

1. Complications include cardiac tamponade and constrictive pericarditis.

2. Stages: effusive, effusive–constrictive, and constrictive

3. Clinical findings

   a. Constitutional signs and symptoms

   b. Signs and symptoms of cardiac tamponade or constrictive pericarditis: dyspnea, orthopnea, chest pain, pulsus paradoxus, neck vein distention, distant heart sounds, edema, ascites, tachycardia, cardiomegaly, hepatomegaly, Ewart's sign

   c. Signs and symptoms of pleural effusion

   d. Pleural or pericardial friction rub

Key Symptoms

- Fever
- Cough
- Cachexia
- Pain
- Sweats
- Sputum
- Anorexia
- Confusion
- Dyspnea
- Hemoptysis
- Diarrhea
- Hematuria

Differential Diagnosis of Pulmonary TB

A. Nontuberculous mycobacterial (NTM) infections: important pathogens include *M. kansasii*, *M. avium*, *M. intracellulare*

B. Other granulomatous diseases: fungal infections, sarcoidosis, berylliosis, foreign body reactions

C. Other cavitary lung diseases: lung abscess, necrotizing pneumonias, Wegener's granulomatosis, fungal infections, cavitary neoplasms, silicosis

D. Other lung diseases with a miliary pattern: fungal infections, sarcoidosis, lymphangitic spread of tumors, histiocytosis X (eosinophilic granuloma), silicosis

Diagnosis

A. Definitive diagnosis is based on culture and identification of *M. tuberculosis*.

1. Clinical specimens: when submitting specify "AFB stain and culture"

   a. Sputum (three single specimens on separate days): may require induction with hypertonic saline aerosol administration

   b. Bronchial washing, bronchoalveolar lavage, and post-bronchoscopy sputum

   c. Pleural fluid: positive only in 20% to 25% of cases

   d. Gastric aspirate: 50 mL aspirated early in morning after 8 to 10 hours of fasting, with patient still in bed

   e. Urine: best if repeated, first-voided early morning, mid-stream urine samples are obtained; may be positive in 5% to 10% of persons with pulmonary TB, 20% of those with extrapulmonary disease, and 25% of patients with miliary TB, even in the absence of clinical, laboratory, or radiologic evidence of genitourinary disease

   f. Other body fluids: pericardial fluid, cerebrospinal fluid (CSF), joint fluid (80% positive yield), ascitic fluid, menstrual blood (first 2 days), endometrial scrapings (end of menstrual cycle)

   g. Tissue: pleura, transbronchial or endobronchial biopsy, tuberculoma, bone, synovium, liver, bone marrow, lymph node, peritoneum, GI tract, GU structures, pericardium

   h. Blood: useful in patients with human immunodeficiency virus infection

   i. Stool

2. Advantages

   a. Provides definitive diagnosis, and allows for antibiotic susceptibility testing

   b. Permits precise species identification (*M. tuberculosis* versus other species of *M. tuberculosis* complex and NTM)

   c. Is 10 times more sensitive than staining and microscopy (see B below)

d. Allows monitoring of the response to therapy

3. Disadvantages

a. Takes time: 1 week to as many as 6 to 8 weeks, depending on technique used

b. Requires approximately 100 organisms/mL for a positive result

c. Requires proficient mycobacteriology laboratory

B. Staining and microscopic examination

1. Acid-fast stain

a. Carbol-fuchsin methods of Ziehl-Neelson or Kinyoun stain bacilli red; appear bright yellow using auramine and rhodamine dyes and fluorescent microscopy.

b. 50% to 80% of patients with pulmonary TB will have positive sputum smears

2. Advantages: rapid and easy, provides quantitative estimate of bacillus shedding, and thus infectiousness of patient

3. Disadvantages: does not differentiate from NTM or other acid-fast bacilli (AFB); less sensitive than culture

C. Histology: when the clinical and radiographic evidence for TB is strong, the tuberculin skin test is positive, or there is a history of exposure, the finding of granulomas, especially with caseation, is presumptive evidence for TB; clinical improvement after anti-TB treatment confirms diagnosis

D. Tuberculin skin testing

1. Identifies individuals with delayed hypersensitivity to mycobacteria by intracutaneous (Mantoux) injection of 5 tuberculin units purified protein derivative (PPD) on the volar surface of the forearm

2. Measure diameter of induration perpendicular to injection 48 to 72 hours later; ignore erythema when interpreting test result.

3. Threshold for interpretation depends on purpose of the test (screening, surveillance, or diagnosis) and consequences of false classification.

a. 5-mm induration: lowest cutting point for those most likely to have TB infection or disease, or those most likely to suffer from failure to identify infection or disease

(1) Recent close contacts of an infectious case

(2) Persons with chest x-ray films consistent with active or old (unchanged for ≥3 months) healed TB

(3) Known HIV infection or, if unknown, risk factors for HIV

(4) Patients with organ transplants or other conditions causing immunosuppression (e.g., persons receiving at least 15 mg/day of prednisone, or its equivalent, for at least 1 month)

b. 10-mm induration: used for all persons with other risk factors for TB infection or disease

(1) Recent immigrants (last 5 years) from high-prevalence countries

(2) Injection drug users who are HIV negative

(3) Residents or employees of long-term care and correctional facilities, homeless shelters, and health care facilities

(4) Mycobacteriology laboratory personnel

(5) Persons with medical conditions that increase risk for TB: silicosis, gastrectomy, jejunoileal bypass, undernutrition (≥10% below ideal body weight), chronic renal failure, diabetes mellitus, some hematologic disorders (lymphoma, leukemia), carcinoma of the head, neck, or lung

(6) Skin test converters (at least 10 mm within the past 2 years)

c. 15 mm (highest threshold)

d. Consider large reactions as positive in BCG-vaccinated persons.

e. Vesiculation and ulceration indicate a positive reaction.

4. Causes of false positive test results

a. Sensitization to cross-reacting antigens (e.g., NTM); reaction is usually smaller than that produced by TB infection

b. Vaccination with BCG

(1) Tuberculin test conversion after vaccination is not invariable.

(2) The mean reaction size is smaller than 10 mm.

(3) Tuberculin sensitivity tends to wane after vaccination.

5. Causes of false negative test results

a. Improper storage of PPD: keep refrigerated, in the dark, and use as soon as possible after filling syringe

b. Impaired delayed (cellular) hypersensitivity

c. Improper administration of PPD or reading of test result

d. Very recent TB infection

e. Need for booster effect: waning over time of the delayed hypersensitivity to PPD, which can be recalled by a second or even a third administration of the test

Key Diagnosis

- Acid-fast stain of sputum
- Culture of sputum for AFB
- Genus and species identification
- Nucleic acid amplification (on AFB⁺ sputum)
- Tuberculin skin test

Laboratory and Other Tests

A. Hematologic abnormalities: anemia, thrombocytopenia, leukopenia, leukocytosis, leukemoid reactions, consumptive coagulopathy, elevated sedimentation rate

B. Serum tests: hypoalbuminemia, elevated alkaline phosphatase, hyponatremia, hypercalcemia

C. Genitourinary disease: azotemia; abacteruric microscopic or gross pyuria or hematuria

D. Central nervous system disease: CSF containing elevated protein, low or normal glucose, modestly elevated white blood cell count (most commonly lymphocytes), presence of mycobacterial antigens

E. Gastrointestinal disease: exudative ascitic fluid with protein concentration greater than 3 g/dL, lactate dehydrogenase level greater than 90 U/L, serum–ascites albumin gradient lower than 1.1 g/dL, total mononuclear cell count elevated, adenosine deaminase elevated

F. Pleural fluid exudate: protein concentration greater than 5 g/dL suggests TB, white blood cell count (WBC) 300 to 3,000 cells/mm³ with more than 50% lymphocytes (predominant polymorphonuclear leukocytes when symptoms present for less than 2 weeks), glucose concentration low or normal, less than 5% mesothelial cells, ADA level greater than 70 U/L; empyema may result from bronchopleural fistula formation

G. Synovial fluid: thick, mucinous, xanthochromic appearance; elevated WBC, 50% to 60% polymorphonuclear leukocytes; elevated protein and very low glucose concentrations; poor mucin clot; low viscosity

H. Studies compatible with adrenal insufficiency

Imaging Studies

A. Chest x-ray and computed tomography (CT): pulmonary and chest involvement
  1. Cavities, thin-walled with little fluid, often accompanied by disseminated nodular densities, and most commonly in upper posterior lung fields
  2. Apical densities, in regions bound by the clavicle, first rib, and sternum; seen best on lordotic films
  3. Retraction of the upper lobes, sometimes with pleural thickening
  4. Hilar or mediastinal lymphadenopathy, often with right paratracheal adenopathy; CT with radiocontrast showing peripheral ring enhancement, central low attenuation, and multiloculation is strongly suggestive of TB
  5. Pleural or pericardial effusions
  6. Small nodule mimicking neoplasm
  7. Small patchy areas of increased density
  8. Consolidation, segmental or lobar atelectasis, calcifications
  9. Miliary pattern: uniformly distributed nodules, 2 to 3 mm in size; early in course of disease may be barely apparent

B. Intravenous pyelogram or GU ultrasound: GU involvement
  1. Calyceal or pelvic dilatation or deformity
  2. Destructive changes: focal calcification, cavities, filling defects, cortical scarring, nonvisualization of calyx, papillary cavities resembling papillary necrosis
  3. Ureteral strictures: "beaded" or "pipe stem"
  4. Autonephrectomy

C. Computed tomography or magnetic resonance imaging (MRI) of brain or spine, with contrast: CNS disease
  1. Tuberculoma: small nodular or ring-enhancing lesions in brain or spinal cord; isointense or hypointense center on T2-weighted images on MRI; mild edema and mass effect
  2. Abscess: larger, solitary, and frequently multilocular, with hyperintense centers on MRI T2-weighted images; significant edema and mass effect
  3. Meningitis: enhancement in basal cisterns and adjacent to the cerebral convexities

D. Skeletal x-ray, CT, MRI: bone and joint disease
  1. Cystic or lytic lesions; metaphyseal and subchondral erosions, joint space narrowing
  2. Anterior vertebral body destruction, spread to adjacent vertebras, disk space narrowing, progressive vertebral collapse and anterior wedging, psoas or paraspinous abscesses, calcification within the abscess

E. Imaging studies for GI involvement

1. Computed tomography or ultrasound of abdomen: hepatosplenomegaly, lymphadenopathy, mesenteric calcifications

2. Barium contrast studies: contraction, retraction of cecum with widening of the ileocecal angle; reflux at ileocecal valve; ulcerative, hyperplastic, and combined mucosal abnormalities of ileum; single or multiple short and concentric small bowel strictures; fistulous tracts

Treatment

See Chapter 186, Antituberculosis Drugs

Bibliography

American Thoracic Society and the Centers for Disease Control. Diagnostic standards and classification of tuberculosis. Am Rev Respir Dis 2000;161:1376–1395.

Barnes PF, Barrows SA. Tuberculosis in the 1990s. Ann Intern Med 1993;119:400–410.

Centers for Disease Control and Prevention. Update: nucleic acid amplification tests for tuberculosis. MMWR 2000;49:593–594.

Iseman MD. A Clinician's Guide to Tuberculosis. Philadelphia: Lippincott, Williams and Wilkins, 2000.

Penner C, Roberts D, Kunimoto D, et al. Tuberculosis as a primary cause of respiratory failure requiring mechanical ventilation. Am J Respir Crit Care Med 1995;151:867–872.

Schluger NW, Rom WN. Current approaches to the diagnosis of active pulmonary tuberculosis. Am J Respir Crit Care Med 1994;149:264–267.

105 Endocarditis

Donald P. Levine

Infective endocarditis almost always comes to the attention of the intensivist because of a complication of the disease. The traditional classification into acute and subacute or chronic forms based on the usual progression of disease has given way to distinctions based on the infecting organism. In a purely clinical sense, patients with "acute" endocarditis have an illness of brief duration that tends to run a more fulminant course. Typically this disease is caused by *Staphylococcus aureus*. The "subacute" form is generally due to *Streptococcus viridans;* infection due to the *Enterococcus* may fall into either group.

Etiology

A. Organisms that usually produce subacute or chronic endocarditis
   1. *Streptococcus viridans, mutans, mitis, mitior, sanguis, salivarius, intermedius, anginosus, morbillorum* (now *Gemella morbillorum*), and nutritionally variant streptococci (*Abiotrophia* spp.)
   2. *Enterococcus* spp.
   3. *Streptococcus bovis*
   4. Coagulase-negative staphylococci: *Staphylococcus epidermidis* and *capitis*)
   5. *Neisseria* spp. (previously associated with fulminant infection)
   6. HACEK group: *Haemophilus* spp., *Actinobacillus actinomycetemcomitans, Cardiobacterium hominis, Eikenella corrodens, Kingella* spp.
   7. *Bacillus* spp.
   8. *Coxiella burnettii* (Q fever)
   9. Anaerobic bacteria (rarely)
B. Organisms that usually produce acute endocarditis
   1. *Staphylococcus aureus*
   2. *Streptococcus:* groups A, B, and G
   3. *Streptococcus pneumoniae*
   4. *Staphylococcus lugdunensis*
   5. Fungi: *Candida* spp. and *Aspergillus* spp.

Key Etiologies

- *Streptococcus viridans*
- *Staphylococcus aureus*
- Coagulase-negative staphylococci
- *Enterococcus* spp.
- HACEK group organisms

Epidemiology

A. Demographics
   1. Mean age older than 50 years
   2. Overall, men more frequently affected than women (up to 70%)
   3. Women predominate in younger age group (<35 years).
   4. Nosocomial endocarditis is commonly secondary to infected intravascular devices.
B. Patients with abnormal valves
   1. Congenital heart disease
      a. Patent ductus arteriosus
      b. Ventricular septal defect
      c. Tetralogy of Fallot
      d. Bicuspid aortic valve
      e. Idiopathic hypertrophic subaortic stenosis
      f. Mitral valve prolapse (with murmur)
   2. Acquired valve disease
      a. Rheumatic heart disease
      b. Degenerative heart disease (aging)
      c. Previous endocarditis
      d. Injection drug users (?)
   3. Prosthetic valve infection
      a. Less than 60 days from insertion
      b. At least 60 days from insertion

Symptoms

A. Constitutional: fever (80%) and chills (40%)
B. Nonspecific (20% to 40%; more common in "subacute" cases)
   1. Malaise, weakness
   2. Anorexia, weight loss, nausea, vomiting
   3. Headache
C. Local (10% to 15%)
   1. Chest pain with or without hemoptysis (right-sided infection)
   2. Congestive heart failure
   3. Abdominal pain
   4. Arthralgia or myalgia
   5. Confusion or delirium
   6. Symptoms related to stroke

Physical Findings

A. Fever (90%)

B. Ophthalmic: Roth spots or conjunctival petechial hemorrhages

C. Chest
   1. Heart murmur (overall ~80%)
      a. New (<10%)
      b. Changing (<5%)
   2. Pericardial friction rub
   3. Pleural friction rub
   4. Rales

D. Abdominal: splenomegaly

E. Extremities
   1. Splinter nail bed hemorrhages
   2. Osler nodes
   3. Janeway lesions
   4. Arthritis

F. Neurologic
   1. Toxic encephalopathy
   2. Focal deficits: e.g., hemiplegia, aphasia, ataxia (from emboli or mycotic aneurysm)
   3. Meningitis

Key Findings

- Fever and chills
- Arthralgia or arthritis
- Weakness
- Confusion or delirium
- Petechiae
- Malaise
- Heart murmur
- Focal neurologic deficits
- Splenomegaly
- Osler nodes or Janeway lesions

Differential Diagnosis

A. Patients presenting with fever and stroke
   1. Endocarditis
   2. Brain abscess
   3. Encephalitis

B. Patients with undifferentiated constitutional signs and symptoms
   1. Atrial myxoma
   2. Connective tissue disorder
   3. Rheumatic fever
   4. Sickle cell disease
   5. Sepsis from noncardiac endovascular source

Diagnosis

A. Compatible history and clinical setting

B. Laboratory evidence: persistently positive blood cultures, histologic evidence

C. Findings on physical examination

D. Duke criteria (most widely accepted)
   1. Definite infective endocarditis
      a. Pathologic criteria
         (1) Microorganisms demonstrated by culture or histology in a vegetation or in infected embolus, or
         (2) Histologic finding of vegetation or intracardiac abscess
      b. Clinical criteria (see Table 105–1)

TABLE 105–1. DEFINITIONS FOR CLINICAL DIAGNOSTIC CRITERIA*

A. Major criteria
   1. Positive blood culture for infective endocarditis
      a. Typical microorganism for infective endocarditis from two separate blood cultures
         (1) Viridans streptococci, *Streptococcus bovis*, HACEK group, or
         (2) Community-acquired *Staphylococcus aureus* or enterococci, in the absence of a primary focus, or
      b. Persistently positive blood culture, defined as recovery of a microorganism consistent with infective endocarditis from:
         (1) Blood cultures drawn more than 12 hours apart, or
         (2) All of three or a majority of four or more separate blood cultures, with first and last drawn at least 1 hour apart
   2. Evidence of endocardial involvement
      a. Positive echocardiogram for infective endocarditis
         (1) Oscillating intracardiac mass, on valve or supporting structures, or both in the path of regurgitant jets, or on implanted material, in the absence of an alternative anatomic explanation, or
         (2) Abscess, or
         (3) New partial dehiscence of prosthetic valve, or
      b. New valvular regurgitation (increase or change in preexisting murmur not sufficient)

B. Minor criteria
   1. Predisposition: predisposing heart condition or IV drug use
   2. Fever: ≥38.0°C (100.4°F)
   3. Vascular phenomena: major arterial emboli, septic pulmonary infarcts, mycotic aneurysm, intracranial hemorrhage, conjunctival hemorrhages, Janeway lesions
   4. Immunologic phenomena: glomerulonephritis, Osler's nodes, Roth spots, rheumatoid factor
   5. Microbiologic evidence: positive blood culture, but not meeting major criterion as noted previously, or serologic evidence of active infection with organism consistent with infective endocarditis
   6. Echocardiogram: consistent with infective endocarditis, but not meeting major criterion as noted previously

*From Durack DT, Lukes AS, Bright DK, et al, New criteria for diagnosis of infective endocarditis: Utilization of specific echocardiographic findings. Am J Med 1994;96:200–209.

(1) Two major criteria, or

(2) One major and three minor criteria, or

(3) Five minor criteria

2. Possible infective endocarditis: findings consistent with endocarditis, but not meeting criteria for either definite or rejected

3. Rejected

   a. Firm alternate diagnosis, or

   b. Resolution of manifestations of endocarditis with up to 4 days of antibiotic therapy, or

   c. Lack of evidence of infective endocarditis at surgery or autopsy after up to 4 days of antibiotic therapy

E. Echocardiogram findings

Laboratory Tests

A. Blood culture is the most important test.

1. Three cultures over 24 hours; allow at least 3 weeks to recover slow-growing organisms

2. Prior antibiotic therapy prevents or slows recovery.

3. Lysis centrifugation method helpful if fungal infection suspected

4. Susceptibility testing (with minimum inhibitory concentrations [MIC]) crucial

B. Hematology

1. Anemia is a constant feature.

2. Leukocytosis common in acute infection, rare in subacute disease

3. Erythrocyte sedimentation rate elevated, but of no diagnostic significance

C. Urinalysis

1. Proteinuria common (>50%)

2. Microscopic hematuria (approximately 50%)

Imaging Tests

A. Chest x-ray

1. Right-sided disease

   a. Multiple, bilateral infiltrates due to septic emboli

   b. Primarily lower lobe

   c. Occasional cavitation

   d. Infiltrates continue to develop despite effective therapy.

   e. Absence of infiltrates is not indicative of absence of right-sided involvement.

2. Left-sided disease indicated by evidence of congestive heart failure

   a. Pulmonary congestion

   b. Acute cardiomegaly in cases of valve rupture or dehiscence

B. Echocardiography

1. Not indicated as a screening tool for febrile patients or bacteremic patients unlikely to have endocarditis

2. Appropriate for all patients suspected to have endocarditis

3. Predictive of disease in patient with high clinical suspicion of endocarditis

4. Excellent negative predictive value when both transthoracic (TTE) and transesophageal (TEE) are negative

5. Transthoracic

   a. Sensitivity 60%, specificity 98%, especially if vegetations larger than 2 mm in size or right-sided infection

   b. May be ineffective if emphysema, obesity, or chest wall deformity

   c. May be inadequate if prosthetic valve infection, periannular abscess, valve leaflet perforation, fistulous track, or for assessment of patients at high risk of complications

   d. Negative test excludes endocarditis in low-risk patients with bacteremia.

6. Transesophageal

   a. Sensitivity and specificity approaches 100%, especially for perivalvular extension, prosthetic valve vegetations, and valvular insufficiency.

   b. Diagnostic method of choice for

     (1) Patients that are difficult to image with TTE

     (2) Possible prosthetic valve infection

     (3) Patients at high risk of complications

     (4) Patients with intermediate or high clinical suspicion of infective endocarditis

   c. False negative tests

     (1) Vegetations too small to be visualized

     (2) Prior embolization of vegetation

     (3) Small abscess

     (4) Obstruction of beam by other structures

   d. False positive tests (for vegetations) are usually due to structural lesions secondary to endocarditis.

C. Angiography

1. Cerebral angiography can demonstrate mycotic aneurysm and intracerebral hemorrhage.

2. Angiography of other areas may be required in the diagnosis extracranial aneurysm.

D. Contrast-enhanced cerebral computed tomography

1. May show ischemic infarction secondary to emboli

2. May reveal multiple ring-enhancing lesions (emboli-induced abscesses)

3. May show hemorrhage from aneurysm (90% to 95% sensitivity)

4. Mycotic aneurysms are usually too small or peripheral to be detected.

E. Magnetic resonance angiogram: may detect mycotic aneurysm larger than 5 mm in diameter

F. Four-vessel angiogram

1. Best method to detect mycotic aneurysm

2. Recommended if severe, localized headache, focal neurologic signs, sterile meningitis

G. Abdominal computed tomography

1. Splenic infarct or abscess

2. Multiple mycotic aneurysms (rare)

Key Test Findings

- Persistently positive blood cultures

- Anemia

- Microscopic hematuria, proteinuria

- Echocardiography showing oscillating intracardiac vegetations

Treatment

A. Obtain blood cultures first.

B. Empiric treatment

1. In noncritical patient, deferred as long as possible (i.e., at least 24 hours) in order to obtain an adequate number of blood cultures

2. Parenteral therapy assures adequate serum concentrations.

3. Bactericidal drugs required

4. Extended duration of therapy required

5. Native valve infection

   a. Nonacute course: cover for *Enterococcus* and *Streptococcus viridans*

   b. Acute course:

   (1) Noninjection drug user: cover for *Staphylococcus aureus*

   (2) Injection drug user: cover for *S. aureus* (some would add gentamicin to cover Gram-negative organisms)

6. Prosthetic valve infection: cover for methicillin-resistant coagulase-negative staphylococci plus *Enterococcus*

C. Definitive treatment

1. Native valve

a. *Streptococcus viridans* and *S. bovis* with penicillin G MIC ≤0.1 μg/mL

(1) Penicillin G, 12 to 18 million U/day IV continuous or divided doses every 4 hours for 4 weeks, or

(2) Penicillin as above, plus gentamicin, 1 mg/kg intravenously every 8 hours, both for 2 weeks, or

(3) Ceftriaxone, 2 g intravenously or intramuscularly 4 times daily for 4 weeks, or

(4) Vancomycin, 15 mg/kg intravenously every 12 hours for 4 weeks

b. *Streptococcus viridans* and *S. bovis* MIC >0.1 μg/mL and <0.5 μg/mL

(1) Penicillin G, 18 million U/day intravenously, continuously or in divided doses every 4 hours for 4 weeks, plus gentamicin 1 mg/kg intramuscularly or intravenously every 8 hours for 2 weeks, or

(2) Vancomycin 15 mg/kg intravenously every 12 hours for 4 weeks

c. Enterococci or streptococci with penicillin MIC at least 0.5 μg/mL

(1) Penicillin G, 18 to 30 million U/day intravenously or ampicillin 12 g/day intravenously, continuously or in divided doses every 4 hours for 4 to 6 weeks, plus gentamicin 1 mg/kg intramuscularly or intravenously every 8 hours for 4 to 6 weeks, or

(2) Vancomycin 15 mg/kg intravenously every 12 hours, plus gentamicin 1 mg/kg intramuscularly or intravenously every 8 hours for 4 to 6 weeks

d. Methicillin-sensitive staphylococci

(1) Nafcillin or oxacillin, 2 g intravenously every 4 hours for 4 to 6 weeks (plus optional gentamicin 1 mg/kg intramuscularly or intravenously every 8 hours for 3 to 5 days), or

(2) Cefazolin 2 g intravenously every 8 hours for 4 to 6 weeks (plus optional gentamicin 1 mg/kg intramuscularly or intravenously for every 8 hours for 3 to 5 days), or

(3) Nafcillin or oxacillin, 2 g intravenously every 4 hours plus gentamicin 1 mg/kg intramuscularly or intravenously every 8 hours for 2 weeks (for uncomplicated right-sided infection in injection drug users), or

(4) Vancomycin 15 mg/kg intravenously every 12 hours for 4 to 6 weeks

e. Methicillin-resistant staphylococci: vancomycin 15 mg/kg intravenously every 12 hours for 4 to 6 weeks

f. HACEK group

(1) Ceftriaxone, 2 g intravenously or intramuscularly 4 times daily for 4 weeks, or

(2) Ampicillin 12 g/day intravenously, continuously or in divided doses every 4 hours, plus gentamicin 1 mg/kg intramuscularly or intravenously every 8 hours, both for 4 weeks (only if not β-lactamase producing organism)

2. Prosthetic valve

a. Methicillin-sensitive staphylococci: nafcillin or oxacillin, 2 g intravenously every 4 hours plus rifampin 300 mg orally every 8 hours, both for at least 6 weeks, plus gentamicin 1 mg/kg intramuscularly or intravenously every 8 hours for the first 2 weeks

b. Methicillin-resistant staphylococci: vancomycin 15 mg/kg intravenously every 12 hours, plus rifampin 300 mg orally every 8 hours, both for at least 6 weeks, plus gentamicin 1 mg/kg or intravenously every 8 hours for the first 2 weeks

Complications

A. Congestive heart failure, cardiogenic shock, pulmonary edema from perforated valve, valve dehiscence, ruptured chordae tendineae, or outlet obstruction by vegetation

B. Perivalvular extension of infection with abscess, fistula, or pericardial effusion

C. Cardiac dysrhythmias and conduction disturbances

D. Respiratory failure secondary to left ventricular failure, septic pulmonary emboli, acute respiratory distress syndrome

E. Mycotic aneurysm: intracranial, intrathoracic, abdominal, peripheral

F. Embolism leading to metastatic infection, abscess, or infarction (e.g., cerebral or splenic abscess or infarction)

G. Septic shock

Bibliography

Bayer AS, Bolger AF, Taubert KA, et al. Diagnosis and management of infective endocarditis and its complications. Circulation 1998;98:2936–2948.

Durack DT, Lukes AS, Bright DK, et al. New criteria for diagnosis of infective endocarditis: Utilization of specific echocardiographic findings. Am J Med 1994;96:200–209.

Lerner PI. Neurologic complications of infective endocarditis. Med Clin North Am 1985;69:385–398.

Levine DP, Fromm BS, Reddy BR. Slow response to vancomycin or vancomycin plus rifampin in methicillin-resistant *Staphylococcus aureus* endocarditis. Ann Intern Med 1991;115:674–680.

Wilson WR, Karchmer AW, Dajani AS, et al. Antibiotic treatment of adults with infective endocarditis due to streptococci, enterococci, staphylococci, and HACEK microorganisms. JAMA 1995;274:1706–1713.

106 Urosepsis

Douglas F. Lindahl
Richard W. Carlson

Urosepsis is a serious urinary tract infection (UTI) with systemic manifestations. Urinary tract infections cause up to 40% of hospital-acquired nosocomial infections and are the most common cause of Gram-negative bacteremia.

Definitions

A. Bacteriuria: presence of a significant concentration of bacteria in urine ($>10^5$ colony forming units/mL)

B. Pyuria
  1. Healthy individuals: more than 5 white blood cells per high power field
  2. Definition is unclear for patients with indwelling urinary catheters or those with preexisting urologic conditions.

C. Uncomplicated UTI: genitourinary infection in an otherwise healthy individual without risk factors, complications, or treatment failure

D. Complicated UTI: genitourinary infection in a patient with anatomic, metabolic, or functional abnormalities that increase the risk of treatment failure

E. Systemic inflammatory response syndrome (SIRS): a syndrome characterized by a systemic response to infection or inflammation that manifests as more than two of the following:
  1. Temperature higher than 100.4°F (38°C) or lower than 96.8°F (36°C)
  2. Heart rate higher than 90 beats/minute
  3. Respiratory rate above 20 breaths/minute or $PaCO_2$ below 32 torr
  4. Peripheral white blood cell count greater than 12,000 or less than 4,000 cells/mm³ or more than 10% immature (band) forms

F. Urosepsis: SIRS, sepsis, or severe sepsis secondary to a UTI

Etiology

A. Mechanical factors: disruption of host defense mechanisms by instrumentation, health care personnel, fecal contamination, or contaminated urinometers or measuring devices

B. Organisms
  1. Aerobic Gram-negative rods, most commonly

Escherichia coli, cause more than 80% of nosocomial UTIs.

2. Other Gram-negative organisms: *Pseudomonas aeruginosa*, *Klebsiella* species, *Proteus mirabilis* (associated with urinary stones), *Enterobacter* and *Serratia* species

3. Gram-positive organisms
  a. Enterococci: *E. faecalis*, *E. faecium*
  b. Staphylococci: especially *Staphylococcus saprophyticus* (periurethral infections)
  c. *Streptococcus agalactiae*: old age, diabetes, HIV infection, malignancy, pregnancy, and youth

Key Etiology and Epidemiology

- *E. coli* is the most common pathogen; it adheres to uroepithelial membranes.

- *Klebsiella, Enterobacter, Proteus,* and *Serratia* are often associated with anatomic defects, obstruction, or prior antimicrobial use.

- Anaerobic organisms and fungi are uncommon causes of urosepsis.

- *S. aureus* in urine suggests a bacteremic source.

- Group B streptococci (*S. agalactiae*) UTI is associated with old age, youth, pregnancy, diabetes, malignancy, and HIV infection.

- There is a rising incidence of nosocomial UTIs caused by enterococci (often multi-drug resistant forms) in critically ill patients with prolonged intensive care unit stays and prior use of antimicrobial agents.

Risk Factors

A. Host risk factors
  1. Diabetes mellitus
  2. Chronic corticosteroid use
  3. Systemic lupus erythematosus
  4. Preexisting renal disease (renal insufficiency, medullary sponge kidney, polycystic kidney disease)
  5. Mechanical obstruction of urinary tract (prostatic disease, other causes of urethral or ureteral obstruction) or reflux

6. Malnutrition

7. Alcoholism

8. Female sex; pregnancy

9. Spinal cord injury or disease; neurogenic bladder

10. Advanced age

11. Prostatic disease

12. Foreign bodies (stones)

13. Transplant recipient

14. Sickle cell disease

15. Critical illness

B. Nosocomial risk factors

1. Urologic instrumentation

2. Urologic surgery

3. Bladder catheterization, especially indwelling catheter use

Key Clinical Findings

- Fever, chills

- Dysuria, frequency, urgency

- Pain—suprapubic, prostatic, costovertebral angle

- Altered mentation

- Cloudy urine

- Tachycardia, tachypnea, hypotension, respiratory distress (SIRS)

Laboratory and Other Tests

A. Urinalysis

1. Pyuria, hematuria, bacteriuria

2. Alkaline urine suggests stones.

3. Distinguish between bacterial colonization and infection.

4. Positive nitrite reduction test or more than 100 leukocytes per high-power field suggests infection.

B. Blood and urine culture

1. Obtain cultures before initiating antimicrobial therapy, if possible.

2. Polymicrobial bacteriuria

a. Suggests contamination of the culture; however, true multiorganism infections occur, often involving *Pseudomonas*

b. Mixed infections carry a worse prognosis.

Key Clinical Tests

- Recovery of the same organism from blood and urine establishes the specific diagnosis of urosepsis.

- Perform ultrasound or computed tomography when obstruction, stone, or abscess is considered.

- Use nuclear studies to assess the function of the involved kidney.

Treatment

A. Antibiotic therapy

1. Start with empiric coverage for both Gram-positive and Gram-negative organisms, including enterococci.

2. Common antibiotic choices

a. Ampicillin or ampicillin-sulbactam, with or without an aminoglycoside

b. Ticarcillin-clavulanate

c. Imipenem-cilastatin

d. Aztreonam

e. Quinolone

f. Second- or third-generation cephalosporins

3. Consider prior culture results and institutional flora susceptibility patterns.

4. Definitive therapy is based on culture and susceptibility results.

5. Begin with parenteral therapy and convert to oral antibiotic after clinical stabilization.

6. Treat for 7 to 14 days, or longer.

B. Supportive

1. Volume resuscitation and hemodynamic stabilization

2. Maintain adequate oxygenation and ventilation.

3. Correct metabolic (acid-base and electrolyte) disturbances.

4. Provide adequate nutrition.

5. Dialysis as indicated

6. General management of sepsis (see Chapter 91, Sepsis and SIRS, and Chapter 92, Septic Shock)

C. Urologic interventions

1. Relieve urinary obstruction.

2. Remove stones, if possible.

3. Ensure supportive care and antibiotic therapy before surgical intervention, if possible.

4. Ureteral stents or percutaneous drainage may provide temporary drainage and stabilization.

5. Suppurative complications frequently require surgical intervention.

> **PEARL**
>
> Consider suppurative complications when patients fail to respond to appropriate antimicrobial therapy and other measures.

Complications

A. Suppurative complications
   1. Renal abscess (emphysematous pyelonephritis)
   2. Perinephric abscess (including infected renal cysts)
B. Septic shock
C. Renal failure
D. Multiple organ failure

Prevention

A. Treat asymptomatic bacteriuria before catheterization or instrumentation.
B. Avoid urinary catheterization, if possible.
C. Remove urinary catheters promptly (consider condom catheters, intermittent catheterization, diapers).
D. Use sterile, closed-system drainage and collection devices.
E. Adhere to proper hand-washing and sterile technique during urinary procedures.

B | Bibliography

Cunha BA. Urosepsis: when to suspect, how to confirm, how to manage. J Crit Illness 1997;12:616–26.

Farley MM, Harvey RC, Stull T, et al. A population-based assessment of invasive disease due to Group B streptococcus in nonpregnant adults. N Engl J Med 1993;328:1807–1811.

Jacobs LG. Fungal urinary tract infections in the elderly: treatment guidelines. Drugs Aging 1996;8:89–96.

Paradisi F, Corti, G, Magnani V. Urosepsis in the critical care unit. Crit Care Clin 1998;14:165–180.

Reed RL II. Contemporary issues with bacterial infection in the intensive care unit. Surg Clin North Am 2000;80:895–909.

Rosser CJ, Bare RL, Meredith JW. Urinary tract infections in the critically ill patient with a urinary catheter. Am J Surg 1999;177:287–290.

Siegman-Igra Y, Kulka T, Schwartz D, et al. Polymicrobial and monomicrobial bacteraemic urinary tract infection. J Hosp Infect 1994;28:49–56.

Stamm WE, Hooton TM. Management of urinary tract infections in adults. N Engl J Med 1993;329:1328–1334.

107 Life-Threatening Infections of the Oropharynx

Remzi Bag

Life-threatening infections of the oropharynx encompass an arbitrary group of infectious diseases involving the oropharynx and neck and caused by bacteria, viruses, and fungi. They have a broad spectrum of clinical findings and a significant risk of fatal complications.

Classification

A. Deep space infections of the neck
   1. Submandibular space infections (Ludwig's angina)
   2. Lateral pharyngeal space infections
   3. Retropharyngeal space infections
   4. Peritonsillar, laryngeal abscess
   5. Masticator space abscess
B. Pharyngeal diphtheria
C. Epiglottis (see Chapter 113, Epiglottitis)
D. Laryngotracheobronchitis (croup)
E. Mucor (see Chapter 96, Non-Candidal Fungal Infections)

Etiology

A. Deep space infections of the neck
   1. Typically polymicrobial infections
   2. Anaerobes usually outnumber aerobes.
   3. Organisms commonly isolated: *Bacteroides, Peptostreptococcus, Veillonella, Actinomyces, Fusobacterium,* and *Clostridium*
   4. Enteric Gram-negative organisms and fungi may also be isolated
B. Pharyngeal diphtheria: etiologic agent is *Corynebacterium diphtheriae.*
C. Laryngotracheobronchitis (croup): respiratory viruses and occasionally *Mycoplasma pneumoniae*

Pathogenesis

A. Deep space infections of the neck
   1. Local infection of odontogenic, oropharyngeal (pharyngitis, tonsillitis, peritonsillar abscess), or traumatic origin
   2. Extension to deep cervical spaces or vascular compartments
   3. Local direct complications
      a. Airway obstruction
      b. Vascular (e.g., carotid, jugular, cortical, cavernous sinus)
         (1) Thrombosis
         (2) Infection
         (3) Rupture
   4. Spread to distant structures via deep cervical spaces
      a. Descending necrotizing mediastinitis
      b. Empyema
      c. Pericardial effusion, pericarditis
      d. Pneumonia
      e. Retroperitoneal extension
      f. Cerebral, epidural abscess
      g. Subdural empyema
      h. Intracranial venous thrombosis
      i. Neurologic complications (e.g., cranial nerve palsies)
   5. Systemic complications
      a. Pulmonary aspiration
      b. Sepsis syndrome
      c. Disseminated intravascular coagulation (DIC)
      d. Acute adrenocortical insufficiency
      e. Death

Epidemiology

A. Deep space infections of the neck
   1. Rare in post-antibiotic era
   2. More common in young adult males
B. Pharyngeal diphtheria: most common in children and young adults
C. Laryngotracheobronchitis: predominantly affects infants and young children

Key Risk Factors (Deep Space Infections of the Neck)	
• Diabetes	• Immunodeficiency
• Renal failure	• Corticosteroid use
• Malignancy	• Radiation therapy
• Alcohol use	• Occasionally occurs in previously healthy subjects
• Intravenous drug abuse	

Clinical Findings

A. Deep space infections of the neck

1. Clinical findings are variable and related to etiology, involved structures, and host factors.

2. Onset may be insidious with minimal findings.

3. May have stormy course with high risk of fatal complications

4. Local findings

   a. Symptoms of upper respiratory infection (early)

   b. Pain, swelling, tenderness, local increased temperature at involved site

   c. Foul breath

   d. Dusky cellulitis, and skin blistering (involvement of overlying skin)

   e. Stiff neck, drooling, dysphagia, trismus, tilting of neck to unaffected side

   f. Cervical adenopathy

   g. Palpable crepitus (subcutaneous necrosis)

5. Systemic findings

   a. Respiratory

      (1) Stridor, cyanosis, respiratory failure

      (2) Pneumonia, pleural effusions

   b. Cardiovascular

      (1) Hypotension

      (2) Tachycardia

      (3) Dysrhythmias

   c. Sepsis syndrome and multiple organ system failure

B. Pharyngeal diphtheria

1. Local findings: tonsillitis, sore throat, dysphagia, membrane formation, bleeding, airway obstruction, cervical lymphadenopathy

2. Systemic findings

   a. Constitutional: fever, malaise, nausea, vomiting

   b. Neurologic: headache; ocular, palatal, ciliary paralysis; motor and sensory changes in the limb

   c. Cardiovascular: myocarditis, dysrhythmias, heart failure, circulatory shock

C. Laryngotracheobronchitis

1. Fever

2. Nasal discharge

3. Barking cough, stridor, hoarseness

4. Respiratory distress

5. Chest wall retractions

Diagnosis

A. Deep space infections of the neck

1. High index of suspicion and awareness of pathophysiology is required.

2. Physical findings are variable and nonspecific.

3. Laboratory findings

   a. Direct Gram stain and culture of extramucosal aspirate (caution: specimens may be contaminated by resident bacteria).

   b. Peripheral neutrophilia with left shift

   c. Blood cultures (negative in 50% of cases)

3. Establishment of local infection

4. Establishment of relationship of distal complications

B. Pharyngeal diphtheria: culture of toxicogenic organism

Imaging Studies

A. Deep space infections of the neck

1. X-ray of the neck

   a. Cervical lordosis

   b. Soft tissue swelling

   c. Subcutaneous emphysema

   d. Displacement of larynx or trachea

   e. May be normal

2. Chest x-ray

   a. Soft tissue thickening at level of thoracic inlet with anterior bulging of posterior wall of trachea on lateral views

   b. Pulmonary infiltrates

   c. Pleural effusion

   d. Widening of mediastinum

   e. Gas collections

   f. Cardiomegaly

3. Computed tomography scanning

   a. Diagnostic in most cases

   b. Differentiates cellulitis from deep space infections

   c. Reveals extent and complications, such as

      (1) Thickening of skin and subcutaneous tissue, fascia, muscles

      (2) Abscess formation and contiguous spread to the thorax and cranium

      (3) Gas collections

   d. Follow-up scans may reveal clinically unsuspected progression.

B. Laryngotracheobronchitis: anteroposterior x-ray of neck may show characteristic funnel-shaped narrowing.

Key Diagnostic Points

- A high index of suspicion is required.

- Deep space infections of the neck must be distinguished from simple, uncomplicated pharyngitis, tonsillitis, or odontogenic infections.

- X-rays of the neck and chest are required.

- Computed tomography scanning can be helpful.

Treatment

A. General
  1. Ensure adequate airway and gas exchange.
  2. Endotracheal intubation or urgent tracheostomy may be necessary.

B. Deep space infections of the neck
  1. Intensive care unit monitoring is required.
  2. Early consultation with surgery
     a. Incision and drainage of abscess
     b. Debridement of necrotic tissue
     c. Thoracotomy or superior mediastinal drainage
  3. Broad-spectrum antibiotics for anaerobes and enteric Gram-negative bacteria:
     a. Extended-spectrum penicillin
     b. Third-generation cephalosporin in combination with clindamycin or metronidazole
  4. Follow-up chest x-rays and computed tomography scanning to detect intrathoracic spread
  5. Close observation and treatment of complications (sepsis, DIC, mediastinitis, adrenal insufficiency, etc.)

C. Pharyngeal diphtheria
  1. Equine diphtheria antitoxin
  2. Antibiotics: penicillin or erythromycin
  3. Hemodynamic and respiratory supportive measures as needed

D. Laryngotracheobronchitis
  1. Management is similar to bacterial epiglottitis.
  2. Use of corticosteroids is controversial.

Key Management of Deep Space Infections of the Neck

- Awareness of the pathophysiology

- Early surgical intervention

- Broad-spectrum antibiotics

- Airway and cardiovascular support

Key Prognosis in Deep Space Infections of the Neck

- Outcome is variable; related to host factors, extent of involvement, timing of intervention.

- Invariably fatal without adequate surgical debridement if descending extension occurs

- Early intervention decreases mortality.

- Mortality in cases of descending necrotizing mediastinitis ranges from 19% to 44%.

Bibliography

Chow AW. Life-threatening infections of the head and neck. Clin Infect Dis 1992;14:991–1002.

Chow AW. Infections of the oral cavity, neck and head. In: Mandell GL, Bennett JE, Dolin R (eds). Mandell, Douglas, and Bennett's Principles and Practice of Infectious Diseases, 5th ed. Philadelphia: Churchill-Livingstone, 2000, pp 689–702.

Epstein JB, Chow AW. Oral complications associated with immunosuppression and cancer therapies. Infect Dis Clin North Am 1999;13:901–921.

Ferguson BJ. Mucormycosis of the nose and paranasal sinuses. Otolaryngol Clin North Am 2000;33:349–365.

Gradon JD. Space-occupying and life-threatening infections of the head, neck and thorax. Infect Dis Clin North Am 1996;10:857–878.

108 Meningitis

Meningitis is characterized by the inflammatory response to infection of the cerebrospinal fluid (CSF) within the subarachnoid space. About 25,000 cases of bacterial meningitis occur each year in the United States, 70% of which occur in children under the age of 5 years. Meningitis can occur in adults and is commonly nosocomial. The mortality rate is as high as 25%. The elderly, those who are obtunded on admission, and patients with seizures within 24 hours of admission are at increased risk of mortality. This chapter focuses on bacterial meningitis, as it is the most likely etiology in critically ill patients.

Etiology

A. Bacteria
1. Community acquired
    a. *Streptococcus pneumoniae*
    b. *Neisseria meningitidis*
    c. *Listeria monocytogenes* (elderly, immunosuppressed hosts)
2. Nosocomial
    a. Gram-negative organisms (neurosurgical, elderly, immunosuppressed hosts)
    b. *Staphylococcus epidermidis* (following neurosurgical procedures, especially with indwelling cerebroventricular shunts)
    c. Streptococci other than pneumococcus (neurosurgical and trauma patients)
B. Viral
C. Tuberculosis
D. Lyme disease
E. Fungi (especially in immunosuppressed hosts)

Clinical Findings

A. Fever
B. Nuchal rigidity
C. Mental status changes
D. Headache
E. Seizures
F. Rash (most common with meningococcal meningitis)
G. Focal neurologic deficits

Laboratory Findings

A. Elevated CSF protein
B. Cerebrospinal fluid pleocytosis (neutrophilic)
C. Hypoglycorrhachia
D. Positive CSF Gram stain, culture, or both
E. Positive CSF bacterial antigens

Key Findings

Clinical	Laboratory
• Headache	• Elevated CSF protein
• Fever	• Cerebrospinal fluid pleocytosis
• Nuchal rigidity	• Hypoglycorrhachia
• Mental status changes	• Positive CSF Gram stain

Complications

A. Seizures
B. Subdural empyema
C. Brain abscess
D. Hydrocephalus
E. Cerebral infarct
F. Thrombosis (cortical vein or sagittal sinus)

Treatment

A. Promptly institute empiric antibiotic therapy, selected according to the most likely pathogen. Antibiotic treatment can be tailored once culture and susceptibility test results are available.
1. Do not delay antibiotics for imaging studies.
2. Broad-spectrum cephalosporin (ceftriaxone 2 g intravenously every 12 hours or cefotaxime 2 g intravenously every 6 hours) plus vancomycin (500 to 750 mg intravenously every 6 hours) for most community-acquired meningitis
3. Add ampicillin if *Listeria* is a consideration (2 g intravenously every 4 hours).
4. Vancomycin plus ceftazidime (2 g intravenously every 8 hours) with head trauma or neurosurgical patients
B. Adjunctive dexamethasone (12 mg intravenously every 12 hours for 3 days) may be considered for pneumococcal pneumonia.
C. Control of seizures

D. Fluid restriction if hyponatremia from syndrome of inappropriate antidiuresis develops

E. Management of increased intracranial pressure

Key Treatment

- Immediate empiric antibiotic therapy

- Ceftriaxone or cefotaxime, plus vancomycin, for community-acquired meningitis

- Vancomycin plus ceftazidime for nosocomial meningitis

- Aggressive supportive care

Special Considerations

A. Respiratory isolation is recommended until 24 hours after initiation of effective antibiotic therapy in the patient with community-acquired meningitis.

B. Prophylaxis of close contacts of patients with meningococcal meningitis with rifampin (600 mg orally every 12 hours for 4 doses) or ceftriaxone (250 mg single IM dose) should be administered within 24 hours of diagnosis.

Bibliography

Cabellos C, Viladrich PF, Corredoira J, et al. Streptococcal meningitis in adult patients: current epidemiology and clinical spectrum. Clin Infect Dis 1999;28:1104–1108.

Durand ML, Calderwood SB, Weber DJ, et al. Acute bacterial meningitis in adults: a review of 493 episodes. N Engl J Med 1993;328:21–28.

Friedland IR, McCracken GH Jr. Management of infections caused by antibiotic-resistant *Streptococcus pneumoniae*. N Engl J Med 1994;331:377–382.

Girgis NI, Farid Z, Mikhail IA, et al. Dexamethasone treatment for bacterial meningitis in children and adults. Pediatr Infect Dis J 1989;8:848–851.

Lonks JR, Medeiros AA. The growing threat of antibiotic-resistant *Streptococcus pneumoniae*. Med Clin North Am 1995;79:523–535.

Quagliarello VJ, Scheld WM. Treatment of bacterial meningitis. N Engl J Med 1997;336:708–716.

109 Encephalitis

Margaret M. Parker

Encephalitis is an acute inflammatory response of the brain, often along with the meninges, usually caused by a viral infection. The etiology of encephalitis is often difficult or impossible to identify, except for herpes simplex encephalitis. Postinfectious encephalomyelitis is an autoimmune process initiated by a viral infection, and follows the acute infection by days to weeks. Acute viral encephalitis is characterized pathologically by inflammation of the cortical vessels, primarily in the gray matter, and perivascular inflammation and demyelination are seen in postinfectious encephalomyelitis.

Etiology

A. Herpes simplex virus (HSV)
B. Arboviruses
   1. St. Louis encephalitis
   2. Eastern equine encephalitis
   3. Venezuelan equine encephalitis
   4. Lacrosse virus
   5. West Nile encephalitis
C. Enteroviruses (echoviruses, coxsackie viruses)
   1. Most commonly cause aseptic meningitis (mild disease)
   2. Encephalitis more common in immunocompromised patients or neonates
   3. Encephalitis is a devastating disease, often with long-term sequelae
D. Rabies
E. Mumps
F. Other herpes viruses
   1. Epstein-Barr virus
   2. Cytomegalovirus
G. Postinfectious encephalomyelitis
   1. Following upper respiratory infections, especially influenza
   2. Varicella
   3. Measles

Clinical Findings

A. Fever (with acute viral encephalitis)
B. Headache
C. Mental status changes
   1. Decreased level of consciousness
   2. Disorientation
   3. Behavioral changes
   4. Speech disturbances
D. Focal neurologic signs (more common with HSV than with other viruses)
E. Seizures

Laboratory and Other Tests

A. Cerebrospinal fluid (CSF)
   1. Pleocytosis, with a predominance of mononuclear cells
   2. Elevated protein
   3. Increased intracranial pressure
   4. Cultures are of little value.
B. Electroencephalography (EEG): high-voltage spike wave activity from temporal regions suggestive of HSV
C. Computed tomography scan: focal findings suggest HSV
D. Magnetic resonance imaging: focal findings suggest HSV
E. Acute and chronic serum antibodies not of practical value
F. Polymerase chain reaction to diagnose HSV or enterovirus
G. Brain biopsy may be considered to diagnose HSV encephalitis or other potentially treatable infections or noninfectious conditions that may mimic HSV.
   1. Abscess
   2. Tuberculosis
   3. Fungal infection
   4. Rickettsial infection
   5. Toxoplasmosis
   6. Tumor
   7. Subdural hematoma
   8. Systemic lupus erythematosus
   9. Adrenal leukodystrophy

Key Findings

- Headache
- Fever
- Mental status changes
- Cerebrospinal fluid pleocytosis
- Elevated CSF protein
- Abnormal EEG

392

Treatment

A. Acyclovir 10 mg/kg intravenously every 8 hours for 3 weeks is effective for HSV encephalitis.

B. No specific therapy for most viral pathogens

C. Diligent supportive care in the intensive care unit

1. Monitoring and control of intracranial pressure
2. Fluid restriction if syndrome of inappropriate antidiuresis develops
3. Fever control
4. Control of seizures
5. Mechanical ventilatory support
6. Nutritional support

Key Treatment

- Early administration of acyclovir for HSV

- Anticonvulsant therapy, if necessary

- Management of fluid and electrolyte imbalances

- Control of intracranial hypertension

- Mechanical ventilatory and nutritional support

Prognosis

A. Outcome in HSV encephalitis is influenced by patient's age, level of consciousness at initiation of treatment, and duration of disease prior to treatment.

B. Glasgow Coma Scale score ≤6 carries a poor prognosis.

C. Sequelae in survivors of HSV

1. 46%: no or minor impairment
2. 12%: moderate impairment
3. 42%: severely impaired

Bibliography

Lakeman FD, Whitley RJ, National Institute of Allergy and Infectious Diseases Collaborative Study Group. Diagnosis of herpes simplex encephalitis: application of polymerase chain reaction to cerebrospinal fluid from brain-biopsied patients and correlation with disease. J Infect Dis 1995; 171:857–863.

Rotbart HA. Enteroviral infections of the central nervous system. Clin Infect Dis 1995:20:971–981.

Whitley RJ. Viral encephalitis. N Engl J Med 1990:323: 242–250.

Whitley RJ, Cobbs CG, Alford Jr CA, et al. Diseases that mimic herpes simplex encephalitis: diagnosis, presentation, and outcome. JAMA 1989:262:234–239.

110 Toxic Shock Syndrome

Susan E. Dantoni

Toxic shock syndrome (TSS) is a serious infectious disease caused by bacterial toxins elaborated by *Staphylococcus aureus*. It has been associated with the use of superabsorbent tampons in young menstruating women. However, as many as 11% to 50% of cases are not related to tampon use, and streptococcal toxic shock has also been recognized. Todd first described TSS in 1978 as "the fatal sequelae to *Staphylococcus aureus* in children." There are multiple presentations, but patients are usually critically ill and require intervention in a critical care setting. The incidence is approximately 6 per 100,000 per year. Multiple organ system involvement is common, and mortality ranges from 2% to 8%.

Pathophysiology

A. Mediated by specific bacteriologic toxins
   1. *Staphylococcus aureus*
      a. Exotoxin 1
      b. Enterotoxin F
      c. Enterotoxin A
   2. Streptococcal exotoxins
B. Main effects of toxins
   1. Increased vascular permeability with fluid leakage from the intravascular compartment to the interstitial space
   2. Profound loss of vasomotor tone with decreased peripheral resistance

Etiology

A. Superabsorbent tampon use
   1. Microulcerations from tampon facilitate toxin entry.
   2. Incidence decreased after superabsorbent tampons were removed from the market.
B. Vaginal contraceptive sponge and diaphragm
   1. Risk increases during menses, the puerperium, or if left in place for longer than 24 hours.
   2. Incidence is 1 per 2 million sponges.
C. Nonmenstrual TSS
   1. Sequelae of focal infection or surgical procedure (usually <48 hours)
   2. The male–female ratio is 1:3.
   3. The streptococcal form is more commonly associated with alcoholism, diabetes, extremes of age, trauma, necrotizing fasciitis, or other local infection.

Clinical Findings

A. Typical presentation in classic staphylococcal TSS
   1. Fever higher than 38.9°C (102°F)
   2. Hypotension (often profound)
   3. Diffuse erythroderma followed by desquamation of palms and soles 1 to 2 weeks after the initial presentation
   4. Involvement of at least three major organ systems (usually gastrointestinal, renal, and neurological)
      a. Gastrointestinal: vomiting or diarrhea at onset of illness
      b. Renal: elevated serum urea nitrogen or creatinine concentration or pyuria (in the absence of urinary tract infection)
      c. Neurologic: altered sensorium or mentation
      d. Genital tract: vaginal mucous membrane inflammation
      e. Hepatic: elevated serum total bilirubin concentration or alanine or aspartate aminotransferase activity
      f. Hematologic: thrombocytopenia
      g. Muscular: severe myalgias or elevated serum creatine phosphokinase activity
B. Abrupt onset and rapid progression in classic staphylococcal TSS
   1. Constitutional
      a. Patients may have prodromal flu-like illness for 24 hours.
      b. Patients may present with low-grade fever and dizziness.
      c. Headache
      d. Myalgias
   2. Mucous membranes
      a. Sore throat
      b. Conjunctival injection
   3. Skin: generalized rash
   4. Cardiovascular
      a. Circulatory shock.
      b. Diffuse capillary leak syndrome
   5. Gastrointestinal

a. Vomiting

b. Watery diarrhea

6. Pulmonary: acute respiratory distress syndrome

7. Renal: acute renal failure

8. Neurologic: altered mental status

9. Hepatic: hepatocellular dysfunction

C. Streptococcal TSS

1. Nonspecific findings

2. Manifestations by stages

a. Early: fever, chills, nausea, vomiting, diarrhea, changes in mentation

b. Mid: tachycardia, respiratory distress, progression of pain at site of primary cutaneous lesion (if present)

c. Last stage: circulatory shock and multiple organ system failure

Physical Examination

A. Skin

1. Initial 48 hours: appears as intense sunburn

2. Subsequently: macular rash develops.

3. Days 12 to 15: fine flaky desquamation develops over face and trunk.

4. Subsequently: sloughing of entire skin thickness of palms and soles

5. May spare the skin where clothing fits tightly

6. Blanches readily with pressure

7. Nikolsky's sign: mild friction of skin produces wrinkling and slough (splitting in glandular layer)

B. Vaginal mucosa

1. Initially hyperemic

2. Tenderness of the external genitalia and vagina

3. Erythema, erosion, or vaginitis sometimes accompanied by purulent exudate

C. Other physical findings

1. Myalgia, vomiting, or diarrhea occur in more than 90% of cases

2. Hyperemia of the conjunctivae or pharyngeal mucous membranes or both

3. Oliguria

4. Hypotension, tachycardia

5. Altered mental function

6. Abdominal or bilateral adnexal tenderness in 50% of cases

7. Strawberry tongue

8. Bleeding from puncture sites

9. Respiratory distress

Key Diagnostic Points

- Consider TSS in women of reproductive age or in postoperative patients with abrupt onset of fever, and skin rash accompanied by shock.

- Presentation may vary, but multiple organ system failure supervenes rapidly.

- Vaginal cultures yield *Staphylococcus* in 75% of cases in the classic form.

Laboratory Findings

A. Vaginal culture: *Staphylococcus aureus* recovered in 75% of women with TSS

B. Blood tests

1. Thrombocytopenia

2. Increased serum creatine phosphokinase activity

3. Decreased serum calcium and phosphorus concentrations

4. Decreased serum albumin concentration

5. Increased circulating levels of calcitonin

6. Abnormal hepatic functional tests

7. Lack of rise in antibody titers to the causative organisms for Rocky Mountain spotted fever, leptospirosis, and rubeola

C. Microbiologic tests

1. Vaginal cultures yield *Staphylococcus* in 75% of cases in the classic form.

2. Blood, pharynx, cerebrospinal fluid, and wound cultures are often negative, but may show growth of *S. aureus* or streptococci.

D. Histologic examination: desquamation of epithelium with underlying subacute vasculitis and perivascular inflammatory infiltrates

Key Differential Diagnosis

- Viral syndromes
- Drug reactions
- Scarlet fever
- Leptospirosis
- Ehrlichiosis
- Gram-negative sepsis

- Meningococcemia
- Toxic epidermal necrolysis
- Rocky Mountain spotted fever
- Staphylococcal scalded skin syndrome

Treatment

A. General measures

1. Intensive care unit admission is usually required.

2. Remove tampon and cleanse vagina with saline or dilute iodine solution to decrease toxin absorption.

3. Remove foreign bodies (non-menstrual form); provide surgical drainage or debridement.

B. Treatment of toxin-induced hypotension

1. Fluid resuscitation: up to 20 L of IV fluids may be required over the initial 24 hours, including crystalloidal and colloidal agents, fresh-frozen plasma and other blood products

2. Vasopressors (see Chapter 27, Cardiogenic Shock, Chapter 92, Septic Shock, and Chapter 161, Vasoactive Catecholamines.

C. Intravenous antibiotic therapy

1. Does not alter initial course but reduces recurrence rate

2. β-Lactamase–resistant antibiotic (oxacillin or nafcillin) for staphylococcal TSS

3. High-dose penicillin G for streptococcal TSS

4. Addition of clindamycin recommended

D. Other pharmacotherapy

1. Intravenous immune globulin reportedly is useful.

2. Corticosteroids are no longer recommended.

E. Supportive measures

1. Correct acid-base, fluid, and electrolyte imbalances.

2. Treat coagulopathy.

3. Provide support for renal and respiratory failure and other organ dysfunction.

Key Treatment

- Supportive care with management of shock and mutisystem organ involvement
- β-Lactamase resistant antibiotics to prevent recurrence
- Primary prevention by changing tampons frequently

Prevention of Recurrence

A. Primary infection
1. Change tampon every 4 to 6 hours.
2. Use pads overnight instead of tampons.

B. Recurrent infection
1. Nonmenstrual toxic shock rarely recurs.
2. Avoid tampons for at least 6 months.

Bibliography

Dinges MM, Orwin PM, Schlievert PM. Exotoxins of *Staphylococcus aureus*. Clin Microbiol Rev 2000;13:16–34.

Drage LA. Life-threatening rashes: dermatologic signs of four infectious diseases. Mayo Clin Proc 1999;74:68–72.

Kain KC, Schulzer M, Chow AW. Clinical spectrum of nonmenstrual toxic shock syndrome (TSS): comparison with menstrual TSS by multivariate discriminant analyses. Clin Infect Dis 1993;16:100–106.

Stevens DL. Streptococcal toxic shock syndrome associated with necrotizing fasciitis. Annu Rev Med 2000;51:271–288.

Todd J, Fishaut M, Kapral F, Welch T. Toxic-shock syndrome associated with phage-group-1 staphylococci. Lancet 1978;2:1116–1118.

Tofte RW, Williams DN. Toxic shock syndrome: evidence of a broad clinical spectrum. JAMA 1981;246:2163–2166.

Waldovogel FA. *Staphylococcus aureus* (including staphylococcal toxic shock). In: Mandell GL, Bennett JE, Dolin R (eds). Mandell, Bennett, and Dolin's Principles and Practice of Infectious Diseases, 5th ed. Philadelphia: Churchill Livingstone, 2000, pp 2080–2082.

111 Nosocomial Sinusitis

Meena Kakarala
Jaya M. Raj
Richard W. Carlson

Nosocomial sinusitis is an important hospital-acquired cause of fever and sepsis in the intensive care unit (ICU), especially in patients with nasotracheal or nasogastric tubes. The associated mortality may exceed 11%.

Key Pathogenesis

- Obstruction of sinus ostia
- Local trauma
- Pathogenic bacterial colonization
- Critical illness

Definitions

A. Infectious sinusitis: optimal diagnostic criteria are signs of sinus infection with identification of pathologic organisms on culture of secretions obtained by transnasal sinus aspiration

B. Radiographic sinusitis: sinus opacification, air-fluid levels, mucosal thickening, or bony changes in patients at risk for sinusitis

C. Presumptive sinusitis (i.e., without identified pathogen by sinus aspiration): nasally cannulated ICU patient with fever of undetermined cause, radiographic sinusitis, and clinical response to therapy

Key Risk Factors

- Nasal (and occasionally oral) cannulation(s)
- Abnormal mental status or sedation
- High degree of illness severity
- Neurosurgery
- Facial trauma
- Colonization with Gram-negative bacteria
- ICU length of stay more than 4 days

Clinical Findings

A. Nonspecific manifestations
   1. Fever
   2. Abnormal mental status
   3. Sepsis
   4. Signs of associated nosocomial pneumonia (?)
B. Other associations
   1. Immunosuppression
   2. Critical illness
   3. Human immunodeficiency virus infection
   4. Diabetes mellitus
   5. Corticosteroid use (?)

PEARL

Signs and symptoms are usually absent or unobtainable, as ICU patients are often sedated or obtunded for other reasons, compared with findings typically seen in ambulatory patients with sinusitis (i.e., headache, facial pain, earache, periorbital edema).

Laboratory Findings

A. Leukocytosis
B. Bacteremia
C. Sinus aspiration culture
   1. Polymicrobial in more than 80% of cultures
   2. Gram-negative bacteria
      a. *Pseudomonas aeruginosa*
      b. *Escherichia coli*
      c. *Proteus mirabilis*
      d. *Acinetobacter* spp.
      e. *Serratia marcescens*
      f. *Enterobacter cloacae*
      g. *Klebsiella* spp.
      h. *Citrobacter* spp.
      i. *Providencia* spp.
      j. *Hemophilus* spp.
   3. Gram-positive bacteria
      a. *Staphylococcus aureus*
      b. *Staphylococcus epidermidis*
      c. *β*-Hemolytic streptococci
      d. Enterococci
      e. *Streptococcus pneumoniae*
      f. Viridans streptococci
   4. Anaerobic bacteria
   5. Fungi

a. *Candida* spp.

b. *Mucor*

c. *Aspergillus*

Key Differential Diagnosis (Mucormycosis versus Bacterial Sinusitis)

- Acute invasive fungal sinusitis (mucormycosis) must be distinguished from bacterial sinusitis in immunocompromised hosts (e.g., those with diabetes, leukemia, HIV, or post-transplant).

- Features of mucormycosis: black discharge, mental obtundation, facial-orbital cellulitis, proptosis, rapid progression

- Mucormycosis sinus involvement requires aggressive management, including wide surgical drainage.

- Rhinocerebral mucormycosis is frequently fatal.

Imaging Studies

A. Portable skull and sinus x-rays are less sensitive than computed tomography (CT) or magnetic resonance imaging for diagnosis.

B. Sinus ultrasonography may also be helpful for diagnosis.

Key Diagnostic Points

- Diagnosis is based on clinical suspicion, fever, and x-ray or CT signs consistent with sinusitis in an ICU patient with nasal cannulation.

- Direct transnasal maxillary sinus puncture with aspiration and culture is the criterion for confirming infectious sinusitis; however, it is unresolved whether maxillary sinus puncture is always required, and it may not detect frontal, ethmoidal, or sphenoidal infections.

Treatment

A. If possible, remove all nasal tubes; consider orogastric or orotracheal tubes or tracheostomy.

B. Elevate head of bed 20 to 30 degrees.

C. Administer topical (intranasal) decongestants.

D. Empirically administer broad-spectrum antibiotics, later guided by sinus aspirate Gram stain and culture results, if available.

E. Do not give antihistamines; they may lead to mucus inspissation and impaired drainage.

Key Complications

- Bacteremia or sepsis
- Nosocomial pneumonia
- Cavernous sinus thrombosis
- Meningitis
- Epidural, subdural, or brain abscess
- Osteomyelitis

Bibliography

George DL, Falk PS, Meduri GU, et al. Nosocomial sinusitis in patients in the medical intensive care unit: a prospective epidemiological study. Clin Infect Dis 1998;217:463–470.

Holzapfel L, Chastang C, Demingeon G, et al. A randomized study assessing the systematic search for maxillary sinusitis in nasotracheally mechanically ventilated patients: Influence of nosocomial maxillary sinusitis on the occurrence of ventilator-associated pneumonia. Am J Respir Crit Care Med 1999;59:695–701.

Holzapfel L, Chevret S, Madinier G, et al. Influence of long-term oro- or nasotracheal intubation on nosocomial maxillary sinusitis and pneumonia: results of a prospective, randomized, clinical trial. Crit Care Med 1993;21:2232–2238.

Rouby J-J, Laurent P, Gosnach M, et al. Risk factors and clinical relevance of nosocomial maxillary sinusitis in the critically ill. Am J Respir Crit Care Med 1994;150:776–783.

Tamor, M, Paul L, Barie PS. Acute paranasal sinusitis in critically ill patients: guidelines for prevention and treatment. Clin Infect Dis 1997;25:1441–1446.

Verschraegen G, Mione S. Difficulties in interpretation of culture results in sinusitis. Rhinology 1998;36:55–58.

112 Necrotizing Soft-Tissue Infections

Mitchell P. Fink

The most common infections involving the skin and soft-tissues are postoperative wound infections and superficial cellulitis. The management of such infections is relatively straightforward, and consists of opening surgical wounds down to the level of the fascia and administering appropriate antibiotics. In contrast to these uncomplicated infections, necrotizing soft-tissue infections are uncommon, but are associated with a substantial risk of mortality. Necrotizing soft-tissue infections are characterized by extensive and rapidly progressive destruction of the skin, subcutaneous tissue, and fascia, with variable involvement of muscle. These infections can affect any part of the body, but most commonly they involve the lower extremities, perineum, buttocks, and lower trunk. Successful treatment depends on very rapid recognition of the problem, leading to early aggressive operative debridement of all devitalized tissue.

Classification and Etiology

A. Cellulitis (infection limited to dermis and epidermis)
1. *Staphylococcus aureus*
2. Group A streptococci
3. Group B streptococci (e.g., *S. agalactiae*), especially in the elderly, and patients with diabetes, underlying malignancy, or human immunodeficiency virus (HIV) infection
4. *Pseudomonas aeruginosa*: cutaneous infections can manifest as ecthyma gangrenosum, nodules, abscesses, vesicles, or cellulitis
5. *Vibrio vulnificus*: occurs in patients who have been in contact with seawater, with breaks in cutaneous integrity due to lacerations, puncture wounds, or bites
6. *Clostridium perfringens*

B. Necrotizing fasciitis: infection involves skin, subcutaneous tissue, and fascia, but muscle is spared
1. In rare cases, infection is monomicrobial
   a. *C. perfringens*
   b. Group A streptococci
   c. *P. aeruginosa*
2. More commonly, infection is polymicrobial and results from the synergistic activity of faculta-

tive aerobes and obligate anaerobes; commonly isolated organisms include
   a. *Bacteroides* spp ≫ *Peptostreptococcus* spp.
   b. *Escherichia coli* > other Enterobacteriaceae
   c. Group A streptococci
   d. *S. aureus*
   e. Enterococci

C. Myonecrosis: infection primarily involves muscle, but may involve more superficial layers as well
1. *C. perfringens* ≫ other *Clostridia* spp.
2. *Bacteroides* spp, Enterobacteriaceae

Risk Factors

A. Common factors that predispose to bacterial contamination of soft tissue structures deep to the epidermis
1. Open fractures
2. Surgical incisions, particularly associated with operations involving the colon, rectum, small intestine, or female genitourinary tract
3. Human bites > animal bites > insect bites or stings
4. Cutaneous burn injury
5. Use of contaminated needles by IV drug users
6. Perirectal abscess
7. Intraperitoneal abscess formation (e.g., due to perforated appendicitis or diverticulitis)

B. Factors that lower host-resistance to the spread of infection within contaminated soft tissues
1. Diabetes mellitus (most important risk factor)
2. Immunosuppression (e.g., as a result of cytotoxic chemotherapy for cancer)
3. Old age or debilitating diseases
4. Peripheral arterial occlusive disease

PEARL

Severe systemic toxicity is often present, and can include any or all of these findings: fever or hypothermia, hypotension, altered mental status, disseminated intravascular coagulation, oliguria, azotemia

---

Clinical Findings

A. Cellulitis
1. Warm, red skin
2. Area of involvement may spread rapidly.
3. Marked systemic toxicity may be present.

B. Necrotizing fasciitis
1. Pain, oftentimes out of proportion to other clinical findings
2. Cutaneous erythema (early), necrosis (later), crepitus (not always present), vesicles (not always present)
3. Cutaneous edema (early), oftentimes extending beyond area of erythema
4. Cutaneous anesthesia
5. Absence of lymphangitis and lymphadenitis

C. Myonecrosis
1. Clostridial myonecrosis is also called "gas gangrene."
2. Pain, oftentimes out of proportion to clinical findings
3. Crepitus

Key Imaging Findings

- Necrotizing infections can manifest radiographically as soft tissue gas formation.
- X-rays can demonstrate subcutaneous gas even in the absence of crepitus on physical examination.
- Evidence of soft tissue gas formation may be present even when the infection is not caused by *C. perfringens* (Enterobacteriaceae and *Bacteroides* spp can produce gas).
- Magnetic resonance imaging may be helpful in excluding necrotizing fasciitis.

Treatment

A. Successful treatment depends on early recognition and prompt and thorough surgical debridement of devitalized tissue.

B. Operative exploration is performed for purposes of both diagnosis and treatment.
1. Devitalization of deeper tissues typically extends beyond the margins of obvious cutaneous involvement.
2. Viability of underlying muscle should be determined at the time of operation (i.e., only at operation is it possible to differentiate necrotizing fasciitis from myonecrosis).
3. Exudate from the wound should be submitted for Gram stain plus aerobic, anaerobic and fungal culture and susceptibility testing.
4. Initial debridement should remove all devitalized tissue.
5. In general, planned re-exploration should be performed approximately 24 hours after the initial procedure, and additional debridement performed as necessary.
6. Wounds should be dressed with gauze moistened with sterile saline solution.
7. For necrotizing fasciitis involving the perineum ("Fournier's gangrene"), a diverting colostomy may be necessary to prevent ongoing fecal contamination of the wound.
8. Amputation may be life-saving in patients with septic shock due to clostridial myonecrosis.

C. Initial antimicrobial chemotherapy should be empiric and instituted as soon as the diagnosis is suspected.
1. The regimen selected should provide excellent coverage against Gram-positive, facultatively aerobic, and obligately anaerobic bacteria.
2. Treatment should be via the IV route.
3. Doses should be adjusted appropriately for renal dysfunction.
4. Satisfactory multiple-drug regimens
   a. Penicillin G, 3 million units every 6 hours + gentamicin, 7 mg/kg every 24 hours + metronidazole, 1 g every 12 hours (preferred regimen)
   b. Third-generation cephalosporin (e.g., cefotaxime, 2 g every 6 hours) + metronidazole, 1 g every 12 hours
   c. Third-generation cephalosporin (e.g., cefotaxime, 2 g every 6 hours) + clindamycin, 600 mg every 8 hours
   d. Fluoroquinolone (e.g., ciprofloxaxin, 400 mg every 12 hours) + metronidazole, 1 g every 12 hours
5. Satisfactory single-drug regimens
   a. Imipenem-cilastin, 1 g every 8 hours (preferred regimen)
   b. Piperacillin-tazobactam, 3 g (piperacillin component) every 6 hours
6. If *P. aeruginosa* is isolated from wound cultures, then the chosen regimen should include two anti-pseudomonal agents in addition to an agent active against obligate anaerobes (e.g., gentamicin, 7 mg/kg every 24 hours + imipenem-cilastin, 1 g every 8 hours).

7. Clostridial myonecrosis should be treated with penicillin G, 3 million units every 6 hours (for penicillin-allergic patients, metronidazole or clindamycin can be substituted).

D. Patients with traumatic wounds should receive tetanus toxoid or human tetanus immune globulin, depending on prior immunization status.

E. Treatment using hyperbaric oxygen has been advocated by some experts, but rigorous data supporting the use of this form of therapy are lacking.

F. Systemic manifestations of sepsis or septic shock should be managed appropriately (see Chapter 91, Sepsis and SIRS and Chapter 92 Septic Shock).

G. When wound sepsis is clearly under control (as evidenced by the presence of healthy granulation tissue), then efforts to provide soft-tissue coverage using split-thickness skin grafting or other approaches should be undertaken.

Key Treatment

- Antimicrobial therapy

- Prompt surgical exploration and debridement

- Tetanus prophylaxis if wound is traumatic

- Management of sepsis and septic shock

 Bibliography

Farley MM, Harvey RC, Stull T, et al. A population-based assessment of invasive disease due to group B *Streptococcus* in nonpregnant adults. N Engl J Med 1993;328: 1807–1811.

Groth D, Henderson SO. Necrotizing fasciitis due to appendicitis. Am J Emerg Med 1999;17:594–596.

Schmid MR, Kossman T, Duewell S. Differentiation of necrotizing fasciitis and cellulitis using MR imaging. Am J Roentgenol 1998:170:615–620.

Urschel JD. Necrotizing soft tissue infections. Postgrad Med J 1999;75:645–649.

113 Epiglottitis

Stacy J. Clark
Richard W. Carlson

Acute epiglottitis is a rapidly progressive and potentially fatal inflammatory process involving the epiglottis and surrounding supraglottic soft tissues (arytenoid cartilage, aryepiglottic folds, true and false vocal cords). Before routine immunization for *Haemophilus influenzae* type b, epiglottitis was most commonly seen in children. Adults now comprise twice as many cases as children. The mortality rate is usually 6% to 7%, but may reach 20%.

Key Epidemiology

- Annual incidence is 1:1,000,000 population.

- Average age is approximately 45 years.

- Occurrence peaks in spring, summer, and fall months.

- Male–female ratio ranges from 2:1 to 4:1.

- African-Americans are affected more than Caucasians.

Etiology

A. Bacterial
  1. Streptococcal and staphylococcal species
  2. *H. influenzae* type b
  3. *Moraxella catarrhalis*
  4. *Klebsiella pneumoniae*
B. Viral
  1. Herpesvirus
  2. Adenovirus
  3. Varicella
  4. Respiratory syncytial viruses
C. Fungal: *Candida albicans*

Key Prevention

- *H. influenzae* type B immunization has reduced incidence in children; impact on adults is uncertain.

- Carrier rate in household and close contacts reduced by 86% with administration of rifampin (20 mg/kg per day, not to exceed 600 mg for 4 days)

Clinical Findings

A. Symptoms
  1. Sore throat
  2. Odynophagia
  3. Dysphagia
  4. Dyspnea
  5. Anterior neck pain
B. Physical findings
  1. Fever
  2. Tachypnea
  3. Tachycardia
  4. Hoarseness
  5. Stridor (usually absent in adults)
  6. Respiratory distress
  7. Lymphadenopathy
  8. Drooling
C. Course
  1. Patients typically present with a 1- to 4-day history of upper respiratory tract infection resembling pharyngitis.
  2. Often initially misdiagnosed
  3. May progress rapidly; acute airway obstruction can occur at any time
  4. Immunocompromised patients have a more rapid and aggressive course.
     a. AIDS
     b. Malignancy
     c. Chronic steroid use

Laboratory Tests

A. Largely nonspecific, other than features of infection and inflammation
B. Complete blood cell count and peripheral smear
  1. Leukocytosis
  2. Atypical lymphocytes suggest Epstein-Barr virus.
C. Throat culture (potential to induce larynospasm and airway obstruction)
D. Blood cultures

Differential Diagnosis

A. Infectious
  1. Pharyngitis
  2. Mononucleosis

3. Diphtheria

4. Pertussis

5. Croup

6. Ludwig's angina

7. Retropharyngeal or peripharyngeal abscess

8. Peritonsillar infection

B. Foreign body

C. Tumor

D. Trauma

E. Laryngospasm

F. Toxic inhalation (e.g., hydrocarbons)

Diagnosis

A. History

B. Physical examination demonstrating erythema and edema of supraglottic area

C. Inspection by indirect laryngoscopy

1. Usually safe in adults

2. Potential for laryngospasm and airway obstruction; be prepared for emergent airway management

D. Lateral neck x-ray may show edematous epiglottis.

1. Known as the "thumb-print" sign

2. Sensitivity: 38%; specificity: 76%

E. If high clinical suspicion, may perform laryngoscopy and bronchoscopy with facilities for emergency airway management

Treatment

A. Respiratory

1. Acute airway management: consider emergent intubation (or tracheostomy) for adults with progressive airway obstruction

2. Humidified supplemental oxygen

B. Antibiotic therapy

1. Second- or third-generation cephalosporins (cefuroxime, cefotaxime, ceftriaxone) to treat ampicillin-resistant *H. influenzae*

2. Ampicillin-sulbactam and trimethoprim-sulfamethoxazole are alternatives.

3. Failure to respond to antibiotics suggests abscess or other underlying cause.

C. Corticosteroids

1. Used by many clinicians

2. No proven effect on outcome

D. Continue observation in the intensive care unit until the airway threat has resolved.

Key Treatment

- Intensive care unit observation
- Provision for emergency airway management
- Humidified supplemental oxygen
- Intravenous hydration and antibiotics

Bibliography

Carey MJ. Epiglottitis in adults. Am J Emerg Med 1996; 14:421–424.

Fontanarosa PB, Polsky SS, Goldman GE. Adult epiglottitis. J Emerg Med 1989;7:223–231.

Hackeling TA, Triana RJ Jr. Disorders of the neck and upper airway. In: Tintanalli, JE, Kelen GD, Stapczynski JS (eds). Emergency Medicine: A Comprehensive Study Guide, 5th ed. New York: McGraw-Hill, 2000, pp 1557–1558.

Kucera CM, Silverstein MD, Jacobson RM, et al. Epiglottitis in adults and children in Olmsted County, Minnesota, 1976 through 1990. Mayo Clin Proc 1996;71:1155–1161.

Mayo-Smith MF, Spinale JW, Donskey CJ, et al. Acute epiglottitis: an 18-year experience in Rhode Island. Chest 1995;108:1640–1647.

Todd JK. The sore throat. Pharyngitis and epiglottitis. Infect Dis Clin North Am 1988;2:149–162.

114 Catheter-Related Bloodstream Infection

Stephen O. Heard

More than 200,000 nosocomial bloodstream infections occur in the United States each year. The consequences of these infections are profound. For the patient who suffers such an infection, the median ICU length of stay is increased by 5 days, and associated direct costs increase by more than $34,000. One of the cornerstones of therapy for catheter-related bloodstream infection (CRBSI) is prevention. A number of strategies to reduce CRBSI have been developed over the last 15 years.

Risk Factors

A. Modifiable
   1. Insertion site
   2. Technical skill
   3. Maintenance of asepsis
   4. Catheter material
   5. Use of venous cutdown
   6. Emergent catheter insertion
B. Non-modifiable
   1. Severity of illness
   2. Age
   3. Gender
   4. Remote infection
   5. Sepsis

Prevention Strategies

A. Use maximum barrier precautions.
   1. Wash hands before insertion.
   2. Wear mask, cap, sterile gown, and gloves.
   3. Use a large fenestrated drape that entirely covers the patient.
B. Use aqueous or alcohol-based chlorhexidine preparation solutions.
C. Choose subclavian insertion site.
D. Insertion by skilled, experienced operators
E. Remove catheters inserted during less than optimal conditions.
F. Preferential use of single-lumen catheters
G. Do not remove or exchange catheters on a routine basis unless clinically indicated.
H. Avoid transparent dressings that are impermeable to moisture.
I. Change IV administration sets no more frequently than every 72 hours.
J. Use catheters with antiseptic surfaces.
   1. Chlorhexidine-silver sulfadiazine
   2. Minocycline-rifampin
   3. Silver-platinum
K. Strategies whose value has not been definitively established
   1. Catheter maintenance teams in the intensive care unit
   2. Use of silver-chelated collagen cuffs

Diagnosis

A. Culture methods
   1. Semiquantitative
      a. Catheter tip or subcutaneous segment removed aseptically and rolled 4 times across a blood agar plate
      b. Colony forming units (CFU) are counted at 24 to 48 hours.
   2. Quantitative
      a. Catheter segment is inserted in broth and sonicated.
      b. Serial dilutions of the broth are cultured on blood agar plates and colonies are counted at 24 to 48 hours.
B. Definitions
   1. Colonized catheter
      a. Growth of at least 15 CFU by semiquantitative culture, or
      b. Growth of at least 1,000 CFU by quantitative culture on the tip or subcutaneous section of the hub of the catheter
   2. Exit site infection
      a. Microbiologic definition: purulent exudate growing microbes in the absence of bloodstream infection
      b. Clinical definition: erythema or induration within 2 cm of the exit site in the absence of purulence or bloodstream infection
   3. Catheter-related bloodstream infection: concordant growth from the catheter hub, subcutaneous catheter segment, catheter tip, or infusate and a peripherally drawn blood culture

Key Tests

- Catheter culture: roll plate method and sonication technique
- Blood culture via peripheral venipuncture

Treatment

A. Suspected infection
1. Do not remove catheter if fever is the only sign of infection.
   a. 90% of the time the catheter will not be the cause of infection.
   b. Draw blood cultures from the catheter and peripheral vein: if culture from the catheter becomes positive more than 120 minutes before the peripheral blood culture, remove the catheter
2. If the catheter is exchanged over a guidewire
   a. Culture the catheter being removed.
   b. If significant CFU growth occurs, remove the new catheter.
B. Proven infection
1. Obvious local infection: remove catheter
2. Positive catheter culture without positive blood culture: remove catheter
3. Catheter-related bloodstream infection
   a. Remove catheter.
   b. Antibiotic therapy based on sensitivity testing
   c. Consider transesophageal echocardiography for *Staphylococcus aureus* CRBSI.
   d. Considerations in persistent bloodstream infection
      (1) Septic thrombosis
      (2) Infective endocarditis
      (3) Metastatic infection
4. Catheter salvage using an antibiotic lock
   a. Should only be used in cases of CRBSI in which vascular access is extremely difficult
   b. Administer systemic antibiotics.
   c. Antibiotic lock

(1) Antibiotic plus heparin (or urokinase)
(2) Minocycline plus ethylenediamine tetra-acetate
d. High concentrations of antibiotic in the catheter lumen can penetrate biofilm to kill microbes.
5. Duration of antibiotic therapy
   a. No evidence of metastatic infection: 7 to 14 days
   b. Metastatic infection or persistent fever: 4 to 6 weeks
   c. Candidemia: 14 days
      (1) Amphotericin B: 0.5 mg/kg per day
      (2) Fluconazole: 400 mg/day

Key Management

- Prevention
- Catheter removal if local infection
- Catheter removal plus systemic antibiotics if CRBSI has occurred

Bibliography

Blot F, Nitenberg G, Chachaty E, et al. Diagnosis of catheter-related bacteraemia: a prospective comparison of the time to positivity of hub-blood versus peripheral-blood cultures. Lancet 1999;354:1071–1077.

Darouiche RO, Raad II, Heard SO, et al. A comparison of two antimicrobial-impregnated central venous catheters. Catheter Study Group. N Engl J Med 1999;340:1–8.

Digiovine B, Chenoweth C, Watts C, et al. The attributable mortality and costs of primary nosocomial bloodstream infections in the intensive care unit. Am J Respir Crit Care Med 1999;160:976–981.

Maki DG, Stolz SM, Wheeler S, et al. Prevention of central venous catheter-related bloodstream infection by use of an antiseptic-impregnated catheter. A randomized, controlled trial. Ann Intern Med 1997;127:257–266.

Maki DG, Weise CE, Sarafin HW. A semiquantitative culture method for identifying intravenous-catheter-related infection. N Engl J Med 1977;296:1305–1309.

Pearson ML. Guideline for prevention of intravascular device-related infections. Part I. Intravascular device-related infections: an overview. The Hospital Infection Control Practices Advisory Committee. Am J Infect Control 1996;24:262–277.

Sherertz RJ, Raad II, Belani A, et al. Three-year experience with sonicated vascular catheter cultures in a clinical microbiology laboratory. J Clin Microbiol 1990;28:76–82.

115 Coagulopathy

Per Thorborg

Pathophysiology

A. Normal hemostasis
   1. Formation of platelet plug (completed within 5 minutes)
   2. Soluble clotting factors are activated to reinforce platelet plug with a fibrin mesh (over a period of hours).
   3. Following tissue repair, fibrinolysis takes place and the clot dissolves within hours to days.
   4. Various mediators modulate the clotting cascade, including
      a. Tissue factor pathway inhibitor
      b. Antithrombin (AT) III
      c. Protein C and protein S system

B. Coagulopathy is an imbalance in the hemostatic system. It can be divided into hypocoagulable and hypercoagulable states (this chapter focuses on hypocoagulable states).

C. Relative downregulation of hemostatic systems, or continuous activation of the coagulation cascade, can lead to an uncontrolled hypercoagulable state, which over time can lead to thrombocytopenia and low clotting factor levels.

D. In sepsis, coagulation is initiated by expression of tissue factor, which leads to consumption of AT-III, protein C, and protein S.
   1. High levels of thrombin–antithrombin complex are found, but the high levels of plasminogen activator inhibitor 1 inhibit plasminogen-induced fibrinolysis.
   2. Disseminated intravascular coagulation (DIC) also occurs commonly in sepsis.
   3. Microembolism is believed to contribute to multisystem organ failure.

E. In massive bleeding and transfusion, both coagulopathy and thrombocytopenia can occur.
   1. Thrombocytopenia typically occurs after 0.8 to 1 blood volume is replaced and usually precedes critical depletion of coagulation factors, which typically occurs after 1 to 2 blood volumes are replaced, depending on starting levels.
   2. Coagulation factors are quickly washed out with massive repetitive red blood cell transfusions, with very low levels (~0.5%) remaining after 3 blood volume replacements.

F. Long hypotensive time may precipitate profound coagulopathy.

G. Factors V and VIII are particularly labile (half-life 5 days) and quickly lose their activity in stored blood.

> **PEARL**
>
> Bleeding from the wound site alone or from surgical drains suggests a technical problem requiring surgical intervention.

Classification

A. Congenital hypocoagulable states (uncommonly encountered in the intensive care unit [ICU] setting)
   1. Hemophilia (A and B)
   2. Von Willebrand's disease
   3. Other specific factor deficiencies

B. Acquired hypocoagulable states (some, e.g., DIC, can be associated with a hypercoagulable state as well)
   1. Sepsis
   2. DIC
   3. Hepatic dysfunction
   4. Uremia
   5. Drugs: anticoagulants (e.g., warfarin, heparin, lepirudin), thrombolytic agents (e.g., streptokinase, tissue plasminogen activator)
   6. Massive transfusion
   7. Transfusion reaction
   8. Vitamin K deficiency
   9. Clotting factor inhibitors (e.g., to factors II, V, VII, VIII, X)
   10. Lupus-type inhibitors
   11. Primary fibrinolysis
   12. Extracorporeal circulation
   13. Dilutional coagulopathy
   14. Hypothermia
   15. Hypocalcemia
   16. Leukemia
   17. Polycythemia vera

Key Etiologies of DIC

- Sepsis and septic shock
- Extensive trauma, surgery, or burn injury
- Circulatory shock or cardiac arrest
- Obstetric emergencies (e.g., abruptio placentae)
- Acute leukemia
- Intravascular hemolysis (e.g., from transfusion reaction)
- Collagen vascular disorders (e.g., acute vasculitis)
- Neoplasms

Clinical Findings

A. Overt bleeding
   1. Hematochezia or melena
   2. Hematemesis or blood from nasogastric tube
   3. Bleeding from surgical incisions
   4. Bleeding from traumatic wounds
   5. Hematuria
   6. Hemoptysis
   7. Vascular catheter sites
   8. Hemarthrosis
   9. Ecchymosis
   10. Epistaxis
   11. Gingival or oral mucous membrane bleeding
B. Occult bleeding
   1. Hemodynamic instability (hemorrhagic shock)
   2. Falling hematocrit
   3. Common scenarios
      a. Retroperitoneal bleeding (check for Cullen's sign or Grey Turner's sign; obtain computed tomography)
      b. Postoperative patient with clotted drains
      c. Hemothorax
      d. Intra-abdominal bleeding
      e. Pelvic or femoral hemorrhage

Key Laboratory Findings in DIC

- Thrombocytopenia of varying degree is present.
- Prothrombin and partial thromboplastin times are usually elevated.
- Fibrinogen level may be low.
- Fibrin(ogen) degradation product levels are elevated.
- D-Dimer level is elevated.
- Fibrin monomer level is elevated.

Treatment

A. Fresh-frozen plasma to replace coagulation factors
   1. Use if prothrombin or partial thromboplastin times are significantly elevated and fibrinogen is normal.
   2. Also consider if overt hemorrhage and coagulation test results are not immediately available.
B. In bleeding patient, replace fibrinogen with cryoprecipitate if less than 125 g/dL; avoid iatrogenic hyperfibrinogenemia.
C. Replace lost red blood cells to restore blood oxygen-carrying capacity.
D. Maintain normal blood volume using crystalloids or colloids, bearing in mind that the resulting dilution of coagulation factors may worsen the coagulopathy.
E. Transfuse platelets if count acutely falls to less than 50,000 platelets/mm³ and there is active bleeding.
F. Give vitamin K to patients with hepatic failure.
G. Consider the possibility of dysfunctional platelets.
   1. Review administered drugs.
   2. Warm patient to maintain body temperature higher than 36°C.
   3. Consider desmopressin or conjugated estrogens for uremic platelet dysfunction.
H. Desmopressin is recommended for type 1 von Willebrand's disease and mild factor VIII deficiency.
I. Consider treatment of ionized hypocalcemia; do not give calcium through the same IV line in which blood is given.
J. Consider need for surgical hemostasis, especially in postoperative patients.
   1. Alternatives to surgical hemostasis include topical fibrin glue and thrombin spray.
   2. Patient with perioperative, uncontrolled, diffuse intra-abdominal bleeding can be towel-packed and the coagulopathy corrected in the ICU before a second-look operation (rescue therapy).
   3. When surgical hemostasis is not possible, consider angiography for localization and therapeutic embolization.
K. If pathological fibrinolysis is suspected (post–coronary artery bypass; tonsillectomy; obstetric, gynecologic, or prostate surgery) consider antifibrinolytic therapy (fibrinolysis in DIC must not be treated with antifibrinolytic drugs).
L. Assess administered drugs for potential effect on coagulation, platelets, or hemostasis (e.g., penicillins, cephalosporins, H₂-receptor antagonists, dex-

Key Treatment in Massive Blood Transfusion

- Guide replacement therapy with frequent laboratory measurements.

- Triggers for transfusion
  Hematocrit less than 30%: 2 units packed red blood cells
  Platelet count less than 50,000 platelets/mm^3: 5 units platelets
  Fibrinogen level less than 125 mg/dL: 10 units cryoprecipitate
  International normalized ratio (INR) greater than 2.0 or partial thromboplastin time greater than 1.5 times normal: 2 to 4 units fresh frozen plasma

- Give blood and plasma through blood warmers.

tran, hetastarch, heparin, warfarin, antiplatelet drugs, nonsteroidal anti-inflammatory drugs).

M. Some patients remain unresponsive to therapy and may have factor inhibitors that require prothrombin complex therapy.

Bibliography

Baglin T. Disseminated intravascular coagulation: diagnosis and treatment. BMJ 1996;312:683–687.

Collins JA. Massive blood transfusion. Clin Haematol 1976;5:201–222.

Fareed J, Hoppenstedt D, Bick RL, et al. Drug-induced alterations of hemostasis and fibrinolysis. Hematol Oncol Clin North Am 1992;6:1229–1245.

Rodgers CRP, Levin J. A critical appraisal of the bleeding time. Semin Thromb Hemost 1990;16:1–20.

Thorborg P. Bleeding and thrombosis problems in critical care patients—an update. Crit Care Shock 2000;1: 4–20.

116 Thrombocytopenia

Per Thorborg

Thrombocytopenia is usually defined as a platelet count under 100,000 (normal typically 150,000 to 400,000) platelets/mm³. Bleeding is rare when the platelet count remains greater than 50,000 platelets/mm³, if the platelets are fully functional. "Pseudo-thrombocytopenia" can occur if ethylenediamine tetra-acetate (EDTA) sampling tubes are used. Intensive care unit patients with thrombocytopenia have a higher mortality rate than unaffected cohorts, with sepsis as the major independent cause. Patients with platelet counts above what usually triggers platelet transfusions can still bleed profusely if platelets are dysfunctional (i.e., thrombocytopathy). The two most common causes of counts lower than 50,000 platelets/mm³ are disseminated intravascular coagulation (DIC) and heparin-induced thrombocytopenia (HIT).

Key Symptoms

- Petechial bleeding
- Spontaneous or easy bruising
- Mucosal membrane bleeding
- Gingival bleeding
- Purpura

Pathophysiology

A. The platelet is involved in primary hemostasis that starts within seconds after injury and is normally completed within 5 minutes.

B. Platelets can adhere to damaged subendothelium by the glycoprotein Ib receptor attaching to a von Willebrand factor (vWF) molecule that in turn attaches to exposed collagen.

C. A plug is formed by activated platelets bound together with fibrinogen, which attach at platelet glycoprotein IIb/IIIa receptors.

D. Secondary hemostasis consists of fibrin reinforcement of the platelet plug.

E. Primary hemostasis can be evaluated on the basis of bleeding time; however, bleeding time does not appear to be a good screening tool in unselected patients.

> **PEARLS**
>
> - If thrombosis: consider HIT and DIC
> - If fever: consider infection and thrombotic thrombocytopenic purpura
> - If afebrile: consider drug reaction and idiopathic thrombocytopenic purpura

Etiology

A. Hereditary or congenital thrombocytopenia (rare)

B. Decreased platelet production (decreased or suppressed megakaryocytes)
   1. Sepsis
   2. Drug-induced
   3. Radiation-induced

C. Increased destruction by immune mechanisms
   1. Thrombotic thrombocytopenic purpura (TTP)
      a. The etiology is unknown.
      b. Prevalence is higher in women and patients with systemic lupus erythematosus.
      c. Can occur during pregnancy, typically at weeks 20 to 22
      d. Related to hemolytic uremic syndrome and HELLP syndrome (hemolytic anemia, elevated liver function tests, and low platelets)
      e. Bone marrow transplant patients may develop TTP; either as an early, fulminant, multiorgan involvement form or as a late form with renal involvement.
      f. Diagnosis rests on finding schistocytes on the peripheral blood smear; bowel ischemia, pancreatitis and cardiac ischemia may also be part of the syndrome.
      g. Drugs related to TTP: cyclosporin, tacrolimus, mitomycin C, cisplatin, ticlodipine
      h. If there is splenomegaly, consider nonimmune thrombocytopenia.
   2. Sepsis
   3. Idiopathic thrombocytopenic purpura (ITP)
      a. Antibodies bind to the platelet glycoprotein IIb/IIIa receptor, and this complex is ingested by macrophages.

b. Patients are usually afebrile.

c. Diagnosis is by exclusion.

4. Heparin-induced thrombocytopenia

a. Type I (nonimmune mechanism)

(1) Occurs in up to 10% of patients receiving heparin

(2) Typically occurs after approximately 7 days of heparin treatment

(3) Usually only mild thrombocytopenia that takes an asymptomatic, benign course without associated thrombosis

(4) Platelet count often normalizes even if heparin is continued.

b. Type II (immune-mediated)

(1) Occurs in 3% of heparin-treated patients; of these, approximately 1/3 develop thrombosis; termed heparin-induced thrombocytopenia and thrombosis syndrome (HITTS) or white clot syndrome

(2) Usually occurs after 5 to 7 days of heparin exposure

(3) Heparin combines with platelet factor 4 (PL4); the Fab domain of an immunoglobulin G binds to the heparin-PL4 complex, and its other domains bind to platelets.

(4) This binding provokes platelet activation and release of proaggregatory substances, typically dropping the count below 50,000 (mean 38,000) platelets/mm³.

(5) Platelet-aggregation tests may have a role in diagnosis (e.g., ELISA method or serotonin-release test).

(6) Heparin is contraindicated.

5. Human immunodeficiency virus infection

6. Drug-related

7. Systemic lupus erythematosus

8. Post-transfusion

D. Increased destruction from nonimmune mechanisms

1. Disseminated intravascular coagulation

a. Excessive activation of the coagulation cascade, leading to thrombin formation and subsequent platelet activation with increased fibrinolysis

b. Continuous activation and consumption of coagulation factors and platelets at a rate that is higher than synthesis can lead to depletion of coagulation factors (including fibrinogen) and thrombocytopenia.

c. The most common causes are sepsis, obstetric emergencies, and malignancies.

d. A low-grade, frequently asymptomatic, form of DIC can occur; typically seen in certain forms of neoplasm.

e. Bleeding is the most common clinical manifestation, especially from surgical and vascular catheter sites.

f. Clinically evident thrombosis occurs less commonly, most often in cancer patients.

g. Purpura with peripheral skin necrosis can be seen in sepsis.

2. Cardiopulmonary bypass (CPB)

a. Activation of the contact pathway results in activation of factor XI, kinins, tissue factor pathway and fibrinolysis, leading to thrombin generation despite heparinization.

b. Cytokine activation prompts endothelial cell tissue factor expression and platelet activation.

c. Platelet receptors either bind to artificial surfaces (glycoprotein Ib) or are destroyed by enzymes (glycoprotein IIb/IIIa).

d. In addition to the above, the underlying pathology—as well as heparinization and, in some cases, large blood loss—sets the scene for coagulopathy, dilutional thrombocytopenia, and dysfunctional platelets.

3. Hypersplenism

E. Massive transfusion (>10 units packed red blood cells during a 24-hour period)

1. Thrombocytopenia as well as coagulation defects may occur from blood loss, from replacement with red cells only, or by dilution from large-volume fluid resuscitation.

2. Dilutional thrombocytopenia after massive transfusions is commonly associated with other deficiencies (low coagulation factor levels, especially factors V and VIII) and anemia, which also may require correction.

3. Predictions regarding the type and extent of the coagulopathy based on lost blood volume are often unreliable.

F. Thrombocytopathy: less common than thrombocytopenia, but can coexist with thrombocytopenia

1. Hereditary causes

a. Congenital absence of glycoprotein Ib receptor (Bernard-Soulier syndrome).

b. Congenital glycoprotein IIb/IIIa receptor absence (Glanzmann's disease)

2. Acquired causes

   a. Dysfunction of the glycoprotein Ib receptor (post-CPB)

   b. Uremia

   c. Myeloproliferative and myelodysplastic disorders

   d. Malignant paraproteinemias (multiple myeloma, Waldenström's macroglobulinemia)

   e. Trauma and surgery

   f. Hypothermia

   g. Anti-platelet drugs (e.g., ticlopidine, clopidogrel, abciximab, tirofiban, eptifibatide)

   h. Other drugs (e.g., COX and thromboxane A_2 inhibitors; β-adrenergic, calcium channel, and H_2-receptor blockers; penicillins and cephalosporins; dextran, starch, and gelatin colloids; heparin; ethanol; nitroprusside; nitroglycerin)

Key Findings in TTP

- Thrombocytopenia
- Fever
- Mental status changes
- Renal failure
- Microangiopathic hemolytic anemia

Treatment

A. Depends on underlying problem

B. Platelet transfusion is not recommended in TTP, HIT, or if there are autoantibodies.

C. Platelet transfusion is otherwise recommended for platelet counts lower than 10,000 platelets/mm³ in stable patients without bleeding, or lower than 50,000 platelets/mm³ in patients with active bleeding.

D. Adjunctive therapy may be warranted in certain conditions.

   1. Consider cryoprecipitate if the fibrinogen level is less than 125 g/dL in the bleeding patient.

   2. Consider desmopressin in the bleeding patient with uremia and in milder cases of von Willebrand's disease.

   3. Consider conjugated estrogens (0.6 mg/kg per day for 1 to 5 days) in uremic thrombocytopathy.

   4. Antifibrinolytic therapy (aprotinin) in selected cases post-CPB

E. If patient continues to bleed, consider drug effect on platelet function and consider the risk–benefit of discontinuing suspect drug(s).

F. Ensure normothermia; coagulopathy is exacerbated by core temperatures lower than 34°C.

G. Idiopathic thrombocytopenic purpura

   1. Prednisone: 1 mg/kg, taper dose by 10 mg/week when platelet count is higher than 50,000 platelets/mm³

   2. Immunoglobulin: 1 g/kg intravenously, repeat in 24 hours if bleeding or very low platelet counts

   3. Splenectomy if relapse occurs

   4. Immunosuppressive therapy for refractory cases

H. Thrombotic thrombocytopenic purpura

   1. Prednisone: 60 to 120 mg/day intravenously

   2. Plasma exchange for at least 5 days (refractory cases may require longer plasma exchange, but check for HIT, folate deficiency, and drug effects)

   3. Avoid platelet transfusions except in life-saving circumstances.

   4. Relapses occur in 30% to 60% but usually respond to therapy.

   5. Chronic TTP is rare and may require immunosuppressive therapy.

   6. Treatment for hemolytic uremic syndrome is renal replacement therapy; residual renal dysfunction is common.

I. Heparin-induced thrombocytopenia

   1. Discontinue all heparin, including heparin-coated central vein catheters.

   2. If anticoagulation is required, consider argatroban or recombinant hirudin (lepirudin); do not use low molecular weight heparin.

   3. Avoid platelet transfusions, which can precipitate thrombosis.

J. Disseminated intravascular coagulation

   1. Address underlying cause.

   2. Give fresh-frozen plasma when prothrombin or partial thromboplastin times are high.

   3. Give platelets when count is lower than 50,000 platelets/mm³.

   4. Give cryoprecipitate when fibrinogen level is low.

   5. Consider heparin if thrombosis is evident; ineffective if antithrombin (AT) III level is low.

   6. Consider exogenous AT-III if blood level is low (investigational).

K. Cardiopulmonary bypass surgery

   1. Aprotinin shown to be effective in controlled trials for reducing blood loss

2. Platelet transfusion justified in selected patients

3. Desmopressin may also help reduce blood loss.

L. Massive blood transfusion

1. Guide replacement therapy with frequent platelet counts.

2. Recommended trigger for transfusion (typically 5 U of platelet) is a level lower than 50,000 platelets/mm³.

M. Primary hemostasis defect

1. Hereditary etiologies: platelet transfusion

2. Acquired etiologies

a. Treatment of underlying problem

b. Fluid resuscitation, if appropriate

c. Warm patient to above 36°C.

d. Avoid drugs listed under Etiology, F. Thrombocytopathy, above.

e. Desmopressin and conjugated estrogens are effective in uremia.

N. Drug-induced

1. Stop offending drug.

2. Transfuse platelets if serious hemorrhage.

Key Treatment

- Platelet transfusions (see Treatment section for trigger values and exceptions)

- Consider cryoprecipitate if fibrinogen level lower than 125 g/dL.

- Desmopressin or conjugated estrogens for thrombocytopathy

- Consider aprotinin for CPB surgery patients.

- Treat hypothermia.

- Consider AT-III administration for DIC (?)

Bibliography

Baglin T. Disseminated intravascular coagulation: diagnosis and treatment. BMJ 1996;312:683–687.

Bick RL. Acquired platelet function defects. Hematol Oncol Clin North Am 1992;6:1203–1228.

Greinacher A. Treatment of heparin-induced thrombocytopenia. Thromb Haemost 1999;82:457–467.

Stéphan F, Hollande J, Richard O, et al. Thrombocytopenia in a surgical ICU. Chest 1999;115:1363–1370.

Thorborg P. Bleeding and thrombosis problems in critical care patients—an update. Crit Care Shock 2000;1:4–20.

117 Hypercoagulable States

Robert I. Parker

Etiology

A. Inherited coagulation disorders
  1. Protein C deficiency
  2. Protein S deficiency
  3. Antithrombin (AT) III deficiency
  4. Factor V Leiden
  5. Prothrombin gene mutation
  6. Thermolabile methylene tetrahydrofolate reductase (MTHFR) variant
  7. Dysfibrinogenemia (with production of fibrinogens that produce fibrin resistant to fibrinolysis)

B. Acquired disorders
  1. Vasculitis, systemic lupus erythematosus
  2. Lupus anticoagulant/anti-phospholipid antibody
  3. Microangiopathy
    a. Disseminated intravascular coagulation (DIC)
      (1) Begins as a microvascular thrombotic disorder with secondary bleeding resulting from activation of fibrinolysis and consumption of platelets and clotting factors
      (2) Approximately 10% of patients present with microthrombotic manifestations without bleeding.
    b. Thrombotic thrombocytopenic purpura (TTP)
    c. Hemolytic uremic syndrome
  4. Disseminated carcinoma (e.g., breast, prostate)
  5. Infections (e.g., meningococcemia)
  6. Paroxysmal nocturnal hemoglobinuria (renal vein thrombosis)
  7. Inhibitors of fibrinolysis
  8. Thrombocytosis (myeloproliferative disorders; e.g., polycythemia vera, essential thrombocythemia)
  9. Surgery, immobilization

C. Drugs
  1. Antifibrinolytic agents (e.g., ϵ-aminocapoic acid)
  2. Heparin (i.e., type II [immunologic] heparin-induced thrombocytopenia [HIT])
    a. Occurs upon re-exposure (or prolonged initial exposure) to heparin
    b. Anti-heparin/platelet factor-4 complex antibodies are produced and lead to in vivo platelet aggregate formation and clearance.
    c. Platelet transfusions are contraindicated in HIT until all heparin has cleared from the circulation.
  3. Warfarin (i.e., warfarin-induced necrosis)
    a. Occurs during the early stages of warfarin anticoagulation in individuals who are heterozygous for protein C or protein S deficiency
    b. The prothrombotic state is due to the rapid fall in protein C or S levels before full anticoagulation is achieved.
    c. Prevented by concomitant heparin therapy
  4. Oral contraceptives
  5. Chemotherapy

Clinical Findings

A. Neurologic
  1. Altered mental status
  2. Focal motor or sensory deficit
B. Cutaneous
  1. Pallor
  2. Cyanosis
  3. Purpura
C. Lungs (due to micropulmonary emboli)
  1. Dyspnea
  2. Tachypnea
  3. Hypoxemia
D. Liver
  1. Jaundice
  2. Ascites
E. Kidneys
  1. Edema
  2. Ascites
  3. Hematuria
  4. Renal insufficiency
F. Extremities
  1. Acrocyanosis
  2. Edema, tenderness
  3. Palpable cord in calf vein or popliteal fossa
  4. Decreased or absent pulse

Key Clinical Findings of Microvascular Thrombosis

- Altered mental status

- Acrocyanosis

- Unexplained hypoxemia

- Renal insufficiency or hematuria

Laboratory Tests

A. Evaluation of a coagulation defect

1. Prothrombin time (PT) and activated partial thromboplastin time (PTT)

   a. Normal in inherited hypercoagulable states

   b. May be prolonged in DIC, TTP, or lupus anticoagulant

2. Fibrinogen

   a. Decreased in microangiopathic processes

   b. May be decreased in dysfibrinogenemia

   c. If dysfibrinogenemia is suspected, obtain an antigenic measure of fibrinogen (in general, functional measurement of fibrinogen should be at least 60% of antigenic fibrinogen).

3. Platelet count

   a. Normal in primary abnormalities of coagulation

   b. Elevated in myeloproliferative disorders

   c. Decreased in microangiopathic disorders

4. Euglobulin clot lysis time

   a. Prolonged with decreased fibrinolysis

   b. Prolonged with lysis-resistant fibrin

5. Specfic assays

   a. Protein C

   b. Protein S

   c. AT-III (functional or antigenic assays)

   d. Gene analysis for factor V Leiden, prothrombin gene mutation, thermolabile variant of MTHFR

B. Lupus anticoagulant evaluation

1. Prothrombin time or PTT mixing study

   a. Assay times do not correct to normal upon addition of an equal volume of normal plasma in the presence of a circulating inhibitor.

   b. If test is positive, obtain specific assays for lupus anticoagulant (e.g., tissue thromboplastin inhibition assay, dilute Russell viper venom time, hexagonal phospholipid neutralization).

2. Anti-phospholipid antibody titers

3. Antinuclear antibody

C. Microangiopathy/DIC

1. Complete blood cell count and peripheral blood smear showing evidence of microangiopathy

   a. Thrombocytopenia

   b. Schistocytes

2. Prothrombin time, PTT, and fibrinogen assays

   a. Prothrombin time and PTT may be normal early on.

   b. May be a modest drop in fibrinogen level early on

3. Fibrin(ogen) degradation products may be elevated.

Treatment

A. Heparin

1. Fast, easy, inexpensive, and appropriate for any cause except heparin-induced thrombocytopenia (in which case the appropriate therapy is to remove all heparin exposure)

2. Dose: 50 to 100 U/kg IV bolus followed by 10 to 20 U/kg per hour by continuous IV infusion

3. Half-life is dose dependent with wide variability.

   a. In general, at a bolus dose of 100 U/kg, $t_{1/2}$ is approximately 1 hour.

   b. $t_{1/2}$ increases to approximately 2.5 hours for bolus doses of 400 U/kg.

   c. $t_{1/2}$ increases to approximately 5 hours for bolus doses of 800 U/kg.

4. Monitoring

   a. Goal is to produce a steady-state heparin concentration of 0.2 to 0.4 U/mL, which generally is achieved by prolonging the PTT to 1.5 to 2.5 times the baseline value.

   b. As reagents become more sensitive to heparin, basing therapy on the PTT may result in significant under-dosing of heparin.

   c. Ideally, one should base therapy on a heparin-sensitivity curve with the goal to keep the heparin concentration between 0.2 to 0.4 U/mL.

   d. Complete blood cell count (with platelet count) should be monitored daily while administering heparin.

   e. Urine and stool should be checked periodically for blood.

B. Warfarin

1. An oral vitamin K antagonist

2. Requires a minimum of 3 to 5 days before anticoagulation is achieved

3. Monitoring

   a. Goal is to achieve an international normalized ratio (INR) within the intended therapeutic range.

   b. Therapeutic range depends on the intensity of anticoagulation desired based on the underlying reason for anticoagulation.

     (1) Uncomplicated venous thrombosis: 1.5 to 2.5

     (2) Recurrent venous thrombosis: 2.5 to 3.0

     (3) Arterial thrombosis: 3.0 to 3.5 (occasionally 4.0)

     (4) Prosthetic heart valves: 3.0 to 3.5

C. Low molecular weight heparins

1. Given subcutaneously or intravenously

2. Longer half-life than unfractionated heparin (up to 36 hours) allows for once or twice daily dosing.

3. Significantly more expensive than unfractionated heparin with similar therapeutic and toxicity profiles (recent studies suggest lower risk of major bleeding)

4. Incompletely neutralized by protamine sulfate

5. Monitoring

   a. Does not affect PTT; must perform specific anti-Xa activity assay

   b. May be dosed by anti-Xa units according to patient weight

D. Newer anticoagulant drugs

1. Usually considered in special circumstances such as in patients with heparin-induced thrombocytopenia

2. Includes danaparoid, argatroban, lepirudin and bivalirudin

3. See Chapter 173, Anticoagulants, for details.

Key Treatment

- Heparin is first choice unless HIT is suspected.

- If HIT is suspected, discontinue all exposure to heparin.

- Thrombin inhibitors are useful if HIT is suspected.

Bibliography

Bates SM, Hirsh J. Treatment of venous thromboembolism. Thromb Haemost 1999;82:870–877.

Bertina RM. Molecular risk factors for thrombosis. Thromb Haemost 1999;82:601–609.

Dahl OE. Mechanisms of hypercoagulability. Thromb Haemost 1999;82:902–906.

Ginsberg JS. Thromboembolism and pregnancy. Thromb Haemost 1999;82:620–625.

Goldhaber SZ. Venous thromboembolism prophylaxis in medical patients. Thromb Haemost 1999;82:899–901.

Rosendaal FR. Risk factors for venous thrombotic disease. Thromb Haemost 1999;82:610–619.

Warkentin TE. Heparin-induced thrombocytopenia: a clinicopathologic syndrome. Thromb Haemost 1999;82:439–447.

118 Deep Venous Thrombosis

Remzi Bag

Deep venous thrombosis (DVT) is the presence of blood clot, composed of fibrin and red blood cells, in the deep veins of the extremities, abdomen, or pelvis. Embolization of the clot can occur, usually to the lungs, with potentially lethal consequences. The spectrum of this syndrome is described by the term *venous thromboembolism* (VTE), often used interchangeably with the terms DVT and pulmonary embolism (PE).

Key Epidemiology

- The incidence of DVT is approximately 400,000 cases per year in the United States.

- Venous thromboembolism is a common undiagnosed fatal disease.

- Venous thromboembolism accounts for approximately 50,000 to 200,000 deaths per year.

- Approximately one-third of DVTs lead to symptomatic PE, and 20% to 30% cause asymptomatic PE.

Risk Factors

A. Inherited thrombophilia
   1. Factor V Leiden mutation
   2. Prothrombin gene mutation (20210A variant)
   3. Protein C deficiency
   4. Protein S deficiency
   5. Antithrombin III deficiency
   6. Sticky platelet syndrome
   7. Hyperhomocysteinemia
   8. Increased factor VIII level
   9. Other rare disorders (e.g., dysfibrinogenemia and deficiencies of factor XII, factor XI, heparin cofactor II, and plasminogen)
B. Acquired disorders
   1. Malignancy (e.g., lung, pancreas, prostate)
   2. Surgery
      a. Particularly high risk: orthopedic and neurosurgery
      b. Procedures longer than 30 minutes
      c. Patients older than 40 years of age
   3. Trauma, especially long bone fractures
   4. Pregnancy and postpartum period
   5. Oral contraceptives, hormone replacement therapy, tamoxifen
   6. Immobilization
   7. Congestive heart failure (CHF)
   8. Hyperhomocysteinemia
   9. Myeloproliferative disorders (e.g., polycythemia vera, myeloid metaplasia, essential thrombocythemia, paroxysmal nocturnal hemoglobinuria)
   10. Nephrotic syndrome
   11. Hyperviscosity
   12. Waldenström's macroglobulinemia
   13. Multiple myeloma
   14. Antiphospholipid antibodies
   15. Indwelling central venous catheters
   16. Obesity
   17. Burns
C. Previous thromboembolism

Key Pathogenesis (Virchow's triad)

- Injury to the vessel wall

- Local hypoxia induced by venous stasis

- Hypercoagulability or decreased fibrinolysis

Differential Diagnosis

A. Muscle tears and pulls
B. Cellulitis
C. Ruptured synovial cyst (Baker's cyst)
D. Venous insufficiency
E. Lymphedema, lymphangitis
F. Extrinsic venous compression (lymph node, tumor, etc.)

Key Clinical Findings

- Limb pain or swelling

- Leg pain on dorsiflexion of the foot (Homan's sign)

- Palpable tender cord

- Warmth and redness of the skin over the area of thrombosis

- Fever

- Evidence of underlying risk factors (e.g., CHF, fracture, malignancy)

Laboratory Tests

A. Impedance plethysmography

1. Detects variability in blood flow of patent and obstructed veins

2. Most useful for thigh DVT

3. High sensitivity and specificity in symptomatic patients; poor sensitivity in asymptomatic cases

4. False positives can occur in conditions with impairment of venous flow.

5. False negatives can occur in nonocclusive thrombi and collateral circulation.

6. Safe to withhold anticoagulation if serial tests are negative over 2 weeks

7. Useful to differentiate recurrent DVT from old DVT, or for follow-up of DVT (where ultrasound is not accurate)

B. D-dimer tests

1. Detects specific fibrin degradation product

2. Methodologies are not standardized.

3. False positives are common in critically ill patients.

4. High negative predictive value for DVT if low level (at least 500 ng/mL by ELISA) or negative erythrocyte agglutination test

5. May be useful in combination with other non-invasive tests

6. Routine use remains controversial.

C. Evaluation of predisposing factors

1. Complete blood count including platelet count

2. Peripheral smear

3. Serum for liver and renal function tests

4. Urinalysis

5. Coagulation studies: prothrombin time and partial thromboplastin time (PTT)

6. For selected cases (e.g., age less than 50 years, unexplained etiology, recurrent thrombosis, familial thrombosis, unusual site)

   a. Protein C and protein S assays (warfarin alters protein C and protein S levels)

   b. Antithrombin III level (heparin and estrogens affect antithrombin III levels)

   c. Anti-phospholipid antibody test

   d. Factor V Leiden (in Caucasians)

   e. Homocysteine (in African Americans)

   f. Prothrombin 20210A variant

   g. Factor VIII level

7. Aggressive search for malignancy is not warranted except in idiopathic recurrent DVT.

Key Diagnostic Points

- Many cases are completely asymptomatic.

- Clinical findings may be misleading.

- High-risk patients may present with sudden, often fatal PE.

- Clinical features are inadequate for diagnosis of DVT or PE.

- Minority of patients suspected of DVT have proven disease.

- If suspected, diagnostic tests are mandatory to establish diagnosis (see Fig. 118–1).

- If diagnosis is established, screen for predisposing factors.

Imaging Studies

A. Contrast venography

1. Gold standard

2. Infrequently performed because of discomfort, risk of morbidity, and alternatives

3. Useful for recurrent DVT or when noninvasive tests are inconclusive

B. Venous ultrasound (US) and color Doppler flow detection (duplex US)

1. Noninvasive

2. High sensitivity and specificity for popliteal and femoral thrombi in symptomatic patients

3. Provides additional information about other causes of leg pain

4. Poor ability to detect calf vein thrombi and indirect evidence for abdominal and pelvic clots

5. Non-compressibility (false-positive results) may occur with venous hypertension from any cause or with intense venoconstriction.

6. Operator dependent

7. Safe to withhold therapy if the initial study is negative; repeat study in 5 to 7 days required

C. Radiolabeled (^{125}I) fibrinogen scan

1. Highly accurate for both symptomatic and asymptomatic patients for active clot formation

2. Not widely available

D. Magnetic resonance imaging

1. Promising new modality, but expensive

2. Most useful for calf and pelvic DVT

3. Differentiates recurrent DVT from old DVT

E. Ventilation–perfusion (V/Q) scan: routine use in established cases of DVT is controversial

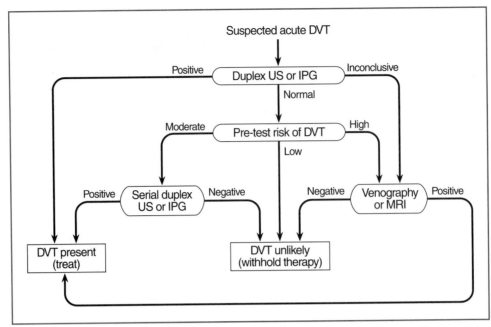

Figure 118–1. Diagnostic algorithm for suspected deep vein thrombosis (DVT). Detection of concurrent pulmonary embolism obviates the evaluation. US = ultrasonography, IPG = impedance plethysmography, MRI = magnetic resonance imaging.

Treatment

A. Prompt, adequate therapy with unfractionated heparin (UH) or low molecular weight heparin (LMWH), followed by oral anticoagulation for longer than 3 months, results in an 80% to 90% risk reduction for recurrent VTE and death.

B. Unfractionated heparin or LMWH should be started when DVT is suspected, continued for 5 to 7 days, overlapping with oral warfarin for approximately 48 hours at doses to keep the international normalized ratio (INR) 2.0 to 3.0.

C. Unfractionated heparin
  1. Loading dose is 80 units/kg.
  2. Maintenance dose is 18 units/kg per hour intravenously or subcutaneously.
  2. Partial thromboplastin time is assayed every 6 hours until therapeutic, then once daily.
  3. Therapeutic PTT: 1.5 to 2.5 times normal (or plasma antifactor Xa level of 0.3 to 0.7 units/mL)
  4. Prognosis is better if therapeutic levels are reached within 24 hours.

D. Low molecular weight heparin
  1. Longer plasma half-life and favorable dose-response relationship; monitoring seldom required
  2. Enoxaparin (1 mg/kg every 12 hours) and dalteparin (120 anti-Xa units/kg every 12 hours or 200 anti-Xa units/kg per day)

E. Warfarin
  1. Start 5 mg daily, after PTT is therapeutic.
  2. Adjust dose to achieve INR between 2.0 and 3.0.
  3. Overlap heparin and warfarin for 2 to 5 days.
  4. The presence of certain comorbidities, diet, and drug interactions can influence warfarin dose effect and dictate careful monitoring of INR.

F. Argatroban: used to treat DVT in patients with heparin-induced thrombocytopenia (HIT)

G. Thrombolytic therapy
  1. Reduces the incidence of post-thrombotic syndrome
  2. Increased risk of bleeding
  3. Routine use is controversial.

Key Treatment

- Start anticoagulation when DVT is suspected.
- Use weight-based dosing for UH.
- Achieve therapeutic anticoagulation within the first 24 hours.
- Start warfarin when PTT is therapeutic.

Complications

A. Pulmonary embolism

B. Chronic thromboembolic pulmonary hypertension

C. Recurrent DVT

D. Post-thrombotic syndrome and chronic venous insufficiency

E. Complications of drug therapy

   1. All anticoagulants: bleeding

   2. Unfractionated heparin

      a. Bone loss

      b. Mild elevations in serum aspartate and alanine aminotransferase activity

      c. Heparin-induced thrombocytopenia

         (1) Early (3 day) or late (5 to 10 days) types

         (2) Incidence is 3% to 4%.

         (3) Thrombocytopenia, bleeding, arterial and venous thrombosis can occur.

         (4) Treatment requires discontinuation of heparin and use of an alternative anticoagulant.

         (5) Plasmapheresis and immune globulin (immunoglobulin G) may be required in severe cases.

   3. Low molecular weight heparin: HIT and bone loss are less common than with UH

   4. Warfarin

      a. Warfarin-induced skin necrosis

         (1) Truncal or extremity skin necrosis occurring within days of anticoagulation

         (2) Risk factors: protein C or protein S deficiency

         (3) Treatment is fresh frozen plasma, vitamin K, and heparin.

      b. Teratogenicity in pregnancy

Prevention

A. Pharmacologic prophylaxis (Table 118–1)

   1. Unfractionated heparin

      a. Low dose: 5,000 units subcutaneously every 8 to 12 hours

      b. Adjusted dose: target PTT at the high end of the normal range

   2. Low molecular weight heparin

      a. Enoxaparin: 40 mg daily or 30 mg every 12 hours subcutaneously

      b. Dalteparin: 5,000 anti-Xa units subcutaneously daily

      c. Nadroparin 2,850 units subcutaneously daily

      d. Tinzaparin 3,500 to 4,500 units subcutaneously daily

   3. Warfarin: adjust dose to achieve INR of 2.5

B. Mechanical prophylaxis methods (Table 118–1)

TABLE 118–1. PREVENTION OF DEEP VENOUS THROMBOEMBOLISM (DVT)*

Risk Group	Recommended Prophylaxis*
Hip fracture or replacement	LMWH or warfarin
Knee replacement	LMWH, warfarin, or ICD
Major trauma	LMWH or ICD
Abdominal or pelvic cancer surgery†	LMWH, ICD, or warfarin
Neurosurgery†	LMWH + ICD, or IPC ± ES, or low-dose UH
Abdominal surgery, coronary artery bypass graft†	UH or LMWH, + ICD or ES; or warfarin in high-risk patients
Urologic surgery†	Low-dose UH, ES, ICD, or LMWH
Acute spinal cord injury†	LMWH, ES, or ICD
Immobilization, medical patients >40 years old	LMWH or UH (ES or ICD if anticoagulation is contraindicated)
Pregnancy with prior idiopathic DVT or hypercoagulability	UH or LMWH

* Abbreviations: ES = graded elastic stockings, ICD = intermittent pneumatic compression devices, LMWH = low molecular weight heparin, UH = unfractionated heparin.

† Combinations of mechanical methods and anticoagulants have additive prophylactic effects in patients undergoing elective abdominal surgery, coronary artery bypass grafting, neurosurgery, elective hip replacement, and urologic surgery, particularly in high-risk groups.

   1. Graded elastic compression hose

   2. Pneumatic compression devices

C. Vena cava filters

   1. Indication

      a. Proximal DVT with contraindication for anticoagulation

         (1) Absolute contraindications: drug allergies, HIT, active major bleeding, refractory thrombocytopenia

         (2) Relative contraindications: severe uncontrolled hypertension, bacterial endocarditis, bleeding disorders, active ulceration and angiodysplastic gastrointestinal disease, recent hemorrhagic stroke, or recent brain, spine or eye surgery

      b. Recurrent DVT or anticoagulation

      c. Before pulmonary endarterectomy

      d. Limited cardiopulmonary reserve and risk of recurrent DVT (e.g., pulmonary hypertension, severe cor pulmonale)

   2. Complications (seen in less than 10%)

      a. Filter misplacement

      b. Filter migration

      c. Penetration of inferior vena cava

      d. Obstruction with venous insufficiency

PEARL

Prophylaxis significantly reduces the incidence of symptomatic DVT and PE and is required in most ICU patients.

Prognosis

A. Proximal DVT
   1. If untreated, one-third to one-half of cases are asymptomatic; another one-third lead to sub-clinical PE.
   2. When treated, fatal PE is rare.
   3. Disruption of deep venous valvular function, with chronic venous insufficiency, may occur in treated patients (post-phlebitic or post-thrombotic syndrome).
   4. Predisposition to recurrent DVT
B. Calf DVT
   1. Most undergo spontaneous fibrinolysis without treatment.
   2. May propagate and cause proximal DVT

Special Considerations

A. Thromboembolism in pregnancy
   1. Pregnancy is a hypercoagulable state due to several factors.
      a. Venous stasis
      b. Reduced physical activity
      c. Increase in circulating coagulation factors
      d. Antithrombin III deficiency
      e. Acquired resistance to activated protein C in the absence of the factor V Leiden mutation
   2. Diagnosis is usually accomplished by duplex US.
   3. Ventilation–perfusion scanning is possible with special precautions.
   4. If serial duplex imaging and V/Q scan are negative, and clinical suspicion remains high, angiography is required.
   5. Subcutaneous heparin (UH or LMWH) is the treatment of choice. Danaparoid is safe.
      a. Convert LMWH to UH 1 to 2 weeks before expected delivery.
      b. Stop UH at delivery.
      c. May require protamine sulfate to reverse markedly prolonged PTT
   6. Use warfarin postpartum for 3 to 6 months.
   7. Can place vena cava filters safely in pregnant women.
B. Subclavian or axillary vein thrombosis
   1. Etiology
      a. Indwelling catheters or pacemaker wires
      b. Hypercoagulability
      c. Post-radiation or post-mastectomy
      d. Idiopathic
      e. Subset of young physically active patients with spontaneous thrombosis
   2. Diagnosis
      a. Signs and symptoms: pain in the axilla, edema of the limb, cyanosis
      b. Laboratory tests: ultrasound and angiography are principal modalities
   3. Treatment
      a. Anticoagulation, as in the treatment of lower extremity DVT
      b. Use of thrombolysis is controversial.

Bibliography

ACCP Consensus Committee on Pulmonary Embolism. Opinions regarding the diagnosis and management of venous thromboembolic disease. Chest 1998;113:499–504.

Aguilar D, Goldhaber SZ. Clinical uses of low-molecular-weight heparins. Chest 1999;115:1418–1423.

Dalen JE, Hirsh J, Guyatt GH (eds). Sixth ACCP Consensus Conference on Antithrombotic Therapy. Chest 2001; 119 (Suppl)1:1S–193S.

Hypers TM. Venous thromboembolism. Am J Respir Crit Care Med 1999;159:1–14.

Kearon C, Julian JA, Newman TE, Ginsburg JS. Noninvasive diagnosis of deep venous thrombosis. McMaster Diagnostic Imaging Practice Guidelines Initiative. Ann Intern Med 1998;128:663–677.

Leroyer C, Mercier B, Escoffre M, et al. Factor V Leiden prevalence in venous thromboembolism patients. Chest 1997;111:1603–1606.

Quinn DA, Fogel RB, Smith CD, et al. D-dimers in the diagnosis of pulmonary embolism. Am J Respir Crit Care Med 1999;159:1445–1449.

Samama MM, Cohen AT, Darmon JY, et al. A comparison of enoxaparin with placebo for the prevention of venous thromboembolism in acutely ill medical patients. N Engl J Med 1999;341:793–800.

Tapson VF, Carroll BA, Davidson BL, et al. The diagnostic approach to acute venous thromboembolism. Clinical practice guideline. American Thoracic Society. Am J Respir Crit Care Med 1999;160:1043–1066.

119 Anemia

Devina Prakash

Pathophysiology

A. Blood loss (acute or chronic)

1. Trauma

2. Disease processes (e.g., peptic ulcer)

3. Iatrogenic (intensive care unit [ICU] diagnostic blood sampling may exceed 70 mL/day)

B. Excessive destruction

1. Intrinsic red blood cell (RBC) defects

   a. Membrane defects: hereditary spherocytosis, hereditary elliptocytosis, hereditary acanthocytosis, hereditary stomatocytosis

   b. Hemoglobinopathies: sickle cell disease and related disorders, thalassemia, unstable hemoglobins, low oxygen-affinity hemoglobinopathies

   c. Enzyme deficiencies: glucose 6-phosphate dehydrogenase (G6PD) deficiency, pyruvate kinase deficiency, porphyria, paroxysmal nocturnal hemoglobinuria

2. Extracorpuscular defects

   a. Immune-mediated defects: naturally occurring isoagglutinins (transfusion reactions), acquired antibodies (autoimmune hemolytic anemia), drug-related (hapten, immune complex, methyldopa, penicillin), disease-associated (e.g., infection or collagen vascular disease)

   b. Non–immune-related: microangiopathic processes (hemolytic-uremic syndrome, thrombotic thrombocytopenic purpura, cardiac prosthesis) or infectious agents (e.g., parasites, bacterial toxins)

3. Hyperactivity of macrophage system: hypersplenism

4. Marrow failure

   a. Aplastic anemia: idiopathic or secondary to drugs and infections

   b. Pure red cell aplasia: Diamond-Blackfan syndrome

5. Marrow replacement: malignancies, osteopetrosis

6. Impaired erythropoietin production: chronic renal disease, chronic inflammation, anemia of critical illness (blunted endogenous erythropoietin response and abnormalities in iron metabolism)

7. Disorders of maturation and ineffective erythropoiesis: deficiency of iron, folate, or B_{12}; primary or secondary dyserythropoietic anemias; heme synthesis defects (sideroblastic anemia)

Classification by Morphology

A. Normocytic, normochromic anemia

1. Acute blood loss

2. Congenital hemolytic anemias: RBC enzyme defects, RBC membrane disorders, hemoglobin mutants

3. Acquired hemolytic anemias: antibody-mediated and microangiopathic anemias

4. Anemia of chronic disease

5. Hypersplenism

B. Microcytic, hypochromic anemia

1. Iron deficiency anemia

2. Chronic lead poisoning

3. Thalassemia

4. Sideroblastic anemias

5. Chronic inflammation

C. Macrocytic, normochromic anemia

1. Megaloblastic bone marrow: vitamin B_{12} or folate deficiency, thiamine-responsive anemia, hereditary orotic aciduria

2. Nonmegaloblastic bone marrow: aplastic anemia, Diamond-Blackfan syndrome, dyserythropoietic anemias, bone marrow infiltration, hypothyroidism, liver disease

D. Spherocytes

1. Hereditary spherocytosis

2. Autoimmune hemolytic anemia

E. Target cells

1. Thalassemia

2. Hemoglobin S, D, C, E

F. Basophilic stippling

1. Lead poisoning

2. Pyrimidine 5'-nucleotidase deficiency

G. Schistocytes and fragmented cells

1. Microangiopathic anemias

2. Disseminated intravascular coagulation

421

Laboratory Tests

A. Blood hemoglobin (Hb) concentration
   1. Normal range (men): 15.7 (14.0 to 17.5) g/dL
   2. Normal range (women): 13.8 (12.3 to 15.3) g/dL

B. Hematocrit
   1. Normal range (men): 0.42 to 0.52
   2. Normal range (women): 0.37 to 0.47

C. Red blood cell count
   1. Normal range (men): 5.21 (4.52 to 5.90) $\times$ 10^{12} cells/L
   2. Normal range (women): 4.60 (4.10 to 5.10) $\times$ 10^{12} cells/L

D. Red blood cell indices
   1. Mean corpuscular volume (Fig. 119–1)
      a. The average volume of individual RBCs
      b. Measured by autoanalyzer or calculated as hematocrit/RBC count
      c. Normal range is 80.0 to 96.1 fL.
   2. Mean corpuscular hemoglobin
      a. The average mass of Hb per individual RBC
      b. Calculated as Hb/RBC count
      c. Normal range is 27 to 32 pg.

3. Mean corpuscular hemoglobin concentration
   a. The average concentration of Hb per individual RBC
   b. Calculated as Hb/hematocrit
   c. Normal range is 33.4 to 35.5 g/dL.

4. Red cell distribution width
   a. A measure of RBC size dispersion, used to detect anisocytosis
   b. Derived from the frequency histogram (MCV on X-axis, relative number of RBCs on Y-axis) that accompanies each automated analysis
   c. Normal range is 11.5% to 14.5%.

E. Reticulocyte count (see Fig. 119–1)
   1. A measure of erythrocyte production, usually expressed as a percentage of circulating erythrocytes; normal range is 0.5% to 1.5%.
   2. The absolute reticulocyte count (the product of the reticulocyte percentage and the RBC count) is a more reliable estimate of total erythropoiesis; normal range is 50 to 100 $\times$ 10^9 cells/L.
   3. The corrected reticulocyte count (reticulocyte index) adjusts for the reduction of red cell count (in anemia), and is calculated as:

$$\text{Reticulocyte index} = \frac{\text{reticulocyte count} \times \text{observed hematocrit}}{\text{normal hematocrit}}$$

The normal index is 1; high values indicate increased erythropoiesis, whereas low values indicate decreased erythropoiesis.
   4. The reticulocyte production index (a reliable measure of RBC production) corrects for both

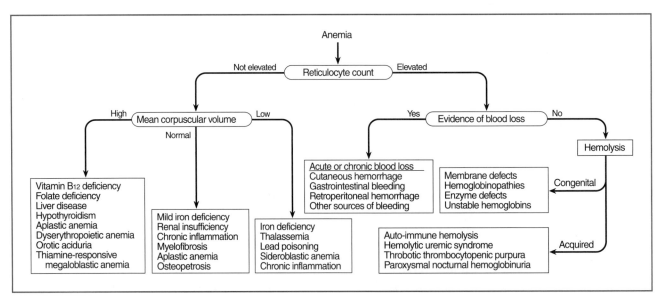

Figure 119–1. Simplified algorithm for the differential diagnosis of anemia.

anemia and reticulocyte maturation time, calculated as:

Reticulocyte production index =

$$\frac{\text{reticulocyte index}}{\text{reticulocyte maturation time}}$$

The normal reticulocyte life span is 1 day and varies inversely with hematocrit.

F. Tests for hemolysis
   1. Elevated serum unconjugated bilirubin concentration
   2. Elevated lactate dehydrogenase activity
   3. Decreased haptoglobin concentration
   4. Hemosiderinemia
   5. Hemoglobinuria

G. Tests for immune-mediated hemolysis
   1. Direct and indirect Coombs' tests
   2. See Chapter 121, Transfusion Reactions.

H. Tests for congenital hemolytic anemias
   1. Membrane defects: osmotic fragility test
   2. Enzyme defects: G6PD and pyruvate kinase activities
   3. Hemoglobinopathies: hemoglobin electrophoresis

I. Tests for nutritional anemia
   1. Iron deficiency anemia
      a. Serum iron level and total iron binding capacity
      b. Serum ferritin concentration
   2. Megaloblastic anemia
      a. Serum B_{12} level
      b. Red blood cell folate level

J. Tests for lead poisoning
   1. Blood lead concentration
   2. Free erythrocyte protoporphyrin

K. Pancytopenia (or blast forms on peripheral blood smear): bone marrow aspiration or biopsy

L. Paroxysmal nocturnal hemoglobinuria
   1. Ham's test
   2. Sucrose lysis test
   3. Flow cytometry

History (Clues to Differential Diagnosis)

A. Race and ethnicity
   1. Hb S and C are more common in blacks.
   2. Thalassemia is more common in whites and people of Mediterranean origin.

B. Sex: consider X-linked disorders, such as G6PD deficiency, in males

C. Diet: nutritional intake deficient in sources of iron, folic acid, or vitamin B_{12}

D. Drugs: drug-induced aplastic, hemolytic, or megaloblastic anemias

E. Infection
   1. Hepatitis-induced aplastic anemia
   2. Infection-induced hemolytic anemia

F. Past medical history: chronic gastritis, peptic ulcer disease, menorrhagia, multiple pregnancies, iron deficiency, chronic malabsorption, vitamin B_{12} deficiency

G. Past surgical history: gastrectomy or surgical removal of ileum

H. Family history: anemia, jaundice, gallstones

Physical Findings (Clues to Differential Diagnosis)

A. Dysmorphic facies, triphalangeal thumbs, and café-au-lait spots: Fanconi's anemia

B. Jaundice, gallstones, splenomegaly: hemolytic anemia

C. Glossitis, angular stomatitis: nutritional anemia

D. Spoon nails: iron deficiency

E. Mucosal and skin bleeding: bone marrow aplasia, leukemia

F. Chronic rheumatologic, immunologic, infectious, or neoplastic disease: anemia of chronic disease, autoimmune hemolytic anemia

Treatment

A. Blood loss: also see Chapters 130, 131, Upper and Lower Gastrointestinal Hemorrhage, and Chapters 137, 138, Chest and Abdominal Trauma
   1. Autologous blood donation for elective surgery
   2. Acute normovolemic hemodilution
   3. Intraoperative and postoperative RBC recovery systems: controversy regarding safety and effectiveness

B. Excessive destruction
   1. Hemolytic anemias: see Chapter 120, Acute Hemolytic Disorders, and Chapter 121, Transfusion Reactions
   2. Sickle cell and other hemoglobinopathies: see Chapter 122, Sickle Cell Crises

C. Other
   1. Ineffective erythropoiesis and maturation: supplementation with iron, folate, and B_{12}
   2. Marrow failure or marrow replacement: specific management for drug-induced, infectious, or malignant process causing marrow failure

Key Prevention (Blood-Conservation Strategies)

- Restrict phlebotomy.
- Use pediatric collection tubes for adults.
- Consolidate blood sampling and testing.
- Monitor phlebotomy volumes.
- Consider use of point-of-care assay devices.
- Employ batch testing and critical care panels of analytes and derived parameters.
- Use blood-conservation devices on indwelling arterial catheters to avoid obligatory discard volumes.

D. Transfusion guidelines: also see Chapter 121, Transfusion Reactions

1. Controversy regarding liberal versus restrictive RBC transfusion threshold strategies

   a. Restrictive strategy appears as effective and safe as liberal approach in many ICU patients.

   b. Patients with cardiovascular disease may require higher hemoglobin levels.

2. Controversy regarding effectiveness of stored blood on oxygen delivery, microcirculation, immune suppression, and risk of infection

E. Erythropoietin

1. Blunted erythropoietin response occurs in many critically ill patients.

2. Transfusion requirements have been shown to be lower in critically ill patients receiving recombinant human erythropoietin as compared to placebo.

F. Blood substitutes

1. Hemoglobin solutions: studies in progress

2. Perfluorocarbon: issues include high PaO_2 requirements, intravascular retention

G. Hyperbaric therapy: limited application for ICU patients

Bibliography

Casutt M, Seifert B, Pasch T, et al. Factors influencing the individual effects of blood transfusions on oxygen delivery and oxygen consumption. Crit Care Med 1999;27:2194–2200.

Corwin HL, Gettinger A, Rodriguez RM, et al. Efficacy of recombinant human erythropoietin in the critically ill patient: a randomized, double-blind, placebo-controlled trial. Crit Care Med 1999;27:2346–2350.

Goodnough LT, Brecher ME, Kanter MH, AuBuchon JP. Transfusion medicine. Second of two parts: blood conservation. N Engl J Med 1999;340:525–533.

Hebert PC, Yetisir E, Martin C, et al. Is a low transfusion threshold safe in critically ill patients with cardiovascular diseases? Crit Care Med 2001;29:227–233.

Smoller BR, Kruskall MS. Phlebotomy for diagnostic laboratory tests in adults: patterns of use and effect on transfusion requirements. N Engl J Med 1986;314:1233–1235.

Smoller BR, Kruskall MS, Horowitz GL. Reducing adult phlebotomy blood loss with the use of pediatric-sized blood collection tubes. Am J Clin Pathol 1989;91:701–703.

Von Ahsen N, Muller C, Serke S, et al. Important role of nondiagnostic blood loss and blunted erythropoietic response in the anemia of medical intensive care patients. Crit Care Med 1999;27:2630–2639.

Weiskopf RB, Viele MK, Feiner J, et al. Human cardiovascular and metabolic response to acute, severe isovolemic anemia. JAMA 1998;279:217–221.

120 Acute Hemolytic Disorders

Devina Prakash

Hemolytic disorders are characterized by a shortened life span of red blood cells (RBCs). Hemolysis can be inferred by the clinical setting and laboratory findings that are seen regardless of the etiology of hemolysis. Hemolysis may be mediated by immune mechanisms or secondary to RBC trapping and destruction in the microvasculature.

PEARL

The magnitude of anemia that follows hemolysis is defined by the balance between the rapidity and severity of RBC destruction, versus the ability of the bone marrow to increase red cell production.

Classification

Hemolytic anemia can be classified broadly as either microangiopathic or immune mediated. The latter is characterized by RBC destruction mediated by immunoglobulins (Ig), complement, or both. The antibody may be an autoantibody or an alloantibody (as in mismatched blood transfusions). In vivo hemolysis is classified as intravascular or extravascular.

A. Intravascular hemolysis

1. Primarily associated with cold-reacting IgM antibodies that activate the complement cascade

2. Maximal activity at temperatures lower than 37°C (usually 4°C); leads to microscopic and macroscopic agglutination

3. Usually directed against the I antigen

4. Direct attachment of C3 to RBC causes cell destruction, with release of free hemoglobin into plasma and urine.

B. Extravascular hemolysis

1. Primarily associated with warm-reacting IgG antibodies

2. Maximal activity at 37°C

3. Not usually associated with complement activation

4. IgG-coated RBCs bind to macrophages by the Fc receptor and are usually cleared by the spleen.

5. Results in hemolytic anemia with spherocytosis

Etiology

A. Autoimmune hemolytic anemia (AIHA; 1 : 80,000 annual incidence)

1. Warm AIHA: approximately 70% of all cases

a. Primary (idiopathic): approximately 75%

b. Lymphoproliferative disease: lymphoma, chronic lymphocytic leukemia

c. Connective tissue disorders: systemic lupus erythematosus, ulcerative colitis

d. Chronic inflammation

e. Immunodeficiency syndromes

f. Drugs

(1) Drug adsorption (hapten) mechanism, e.g., penicillin

(2) Immune complex disease, e.g., quinine, sulfonamides

(3) Antibody induction type, e.g., α-methyldopa

B. Cold hemagglutinin disease: approximately 20% of all cases

1. Idiopathic (~30%)

2. Acute form

a. Common in children

b. Tends to be transient and usually secondary to infectious diseases

(1) *Mycoplasma pneumoniae* (cold autoantibody seen in 33% to 76% of patients)

(2) Epstein-Barr virus

(3) Parvovirus B19

3. Chronic form

a. More common in middle-aged and elderly patients

b. Secondary to lymphoproliferative disorders

C. Paroxysmal cold hemoglobinuria (2% in adults; 5% in children)

1. Viral infections: measles, mumps, chickenpox, Epstein-Barr virus, cytomegalovirus

2. Bacterial infections: syphilis, *M. pneumoniae, Klebsiella pneumoniae, Escherichia coli*

D. Microangiopathic hemolytic anemia

1. Thrombotic thrombocytopenic purpura (TTP); clinical associations include

a. Drug exposures, e.g., oral contraceptives, chemotherapy

b. Pregnancy

c. Collagen vascular diseases

d. Infections, especially human immunodeficiency virus

2. Hemolytic uremic syndrome

3. Disseminated intravascular coagulation

4. Kasabach-Merritt syndrome

5. Pre-eclampsia and eclampsia

6. Malignant hypertension

7. Immunologic vasculitides

E. Miscellaneous causes of acute hemolysis

1. Paroxysmal nocturnal hemoglobinuria

2. March hemoglobinuria

3. Other infections: malaria, *Clostridium perfringens*

4. Patients with glucose-6-phosphate dehydrogenase deficiency, on exposure to certain drugs, infectious agents, toxins, or foods

Pathophysiology

A. Warm AIHA: IgG-coated RBCs with extravascular clearance

B. Cold hemagglutinin disease

1. Autoantibody is usually a polyclonal IgM, and usually reacts with I antigen.

2. Antibody has optimum reactivity at 0° to 4°C, but also reacts at 28° to 31°C.

3. IgM–RBC complexes form in periphery at low temperature.

4. Immune complex binds complement, leading to hemolysis with central warming.

C. Paroxysmal cold hemoglobinuria

1. Biphasic IgG antibody that reacts with RBC at low temperatures and initiates complement cascade, hemolysis completed on warming: Donath-Landsteiner antibody

2. Autoantibody of anti-P specificity

D. Microangiopathic hemolytic anemia

1. Formation of thrombi in arterioles and capillaries

2. RBCs are caught in fibrin strands during passage through these vessels, causing cell fragmentation.

3. Thrombocytopenia occurs because of underlying pathophysiology causing formation of platelet thrombi.

4. Occasionally may have procoagulant activation and disseminated intravascular coagulation (DIC)

5. Schistocytes (fragmented RBCs) are seen on the peripheral blood smear and are a hallmark of the disorder.

6. Thrombotic thrombocytopenic purpura

a. Annual incidence is 1 : 1,000,000

b. Etiology remains unclear.

c. Abnormalities in the von Willebrand factor (vWF) have been demonstrated at diagnosis and recovery, with loss of large multimers of vWF in plasma.

Clinical Findings

A. Warm AIHA

1. Clinical features are related to the degree of anemia.

2. Jaundice

3. Splenomegaly

B. Cold hemagglutinin disease

1. Acute form

a. Hemolysis is seen in third to fourth week of infection.

b. Acrocyanosis may occur during cold exposure.

c. Hemolysis may be severe and lead to renal failure.

d. Usually subsides spontaneously in 1 to 2 weeks

2. Chronic form

a. Symptoms and signs of chronic anemia are seen.

b. Episodic hemolysis occurs during cold exposure.

c. Acrocyanosis occurs on exposure to cold.

d. Raynaud's phenomenon

C. Paroxysmal cold hemoglobinuria

1. Acute attacks, usually during convalescence from viral illness

2. Sudden onset of shaking chills, fever, and hemoglobinuria

3. Back and leg pains

4. Occasionally, renal failure occurs.

5. Full recovery occurs in a few days to several weeks.

D. Thrombotic thrombocytopenic purpura

1. Central nervous system manifestations (most common): e.g., headache, behavioral changes, coma

2. Constitutional symptoms: fever, malaise

3. Hemorrhagic complications: e.g., skin or mucosal bleeding

4. Renal dysfunction: hematuria (gross or microscopic), azotemia, oliguria, anuria

E. Hemolytic-uremic syndrome

1. Usually seen in previously healthy children, but may occur in adolescents and adults; may be familial

2. Follows infections with *E. coli* O157:H7, *Shigella,* and pneumococcus

3. Triad of anemia, thrombocytopenia, and renal failure

4. May have neurologic symptoms, especially seizures

Key Laboratory Findings of Hemolysis

- Increased blood reticulocyte count

- Increased serum indirect bilirubin concentration

- Increased serum lactate dehydrogenase activity

- Decreased serum haptoglobin level (<50 mg/dL)

Laboratory Findings

A. Warm AIHA

1. Positive direct Coombs test

2. Spherocytosis

3. Other features common for hemolysis

B. Cold hemagglutinin disease

1. Direct Coombs test is positive with anti-C3, absent with IgG.

2. Presence of cold agglutinin with reactivity up to at least 30°C (clinically significant)

C. Paroxysmal cold hemoglobinuria

1. Low hemoglobin level and increased serum unconjugated bilirubin level

2. Direct Coombs test is positive for complement, as Ig elutes at higher temperatures.

3. Low serum complement levels during attack

4. Biphasic Donath-Landsteiner test is positive.

D. Thrombotic thrombocytopenic purpura

1. There is no specific diagnostic test.

2. Anemia is present, but usually mild.

3. Thrombocytopenia is present and usually severe.

4. Direct Coombs test is negative.

5. Prothrombin and partial thromboplastin times are usually normal despite bleeding.

**Key Laboratory Test
The Direct Coombs Test**

- The sine qua none of immune-mediated hemolysis is demonstration of bound Ig and complement components on the RBC surface by the direct Coombs test.

- The patient's RBCs are incubated with broad-spectrum anti-human globulins containing antibodies to IgG and the C3d component of complement.

- If IgG or C3 are bound to the patient RBCs, there is cross-linkage and agglutination.

- Sera containing monospecific anti-human globulins against IgG, C3b, and C3d is then used to confirm the diagnosis.

Therapy

A. Warm AIHA

1. Prednisone: 1 to 2 mg/kg, continued until response occurs (usually 3 weeks); 75% are responsive, then slow taper

2. Splenectomy performed for refractory cases

3. Intravenous Ig is effective in patients with associated lymphoproliferative disorder.

4. Immunosuppressive agents (e.g., azathioprine)

5. Transfusion therapy

a. Transfuse with caution and only in patients with severe anemia and high-output congestive heart failure.

b. Autoantibodies and panagglutinins can make it difficult to find compatible donor cells.

c. Co-existing alloantibody is difficult to exclude; observed in 20% to 40% of patients, especially those with a history of prior transfusion and pregnancies.

d. Transfusion can accelerate hemolysis at a rate proportional to the amount of blood transfused.

e. Transfuse with blood that is "least incompatible."

f. Transfuse the smallest amount needed to ameliorate symptoms.

B. Cold hemagglutinin disease

1. Keep the patient warm.

2. Corticosteroids and splenectomy are not helpful.

3. Transfuse only for clinical symptoms.

4. In chronic cases may try chlorambucil and cyclophosphamide

5. Watchful waiting for resolution in acute cases

C. Paroxysmal cold hemoglobinuria
1. Avoidance of cold temperatures
2. Transfusions as needed
3. Supportive care

D. Thrombotic thrombocytopenic purpura
1. Plasmapheresis and plasma exchange
2. Methylprednisolone 0.75 mg/kg every 12 hours until recovery
3. Red blood cell transfusions given if anemia is symptomatic
4. Platelet transfusions should be avoided because they may exacerbate the thrombocytopenia.
5. Antiplatelet drugs may be tried.
6. Vincristine or splenectomy for refractory patients

E. Hemolytic-uremic syndrome
1. Care is supportive.
2. Manage renal failure.
3. Treat hypertension.
4. Give RBC transfusions.
5. Avoid platelet transfusions unless life-threatening bleeding occurs, because platelet transfusions may worsen the thrombotic process.
6. Plasma exchange: no documented benefit except in the familial form
7. Anecdotal reports of response to IV Ig therapy
8. No role for corticosteroids, fibrinolytic drugs, or antiplatelet agents

Key Prognosis

Thrombotic Thrombocytopenic Purpura

- Mortality if untreated is 90%.

- Survival with early institution of plasmapheresis is 80%.

- Relapse occurs in 10% to 60% of patients.

Hemolytic-Uremic Syndrome

- Mortality is 5% to 10% during the acute illness.

- Complete recovery occurs in 65% to 85% of patients.

- Some patients develop progressive renal failure and end-stage renal disease.

Bibliography

Chang JC, Aly ES. Acute respiratory distress syndrome as a major clinical manifestation of thrombotic thrombocytopenic purpura. Am J Med Sci 2001;321:124–128.

Domen RE. An overview of immune hemolytic anemias. Cleve Clin J Med 1998;65:89–99.

Jefferies LC. Transfusion therapy in autoimmune hemolytic anemia. Hematol Oncol Clin North Am 1994;8:1087–1104.

Ruggenenti P, Remuzzi G. Pathophysiology and management of thrombotic microangiopathies. J Nephrol 1998;11:300–310.

121 Transfusion Reactions

Devina Prakash

Transfusion reactions include any adverse effect from administration of blood products. Adverse events can be caused by immune or non–immune-mediated mechanisms. The severity of such reactions ranges from mild to immediately life-threatening, although the overall fatality rate is approximately 1:100,000 transfusions.

Incidence

A. Immune-mediated transfusion reactions
1. Acute intravascular hemolytic transfusion reactions: approximately 1:50,000 transfused units
2. Delayed extravascular hemolytic reactions: 1:2,000 to 1:4,000
3. Febrile nonhemolytic reactions: approximately 1:100 to 1:200 (most common after multiple transfusions or in multiparous recipients)
4. Anaphylactic reactions: 1:50,000 to 1:100,000
5. Urticarial transfusion reactions: approximately 1:100
6. Transfusion-related acute lung injury: approximately 1:5,000
7. Transfusion associated graft-versus-host disease: incidence unknown
8. Post-transfusion purpura: rare, but more common in multiparous women

B. Transfusion-associated infections
1. Hepatitis B: 1:65,000 transfused units
2. Hepatitis C: 1:100,000 (pre-nucleotide testing) and 1:500,000 (post-nucleotide testing)
3. Human immunodeficiency virus: 1:500,000 to 1:750,000
4. Human T-cell lymphocyte virus: 1:650,000
5. Cytomegalovirus: 1% to 17% of seronegative recipients
6. Syphilis: rare
7. Other bacterial contamination: 1:1,500 to 1:2,500
8. Malaria: rare

Pathophysiology

A. Immune-mediated transfusion reactions
1. Acute intravascular hemolytic transfusion reactions (transfusing the wrong blood to the patient)

a. Presence of alloantibody: immunoglobulin (Ig) M anti-A or anti-B isoantibodies of recipient producing antigen–antibody complex with transfused red blood cells (RBCs)
b. ABO incompatibility is the most common cause.
c. Involved mediators
(1) Activation of classical complement pathway with release of C3a and C5a anaphylatoxins, plus activation of C9 with hemolysis
(2) Release of thromboplastic materials by activated complement, activating coagulation cascade with disseminated intravascular coagulation
(3) Bradykinin elaboration leading to hypotension
(4) Cytokine (e.g., IL-1, TNFα) and chemokine (e.g., IL-8) elaboration
2. Extravascular hemolytic reactions
a. Acute extravascular hemolytic reactions
(1) Caused by Rh, IgG, or other antibodies
(2) Recipient's antibodies coat donor RBCs resulting in complement (C3b)-mediated extravascular hemolysis.
b. Delayed extravascular hemolytic reactions
(1) Caused by antibodies to Rh, Kidd, Duffy, Kell, and MNSs antigens
(2) Result in extravascular hemolysis of IgG and C3b-coated RBCs
3. Febrile nonhemolytic reactions
a. Antibodies in recipient against human leukocyte antigen or other leukocyte-specific antigens on donor white cells or platelets, or both
b. Mediated by release of endogenous pyrogens (e.g., IL-1, IL-6, TNFα)
4. Anaphylactic reactions
a. Recipients with IgA deficiency with antibodies directed against IgA or subclass of IgA
b. Activation of complement and release of anaphylatoxins
5. Other allergic transfusion reactions: IgE-mediated reactions to donor plasma proteins
6. Transfusion-related acute lung injury
a. From donor anti-leukocyte alloantibody,

429

which activates or destroys recipient neutrophils in the lung

  b. Reactive lipid components derived from cell membranes during blood storage and complement activation are also implicated.

  c. Mortality rate is as high as 6%, although most patients recover within 3 to 4 days.

7. Transfusion-associated graft-versus-host disease

  a. Transfusion of immunocompetent lymphocytes into immunodeficient recipients or individuals tolerant of donor lymphocyte antigens

  b. Immunocompetent lymphocytes engraft and attack host tissues.

  c. In contrast to bone marrow transplant graft-versus-host disease, recipient bone marrow is a target, resulting in aplasia.

  d. Risk factors: bone marrow and stem cell recipients, congenital immunodeficiency syndromes, intrauterine transfusion, transfusion from first-degree relatives, Hodgkin's disease, hematologic malignancies, solid tumors with high-dose chemotherapy

  e. High (greater than 90%) fatality rate

8. Post-transfusion purpura

  a. Presence of alloantibody in recipient's serum against platelet antigens

  b. Destroys both donor and recipient platelets

B. Transfusion reactions not mediated by the immune system

1. Bacterial reactions

  a. Bacterial contamination of blood product, most commonly *Pseudomonas* spp., *Citrobacter freundii, Escherichia coli*; or (rarely) *Yersinia enterocolitica*

  b. Most organisms do not survive cold storage but release endotoxin and other pyrogens.

2. Viral contamination

3. Miscellaneous reactions

  a. Non-immune hemolysis

    (1) Thermal: warming (greater than 45°C) or freezing

    (2) Osmotic

      (a) Infusion with dextrose solution

      (b) Addition of drugs to infused unit

      (c) Mechanical: rapid infusion through small needle

  b. Storage lesions

    (1) Shortened RBC viability

    (2) Depletion of 2,3-diphosphoglycerate

    (3) Depletion of coagulation factors V and VIII

    (4) Depletion of other essential components

    (5) Increased concentration of potentially toxic substances (e.g., potassium, citrate, lactate, adenine)

4. Volume overload

Clinical Findings

A. Immune-mediated transfusion reactions

1. Acute intravascular hemolytic transfusion reactions

  a. Fever and chills

  b. Burning pain at infusion site, back pain, flushing

  c. Hypotension, dyspnea, bleeding, oliguria, renal failure, jaundice

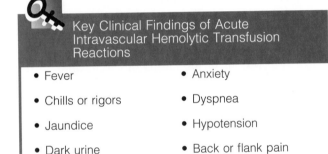

Key Clinical Findings of Acute Intravascular Hemolytic Transfusion Reactions

• Fever	• Anxiety
• Chills or rigors	• Dyspnea
• Jaundice	• Hypotension
• Dark urine	• Back or flank pain

2. Delayed extravascular hemolytic reactions: manifestations occur 7 to 21 days after transfusion

3. Febrile nonhemolytic reactions

  a. Fever, chills, anxiety, dyspnea

  b. Usually self-limited and lasting less than 8 hours

4. Anaphylactic reactions

  a. Shock, bronchospasm, laryngeal edema, nausea, vomiting, abdominal pain

  b. See Chapter 150, Anaphylaxis.

5. Other allergic transfusion reactions: pruritus, urticaria, or both, without fever; occasionally anaphylaxis

6. Transfusion-related acute lung injury

  a. Respiratory symptoms due to noncardiogenic pulmonary edema occur within 4 hours.

  b. Accompanied by fever, hypoxemia, hypotension, diffuse pulmonary infiltrates

7. Transfusion-associated graft-versus-host disease

  a. Occurs 20 to 30 days post-transfusion

b. Central erythematous maculopapular eruption spreading to extremities, which may lead to generalized erythroderma with bullae

c. Fever, hepatic dysfunction, gastrointestinal disturbances, and pancytopenia are also characteristic.

d. Risk of sepsis

8. Post-transfusion purpura: thrombocytopenia and bleeding

B. Transfusion reactions not mediated by the immune system

1. Bacterial reactions

a. High fever (usually within minutes of initiating transfusion)

b. Abdominal pain, cramping, diarrhea

c. Septic shock, bleeding, and acute renal failure can occur.

2. Viral contamination: seropositivity, viral hepatitis, etc.

3. Volume overload: dyspnea, rales, respiratory distress

Laboratory Findings

A. Immune-mediated transfusion reactions

1. Acute intravascular hemolytic transfusion reactions

a. Positive direct antiglobulin (Coombs') test: detects antibody or complement bound to RBC in vitro

b. Coagulopathy

c. Hemoglobinuria

d. Hypoxemia

e. Hyperbilirubinemia

f. Azotemia

2. Acute extravascular hemolytic reactions

a. Positive direct antiglobulin test

b. Increase in serum indirect bilirubin concentration, lactate dehydrogenase activity, and urine urobilinogen concentration

c. Usually no hemoglobinuria

3. Delayed extravascular hemolytic reactions: positive direct and indirect antiglobulin tests

4. Febrile nonhemolytic reactions: direct antiglobulin test should be negative

5. Post-transfusion purpura: thrombocytopenia occurs 5 to 10 days post-transfusion

B. Bacterial reactions

a. Positive blood cultures

b. Laboratory evidence of disseminated intravascular coagulation

Key Laboratory Findings of Immune-Mediated Transfusion Reactions

- Positive direct or indirect Coombs' test
- Hypoxemia
- Hemolysis
- Falling hematocrit
- Hemoglobinuria
- Disseminated intravascular coagulation
- Increased serum indirect bilirubin level
- Increased lactate dehydrogenase activity
- Increased urine urobilinogen concentration

Treatment

A. Immune-mediated transfusion reactions

1. Acute intravascular hemolytic transfusion reactions

a. Stop transfusion immediately.

b. Provide IV volume loading.

c. Give diuretics to maintain urine output greater than 100 mL/hr.

d. Vasoactive drugs may be necessary.

e. Provide factor replacement for coagulopathy with bleeding.

f. Send recipient blood, transfusion blood, and urine samples to laboratory for evaluation.

g. Repeat cross-match, ABO, and Rh testing.

h. Review laboratory and medical records to establish appropriate donor/recipient match.

i. Follow renal function, urine hemoglobin, serum lactate dehydrogenase activity, bilirubin and haptoglobin concentrations, and coagulation profile.

2. Delayed extravascular hemolytic reactions

a. Usually benign

b. Specific treatment usually not required

3. Febrile nonhemolytic reactions

a. Stop transfusion.

b. Provide IV hydration.

c. Give acetaminophen for fever.

d. Administer corticosteroids.

e. Meperidine may be helpful for rigors.

f. Send samples to laboratory for analysis; assess serum for hemolysis.

g. Suspect sepsis if reaction persists.

h. Reassess ABO compatibility of donor and recipient.

i. Antihistamines are not useful.

j. Prevention

(1) Pre-medicate with acetaminophen and antihistamines, if prior allergic reaction.

(2) Use leukocyte reduced transfusion if fewer than 2 prior reactions.

(3) Leukoreduction filters may be helpful.

4. Anaphylactic reactions

a. See Chapter 150, Anaphylaxis.

b. Prevention for future transfusions: use IgA-negative donors or washed RBCs free of plasma

5. Other allergic transfusion reactions

a. Antihistamines

b. May continue transfusion if symptoms resolve with treatment

c. If severe reaction, use washed cell preparations for future transfusions.

6. Transfusion-related acute lung injury

a. Provide supplemental oxygen and respiratory support (see Chapter 8, Acute Respiratory Distress Syndrome; Chapter 222, Oxygen Therapy; Chapters 223 and 224, Mechanical Ventilation; and Chapter 225, Positive End-Expiratory Pressure).

b. Filtering to remove cellular components is of unproven preventive value.

7. Transfusion-associated graft-versus-host disease

a. Treatment is supportive.

b. Prevention: irradiation of donor blood; leukocyte reduction filters do not provide effective protection

8. Post-transfusion purpura

a. High-dose intravenous Ig is the treatment of choice.

b. Platelet transfusions are not useful (transfused platelets are destroyed).

c. Usually self-limiting within days

B. Bacterial reactions

1. Stop transfusion.

2. Send blood samples for transfusion evaluation.

3. Obtain blood cultures.

4. Give antibiotics.

5. Administer IV fluids and vasopressors, as needed (see Chapter 91, Sepsis and SIRS; Chapter 92, Septic Shock).

6. Preventive measures include storage at appropriate temperature, and visual inspection of product for abnormal color, cloudiness, or hemolysis.

C. Volume overload (see Chapter 7, Pulmonary Edema; Chapter 24, Left Ventricular Failure)

Bibliography

Anderson KC, Weinstein HJ. Transfusion-associated graft-versus-host disease. N Engl J Med 1990;323:315–321.

Capon SM, Goldfinger D. Acute hemolytic transfusion reaction, a paradigm of the systemic inflammatory response: new insights into pathophysiology and treatment. Transfusion 1995;35:513–520.

Goodnough LT, Brecher ME, Kanter MH, AuBuchon JP. Transfusion medicine. First of two parts: blood transfusion. N Engl J Med 1999;340:438–447.

Heddle NM. Pathophysiology of febrile nonhemolytic transfusion reactions. Curr Opin Hematol 1999;6:420–426.

Popovsky MA. Transfusion-related acute lung injury. Curr Opin Hematol 2000;7:402–407.

Schreiber GB, Busch MP, Kleinman SH, Korelitz JJ. The risk of transfusion-transmitted viral infections. N Engl J Med 1996;334:1685–1690.

122 Sickle Cell Crises

Devina Prakash

Pathophysiology

A. Aplastic crisis
1. Caused by diminished RBC production superimposed on usual rapid RBC destruction
2. Usually secondary to infections (e.g., parvovirus B19, severe bacterial infections)

B. Acute sequestration crisis
1. Caused by sudden pooling of blood in the spleen
2. Occurs prior to auto-infarction of spleen
   a. Seen in infants and young children
   b. Not seen in adults unless they have sickle cell variants in which the spleen remains enlarged into adulthood (e.g., hemoglobin SC)

C. Vaso-occlusive (pain) crisis
1. Due to intravascular sickling, leading to microvascular occlusion and tissue infarction
2. The most common form of sickle cell crisis

D. Acute chest syndrome
1. Fat embolism is probably involved in many cases.
2. Pulmonary infection is commonly implicated.
   a. *Chlamydia pneumoniae* (most common isolate)
   b. *Mycoplasma pneumoniae*
   c. Viral pneumonia
   d. *Streptococcus pneumoniae*

E. Stroke
1. Overall incidence in patients with sickle cell disease is 0.46 per 100 patient years; age-adjusted prevalence is 4.9%.
2. Most strokes (70% to 80%) are bland infarctions secondary to thrombosis.
3. Approximately 20% are hemorrhagic infarcts, which are more common in adults than in children.

Clinical Features

A. Aplastic crisis
1. Severe anemia (hemoglobin concentration may be as low as 2 g/dL)
2. Congestive heart failure can occur.
3. Other laboratory features include low reticulocyte count, presence of nucleated RBCs, decreased serum bilirubin concentration.
4. May be fatal

B. Acute sequestration crisis
1. Acute onset of pallor, dyspnea, abdominal distention, vomiting, and pain
2. Massive splenomegaly can occur.
3. Precipitous drop in hemoglobin
4. Hypovolemic shock
5. May be fatal within hours

C. Vaso-occlusive crisis
1. Acute, painful episodes may be precipitated by dehydration, exposure to cold, infections, fever, physical fatigue, or may occur spontaneously.
2. Common sites of pain include extremities and joints, flat bones (e.g., skull), or abdominal viscera.

D. Acute chest syndrome
1. Episodes of acute chest pain, tachypnea, fever, wheezing, and cough, associated with new infiltrate(s) on chest x-ray
2. Respiratory distress and hypoxemia may require mechanical ventilation.
3. Approximately 50% of patients are initially admitted for uncomplicated pain crisis or another diagnosis.
4. Some 10% have neurologic events; e.g., altered mental status or seizures. These patients are more likely to develop respiratory failure.

Key Pathophysiology

- Sickle cell hemoglobin is due to substitution of valine for glutamic acid in the sixth position on the β-chain of hemoglobin.

- Sickle hemoglobin forms polymers when deoxygenated, resulting in sickling of erythrocytes (RBCs).

- Sickle RBCs have increased adhesion to the endothelium of post-capillary venules.

- Sickle RBCs have a decreased life span (10 to 20 days compared to the normal average of 120 days).

5. Older patients, particularly those over 20 years old, are at greater risk of death.

E. Stroke

1. Cerebral infarction: hemiparesis, coma, seizures, speech defects, visual impairment

2. Hemorrhagic infarction: neck stiffness, photophobia, severe headache

3. Recurrence rate is approximately 90% in patients who do not receive subsequent preventive measures (such as hypertransfusion therapy) and occurs within 3 years of initial stroke.

F. Priapism

1. Painful, sustained, non-sexual erection

2. May have recurrent short episodes of "stuttering" priapism

3. Ultimate sequela is impotence.

PEARL

Acute chest syndrome is a leading cause of death in patients with sickle cell disease.

Treatment

A. Aplastic crisis

1. Judicious transfusion of packed RBCs (e.g., 2 to 3 mL/kg every 6 to 8 hours until hemoglobin exceeds 5 g/dL)

2. To ensure adequate levels of 2,3-diphosphoglycerate, use fresh packed RBCs when the anemia is severe.

3. Partial exchange transfusion in patients with congestive heart failure secondary to severe anemia

B. Acute sequestration crisis

1. Prompt correction of hypovolemia with plasma expanders and blood transfusions

2. Elective splenectomy after two sequestration episodes (high risk of recurrence)

C. Vaso-occlusive crisis

1. Assess pain using visual-analog or other pain scale.

2. Select analgesic based on past history of response.

a. Morphine and hydromorphone are the preferred narcotic analgesics in acute crises.

b. Meperidine is not recommended as it is associated with central nervous system toxicity.

c. Oral analgesics are not recommended in early crisis, but may be used once the crisis is over and analgesia is being tapered.

d. Narcotic dependence may develop and dosing may need to be tapered to prevent withdrawal, but patients with sickle cell disease do not have a higher incidence of drug addiction than the general population.

3. Begin analgesics promptly; administer around the clock, not "as needed."

4. Titrate drug dose to relief of pain, with frequent reassessment of response.

5. Patient-controlled analgesia can be used for severe pain.

6. Hydrate with 1.5 to 2 times maintenance fluid requirements.

7. Adjunctive use of non-steroidal anti-inflammatory drugs and muscle relaxants (e.g., baclofen, methocarbamol) may be helpful.

8. Hydroxyurea is cost effective for patients experiencing multiple crises yearly.

D. Acute chest syndrome

1. Obtain appropriate specimens for culture.

2. Administer antibiotic therapy (e.g., a macrolide plus a cephalosporin) to ensure coverage for atypical, Gram-negative, and Gram-positive organisms.

3. Provide adequate hydration with IV fluids at 1 to 1.5-times daily maintenance requirements.

4. Give analgesics for pain (both narcotic and non-steroidal).

5. Provide supplemental oxygen for hypoxemia.

6. Administer bronchodilators for wheezing.

7. Careful monitoring of respiratory status; mechanical ventilation as needed

8. If no response to other therapies, give packed RBCs using partial exchange transfusion to achieve sickle hemoglobin proportion less than 40%.

9. Red blood cell exchange transfusion has advantages over simple transfusion during acute chest syndrome as both hematocrit and hemoglobin S can be adjusted simultaneously, lowering the risk of increased viscosity.

a. Blood used should be negative for hemoglobin S trait.

b. Patients with sickle cell disease have a high risk of alloimmunization to RBC antigens (as high as 50% in multiply transfused adults). To prevent this, type patient for C, E, and Kell antigens and given type-specific blood.

c. Leukocyte-depleted blood should be used to prevent nonhemolytic febrile reactions.

10. Hydroxyurea has been found to decrease the frequency of acute chest syndrome.

E. Acute cerebral infarction

1. Provide immediate exchange transfusion to lower hemoglobin S level to less than 30% of total hemoglobin.

2. Maintain patient with chronic transfusion therapy because of risk of recurrence.

3. See Chapter 80, Cerebral Infarction, for specific treatment.

F. Priapism

1. Hydration

2. Analgesia

3. Transfusion, if no response in 4 to 6 hours

4. Exchange transfusion, if no response in 24 hours

5. Corporal irrigation with α-adrenergic agent if no response to prior measures

6. Surgical drainage procedure if irrigation fails

Bibliography

Claster S, Vichinsky E. Acute chest syndrome in sickle cell disease: pathophysiology and management. J Intensive Care Med 2000;15:159–166.

Maitre B, Habibi A, Roudot-Thoraval F, et al. Acute chest syndrome in adults with sickle cell disease. Chest 2000; 117:1386–1392.

Moore RD, Charache S, Terrin ML, et al. Cost-effectiveness of hydroxyurea in sickle cell anemia. Am J Haematol 2000;64:26–31.

Steinberg MH. Management of sickle cell disease. N Engl J Med 1999;340:1021–1030.

Vichinsky EP, Neumayr LD, Earles AN, et al. Causes and outcome of the acute chest syndrome in sickle cell disease. N Engl J Med 2000;342:1855–1865.

123 Graft Versus Host Disease

Lisa Mueller

Graft-versus-host disease (GVHD) is a major cause of morbidity and mortality following allogeneic bone marrow transplant. It occurs in the setting of infusion into the host of immunologically competent donor T cells, histoincompatibility between donor and host, and the immunocompromised host's inability to reject donor cells. There are two basic forms of GVHD: alloreactive (acute post-transplant and transfusion-induced GVHD) and autoreactive or autoimmune (chronic GVHD and autologous transplantation). All forms require the primary effector cell, i.e., the T cell, to induce GVHD by attacking various organ systems, typically the skin, gastrointestinal tract, and liver. Acute GVHD is due to donor T cell recognition of host antigen(s) as foreign.

Post-Transplant Acute GVHD

Clinical Findings (Table 123–1)

A. Skin

  1. Maculopapular rash

    a. May be pruritic or sunburn-like

    b. Distribution initially involves palms, soles and ears.

    c. Spreads to face, trunk, extremities

    d. Can become confluent

    e. Bullous lesions and epidermal necrolysis occur in severe cases.

B. Gastrointestinal tract

  1. Watery diarrhea

  2. Progresses to bloody diarrhea with severe abdominal cramping in lower tract disease (worse prognosis)

  3. Nausea and vomiting in upper tract disease

C. Liver

  1. Presents with abnormal liver function tests (usually elevated serum conjugated bilirubin level)

  2. Typically asymptomatic

  3. Hepatitis-like picture

  4. Leads to biliary cirrhosis, hepatocellular necrosis, and hepatic failure

Key Risk Factors

- HLA mismatch
- Unrelated donor
- Sex mismatch
- Disease status
- Increasing age of recipient or donor
- Prior donor pregnancies
- Prior herpesvirus infections
- Seropositivity (donor or recipient)

Prophylaxis

A. Immunosuppressive medications

  1. Common

    a. Methotrexate

    b. Cyclosporin A

    c. Prednisone

  2. Other

    a. Tacrolimus (FK506)

    b. Mycophenolate mofetil

B. Graft manipulation

  1. T cell depletion

  2. CD 34 selection

C. Patient decontamination

D. Treatment in a protective, germ-free environment (gnotobiosis)

Treatment

A. Severe acute GVHD despite prophylaxis is life-threatening, requiring prompt intervention.

B. Standard therapy

  1. Addition of methylprednisolone (2 to 3 mg/kg per day)

  2. 20% to 30% of patients respond

  3. Steroid refractory acute GVHD has a very poor outcome.

C. Investigational therapy

  1. Very high doses of steroids

  2. Antithymocyte globulin

  3. Thalidomide

  4. Immunotoxin conjugate (anti-CD5 antibody)

  5. Anti-Tac (anti-CD 25 antibody)

TABLE 123–1. CLINICAL GRADING OF ACUTE GVHD

GRADE*	SKIN (BODY SURFACE (AREA AFFECTED, %)	GASTROINTESTINAL TRACT (DIARRHEA, L/DAY)	LIVER FUNCTION (BILIRUBIN, MG/DL)
I	<25	<0.5	<3
II	25 to 50	0.5 to 1.0	3 to 6
III	>50	>1.0	7 to 15
IV	Desquamated, bullae, bleeding	Ileus or bloody diarrhea	>15 or ↑ in serum transaminase activity

*Patients with stage II to IV acute GVHD and involvement of at least 2 organ systems have clinically significant disease.

6. Anti-TNF antibody

7. IL-1 receptor antagonist

D. Often fatal despite treatment (up to 50%)

Transfusion-Induced GVHD

> **PEARL**
>
> Prevent transfusion-induced GVHD in susceptible patients by irradiation of all blood products to kill T cells.

Etiology

A. Caused by recipient's inability to reject viable T cells in a transfusion product

B. Settings
   1. Severe combined immunodeficiency
   2. Wiskott-Aldrich syndrome
   3. Acquired T cell defects
      a. Hodgkin's disease
      b. Non-Hodgkin's lymphoma
      c. Neuroblastoma
      d. Transfusion from a donor (usually related) who is homozygous for one of the recipient's HLA haplotypes

Key Findings in Transfusion-Induced GVHD

- Rash
- Pancytopenia
- Bone marrow aplasia
- Abnormal liver function tests
- Course usually fulminant
- Death due to complications of marrow failure

Treatment

A. Immunosuppressive therapy

B. Corticosteroids
   1. Frontline therapy
   2. Methylprednisolone: 2 to 3 mg/kg per day

Post-transplant Chronic GVHD

Etiology

A. Usually a progression from acute GVHD

B. Also can occur de novo

C. Represents an autoimmune-type process with a dysregulated immune system

D. Occurs more than 100 days post-transplant

Clinical Findings

A. History
   1. Hair loss
   2. Anorexia
   3. Weight loss
   4. Nausea
   5. Vomiting
   6. Arthralgia
   7. Myalgia

B. Physical examination
   1. Skin
      a. Sclerodermatous changes
      b. Hypo- or hyperpigmentation
      c. Loss of hair follicles and sweat glands
   2. Musculoskeletal
      a. Arthritis
      b. Polymyositis
   3. Gastrointestinal
      a. Malabsorption
      b. Esophageal web formation
      c. Fibrosis of submucosa and serosa
   4. Liver

a. Obstructive jaundice picture

b. Cirrhosis

5. Lung

a. Bronchiolitis obliterans

b. Pulmonary fibrosis

6. Other

a. Keratoconjunctivitis

b. Sicca (dry mouth with or without ulceration)

c. Serositis

C. Clinical grading

1. Limited: localized skin or hepatic dysfunction

2. Extensive (usually progressive and often fatal)

a. Skin (local or generalized) plus

b. Hepatic: chronic hepatitis with bridging necrosis or cirrhosis

c. Eye: keratoconjunctivitis, Schirmer's test less than 5 mm wetting

d. Mucosal: sicca syndrome

e. Any other organ involvement

Key Laboratory Findings

- Hyperbilirubinemia

- Chronic hepatitis, elevated serum transaminase activity

- Autoantibodies (e.g., antinuclear antibody positive)

- Hemolytic anemia

Treatment

A. Treatment is similar to acute GVHD because the same effector cells (T cells) are involved.

B. Prednisone

C. Other treatment

1. Cyclosporin A

2. Thalidomide

3. Beclomethasone (oral)

4. Ursodeoxycholic acid (for hepatic involvement)

5. Psoralens plus long-wave ultraviolet light therapy (for skin involvement)

6. Azathioprine

7. Etretinate

8. Extracorporeal phototherapy

Bibliography

Billingham RE. The biology of graft versus host reactions. Harvey Lectures 1966;62:21–78.

Ferrara JL, Levy R, Chao NJ. Pathophysiologic mechanisms of acute graft-vs-host disease. Biol Blood Marrow Transplant 1999;5:347–356.

Gerber M, Gmeinhart B, Volc-Platzer B, et al. Complete remission of lichen-planus-like graft-versus-host disease (GVHD) with extracorporeal phototherapy (ECP). Bone Marrow Transplant 1997;19:517–519.

Marcellus DC, Altomonte VL, Farmer ER, et al. Etretinate therapy for refractory sclerodermatous chronic graft-versus-host disease. Blood 1999;93:66–70.

Saigo K, Ryo R. Therapeutic strategy for post-transfusion acute graft-vs-host disease. Int J Hematol 1999;69:147–151.

Tse JC, Moore TB. Monoclonal antibodies in the treatment of steroid-resistant acute graft-versus-host disease. Pharmacotherapy 1998;18:988–1000.

Vogelsang GB. Advances in the treatment of graft-versus-host disease. Leukemia 2000;14:509–510.

124 Acute Abdominal Pain

Mitchell P. Fink

Patients with acute onset of abdominal pain are said to have an "acute abdomen." Although the clinician (surgeon, emergency physician, or intensivist) should try to establish the correct and precise diagnosis, the most important issue is to determine whether urgent operative intervention (laparoscopy or laparotomy) is indicated. When an emergency operation is warranted, failure to provide such therapy in a timely fashion can have dire consequences for the patient, and even lead to death.

Classification

A. General categorization
   1. Visceral pain
      a. Arises from the organs within the peritoneal cavity and travels to the central nervous system via the autonomic nervous system and the somatic nerves innervating the body wall and the diaphragm
      b. Is induced by these stimuli: strong contractions of smooth muscle elements in the walls of hollow organs (bile ducts, ureters, stomach, intestine, colon, bladder); acute distention of hollow organs; chemical irritation and inflammation of the visceral peritoneum
      c. Is deep pain
   2. Pain arising from irritation of the parietal peritoneum
      a. Pain is sharp and often triggers spasm of the abdominal musculature (referred to as "involuntary guarding" or rigidity).
      b. "Rebound (percussion) tenderness" is thought to be caused by transient irritation of the parietal peritoneum.
   3. Pain arising from skeletal muscles
   4. Pain arising from the skin
B. Location of abdominal pain (can provide clues to its origin)
   1. Biliary tract: right upper quadrant or epigastric abdominal pain; referred pain to right shoulder
   2. Duodenal ulcer without perforation: epigastric pain
   3. Posterior penetrating duodenal ulcer and/or pancreatitis: back pain

   4. Small intestine: poorly localized periumbilical abdominal pain
   5. Colon: poorly localized abdominal pain
   6. Ureter: pain radiating to the groin

History

A. History of the present illness
   1. Pain
      a. Define time of onset and location of pain; severe pain of longer than 6 hours duration is likely to warrant operative intervention.
      b. Pain that is sharp and sudden in onset suggests a perforated viscus.
      c. Upper abdominal pain favors peptic ulceration, biliary colic or acute cholecystitis, or pancreatitis.
      d. Lower abdominal pain favors ruptured tubo-ovarian abscess, colonic diverticulitis, ruptured ovarian cyst.
      e. Early epigastric pain followed later by right lower quadrant discomfort suggests appendicitis.
      f. Acute severe back pain suggests acute pancreatitis or expansion/contained leakage of an abdominal aortic aneurysm.
      g. Colicky pain (i.e., pain that comes in waves with periods of partial or complete relief between each new bout) suggests ureteral or small bowel obstruction.
   2. Vomiting
      a. Vomiting can be triggered by severe pain (as with ureteral colic).
      b. Vomiting occurs commonly in acute cholecystitis
      c. Vomiting always occurs with small bowel obstruction (unless nasogastric decompression is already being provided when the obstruction develops).
      d. Vomiting that starts prior to the onset of pain suggests gastroenteritis.
      e. Absence of bile in emesis suggests obstruction proximal to the pylorus.
      f. Feculent emesis suggests distal small bowel or colonic obstruction.

g. If vomiting temporarily relieves abdominal cramping, then intestinal obstruction is the most likely diagnosis.

3. Anorexia

a. A virtually universal finding in patients with peritonitis

b. Often precedes the onset of pain in patients with appendicitis

4. Bowel habits

a. Profuse watery diarrhea for more than 12 hours suggests gastroenteritis, although diarrhea can also be a symptom of partial bowel obstruction.

b. A history of a recent change in stool frequency or caliber may suggest the presence of colon or rectal carcinoma.

c. Failure to pass flatus for more than 12 hours in association with crampy abdominal pain suggests complete bowel obstruction.

5. Females

a. Recent menstrual history

b. Sexual activity and use of contraceptives

c. Helpful to exclude diagnosis of ruptured ectopic pregnancy

B. Past history and family history

1. History of previous abdominal operations (increases risk for bowel obstruction secondary to intraperitoneal adhesion formation)

2. History of gallstones, acute cholecystitis, kidney stones, pelvic inflammatory disease

3. Concurrent illnesses and medications

a. May determine need for ICU care during preoperative period for resuscitation, or need for invasive intraoperative monitoring and postoperative ICU care

b. May suggest alternative diagnoses (e.g., known history of coronary artery disease may increase suspicion of acute myocardial ischemia as a cause of upper abdominal pain)

c. May alter therapeutic plan (e.g., suggest the need for "stress" doses of hydrocortisone in a patient receiving chronic glucocorticoid therapy for a chronic disease)

4. History of rare heritable illnesses associated with abdominal pain (e.g., familial Mediterranean fever)

Physical Examination

A. General

1. Fever and tachypnea are nonspecific findings,

but ones that are consistent with peritoneal inflammation.

2. Patients with peritonitis tend to avoid movement, lying on their sides with knees and hips flexed.

3. Assess the patient's hydration status by examining mucous membranes and skin turgor; dehydration is common with peritonitis because of "third space" sequestration of fluid, as well vomiting or decreased oral intake of liquids.

4. Assess the patient for evidence of jaundice.

B. Abdomen

1. Inspect for previous scars, obvious masses, and hernias.

2. Auscultation of the abdomen is useful.

a. High-pitched bowel sounds suggest intestinal distention proximal to a site of partial or complete obstruction.

b. Peritonitis commonly leads to ileus and, hence, absent bowel sounds.

3. Palpation and percussion

a. Should be done gingerly and started away from the region described as being painful

b. Assess for the presence of rebound (or, better, percussion) tenderness.

c. The presence of muscular rigidity supports the diagnosis of peritonitis.

d. Pelvic and rectal examination are mandatory (but generally should be performed only once, and by the surgeon who will make the final decision regarding the need for urgent operation).

PEARL

Documentation of the presence of rebound (or, better, percussion) tenderness is important, but this finding often can be elicited in a way that is less painful for the patient by asking the patient to cough.

Laboratory Tests

A. Laboratory studies are much less important than either the history or physical examination for establishing a diagnosis; only a few simple laboratory tests are generally warranted.

B. Complete blood cell count

1. Leukocytosis, especially with a left-shift of the differential white blood cell (WBC) count, is common in peritonitis.

2. Rarely, leukopenia will be present in patients

with severe sepsis secondary to intraperitoneal infection; this finding is a grave prognostic sign.

3. Hemoconcentration is common in peritonitis or bowel obstruction secondary to "third-space" sequestration of fluid.

C. Serum amylase activity level

1. Differential diagnosis of elevated serum amylase activity

  a. Acute pancreatitis

  b. Pancreatic trauma

  c. Biliary tract disease (with or without evidence of pancreatitis)

  d. Pancreatobiliary instrumentation (e.g., endoscopic retrograde pancreatocholangiography)

  e. Perforated duodenal ulcer, peritonitis, intestinal obstruction or infarction, and recent abdominal surgery (9% to 32% of cases)

  f. Acute salivary gland disease

  g. Macroamylasemia

  h. Renal failure (although roughly half of cases have normal circulating amylase levels)

  i. Miscellaneous: severe cardiac circulatory failure (29% of cases), diabetic ketoacidosis in the recovery phase (41% to 80% of cases), pregnancy

2. Very high amylase activities are common in cases of gallstone pancreatitis, but this finding is not sufficiently reliable to establish the diagnosis.

D. Serum lipase activity

1. Because it has equal sensitivity but better specificity, measurement of serum lipase activity is preferable to measurement of serum amylase activity as a test for acute pancreatitis.

2. The serum lipase level is invariably elevated on the first day of acute pancreatitis and remains elevated somewhat longer than the serum amylase level.

3. Differential diagnosis of elevated serum lipase activity is the same as for elevated serum amylase activity, but it does not include macroamylasemia or salivary gland disease.

4. Almost all patients with increased serum lipase activity from nonpancreatic causes of abdominal pain have levels less than three times the upper limit of normal.

E. Serum bilirubin concentration

1. Differential diagnosis of elevated total bilirubin concentration

  a. Fasting (Even in normal individuals, fasting for 24 hours increases total bilirubin by about 0.5 mg/dL.)

  b. Hemolysis

    (1) Most of the increase in bilirubin concentration from hemolysis is in the unconjugated ("direct") fraction.

    (2) Causes of hemolysis include congenital hemolytic anemias (e.g., sickle cell disease), drug-induced red cell destruction, autoimmune diseases, and transfusion reactions.

  c. Extrahepatic biliary tract obstruction (e.g., from tumor or choledocholithiasis)

  d. Uncomplicated acute cholecystitis (total bilirubin concentration rarely exceeds 4 mg/dL)

  e. Congenital disorders

    (1) Gilbert's syndrome

    (2) Crigler-Najjar syndrome (type I or II)

    (3) Dubin-Johnson syndrome

    (4) Rotor syndrome

  f. Intrahepatic cholestasis

    (1) Acute hepatitis (including viral hepatitis and alcoholic hepatitis)

    (2) Multiple organ dysfunction syndrome

    (3) Drug-induced

  g. Severe congestive heart failure

2. With few exceptions (notably hemolysis and certain congenital disorders of bilirubin metabolism), elevations of serum bilirubin concentration are associated with increased levels of direct and indirect fractions.

F. Serum alkaline phosphatase activity level

1. Mild elevations are common with many forms of liver disease.

2. Marked elevation is indicative of extrahepatic (or less commonly intrahepatic) cholestasis.

G. Urinalysis

1. Patients with appendicitis have pyuria in approximately 20% of cases.

2. Hematuria (macroscopic or microscopic) in a spontaneously voided specimen

  a. Suggests a urinary tract source for abdominal pain (e.g., ureterolithiasis)

  b. Caution must be exercised when interpreting a specimen obtained from a menstruating female.

H. Tests for pregnancy

1. When the patient is a female with childbearing potential, a test for pregnancy should be obtained to exclude the possibility of pregnancy or a pregnancy-related disorder (e.g., ruptured ectopic pregnancy).

2. Accurate and sensitive pregnancy tests include radioimmunoassay and enzyme-linked immunoabsorbent assay of serum or urine for the

presence of the beta-subunit of human chorionic gonadotropin (HCG).

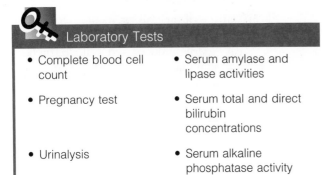

Laboratory Tests

- Complete blood cell count
- Pregnancy test
- Urinalysis

- Serum amylase and lipase activities
- Serum total and direct bilirubin concentrations
- Serum alkaline phosphatase activity level

Imaging Studies

A. Plain abdominal x-rays
1. Upright (if possible) and supine films should be obtained routinely.
2. Free air under the hemi-diaphragms indicates the presence of a perforated viscus (except in patients who have undergone laparotomy within the past few days).
3. Abnormal calcific densities can support the diagnosis of certain conditions, such as appendicitis (appendicolith), gallstone pancreatitis, gallstone ileus, renal or ureteral calculi, or leaking abdominal aneurysm (calcification of dilated aortic wall).
4. Look for the presence of air–fluid levels on the upright film (indicative of bowel obstruction).
5. Presence of gas in the small intestine and colon suggests ileus rather than mechanical obstruction.

B. Chest x-ray
1. Obtain routinely.
2. Pneumonia, particularly involving the basilar segments, can present as upper abdominal pain.
3. Look for the presence of free air.

C. Excretory urogram ("IVP") is indicated when the history, physical examination, and urinalysis support the diagnosis of renal or ureteral colic.

D. Ultrasonography (US)
1. Is most useful for rapid evaluation of the liver, biliary tree, spleen, ovaries and adnexa, and uterus
2. Can be used to diagnose appendicitis, but computed tomography (CT) is a preferable test in most cases.
3. Is the diagnostic imaging procedure of choice when acute cholecystitis is the most probable diagnosis

E. Abdominal CT
1. Is the imaging procedure of choice in most cases of acute abdomen
2. Useful for diagnosing a very long list of conditions, ranging from appendicitis to leaking abdominal aortic aneurysm
3. Computed tomography should be performed with both enteral and IV contrast.

F. Arteriography
1. Is rarely indicated
2. May be useful to establish or exclude mesenteric vascular occlusion due to embolization or thrombosis
3. May be useful for both diagnosis and therapy of very unusual conditions (e.g., ruptured intrahepatic arterial aneurysm)

Key Imaging Studies

- Plain abdominal x-rays (routinely obtained)
- Chest x-ray (routinely obtained)
- Excretory urogram (if renal or ureteral colic is suspected)
- Ultrasonography (study of choice for suspected acute cholecystitis)
- Abdominal computed tomography (study of choice in most cases)
- Arteriography (rarely indicated)

Electrocardiogram

A. Should be obtained routinely
B. Inferior acute myocardial infarction can present as epigastric pain.

Differential Diagnosis

A. Peritonitis
1. Spontaneous bacterial peritonitis in adults occurs predominantly in patients with ascites secondary to cirrhosis.
2. Secondary peritonitis occurs after perforation of hollow viscus, leading to chemical irritation of the peritoneum and microbial contamination.

B. Perforated peptic ulcer
1. Sudden onset of epigastric pain is the typical history.
2. Guarding and rebound tenderness are usually present.
3. Most patients have free intraperitoneal air that is detectable on plain films.

C. Acute cholecystitis

1. Most patients complain of dull right upper quadrant pain, sometimes with radiation to the back or right shoulder.

2. Low-grade fever is commonly present (temperature higher than 39°C suggests cholangitis).

3. Right upper quadrant tenderness is present on physical examination.

4. Laboratory evaluation shows leukocytosis and mildly elevated bilirubin concentration. Commonly, serum amylase activity is also mildly elevated.

5. Both abdominal US and CT can establish the diagnosis.

D. Acute pancreatitis

1. Severe epigastric pain with radiation to the back is the common presentation.

2. Past history is commonly significant for ethanol abuse or biliary tract disease.

3. In severe cases associated with retroperitoneal hemorrhage, the patient may present with Grey Turner's sign (flank ecchymosis) or Cullen's sign (discoloration of the periumbilical skin).

4. Most patients look acutely ill and manifest marked abdominal tenderness; signs of dehydration, and even hypotension, may be present.

5. Laboratory evaluation

a. Leukocytosis and, as the disease progresses leading to sequestration of "third-space" fluids, hemoconcentration

b. Serum lipase and amylase levels are increased.

c. Serum bilirubin concentration may be elevated as well (either as a result of concomitant biliary tract pathology or as a result of nonspecific spasm of the sphincter of Oddi).

6. Computed tomography is commonly diagnostic, showing pancreatic edema with or without intrapancreatic or peripancreatic fluid collections and other findings indicative of intraperitoneal inflammation.

E. Acute appendicitis

1. Most commonly, abdominal pain begins in the epigastrium and migrates to the right lower quadrant.

2. Physical examination typically reveals tenderness, rebound (or percussion) tenderness, and guarding in the right lower quadrant of the abdomen.

3. Laboratory findings are variable.

a. If leukocytosis is present, the total WBC count is rarely higher than 15,000 cells/μL.

b. Urinalysis sometimes reveals pyuria, presumably because of inflammation in the ureter or the bladder, caused by contact with the inflamed appendix.

4. Although both US and CT can be diagnostic, the latter test is probably somewhat more accurate.

F. Meckel's diverticulitis

1. Signs and symptoms are similar to those observed in acute appendicitis.

2. Diagnosis is usually made at the time of operation.

G. Acute (colonic) diverticulitis

1. The most common presentation is left lower quadrant abdominal pain; vomiting is uncommon.

2. Physical examination

a. Fever

b. Left (or, rarely, even right) lower quadrant abdominal tenderness

c. A left lower quadrant mass is often palpable.

3. Laboratory evaluation reveals leukocytosis with a left shift.

4. Abdominal CT often confirms the presence of an inflammatory mass in the left lower quadrant, although differentiating diverticulitis from perforated colonic carcinoma may be impossible.

H. Mechanical small bowel obstruction

1. The typical presentation is intense, but intermittent, bouts of abdominal pain; vomiting is common, and vomiting sometimes provides transient relief from symptoms.

2. Physical examination

a. Abdominal distention

b. Scars from prior intra-abdominal procedures are often present.

c. A careful search should be made for evidence of an incarcerated (inguinal, umbilical, incisional) hernia.

d. High-pitched bowel sounds, caused by peristalsis of acutely distended fluid-filled and air-filled segments of bowel, usually are audible when the abdomen is auscultated.

e. Tenderness is not a prominent feature unless bowel obstruction has proceeded to intestinal strangulation, and hence, peritonitis.

3. Laboratory evaluation

a. Typically reveals hemoconcentration and leukocytosis

b. The serum amylase level may be moderately elevated.

4. Plain x-rays

   a. Reveal dilated segments of intestine (unless the site of obstruction is very proximal) and multiple air-fluid levels

   b. Often, plain flat and upright x-rays of the abdomen and a chest x-ray are the only imaging studies necessary or warranted prior to taking the patient for operative intervention.

5. If plain films are nondiagnostic or there is a suspicion of a colonic process as the source of the obstructive pattern, then additional imaging studies may be needed; options include barium enema and abdominal CT.

6. Differentiating paralytic ileus from mechanical obstruction can be difficult; absence of bowel sounds supports the diagnosis of ileus unless the mechanical obstruction has progressed to the point of bowel infarction and peritonitis.

I. Mechanical large intestinal obstruction

1. Compared to small intestinal obstruction, pain due to colonic obstruction is less severe and occurs later in the process.

2. A recent change in bowel habits can suggest carcinoma of the colon as the source of obstruction.

3. Vomiting, if it occurs at all, occurs late and is feculent in character.

4. Often the patient does not appear to be as sick as many patients with small bowel obstruction.

5. Although abdominal distention is present, tenderness is usually absent, unless obstruction co-exists with perforation.

6. Laboratory evaluation can reveal findings similar to those of small bowel obstruction, or can yield entirely normal results.

7. Abdominal x-rays

   a. Show dilatation of the colon to the point of obstruction

   b. As cecal dilation progresses and leads to incompetence of the ileocecal valve, distended ileal segments can be appreciated, a finding that persists later in the course of the process.

   c. When obstruction is due to sigmoid volvulus, plain x-rays can reveal a characteristic pattern.

8. A barium or water-soluble contrast enema is often diagnostic.

9. Sigmoidoscopy or colonoscopy sometimes reveals an obstructing carcinoma or a point of obstruction due to volvulus; by relieving the torsion of the bowel, sigmoidoscopy is sometimes also therapeutic in cases of volvulus.

10. Fecal impaction

    a. Is sometimes the cause of large intestinal obstruction

    b. Most patients are elderly, and have a history of chronic constipation.

    c. Rectal examination is diagnostic; disimpaction is therapeutic.

11. Pseudo-obstruction of the colon (Ogilvie's syndrome) generally occurs in elderly patients with other serious medical conditions; marked abdominal distention is a prominent feature.

J. Rapid expansion or contained rupture of abdominal aortic aneurysm

1. Presentation is back and abdominal pain, sometimes of several days duration.

2. If the patient is hemodynamically unstable, the diagnosis of ruptured abdominal aortic aneurysm may be obvious, and no time should be wasted obtaining further diagnostic studies.

3. Physical examination often reveals a tender, pulsatile abdominal mass.

4. Plain x-rays of the abdomen may demonstrate the calcified border of the aneurysm.

5. Ultrasound is usually diagnostic, although in very obese patients, CT is probably the imaging study of choice.

K. Acute gynecological conditions presenting with abdominal pain

1. Acute salpingitis

   a. A menstruating, sexually active woman

   b. Suprapubic pain with radiation to the right and left lower quadrants

   c. Right and left lower quadrant tenderness and rebound tenderness

   d. Movement of the cervix causes severe pain.

   e. Smear and culture of cervical discharge is often diagnostic.

   f. Ultrasound should be obtained to exclude hydrosalpinx or tubo-ovarian abscess.

2. Acute torsion or rupture of an ovarian tumor

   a. Sudden ipsilateral lower quadrant pain

   b. Signs of generalized peritonitis (due to hemoperitoneum)

   c. Palpable mass on pelvic examination

   d. Ultrasound is the initial imaging study of choice.

3. Ruptured ectopic pregnancy

a. Acute lower abdominal pain

b. Signs of generalized peritonitis (secondary to hemoperitoneum)

c. Pelvic examination may reveal blood in the vagina or cervical os.

d. An adnexal mass may be present.

e. Positive HCG test

f. Ultrasound is the imaging study of choice.

L. Acute abdominal pain in patients with acquired immunodeficiency syndrome

1. Differential diagnosis includes gastrointestinal mucosal infection and hepatosplenomegaly, among many other causes.

2. Physical examination typically reveals generalized tenderness in the absence of signs of peritonitis.

3. Computed tomography is the imaging procedure of choice.

Bibliography

Martin RF, Flynn P. The acute abdomen in the critically ill patient. Surg Clin North Am 1997;77(6):1455–1464.

Merrell RC. The abdomen as source of sepsis in critically ill patients. Crit Care Clin 1995;11(2):255–272.

Roy S, Weimersheimer P. Nonoperative causes of abdominal pain. Surg Clin North Am 1997;77(6):1433–1454.

Urban BA, Fishman EK. Targeted helical CT of the acute abdomen: appendicitis, diverticulitis, and small bowel obstruction. Semin Ultrasound, CT, MR 2000;21:20–39.

125 Acute Pancreatitis

Mitchell P. Fink

Definitions

A. Acute pancreatitis: an acute inflammatory process that involves the pancreas and may involve other nearby or remote tissues and organs

B. Pancreatic necrosis: focal or diffuse areas of nonviable pancreatic parenchyma and peripancreatic fat characterized by failure to enhance like normal pancreatic tissue when visualized using dynamic IV contrast-enhanced computed tomography (CT)

C. Pancreatic pseudocyst: fluid collection enclosed by fibrous or organizing inflammatory tissue
    1. Contains high concentrations of pancreatic enzymes
    2. Sterile collection

D. Pancreatic abscess: collection of pus within or near the pancreas and associated with acute pancreatitis

Key Risk Factors

- Gallstones (30% to 70% of cases)

- Alcohol abuse (~30% of cases)

- Hypertriglyceridemia (~4% of cases)

- Hyperparathyroidism or (rarely) other causes of hypercalcemia (<1% of cases)

- Drugs, including sulfonamides, furosemide, and azathioprine

- Instrumentation of the sphincter of Oddi (i.e., endoscopic retrograde cholangiopancreatography—ERCP)

- Infections

- Surgery (i.e., postoperative pancreatitis)

- Trauma

- Idiopathic (many cases of "idiopathic" pancreatitis may be related to small gallstones or a poorly documented history of ethanol abuse)

- Hereditary risk

Clinical Findings

A. Symptoms
    1. Pain
        a. Moderate to very severe
        b. Epigastric or upper abdominal in location, often with radiation to the back
    2. Vomiting

B. Physical examination
    1. Abnormal vital signs (low-grade to moderate hyperthermia, tachycardia, tachypnea, and, after the development of hypovolemia, hypotension)
    2. Jaundice is sometimes present when pancreatitis is caused by partial or complete occlusion of the sphincter of Oddi by gallstone(s).
    3. Upper abdominal tenderness
    4. Signs of peritoneal irritation: guarding and rebound (or percussion) tenderness
    5. Later in the course of the disease, there may be signs of extravasation of blood and fluid into retroperitoneal tissues.
        a. Grey Turner's sign (ecchymoses involving the flanks)
        b. Cullen's sign (periumbilical ecchymoses)

Laboratory Tests

A. Serum amylase activity
    1. Elevated early in the course of most cases of pancreatitis, but may be normal when hypertriglyceridemia is the predisposing factor or in patients with an acute exacerbation of chronic (alcoholic) pancreatitis
    2. Hyperamylasemia can be associated with many other conditions in addition to pancreatitis; i.e., this finding lacks specificity.

B. Serum lipase activity is a better test than serum amylase activity for acute pancreatitis.
    1. Sensitivity is similar to serum amylase activity.
    2. Hyperlipasemia is a relatively specific indicator of acute pancreatitis.
    3. The only important causes of hyperlipasemia other than acute pancreatitis are renal failure and perforation or acute inflammation of the intestine.

C. Leukocytosis with left shift

D. Hemoconcentration and azotemia (secondary to sequestration of "third space" fluid) are often present in advanced cases of severe pancreatitis.

E. Hypocalcemia

Imaging Studies

A. Plain x-rays of the abdomen

1. Findings are nonspecific

2. Localized ileus of segments of small intestine ("sentinel loop")

3. Dilation of ascending colon with abrupt narrowing in the transverse colon ("colon cutoff sign")

4. Calcified gallstones

5. Calcified pancreatic stones

B. Chest x-ray

1. Findings are nonspecific

2. Pleural effusion (left-side only or bilateral)

3. Diffuse pulmonary infiltrates consistent with acute respiratory distress syndrome (ARDS) may be present in some cases

C. Abdominal ultrasonography

1. Should be performed as part of the initial evaluation

2. Useful to detect gallstones, determine caliber of the common bile duct, and diagnose presence of ascites

D. Abdominal CT

1. Important diagnostic study that should be obtained routinely in cases of proven or suspected acute pancreatitis

2. Useful to rule out other conditions that can present with findings similar to those of acute pancreatitis, but, unlike acute pancreatitis, mandate early operative intervention

3. Images should be obtained after administration of an oral contrast agent.

4. Intravenous contrast agent should be administered rapidly by pump during the acquisition of images ("dynamic contrast-enhanced CT").

5. The severity of pancreatitis can be assessed based on the findings observed on CT, using the scoring system proposed by Balthazar and Ranson (Table 125–1).

6. Additional information regarding the severity of pancreatitis can be assessed based on the extent of necrosis as assessed by dynamic contrast-en-

TABLE 125–1. SYSTEM OF BALTHAZAR AND RANSON FOR GRADING PANCREATITIS BY CT FINDINGS

Grade A:	Normal pancreas
Grade B:	Focal of diffuse enlargement of the pancreas
Grade C:	Mild peripancreatic inflammatory changes
Grade D:	Fluid collection in a single location
Grade E:	Multiple fluid collections or gas within the pancreas or peripancreatic inflammation

TABLE 125–2. RANSON'S SIGNS OF A GRAVE PROGNOSIS IN ACUTE PANCREATITIS

- Signs that can be assessed at the time of admission
  - Age >55 years
  - White blood cell count >16,000 cells/μL
  - Serum glucose concentration >200 mg/dL
  - Serum lactate dehydrogenase activity >350 U/L
  - Serum aspartate aminotransferase activity >250 U/L
- Signs that can be assessed after 48 hours of therapy
  - Decrease in absolute hematocrit >10%
  - Increase in serum urea nitrogen concentration >5 mg/dL
  - Serum calcium concentration <8 mg/dL
  - PaO_2 <60 mm Hg
  - Base deficit >4 mEq/L
  - Positive fluid balance >6 L

hanced CT (<33% of the gland nonviable, 33% to 50% of the gland nonviable, >50% of the gland nonviable).

Differential Diagnosis

A. Acute pancreatitis is in the differential diagnosis for most causes of acute upper abdominal pain.

B. Conversely, at least some of the features of acute pancreatitis can be mimicked by many causes of acute upper abdominal pain, including

1. Acute cholecystitis

2. Perforated peptic ulcer

3. Rapidly expanding or leaking abdominal aortic aneurysm

4. Mesenteric vascular catastrophe

5. Inferior wall acute myocardial infarction

Prognosis

A. It is important to make an early and reliable assessment of the severity of acute pancreatitis to ensure that patients are appropriately resuscitated and cared for in the proper environment (i.e., intensive care unit [ICU] versus ward).

B. The most widely employed scoring system for severity of illness in acute pancreatitis is the one devised by Ranson and colleagues (Table 125–2).

1. Patients with fewer than three of Ranson's signs have mild pancreatitis, and the risk of mortality is low.

2. Patients with more than six of Ranson's signs have very severe pancreatitis, and the risk of serious complications (e.g., ARDS or sepsis) and death is high (predicted mortality >60%).

C. Other ICU outcome prediction systems (e.g., APACHE II, APACHE III, or SAPS) may be as effective as, or even more predictive than, Ranson's signs for predicting outcome in patients with acute pancreatitis.

Management of Severe Acute Pancreatitis

A. Multidisciplinary approach

   1. Intensivist

   2. Surgeon

   3. Gastroenterologist

B. Fluid resuscitation guided by appropriate invasive hemodynamic monitoring and measurements of urine output

C. Mechanical ventilation as indicated by standard criteria

D. Endoscopic retrograde cholangiopancreatography (ERCP) to remove stones from the common bile duct should be performed within the first 2 to 3 days of hospitalization in cases of acute gallstone-induced pancreatitis associated with biliary sepsis or dysfunction.

E. Infection

   1. In cases of very severe pancreatitis (>50% necrosis by CT plus evidence of remote organ dysfunction), the risk of pancreatic infection is high (20% to 50% of cases).

   2. Accordingly, many authorities recommend providing prophylaxis against pancreatic infection by systemically administering an antibiotic that penetrates effectively into pancreatic tissue and provides good coverage against enteric Gram-negative bacilli (e.g., imipenem, meropenem, ciprofloxacin, ofloxacin, or levofloxacin).

   3. Pancreatic infection can be diagnosed by performing percutaneous aspiration of the inflammatory retroperitoneal mass under CT guidance.

   4. When infection is confirmed by culture or Gram's stain, then appropriate antibacterial (and, possibly, antifungal) chemotherapy should be instituted if the patient is not already receiving it.

F. Nutrition

   1. Total parenteral nutrition (TPN) should be used for nutritional support during the acute phase of the illness.

      a. Monitor serum triglyceride levels.

      b. If the serum triglyceride concentration is greater than 500 mg/dL, do not administer lipids.

   2. Enteral nutrition should be reinstituted when ileus resolves; i.e., it is unnecessary to wait for normalization of serum amylase or lipase concentration or resolution of all CT findings of pancreatic inflammation.

G. Other supportive measures

   1. Treat pain with meperidine.

   2. H_2-receptor antagonist, sucralfate, or antacids for prophylaxis against erosive gastritis for patients requiring mechanical ventilation

   3. Control hyperglycemia with IV insulin.

   4. Correct derangements in serum electrolyte concentrations, including magnesium and ionized calcium.

H. Surgical debridement

   1. Only indicated for patients with extensive pancreatic necrosis complicated by pancreatic infection

   2. The proper timing of surgical intervention is controversial, but ongoing distant organ system

Key Management of Severe Acute Pancreatitis

- Fluid resuscitation should be guided by appropriate invasive hemodynamic monitoring and measurements of urine output.

- In cases of acute gallstone-induced pancreatitis associated with biliary sepsis or dysfunction, ERCP to remove stones from the common bile duct should be performed within the first 2 to 3 days of hospitalization.

- Many authorities recommend providing prophylaxis against pancreatic infection using an IV antibiotic that effectively penetrates into pancreatic tissue and provides good coverage against enteric Gram-negative bacilli (use imipenem, meropenem, ciprofloxacin, ofloxacin, or levofloxacin).

- Pancreatic infection can be diagnosed by performing percutaneous aspiration of the inflammatory retroperitoneal mass under CT guidance; when infection is confirmed by culture or Gram's stain, then appropriate antibacterial (and, possibly, antifungal) chemotherapy should be instituted if the patient is not already receiving it.

- Total parenteral nutrition should be used for nutritional support during the acute phase.

- Enteral nutrition should be reinstituted when ileus resolves; i.e., it is unnecessary to wait for normalization of serum amylase or lipase activities or resolution of all CT findings of pancreatic inflammation.

- Surgical debridement is indicated only for patients with extensive pancreatic necrosis complicated by pancreatic infection.

dysfunction despite aggressive medical management of confirmed pancreatic infection should prompt operation to remove necrotic and infected tissue.

3. After surgical debridement of nonviable tissue, some centers advocate packing the abdomen open to facilitate repetitive debridement (either at the bedside in the ICU or in the operating room).

4. Other centers close the abdomen (with or without leaving closed suction drains in place) and take the patient back to the operating room as needed for further debridement.

5. Still other centers close the abdomen but leave drains in place for continuous or intermittent peritoneal lavage.

I. Ineffective therapeutic approaches

1. Pharmacological measures to decrease secretion of enzymes by the pancreas (e.g., treatment with octreotide or H_2-receptor antagonists) have not been shown to improve outcome.

2. Although widely used, there is no evidence that nasogastric suction improves outcome; however, it may provide some symptomatic relief for nausea and decrease the risk of aspiration.

3. Treatment with protease inhibitors (aprotinin or gabexate mesilate) has not been shown to improve outcome.

4. Continuous peritoneal lavage is ineffective.

5. Treatment with a platelet activating factor antagonist failed to improve outcome.

Bibliography

Balthazar EJ, Robinson DL, Megibow AJ, et al. Acute pancreatitis: Value of CT in establishing prognosis. Radiology 1990;174:331–336.

Bassi C, Falconi M, Talamini G, et al. Controlled clinical trial of pefloxacin versus imipenem in severe acute pancreatitis. Gastroenterology 1998;115:1513–1517.

Ho HS, Frey CF. The role of antibiotic prophylaxis in severe acute pancreatitis. Arch Surg 1997;132:487–492.

Pederzoli P, Bassi C, Vesentini S, et al. A randomized multicenter clinical trial of antibiotic prophylaxis of septic complications in acute necrotizing pancreatitis with imipenem. Surg Gynecol Obstet 1993;176:480–483.

Ranson JH, Rifkind KM, Roses DF, et al. Prognostic signs and the role of operative management in acute pancreatitis. Surg Gynecol Obstet 1974;139:69–81.

Sarr MG, Sanfey H, Cameron JL. Prospective, randomized trial of nasogastric suction in patients with acute pancreatitis. Surgery 1986;100:500–504.

Simchuk EJ, Traverso LW, Nukui Y, et al. Computed tomography severity index is a predictor of outcomes for severe pancreatitis. Am J Surg 2000;179:352–355.

Uhl W, Buchler MW, Malfertheiner P, et al. A randomised, double blind, multicentre trial of octreotide in moderate to severe acute pancreatitis. Gut 1999;45:97–104.

126 Acute Cholecystitis

Mitchell P. Fink

The vast majority of cases of acute cholecystitis are caused by obstruction of the cystic duct by a gallstone. Most cases of acute calculous cholecystitis either resolve spontaneously or resolve after surgical or medical interventions (cholecystectomy, antibiotics, and intravenous fluids). Acute acalculous cholecystitis is often a more severe form of the disease, and it frequently progresses to necrosis of the gallbladder wall or empyema of the gallbladder. It typically occurs in patients who are already critically ill as a result of another serious medical problem (e.g., pneumonia) or other conditions, such as major trauma, burn injury, or extensive surgery. The pathophysiology underlying the development of acute acalculous cholecystitis is not completely understood, but ischemia and stasis of bile within the gallbladder have been implicated as important causative factors. Stasis of bile in the gallbladder is common in critically ill patients, particularly those not receiving enteral nutrition. Stasis can foster colonization of bile within the lumen of the gallbladder by bacteria. Gallbladder ischemia may be caused by microcirculatory derangements that are thought to be a characteristic of certain critical illnesses (e.g., sepsis) or a more global decrease in hepatosplanchnic perfusion that is thought to occur when cardiac output is compromised.

PEARL

Acute acalculous cholecystitis accounts for 5% to 10% of cases of acute cholecystitis.

Clinical Findings

A. Symptoms
   1. Right upper quadrant abdominal pain
   2. Nausea and vomiting

B. Signs
   1. Fever
   2. Right upper quadrant abdominal tenderness and guarding
   3. A palpable right upper quadrant mass may be present.
   4. Murphy's sign (inspiration during deep palpation of the right upper quadrant elicits pain)

Key Laboratory Findings

- Leukocytosis
- Mild hyperbilirubinemia (serum total bilirubin concentration <4 mg/dL) is common.
- Mildly elevated circulating levels of alkaline phosphatase or amylase are sometimes present.

Diagnostic Imaging

A. Ultrasonography
   1. The most useful diagnostic test; should be the first diagnostic study ordered in most cases of suspected calculous or acalculous cholecystitis
   2. A sensitive and specific means for establishing the presence or absence of cholelithiasis
   3. Findings indicative of acute cholecystitis include
      a. Thickened gallbladder wall (>4 mm)
      b. Pericholecystic fluid

B. Technetium 99m-hepato-iminodiacetic acid (HIDA) radionuclide scan
   1. In patients without critical illness, non-filling of the gallbladder indicates obstruction of the cystic duct by a gallstone and strongly supports the diagnosis of acute calculous cholecystitis.
   2. In patients with critical illness, however, absence of gallbladder filling by HIDA scan may simply reflect stasis of bile and cannot be relied upon as a sign of cystic duct obstruction.

C. Computed tomography (CT)
   1. Used primarily for the evaluation of critically ill patients when calculous or acalculous cholecystitis is part of the differential diagnosis for unexplained fever in the presence of abdominal pain, tenderness, mass, or distention.
   2. Findings indicative of acute cholecystitis are the same as those with ultrasound, namely
      a. Thickened gallbladder wall
      b. Pericholecystic fluid

Treatment

A. Acute calculous cholecystitis
   1. Supportive medical care

a. Nothing by mouth and IV fluids

b. Analgesia (preferably a nonsteroid anti-inflammatory agent rather than a narcotic)

c. Antibiotics (e.g., ampicillin-sulbactam, piperacillin-tazobactam, or a fluoroquinolone + metronidazole) active against the most common biliary tract pathogens (*Escherichia coli, Enterococcus, Klebsiella, Clostridia*)

2. Cholecystectomy

a. Most can be successfully performed laparoscopically.

b. Rate of conversion to open cholecystectomy is higher for acute intervention than for elective operation.

c. Most patients should undergo operation early in the course of their illness.

B. Acute acalculous cholecystitis (or acute calculous cholecystitis in patients with major comorbid conditions)

1. Supportive care as described above

2. Surgical management options

a. Cholecystectomy (laparoscopic or open)

b. Percutaneous transhepatic cholecystostomy (under CT guidance)

Complications

A. Empyema of the gallbladder (pus-filled gallbladder)

1. Caused by bacterial proliferation behind an obstructed cystic duct

2. Patients can present with symptoms and signs of sepsis or septic shock.

B. Emphysematous cholecystitis (gas within the gallbladder wall or lumen)

1. Caused by proliferation of gas-forming bacteria

2. More common in men and in diabetics

C. Perforation

1. Caused by ischemic necrosis of the gallbladder wall

2. Usually leads to local abscess formation or formation of a fistula between the gallbladder and another hollow viscus (e.g., duodenum or colon)

3. Occasionally free perforation leads to generalized peritonitis.

Bibliography

Boggi U, Di Candio G, Campatelli A, et al. Percutaneous cholecystostomy for acute cholecystitis in critically ill patients. Hepato-Gastroenterol 1999;46:121–125.

Lilliemoe KD. Surgical treatment of biliary tract infections. Am Surg 2000;66:138–144.

Prevot N, Mariat G, Mahul P, et al. Contribution of cholescintigraphy to the early diagnosis of acute acalculous cholecystitis in intensive-care-unit patients. Eur J Nucl Med 1999;26:1317–1325.

Westphal JF, Brogard JM. Biliary tract infections: a guide to drug treatment. Drugs 1999;57:81–91.

127 Acute Alcoholic Hepatitis

David J. Kramer

Alcohol abuse, usually defined as a pattern of alcohol consumption that leads to dysfunctional social interactions, affects 7% of the U.S. population. Acute ethanol intoxication injures hepatocytes, leading to inflammation and necrosis. Steatosis can develop after acute injury. Susceptibility to the injurious effects of ethanol differs among individuals, and only about 15% of heavy alcohol users develop cirrhosis. Several factors predispose patients to the hepatotoxic effects of alcohol. Cirrhosis is more likely in women than men. The threshold daily dose of ethanol for the development of cirrhosis is approximately 20 g for women and 60 g for men. Cirrhosis is also more likely to develop in people with poor nutrition. Coexisting hepatic injury, such as hepatitis C infection, renders the liver much more susceptible to the toxic effects of alcohol.

The mechanisms responsible for alcohol-induced hepatic injury are not yet fully elucidated. Lipopolysaccharide, presumably derived from Gram-negative bacteria in the gut, seems to be an important factor. Plasma LPS levels increase following acute ingestion of alcohol and correlate with the severity of liver injury. In animal models, pharmacological agents that neutralize the effects of LPS ameliorate hepatic injury. Circulating concentrations of proinflammatory cytokines (e.g., tumor necrosis factor and interleukin-1, -6, and -8) are elevated in patients with alcoholic hepatitis.

Clinical Findings

A. History
1. Patients may not provide a reliable estimate of alcohol use.
2. Often it is difficult to elicit a history of increased ethanol consumption; a change in the pattern of alcohol consumption is probably typical.
3. Anorexia accompanies alcohol use as nonprotein calories are provided, and alcohol may be used for self-treatment of depression or may accompany eating disorders.
4. Weight loss is sometimes masked by salt and water retention as patients develop features of chronic liver disease, such as ascites and edema.
5. Malaise is nearly a universal finding, but it may be difficult to distinguish from the symptoms of depression.

B. Physical examination
1. Patients may present with signs typically associated with chronic liver disease.
   a. Feminization
   b. Parotid enlargement
   c. Palmar erythema
   d. Dupuytren's contracture
   e. Jaundice
   f. Hepatomegaly
   g. Right upper quadrant abdominal tenderness
2. Less commonly (and usually only after significant fibrosis or frank cirrhosis has developed), patients have spider angiomata.

> **PEARL**
>
> Severity of alcoholic hepatitis is related to the extent of the toxic injury and the presence of pre-existing liver disease, such as concurrent hepatitis C infection.

Laboratory Findings

A. No particular set of laboratory findings uniquely characterizes acute alcoholic hepatitis.
B. The complete blood cell count (CBC) is often abnormal.
1. Anemia with macrocytic indices is typical.
2. Thrombocytopenia (secondary to bone marrow depression)
3. Leukopenia (secondary to bone marrow depression)
4. Rebound leukocytosis with left shift is sometimes observed when patients have been abstinent for one week.
5. Hypersegmentation of polymorphonuclear leukocytes is absent unless vitamin B_{12} deficiency is a concurrent problem.
C. Patients are rarely iron deficient unless significant bleeding has occurred; because alcohol increases iron absorption by the intestine secondary hemochromatosis is a possibility.
D. Electrolyte abnormalities
1. Hypomagnesemia, hypophosphatemia, and hypokalemia are common.
2. Electrolyte abnormalities can be temporarily obscured if the patient is severely dehydrated or

acidemic, but they can manifest later, after resuscitation.

3. Patients who have recently discontinued alcohol use may present with acidemia and ketosis related to alcoholic ketoacidosis.

E. Liver function tests are of limited value in determining the extent of injury and the prognosis.

1. Serum aspartate aminotransferase activity is increased and is usually greater than the serum alanine aminotransferase activity; this pattern is uncommon with nonalcoholic hepatitis.

2. Direct hyperbilirubinemia develops in many patients.

3. Circulating γ-glutamyl transpeptidase activity is typically elevated to a greater extent than alkaline phosphatase activity.

4. Hypoalbuminemia

5. Prolongation of prothrombin time (PT) occurs before prolongation of partial thromboplastin and bleeding times becomes apparent.

Treatment

A. Abstinence from alcohol is essential.

B. Fluid and blood products for active bleeding

1. Fluid resuscitation

2. Transfusion of fresh frozen plasma or cryoprecipitate to treat coagulopathy

3. Transfusion of platelets to treat thrombocytopenia

4. Transfusion of packed red blood cells to treat anemia

5. Rarely, ε-aminocaproic acid may be used judiciously if fibrinolysis is a dominant cause of bleeding.

6. Elevated central venous pressure may cause ongoing variceal hemorrhage; avoid over-resuscitation with fluid and treat refractory hypotension secondary to vasodilation with norepinephrine.

C. Maintain euglycemia; perform capillary glucose determinations every 2 hours during the acute phase.

D. Support for failing organs

1. Endotracheal intubation and mechanical ventilation to prevent aspiration (from coma and failure to protect the airway) and support gas exchange in the setting of respiratory failure

2. Renal replacement therapy as indicated for treatment of refractory hyperkalemia, uremia, or volume overload from acute renal insufficiency

E. Control infection.

1. Exclude active infection.

2. Obtain surveillance cultures (blood, urine, ascites, sputum).

3. Establish a low threshold for instituting antimicrobial chemotherapy.

F. Corticosteroids

1. May benefit selected patients with acute alcoholic hepatitis who are not infected

2. Shown to reduce mortality by 50% at one month in patients with a discriminant function value higher than 32 (see below)

3. Methylprednisolone: 32 mg/day in divided doses

G. Nutritional support should be provided.

H. Monitor for electrolyte imbalances.

1. Particularly likely to occur during refeeding

2. Can provoke malignant ventricular arrhythmias

I. Orthotopic liver transplantation

1. Use of this therapeutic option is controversial for patients with acute alcoholic decompensation due to active (ongoing) ethanol abuse.

2. Compared to abstinent patients, results for patients with acute alcoholic liver decompensation are poorer in both the immediate postoperative period and over the long term.

3. Recidivism and noncompliance are much greater concerns in the latter group, particularly for those in hepatic coma at the time the decision is made for transplantation.

4. Abstinence is required for 6 months by most transplant programs.

5. Exceptions are entertained when the predicted survival is much shorter than 6 months and abstinence after transplant seems probable.

J. Investigational agents (role, if any, not defined)

1. Propylthiouracil

2. D-penicillamine

3. Colchicine

4. Pentoxifylline

Key Treatment

- Routine supportive measures include intravascular volume expansion, correction of electrolyte abnormalities, maintenance of euglycemia, and early detection and treatment of infection.

- Patients often require support for multiple failing organ system functions until hepatic function returns.

Prognosis

A. Mortality depends on the severity of the underlying liver disease and malnutrition, and the extent of extrahepatic organ dysfunction.

B. In most cases, recovery from multisystem organ failure depends on recovery of adequate liver function.

C. Mortality can be predicted by a discriminant function based on prothrombin time and the serum total bilirubin measurement (see box).

1. Mortality exceeds 50% when the discriminant function result is higher than 32

Key Prognostic Evaluation

Mortality risk exceeds 50% when the following discriminant function (DF) solves to higher than 32

$$DF = 4.6 \times (PT_{pt} - PT_{ctl}) + Bili$$

where PT_{pt} is the patient's prothrombin time (in seconds), PT_{ctl} is the laboratory's control prothrombin time (in seconds), and $Bili$ is the serum total bilirubin concentration (mg/dL).

2. Discrimination is too crude to dictate withdrawal of life support.

D. Cirrhosis develops in 10% of patients per year after an index episode of acute alcoholic hepatitis.

1. Overall, 70% of patients can be expected to develop cirrhosis.

2. Cirrhosis is more likely to develop in women and in patients with more severe histopathologic abnormalities.

Bibliography

Abittan CS, Lieber CS. Alcoholic liver disease. Curr Treat Options Gastroenterol 1999;2:72–80.

Carithers RL Jr, Herlong HF, Diehl AM, et al. Methylprednisolone therapy in patients with severe alcoholic hepatitis. A randomized multicenter trial. Ann Intern Med 1989;110:685–690.

Conjeevaram HS, Hart J, Lissoos TW, et al. Rapidly progressive liver injury and fatal alcoholic hepatitis occurring after liver transplantation in alcoholic patients. Transplantation 1999;67:1562–1568.

Ramond MJ, Poynard T, Rueff B, et al. A randomized trial of prednisolone in patients with severe alcoholic hepatitis. N Engl J Med 1992;326:507–512.

Taieb J, Mathurin P, Elbim C, et al. Blood neutrophil functions and cytokine release in severe alcoholic hepatitis: effect of corticosteroids. J Hepatol 2000;32:579–586.

128 Viral Hepatitis

David J. Kramer

Viral hepatitis infections caused by hepatitis A virus (HAV), hepatitis B virus (HBV) and hepatitis C virus (HCV) are a major public health concern in the United States. The intensivist is called upon to care for patients with acute viral hepatitis, particularly when fulminant hepatic failure (FHF) develops. This is a feared complication that occurs in approximately 1% of patients with HBV. In countries with a high standard of living, childhood infection with HAV is relatively uncommon. Consequently, adults are infected primarily and often have a much more severe course. Fulminant hepatic failure is much more lethal in patients older than 40 years of age. Hepatitis C is not an important cause of FHF. The intensivist should also be aware of recommendations for post-exposure prophylaxis, which may be necessary in health care workers who sustain contaminated needle injury.

Epidemiology

A. Nearly 500,000 patients are infected annually.

B. Chronic liver disease accounts for more than 25,000 deaths annually and is the tenth leading cause of death.

C. The Centers for Disease Control and Prevention (CDC) estimates that 5% of the U.S. population will be infected with HBV during their lifetime.

D. Although the CDC estimates that the incidence of HCV is decreasing, from an annual incidence of 230,000 in the 1980s to 36,000 more recently, nearly 1.8% of the population has been infected with HCV.

  1. Approximately 40% of patients with chronic liver disease have HCV.

  2. Because most patients with HCV infections are younger than 50 years of age, the morbidity, mortality, and associated health care costs are expected to increase dramatically in the next decades.

  3. Hepatitis C is already the most common indication for orthotopic liver transplantation in adults.

Clinical Findings

A. Hepatitis A infection

  1. Symptoms develop approximately 30 days after exposure.

  2. Patients are infectious during the 2 weeks preceding the onset of jaundice.

  3. Symptoms

    a. Malaise

    b. Anorexia

    c. Nausea

    d. Abdominal fullness

    e. Distaste for tobacco

  4. Physical examination

    a. Low-grade fever

    b. Icterus

    c. Dehydration

    d. Abdominal tenderness of the liver edge in the right upper quadrant (Murphy's sign is usually absent)

    e. Smokey urine

B. Hepatitis B infection

  1. History of factor(s) that increase the risk of HBV infection

    a. Blood transfusion

    b. Intravenous drug use

    c. Cohabitation with a patient chronically infected with HBV

    d. Sexual intercourse with a patient infected with HBV

    e. Multiple sex partners

    f. Parents born in Southeast Asia, Africa, the Amazon Basin, the Pacific Islands, or the Middle East

    g. Lives or works in an institution for the developmentally disabled

    h. Hemophilia

    i. International travel to areas with a high prevalence of hepatitis B

  2. Patients with HBV develop symptoms approximately 90 days after exposure.

  3. Symptoms

    a. When present, symptoms are similar to those described above for HAV.

    b. Approximately 10% to 20% of patients with HBV are asymptomatic.

C. Hepatitis C infection

  1. History

    a. If symptoms develop, patients typically

present approximately 60 days after exposure.

   b. Many patients have no symptoms.

2. Risk factors for HCV infection

   a. Similar to those for HBV

   b. The question of whether HCV can be transmitted via sexual contact remains controversial.

Key Differential Diagnosis for Acute Hepatitis Versus Acute Cholecystitis

- Fever and leukocytosis are typically higher in acute cholecystitis.

- In acute cholecystitis, total bilirubin concentration is often mildly elevated (<4 mg/dL), and serum transaminase activities are normal or only minimally increased; γ-glutamyl transpeptidase is more elevated.

- Ultrasonographic findings indicative of acute cholecystitis (e.g., thickened gallbladder wall, pericholecystic fluid, gallstones) are useful for establishing this diagnosis.

- Confusion can result when ischemic hepatitis is precipitated by septic shock.

Laboratory Findings

A. Hepatitis A infection

1. Immunoglobulin M (IgM) anti-HAV antibodies develop early, then decrease and disappear during the first year.

2. Immunoglobulin G (IgG) anti-HAV antibodies develop later, but persist for life.

B. Hepatitis B infection

1. Most patients with HBV infection seroconvert, no longer have active HBV replication, and are no longer infectious.

2. Initial infection with HBV is associated with circulating HBV surface antigen (HbsAg).

3. The initial antibody response is production of IgM antibodies directed against the core antigen (HBcAb-IgM).

4. This is followed by a decrease in circulating levels of HBsAg and a time window during which only IgG antibodies against the core antigen (HBcAb-IgG) are present in the circulation; patients are still infectious during this period.

5. Subsequently, IgG antibodies to the surface antigen (HBsAb) develop; once HBsAb is detectable, patients are no longer infectious.

6. Persistent antigenemia

   a. Approximately 10% of patients with HBV have ongoing viral replication and fail to develop HBsAb; these patients are infectious.

   b. Evidence of HBV viral replication is determined by detecting HBV DNA using a polymerase chain reaction assay.

   c. A surrogate marker for HBV replication is the presence of e-antigenemia.

   d. Patients with e-antigen (HBeAg) have active viral replication and are infectious, whereas those with anti-e-antigen antibody (HBeAb) are much less infectious.

   e. Patients with active viral replication at the time of liver transplantation (HBV-DNA and HbeAg positive) are more likely to lose the transplanted organ because of HBV recurrence.

C. Hepatitis C infection

1. Patients with HCV antibodies often (~80%) have active viral replication and must be considered infectious.

2. More than 90% of patients develop IgG anti-HCV antibodies within 6 months.

3. HCV RNA is not detectable in about 20% of patients who are anti-HCV positive but have no transaminase elevation and no inflammation or fibrosis on liver biopsy; these patients presumably are not infectious and are not at risk for chronic sequelae such as cirrhosis and hepatocellular carcinoma.

4. The remaining 80% of patients develop chronic active hepatitis manifested by waxing and waning increases in circulating transaminase levels and varying degrees of clinical symptomatology.

5. Approximately 50% of patients develop cirrhosis, and hepatocellular carcinoma develops in a significant proportion of these patients.

Key Laboratory Findings

- Serum transaminase activity levels are typically elevated to approximately 10 times the upper limit of normal.

- Serum total and direct bilirubin concentrations are increased.

- Serum activity levels of the canalicular enzymes alkaline phosphatase and γ-glutamyl transpeptidase are typically normal or only slightly increased.

- Serological tests may be positive (see text).

Treatment

A. Treatment options for HBV and HCV are rapidly evolving.

B. Most patients with HBV seroconvert and require no active intervention.

C. Treatment should be considered for patients who are at high risk of developing the lethal complication of FHF such as recipients of solid organ transplants and patients with chronic HBV who require chemotherapy.

D. Treatment with lamivudine, a nucleoside analogue reverse transcriptase inhibitor, is efficacious.

1. Treatment with 100 mg daily for 1 year is associated with suppression of HBV replication and is well tolerated.

2. Hepatitis B resistance may develop on therapy.

E. α-Interferon (5 million U/day or 10 million U three times weekly)

1. Effective in ⅓ of patients in eliminating viral replication

2. Relapse after treatment is common.

3. Side effects

a. Influenza-like symptoms

b. Risk of acute hepatic decompensation in patients with advanced liver disease

F. Prolonged treatment of patients with active hepatitis and bridging fibrosis with interferon and ribaviron is recommended.

1. Unfortunately, relapse is common after treatment is stopped.

2. Side effects of both agents preclude their long-term administration.

Special Consideration (Health Care Worker Exposure)

A. Risk reduction

1. Observe universal precautions; consider all patients as infectious.

2. Follow strict hand-washing precautions.

3. Wear gloves for all contact with surfaces or materials contaminated with bodily secretions.

B. Intensivists should be considered "at-risk" specialists as they are routinely exposed to blood and bodily secretions.

1. In 1994 the CDC reported that more than 1,000 health care workers were infected with HBV.

2. More than 100 health care workers die annually from complications of chronic HBV.

3. Up to 30% of percutaneous injuries from patients with active HBV result in infection of the health care worker.

C. Vaccination against HBV

1. Mandated by OSHA for all health care workers exposed in their occupations to blood, bodily secretions, and vectors of infection such as sharps.

2. Three intramuscular doses of HBV vaccine are required.

3. More than 95% of vaccinees develop protective levels of HBsAb; half of the remainder will mount an adequate response with another course of HBV vaccination.

D. Vaccination against HAV

1. Two HAV vaccines are available for pre-exposure immunization.

2. Vaccination should be considered for the following "at-risk" populations.

a. Men who have sex with men

b. Patients with chronic liver disease

c. Health care workers from areas with low or intermediate prevalence of HAV who are seronegative and who care for patients with acute HAV

E. Vaccination against HCV is not available.

F. Post-exposure prophylaxis

1. Individuals exposed to HAV without prior infection or vaccination benefit from immune globulin (0.02 mL/kg intramuscularly) within 2 weeks of exposure.

2. Unvaccinated health care workers who sustain a needle stick from an HBV-infected patient should be treated with hepatitis B immune globulin.

3. Treatment with immunoglobulin does not appear to affect the post-exposure risk of HCV and is not recommended.

B Bibliography

Advisory Committee on Immunization Practices. Prevention of hepatitis A through active or passive immunization. MMWR Morb Mortal Wkly Rep 1996;45(RR15):1–30.

Andreone P, Caraceni P, Grazi GL, et al. Lamivudine treatment for acute hepatitis B after liver transplantation. J Hepatol 1998;29:985–989.

Centers for Disease Control and Prevention. Recommendations for prevention and control of hepatitis C virus (HCV) infection and HCV-related chronic disease. MMWR Morb Mortal Wkly Rep 1998;47(RR19):1–39.

Dodd RY. Current viral risks of blood and blood products. Ann Med 2000;32:469–474.

Lin OS, Keeffe EB. Current treatment strategies for chronic hepatitis B and C. Annu Rev Med 2001;52:29–49.

Weston SR, Martin P. Serological and molecular testing in viral hepatitis: an update. Can J Gastroenterol 2001;15: 177–184.

Williams R, Riordan SM. Acute liver failure: Established and putative hepatitis viruses and therapeutic implications. J Gastroenterol Hepatol 2000;15(Suppl):G17–G25.

129 Fulminant Hepatic Failure

David J. Kramer

Fulminant hepatic failure (FHF) is defined as acute liver failure that is associated with coagulopathy and encephalopathy and that develops within 8 weeks of onset, in the absence of prior liver disease. It is the onset of encephalopathy or moderate coagulopathy that marks the transition between acute hepatitis or hepatic injury and fulminant hepatic failure.

Etiology

A. Viral
1. Hepatitis A virus (HAV)
2. Hepatitis B virus (HBV)
3. Hepatitis C virus
4. Hepatitis E virus
5. Herpes simplex virus
6. Herpes zoster
7. Epstein-Barr virus
8. Cytomegalovirus
9. Other viruses (e.g., Adenovirus)

B. Drugs and toxins
1. Acetaminophen
2. Carbon tetrachloride
3. Yellow phosphorus
4. Poison mushroom (*Amanita phalloides*) ingestion
5. Sea anenome sting
6. HMG coenzyme-A reductase inhibitors
7. Isoniazid
8. Valproic acid
9. Nortriptyline
10. Gold compounds
11. Halothane
12. Certain herbal medicines (e.g., chaparral, germander)
13. Other rare drug reactions

C. Cardiovascular
1. Hepatic ischemia
2. Circulatory shock
3. Budd-Chiari syndrome
4. Hepatic veno-occlusive disease

D. Miscellaneous causes
1. Autoimmune hepatitis
2. Fatty liver of pregnancy
3. Neoplastic infiltration
4. Nonfunctioning graft post-liver transplant

5. Reye's syndrome
6. Wilson's disease

Pathophysiology of Hepatic Encephalopathy

A. It is a completely reversible metabolic encephalopathy characterized by progressive impairment of cerebration and level of consciousness.
B. Although circulating ammonia concentration is often elevated, ammonia alone is insufficient to explain the clinical findings.
C. High plasma levels of aromatic amino acids represent an epiphenomenon, not the cause of encephalopathy.
D. The density of γ-aminobutyric acid receptors in brain tissue is increased in patients with end-stage liver disease and may explain why hepatic failure patients are extremely sensitive to oversedation with benzodiazepines or barbiturates.

Key Clinical Findings

- Nausea, vomiting
- Malaise, fatigue
- Jaundice
- Encephalopathy, coma
- Manifestations related to complications (see text)

Classification of Hepatic Encephalopathy

A. Grade I
1. Subtle change in character
2. Disorders of the sleep–wake cycle
3. Difficulty performing arithmetic computations such as serial sevens

B. Grade II
1. Frank confusion
2. Inappropriate behavior
3. Asterixis

C. Grade III
1. Obtundation
2. Severe confusion following arousal
3. Asterixis

D. Grade IV (frank coma)
1. Grade IVa: decerebrate or decorticate posturing in response to stimulation
2. Grade IVb: no response in any way to stimulation

Key Laboratory Findings

- Elevated serum transaminase and lactate dehydrogenase activities
- Hyperbilirubinemia
- Elevated plasma ammonia concentration
- Prolonged prothrombin time
- Laboratory abnormalities secondary to complications (see text)

Complications

A. Coagulopathy

B. Cerebral edema (~60% of cases of FHF; very rarely in chronic liver disease)

C. Infection, sepsis

D. Fluid and electrolyte disturbances (e.g., hyponatremia, hypokalemia)

E. Acid-base disturbances (especially respiratory alkalosis)

F. Cardiac dysrhythmias (common, even early in the course of the disease)

G. Hypoglycemia

H. Hypotension

    1. Advancing liver failure is associated with progressive vasodilation and increased cardiac output.

    2. Echocardiography often reveals four-chamber enlargement and reduced ejection fraction, despite increased cardiac output.

    3. Hemodynamic instability is rare until encephalopathy is advanced.

I. Seizures

J. Pulmonary edema

    1. Mechanism is increased pulmonary vascular permeability (i.e., a form of acute respiratory distress syndrome).

    2. Often accompanies cerebral edema

K. Gastrointestinal bleeding

L. Pancreatitis

M. Acute renal failure

PEARLS

- Clotting may be normal despite a prolonged prothrombin time secondary to acetaminophen-induced FHF.
- Disseminated intravascular coagulation may complicate the course of FHF.

Treatment

A. During the acute phase, medical care should be provided in a setting where complications can be rapidly identified and addressed.

B. Monitor blood or serum glucose and give IV dextrose continuously.

C. Avoid sedation, if at all possible, to minimize confounding the assessment of encephalopathy.

D. Administer *N*-acetylcysteine (NAC) to patients with acetaminophen-induced hepatotoxicity.

    1. Administer a loading dose of 140 mg/kg followed by 70 mg/kg every 4 hours for a total of 17 doses (recommended by the Centers for Disease Control and Prevention).

    2. Route of administration

        a. Only the oral formulation is approved in the United States; an IV formulation is available in Europe and is investigational in the United States.

        b. Pancreatitis often complicates FHF, and NAC administered orally may not be adequately absorbed under these conditions.

        c. In these cases, the sterile oral formulation of NAC has been administered intravenously after passage through a pyrogen filter.

    3. *N*-acetylcysteine should be used even when patients present late after acetaminophen ingestion.

    4. *N*-acetylcysteine may be beneficial in cases of FHF from causes other than acetaminophen.

E. Transportation and consultation

    1. Consultation should be obtained with a referral center where liver transplantation is offered.

    2. Selection of such a center should be guided in part by the center's willingness and ability to consider transplantation in very high acuity patients.

    3. Patients who have a severe coagulopathy (international normalized ratio [INR] >2.0) or encephalopathy grade II or higher should be referred.

    4. Patients should be transferred before intracranial hypertension develops.

    5. Transport for many of these patients is risky.

    6. Endotracheal intubation prior to transport is mandatory for patients who are unable to protect their airway and prevent aspiration.

    7. Maintain normocarbia.

F. Coagulopathy

    1. Do not transfuse clotting factors prophylactically, except prior to certain invasive procedures, such as placement of an intracranial

pressure monitor or obtaining a transjugular liver biopsy.

2. Treat excessive fibrinolysis with ε-aminocaproic acid.

G. Fulminant hepatic failure due to viral hepatitis

1. Hepatitis A and B infections do not respond to available anti-viral interventions.

2. Viral hepatitis caused by the herpesviruses such as cytomegalovirus, Epstein-Barr virus, and herpes simplex may respond to treatment with acyclovir or ganciclovir.

H. Cardiovascular support for hypotension

1. When the encephalopathy progresses to stage III or IV, institute invasive monitoring using systemic and pulmonary artery catheterization.

2. Use volume expansion judiciously, titrated to avoid increasing intracranial pressure or exacerbating pulmonary edema.

3. Use norepinephrine to restore vasomotor tone.

I. Neurologic monitoring and support

1. The best way to monitor neurologic status is to assess mental status; therefore, all sedatives and drugs with sedating effects should be withheld.

2. Lactulose (less beneficial in FHF than in chronic hepatic disease)

3. Intracranial hypertension

a. Fulminant hepatic failure is associated with increased intracranial blood volume and cerebral hyperemia early in the course, followed later by the development of cerebral edema and decreased cerebral blood flow.

b. Ultimately, herniation can occur.

c. Cerebral monitoring includes placement of an intracranial pressure monitor when the encephalopathy is at least grade III.

d. Cerebral blood flow can be measured at some centers using xenon-enhanced computed tomography, among other techniques.

e. Minute-to-minute changes in cerebral blood flow can be estimated by monitoring arterial-jugular venous oxygen content difference by assuming that cerebral oxygen consumption remains constant.

(1) This requires jugular bulb catheterization for simultaneous sampling of arterial and jugular venous oxygen content.

(2) Cerebral blood flow is inversely proportional to the arterial-jugular venous oxygen content difference.

J. Renal support

1. Renal failure is common in FHF and appears to be functional (a form of hepatorenal syndrome), except in cases of acetaminophen poisoning (acetaminophen is directly nephrotoxic).

2. Renal function recovers as liver function improves.

3. Renal replacement therapy in the interim is often required to treat volume overload or acid-base disturbances.

a. Continuous renal replacement therapy (CRRT) is preferable to intermittent hemodialysis.

b. Continuous renal replacement therapy is less likely to precipitate rapid osmolar shifts that can result in abrupt worsening of cerebral edema and intracranial hypertension, and may even precipitate herniation.

c. Continuous renal replacement therapy offers more time for correction of fluid and electrolyte imbalances, minimizing the chance of other organ damage from hypoperfusion.

d. Although the prothrombin time is often very prolonged, regional or systemic heparinization is often required to prevent clotting of the hemofiltration cartridge.

K. Respiratory support

1. Endotracheal intubation is usually not necessary for airway protection until grade III encephalopathy develops.

2. Acute respiratory distress syndrome is common in patients with FHF.

a. Initially, use a low tidal volume, low airway pressure approach for mechanical ventilation.

b. Be aware that hypercarbia worsens cerebral hyperemia and often is poorly tolerated in patients with intracranial hypertension.

c. Use tromethamine to buffer acidosis.

L. Infectious disease considerations

1. Virtually all patients with advanced FHF develop bacterial infections before or after hepatic transplantation.

2. Staphylococci and enteric organisms are typical pathogens.

3. Fungal infections are also common, affecting nearly 40% of patients.

4. Many centers routinely treat patients with FHF with ampicillin-sulbactam and fluconazole; some centers add selective decontamination of the digestive tract.

M. Hepatic transplantation

1. Liver transplantation offers the only chance of survival for many patents with FHF.

2. The following categories of patients are candi-

dates for orthotopic liver transplantation because of high risk of death.

    a. Patients younger than 30 years of age with factor V levels 30% of normal or lower

    b. Patients at least 30 years of age with factor V levels 20% of normal or lower

    c. Patients who meet King's College criteria (see below)

      (1) Acetaminophen intoxication and acidemia

      (2) Age younger than 10 or older than 40 years

      (3) Non-acetaminophen cause plus severe coagulopathy (INR >6)

3. In contrast to the careful selection of candidates that occurs among patients with chronic liver disease, in which social factors may be considered and appropriate interventions are planned or initiated, patients with FHF require an emergent evaluation and decision regarding the feasibility of liver transplantation.

4. The role of transplantation for patients with FHF who are active substance abusers is controversial.

5. Morbidity and mortality are higher for transplantation carried out for FHF as compared to chronic end-stage liver disease.

6. Auxiliary transplantation is an alternative approach gaining favor in Europe.

    a. A left lateral segment from either a split cadaveric organ or a living donor is implanted into the recipient with FHF, who also undergoes left lateral segmentectomy.

    b. When the native liver regains spontaneous function, immunosuppression can be stopped and the native liver allowed to wither.

N. Bio-artificial liver support

1. Hollow fiber cartridges loaded with porcine or cultured human hepatocytes are perfused with the patient's blood.

2. Investigational; no device currently in trials has favorably impacted survival.

Prognosis

A. Overall mortality is 75% despite aggressive intensive care.

B. Risk stratification

1. By etiology

    a. Acetaminophen overdose is associated with the best survival: 70%

    b. Hepatitis A and B infections: 50% to 60% survival

    c. Toxic reactions from medications or poisons other than acetaminophen: 5% to 20% survival

    d. Viral hepatitides other than HAV and HBV: very low survival unless promptly recognized and treated with acyclovir or ganciclovir

2. By age: patients younger than 10 and older than 40 years of age have much lower survival than other age groups

3. By grade of hepatic encephalopathy: if the worst grade is grade II, then the prognosis is better

4. By presence of cerebral edema

    a. Herniation was the cause of death in more than ⅔ of patients who died, but improved monitoring techniques (including intracranial pressure and cerebral blood flow measurement) have reduced the frequency of neurologic death.

    b. Multiple organ dysfunction syndrome is now the most common cause of death.

5. By severity of coagulopathy

6. By interval between onset of jaundice and development of encephalopathy

    a. Survival is inversely related to the interval between the onset of jaundice and the development of encephalopathy.

    b. Life-threatening cerebral edema is most common when this interval is 2 weeks or less and rare if the interval is longer.

    c. Patients with delayed onset of jaundice behave more like patients with chronic end-stage liver failure.

    d. As liver function deteriorates, survival without transplantation approaches zero.

C. King's College Hospital prognostic criteria for non-survival in patients with acute liver failure

1. Acetaminophen-related

    a. Arterial pH <7.30 after 24 hours of resuscitation, or

    b. Grade III or IV encephalopathy, INR >6.5, and serum creatinine concentration higher than 3.4 mg/dL

2. Unrelated to acetaminophen overdose

    a. INR >6.5, or

    b. Any three of the following

      (1) Age younger than 10 or older than 40 years

      (2) Etiology not related to acetaminophen, HAV or HBV (i.e., either the cause cannot be determined or it is an idiosyn-

cratic drug reaction or exposure to a toxin)

(3) Duration of jaundice before onset of encephalopathy longer than 7 days

(4) INR >3.5

(5) Serum total bilirubin level higher than 17.5 mg/dL

Key Prognosis

The availability of orthotopic liver transplantation increases overall survival from 20% to 70%.

Bibliography

Aggarwal S, Kramer DJ, Yonas H, et al. Cerebral hemodynamic and metabolic changes in fulminant hepatic failure. A retrospective study. Hepatology 1994;19: 80–87.

Harrison PM, Wendon J, Gimson AES, et al. Improvement by acetylcysteine of hemodynamics and oxygen transport in fulminant hepatic failure. N Engl J Med 1991;324: 1852–1857.

Klein AS, Hart J, Brems JJ, et al. Amanita poisoning: Treatment and the role of liver transplantation. Am J Med 1989;86:187–193.

O'Grady JG, Alexander GJ, Hayllar KM, et al. Early indicators of prognosis in fulminant hepatic failure. Gastroenterology 1989;97:439–445.

130 Upper Gastroenteral Hemorrhage

Mitchell P. Fink

Epidemiology

A. Upper gastrointestinal (UGI) hemorrhage accounts for approximately 100 hospital admissions annually per 100,000 adults in the United States.

B. Male : female = 2 : 1

C. Incidence increases with age.

D. Mortality is less than 1% for patients younger than 60 years old without malignancy as a predisposing cause.

E. Overall mortality is approximately 10%.

Key Clinical Findings

- Hematemesis and melena are the most common presenting manifestations of UGI bleeding.

- Hematochezia is usually a sign of lower gastrointestinal (LGI) bleeding; if hematochezia is due to UGI hemorrhage, then it indicates major bleeding and a substantial risk of death (~18% to 29%).

- Hypotension is a late sign of hemorrhagic shock; tachycardia and delayed capillary refill are more sensitive signs of hypovolemia.

Diagnosis

A. Historical findings favoring an UGI rather than a LGI source for hemorrhage
  1. Use of nonsteroidal anti-inflammatory drugs (NSAIDs)
  2. Ethanol abuse
  3. Prior episodes of UGI bleeding
  4. Predisposing conditions
    a. Peptic ulcer disease
    b. Cirrhosis and/or portal hypertension
    c. Gastric cancer
  5. Epigastric abdominal pain
  6. Hematemesis or melena

B. Physical examination
  1. Cutaneous stigmata of cirrhosis and/or portal hypertension
  2. Hepatomegaly, splenomegaly, or both

C. Bloody aspirate from nasogastric tube

  1. Presence of only occult blood is of no diagnostic significance.
  2. Asanguinous nasogastric aspirate does not exclude a UGI source of bleeding that is distal to the pylorus.

D. Upper GI endoscopy
  1. Virtually all patients with suspected UGI bleeding should undergo UGI endoscopy.
  2. Upper GI endoscopy is more sensitive and specific than UGI barium radiographs.
  3. Upper GI endoscopy provides prognostic information regarding risk of rebleeding.

E. Angiography
  1. Rarely indicated in cases of UGI hemorrhage
  2. May be indicated for rare cases of massive bleeding when surgical therapy is contraindicated

Key Laboratory Findings

- Initially, hematocrit and hemoglobin concentration do not change with hemorrhage.

- Hematocrit and hemoglobin concentration decrease later, either as a result of intravascular recruitment of volume ("transcapillary refill") or from intravenous infusion of asanguinous fluids for resuscitation.

Treatment

A. General resuscitative measures
  1. Guidelines for resuscitation are essentially the same as for trauma.
  2. Initial efforts should be directed at assuring that airway and breathing are adequate.
  3. Initial fluid resuscitation
    a. Insert (at least) two large-bore (≥16-gauge) IV catheters.
    b. Infuse at least 2 L Ringer's lactate or normal saline solution, titrated to stabilize hemodynamic parameters.
  4. Indications for transfusion of packed red blood cells

a. Persistent hemodynamic instability after infusion of 2 L of crystalloid solution

b. Low hematocrit (<25%)

c. Signs or symptoms of inadequate tissue oxygenation (e.g., angina pectoris)

B. Esophagitis

1. Rare cause of clinically significant UGI hemorrhage (<8% of cases)

2. Most bleeding stops spontaneously.

C. Mallory-Weiss tears

1. Mucosal lacerations at the gastroesophageal junction that are associated with vomiting or retching, typically in patients with a history of ethanol abuse

2. Relatively rare cause of UGI hemorrhage (5% to 15% of cases)

3. Bleeding stops spontaneously in most cases.

4. Endoscopic interventions (bipolar coagulation, heater probe) are effective in stopping bleeding.

5. Angiographic intervention (superselective arterial embolization) is also effective in refractory cases.

6. Surgical intervention to oversew the site of bleeding, while effective, is rarely indicated.

D. Gastric and esophageal varices due to portal hypertension

1. Variceal bleeding accounts for 10% to 33% of cases of significant UGI hemorrhage, the actual rate being dependent on the incidence of ethanol abuse in the population served by the institution.

2. Mortality after a variceal bleed ranges from 40% to 70%.

3. Endoscopic therapeutic approaches (sclerotherapy or ligation of varices) for acute control of bleeding due to esophageal varices are effective in about 90% of cases.

4. Infusion of octreotide (e.g., 100 μg bolus followed by 50 μg/hour for 48 hours, followed by 100 μg subcutaneously every 8 hours for 72 hours) is also effective, and may be especially so in combination with endoscopic sclerotherapy.

5. Balloon tamponade

a. Useful only as a temporizing measure pending more definitive therapy in patients with active, life-threatening hemorrhage refractory to endoscopic and pharmacological approaches.

b. The four-lumen Minnesota tube is the safest of the available devices because it allows continuous aspiration of secretions that tend to collect proximal to the esophageal balloon.

c. Patients should be endotracheally intubated for airway protection before insertion of the Minnesota tube, and the position of a partly inflated gastric balloon should be confirmed radiographically before full inflation.

d. The tube should be removed as soon as possible, with 24 hours being the longest period of continuous inflation allowable.

6. Transjugular intrahepatic portosystemic shunt (TIPS)

a. Nonsurgical approach for achieving portal decompression

b. In experienced hands, TIPS placement is successful in more than 95% of patients.

c. Acute variceal bleeding is controlled in almost all patients after a technically successful TIPS.

E. Peptic ulcer

1. Most common cause of UGI bleeding (~50% of cases)

2. Bleeding is more often a problem with duodenal ulcers than with gastric ulcers.

3. Nonsteroidal anti-inflammatory drugs (NSAIDs) are a major risk factor for bleeding (and other complications) associated with peptic ulceration.

4. General risk factors for mortality

a. Hemodynamic instability

b. Requirement for transfusion of multiple units of blood or red cells

c. Bright-red emesis or nasogastric aspirate

d. Age greater than 60 years

e. Coagulopathy

5. Findings at endoscopy that are associated with increased risk of rebleeding and mortality

a. Ulcer diameter larger than 1 cm

b. Clot in base of ulcer

c. Visible vessel in base of ulcer

d. Active bleeding from ulcer

6. If the ulcer has a clean base, then only pharmacological therapy is generally indicated, and patients can be discharged from the ICU after resuscitation and stabilization and observation for approximately 24 hours.

7. If the ulcer base shows clot, a visible vessel, or active bleeding, then endoscopic hemostatic therapy should be performed.

a. Bipolar or multipolar electrocoagulation

b. Heater probe

c. Injection therapy using epinephrine, ethanol, or other sclerosing agent

8. Pharmacological agents

   a. H$_2$-receptor antagonists, although widely used, do not decrease the risk of rebleeding from duodenal ulcers.

   b. Treatment with a proton pump inhibitor (e.g., omeprazole) may decrease the risk of recurrent bleeding.

   c. Treatment with octreotide seems to control bleeding and decrease the risk of recurrent hemorrhage.

9. Angiographic embolization of a bleeding vessel

   a. Indicated only in cases of intractable hemorrhage when surgical intervention is contraindicated

   b. Initial control of hemorrhage is usually good, but rebleeding is common.

10. Surgery is indicated when bleeding persists despite endoscopic and pharmacological interventions.

F. Stress-related mucosal injury

1. Among a general population of medical and surgical ICU patients, the major risk factors are requirement for mechanical ventilation and coagulopathy.

2. Other risk factors are renal dysfunction and absence of enteral nutrition.

3. The best "treatment" is prophylaxis using H$_2$-receptor antagonists, sucralfate, or antacids.

4. Clinically significant bleeding from erosive gastritis that persists despite alkalinization is probably best treated pharmacologically using octreotide or vasopressin infusion.

5. Surgical therapy (total or near-total gastrectomy) is rarely, if ever, indicated.

G. Aortoenteric fistula

1. The most common site is the third portion of the duodenum.

2. Most cases occur several years after aortic aneurysmorrhaphy using a prosthetic graft.

3. Many, but certainly not all, cases have a history of a "sentinel bleed" that stops spontaneously hours or days before the onset of massive hemorrhage.

4. Initial evaluation consists of UGI endoscopy followed by abdominal computed tomography.

5. Surgical intervention should be carried out as soon as the diagnosis is confirmed or even strongly suspected.

H. Dieulafoy's lesion

1. Submucosal gastric artery of unusually large caliber that compresses the overlying mucosa, eventually leading to erosion and rupture of the vessel into the lumen

2. Treatment is endoscopic (e.g., bipolar coagulation).

Bibliography

Bildozola M, Kravetz D, Argonz J, et al. Efficacy of octreotide and sclerotherapy in the treatment of acute variceal bleeding in cirrhotic patients. A prospective, multicentric, and randomized clinical trial. Scand J Gastroenterol 2000;35:419–425.

Cook D, Heyland D, Griffith L, et al. Risk factors for clinically important upper gastrointestinal bleeding in patients requiring mechanical ventilation. Canadian Critical Care Trials Group. Crit Care Med 1999;27:2812–2817.

Cook DJ, Fuller HD, Guyatt GH, et al. Risk factors for gastrointestinal bleeding in critically ill patients. Canadian Critical Care Trials Group. N Engl J Med 1994;330:377–381.

Lin HJ, Perng CL, Wang K, et al. Octreotide for arrest of peptic ulcer hemorrhage—A prospective, randomized controlled trial. Hepatogastroenterology 1995;42:856–860.

Zuberi BF, Baloch Q. Comparison of endoscopic variceal sclerotherapy alone and in combination with octreotide in controlling acute variceal hemorrhage and early rebleeding in patients with low-risk cirrhosis. Am J Gastroenterol 2000;95:768–771.

131 Lower Gastroenteral Hemorrhage

Murray N. Ehrinpreis

Lower gastrointestinal bleeding (LGIB) is defined as bleeding arising distal to the ligament of Treitz. While most such bleeding has a colonic source, small intestinal bleeds also occur. Upper gastrointestinal bleeding (UGIB) without hematemesis and with rapid intestinal transit may appear to be lower gastrointestinal in nature. Bleeding may be acute, chronic, recurrent, occult, or clinically obvious. This chapter focuses on the latter, especially those cases occurring with hemodynamic changes.

Etiologies

A. Colonic (85% of LGIB)
   1. Diverticulosis
   2. Angiodysplasia (vascular ectasias)
   3. Neoplasm
      a. Carcinoma
      b. Adenoma
      c. Hemangioma
   4. Colitis
      a. Ulcerative colitis
      b. Crohn's colitis
      c. Radiation proctitis or colitis (proctopathy or colopathy)
      d. Ischemic
      e. Infectious
   5. Ulcers
      a. Drug-induced (e.g., nonsteroidal anti-inflammatory drugs [NSAIDs])
      b. Vasculitic (e.g., systemic lupus erythematosus)
   6. Other colonic etiologies
      a. Portal hypertensive colopathy
      b. Postpolypectomy bleeding
      c. Non-neoplastic polyps
B. Anorectal
   1. Hemorrhoids
   2. Rectal varices
   3. Fissure-in-ano
   4. Rectal ulcer
C. Small intestinal (<10% of LGIB)
   1. Angiodysplasia

2. Neoplasm (leiomyoma, carcinoma)
3. Crohn's disease
4. Ulcer (drug-induced, ischemic, vasculitic)
5. Meckel's diverticulum
6. Aortoenteric fistula
7. Intussusception

Risk Factors

A. Co-morbid conditions
   1. Liver disease (portal hypertension, coagulopathy)
   2. Renal failure (angiodysplasia)
   3. Idiopathic inflammatory bowel disease (IBD)
   4. Acquired immunodeficiency syndrome (AIDS)
   5. Aortic graft
   6. Collagen vascular disease
   7. Coagulopathy
   8. Peripheral vascular disease (ischemia)
   9. Coronary artery disease (concurrent cardiac ischemia)
   10. Radiation therapy
   11. Chemotherapy
   12. Peptic ulcer disease or previous UGIB
B. Drugs
   1. Anticoagulants
   2. NSAIDs
   3. Antibiotics
   4. Immunosuppressants
C. Social history
   1. Travel history (infectious, parasitic colitis)
   2. Country of origin (intestinal tuberculosis)
   3. Illicit drug use (endocarditis, cocaine-induced ischemia)

Symptoms

A. Stool characteristics
   1. Hematochezia: high-volume bright-red blood or clots per rectum without stool (anorectal or massive GI bleeding)

2. Blood mixed with stool: left colon source

3. Maroon stools: small bowel or colonic

4. Melena: small bowel or right colon, slow transit

5. Bloody diarrhea: colitis

B. Hemodynamic-related symptoms

  1. Dizziness, lightheadedness, postural symptoms

  2. Fatigue

  3. Diaphoresis

  4. Dyspnea

  5. Chest pain, palpitations

C. Other gastrointestinal symptoms

  1. Painless presentation: diverticulosis, angiodysplasia, hemorrhoids, colopathy

  2. Abdominal pain or cramps: colitis, ileitis, ulcer, aortoenteric fistula, ischemia

  3. Anorectal pain or urgency: fissure-in-ano, proctitis, rectal tumor

  4. Constipation: colon cancer (left colon or rectum), fissure-in-ano, hemorrhoids, ulcer

Physical Findings

A. General

  1. Pallor

  2. Jaundice

  3. Fever

B. Hemodynamic

  1. Tachycardia (supine or orthostatic)

  2. Hypotension (supine or orthostatic)

C. Localized

  1. Bowel sounds

  2. Tenderness

  3. Mass

  4. Bruits

  5. Ascites, splenomegaly, accentuated abdominal vasculature

  6. Rectal tenderness, mass, blood

  7. Other

    a. Ecchymoses, petechiae

    b. Hyperpigmentation or telangiectases of buccal mucosa or skin

    c. Heart murmur

Laboratory and Other Tests

A. Hematologic (initial tests)

  1. Hemoglobin, hematocrit: may be normal despite massive blood loss

2. Coagulation studies: platelet count, prothrombin time, partial thromboplastin time

3. Type and cross-match for possible red blood cell (RBC) transfusion

B. Biochemical tests

  1. Blood urea nitrogen (BUN) and creatinine: BUN:creatinine ratio greater than or equal to 25:1 is highly suggestive of UGIB

  2. Liver function tests

C. Other examinations

  1. Electrocardiogram (patients older than 50 years)

  2. Abdominal x-ray, if significant abdominal findings (e.g., pain, tenderness, distention, mass)

Key Findings

- Tachycardia, hypotension, or postural changes reflect 10% to 30% blood volume loss.

- Abdominal pain and tenderness are important diagnostic clues.

- Upper GI bleeding may present with hematochezia.

- Melena may occur with right colon or small bowel bleeding.

- Nasogastric tube aspirate may be negative in a significant proportion of UGIB.

- Hemoglobin and hematocrit may not reflect severity of GI bleeding.

Diagnosis

A. Upper vs. lower GI bleeding

  1. Nasogastric tube aspirate

    a. Gross blood, clots, "coffee grounds" suggest upper GI source.

    b. Clear bile makes upper GI source unlikely, but not impossible.

    c. There is no value in testing gastric aspirate for occult blood (false positives are common from nasogastric tube trauma; negative result does exclude upper GI bleeding source).

  2. Esophagogastroduodenoscopy (EGD): best way to exclude upper GI source if there is any doubt

B. Identification of bleeding site and etiology

  1. Anoscopy, sigmoidoscopy: if anorectal source strongly suggested

  2. Colonoscopy following polyethylene glycol lav-

age preparation, once patient is stabilized hemodynamically

    a. Lavage may be given via nasogastric tube if necessary.

    b. Diagnostic yield: 70% to 80%

3. Arteriography if continued active bleeding (diagnostic yield: 40% to 70%)

4. Computed tomography scan: if aortoenteric fistula suspected (after EGD with evaluation of distal duodenum)

5. Surgery, if continued active bleeding with hemodynamic instability; intraoperative endoscopy may be helpful

6. Radionuclide-tagged RBC scans may help localize bleeding site, but usually are not reliable enough to guide surgery.

7. Meckel's scan indicated in young patients with normal colonoscopy and EGD

8. No role for barium contrast studies in the evaluation of active GI bleeding

Treatment

A. Resuscitation

1. Assure adequate IV access (2 sites, at least 18 gauge).

2. Infuse isotonic crystalloids for volume expansion (normal saline or lactated Ringer's).

3. Transfuse packed RBCs as indicated.

4. Transfuse platelets, fresh-frozen plasma, clotting factors as indicated.

5. Vasopressors generally not indicated

B. Monitor in intensive care unit.

C. Consult endoscopist and surgeon for consultation and follow-up.

D. Treat based on diagnosis and severity.

E. Urgent treatment for continuing or recurrent bleeding

1. Colonoscopic

    a. Angiodysplasia: thermal coagulation (heater probe, bipolar or multipolar electrocoagulator, laser, argon plasma coagulator), injection sclerosis or vasoconstriction of bleeding lesions

    b. Diverticulosis: injection vasoconstriction and thermal coagulation of the bleeding diverticulum

    c. Polyp bleeding: polypectomy

    d. Postpolypectomy bleeding: injection vasoconstriction, thermal coagulation, or metallic clip application, if necessary

    e. Hemorrhoids: band ligation, injection sclerosis

    f. Radiation proctopathy or colopathy: argon plasma coagulator, laser

2. Angiographic: intra-arterial vasopressin or embolization of bleeding vessels, if feasible, especially in high-risk surgery patients

3. Medical treatment

    a. Inflammatory bowel disease: steroids

    b. Portal hypertensive bleeding: octreotide

    c. Uncontrolled portal hypertensive bleeding: transjugular intrahepatic portosystemic shunt (TIPS)

    d. Infectious colitis: antibiotics, antiviral therapy

4. Surgery for uncontrolled bleeding; localization of bleeding area prior to surgery desirable

    a. Diverticulosis or angiodysplasia: limited colonic resection safer and more effective than subtotal colectomy or "blind" right hemicolectomy

    b. Aortoenteric fistula: vascular procedure

    c. Meckel's diverticulum or intussusception: resection

Key Treatment

- Vigorous resuscitation

- Nasogastric tube placement to check for UGIB

- Low threshold for performing EGD to exclude UGIB

- Anoscopy or flexible sigmoidoscopy often helpful

- Colonoscopy after preparation is best examination in stabilized patient.

- Arteriography or surgery if bleeding too active for colonoscopic preparation

- No barium studies for evaluation of acute bleeding

- Surgeon must be involved in management.

Prognosis

A. In 80% to 85% of LGIB cases bleeding stops spontaneously.

B. Recurrence rate for diverticular bleeding is 38%.

C. Colonoscopic hemostasis may be very successful in the 20% of patients with LGIB and diverticulosis, where a bleeding diverticulum is definitely identified.

D. Arteriographic treatment is 70% successful where a bleeding lesion is identified.

E. Surgical morbidity and mortality depend on type of surgery, patient age, co-morbid illnesses.

Bibliography

DeMarkles MP, Murphy JR. Acute lower gastrointestinal bleeding. Med Clin North Am 1993;77:1085–1100.

Jensen DM, Machicado GA. Diagnosis and treatment of severe hematochezia. The role of urgent colonoscopy after purge. Gastroenterology 1988;95:1569–1574.

Jensen DM, Machicado GA, Jutabha R, et al. Urgent colonoscopy for the diagnosis and treatment of severe diverticular hemorrhage. N Engl J Med 2000;342:78–82.

Lieberman D. Gastrointestinal bleeding: initial management. Gastroenterol Clin North Am 1993;22:723–736.

McGuire HH Jr. Bleeding colonic diverticula. A reappraisal of natural history and management. Ann Surg 1994;220: 653–656.

Setya V, Singer JA, Minken SL. Subtotal colectomy as a last resort for unrelenting, unlocalized, lower gastrointestinal hemorrhage: experience with 12 cases. Am Surgeon 1992;58:295–299.

Zuccaro G Jr. Management of the adult patient with acute lower gastrointestinal bleeding. Am J Gastroenterol 1998;93:1202–1208.

132 Diarrhea

Murray N. Ehrinpreis

Definitions

A. Diarrhea is physiologically defined as greater than 250 g/day on an "average" American diet.

B. Acute diarrhea: present for fewer than 3 weeks

C. Chronic diarrhea: present for at least 3 weeks

Etiologies

A. Acute
   1. Infectious (immunocompetent patient)
      a. Bacterial
         (1) Invasive or enterotoxigenic (rarely hospital acquired)
            (a) *Escherichia coli*: enterotoxigenic, enteroinvasive, enteroadherent, or enterohemorrhagic
            (b) *Shigella*
            (c) *Salmonella*
            (d) *Campylobacter*
            (e) *Yersinia*
            (f) *Vibrio*
            (g) *Aeromonas hydrophila*
            (h) *Pleisiomonas shigelloides*
            (i) *Listeria monocytogenes*
         (2) Cytotoxin: *Clostridium difficile*
         (3) Pre-formed toxin (food poisoning)
            (a) *Staphylococcus aureus*
            (b) *Bacillus cereus*
            (c) *Clostridium perfringens*
      b. Viral
         (1) Rotavirus
         (2) Norwalk virus
         (3) Enteric adenovirus
         (4) Calcivirus
         (5) Astrovirus
      c. Protozoal and parasitic agents
         (1) *Giardia lamblia*
         (2) *Entamoeba histolytica*
         (3) *Strongyloides stercoralis*
      d. Fungal: *Candida* overgrowth (especially in critically ill patients)
   2. Infectious (immunocompromised patient)
      a. Bacterial
         (1) Usual stool bacterial pathogens (see above)
         (2) *Mycobacterium avium intracellulare* complex (MAI)
      b. Viral
         (1) Usual viral pathogens (see above)
         (2) Cytomegalovirus (CMV)
         (3) Herpes simplex (HSV)
         (4) Human immunodeficiency virus (HIV)
      c. Protozoal
         (1) Usual protozoal pathogens (see above)
         (2) *Cryptosporidium parvum*
         (3) *Microsporidia*
         (4) *Isospora belli*
         (5) *Cyclospora*
   3. Noninfectious
      a. Mesenteric ischemia
      b. Idiopathic inflammatory bowel disease (IBD)
      c. Fecal impaction
      d. Drug-induced
         (1) Antibiotics (account for 25% of drug-induced diarrhea)
         (2) Laxatives: e.g., lactulose, sorbitol, polyethylene glycol cathartics, stimulant laxatives, milk of magnesia
         (3) Magnesium-based antacids
         (4) Oral phosphate supplements
         (5) Proton pump inhibitors
         (6) H_2 receptor antagonists
         (7) Other drugs: e.g., digoxin, quinidine, theophylline, cancer chemotherapy, misoprostol, α-glucosidase inhibitors, colchicine, cholinesterase inhibitors, gold
      e. Environmental toxins: e.g., insecticides

B. Chronic
   1. Infectious, including parasitic
      a. Immunocompetent patient: relapsing *C. difficile*, yersiniosis, Whipple's disease, giardiasis, amebiasis
      b. Immunocompromised: yersiniosis, salmonellosis, shigellosis, *Campylobacter*, MAI, giardiasis, amebiasis, cryptosporidiosis, microsporidiosis, *Isospora belli*, *Cyclospora*, CMV, HSV, adenovirus, HIV
   2. Inflammatory
      a. Inflammatory bowel disease
      b. Celiac sprue
      c. Tropical sprue

    d. Radiation

    e. Graft-versus-host disease (GVHD)

    f. Collagen vascular disease

  3. Neoplastic

    a. Colon carcinoma

    b. Large villous adenoma of colon

    c. Intestinal lymphoma

    d. Secretogogue-producing neuroendocrine tumors

      (1) Gastrinoma (Zollinger-Ellison syndrome)

      (2) Vasoactive intestinal polypeptide (VIP) secreting tumor (VIPoma): watery diarrhea–hypokalemia–achlorhydria (WDHA) syndrome, pancreatic cholera

      (3) Carcinoid tumor

      (4) Medullary thyroid carcinoma

  4. Endocrine etiology

    a. Thyrotoxicosis

    b. Adrenal insufficiency

    c. Diabetes mellitus

  5. Structural organ abnormality

    a. "Short bowel" syndrome

    b. Fistula: enteroenteric, enterocolic, gastrocolic

    c. Ileal resection (due to bile salt malabsorption and fatty-acid diarrhea)

    d. Intestinal lymphangiectasia

    e. Pancreatic exocrine insufficiency

    f. Intestinal bacterial overgrowth

    g. Partial bowel obstruction

  6. Others

    a. Tube feeding

    b. Chronic mesenteric insufficiency

Risk Factors

A. Significant travel history

B. Infection exposure: e.g., day care center, institution for mentally challenged, recent epidemics (community exposure)

C. Immunosuppression: e.g., acquired immunodeficiency syndrome, bone marrow or other organ transplantation, cancer chemotherapy

D. Other critical illnesses: e.g., sepsis, respiratory failure, multisystem organ failure

E. Antibiotic use

F. Polypharmacy

G. Family history: malabsorption, IBD, endocrinopathies

H. Enteral feeding

I. Chemical exposure

J. Lifestyle: alcoholism, oral-anal or anal receptive intercourse, prostitution, IV drug use

K. Diabetes mellitus

Symptoms

A. Loose, watery, frequent stools

  1. High volume: suggests small bowel disease or intestinal secretogogue

  2. Small volume: suggests colonic disease

B. Urgency, incontinence: rectal disease

C. Bloody stools: invasive infection, ischemia, IBD

D. Crampy abdominal pain

E. Nausea, vomiting: suggest toxin ingestion

F. Postural dizziness: due to volume depletion

G. Prostration, weakness: volume depletion, electrolyte abnormalities

H. Weight loss: malabsorption, IBD, dehydration

I. Ecchymoses: coagulopathy due to fat-soluble vitamin malabsorption

J. Skin rash: infection, IBD, malabsorption

K. Muscle cramps, tetany: Mg^{2+}, Ca^{2+} depletion

Physical Findings

A. Vital signs: tachycardia, hypotension, orthostatic hypotension

B. Cardiovascular: flat neck veins

C. Abdomen: bowel sounds variable, distention, tenderness

D. Skin: tenting, decreased turgor, rash, ecchymoses, hyperpigmentation (Addison's disease)

E. Rectum: mass, decreased tone

Laboratory Findings

A. Hematologic tests

  1. Hemoglobin and hematocrit: to detect hemoconcentration from fluid loss, anemia from chronic bloody diarrhea

  2. White blood cell (WBC) count: elevated with IBD and some infectious diarrheas

  3. Platelet count: rectal bleeding due to thrombocytopenia

B. Serum biochemical tests

  1. Electrolyte and acid-base related: non-anion gap metabolic acidosis, hyponatremia or hypernatremia, hypokalemia, hypomagnesemia

  2. Pre-renal azotemia: due to volume depletion

  3. Albumin: low in malabsorption, protein-losing enteropathy, chronic illness; high with hemoconcentration

  4. Iron studies: low levels suggest chronic blood loss or Fe malabsorption

C. Stool tests

  1. Fecal WBCs: present with bacterial diarrheas and IBD; suggests mucosal invasion

2. Positive test for fecal occult blood, or frank bleeding: suggests mucosal ulceration

3. *C. difficile* toxin: antibiotic-induced (pseudomembranous colitis); several specimens may be required

4. Cultures

   a. Bacterial cultures may require special laboratory techniques.

   b. Perform fungal cultures; do not ignore yeast overgrowth.

5. Examination for ova and parasites

6. Stool assays for electrolytes and osmolality (must be fresh specimen)

   a. Fecal Na^+ increased with secretory diarrhea

   b. Osmolality of diarrheal stool should approximate serum (normally ~290 mOsm/kg H_2O).

   c. Occult stool osmoles detected by stool osmole gap

      (1) Calculated from stool osmolality (mOsm/kg H_2O), Na^+ and K^+ concentration (mmol/L) by the following formula:

$$\text{stool osmole gap} = \text{stool osmolality} - 2 \times (Na^+ + K^+)$$

      (2) Gap greater than 40 to 60 mOsm/kg H_2O suggests osmotic diarrhea: carbohydrate malabsorption or osmotic laxative, e.g., $Mg(OH)_2$.

7. Alkalinization test with NaOH: red color suggests phenolphthalein laxative abuse

8. Stool volume greater than 1 to 2 L/day suggests secretory diarrhea.

D. Serologic tests: ameba, *Giardia,* antiendomysial antibodies, antigliadin antibodies (celiac sprue)

E. Serum secretogogue levels: gastrin, thyrocalcitonin, VIP, serotonin

F. Blood prothrombin time: prolonged with vitamin K malabsorption

Key Diagnostic Questions

- Acute or chronic?
- Community or hospital acquired?
- Large volume or small volume?
- Any current or recent medications?
- Bloody or non-bloody?
- Systemic symptoms or not?
- Fecal WBCs present or not?
- Immunocompetent or immunocompromised?

Diagnosis

A. Stool analysis and serologic tests (see D. above)

B. Sigmoidoscopy or colonoscopy with biopsy

C. Small bowel aspirate and biopsy (when colon normal)

D. Imaging studies

1. Abdominal flat x-ray films: obstruction, perforation, ischemic changes, abnormal calcifications (e.g., chronic pancreatitis)

2. Small bowel x-ray series: should not be done until complete stool examination studies have been performed

Treatment

A. Nonspecific measures

1. Rehydration: replace fluid deficits and ongoing losses

   a. Intravenous: may require potassium and alkali supplementation, e.g.,

      (1) Lactated Ringer's solution

      (2) 0.45% saline with added $NaHCO_3$ (25 mEq/L) and KCl (20 mEq/L)

   b. Oral (unusual in the hospital setting): World Health Organization solution or similar (Na^+ 60 to 90 mEq/L, K^+ 20 mEq/L, Cl^- 80 mEq/L, citrate 30 mEq/L, glucose 20 g/L)

2. Correction of electrolyte (Na^+, K^+, Mg^{2+}, Ca^{2+}, phosphate) and acid-base disturbances

3. Monitor intake and output carefully; assure adequate urine output.

4. Blood transfusion, vitamin K, fresh-frozen plasma (if appropriate)

5. Antidiarrheal agents

   a. Bismuth (Pepto-Bismol)

   b. Anticholinergic drugs (tincture of belladonna, hyoscyamine)

   c. Opiates (loperamide, codeine, paregoric)

   d. Octreotide

   e. Cholestyramine

6. Antidiarrheal agents inappropriate or contraindicated

   a. Bowel obstruction

   b. Certain bacterial infections (*Shigella, Salmonella, Campylobacter,* enterohemorrhagic *E. coli*)

B. Specific measures

1. Infectious etiology

   a. Antibiotics

      (1) Invasive (e.g., *Shigella,* systemic *Salmonella, Campylobacter, Yersinia, E. coli* [possibly], MAI, Whipple's disease): typi-

cal antibiotics are quinolones, trimethap-rim/sulfamethoxazole, erythromycin, tetracycline, and others depending on infecting organism

    (2) Cytotoxic due to *C. difficile*

       (a) Antibiotic choices are metronidazole or vancomycin.

       (b) Recurrence occurs in approximately 20%.

       (c) Often responds to repeat or longer-term treatment, change in antibiotic, use of cholestyramine or probiotics (e.g., *Lactobacillus*)

  b. Antiviral agents: for CMV and HSV (primarily immunocompromised patients)

  c. Antiprotozoal and antihelmintic agents: for *Giardia, Strongyloides,* ameba

  d. Antifungal agents: *Candida* overgrowth

2. Inflammatory etiology

  a. Inflammatory bowel disease

    (1) Corticosteroids

    (2) Mesalamine

    (3) Antibiotics

    (4) Cyclosporin

    (5) Surgical resection

  b. Celiac sprue

    (1) Gluten-free diet

    (2) Corticosteroids

  c. Tropical sprue: antibiotics, folate

  d. Radiation-induced: ablation techniques for bleeding; surgery

  e. Graft-versus-host disease: corticosteroids, cyclosporin, tacrolimus, others

  f. Collagen vascular disease: corticosteroids, antimetabolites, other treatments

3. Neoplastic etiology

  a. Surgical resection (e.g., lymphoma, solid tumors)

  b. Chemotherapy (e.g., lymphoma)

  c. Neuroendocrine tumors

    (1) Gastrinoma: proton pump inhibitors

    (2) Others: octreotide

4. Endocrine etiology

  a. Thyrotoxicosis: propylthiouracil, radioactive iodine, surgery

  b. Adrenal insufficiency: glucocorticoids

  c. Diabetes mellitus: glucose control, antibiotics (bacterial overgrowth), antidiarrheal agents, clonidine

5. Structural abnormality (various treatments depending on lesion)

  a. Surgery

  b. Total parenteral nutrition (TPN)

  c. Dietary measures

  d. Antidiarrheal agents

  e. Antibiotics

  f. Proton pump inhibitors

  g. Cholestyramine

  h. Pancreatic enzyme replacement

6. Other etiologies

  a. Tube feeding: antidiarrheal agents, change in formula, change in infusion rate, check for feed contamination

  b. Ischemia: revascularization, surgery

Key Treatment

- Aggressively replenish fluid deficits and provide for ongoing losses.

- Monitor serum electrolytes, especially Na^+, K^+, Mg^{2+}, HCO_3^-) and correct disturbances.

- Perform stool examination and laboratory studies on fresh specimens.

- Practice universal precautions.

- Provide specific therapy depending on etiology.

- Patience, persistence, and attention to detail are required for successful tube feeding.

- Occasionally TPN may be required for severely debilitated patients.

Bibliography

American Gastroenterological Association medical position statement. Guidelines for the evaluation and management of chronic diarrhea. Gastroenterology 1999;116:1461–1463.

Brinson RR, Kolts BE. Hypoalbuminemia as an indicator of diarrheal incidence in critically ill patients. Crit Care Med 1987;15:506–509.

DuPont HL, The Practice Parameters Committee of the American College of Gastroenterology. Guidelines on acute infectious diarrhea in adults. Am J Gastroenterol 1997;92:1962–1975.

Gupta TP, Ehrinpreis MN. *Candida*-associated diarrhea in hospitalized patients. Gastroenterology 1990;98:780–785.

Kelly CP, Pothoulakis C, LaMont JT. *Clostridium difficile* colitis. N Engl J Med 1994;330:257–262.

Wolf DC, Giannella RA. Antibiotic therapy for bacterial enterocolitis: a comprehensive review. Am J Gastroenterol 1993;88:1667–1683.

133 Toxic Megacolon

Murray N. Ehrinpreis

Inflammatory diseases of the colon, when severe, may result in substantial systemic effects and loss of colonic motor tone. The result of such fulminant colitis is referred to as "toxic megacolon." It is usually a complication of idiopathic inflammatory bowel disease (IBD), but other colitides may also result in this dangerous condition. For toxic megacolon, dilation of the colon must be present, but toxicity must be evident as well. Toxicity in this context is usually defined as the presence of at least three of the following: temperature higher than 101.5°F, tachycardia at least 120 beats/min, white blood cell count higher than 10,500 cells/mm^3, and a substantial drop in blood hemoglobin concentration. There is often associated dehydration, hypotension, electrolyte disturbances, and mental status changes.

Etiology

A. Idiopathic inflammatory bowel disease
1. Ulcerative colitis (usually pancolitis)
2. Crohn's disease (colitis)
B. Ischemic colitis
C. Infectious
1. Bacterial
a. *Salmonella*
b. *Shigella*
c. *Campylobacter*
d. *Clostridium difficile* (pseudomembranous colitis)
e. *Yersinia enterocolitica*
2. Viral (especially with immunosuppression)
a. Cytomegalovirus (CMV)
b. Self-limited (culture negative)
3. Parasitic
a. *Entamoeba histolytica*
b. *Strongyloides stercoralis*
D. Drug-induced
1. Imipramine
2. Loperamide
3. Methotrexate
4. Cancer chemotherapy
E. Neoplastic
1. Kaposi's sarcoma
2. Lymphoma

F. Precipitating factors in IBD
1. Barium enema
2. Opioids
3. Anticholinergics
4. Antidepressants
5. Hypokalemia
6. Rapid steroid tapering

Symptoms

A. Prostration
B. Abdominal pain, cramps
C. Diarrhea (diminishing diarrhea may suggest decreased evacuation and megacolon)
D. Tenesmus
E. Hematochezia
F. Abdominal distention

Physical Findings

A. General
1. Fever
2. Tachycardia
3. Hypotension
4. Lethargy
5. Pallor
6. Altered mental status
B. Abdominal (patients on steroids may demonstrate attenuated signs)
1. Distention
2. Hypoactive bowel sounds
3. Tympany
4. Colonic tenderness
5. Diffuse tenderness with or without rebound tenderness (peritonitis)
6. Absent hepatic dullness (colonic perforation)

Laboratory Findings

A. Hematologic
1. Anemia
2. Leukocytosis with left shift
3. Elevated erythrocyte sedimentation rate
B. Biochemical

1. Hypokalemia
2. Metabolic akalosis
3. Hypomagnesemia
4. Pre-renal azotemia
5. Hypoalbuminemia

C. Stool studies
   1. Blood
   2. Leukocytes
   3. *C. difficile* toxin (present with pseudomembranous colitis)
   4. Culture (positive for *Salmonella, Shigella, Campylobacter,* or *Yersinia* in bacterial colitis)
   5. Wet mount for ameba
   6. *Cryptosporidium*

D. Human immunodeficiency virus testing and acquired immunodeficiency syndrome (AIDS) status

---

Key Findings

- Prostration
- Altered sensorium
- Fever (>38°C [101.5°F])
- Tachycardia (>120 beats/minute)
- Hypotension

- Toxic general appearance
- Colonic dilation (right or transverse) to at least 6 cm
- Leukocytosis (>10,500 cells/mm³ with left shift)
- Anemia
- Electrolyte disturbances

Diagnosis

A. Radiologic
   1. Abdominal (plain and obstructive series) x-rays
      a. Dilation of transverse or right colon (diameter ≥6 cm)
      b. Absent or edematous haustral pattern
      c. Scalloped, nodular, polypoid wall margins
      d. Intramural gas (pre-perforation), subcutaneous emphysema
      e. Pneumoperitoneum (perforation)
      f. Small bowel gas
   2. Computed tomography may be helpful
      a. Diffuse colonic thickening in pseudomembranous colitis
      b. Pneumoperitoneum, abscess
      c. AIDS patients

B. Endoscopic
   1. Flexible sigmoidoscopy with or without biopsy may be performed safely, with no preparation and minimal air insufflation, for diagnostic confirmation of colitis.
   2. Colonoscopy should be avoided unless deemed crucial for decision making.

C. Laboratory
   1. Stool studies crucial in diagnosis of infectious or *C. difficile* toxin colitis
   2. Severe exacerbations of IBD may result from *C. difficile* toxin or CMV infection.

Treatment

A. General measures
   1. Nothing by mouth
   2. Nasogastric (NG) or long intestinal tube to suction
   3. Intravenous fluid for volume repletion
   4. Correction of electrolyte disturbances, especially K^+ and Mg^{2+}
   5. Packed red blood cell (PRBC) transfusion for anemia, as indicated
   6. Turn patient every few hours: sides, prone, knee-chest (if possible)
   7. Deep-vein thrombosis prophylaxis
   8. Surgical consultation

B. Monitoring
   1. Abdominal x-ray at least daily
   2. Serial abdominal examination
      a. Check bowel sounds, distention, hepatic dullness, peritoneal signs
      b. Perform at least twice daily
   3. Daily serum electrolyte assays and complete blood cell count

C. Specific measures and drugs
   1. Specific antimicrobial treatment for *C. difficile*, ameba, CMV, other infectious agents
   2. Hydrocortisone 300 to 400 mg/day, or methylprednisolone 60 to 80 mg/day, intravenously in divided doses (if due to IBD)
   3. Broad-spectrum antibiotics: ampicillin, aminoglycoside, and metronidazole; may use third-generation cephalosporin alone
   4. No antidiarrheal, opiate, or anticholinergic (including anticholinergic antidepressant) drugs
   5. Mesalamine and sulfasalazine are not indicated acutely.
   6. Consider cyclosporine 4 mg/kg intravenously if little improvement in 7 to 10 days and no surgical indications.

D. Indications for surgery (subtotal colectomy, end ileostomy, retention of rectal stump)
   1. Perforation
   2. Peritonitis

Key Treatment

- Give nothing by mouth and maintain NG suction.

- Position patient for flatus passage.

- Monitor for and correct fluid and electrolyte disorders.

- Consider PRBC transfusion.

- Perform stool studies for *C. difficile*, pathogenic bacteria, ova, and parasites.

- Consider diagnostic flexible sigmoidoscopy with biopsy (safe and valuable).

- Give corticosteroids and broad-spectrum antibiotics for IBD.

- Give appropriate antibacterial or antiviral drugs for infectious colitis.

- Do not give opiate, antidiarrheal, or anticholinergic drugs.

- Repeat abdominal examinations frequently.

- Obtain abdominal x-ray at least once daily.

- Consult surgeon for participation in management (mandatory).

- Make decision regarding surgery in 48 to 72 hours.

3. Continued hemorrhage
4. No improvement in 48 to 72 hours and
   a. Worsening toxicity
   b. Increasing dilation
   c. If patient stable, consider continuation of treatment for 7 to 10 days (parenteral nutrition may be indicated).

Prognosis

A. 70% to 80% of patients may require surgery during admission for toxic megacolon from IBD.

B. 30% to 50% of patients responding to medical therapy will require colectomy within a year.

C. 0 to 45% mortality rates reported, with the highest surgical mortality seen in patients who perforate

D. Early surgical intervention is associated with the best prognosis.

E. Colectomy in AIDS patients with infectious toxic megacolon appears to be associated with a poor prognosis.

 Bibliography

Beaugerie L, Ngô Y, Goujard F, et al. Etiology and management of toxic megacolon in patients with human immunodeficiency virus infection. Gastroenterology 1994; 107:858–863.

Lichtiger S, Present DH, Kornbluth A, et al. Cyclosporine in severe ulcerative colitis refractory to steroid therapy. N Engl J Med 1994;330:1841–1845.

Present DH. Toxic megacolon. Med Clin North Am 1993; 77:1129–1148.

Roy MA. Inflammatory bowel disease. Surg Clin North Am 1997;77:1419–1431.

Sheth SG, LaMont JT. Toxic megacolon. Lancet 1998;351: 509–513.

134 Acute Renal Failure

James Sullivan
Richard W. Carlson

Acute renal failure (ARF) affects one-fourth of intensive care unit (ICU) patients and significantly increases mortality and morbidity, particularly in the setting of multiorgan failure and refractory hypotension. Early recognition and treatment of ARF may limit progression of renal dysfunction and complications. Causes of ARF in this setting are usually multifactorial, but often include decreased effective renal perfusion and exogenous or endogenous nephrotoxins.

Terminology

A. Acute renal failure
1. Rapid decline of glomerular filtration rate (GFR) with retention of nitrogenous wastes
2. Manifests as a rise in serum creatinine concentration by more than 0.5 mg/dL or 50% above baseline, or complications requiring dialysis
B. Oliguric renal failure: ARF with urine output of less than 400 mL/day or less than 20 mL/hour (see Chapter 3, Oliguria)
C. Nonoliguric renal failure
1. Acute renal failure with urine output greater than 400 mL/day
2. Prognosis is better than in oliguric renal failure
D. Serum creatinine concentration
1. The best indicator of renal function
2. Correlates inversely with GFR
E. Serum urea nitrogen (BUN)
1. A common indicator of renal function
2. Affected by multiple factors such as corticosteroids, tetracycline, gastrointestinal (GI) bleeding

Classification

A. Pre-renal failure
1. Solute clearance limited by renal perfusion; GFR and tubular function initially intact
2. Causes
   a. Hypovolemia
      (1) Blood loss: trauma, GI or other bleeding
      (2) Third space fluid sequestration: burns, peritonitis, pancreatitis, bowel obstruction, hypoalbuminemia, nephrotic syndrome, cirrhosis
      (3) Gastrointestinal: diarrhea, vomiting, nasogastric suction
      (4) Renal loss: diabetic ketoacidosis, mannitol, diabetes insipidus, hypokalemia, hypercalcemia
      (5) Skin loss: sweating, burns, exfoliative dermatitis, disordered thermoregulation
   b. Cardiovascular (reduced cardiac output): myocardial infarction, cardiogenic shock, pericardial tamponade, pulmonary embolism, cardiopulmonary bypass, dysrhythmias
   c. Renal vascular obstruction: occlusion, constriction, emboli, thrombosis, vasculitis, atherosclerosis, abdominal aortic dissection
   d. Renal vascular dysregulation
      (1) Prostaglandin or angiotensin converting enzyme (ACE) inhibitors
      (2) Sepsis
      (3) Hepatorenal syndrome
         (a) Features include hypotension (systemic vasodilation) and oliguria (renal vasoconstriction) in association with severe hepatic dysfunction.
         (b) Pathogenesis is unknown.
         (c) Reversible alternative causes (e.g., hypovolemia) must be excluded.
         (d) High mortality
B. Intrinsic renal failure
1. Tubulointerstitial insult with decreased GFR and solute filtration (may be reversible)
2. Etiologies
   a. Tubular: acute tubular necrosis
   b. Ischemic: prolonged pre-renal azotemia
   c. Toxin: antibiotic use (e.g., aminoglycosides), contrast dye, heavy metals
   d. Pigment-related: rhabdomyolysis, hemolysis, heat injuries, transfusion reactions
   e. Pregnancy: eclampsia, uterine hemorrhage, septic abortion, amniotic fluid embolism
   f. Interstitial nephritis
      (1) Infectious: bacteria, fungi, viruses
      (2) Infiltrative: lymphoma, sarcoidosis
      (3) Antibiotics: penicillins, rifampin, sulfa,

vancomycin, quinolones, cephalosporins, erythromycin, acyclovir, ethambutol
   (4) Diuretics: thiazides, furosemide, triamterene
   (5) Other: nonsteroidal antiinflammatory agents (NSAIDs), ACE inhibitors, H₂-receptor blocking agents, phenobarbital, phenytoin, allopurinol, interferon, α-methyldopa
g. Glomerular causes
   (1) Antiglomerular basement membrane antibody (anti-GBM): Goodpasture's syndrome
   (2) Antineutrophil cytoplasmic antibodies (ANCA): Wegener's granulomatosis, microscopic polyarteritis nodosa
   (3) Glomerular immune complexes and hypocomplementemia: postinfectious and membranoproliferative glomerulonephritis, subacute bacterial endocarditis, systemic lupus erythematosus
   (4) Absence of anti-GBM, ANCA and hypocomplementemia: Henoch-Schönlein purpura, immunoglobulin A nephropathy, classic polyarteritis nodosa, radiation injury
   (5) Hyperviscosity syndrome: multiple myeloma, Waldenström's macroglobulinemia, polycythemia
   (6) Drugs: cyclosporine, amphotericin B, oral contraceptives, mitomycin, cisplatin, bleomycin, radiocontrast agents
   (7) Other: hemolytic-uremic syndrome, thrombotic thrombocytopenic purpura, malignant hypertension, scleroderma crisis, toxemia
C. Post-renal disorders (outflow obstruction)
   1. Intrarenal obstruction: clots, stones, papillary necrosis, fungus balls, crystals (acyclovir, methotrexate, sulfa, oxalate, or urate)
   2. Extraureteral obstruction: malignancy, endometriosis, retroperitoneal processes
   3. Lower tract obstruction: urethral stricture, prostate disease, bladder masses, neurogenic bladder

---

Key Clinical Findings

- Findings are nonspecific and may be minimal until renal dysfunction becomes severe.
- Symptoms correlate with rapidity of progressive renal dysfunction.
- Common signs and symptoms include malaise, nausea and vomiting, weakness, altered sensorium, dyspnea, chest pain (pericarditis), anasarca, oliguria, and asterixis.

Special Considerations

A. Assess vascular volume.
   1. Exclude hypovolemia.
   2. Consider hemodynamic monitoring if fluid and cardiac status uncertain.
B. Exclude toxin-induced injury.
C. Exclude obstruction.
   1. Insert urinary catheter.
   2. Perform ultrasonography.
      a. May be negative in the presence of hypovolemia or retroperitoneal fibrosis
      b. Useful to identify both kidneys
D. Renal biopsy
   1. Limited value except in ARF with unknown intrinsic cause (e.g., nephritis or ARF with renal transplant)
   2. May help guide therapy (e.g., use of corticosteroids)

PEARLS—DRUG-INDUCED ACUTE INTERSTITIAL NEPHRITIS

- May present with bilateral flank pain, fever, sterile pyuria, eosinophilia, hematuria, rash
- Peripheral eosinophilia may be transient.
- Common with penicillins
- Typically occurs after several days of treatment with the offending agent

---

Laboratory and Other Tests (see Table 134–1)

A. Fractional excretion of sodium (FENa)
   1. Calculated from urine sodium (Na_u), serum sodium (Na_s), urine creatinine (Cr_u), and serum creatinine (Cr_s) concentrations as:

   $$FENa = 100\% \times \frac{Na_u \div Na_s}{Cr_u \div Cr_s}$$

   2. Assesses ability of tubules to excrete or absorb sodium in relationship to GFR (creatinine filtration)
   3. Helps distinguish pre-renal, renal, and post-renal causes
   4. Less predictive with diuretic use, chronic renal insufficiency, high aldosterone levels, or metabolic alkalosis
B. Other tests: calcium and uric acid concentration, creatine phosphokinase activity, protein electrophoresis, anion and osmole gaps, complement, anti-GBM, c-ANCA, p-ANCA, rheumatoid factor

TABLE 134-1. DISTINGUISHING ETIOLOGY USING LABORATORY FEATURES

Condition	FE_{Na}	Urine Osmolality (mOsm/kg H_2O)	BUN: Creatinine	Urine Sodium (mmol/L)	Proteinuria	Urine Sediment	Clinical Correlates
Pre-renal failure	<1	>500	>10:1	<20	Trace to none	Normal, hyaline or granular casts	CHF, cirrhosis, nephrosis
Renal tubular injury	≫1	<350	<15:1	>20	Mild to moderate	Pigmented or granular casts	Trauma, shock, postoperative, sepsis, ischemia
Interstitial disorders	≫1	<350	<15:1	>20	Mild to moderate	WBCs, WBC casts, eosinophils, RBCs	Contrast dye, lymphoma, infection, chemotherapy

FE_{Na} = fractional excretion of sodium, BUN = serum urea nitrogen, CHF = congestive heart failure, WBC = white blood cell, RBC = red blood cell.

CAUTION

Acute obstruction of one kidney should not alter renal function. However, if obstruction is suspected, both kidneys should be identified because obstruction with only one functioning kidney will cause renal failure.

Complications

A. Metabolic
   1. Metabolic acidosis
   2. Hyperkalemia
   3. Hyponatremia
   4. Hyperphosphatemia
   5. Hyperuricemia
   6. Hypocalcemia
   7. Hypermagnesemia
   8. Disturbances of salt and water balance
   9. Catabolic state
B. Cardiovascular
   1. Volume overload, cardiogenic pulmonary edema
   2. Uremic (permeability) pulmonary edema
   3. Pericarditis
   4. Hypertension
   5. Cardiac dysrhythmias
C. Neurologic
   1. Uremic syndrome: neuropsychiatric alterations, asterixis, myoclonus, hyperreflexia, obtundation, coma
   2. Focal neurologic defects, seizures
D. Gastrointestinal
   1. Bleeding
   2. Nausea, vomiting, anorexia, malnutrition
   3. Gastritis, pancreatitis, ileus

E. Hematologic
   1. Coagulopathy, platelet dysfunction
   2. Anemia
F. Infectious
   1. Immunosuppression
   2. Increased risk of sepsis

PEARLS—IMMUNE-RELATED RENAL FAILURE

- Prompt recognition is crucial.
- Early use of immunosuppressants or plasmapheresis lowers risk of progressing to end-stage renal failure.

Treatment

A. Hemodynamic
   1. Hypovolemia: volume load with crystalloids (see Chapter 208, Fluid Challenge)
   2. Hypervolemia: attempt diuresis, restrict fluids, provide dialysis
      a. Loop diuretics: after excluding hypovolemia, consider trial of escalating doses of IV furosemide to 400 mg, or IV infusion 10 to 20 mg/hour (see Chapter 166, Diuretics)
      b. Low-dose dopamine (<5 μg/kg per minute): dilates renal arterioles, increases renal blood flow and GFR; however, not proven to be efficacious in reversing renal failure
   3. Optimize cardiac output.
B. Metabolic
   1. Maintain acid-base balance.
      a. Restrict phosphate intake and give oral phosphate-binding agents (aluminum hydroxide or calcium carbonate).
      b. Treat severe or symptomatic hypocalcemia.
   2. Treat hyperkalemia (see Chapter 40).

a. Moderate hyperkalemia (5.5 to 6.5 mmol/L)

   (1) Ion-exchange resin (sodium polystyrene sulfonate 15 to 30 g every 3 to 4 hours, with sorbitol 50 to 100 mL 20% solution)

   (2) Consider loop diuretics.

   (3) Potassium restriction

b. Severe hyperkalemia (>6.5 mmol/L)

   (1) Glucose and insulin

   (2) Intravenous sodium bicarbonate

   (3) Intravenous calcium salts

   (4) Nebulized β-adrenergic agent (albuterol 10 to 20 mg)

   (5) Intravenous hypertonic saline

3. Provide nutritional support.

C. Hematologic

1. Anemia: antacids, H_2-receptor blocking agents, recombinant erythropoietin

2. Platelet dysfunction: desmopressin

D. Infectious

1. Strict catheter and vascular access management

2. High index of suspicion for sepsis

E. Dialysis (see Chapter 203, Hemodialysis)

1. Does not alter mortality

2. Short-term dialysis may be required; does not predict need for chronic dialysis.

Key Indications for Acute Hemodialysis

- Symptomatic volume overload (congestive heart failure, pulmonary edema)

- Refractory metabolic derangements (e.g., metabolic acidosis, hyperkalemia)

- Symptomatic uremia (bleeding diathesis, encephalopathy)

- Uremic pericarditis

F. Continuous renal replacement therapy (see Chapter 204, Continuous Renal Replacement Therapies)

1. Alternative to standard, intermittent dialytic therapy in selected critically ill patients

2. Advantages: continuous (reduces hemodynamic perturbations with control of fluid and electrolytes); facilitates nutritional support; improves removal of large molecular weight solutes

3. Disadvantages: complicates dosing of vasoactive agents, antibiotics, and protein-bound drugs; anticoagulation requirements; increased requirement for bedside personnel

G. Pharmacology

1. Avoid nephrotoxic drugs.

2. Adjust medications for renal dysfunction.

H. Prevention

1. Radiocontrast dye

a. Increased risk: diabetes; preexisting renal dysfunction

b. Ensure adequate vascular volume: 0.45% saline 0.5 to 2.0 m/kg per hour before procedure.

c. Consider *N*-acetylcysteine (600 mg orally every 12 hours) prior to contrast.

d. Avoid NSAIDs.

2. Meticulous dosing of nephrotoxic agents

3. Vigorous management of myoglobinuria and hemoglobinuria (see Chapter 153, Rhabdomyolysis and Chapter 121, Transfusion Reactions)

Key Prognosis

- Overall mortality is approximately 50% to 60% for ICU patients.

- Mortality is increased in patients with sepsis and multiple organ dysfunction, trauma, postoperative state, maximum creatinine greater than 3 mg/dL, advanced age, and prior renal dysfunction.

Bibliography

Briglia A, Paganini EP. Acute renal failure in the intensive care unit. Therapy overview, patient risk stratification, complications of renal replacement, and special circumstances. Clin Chest Med 1999;20:347–366.

De Mendonca A, Vincent J–L, Suter PM, et al. Acute renal failure in the ICU: risk factors and outcome evaluated by the SOFA score. Intensive Care Med 2000;26:915–921.

Green J, Abassi Z, Winaver J, Skorecki KL. Acute renal failure: Clinical and pathophysiologic aspects. In: Seldin DW, Giebisch G (eds). The Kidney: Physiology and Pathophysiology, 3rd ed. Philadelphia: Lippincott Williams & Wilkins, 2001, pp 2329–2363.

Hladunewich M, Rosenthal MH. Pathophysiology and management of renal insufficiency in the perioperative and critically ill patient. Anesthesiol Clin North Am 2000;18:773–789.

Ichai C, Soubielle J, Carles M, et al. Comparison of the renal effects of low to high doses of dopamine and dobutamine in critically ill patients: A single-blind randomized study. Crit Care Med 2000;28:921–928.

Sladen RN. Oliguria in the ICU: systemic approach to diagnosis and treatment. Anesthesiol Clin North Am 2000;18:739–752.

Tepel M, van der Giet M, Schwarzfeld C, et al. Prevention of radiographic-contrast-agent-induced reductions in renal function by acetylcysteine. N Engl J Med 2000;343:180–184.

Vanholder R, Van Biesen W, Lameire N. What is the renal replacement method of first choice for intensive care patients? J Am Soc Nephrol 2001;12(Suppl 17):S40–S43.

135 Chronic Renal Failure

James Sullivan
Richard W. Carlson

There are over 280,000 patients in the United States with end-stage renal disease. Thus, patients with diverse etiologies of chronic renal insufficiency are commonly encountered in the intensive care unit (ICU). Impairment may range from mild dysfunction to end-stage renal disease. Critical illness or injury is associated with the risk of progressive renal dysfunction, as well as increased morbidity and mortality in this population.

Terminology

A. Chronic renal failure
1. Progressive, long-term loss of renal function from any cause
2. End-stage renal disease
B. Uremic pulmonary edema
1. Excessive interstitial or alveolar lung water accumulation from uremia
2. Mechanism is increased permeability of the pulmonary vascular endothelium; i.e., noncardiogenic or low-pressure pulmonary edema.
C. Uremic pericarditis
1. Acute pericardial inflammation that occurs as a complication of uremia
2. Often occurs within the initial weeks of starting dialysis
D. Dialysis-associated pericarditis: pericarditis occurring during chronic dialysis
E. Permanent arteriovenous access for chronic dialysis
1. Native vein fistula: surgically created, direct communication between a peripheral artery and a peripheral vein
2. Arteriovenous graft: surgically created communication between a peripheral artery and a peripheral vein using a synthetic conduit
F. Dry ultrafiltration
1. Hemodialysis without dialysate
2. Uses negative pressure for fluid removal, without solute removal

Key Etiologies

- Diabetes
- Hypertension
- Glomerulonephritis
- Cystic disease

Classification

A. Stage 1: decreased renal reserve
1. Glomerular filtration rate (GFR) is approximately 100 to 120 mL/minute.
2. Usually asymptomatic
3. Glomerular filtration rate declines in response to physiologic change (e.g., pregnancy), but remains near normal.
B. Stage 2: renal insufficiency
1. GFR is approximately 40 to 100 mL/minute.
2. Serum urea nitrogen and creatinine concentrations increase.
3. Usually asymptomatic
4. Calcium, phosphate, and potassium homeostasis are intact but altered by changes in regulatory hormones (e.g., parathormone, insulin).
C. Stage 3: renal failure
1. GFR is approximately 10 to 50 mL/minute.
2. Symptoms from declining renal function manifest (e.g., fatigue, malaise).
3. Electrolyte disturbances occur in association with progressive failure of compensatory mechanisms.
4. Normochromic, normocytic anemia is often present.
D. Stage 4: uremia
1. GFR is lower than 10 mL/minute.
2. Symptoms are present.
3. Treatment: extracorporeal renal replacement or transplantation

Key Symptoms

- Malaise
- Nausea
- Fatigue
- Dyspnea on exertion
- Edema
- Oliguria

Laboratory Tests

A. Serum creatinine concentration
1. Key test for monitoring renal function
2. Allows estimation of creatinine clearance

481

B. Key serum electrolyte concentrations
1. Potassium
2. Sodium
3. Phosphate
4. Calcium
5. Magnesium
C. Acid-base balance
1. Total serum CO_2 content
2. Serum anion gap
3. Arterial blood gases and pH
D. Hemoglobin or hematocrit
1. Anemia is universal.
2. There is altered red cell rheology and nitric oxygen scavenger function.
E. Uremic platelet dysfunction
1. Defects include decreased platelet factor III and glycoprotein Ib, increased cyclic adenosine monophosphate and guanosine monophosphate, decreased adenosine diphosphate and serotonin, cyclooxygenase defects, and decreased platelet adhesiveness.
2. Practical functional tests for routine use are lacking.
F. Coagulation profile
1. Prothrombin time and partial thromboplastin time assays
2. Von Willebrand factor and receptor defects
G. Serum creatine phosphokinase (total and MB fraction) activity and plasma troponin concentration (prolonged elevation can occur with renal insufficiency)
H. Drug levels
1. Renal patients typically receive 7 to 10 medications; thus, they have a high incidence of adverse drug reactions.
2. Adjust dose and interval for renal dysfunction.
3. Monitor drug levels.

PEARL

Clinical manifestations may be absent or nonspecific, but they generally correlate with the degree of renal dysfunction.

Complications

A. Cardiovascular
1. Hypotension
a. May aggravate renal dysfunction
b. Etiologies include hypovolemia, depressed left ventricular function, cardiac tamponade, myocardial infarction, autonomic dysfunction, and adrenal insufficiency.
c. Hypovolemia may be due to acute illness (e.g., bleeding, trauma, third-space fluid collections), inadequate fluid intake, overaggressive dialysis or diuretic use.
2. Fluid overload
a. Excessive fluid intake
b. Inadequate diuresis or dialysis
3. Ischemic heart disease and acute myocardial infarction
a. Common in this patient population; related to hypertension, accelerated atherosclerosis, diabetes, lipid disorders
b. Indications for thrombolytic therapy are similar to nonrenal patient.
c. Higher postangioplasty re-stenosis rate and higher perioperative bypass mortality
4. Left ventricular hypertrophy is also common.
5. Pericarditis and pericardial effusion (with risk of tamponade)
6. Thrombosis of vascular access
B. Infectious
1. Uremia poses an increased risk of infection.
a. Immunosuppression; blunted graft-versus-host reaction
b. Neutrophil dysfunction; decreased responsiveness to viral antigens
2. Dialysis access sites and devices are commonly implicated.
a. *Staphylococcus aureus* or *Staphylococcus epidermidis*
b. *Escherichia coli* from urinary source in hemodialysis patients
c. *Pseudomonas aeruginosa* or *Staphylococcus* in peritoneal dialysis patients
C. Neurologic
1. Uremic encephalopathy and neuropsychiatric changes
a. Progressive encephalopathic: fatigue, sleep-wake disturbances, loss of concentration, confusion, delirium, coma, electroencephalographic changes, parathyroid disturbances, aluminum dialysate toxicity
b. Musculoskeletal features: hyperreflexia, twitching, asterixis
c. Depression
2. Autonomic nervous system dysfunction
a. Common; multifactorial causes
b. Manifestations: orthostatic hypotension, altered blood pressure and circadian rhythm, reduced responsiveness to vasopressors, car-

diac dysrhythmias, altered baroreceptor sensitivity, gastrointestinal motility defects

3. Disequilibrium syndrome
   a. Onset is usually after initiation of dialysis, but may occur during chronic dialysis.
   b. More common in elderly patients
   c. Probably a consequence of fluid and solute shifts related to idiogenic osmoles
   d. Features: nausea, vomiting, seizures, altered mentation
   e. Management: shorter, more frequent dialysis; reduced flow rate

4. Dialysis dementia
   a. Manifests as progressive cognitive deterioration, myoclonus, seizures
   b. Results from aluminum in dialysate or phosphate binders
   c. May be irreversible
   d. Management: eliminate excess aluminum; deferoxamine

5. Wernicke's encephalopathy: thiamine loss in dialysate

6. Cerebrovascular events: hypertension, accelerated atherosclerosis, anticoagulation, uremic coagulopathy

D. Pulmonary
   1. Pulmonary edema
      a. Cardiogenic (volume overload)
      b. Noncardiogenic (uremic)
   2. Pneumonia
   3. Pulmonary emboli
   4. Pulmonary–renal syndromes
      a. Antiglomerular basement membrane
      b. Wegener's granulomatous vasculitis

Bibliography

Bennett WM, Aronoff GR, Golper TA, et al. Drug Prescribing in Renal Failure: Dosing Guidelines for Adults, 3rd ed. Philadelphia: American College of Physicians, 1994.

Goldman M, Vanherwegham JL. Bacterial infections in chronic hemodialysis patients: epidemiologic and pathophysiologic aspects. Adv Nephrol 1990, 19:315–332.

Goodman WG, Goldin J, Kuizon BD, et al. Coronary-artery calcification in young adults with end-stage renal disease who are undergoing dialysis. N Engl J Med 2000; 342:1478–1483.

Kaul TK, Fields BL, Reddy MA. Cardiac operations with end-stage renal disease. Ann Thorac Surg 1994;57:691–696.

Kimmel PL. Management of the patient with chronic renal disease. In: Greenberg A (ed). Primer on Kidney Diseases, 2nd ed. San Diego: National Kidney Foundation, Academic Press, 1998:433–440.

Laski ME, Kurtzman NA, Sabatini S. Chronic renal failure. In: Seldin DW, Giebisch G (eds). The Kidney, 3rd ed. Philadelphia: Lippincott Williams and Williams, 2001: 2375–2409.

Remuzzi G, Bertani T. Pathophysiology of progressive nephropathies. N Engl J Med 1998;339:1448–1456.

Sagripanti A, Barsotti G. Bleeding and thrombosis in chronic uremia. Nephron 1997;75:125–139.

Weigert AL, Schafer AI. Uremic bleeding: pathogenesis and therapy. Am J Med Sci 1998;316:94–104.

136 Preoperative Evaluation of the Critically Ill Patient

Stephen O. Heard

Preoperative evaluation of the critically ill patient can be challenging. Many times, the evaluation must be brief because it coincides with resuscitation. Perioperative mortality for elective procedures ranges from 0.001% to 1.9%, but can increase twofold to fivefold for emergency procedures. For patients with underlying disease, the mortality increases even further. The preoperative evaluation should focus on several areas: presence of concurrent diseases and opportunities for improving the patient's condition before the procedure.

Key Cardiac Risk Factors

- Recent myocardial infarction (<3 months)
- Unstable angina
- Decompensated congestive heart failure
- Severe cardiac dysrhythmia or high-grade atrioventricular block
- Aortic stenosis or other severe valvular disease
- Emergency operation or critical illness

History

A. Present illness
   1. Reason for admission to the hospital
   2. Reason for surgery
   3. Complications that have occurred during this hospitalization that could have an impact on conduct of anesthesia and surgery
B. Past history of surgery and anesthesia
   1. Airway problems
   2. Malignant hyperthermia
   3. Prolonged paralysis following succinylcholine
   4. Respiratory or cardiac complications
C. Drugs
   1. Cardiovascular drugs
      a. Vasopressors and inotropes
      b. Antidysrhythmics
      c. β-Adrenergic blockers
   2. Sedatives and analgesics
   3. Antibiotics and time of next dose
D. Allergies
   1. Drugs
   2. Latex
E. Social history
   1. Tobacco
   2. Alcohol (potential for perioperative withdrawal)
   3. Recreational drugs
   4. Toxicologic screening results from admission, if relevant
F. Review of systems
   1. Neurologic
      a. Spinal cord injury and level of deficit
         (1) Hyperkalemia with use of succinylcholine
         (2) Autonomic hyperreflexia
      b. Head injury
         (1) Intracranial hypertension and cerebral perfusion pressure.
         (2) Presence of pneumocephalus mandates avoidance of nitrous oxide as an anesthetic.
      c. All neurologic deficits should be documented, especially if regional anesthesia is to be used.
   2. Cardiovascular
      a. Coronary artery disease
         (1) Frequency and precipitating factors for angina pectoris
         (2) Previous myocardial infarction(s) and date(s)
         (3) History of congestive heart failure
         (4) Physical activity and functional status
      b. Hypertension
         (1) Severity
         (2) Adequacy of treatment
      c. History of dysrhythmias
      d. Valvular dysfunction
      e. Pacemaker
   3. Pulmonary

a. Tobacco use
b. Asthma
  (1) Frequency of attacks and need for hospitalization
  (2) Drug therapy and need for systemic corticosteroids
  (3) Adequacy of treatment
c. Chronic lung disease
  (1) Change in sputum production
  (2) Recent infections
4. Gastrointestinal
  a. Record time of last meal.
  b. Gastroesophageal reflux disease (increases the risk for aspiration)
  c. Bowel obstruction
    (1) Increases the risk for aspiration
    (2) Mandates avoidance of nitrous oxide
  d. Presence of liver dysfunction
    (1) Portal hypertension
    (2) Synthetic function
      (a) Hypoproteinemia
      (b) Coagulopathy
      (c) Altered volume of distribution and clearance of drugs
5. Genitourinary
  a. Renal function
    (1) Urine volume
    (2) Nature of dysfunction
      (a) Prerenal
      (b) Intrinsic
      (c) Obstructive
    (3) Dialysis
      (a) Hemodialysis (time of last dialysis, location of shunt or fistula)
      (b) Continuous venovenous or arteriovenous hemofiltration
    (4) Altered clearance of drugs
  b. Pregnancy
    (1) Duration
    (2) Preeclampsia
    (3) HELLP (hemolysis, liver dysfunction and thrombocytopenia) syndrome
    (4) Risk of hypotension in supine position from gravid uterus pressing on inferior vena cava
6. Endocrine
  a. Diabetes
    (1) Drug therapy: oral hypoglycemic agents or insulin
    (2) Dose and route of administration
    (3) End-organ sequelae
  b. Adrenal insufficiency
    (1) Relative versus absolute
    (2) History of steroid use (type, dose, dosing frequency, date of last use)
    (3) Assessment of adrenal function by stimulation testing
  c. Hypothyroidism (discriminate from sick euthyroid syndrome)
  d. Syndrome of inappropriate antidiuretic hormone secretion
7. Hematologic
  a. Anemia
    (1) Severity
    (2) Potential for blood loss
    (3) Need for blood transfusion perioperatively
    (4) Assurance that blood is available for surgery
    (5) Techniques for blood conservation
      (a) Normovolemic hemodilution
      (b) Autologous preoperative donation
      (c) Cell saver
      (d) Perioperative erythropoietin
  b. Thrombocytopenia
    (1) Etiology
    (2) Severity
    (3) Need for correction perioperatively
8. Dermatologic
  a. Burns
    (1) Adequacy of resuscitation
    (2) Large-bore IV catheters
    (3) Neuromuscular blocking agents
      (a) Succinylcholine: hyperkalemia
      (b) Nondepolarizing agents: resistance to effect
  b. Potential for skin breakdown in debilitated patients during long procedures

Physical Findings

A. General
  1. Vital signs
  2. Presence and size of IV catheters
  3. Presence and types of invasive hemodynamic monitoring catheters
  4. Assessment of volume status
B. HEENT
  1. Airway
    a. Mallampati classification
    b. Mouth opening

c. Range of motion of neck

d. Teeth

e. If patient already intubated

(1) Route of intubation

(2) Size of endotracheal tube and depth of placement

2. Nasogastric tube

C. Neck

1. Status of cervical spine, if trauma patient

2. Other limitation in range of motion (e.g., cervical spine arthritis)

D. Lungs

1. Breath sounds

2. Presence of wheezing or rhonchi

3. Ventilator settings

a. Mode of ventilation

b. Tidal volume

c. FIO_2

d. Positive end-expiratory pressure

4. Adequacy of anesthesia machine ventilator to support patient

5. Chest tubes

E. Heart

1. Rhythm

2. Murmurs

3. Rubs

4. Pacemaker

a. Type

b. Preoperative interrogation

F. Abdomen

1. Distention and potential for interference with ventilation

2. Ascites (need for increased intraoperative fluids if drained)

3. Hepatomegaly (potential altered volume of distribution of drugs and diminished clearance)

G. Extremities

1. Range of motion (intraoperative positioning)

2. Pulses (contemplating arterial catheters)

3. Peripheral IV catheters

H. Central nervous system

1. Mental status

2. Pupillary response

3. Motor and sensory function (regional anesthesia technique)

4. Intracranial pressure

a. Type of monitoring device

b. Frequency of drainage, if ventriculostomy

Laboratory and Other Tests

A. Blood tests

1. Complete blood cell and platelet counts

2. Serum biochemical tests

a. Sodium, potassium, and chloride concentrations and total CO_2 content

b. Urea nitrogen and creatinine concentrations

c. Glucose

3. Prothrombin and partial thromboplastin times

4. Determination of serum drug concentrations: assay if there is recent change in dose or condition of patient

5. Further blood testing should be performed only if the results will change the preparation or management of the patient perioperatively.

B. Pulmonary

1. Chest x-ray

2. Arterial blood gases

3. Spirometry: no better than clinical examination and blood gases in predicting complications and need for postoperative mechanical ventilation, except for

a. Pneumonectomy

b. As a means to assess adequacy bronchodilator therapy

C. Cardiovascular

1. Routine: 12-lead electrocardiogram

2. Further evaluation is predicated on the following.

a. Clinical markers of risk

b. Functional capacity of the patient

c. Risk of the surgical procedure

3. Noninvasive testing

a. Treadmill testing

b. Dipyridamole-thallium or adenosine-thallium testing

c. Dobutamine stress echocardiography

d. Echocardiography

e. Gated radionuclide angiography

4. Coronary angiography

D. Microbiologic cultures, if relevant

E. Pulmonary artery catheterization

1. Use for preoperative monitoring is controversial.

2. Few data support preoperative insertion (>1 day) in high-risk patients.

3. Use should not be predicated on the surgical procedure alone, but on the procedure along with the patient's condition and underlying disease states.

Key Tests

- Chest x-ray

- 12-Lead electrocardiogram

- Complete blood cell and platelet counts

- Serum electrolytes, glucose, urea nitrogen and creatinine concentrations

- Prothrombin and partial thromboplastin times

- Arterial blood gases

- Selection of other tests is based on condition of patient and the proposed surgery.

- Further testing is performed if the results will change the preparation or management of the patient perioperatively.

Preoperative Drug Treatment

A. Sedatives and analgesics
   1. Sedatives employed to calm the patient
   2. Analgesics employed to treat pain
B. Cardiovascular drugs
   1. Continue antihypertensives
   2. Stop diuretics
C. Bronchodilators: administer metered dose inhalers before start of surgery
D. Hypoglycemic agents
   1. Insulin
      a. Give one-half the usual dose of insulin the morning of surgery.
      b. Provide a basal IV infusion using a crystalloid solution containing 5% dextrose.
   2. Stop oral hypoglycemic agents (increase risk of asymptomatic hypoglycemia).
E. Corticosteroids
   1. Patients with recent steroid therapy should receive stress dose steroid coverage.
   2. Hydrocortisone: 200 to 300 mg/day

F. Aspiration prophylaxis (unintubated patient)
   1. Nonparticulate antacid
   2. H_2-blocker (or proton pump inhibitor), metoclopramide (if no bowel obstruction)
G. Prophylaxis for venous thrombosis
   1. Venous compression boots
   2. Low-dose unfractionated heparin
   3. Low molecular weight heparin
   4. Dextran
   5. Adjusted dose warfarin
H. Antibiotics
   1. Prophylaxis for endocarditis, if relevant
   2. Prophylaxis for surgical wound infections (antibiotic should be administered 30 minutes before incision to maximize effectiveness)

Bibliography

Bourke ME. The patient with a pacemaker or related device. Can J Anaesth 1996;43:R24–R41.

Dajani AS, Taubert KA, Wilson W, et al. Prevention of bacterial endocarditis. Recommendations by the American Heart Association. JAMA 1997;277:1794–1801.

Eagle KA, Brundage BH, Chaitman BR, et al. Guidelines for perioperative cardiovascular evaluation for noncardiac surgery. Report of the American College of Cardiology/American Heart Association Task Force on Practice Guidelines. Committee on Perioperative Cardiovascular Evaluation for Noncardiac Surgery. Circulation 1996;93:1278–1317.

Fischer SP. Cost-effective preoperative evaluation and testing. Chest 1999;115:96S–100S.

Mallampati SR, Gatt SP, Gugino LD, et al. A clinical sign to predict difficult tracheal intubation: a prospective study. Can Anaesth Soc J 1985;32:429–434.

Mangano DT, Layug EL, Wallace A, et al. Effect of atenolol on mortality and cardiovascular morbidity after noncardiac surgery. Multicenter Study of Perioperative Ischemia Research Group [published erratum appears in N Engl J Med 1997;336:1039] N Engl J Med 1996;335:1713–1720.

McCulloch HA, Sprague DH. Myths in vascular anesthesia. Probl Anesth 1991;5:453–467.

Schlaghecke R, Kornely E, Santen RT, et al. The effect of long-term glucocorticoid therapy on pituitary-adrenal responses to exogenous corticotropin-releasing hormone. N Engl J Med 1992;326:226–230.

Smetana GW. Preoperative pulmonary evaluation. N Engl J Med 1999;340:937–944.

Smith MS, Muir H, Hall R. Perioperative management of drug therapy, clinical considerations. Drugs 1996;51:238–259.

137 Chest Trauma

Keith D. Clancy
Mitchell P. Fink

Chest injuries are responsible for 20% to 25% of all deaths due to trauma in the United States. Injuries to the chest wall or the visceral contents of the thoracic cavity can result from both blunt trauma and penetrating trauma. Successful management depends on prompt recognition of life-threatening injuries and timely institution of appropriate therapeutic measures.

Classification and Diagnosis

A. Injuries to the trachea or bronchi
   1. The index of suspicion for these injuries should be raised by the presence of subcutaneous air in the neck or upper chest, or evidence of mediastinal air on chest x-ray.
   2. The diagnosis is often confirmed using bronchoscopy.

B. Injuries to the lung parenchyma
   1. Laceration of the parenchyma causes hemorrhage or air leak.
      a. Bleeding leads to hemothorax.
      b. Air leak causes pneumothorax.
   2. Contusion
      a. Initial chest x-rays may be normal.
      b. Diagnosis is made by seeing unilateral infiltrates on chest x-ray (sometimes associated with rib fractures) or areas of increased density in the lungs on computed tomography (CT) of the chest.

C. Pneumothorax and hemothorax
   1. Simple pneumothorax
      a. Visible on chest x-ray in most cases
      b. Very small or anterior pneumothoraces may be missed on plain films of the chest but will be detected by chest CT.
   2. Tension pneumothorax
      a. Tension pneumothorax should be part of the differential diagnosis for hypotension in patients with chest or multiple trauma.
      b. This diagnosis is suggested by presence of tracheal deviation.
      c. Neck veins may be distended.
      d. Hyper-resonance to percussion is a "textbook" physical examination finding, but is rarely appreciated in clinical practice.
      e. The chest x-ray reveals characteristic findings.
         (1) Absent lung markings on the affected side
         (2) Widening of the intercostal spaces on the affected side
         (3) Shift of the mediastinum away from the affected side
   3. Hemothorax
      a. Can be caused by pulmonary parenchymal injury or laceration of intercostal vessels
      b. Suggested by the presence of pleural fluid on a chest x-ray or CT scan
      c. Diagnosis is confirmed by placing a chest tube.

D. Rib fractures
   1. Diagnosis is made by inspection of the chest x-ray.
   2. Fractures of the first or second rib signify that the chest has absorbed considerable energy; accordingly, presence of this finding should increase the index of suspicion for aortic injury.
   3. A "flail segment" occurs when at least three adjacent ribs are fractured in at least two places.

E. Diaphragmatic laceration
   1. Traumatic injury to the diaphragm usually is limited to the left hemidiaphragm.
   2. Chest x-ray may show elevated left hemidiaphragm or the presence of a (gastric) air bubble in the left pleural space.
   3. CT is the diagnostic study of choice.

F. Cardiac injuries and pericardial tamponade
   1. Types of cardiac injury
      a. Blunt trauma
         (1) Myocardial contusion
         (2) Chamber rupture
         (3) Coronary artery dissection
         (4) Valvular disruption
      b. Penetrating trauma
         (1) Chamber laceration
         (2) Coronary artery laceration
   2. Pericardial tamponade should be part of the differential diagnosis for hypotension in patients with chest trauma or multiple trauma.
      a. Distended neck veins
      b. Distant heart sounds

c. Pericardial fluid detected by ultrasound or transesophageal echocardiography

G. Injuries to the aorta and arch vessels

1. Physical examination findings that suggest injury to the aorta or arch vessels include

   a. Hypotension

   b. Unequal blood pressure measurements in the upper extremities

   c. External evidence of major chest trauma

   d. Palpable sternal fracture

   e. Neurologic findings (e.g., hemiparesis due to injury to the contralateral carotid artery)

2. Chest x-ray findings that suggest injury to the aorta or arch vessels

   a. Massive hemothorax

   b. Loss of the aortic knob

   c. Wide mediastinum (>8 cm on anterior–posterior view)

   d. Depression of the left mainstem bronchus by more than 140° relative to the trachea

   e. Rightward deviation of a nasogastric tube in the esophagus

   f. Rightward displacement of the trachea

3. Chest CT

   a. Hemomediastinum suggests the possibility of aortic or arch vessel injury.

   b. Conversely, absence of hemomediastinum makes it highly unlikely that such injuries are present.

   c. Helical CT angiography can provide images comparable to those obtained by angiography, and can be used to provide a definitive diagnosis.

4. Transesophageal echocardiography

   a. Excellent means for diagnosing injuries to the thoracic aorta

   b. May be less reliable for excluding injuries to the arch vessels

5. Arteriography remains the "gold standard" for diagnosis.

H. Esophagus

1. Esophageal injury due to blunt trauma is uncommon.

2. Penetrating injuries to the esophagus can be diagnosed using either of the following approaches.

   a. Esophagoscopy

   b. Gastrograffin contrast study

Key Diagnosis

- If not recognized and treated immediately, six thoracic injuries can lead to death immediately: (1) acute airway obstruction; (2) open pneumothorax ("sucking chest wound"); (3) tension pneumothorax; (4) massive hemothorax; (5) massive flail chest; (6) cardiac tamponade.

- Six other thoracic injuries also can cause mortality, albeit later: (1) pulmonary contusion; (2) myocardial contusion; (3) aortic disruption; (4) diaphragmatic injury; (5) disruption of the tracheobronchial tree; (6) esophageal injury.

Treatment

A. Injuries to the trachea or bronchi

1. Minor tracheal injuries may be managed with endotracheal intubation only.

2. Major tracheal injuries require operative repair.

3. Major bronchial injuries can lead to persistent air leak from chest tubes (bronchopleural fistula) that can compromise ventilation.

   a. Efforts should be made to avoid high airway pressures.

   b. Bronchopleural fistula is an accepted indication for special modes of mechanical ventilation (jet ventilation or high-frequency oscillation).

   c. Persistent air leak may warrant operative intervention.

B. Injuries to the lung parenchyma

1. Many patients can be managed without intubation and mechanical ventilation.

2. Noninvasive mechanical ventilation using bi-level positive airway pressure may obviate the need for endotracheal intubation in selected cases.

3. Provide aggressive pulmonary toilet.

4. Provide adequate pain control for associated rib fractures.

C. Pneumothorax and hemothorax (see Chapter 202, Chest Tube Thoracostomy)

1. Simple pneumothorax: treatment is placement of a chest tube (fourth or fifth intercostal space at the mid-axillary line)

2. Tension pneumothorax

   a. Tension pneumothorax is potentially life-threatening, and appropriate intervention must be performed immediately.

   b. Initial treatment is pleural decompression using an 18-gauge needle inserted into the ipsilateral pleural space in the second intercostal space at the midclavicular line.

   c. Needle thoracostomy should be followed by placement of a chest tube (fifth intercostal space at the mid-axillary line).

3. Hemothorax

   a. Massive hemothorax can be life-threatening.

   b. Indications for operative intervention

      (1) Initial drainage of more than 1,500 mL of blood after placement of a chest tube

      (2) Ongoing drainage of blood at a rate higher than 250 mL per hour for more than 2 hours after placement of the chest tube

   c. It is important to ensure that all blood is evacuated from the pleural cavity to decrease the risk of entrapped lung, infected hemothorax, or empyema.

D. Rib fractures

1. Pain control is important to avoid the development of complications related to low tidal volumes and impaired clearance of secretions.

   a. Narcotics

   b. Ketorolac or other nonsteroidal anti-inflammatory agent

   c. Thoracic epidural catheter

   d. Local anesthetic infused using an intrapleural catheter

2. Most treatment issues are related to pulmonary contusion that often accompanies rib fractures.

E. Diaphragmatic laceration

1. Operative repair

2. Delay increases morbidity.

F. Cardiac injuries and pericardial tamponade

1. Pericardial tamponade is a life-threatening emergency, and prompt recognition and treatment is imperative; treatment options include

   a. Pericardiocentesis

   b. Creation of a subxyphoid pericardial window

2. See Chapter 23, Myocardial Contusion, for its management.

3. Penetrating or blunt injuries to cardiac chambers require emergency operative repair.

G. Injuries to the aorta and arch vessels

1. Penetrating injuries to the aorta or arch vessels require emergency operative repair.

2. Injury to the aorta due to blunt thoracic trauma

   a. Indications for delaying operative management include

      (1) Severe multisystem trauma associated (in particular) with severe pulmonary dysfunction (i.e., acute respiratory distress syndrome) or marked hemodynamic instability

      (2) Severe head trauma

   b. Temporizing measures to avoid frank aortic rupture while awaiting operative management include tight control of blood pressure to avoid hypertension and administration of β-adrenergic blocking agents to decrease aortic wall stress.

   c. Endovascular stenting also may be an option in selected cases at some centers.

   d. Standard management, however, is surgical repair using a prosthetic graft to replace the damaged aorta.

H. Esophagus

1. Surgical repair

2. Morbidity and mortality are lessened with prompt recognition and treatment.

PEARL

Most thoracic injuries can be managed with only a chest tube; approximately 10% to 15% require thoracotomy.

 Bibliography

Ferguson M, Luchette FA. Management of blunt chest trauma. Respir Care Clin North Am 1996;2:449–466.

Haenel JB, Moore FA, Moore EE. Pulmonary consequences of severe chest trauma. Respir Care Clin North Am 1996;2:401–424.

Madiba TE, Thomson SR, Mdlalose N. Penetrating chest injuries in the firearm era. Injury 2001;32:13–16.

Wicky S, Wintermark M, Schnyder P, et al. Imaging of blunt chest trauma. Eur Radiol 2000;10:1524–1538.

138 Abdominal Trauma

Samuel A. Tisherman

Abdominal injury is a frequent cause of morbidity and mortality in trauma victims. The physical examination of the abdomen is frequently unreliable in blunt trauma victims because of concomitant alcohol or drug intoxication, closed head injury, spinal cord injury, or confounding findings caused by extraabdominal injuries. Consequently, given an appropriate mechanism of injury, adjunctive tests are frequently required to determine if an intra-abdominal injury is present. Management often involves observation. Evaluation of the victim with penetrating trauma is more often dependent upon physical examination. Management more frequently necessitates laparotomy.

Etiology

A. Blunt abdominal injury
  1. Mechanisms of injury
    a. Motor vehicle accident
    b. Motorcycle or bicycle accidents
    c. Falls
    d. Pedestrian struck by a motor vehicle
    e. Assaults
    f. Sports injuries
  2. Commonly injured organs
    a. Liver
    b. Spleen
    c. Kidney
    d. Large and small bowel
    e. Pancreas
B. Penetrating injuries
  1. Mechanisms of injury
    a. Gunshot wounds
    b. Shotgun wounds
    c. Stab wounds
    d. Impalement injuries
  2. Commonly injured organs
    a. Small bowel
    b. Liver
    c. Colon
    d. Stomach

Physical Findings

A. Blunt abdominal injury
  1. Look for ecchymoses and abrasions of the abdominal wall (suggesting, e.g., lap belt injury).
  2. Abdominal distention
    a. Is often caused by swallowing air
    b. May be absent, even in the presence of significant hemoperitoneum
  3. Signs of peritoneal irritation
B. Penetrating abdominal injury
  1. Physical examination is critical for determining trajectory.
  2. Need to "log roll" the patient and examine all creases.
  3. Attempt to elicit peritoneal signs.

PEARL

The peritoneal cavity extends from the nipple line to the buttocks.

Imaging Studies

A. Blunt abdominal injury
  1. Plain x-rays
    a. Chest x-ray may reveal a ruptured diaphragm or pneumoperitoneum.
    b. Pelvic x-ray may reveal pelvic fractures, which are frequently associated with intraabdominal injuries.
    c. Plain x-rays of the abdomen are rarely indicated.
    d. A cystogram is indicated for evaluation of hematuria.
  2. Focused abdominal sonogram for trauma (FAST)
    a. Indications
      (1) Evaluation of hemodynamically unstable patients without obvious need for laparotomy
      (2) Evaluation of patients with an unreliable physical examination (secondary to alcohol or drug intoxication, closed head injury, or spinal cord injury)
      (3) Evaluation of patients requiring prompt transfer to the operating room for nonabdominal procedures (e.g., craniotomy, thoracotomy, amputation of a limb)
      (4) Evaluation of patients with an equivocal physical examination

b. Contraindications
  (1) Obvious need for laparotomy
  (2) Lack of a team member with training and experience with the procedure
c. Examination
  (1) Look for the presence of blood in the peritoneal cavity (hemoperitoneum) in these areas: right upper quadrant (Morrison's pouch), left upper quadrant, pelvis
  (2) Look for the presence of blood in the pericardial sac (hemopericardium) from the subxyphoid view.
3. Computed tomography (CT)
  a. Indications
    (1) Patients with an unreliable physical examination (secondary to alcohol or drug intoxication, closed head injury, or spinal cord injury)
    (2) Hemodynamically stable patients requiring prompt transfer to the operating room for nonabdominal procedures (e.g., craniotomy, thoracotomy, amputation of a limb)
    (3) Patients with an equivocal physical examination
    (4) Patients with an injury to an adjacent structure (e.g., pelvic fracture)
    (5) Patients with a need for prolonged general anesthesia for repair of other injuries
  b. Contraindications
    (1) Hemodynamically unstable patient
    (2) Obvious indication for emergency laparotomy
    (3) Lack of availability of a scanner with adequate resolution
    (4) Lack of personnel on site with the necessary expertise to interpret the scan
  c. Technique
    (1) Oral and IV contrast is standard practice.
    (2) Oral contrast may be omitted if there is a significant risk of aspiration.
    (3) Intravenous contrast may be omitted if the patient has an allergy to contrast agents.
B. Penetrating abdominal injury
  1. Plain x-rays
    a. Obtain chest and abdominal x-rays.
    b. The sum of the number of bullet holes and bullets remaining in the patient must be an even number.

2. Computed tomography
  a. Useful for posterior or flank wounds
  b. Use triple contrast (oral, IV, and rectal).

Diagnostic Procedures and Treatment

A. Local wound exploration for penetrating injury
  1. Use local anesthesia.
  2. Enlarge the initial wound.
  3. Follow the track down to the fascia.
  4. Perform laparotomy if the fascia has been violated.
  5. Discharge the patient if the fascia is intact.
B. Diagnostic peritoneal lavage (DPL)
  1. Indications
    a. In blunt injury, indications are similar to those for ultrasound.
    b. In penetrating injury, DPL is sometimes used after a positive local wound exploration.
  2. Contraindications
    a. Indication for emergency laparotomy
    b. Multiple previous abdominal procedures (relative contraindication)
    c. Pregnancy (relative contraindication)
  3. Technique
    a. Open versus semi-open versus closed
    b. Infraumbilical incision, except for patients with pregnancy or pelvic fracture
    c. Advance the catheter toward the pelvis.
    d. Aspirate any fluid that is present.
    e. If the aspirate is negative, instill 1 L of warm crystalloid solution.
  4. Positive findings in blunt trauma
    a. At least 10 mL gross blood aspirated
    b. At least 100,000 red blood cells/mm^3 in lavage fluid
    c. At least 500 white blood cells/mm^3 in lavage fluid
    d. Bacteria in lavage fluid
    e. Bile in lavage fluid
    f. Food particles in lavage fluid
    g. Stool in lavage fluid
  5. Positive findings for penetrating trauma are similar to those for blunt trauma, except that the threshold for positive red blood cell count is decreased from 100,000 to 10,000 cell/mm^3.
C. Diagnostic laparoscopy for penetrating injury
  1. Use to determine if there has been occult diaphragmatic injury.
  2. Use to determine if tangential gunshot wounds entered the peritoneal cavity.

D. Indications for laparotomy in blunt abdominal injury
  1. Peritoneal signs
  2. Hemodynamic instability (with or without positive FAST or DPL)
  3. Specific injuries (e.g., ruptured diaphragm, pancreatic transection)
  4. Free fluid in the peritoneal cavity without solid organ injury
  5. Hollow viscus injury

E. Gunshot wounds
  1. Exploratory laparotomy is almost always indicated.
  2. Evaluation of tangential wounds may include laparoscopy or triple-contrast CT.
  3. Shotgun wounds
    a. Close-range wounds should be managed in the same way as other gunshot wounds.
    b. Laparotomy is required for peritoneal penetration.

F. Stab wounds
  1. Immediate exploratory laparotomy is indicated for hypotension, peritoneal signs, and evisceration (controversial).
  2. Anterior stab wounds
    a. One-third do not penetrate the peritoneum, one-third enter the peritoneum but do not cause injury, one-third cause an intra-abdominal injury that requires operative repair.
    b. Negative local wound exploration may allow the patient to be discharged home.
    c. Serial physical examinations are appropriate.
    d. Diagnostic peritoneal lavage may be appropriate for patients with an equivocal examination or positive wound exploration.
  3. Back or flank stab wounds
    a. Obtain triple-contrast CT.
    b. Consider diagnostic laparoscopy.
  4. Thoracoabdominal stab wounds
    a. Obtain triple-contrast CT.
    b. Consider diagnostic laparoscopy.

G. Impalement injury: the impaled object should not be removed until the patient is in the operating room and the abdomen is open

H. Angiographic embolization for selected blunt injuries

  1. Solid organ injuries with extravasation on CT (liver, spleen, kidney)
  2. Massive and unrelenting pelvic hemorrhage

I. Damage control laparotomy
  1. Indications
    a. Combination of hypothermia, coagulopathy, and acidosis
    b. Planned second-look laparotomy
    c. Need for urgent extra-abdominal procedure (e.g., thoracotomy for aortic injury, craniotomy for intracranial injury)
  2. Patient management
    a. Mechanical ventilation
    b. Circulatory support with fluids, vasopressor, or inotropic agent, as indicated
    c. Correct coagulopathy.
    d. Actively rewarm patient.
    e. Sedation with or without neuromuscular blockade
    f. Beware of possible abdominal compartment syndrome.

Key Diagnosis and Treatment

- Diagnosis of blunt injury frequently requires adjunctive tests.
- Gunshot wounds almost always mandate laparotomy.
- Damage control laparotomy should be considered in the presence of hypothermia, coagulopathy, and acidosis.

Bibliography

Fabian TC, Croce MA, Stewart RM, et al. A prospective analysis of diagnostic laparoscopy in trauma. Ann Surg 1993;217:557–565.

Feliciano DV. Diagnostic modalities in abdominal trauma: Peritoneal lavage, ultrasonography, computed tomography scanning, and arteriography. Surg Clin North Am 1991;71:241–256.

Rozycki GS, Ochsner MG, Jaffin JH, et al. Prospective evaluation of surgeons' use of ultrasound in the evaluation of trauma patients. J Trauma 1993;34:516–527.

Schurr MJ, Fabian TC, Gavant M, et al. Management of blunt splenic trauma: computed tomography contrast vascular blush predicts failure of nonoperative management. J Trauma 1995;39:507–513.

Shorr RM, Gottlieb MM, Webb K, et al. Selective management of abdominal stab wounds: importance of the physical examination. Arch Surg 1988;123:1141–1145.

139 Traumatic Brain Injury

Joseph M. Darby

The principal goal in the management of patients with severe traumatic brain injury (TBI) in the intensive care unit (ICU) is to prevent and treat secondary brain injury. This goal is met principally through intensive monitoring, life support, and therapeutic interventions directed at the restoration and maintenance of systemic hemodynamics, oxygen transport, and control of intracranial pressure.

Definitions

A. Glasgow coma scale (GCS): the main clinical scoring system used to assess severity of injury and monitor clinical neurologic condition in patients with severe TBI (see Table 4–1)

B. Severe TBI
   1. A coma-producing head injury (GCS ≤8)
   2. Approximately 10% of all admissions to the hospital for TBI are severe

C. Primary injury: the direct mechanical injury to the brain

D. Secondary injury: any process occurring after TBI that has the potential to produce additional neuronal injury or exacerbate the primary brain injury

E. Intracranial pressure (ICP): the pressure measured within the intracranial vault (normally <10 mm Hg)

F. Cerebral perfusion pressure (CPP)
   1. The principal determinant of cerebral blood flow
   2. Calculated as the difference between the mean arterial pressure (MAP) and ICP
   3. Used as an end point in the management of intracranial hypertension

Key Epidemiology

- Common causes are motor vehicle crashes, falls, and gunshot wounds.

- The age distribution for mortality is bimodal (15 to 24 years and older than 70 years).

- More than 50,000 deaths/year in the United States are caused by TBI.

- Approximately 40% of all trauma-related deaths are due to TBI.

- Traumatic brain injury is responsible for approximately 50% of all in-hospital trauma-related mortality.

Pathophysiology

A. Primary injury
   1. Contusion
   2. Hematoma (epidural, subdural)
   3. Shearing
   4. Vascular injuries

B. Secondary injury
   1. Systemic
      a. Hypotension
      b. Hypoxia
      c. Extreme hypocarbia
      d. Fever
      e. Hyponatremia
      f. Hyperglycemia
   2. Mediators
      a. Excitatory amino acids (glutamate, aspartate)
      b. Free radicals
      c. Lactic acid
      d. Leukotrienes
      e. Pro-inflammatory cytokines
      f. Calcium
      g. Nitric oxide and peroxynitrite
   3. Intracranial
      a. Elevated ICP
      b. Brain edema
      c. Vasospasm
      d. Seizures
      e. Central nervous system infection

C. Contributors to intracranial hypertension
   1. Mass
   2. Vascular congestion
   3. Edema
   4. Impaired cerebrospinal fluid (CSF) drainage

Key Clinical Evaluation

- Glasgow coma score (GCS)

- Pupillary reflexes

- Open fractures

- Cerebrospinal fluid leak (otorrhea or rhinorrhea)

494

Monitoring

A. Systemic
1. Arterial blood pressure
2. Central venous pressure
3. Arterial oxyhemoglobin saturation
4. Body temperature
5. Arterial blood gases
6. Serum electrolyte concentrations
7. Serum or blood glucose concentration

B. Intracranial pressure monitoring (see Chapter 220)
1. Should be considered for all patients in coma with an abnormal computed tomography (CT) scan
2. Should be considered for all patients in coma with a normal head CT scan and at least 2 of the following
   a. Hypotension on admission
   b. Age older than 40 years
   c. Posturing
3. Ventriculostomy is the preferred method.
   a. A catheter is placed within the lateral ventricle of the brain to monitor ICP through a fluid-coupled system.
   b. Considered the criterion standard for ICP monitoring
   c. Can also be used therapeutically to treat intracranial hypertension by allowing drainage of CSF

C. Adjunctive measures of unproven benefit
1. Jugular venous oximetry
   a. Blood samples are obtained from a catheter advanced in a retrograde fashion into the jugular bulb of the internal jugular vein for measurement of oxyhemoglobin saturation ($SjvO_2$) or oxygen tension ($PjvO_2$).
   b. Measurements reflect the value of mixed cerebral venous blood.
   c. Low $SjvO_2$ or $PjvO_2$ values suggest impairment in cerebral blood flow relative to metabolism, whereas high $SjvO_2$ or $PjvO_2$ values suggest excess of flow relative to metabolism (luxury perfusion).
   d. Normal $SjvO_2$ averages approximately 0.62; normal $PjvO_2$ averages approximately 37 torr.
2. Continuous electroencephalography (for use with high-dose barbiturate therapy)

Treatment

A. Restore and maintain systemic tissue oxygenation.
1. Fluid resuscitation and blood transfusion as required

a. Maintain MAP above 80 to 90 mm Hg.
   b. Maintain hematocrit above 30%.
2. Oxygenation and ventilation
   a. Ensure a secure airway.
   b. Adjust FIO_2 and positive end-expiratory pressure (PEEP) as required to maintain arterial saturation above 0.95.
   c. Positive end-expiratory pressure levels up to 15 cm H_2O are safe.
   d. Adjust ventilation to establish and maintain low–normal $PaCO_2$ (~35 mm Hg).

B. Monitor and control ICP and CPP
1. Seek to maintain ICP below 20 to 25 mm Hg.
2. Seek to maintain CPP above 60 to 70 mm Hg.

C. Monitor and correct coagulopathy and thrombocytopenia.

D. Fluids and electrolytes
1. Use isotonic fluids (0.9% saline) as long as ICP control is problematic.
2. Use dextrose-free fluids for the first 24 hours.
3. Normal serum sodium concentration, or mild hypernatremia, is desirable.
4. Keep serum or blood glucose concentration above 100 mg/dL and below 200 mg/dL.

E. Computed tomographic imaging
1. Obtain a routine follow-up CT scan within 24 hours to detect delayed or expanding hematoma formation.
2. Obtain a repeat head CT as indicated to evaluate refractory intracranial hypertension.

F. Prophylactic measures
1. Until risk of intracranial bleeding is minimal, external pneumatic compression devices are preferred over prophylactic heparin to prevent deep venous thrombosis.
2. H_2-receptor blockers are a preferred method for preventing stress-related bleeding due to erosive gastritis.
3. Phenytoin is commonly used for 7 days postinjury as seizure prophylaxis.
4. Prophylactic antibiotics are used for penetrating injuries and open skull fractures; no prophylaxis is required for CSF leaks.

G. Enteral nutrition is started as soon as tolerable, within 7 days of injury.

H. Consider early tracheostomy for airway maintenance in patients remaining in coma longer than 3 days.

I. Management of intracranial hypertension (see Chapter 84)

J. Neuroprotection
1. The goal is prevention of secondary brain injury.

2. Thus far there is no conclusive evidence for efficacy in improving outcome following TBI in human trials of the following treatments.
   a. Moderate hypothermia
   b. Corticosteroids
   c. Barbiturates
   d. Hyperventilation
   e. Free radical scavengers
   f. Arachidonic acid metabolism inhibitors
   g. Calcium channel blockers
   h. N-methyl-D-aspartate (NMDA) antagonists

Pitfalls

A. Inadequate treatment of fever
   1. Elevation in body temperature enhances neuronal loss and injury, increases brain oxygen consumption, and has the potential to increase ICP.
   2. Cooling blankets and antipyretics are employed to maintain normothermia.
B. Rapid correction of hypernatremia
   1. Rapid correction of hypernatremia with free water can promote brain edema and worsening intracranial hypertension.
   2. When indicated, hypernatremia should be corrected at less than 5 mmol/L per day while intracranial hypertension remains problematic.
C. Large reductions in minute ventilation
   1. Rapid increases in $PaCO_2$ can increase ICP.
   2. When indicated, reductions in minute volume should be gradual; do not allow the $PaCO_2$ to rise by more than 5 torr every 6 hours while ICP remains problematic.
D. Withholding PEEP therapy
   1. Withholding PEEP therapy in patients with elevated ICP for fear of increasing ICP is unwarranted.
   2. Positive end-expiratory pressure levels up to 15 cm H_2O are safe in patients with intracranial hypertension when necessary to maintain systemic oxygenation in patients with concomitant severe respiratory failure.
E. Inadequate ventilation during transport
   1. Intracranial pressure may rise during intrahospital transport if adequate ventilation is not maintained.
   2. Intracranial pressure should be monitored during transport and attention focused on maintaining ICP control through proper ventilation as indicated by either end-tidal PCO_2 measurements or, indirectly, by assessment of ICP response.

F. Excessive hyperventilation (hypocapnia), especially within the first 24 hours after injury, has the potential to produce cerebral ischemia and should be avoided.
G. Use of vasodilators or antihypertensives
   1. Antihypertensive drugs, especially agents that are primary vasodilators, can produce sudden and sustained elevations in ICP (plateau waves) if systemic arterial pressure falls precipitously.
   2. Current management strategies avoid the use of antihypertensives in patients with intracranial hypertension.
H. Dehydration
   1. Excessive diuretic use in the management of intracranial hypertension can produce volume depletion, hypotension, and impaired renal function.
   2. Supplemental fluid boluses should be administered as required to maintain euvolemia while osmotic diuretics are being administered.
I. Delaying tracheostomy
   1. Delayed tracheostomy in patients with persistent coma increases ICU length of stay.
   2. Tracheostomy should be considered early in patients who remain in coma for more than 3 or 4 days after injury, provided ICP is under control.

Complications

A. Intracranial complications
   1. Delayed hematoma formation
   2. Central nervous system infection
   3. Hydrocephalus
   4. Unrecognized vascular injury
   5. Seizures
B. Extracranial complications
   1. Electrolyte disturbances
      a. Hyponatremia: from inappropriate antidiuresis syndrome or cerebral salt-wasting syndrome
      b. Hypernatremia: from diabetes insipidus (<1%) or osmotic diuretics
      c. Hypokalemia
      d. Hypomagnesemia
   2. Pneumonia
   3. Coagulopathy
   4. Ileus or gastroparesis
   5. Pancreatitis
   6. Stress gastritis
   7. Deep venous thrombosis
   8. Adrenergic surges

TABLE 139–1. COMPUTED TOMOGRAPHY (CT) CLASSIFICATION FOR HEAD INJURIES

CT CATEGORY	DEFINITION	MORTALITY (%)
Diffuse I	No visible CT-defined pathology	9.6
Diffuse II	Basal cisterns present with midline shift of 0 to 5 mm, or lesion densities present; no high- or mixed-density lesions greater than 25 cc	13.5
Diffuse III	Basal cisterns compressed or absent with midline shift of 0 to 5 mm; no high- or mixed-density lesions greater than 25 cc	34.0
Diffuse IV	Midline shift greater than 5 mm; no high- or mixed-density lesion greater than 25 cc	56.2
Evacuated mass lesion	Any lesion surgically evacuated	38.8
Non-evacuated mass lesion	High- or mixed-density lesion greater than 25 cc not surgically evacuated	52.8

Adapted from Marshall LF, Bowers-Marshall S, Klauber MR, et al. A new classification of head injury based on computerized tomography. J Neurosurg 1991;75:S14–S20.

a. Manifestations: hypertension, fever, tachycardia, diaphoresis, posturing, hyperventilation

b. Treatment: narcotics, thorazine, clonidine, β-adrenergic blockers

9. Contractures

  a. Physical therapy to maintain range of motion

  b. Orthotics: splints and casts as required

Prognosis

A. Individual prognostication for severe TBI is difficult, especially early after injury.

B. However, certain factors identifiable early after injury tend to portend a poor outcome.

  1. Closed head injury

    a. Advanced age

    b. Low GCS score

    c. Impaired pupillary reflexes

    d. Sustained ICP higher than 20 mm Hg

    e. Hypotension or hypoxemia

    f. Diffuse type IV and surgical mass lesions by CT (see Table 139–1)

    g. Lesions involving deep, midline structures (basal ganglia, corpus callosum, hippocampus, upper brain stem), as defined by magnetic resonance imaging

2. Traumatic brain injury due to gunshot wounds in patients with

  a. Glasgow coma scale score of 3 to 5

  b. Unreactive pupils

  c. Bihemispheric involvement

  d. Intraventricular or parenchymal hemorrhage

  e. Coagulopathy

Key Prognosis

- Mortality variable ranges from 25% to 40%.

- Most deaths occur within 3 days of admission.

- Prognostication in severe TBI is difficult, especially early after injury.

Bibliography

Bullock R, Chestnut RM, Clifton G, et al. Guidelines for the management of severe head injury. Eur J Emerg Med 1996;3:109–127.

Kraus JF, McArthur DL. Epidemiologic aspects of brain injury. Neurol Clin 1996;14:435–450.

Marshall LF, Bowers-Marshall S, Klauber MR, et al. A new classification of head injury based on computerized tomography. J Neurosurg 1991;75:S14–S20.

Piek J. Medical complications in severe head injury. New Horizons 1995;3:534–538.

Prough DS, Lang J. Therapy of patients with head injuries: Key parameters for management. J Trauma 1997;42:S10–S18.

Reinert MM, Bullock R. Clinical trials in head injury. Neurol Res 1999;21:330–338.

140 Post-Craniotomy Management

Lakshmipathi Chelluri

Patients undergoing craniotomy for cerebrovascular procedures or tumor resection are usually admitted to an intensive care unit (ICU) for postoperative monitoring and management. The primary goal is to provide early detection of and intervention for neurologic complications, but, of course, other aspects of care, including respiratory and metabolic support, are important as well.

Key Indications for Prolonged Monitoring after Neurosurgery

- Resection of supratentorial glioma or meningioma with marked cerebral edema
- Resection of posterior fossa tumor
- Aneurysm clipping
- Traumatic brain injury
- Complicated operative course
- Significant cardiac or pulmonary co-morbidity

Monitoring

A. All patients should be monitored for 12 to 24 hours after craniotomy.

B. Frequent and detailed neurologic physical examination is crucial.
  1. All new neurologic deficits or alterations in responsiveness should be evaluated immediately by computed tomography (CT) of the head to exclude hematoma formation or brain edema as correctable problems.
  2. Glasgow coma score should be assessed and recorded hourly on the ICU flow sheet.
  3. Level of consciousness
  4. Pupillary reflexes
    a. Unilateral anisocoria or a sluggishly reactive pupil may indicate uncal herniation.
    b. Bilateral pupillary abnormalities may indicate transtentorial herniation.
  5. Extraocular eye muscle function
  6. Motor examination
    a. Pronator drift is an early indication of evolving hemiparesis or supratentorial mass lesion.

b. Dysarthria + ataxia + progressive somnolence can be an early indication of infratentorial mass lesion.

C. Intracranial pressure (ICP) monitoring
  1. Indicated in patients at significant risk of developing cerebral edema postoperatively
  2. If monitoring is provided using an intraventricular catheter, then drainage of cerebrospinal fluid (CSF) can be used to treat elevated ICP.
  3. Seek to maintain ICP below 20 mm Hg and cerebral perfusion pressure (mean arterial pressure − ICP) above 60 mm Hg.

D. Techniques for estimating cerebral blood flow monitoring (employed at some centers)
  1. Transcranial Doppler
  2. Xenon 133 enhanced computed tomography
  3. Jugular venous oxygen saturation monitoring
  4. Cerebral oximetry

E. Postoperative CT showing absence of cerebral edema or hydrocephalus supports the decision to discharge the patient from the ICU back to the ward.

Management

A. Prevention and treatment of seizures
  1. Prophylaxis is indicated for all patients undergoing supratentorial craniotomy.
  2. Agent of choice for prophylaxis and treatment is phenytoin.
    a. 18 to 20 mg/kg loading dose by IV infusion at a maximum rate of 50 mg/minute
    b. Target total serum level is 15 to 20 μg/mL.
  3. Identify and correct possible underlying causes.
    a. Electrolyte (sodium, calcium, magnesium) abnormalities
    b. Hypoglycemia
    c. Hypoxemia
    d. Ethanol withdrawal
    e. Intracranial mass lesion
    f. Drug (e.g., penicillin) toxicity
  4. If available, use continuous encephalographic monitoring for status epilepticus.
  5. Optimize phenytoin serum level by administering additional drug as indicated.
  6. Use additional anticonvulsants, as needed.

B. Pulmonary system

1. Protect airway and clear secretions.

2. Extubate most patients in the early postoperative period when level of consciousness is adequate and presence of protective airway reflexes has been verified.

3. Consider early tracheotomy for patients with persistent decreased level of consciousness.

C. Cardiovascular system

1. Invasive hemodynamic monitoring using a pulmonary artery catheter is rarely indicated.

2. Patients with intracranial hypertension may need central venous pressure monitoring.

D. Renal system

1. Usual maintenance IV fluid is normal saline.

2. Monitor electrolytes (sodium, potassium, chloride, ionized calcium, magnesium, and phosphate).

3. Hyponatremia is usually due to the syndrome of inappropriate antidiuretic hormone or cerebral salt-wasting syndrome.

4. Diabetes insipidus

a. Occurs commonly after pituitary surgery

b. Portends a bad outcome in patients with head trauma or subarachnoid hemorrhage

c. Treatment (see Chapter 53, Diabetes Insipidus)

E. Nutrition

1. The enteral route is preferred.

a. Oral feeding for patients with adequate mental status, cough reflex, and gag reflex

b. Nasoenteric feeding for most other patients

2. Hyperglycemia can worsen brain injury due to hypoxia; maintain blood glucose concentration between 100 and 200 mg/dL.

F. Anticoagulation and prophylaxis against deep venous thrombosis

1. Anticoagulation in the perioperative period increases the risk for intracranial hemorrhage.

2. For patients requiring long-term therapeutic anticoagulation for chronic atrial fibrillation or prosthetic heart valves

a. Warfarin is stopped prior to operation and heparin is started 3 to 7 days postoperatively.

b. The duration of the unprotected interval depends on the perceived risk of thrombotic complications, and on the perceived risk of intracranial bleeding complications.

3. Deep venous thrombosis prophylaxis is provided with pneumatic compression devices.

G. Stress ulcer prophylaxis should be provided using one of the following agents.

1. H_2-receptor antagonist

2. Sucralfate

3. Proton pump inhibitor

H. Infection

1. Perioperative antibiotic prophylaxis is routinely provided.

2. In patients with a ventriculostomy catheter, CSF should be monitored daily for cell count, protein concentration, and glucose concentration in an effort to detect infections early.

PEARL

Extubation is contraindicated in patients with or at high risk for intracranial hypertension.

B Bibliography

Balestrieri FJ, Chernow B, Rainey TG. Postcraniotomy diabetes insipidus: who's at risk? Crit Care Med 1982;10:108–110.

Barker FG II. Efficacy of prophylactic antibiotics for craniotomy: a meta-analysis. Neurosurgery 1994;35:484–492.

Kelly DF. Neurosurgical postoperative care. Neurosurg Clin North Am 1994;5:789–810.

Lazio BE, Simard JM. Anticoagulation in neurosurgical patients. Neurosurgery 1999;45:838–848.

Lu WY, Rhoney DH, Boling WB, et al. A review of stress ulcer prophylaxis in the neurosurgical intensive care unit. Neurosurgery 1997;41:416–426.

Wong MF, Chin NM, Lew TW. Diabetes insipidus in neurosurgical patients. Ann Acad Med Singapore 1998;27:340–343.

141 Post-Cardiac Surgery Management

Alan Lisbon
Mitchell P. Fink

During the first few hours after cardiac surgery, most patients require close monitoring and many are dependent on pharmacological or mechanical support for dysfunctional organ systems. However, within 24 to 48 hours, most of these patients are ready to be discharged from the intensive care unit (ICU) setting to a surgical ward. Patients who remain in an ICU longer than 48 hours have preexisting organ dysfunction, have undergone a particularly complex operation, or have sustained perioperative complications.

Management (Admission to ICU Post-Cardiac Surgery)

A. Transfer operating room monitors.
   1. Electrocardiogram (ECG)
   2. Intra-arterial catheter
   3. Pulse oximeter
   4. Central venous pressure or pulmonary artery catheter
   5. Left atrial catheter (if present)
   6. Intra-aortic balloon pump (if present)
B. Reconnect chest tubes to suction, and note the amount of drainage at the time of admission.
C. Connect the endotracheal tube to a mechanical ventilator with these initial settings.
   1. FIO_2: 1.00
   2. Mode: assist-control or synchronized intermittent mandatory ventilation
   3. Rate: 14 to 16 breaths/minute
   4. Tidal volume: 8 to 10 mL/kg
   5. Positive end-expiratory pressure: 5 cm H_2O
D. Transfer infusions of vasoactive drugs to IV pumps used in the ICU and adjust infusion rates to those used to ensure stability during transport.
E. Re-zero pressure transducers.
F. Obtain report from operating room staff.
G. Obtain admission laboratory tests.
H. Obtain atrial electrogram (using atrial pacing leads) and 12-lead ECG.
I. Obtain chest x-ray to
   1. Assess endotracheal tube position.
   2. Rule out pneumothorax.
   3. Assess intravascular line placement.
   4. Assess gastric tube position.
   5. Evaluate mediastinal silhouette and size.
J. Perform a brief physical examination focusing on skin temperature and color, peripheral pulses, and auscultation of the chest for mechanical valve sounds and murmurs.

Key Laboratory Test (Postoperative)

- Hemoglobin and hematocrit

- Serum electrolytes, including magnesium and ionized calcium

- Prothrombin time, partial thromboplastin time, and platelet count

- Arterial blood gases

- Blood lactate concentration

Management (First 12 to 24 Hours)

A. Cardiovascular system
   1. Most patients coming directly from the operating room are vasoconstricted because of the hypothermia caused by intentional cooling during cardiopulmonary bypass.
   2. Over the succeeding few hours, peripheral vasodilation is common as core temperature rises, leading to relative hypovolemia.
   3. Ventricular compliance is typically decreased.
   4. If there is evidence of myocardial ischemia (ST segment changes on the precordial monitor or 12-lead ECG), consider these diagnoses.
      a. Graft failure
      b. Coronary artery spasm
      c. Thrombosis of native coronary vessels
   5. Seek to maintain a cardiac index greater than 2 L/minute per m^2 of body surface area (as assessed using thermodilution pulmonary artery catheter or Doppler intraesophageal monitoring) and mixed venous (or central venous) oxygen saturation greater than 60%.
   6. If cardiac output is low or the patient is hypotensive (mean arterial pressure lower than 65 mm Hg), consider these interventions.

a. Increase heart rate to 90 to 100 beats/minute (with pacing, if necessary).

b. Increase cardiac preload using Ringer's lactate solution, colloid solutions (e.g., 6% hetastarch solution or 5% human serum albumin solution), or (if hemoglobin concentration is low) packed red blood cells.

c. The optimal approach for titrating preload is controversial, but if invasive monitoring is available, one approach is to increase preload as needed until one of these criteria are satisfied.

   (1) Cardiac index is adequate.

   (2) There is no further increment in stroke volume.

   (3) Pulmonary artery occlusion pressure is 20 to 24 mm Hg.

d. If a dysrhythmia is present, use cardioversion or drugs to restore and maintain sinus rhythm.

e. If cardiac output is low and blood pressure is normal or high, then pharmacological afterload reduction may be appropriate; in the early postoperative period, short-acting and easily titratable agents (sodium nitroprusside or nitroglycerine) are preferred for this purpose.

f. If cardiac output is adequate but the patient is hypotensive, α-adrenergic agents (norepinephrine or phenylephrine) are most commonly employed.

g. If cardiac output and stroke volume are low despite optimization of preload and heart rate, then most patients benefit from therapy with an inotropic agent (milrinone, amrinone, and dobutamine are the most commonly used drugs for this purpose).

h. When both peripheral vasoconstriction and inotropic support are needed, norepinephrine is the most commonly employed vasoactive agent.

i. Transesophageal echocardiography can be invaluable in patients with refractory cardiogenic shock to rule out tamponade, new regional wall motion abnormalities (suggestive of graft failure), or diastolic dysfunction.

B. Pulmonary system

1. Pulmonary function is reduced after cardiac surgery because of

   a. Decreased functional residual capacity

   b. Increased lung water

   c. Ventilation/perfusion mismatching

2. Maintain full mechanical ventilatory support until the patient's core temperature has normalized, hemodynamic stability is assured, and there is no evidence of ongoing bleeding.

3. Begin weaning from mechanical ventilation when the patient is awake.

4. Weaning should be protocol-driven, using arterial oxygen saturation monitoring and physical examination findings to guide the process.

5. Arterial blood gases should be evaluated prior to extubation.

6. If patient is awake and warm on admission, then many centers routinely reverse residual neuromuscular blockade using glycopyrolate and neostigmine.

C. Renal system

1. The primary determinant of renal function is usually cardiac function.

2. Low urine output maybe secondary to low cardiac output, low blood pressure, obstructed renal arteries (rare), or an obstructed urinary catheter.

3. Polyuria is common in the early postoperative period secondary to hypothermia (leads to decreased tubular concentrating ability), increased circulating levels of atrial natriuretic factor, and prior intraoperative administration of a potent loop diuretic (e.g., furosemide) or osmotic diuretic (mannitol).

4. Polyuria also can be caused by glycosuria secondary to hyperglycemia.

D. Sedation and pain management

1. During warming, short-term sedation is best provided with propofol or a short-acting benzodiazepine.

2. Pain control is usually provided by administering a narcotic, such as fentanyl, as needed.

3. Shivering may be treated with meperidine or a neuromuscular blocking agent, such as vecuronium.

Management (Second 12 to 24 Postoperative Hours)

A. Cardiac system

1. In uncomplicated cases, cardiac performance should be improving during this interval.

2. Intravenous vasoactive drugs and inotropic agents generally are tapered and discontinued.

3. The patient begins to mobilize "third-space" fluids.

   a. This process can (and should) be facilitated by carefully titrated doses of furosemide or another potent diuretic agent.

   b. Care should be taken to monitor serum potassium and magnesium concentrations and replace these electrolytes as needed.

   4. Atrial dysrhythmias are common.

B. Respiratory system

   1. Wean the patient from mechanical ventilation and extubate, if this has not already been done.

   2. Provide supplemental oxygen by face mask or nasal prongs.

   3. Provide incentive spirometry.

C. "De-intensify" therapy.

   1. Change IV drugs to the oral route; resume preoperative medication regimen.

   2. Begin oral feeding.

   3. Remove intravascular monitoring catheters and prepare the patient for transfer to a surgical or cardiac surgical ward.

Complications

A. Tamponade should be suspected (and the diagnosis excluded by echocardiography or in a true emergency by mediastinal exploration at the bedside) when specific signs are present.

   1. Excessive bleeding from mediastinal tubes, which stops abruptly

   2. Clotted chest tubes

   3. Rising central venous pressure

   4. Equalization of (high) right- and left-sided filling pressures

   5. Exaggerated decrease in systolic arterial pressure (by >10 mm Hg)

   6. Hypotension, tachycardia, and low cardiac output

B. Cardiac dysrhythmias

   1. Sinus bradycardia: treatment is atrial pacing

   2. Sinus tachycardia

     a. Predisposing factors include hypovolemia, hypervolemia, anemia, inadequate sedation, pain, diminished left or right ventricular contractility.

     b. After correcting predisposing factors, sinus tachycardia should be managed by titrating therapy with a short-acting β-adrenergic blocker (esmolol).

   3. Complete heart block: treatment is atrioventricular pacing

   4. Premature ventricular contractions (PVCs)

     a. Occasional unifocal PVCs (<6 beats/minute) are common.

     b. Frequent or multifocal PVCs may be caused by myocardial ischemia (due to incomplete revascularization or graft occlusion); hypox-

emia; electrolyte derangement (particularly, hypokalemia or hypomagnesemia); pro-arrhythmic effects of vasoactive catecholamines (e.g., dobutamine or epinephrine) used to support blood pressure or cardiac output.

     c. Treatment options

       (1) Give 2 g magnesium sulfate empirically.

       (2) Overdrive suppression by pacing

       (3) Intravenous lidocaine, amiodarone, or other antidysrhythmic agents

   5. Ventricular tachycardia

     a. Evaluate for potential causes (see section on PVCs above).

     b. If the patient is hemodynamically stable, treat with lidocaine or amiodarone.

     c. If the patient is hemodynamically unstable, perform synchronized direct current cardioversion.

   6. Ventricular fibrillation requires emergency electrical defibrillation.

   7. Atrial flutter

     a. Seek potential causes (e.g., hypoxemia, intravascular volume overload, hypokalemia, hypomagnesemia).

     b. If the patient is hemodynamically stable, there are several treatment options, including

       (1) Overdrive pacing

       (2) Slowing the ventricular rate by infusing a calcium channel antagonist (diltiazem) or a short-acting β-adrenergic blocker (esmolol), but not both together (because of the risk of complete heart block)

       (3) Chemical conversion with procainamide or amiodarone

     c. If the patient is hemodynamically unstable, the treatment is synchronized direct current cardioversion; because atrial flutter typically responds to relatively low energy levels, the first attempt at cardioversion should use 50 to 100 joules.

   8. Atrial fibrillation

     a. This dysrhythmia occurs commonly after cardiac surgery.

     b. Treatment options are the same as for atrial flutter.

C. Bleeding

   1. Serious bleeding requiring exploration occurs in 3% to 5% of patients.

   2. Causes

     a. Inadequate surgical hemostasis

     b. Thrombocytopenia (from platelet destruction during cardiopulmonary bypass or immune destruction of cells triggered by heparin-dependent antibodies)

  c. Platelet dysfunction (e.g., from treatment with aspirin or other drugs)

  d. Inadequate reversal of heparin administered during operation

  e. Excessive fibrinolysis

  f. Congenital coagulopathy

  g. Acquired coagulopathy

  h. Disseminated intravascular coagulation

3. Initial laboratory evaluation should include these studies: prothrombin time, partial thromboplastin time, platelet count, activated clotting time, fibrinogen concentration, circulating levels of fibrin degradation products or D-dimers.

4. Treatment options

  a. Heparin excess: give additional protamine sulfate

  b. Thrombocytopenia: transfuse platelets

  c. Excessive fibrinolysis: give ϵ-aminocaproic acid

  d. Dilution of clotting factors or low fibrinogen concentration: give thawed fresh frozen plasma or cryoprecipitate

5. Operative intervention to control bleeding is usually warranted when drainage from chest tubes is more than

  a. 400 mL in 1 hour

  b. 300 mL per hour for 2 successive hours

  c. 200 mL per hour for 3 successive hours

  d. 100 mL per hour for 6 successive hours

Key Complications

- Myocardial ischemia
- Cardiac dysrhythmias
- Cardiac tamponade
- Hemorrhage
- Hypotension
- Graft failure
- Oliguria or polyuria
- Respiratory failure

Bibliography

Cheng DC, Karski J, Peniston C, et al. Morbidity outcome in early versus conventional tracheal extubation after coronary artery bypass grafting: A prospective randomized controlled trial. J Thorac Cardiovasc Surg 1996;112: 755–764.

Fairman RM, Edmunds LH Jr. Emergency thoracotomy in the surgical intensive care unit after open cardiac operation. Ann Thorac Surg 1981;32:386–391.

Higgins TL, Yared J-P, Ryan T. Immediate post-operative care of cardiac surgical patients. J Cardiothorac Vasc Anesth 1996;10:643–658.

Huffman SM, Stammers AH. Methods for monitoring hemostasis during and following cardiac surgery. Int Anesthesiol Clin 1996;34:123–139.

142 Post-Peripheral Vascular Bypass Management

Alan Lisbon

Patients undergoing peripheral vascular surgery typically are elderly. Many suffer from diabetes mellitus and have other cardiovascular and pulmonary co-morbid conditions. A limb salvage operation may take precedence over definitive therapy of these other concurrent diseases.

Risk Factors for Postoperative Complications

A. Predisposing causes of cardiovascular morbidity
1. Advanced age
2. Coronary artery disease
   a. Angina pectoris
   b. Prior myocardial infarction
   c. Underlying silent coronary disease
3. Congestive heart failure
4. Valvular heart disease
5. Dysrhythmias, including paroxysmal atrial fibrillation, multifocal premature ventricular contractions
6. Tobacco smoking
7. Diabetes mellitus
B. Predisposing causes of pulmonary morbidity
1. Advanced age
2. Chronic obstructive pulmonary disease
3. Tobacco smoking

 Key Risk Factor

Coronary artery disease is present in more than 50% of patients undergoing peripheral vascular surgery and causes the majority of perioperative complications.

Complications

A. Postoperative cardiovascular complications
1. Myocardial ischemia or infarction
2. Congestive heart failure
3. Cardiac dysrhythmias
B. Postoperative respiratory insufficiency
1. Respiratory depression
   a. Central nervous system depression
   b. Intravenous narcotics
   c. Epidural narcotics
   d. Sedatives
2. Atelectasis
3. Pulmonary edema secondary to heart failure
4. Pneumonia
5. Acute respiratory distress syndrome (rare)
C. Bleeding
1. Surgical bleeding (i.e., uncontrolled hemorrhage from a major blood vessel)
2. Dilution of clotting factors
3. Hypothermia
4. Excessive (or residual) heparinization
D. Thrombosis
1. Long-term patency is reduced if graft thrombosis occurs in the early postoperative period.
2. Most cases are due to errors in surgical technique.
3. Medical causes
   a. Low cardiac output
   b. Low circulating concentration of natural anticoagulants (antithrombin III, protein C, protein S)
   c. Lupus anticoagulant
   d. Heparin-induced thrombocytopenia
E. Compartment syndrome
1. Should be considered in patients with prolonged ischemia (>6 hours)
2. The diagnosis requires a high index of suspicion.
3. Signs and symptoms include
   a. Pain on passive stretch of limb
   b. Loss of sensation
   c. Loss of motor function
   d. Tense extremity
   e. Pressure in compartment greater than 25 mm Hg
F. Renal dysfunction
1. Hypovolemia
2. Low output cardiac failure
3. Drug-induced renal injury (e.g., aminoglycosides)
4. Radiocontrast agents
   a. More common with preexisting renal disease

b. Incidence is decreased when patients are actively volume loaded with normal saline or given *N*-acetylcysteine.

c. Recovery of renal function is common.

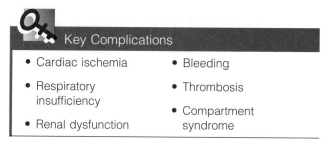

Key Complications

- Cardiac ischemia
- Respiratory insufficiency
- Renal dysfunction
- Bleeding
- Thrombosis
- Compartment syndrome

Monitoring

A. Patients usually arrive from the operating room with the following devices and monitors, which should be continued in the postoperative unit.

1. Continuous electrocardiographic (ECG) monitoring with ST segment analysis
2. Pulse oximetry
3. Arterial catheter for continuous intra-arterial blood pressure monitoring
4. Foley catheter for monitoring urine output
5. Pulmonary artery catheter (commonly used, but not shown to affect outcome in prospective studies)

B. Serial evaluation of pulses

1. For the first 12 to 24 hours postoperatively, distal pulses in operated limb(s) should be assessed at least hourly to detect graft thrombosis or embolization.
2. A decrement or loss of pulse or Doppler signal indicates the need for urgent reevaluation by the surgical team and consideration for reoperation.

C. Coronary ischemia may manifest in the postoperative period as

1. ST segment changes on the ECG monitor or 12-lead electrocardiogram
2. Angina pectoris (myocardial ischemia is frequently silent)
3. Symptoms or signs of myocardial infarction
4. Symptoms or signs of heart failure
5. Hypotension
6. Serious cardiac dysrhythmias

Treatment

A. Pain management

1. Epidural analgesia

a. Can be provided with an epidural catheter placed at the time of operation

b. Should be provided by continuous infusion of a mixture of local anesthetic and a narcotic

c. May be associated with better graft patency in the perioperative period, possibly due to

(1) Increased plasminogen activator inhibitor

(2) Improved fibrinolysis

d. May modify the stress response to surgery and improve pulmonary function

e. May prevent rapid changes in blood pressure and heart rate

f. Is preferred by patients when compared to patient-controlled analgesia

2. Patient-controlled analgesia

a. Well tolerated and is a good alternative to epidural analgesia

b. A basal infusion rate is not recommended.

B. Prevention and treatment of cardiovascular complications

1. Prevention of cardiac complications is easier than treatment.
2. Perioperative treatment with a β_1-adrenergic receptor blocker may reduce adverse cardiac events.

a. A cardioselective β-adrenergic blocker, such as atenolol, should be administered preoperatively.

b. Postoperatively, IV or oral metoprolol should be given to maintain heart rate between 55 to 80 beats/minute.

3. Blood pressure should be maintained within 20% of normal values by infusing IV nitroglycerine or phenylephrine as necessary.
4. The patient's usual cardiac drugs should be restarted as soon as possible after operation.
5. Treat coronary ischemia with nitrates and a β_1-adrenergic blocker.
6. If coronary ischemia develops in the postoperative period, consider

a. Aspirin, IV heparin, or both

b. Cardiology consultation (urgent cardiac catheterization may be warranted in selected cases)

C. Routine prevention of pulmonary complications

1. Incentive spirometry
2. Early ambulation, if possible

D. Treatment of bleeding

1. Seek to exclude surgical bleeding; obtain surgical consultation.
2. Measure coagulation parameters: prothrombin and partial thromboplastin times, platelet count.

3. Warm the patient.

4. Provide clotting factors (fresh-frozen plasma) and platelets as guided by laboratory studies.

E. Treatment of thrombosis

1. Reexploration

2. Local or systemic heparinization

3. Low molecular weight dextran

4. Intra-arterial infusion of nitroglycerin

F. Treatment of compartment syndrome

1. Treatment is fasciotomy.

2. See Chapter 153, Rhabdomyolysis.

G. Treatment of renal dysfunction

1. Maintain intravascular volume.

2. Maintain adequate cardiac output.

3. Avoid nephrotoxic agents.

Bibliography

American College of Cardiology/American Heart Association Task Force on Practice Guidelines. Special report: guidelines for perioperative cardiovascular evaluation for noncardiac surgery (common perioperative cardiovascular evaluation for noncardiac surgery). J Cardiothorac Vasc Anesth 1996;10:540–552.

Boylan JF, Katz J, Kavanagh BP, et al. Epidural bupivacaine-morphine analgesia versus patient-controlled analgesia following abdominal aortic surgery. Anesthesiology 1998;89:585–593.

Poldermans D, Boersma E, Bax JJ, et al. The effect of bisoprolol on perioperative mortality and myocardial infarction in high-risk patients undergoing vascular surgery. Dutch Echocardiographic Cardiac Risk Evaluation Applying Stress Echocardiography Study Group. N Engl J Med 1999;341:1789–1794.

Raby KE, Brull SJ, Timimi F, et al. The effect of heart rate control on myocardial ischemia among high-risk patients after vascular surgery. Anesth Analg 1999;88:477–482.

143 Acute Peripheral Arterial Occlusion

T.J. Bunt

Etiology

A. Embolus
1. Common
   a. Atrial fibrillation
   b. Recent (≤6 weeks) myocardial infarction with mural thrombus
2. Uncommon
   a. Endocarditis
   b. Prosthetic valve
   c. Abdominal aortic aneurysm
   d. Popliteal or femoral aneurysm
   e. Pseudoaneurysm
   f. Cardiac myxoma
   g. Paradoxical embolus (patent foramen ovale)
   h. Iatrogenic (e.g., arterial catheterization, intra-aortic balloon counterpulsation)

B. Thrombosis
1. Common
   a. Prior arterial graft
   b. Prior clinical (i.e., with claudication) or subclinical arterial stenosis
2. Uncommon
   a. Popliteal or femoral aneurysm
   b. Popliteal entrapment syndrome
   c. Cystic adventitial disease
   d. Heparin-induced thrombocytopenia and thrombosis syndrome
   e. Hypercoagulable states

Differential Diagnosis

A. Phlegmasia cerulea dolens
1. Limb edema
2. Intact pulses, although 25% may be detectable only by Doppler ultrasound

B. Acute lumbar plexopathy
1. Radicular pain rather than stocking distribution
2. Intact pulses

C. Cholesterol emboli syndrome
1. Livedoreticularis
2. Pulses usually intact
3. Multiple patchy ischemic areas

D. Blue toe syndrome
1. Variant of embolus
2. Ischemic painful toe(s)
3. Intact pedal pulses

Key Symptoms

- Pain
- Paresis or paralysis
- Pallor
- Pulse deficit
- "Polar" (i.e., cold distal extremity)

Diagnosis

A. The most important diagnostic goal is to determine the degree of ischemia, which will then indicate the urgency and choice of revascularization.
1. Class I ischemia: intact sensory and motor function at distal extremity, with pulses detectable by Doppler ultrasound
2. Class II: loss of sensorimotor function at distal extremity
3. Class III: a cadaveric extremity without motor function or distal flow detectable by Doppler ultrasound
4. Class IV: nonsalvageable due to rigor or doughy edema of the extremity

B. Urgent assessment
1. Determine clinical ischemic class.
2. Perform Doppler pulse examination.
3. Assay serum creatine phosphokinase activity.
4. Perform 12-lead electrocardiogram.
5. Consider angiography.
   a. Angiography is not always necessary nor indicated.
   b. In lesser degrees of ischemia (with intact function) it may be diagnostic and allow immediate thrombolytic therapy.
   c. The more severe the ischemic class, the more urgent the need for revascularization, which

usually indicates surgical intervention: therefore, angiography not indicated

C. Other assessment

1. Transthoracic echocardiography
2. Transesophageal echocardiography (selected cases)
3. Holter monitoring

Treatment

A. Anticoagulation

1. Bolus with 5,000 to 10,000 units intravenously followed by a continuous infusion, unless there is a contraindication to heparin specifically or anticoagulation in general.
2. If contraindication to heparin (e.g., due to heparin-induced thrombocytopenia) but not to anticoagulation, consider use of thrombin inhibitor (e.g., argatroban or lepirudin).
3. Angiography can be performed while the patient is anticoagulated.
4. Consider using the angiography puncture site for thrombolysis, or as an arterial line.

B. Thrombolysis

1. Thrombolytic therapy may be elected if the patient does not have a severely threatened limb and if angiography demonstrates suitable anatomy.
2. Surgery is required for threatened or nonviable limbs.

C. Surgical thromboembolectomy or bypass

1. Acute thrombotic ischemia usually requires surgical intervention.
2. Patients with acute thrombotic ischemia may initially respond to thrombolytic treatment, but 75% require further surgical care (e.g., bypass surgery or correction of vascular stenosis).

D. Further evaluation

1. Once acute embolic ischemia is relieved, further delineation of the source of the embolus may be necessary.
2. Use Holter monitor to detect paroxysmal cardiac dysrhythmias.

3. Use transthoracic or transesophageal echocardiography to look for intracardiac clot or aneurysm.
4. Formal aortic angiography may be indicated if an aneurysm is suspected.
5. Correction of surgical causes of embolus follow their detection.
6. Most emboli can be removed locally with Fogarty thromboembolectomy catheters, but on occasion multiple site (popliteal, tibial, pedal) embolectomy becomes necessary.

E. Long-term anticoagulation with warfarin

1. Long-term anticoagulation is unnecessary for thrombosis once the causative problem is corrected.
2. Indicated for embolus if no definite cause identified or if a cardiac source is found
3. Duration of therapy is at least 6 months.
4. There is a 10% recurrent embolus rate at cessation of anticoagulation.

Key Complications

- Compartment syndrome may be prevented by early relief of ischemia, liberal use of fasciotomy, and IV mannitol therapy for 12 to 24 hours.
- Acute renal failure, secondary to rhabdomyolysis
- Acute respiratory distress syndrome, secondary to rhabdomyolysis
- Amputation (major amputation rate of 20% to 30%)
- Death (associated mortality is 15% to 30%)

Bibliography

Dormandy J, Heeck L, Vig S. Acute limb ischemia. Semin Vasc Surg 1999;12:148–153.

Jenkins DM, Newton WD. Atheroembolism. Am Surgeon 1991;57:588–590.

Ouriel K, Veith FJ. Acute lower limb ischemia: determinants of outcome. Surgery 1998;124:336–341.

Pilger E. Thrombolytic therapy in acute lower limb ischemia. Semin Thromb Hemost 1996;22:61–67.

Yeager RA, Moneta GL, Taylor LM, et al. Surgical management of severe acute lower extremity ischemia. J Vasc Surg 1992;15:385–393.

144 Abdominal Aortic Aneurysm

Samuel A. Tisherman

The natural history of abdominal aortic aneurysms (AAA) is to progressively enlarge and eventually rupture. Whereas the mortality rate for elective abdominal aortic aneurysmorrhaphy is about 1% to 3%, only about 50% of patients with a ruptured AAA make it to the hospital alive, and of those only about 20% survive. Accordingly, optimal management of AAA consists of early recognition and timely surgical intervention to repair or stabilize the aneurysm before it ruptures. Most patients with an AAA larger than 5 cm in diameter should undergo operative repair, unless comorbid conditions make the risk of operation excessively high or overall life expectancy is thought to be less than two years. Patients with smaller aneurysms (>4 cm in diameter) with evidence of rapid enlargement (>0.5 cm over 6 months) also should be considered candidates for aneurysmorrhaphy. Patients with evidence of rapid expansion by ultrasound examination or the presence of symptoms (back or abdominal pain) should undergo urgent operation, as rupture is probably imminent. Patients with AAA often have serious comorbid conditions that can complicate the perioperative course. The same atherosclerotic process that leads to development of AAA can lead to coronary or carotid arterial occlusive disease.

Nonruptured AAA

Key Clinical Findings of Nonruptured AAA

- Patients are usually asymptomatic.
- Physical examination often reveals a pulsatile abdominal mass.
- The presence of AAA is often an incidental finding during radiologic tests performed for other reasons.

Diagnostic Imaging Studies

A. Plain abdominal x-rays: sometimes show evidence of a calcified aortic wall (minority of cases)

B. Ultrasonography
  1. Most widely used test for establishing the diagnosis and following progression of the disease
  2. Measurements of diameter correlate well with measurements made by computed tomography (CT) or at the time of operation.

C. Computed tomography
  1. Dynamic helical CT using timed injection of IV contrast provides detailed information not only about AAA diameter but other issues as well (e.g., presence of left renal vein anomaly or renal artery stenosis).
  2. In general, this test has replaced angiography for preoperative planning.

D. Magnetic resonance imaging can yield high-quality images.

E. Aortography can underestimate the size of the aneurysm because of intravascular clot.

Preoperative Evaluation

A. History and physical examination

B. Common comorbid conditions
  1. Coronary artery disease
  2. Carotid artery disease
  3. Hypertension
  4. Diabetes mellitus
  5. Chronic obstructive pulmonary disease

C. Electrocardiogram

D. Chest x-ray

E. Noninvasive cardiac testing
  1. Exercise stress thallium scan
  2. Dipyridamole thallium scan
  3. Adenosine thallium scan
  4. Stress dobutamine echocardiogram

F. Pulmonary evaluation
  1. Pulmonary function tests
  2. Baseline arterial blood gas analysis
  3. Severe chronic obstructive pulmonary disease does not preclude repair

G. Arteriography is required only if peripheral, renal, or mesenteric arterial disease is suspected (and may not be needed even in these cases if dynamic helical CT is employed).

Management (Perioperative)

A. Minimize risk of myocardial infarction
  1. Begin therapy with a β-adrenergic antagonist preoperatively and continue postoperatively, unless contraindicated by very severe left ven-

tricular dysfunction or presence of active wheezing on physical examination.

2. Consider using topical, IV, or oral nitrate.

B. Intraoperative monitoring

1. Arterial catheterization for continuous blood pressure monitoring

2. Consider pulmonary arterial catheterization, although several small randomized prospective studies have questioned its role.

3. Consider transesophageal echocardiography.

C. Postoperative monitoring

1. Cardiac (ECG) monitoring

2. It is not clear that routine care in an intensive care unit improves outcome for these patients.

Complications

A. Cardiac

1. Myocardial ischemia or infarction

2. Congestive heart failure

3. Dysrhythmias

B. Pulmonary

1. Respiratory failure (i.e., prolonged requirement for mechanical ventilation)

2. Bronchospasm

C. Postoperative bleeding

1. Anastomosis

2. Aorto-enteric fistula

   a. Usually occurs months to years after placement of a prosthetic aortic graft

   b. Diagnosis is made by CT with or without upper gastrointestinal endoscopy.

   c. Treatment usually entails removal of the graft.

D. Distal atheromatous embolization

E. Infection

1. Pneumonia

2. Urinary tract infection

3. Wound infection

4. Graft infection (late)

F. Gastrointestinal

1. Ischemic colitis

   a. Abdominal pain and tenderness

   b. Fever

   c. Leukocytosis

   d. Bloody diarrhea

   e. Diagnosis is made using sigmoidoscopy.

   f. If only the mucosa is involved, treatment with antibiotics active against Gram-negative

rods and obligate anaerobes may be sufficient; if transmural infarction is suspected, then reoperation and colonic resection are necessary.

2. Bowel obstruction

3. Acute cholecystitis

   a. Calculous

   b. Acalculous

4. Acute pancreatitis

G. Renal insufficiency

1. Inadequate intravascular volume loading during the intraoperative and early postoperative period contributes to the risk of this complication.

2. Renal ischemia secondary to suprarenal clamping of the aorta (necessary when the neck of the aneurysm is proximal to the origin of the renal arteries) greatly increases the risk of this complication.

H. Endovascular repair may decrease complication rate.

Ruptured Abdominal Aortic Aneurysm

Key Clinical Findings of Ruptured Abdominal Aortic Aneurysm

- Abdominal or back pain may herald impending rupture.

- Abdominal tenderness

- Pulsatile abdominal mass

- Circulatory shock

- Flank or periumbilical ecchymosis

- Syncope

Management

A. It is essential that the operation not be delayed by obtaining unnecessary tests or imaging studies.

B. If the diagnosis is obvious based on history and physical examination findings, the patient should be moved immediately from the emergency department to the operating room.

C. Fluid resuscitation

1. Aggressive fluid resuscitation in hypotensive patients should be delayed until proximal control of the aorta can be achieved at operation.

2. Sufficient volume of fluid should be infused, however, to prevent cardiac arrest.

D. In hemodynamically stable patients with a questionable diagnosis, abdominal CT should be performed as an emergency procedure to establish or exclude the diagnosis of ruptured or leaking AAA.

Key Management

- For elective aneurysm repair, provide perioperative treatment with a β-adrenergic antagonist unless there is an absolute contraindication.

- Aggressive intraoperative and early postoperative resuscitation of intravascular volume is important to decrease the risk of postoperative renal dysfunction.

- Although pulmonary artery catheterization is common in many centers, routine use of this form of monitoring is of unproven value.

Bibliography

American Society of Anesthesiologists and the Society of Cardiovascular Anesthesiologists Task Force on Transesophageal Echocardiography. Practice guidelines for perioperative transesophageal echocardiography. Anesthesiology 1996;84:986–1006.

Bender JS, Smith-Meek MA, Jones CE. Routine pulmonary artery catheterization does not reduce morbidity and mortality of elective vascular surgery: results of a prospective, randomized trial. Ann Surg 1997;226:229–236.

Cunneen SA, Wagner WH, Shabot MM. Outcomes from abdominal aortic aneurysm resection: does surgical intensive care unit length of stay make a difference? Am Surgeon 1998;64:196–199.

Eskandari MK, Rhee RY, Steed DL, et al. Oxygen-dependent chronic obstructive pulmonary disease does not prohibit aortic aneurysm repair. Am J Surg 1999;178:125–128.

Sandison AJ, Wyncoll DL, Edmondson RC, et al. ICU protocol may affect the outcome of non-elective abdominal aortic aneurysm repair. Euro J Vasc Endovasc Surg 1998;16:356–361.

Valentine RJ, Duke ML, Inman MH, et al. Effectiveness of pulmonary artery catheters in aortic surgery: a randomized trial. J Vasc Surg 1998;27:203–211.

White GH, May J, McGahan T, et al. Historic control comparison of outcome for matched groups of patients undergoing endoluminal versus open repair of abdominal aortic aneurysms. J Vasc Surg 1996;23:201–211.

145 Thermal Burn Injury

Jai K. Prasad

Epidemiology

A. As many as 1.5 to 2 million burn injuries are sustained annually in the United States.

B. Most of these involve less than 20% of total body surface area (TBSA).

C. Approximately 70,000 individuals per year sustain burns that require hospital admission because of the severity of the burns and the presence of co-morbid conditions.

D. Careless smoking combined with alcohol and drug intoxication accounts for 40% of residential fire deaths.

E. Approximately 20,000 burn patients have severe injuries and are optimally managed in a specialized burn intensive care unit.

Pathophysiology

A. Burn injury causes breakdown of cell membranes and an ensuing local and systemic inflammatory response.

B. Production of peroxides and oxygen-free radicals leads to protein destruction and coagulation necrosis that, when complete, manifests as third-degree burns.

C. Lying deep and peripheral to the zone of coagulation necrosis is the zone of stasis.

D. Impairment of perfusion begins with events occurring in the microvascular circulation, including platelet aggregation, neutrophil margination, fibrin deposition, and endothelial swelling, resulting in a zone of edema formation that manifests clinically as second-degree burn injury.

Assessment

A. Accurate estimation of burn size and depth assists in determining severity, fluid needs, nutritional support, wound care, surgical intervention, and prognosis.

B. Estimation of burn area:

   1. The size of the burn wound is estimated as percentage of TBSA.

   2. This estimate is most commonly performed using the rule-of-nines (Fig. 145–1).

C. Classification of burn depth:

   1. First-degree burns

     a. Involve the epidermal layer

     b. Manifest as erythema and hyperemia (sunburn is an example)

     c. Are characterized by intact sensations of pain, touch, and temperature

     d. Heal in less than 10 days, although the wounds may be quite painful during the first 3 days

   2. Second-degree burns

     a. Destroy the entire epidermis and variable depths of the dermis

     b. Are marked by a zone of stasis caused by extensive plasma leakage into the interstitial space

     c. Involve superficial partial-thickness injury

       (1) Involvement of papillary dermis

       (2) Erythema, blisters, bullae

       (3) Intact pain sensation

       (4) Epithelium is usually reestablished in 1 to 3 weeks.

       (5) Full functional recovery is expected.

     d. Deep partial-thickness injury

       (1) Involvement of reticular dermis

       (2) Blisters, pale white or yellow color

       (3) Sensation impaired to some degree

       (4) Epithelium is usually reestablished in 3 to 8 weeks (without surgical intervention).

       (5) Hypertrophic scar formation can occur.

   3. Third-degree burns

     a. Full-thickness injury with destruction of the entire epidermis and dermis

     b. Involvement of subcutaneous fat, fascia, muscle, and bone

     c. Wrinkled, leather-like appearance over bony eminences

     d. Complete lack of sensation (although there can be interspersed areas of partial-thickness injury with some intact sensation)

     e. The eschar is usually waxy-white in color.

     f. Prolonged contact with hot water (>125°F) can lead to third-degree burns that result in

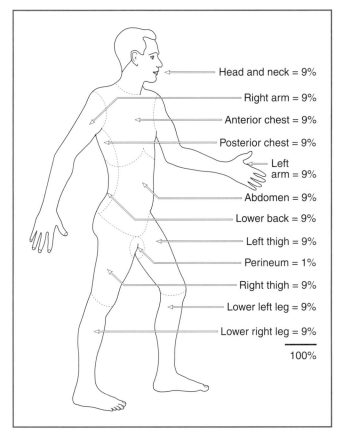

Head and neck = 9%
Right arm = 9%
Anterior chest = 9%
Posterior chest = 9%
Left arm = 9%
Abdomen = 9%
Lower back = 9%
Left thigh = 9%
Perineum = 1%
Right thigh = 9%
Lower left leg = 9%
Lower right leg = 9%

100%

Figure 145–1 Estimation of burn area expressed as a percentage of total body surface area using the "rule of nines."

substantial hemolysis and have the appearance of a dark-red wound.

    g. Hypertrophic scar formation is common.

    h. Functional limitation is common.

  4. Burn depth can increase somewhat over the first 2 to 3 days after injury as a result of fluid loss and inflammation.

D. Inhalation injury (also see Chapter 16, Smoke Inhalation)

  1. The leading cause of mortality in burn patients

  2. Approximately 80% of fire-related deaths result not from burn injury but from inhalation of toxic products of combustion.

  3. Classification

    a. Inhalation injury above the glottis

      (1) Check nares for carbonaceous material and singed hair.

      (2) Assess airway as inflammation-induced swelling of the epiglottis and supraglottic tissues caused by inhaled hot gases can rapidly lead to airway compromise.

    b. Inhalation injury inferior to glottis (primary pulmonary damage)

      (1) Lung injury occurs when noxious gases containing carbon monoxide (CO), hydrogen cyanide, hydrogen chloride, aldehydes, oxides of sulfur and nitrogen, other toxins, and smoke particles, make contact with and damage lower airway mucosa and alveoli.

      (2) An intense inflammatory reaction to bronchial mucosa occurs, leading to distal airway obstruction, micro-atelectasis, and denaturation of surfactant.

      (3) Acute respiratory distress syndrome, respiratory failure, and secondary pneumonia can result.

      (4) Assessed by chest x-ray, arterial blood gases, CO-oximetry, bronchoscopy, and Xenon 133 lung scanning

    c. Carbon monoxide poisoning

      (1) A leading cause of death at the site of the accident as well as during the early resuscitation period

      (2) Carbon monoxide, a colorless, odorless gas, that is lighter than air, can be generated in any fire within an enclosed space where oxygen is rapidly used.

      (3) Obtain carboxyhemoglobin level (see Chapter 71, Carbon Monoxide Poisoning for additional diagnostic considerations).

    d. Cyanide intoxication

      (1) Hydrogen cyanide gas is commonly produced in house and motor vehicle fires from burning polyurethane.

      (2) Clinical findings: similar to CO poisoning

      (3) Diagnosis: confirmed by finding elevated blood cyanide levels (also see Chapter 70, Cyanide Poisoning)

E. Evaluate for trauma

  1. Primary and secondary assessments for trauma per Advanced Trauma Life Support guidelines

  2. Cervical spine x-ray, if indicated

  3. Consider other skeletal x-rays, as indicated.

F. Risk factors for severity and death

  1. Age greater than 60 years

  2. Burns involving more than 40% TBSA

  3. Inhalation injury

  4. Preexisting comorbid factors

Key Diagnostic Criteria for Major Burn Injury

- Second- and third-degree burns involving more than 20% TBSA

- Burns involving less than 20% TBSA in the elderly (≥60 years old)

- Smoke-inhalation injury

- Significant electrical or chemical injury

- Burns associated with significant concomitant trauma

- Burn patients with a significant preexisting medical disorder

- Significant burns involving the face, hands, perineum, genitalia, or skin overlying major joints

Treatment

A. Combine initial assessment with resuscitation.

B. Resuscitation

  1. Airway

    a. Endotracheal intubation should be performed early, before edema obliterates the anatomy of the area.

    b. Progressive hoarseness is a sign of impending airway obstruction.

  2. Breathing: mechanical ventilation may be indicated

  3. Circulation: circulatory shock necessitates emergency fluid resuscitation

    a. Establish at least two large-bore IV catheters.

    b. Begin rapid infusion of lactated Ringer's immediately.

    c. Calculate fluid requirements for the first 24 hours as 4 mL/kg, multiplied by the burn area expressed as a percentage of TBSA.

    d. Administer half of the calculated fluid volume over the first 8 hours, and the remainder over the next 16 hours.

    e. These are average requirements, useful as a starting point; actual requirements can vary substantially.

    f. Usually change to hypotonic fluids after the first 24 hours.

    g. Fluid needs during the second 24 hours are typically about half of that required during the first day.

  4. Ensure cervical spine immobilization, if indicated.

C. Following the above measures, perform a secondary survey of the patient, including head-to-toe evaluation and complete neurologic examination.

D. Smoke-inhalation injury (also see Chapter 16, Smoke Inhalation)

  1. Early endotracheal intubation and positive pressure ventilation may be necessary to protect the airway and provide respiratory support.

  2. Provide adequate pulmonary toilet.

  3. See Chapter 71, Carbon Monoxide Poisoning.

  4. See Chapter 70, Cyanide Poisoning.

  5. Systemic antibiotic therapy

    a. Indicated if secondary pneumonia develops; not given prophylactically

    b. Selection is guided by bacterial culture and susceptibility testing of sputum.

E. Pain Management

  1. Burn injury is probably one of the most painful conditions encountered.

  2. Pain control should be initiated before wound manipulation is considered.

  3. A narcotic analgesic (morphine or fentanyl) given intravenouly is the best choice since erratic absorption from gut, muscle, or subcutaneous tissue renders these routes less effective.

  4. Two types of pain

    a. Background pain: treated with a narcotic analgesic given either by standard continuous IV infusion or using patient-controlled analgesia

    b. Procedure pain: treated with either morphine or fentanyl, in adequate dosages, given prior to the procedure and titrated to effect

F. Wound care and infection control

  1. Closed sterile gauze dressings

  2. Tetanus prophylaxis indicated

  3. Topical antibiotic agents: routinely used for prophylaxis of second- and third-degree burns

    a. Silver sulfadiazine (Silvadene) cream: low toxicity, but can cause leukopenia

    b. 0.5% $AgNO_3$ solution: stains anything it contacts

    c. Mafenide acetate (Sulfamylon) cream: good wound penetration; effective against *Pseudomonas aeruginosa*; may cause non-anion gap metabolic acidosis

    d. Acticoat (elemental Ag membrane)

  4. Temporary skin substitutes

    a. Use of skin substitutes (e.g., Biobrane or Transcyte) to occlude partial-thickness burns has several advantages.

(1) Wounds epithelialize more rapidly.

(2) Wounds are less painful.

(3) Wounds do not desiccate.

(4) Heat loss and evaporative water loss are minimized, offering a more favorable environment for healing.

b. The wound must be thoroughly cleaned before it can be covered by skin substitutes; otherwise, infection will likely occur.

5. Surgery

a. Initial debridement and cleaning of wound should be done once the patient's airway, breathing, and circulation have been stabilized.

b. Loose skin and blisters as well as soot and dirt should be removed with soap and water or a diluted detergent (e.g., chlorhexidine).

c. A hydrotherapy tank should be used only if the patient is hemodynamically stable (hemodynamic monitoring in a hydrotherapy tank may be impossible or risky).

d. Wound excision and grafting considered for deep partial-thickness and full-thickness wounds

e. All circumferential third-degree burns to extremities should be evaluated for the need for escharotomy.

f. Peripheral pulses should be monitored in the hands and feet (with a Doppler probe, if necessary) to detect the need for escharotomy.

g. Circumferential burns of chest wall may interfere with respiration and require escharotomy.

6. Sepsis

a. Common in major burn injury

b. Common sources are burn wound infection and pneumonia.

c. Can lead to multiple organ system failure and septic shock, with high attendant mortality

d. Necessitates parenteral antibiotic therapy

G. Nutritional support

1. High protein, high calorie alimentation (enteral if possible; parenteral otherwise) is necessary.

2. Ideally, nutritional support is titrated by determination of caloric requirements from expired gas analysis (see Chapter 213, Nutritional Assessment) and assessment of nitrogen balance.

H. Physical therapy

Key Treatment

- Average fluid requirements in first 24 hours are 4 mL/kg multiplied by percentage of TBSA.

- Early endotracheal intubation and mechanical ventilation may be necessary.

- Adequate analgesia must be provided.

- Topical antibiotic therapy is necessary: e.g., silver sulfadiazine or mafenide.

- Protein and calorie requirements are high and proportional to the extent of burn injury.

Monitoring (integrate with treatment)

A. Vital signs

1. Heart rate

a. Tachycardia is the rule in burn patients because of hypovolemia, catecholamine release, and pain.

b. Heart rate lower than 120 beats/minute usually indicates adequate intravascular volume.

2. Mean arterial blood pressure

a. Assure adequate perfusion pressure (usually >90 mm Hg).

b. Insertion of an arterial catheter may be necessary for continuous blood pressure monitoring.

c. Not a sensitive parameter of the adequacy of intravascular volume, in part because of increased sympathetic tone in the early post-burn period

3. Body temperature

a. Hypothermia can be a major complication of burn injury.

b. Body temperature must be monitored and, if necessary, controlled.

B. Continuous electrocardiographic monitoring: necessary in early post-burn period for patients with major burn injury

C. Pulse oximetry

1. Allows continuous monitoring of arterial oxygenation status

2. Not accurate in carbon monoxide intoxication

D. Intake and output

1. Intake will far exceed output in the first 48 hours post-burn.

2. The single best parameter for monitoring the adequacy of fluid replacement is urine output.

3. Urine output of 0.5 mL/kg per hour should be targeted.

4. Higher output (e.g., 100 mL/hour) should be targeted in patients with myoglobinuria or hemoglobinuria, along with attempts to alkalinize the urine using IV sodium bicarbonate.

E. Central venous pressure (CVP): normal to low (usually 0 to 3)

F. Pulmonary artery catheterization

1. Not routinely employed, but helpful in titrating resuscitation in patients with severe burn injury

2. Key relevant indications for pulmonary artery catheterization

   a. Elderly patients with more than 30% TBSA burn

   b. Patients with preexisting heart disease and massive burns

   c. Substantial smoke inhalation injury

   d. Patients with massive burns and inadequate urine output despite vigorous fluid administration

G. Laboratory tests

1. Hematocrit: usually substantially elevated initially due to hemoconcentration, but may fall precipitously during resuscitation

2. Arterial blood gases

   a. Allows assessment of gas exchange

   b. Detects hypoxemia and acid-base abnormalities

   c. CO-oximetry should be performed to allow detection and quantification of carbon monoxide intoxication.

3. Arterial blood lactate concentration: elevations usually indicate severe hypoperfusion and tissue hypoxia

4. White blood cell count: may be elevated initially due to stress response

5. Blood glucose concentration: hyperglycemia can occur secondary to stress hormone release (e.g., catecholamines, cortisol, glucagon)

6. Plasma protein levels: a marked decrease can occur due to albumin loss from wound surface and into the interstitial space

Key Complications

- Hypovolemic shock
- Electrolyte disturbances
- Rhabdomyolysis
- Compartment syndrome
- Myoglobinuric renal failure
- Wound infections and sepsis
- Severe pain
- Smoke inhalation
- Airway obstruction
- Carbon monoxide poisoning
- Cyanide intoxication
- Respiratory failure

Bibliography

Deitch EA. The management of burns. N Engl J Med 1990;323:1249–1253.

Dziewsulski P. Burn wound healing: James Ellsworth Laing memorial essay for 1991. Burns 1992;18:466–478.

Monafo WW. Initial management of burns. N Engl J Med 1996;335:1581–1586.

Purdue GF, Hunt JL, Still Jr JM, et al. A multicenter clinical trial of a biosynthetic skin replacement, Dermagraft-TC, compared with cryopreserved human cadaver skin for temporary coverage of excised burn wounds. J Burn Care Rehabil 1997;18:52–57.

Ryan CM, Schoenfeld DA, Thorpe WP, et al. Objective estimates of the probability of death from burn injuries. N Engl J Med 1998;338:362–366.

Saffle JR, Davis B, William P, et al. Recent outcomes in the treatment of burn injury in the United States: a report from the American Burn Association patient registry. J Burn Care Rehabil 1995;16:219–232.

146 Electrical and Lightning Injuries

Jai K. Prasad
James A. Kruse

Definitions

A. Voltage (V)
   1. An electromotive force that propels electrons through a conductor
   2. The standard unit of measure is the volt.
   3. High voltage (or tension) is defined as ≥1,000 volts.
   4. Low voltage (or tension) is defined as <1,000 volts.

B. Current (I)
   1. The flow of electrons through a conductor
   2. Direct current (DC) is unidirectional and the polarity of the associated voltage is invariate; DC sources can thus be designated as positive and negative.
   3. Alternating current (AC) changes direction many times each second (60 for residential current sources in the United States), and the polarity of its associated voltage cycles correspondingly.
   4. The standard unit of measure is the ampere (A).
   5. Low values are commonly expressed in milliamperes (mA).

C. Resistance (R)
   1. Opposition to electrical current flow
   2. The standard unit of measure is the ohm (Ω).
   3. Opposition to flow of AC is better described as impedance.

D. Ohm's law
   1. Quantifies the relationship among the above parameters
   2. $V = I \times R$

E. Electrical power (P)
   1. Quantified as $P = V \times I$
   2. Alternatively expressed as $P = I^2 \times R$
   3. The standard unit of measure is the watt.

Pathophysiology

A. Contact with electricity can cause bodily injury in three ways.
   1. Flash injury
      a. Usually manifests as minor burn injury to the face and hands
      b. Clothes may catch fire, leading to additional flame burns.
   2. Arc injury
      a. Only occurs with high-voltage contact
      b. Arc manifests as an intense violet light and consists of ionized particles driven by high voltage.
      c. Arc temperature is very high (>1000°C).
   3. Current injury
      a. Electric current passes through the body from the point of contact with the body (entrance site) to the point of exit from the body (exit site), usually to ground.
      b. Current follows the shortest path between contact points and can cause devastating injury to intervening tissues and vital structures by generation of heat in proportion to the resistance of the tissues traversed.

B. The extent of damage from current injury depends on multiple factors.
   1. Type of current (AC or DC)
      a. Low-voltage AC can cause tetanic skeletal muscle contractions, including inability to let go of manual contact with electrical source.
      b. Relatively low-level AC can cause ventricular fibrillation and respiratory arrest.
      c. Direct current can cause a single strong muscle contraction, often thrusting the victim away from the source of electricity (high-voltage AC shock can also have this effect) and may result in fractures or asystole.
      d. Lightning is a form of high-voltage direct current.
   2. Magnitude of voltage: i.e., low tension or high tension
   3. Electrical resistance of the body: determines the magnitude of current passing through the body at a given voltage, as specified by Ohm's law
   4. Magnitude of electrical current (examples are representative responses to cutaneously applied AC with typical skin resistance)
      a. <1 mA: imperceptible
      b. 1 to 10 mA: unpleasant tingling sensation

c. 10 to 15 mA: pain

d. >15 mA tetanic muscle contraction

e. >30 to 50 mA: tetanic contraction of respiratory muscles (respiratory arrest)

f. >50 to 100 mA: ventricular fibrillation

g. >10 A: ventricular asystole

5. Internal path of current through body

a. Flow through thorax can cause respiratory or cardiac arrest.

b. Flow through the brainstem can cause respiratory arrest.

c. Flow through specific areas can cause current injury to underlying structures.

6. Duration of contact

7. Extent of contact area

C. Common sources of electrical contact

1. Low tension: usually from contact with domestic current (usually 110 to 240 volts AC)

2. High-voltage sources

a. Industrial and power distribution sources: factory, electrical utility, power plant, construction workers, and electricians are at risk.

b. Lightning

(1) Causes more deaths annually in the United States than all other weather-related phenomena combined

(2) Voltage can be $>10^8$ volts DC; current $>10^4$ A.

(3) Can cause electrothermal injury from direct strike, side flash, splash, arc, or step current; can also result in cardiorespiratory arrest

(4) Step (or stride) current injury is due to an electrical potential difference between the subject's feet at point of contact with the ground, causing current flow up one leg and down the other.

PEARL

Regard all patients with electrical or lightning injury as potentially having sustained multiple traumatic injuries.

Clinical Findings

A. Skin

1. Presents an initial barrier (resistance) to the flow of current

2. Cutaneous damage can manifest as first-, second-, or third-degree burns.

3. Damage to the skin apparent at the entrance and exit sites may be like the tip of an iceberg, with extensive internal damage comparable to a crush injury.

4. May be little or no apparent skin damage, especially if contact made over a large area, such as electrical injuries associated with water immersion

5. High-voltage contact can result in arcing across limbs that manifests as burns at flexion creases.

6. Cutaneous lightning injury patterns

a. Feathering burns: fern-like pattern appears on skin within hours of the injury and resolves spontaneously within approximately 24 hours

b. Flame or thermal burns from burning clothing or secondary heating of adjacent metallic conductors

c. Linear partial-thickness burns, commonly over axilla and groin

d. Discrete, circular, punctate partial- or full-thickness burns, usually multiple and closely spaced

B. Musculoskeletal and extremities

1. General effects

a. Bone has the highest resistance and, therefore, yields large amounts of heat, transforming the skeleton into a heat source that damages tissues overlying the bone.

b. Heat affects muscles in a centrifugal manner; i.e., muscles in the deeper compartment are damaged the most.

2. Extremities

a. Fractures

b. Dislocations

c. Rhabdomyolysis (see Chapter 153, Rhabdomyolysis)

d. Coagulation necrosis

e. Compartment syndrome

C. Cardiovascular

1. Hypovolemic shock: vascular permeability is increased, resulting in depletion of intravascular volume

2. Myocardial infarction

3. Ventricular fibrillation

4. Other cardiac dysrhythmias

5. Asystole (lightning and other DC sources)

6. Myocardial perforation

7. Late-onset myocardial damage

8. Pericardial effusion or pericarditis

9. Transient autonomic instability

10. Arterial or venous thrombosis

D. Respiratory
   1. Respiratory arrest
   2. Pneumothorax
   3. Atelectasis
   4. Pulmonary contusion

E. Renal and metabolic
   1. Myoglobinuria
   2. Hemoglobinuria (from intravascular hemolysis)
   3. Acute tubular necrosis
   4. Electrolyte abnormalities secondary to rhabdomyolysis and renal failure

F. Neurologic
   1. Transient loss of consciousness or coma
   2. Disorientation, agitation, confusion, personality changes, amnesia
   3. Seizures
   4. Aphasia
   5. Intracerebral injury, including hemorrhage and edema
   6. Associated head injury
   7. Early-onset, transient paralysis, most commonly paraplegia, is common with step injuries from lightning.
   8. Late-onset spinal cord injury resulting in paraplegia has been described; may be due to perivascular injury or demyelination.
   9. Peripheral neuropathy: can be due to local electrothermal injury, ischemia, or compartment syndrome

G. Gastrointestinal
   1. Damage to abdominal viscera (e.g., intestinal perforation, blunt hepatic injury)
   2. Paralytic ileus
   3. Stress ulcers

H. Ocular
   1. Acute ocular injury (retinal detachment, optic nerve injury, vitreous hemorrhage)
   2. Late-onset cataracts (>6 months postinjury)

I. Otic
   1. Ruptured tympanic membrane (lightning injury)
   2. Transient sensorineural hearing loss (lightning injury)

Laboratory Findings

A. Electrolyte and acid-base disturbances
   1. Hyperphosphatemia
   2. Hypocalcemia (early)
   3. Hypercalcemia (late)
   4. Hyperkalemia
   5. Metabolic (lactic) acidosis

B. Elevated plasma markers of myocardial and skeletal muscle damage
   1. Total creatine phosphokinase
   2. Creatine phosphokinase MB fraction
   3. Creatine phosphokinase MM fraction
   4. Troponin
   5. Lactate dehydrogenase
   6. Transaminases
   7. Aldolase
   8. Myoglobin

Electrocardiographic Findings

A. Dysrhythmias
   1. Asystole
   2. Ventricular fibrillation
   3. Sinus tachycardia
   4. Atrial fibrillation
   5. Other dysrhythmias

B. Signs of myocardial injury or infarction
   1. ST-segment changes
   2. T wave changes
   3. QT interval prolongation
   4. Q waves

Key Tests

- X-ray films: chest + consider cervical spine and other skeletal x-rays

- Serial 12-lead electrocardiograms

- Serial serum creatine phosphokinase (total and MB fraction) activity

- Serial plasma troponin levels

- Consider computed tomography of brain, if neurologic findings.

- Consider ^{99m}Tc scan to elucidate muscle damage.

- Consider angiogram to delineate vascular damage.

Treatment

A. Resuscitation
   1. Basic life support, per American Heart Association guidelines
      a. Airway: endotracheal intubation, if necessary
      b. Breathing: assisted ventilation, if necessary

c. Circulation: chest compressions, defibrillation, cardioversion, etc., as indicated

2. Advanced cardiac life support, per American Heart Association guidelines

3. Advanced trauma life support, per American College of Surgeons guidelines

4. Continuous electrocardiographic monitoring

5. Fluid resuscitation, as required

   a. Hypovolemia can occur secondary to associated trauma, rhabdomyolysis, transcapillary leak.

   b. Initiate with isotonic crystalloid (lactated Ringer's or normal saline) and titrate to usual indicators of volume status and perfusion.

B. Rhabdomyolysis: see Chapter 153, Rhabdomyolysis

C. Myoglobinuria or hemoglobinuria

1. Both can result in acute tubular necrosis and renal failure.

2. Renal failure may be prevented or minimized by giving generous volumes of IV crystalloid, titrated to maintain a urine output of 100 mL/hour.

3. Sodium bicarbonate given to alkalinize the urine (see Chapter 153)

4. Consider use of mannitol once hypovolemia is corrected and urine output is established.

D. Electrolyte disturbances may be present (see Chapter 153).

E. Treat cutaneous electrical burn injuries.

1. Topical antibiotic treatment (e.g., mafenide or silver sulfadiazine)

2. Systemic antibiotic treatment, if indicated

3. Surgical debridement and exploration, as necessary

4. Tetanus prophylaxis

F. Compartment syndrome

1. Compartment pressure should be monitored in all suspicious or tense muscle compartments.

2. Compartment pressures greater than 40 mm Hg are an indication for decompression surgery.

3. Fasciotomy may be required early on (first 4 hours).

4. Digital escharotomy may be needed for circumferential burns of the fingers.

5. Carpal tunnel decompression may be needed if the median nerve is involved in the injury.

6. Accompanying injury to the intrinsic muscles of the hand can occur, resulting in pain on passive abduction and adduction; in such cases, decompression of interosseous compartment may be needed.

7. Entire limbs may become ischemic and necrotic, necessitating amputation (commonly encountered in high-tension injuries involving either the forearm or the lower leg).

Bibliography

Brown BJ, Gaasch WR. Electrical injuries and lightning. Emerg Med Clin North Am 1992;10:211–229.

Christensen JA, Sherman RT, Balis GA, et al. Delayed neurologic injury secondary to high voltage current with recovery. J Trauma 1980;20:166–168.

Fontanarosa PB. Electrical shock and lightning strike. Ann Emerg Med 1993;22:378–387.

Grube BJ, Heimbach DM, Engrav LH, et al. Neurologic consequences of electrical burns. J Trauma 1990;30:254–258.

Housinger TA, Green L, Shahangian S, et al. A prospective study of myocardial damage in electrical injuries. J Trauma 1985;25:122–123.

Hunt JL, Sato RM, Baxter CR. Acute electric burns: current diagnostic and therapeutic approaches to management. Arch Surg 1980;115:434–438.

Lichtenberg R, Dries D, Ward K, et al. Cardiovascular effects of lightning strikes. J Am Coll Cardiol 1993;21:531–536.

147 Kidney Transplantation

Stephen A. Bowles

Overview

A. Kidney transplantation is performed for the following conditions.
   1. Diabetes mellitus (31%)
   2. Chronic glomerulonephritis (28%)
   3. Polycystic kidney disease (12%)
   4. Nephrosclerosis (9%)
   5. Systemic lupus erythematosus (3%)
   6. Interstitial nephritis (3%)
   7. Immunoglobulin A nephropathy (2%)
   8. Alport's syndrome (1%)
   9. Recurrent disease in a previously transplanted allograft

B. Assessment of potential recipients
   1. No age restriction
   2. Evaluate medical conditions that may cause surgical or postoperative complications.
      a. A thorough cardiac evaluation is essential in patients with diabetes because of a high incidence of coronary artery disease.
      b. Viral serology testing: cytomegalovirus (CMV), hepatitis B, hepatitis C
      c. Tuberculin skin test and anergy panel
   3. The kidney is matched to potential recipients using an algorithm that considers
      a. The match between donor and recipient for HLA antigens A, B, and DR
      b. The time spent on the waiting list
      c. Panel reactive antibody test (a measure of the extent of the sensitization of a recipient to a panel of HLA antigens)
   4. A cross-match is performed with potential recipients.
      a. Tests are performed to assess complement activation when recipient serum is incubated with donor lymphocytes.
      b. The cross-match must be negative for transplantation to be performed.

C. Surgical procedure
   1. Heterotopic transplant
   2. In adults, the allograft is placed extraperitoneally in the iliac fossa.
   3. The donor renal artery is anastomosed to the recipient's hypogastric or common iliac artery.
   4. The donor renal vein is anastomosed to the recipient's iliac vein.
   5. The donor ureter is passed though a submucosal tunnel in the wall of the bladder and sutured to the mucosa.

Key Contraindications

- Active infection
- Malignancy

Treatment (Early Postoperative Period)

A. Immunosuppressive regimens usually include the following agents.
   1. An inhibitor of calcineurin-dependent cytokine synthesis in activated lymphocytes: cyclosporin or tacrolimus
      a. Side effects include hypertension, hyperlipidemia, central nervous system (CNS) changes, nephropathy, and diabetes.
      b. Cimetidine, diltiazem, macrolide antibiotics, and azole antifungals may increase drug levels.
      c. Improved absorption seen with a microemulsion preparation of cyclosporin (Neoral)
   2. Prednisone or methylprednisolone
      a. A large bolus of methylprednisolone is given at induction, and the dose is rapidly titrated downward.
      b. The initial maintenance dose of prednisone is 10 to 20 mg/day; the dose is lowered as tolerated.

B. Additional immunosuppressive agents are sometimes used.
   1. Mycophenylate mofentil inhibits T and B cell proliferation by blocking guanosine nucleotide synthesis; the usual dose is 1 g every 12 hours.
   2. Azathioprine
      a. Mechanism of action is unclear.
      b. The usual dose is 3 to 5 mg/kg for induction followed by 1 to 2 mg/kg per day for maintenance.
   3. Antilymphocyte immunoglobulins are used for induction therapy at some centers and reserved for steroid-resistant rejection at others.

521

a. Murine monoclonal antibody (OKT3)

b. Polyclonal antithymocyte globulin

C. Prophylaxis against infections

1. *Pneumocystis carinii*: trimethoprim-sulfamethoxazole, dapsone, or inhaled pentamidine

2. Cytomegalovirus

a. Use ganciclovir or hyperimmune globulin therapy in CMV-negative recipients receiving CMV-positive allografts and in patients who have received antilymphocyte immunoglobulins.

b. All patients receive routine monitoring for active CMV infection.

3. Epstein-Barr virus: acyclovir

4. *Candida* involving the oropharynx and esophagus: nystatin (swish and swallow)

D. Hydration

E. Prophylaxis against stress ulceration and deep venous thrombosis

F. Calcium channel blockers are used in some centers in an effort to reduce intrarenal vasospasm and reperfusion injury.

Complications

A. Early allograft dysfunction

1. Causes

a. Hypovolemia

b. Ischemic injury prior to procurement

c. Preservation injury

d. Excessively elevated cyclosporin or tacrolimus levels

e. Vascular thrombosis

(1) Evaluate using Doppler ultrasonography.

(2) Salvage therapy usually fails.

f. Ureteral obstruction

(1) Evaluate using ultrasonography.

(2) Treat with nephrostomy tubes, surgery, or transurethral balloon dilation.

2. More than 20% of recipients require dialysis in the first postoperative week.

3. The necessity for early dialysis is associated with a 15% to 20% reduction in one-year graft survival rate.

B. Rejection

1. Hyperacute

a. Very rare

b. Humorally mediated (due to cross-match error)

c. Diagnosed intraoperatively

d. Immediate removal of the (newly) transplanted kidney is required.

2. Accelerated

a. Rare

b. Cell-mediated rejection that occurs within the first three days after transplantation

c. Allograft usually fails.

d. Treatment is the same as for acute cellular rejection (see below).

3. Acute cellular rejection

a. Occurs in at least 50% of patients 1 week to several months after transplantation

b. Characterized by declining renal function, which may be accompanied by fever, tenderness at the allograft site, and eosinophilia

c. Definitive diagnosis requires biopsy (mononuclear interstitial infiltrate).

d. Initial therapy is usually high-dose pulse steroids (85% response rate).

e. Patients with refractory disease receive antilymphocyte therapy.

4. Chronic rejection

a. Occurs after 3 months

b. Characterized by proteinuria

c. Histopathological findings are nonspecific.

d. Increased incidence in recipients with prior acute cellular rejection

e. Poorly responsive to therapy

f. Graft loss occurs eventually.

C. Common reasons for intensive care unit admission in the early postoperative period

1. Myocardial dysfunction (by history or as current problem)

2. Pulmonary edema

a. May be due to volume overload

b. Cardiac ischemia should be considered a potential cause.

c. OKT3 often causes transient pulmonary edema after administration of the first dose.

3. Hyperkalemia

a. Cation exchange resins are associated with bowel perforation and should be avoided.

b. Dialysis is the treatment of choice.

4. Hemorrhage

a. Can arise from the vascular anastomoses or from small vessels on the surface of the kidney or in the transplantation bed

b. Uremic coagulopathy can contribute to the problem and can be treated with

(1) Desmopressin: 0.3 μg/kg

(2) A conjugated estrogen (e.g., Premarin, 0.7 mg/kg)

(3) Maintaining the hematocrit near 30%

(4) Fibrinogen provided by infusing cryoprecipitate

(5) Dialysis

5. Infections in the first month after transplantation

   a. Usually are routine postoperative nosocomial infections

   b. The pathogens encountered are those typically seen in postoperative patients.

D. Late infections after renal transplantation

  1. Viral infections

    a. Cytomegalovirus

     (1) The most severe cases occur in patients who were seronegative for CMV prior to transplantation.

     (2) There is an increased incidence after antilymphocytic therapy.

     (3) Cytomegalovirus infection can cause pneumonia, enteritis, hepatitis, or CMV syndrome.

     (4) Diagnosis is by serologic testing for CMV antigenemia or polymerase chain reaction testing.

     (5) Cytomegalovirus infections are treated with ganciclovir.

     (6) The immunomodulating effects of CMV infection predispose patients to later opportunistic infections.

    b. Herpes simplex virus

     (1) Mucocutaneous disease

     (2) Treat with acyclovir.

    c. Herpes varicella zoster: rarely causes disseminated infection

    d. Epstein-Barr virus

     (1) Causes post-transplant lymphoproliferative disease (PTLD), which is most often a B cell lymphoma

     (2) Treatment consists of discontinuing immunosuppression, providing antiviral therapy with high doses of acyclovir or ganciclovir, and, in some cases, using chemotherapy.

    e. Hepatitis B and C

  2. Fungal infections

    a. *Candida*: oropharyngeal, esophageal, or urinary tract

    b. *Aspergillus*: lungs, skin, central nervous system (CNS)

    c. *Cryptococcus*: CNS, skin, urinary track

    d. *Mucor*: sinuses, lungs

    e. *Pneumocystis*: virtually never seen in patients taking prophylaxis

3. Protozoal infections: toxoplasmosis and strongyloidiasis are rare

4. Bacterial infections

    a. Increased incidence of common infections

    b. Other significant infections include

     (1) *Listeria*: CNS

     (2) *Clostridium difficile*: antibiotic-associated colitis

     (3) *Legionella*: lungs

     (4) *Mycobacterium tuberculosis*: most infections are restricted to the lungs, but 30% to 40% are disseminated or extrapulmonary

     (5) *Salmonella*: gastroenteritis, endovascular

     (6) *Nocardia*: skin, bones, lungs, CNS

5. General principles of management

    a. Atypical infections occur most commonly 1 to 6 months after transplantation.

    b. Identification of the source of infections must be aggressively pursued using techniques such as bronchoalveolar lavage, protected brushing of endobronchial surfaces, endoscopy, lumbar puncture.

    c. Early therapy should be started empirically.

    d. In serious infections, immunosuppression should be reduced or stopped; it is more important to save the patient than the graft.

E. Other common problems following renal transplantation

  1. Cardiovascular disease

    a. Next to infections, coronary artery disease is the most common cause of death in renal transplant recipients.

    b. Immunosuppressive medications may accelerate the development of coronary artery disease by inducing hyperlipidemia and hypertension.

  2. Hypertension

    a. Develops in more than 50% of transplant recipients

    b. In the presence of declining renal function or an abdominal bruit, renal artery stenosis should be considered; the diagnosis is made using ultrasound or captopril-radionuclide renal flow scans.

  3. Gastrointestinal complications are common.

    a. Esophageal: viral and fungal infections

    b. Stomach and duodenum: immunosuppressive therapy may increase the incidence of ulcer disease

    c. Pancreatitis

     (1) Trimethoprim-sulfamethoxazole, azathio-

prine, and steroids may increase the incidence of this complication.

(2) Mortality is high in this population.

d. Bowel complications

(1) Immunosuppression may exacerbate underlying diseases such as diverticulitis.

(2) Oglivie's syndrome (pseudo-obstruction of the colon): usually occurs within 5 days after surgery; colonoscopic decompression is indicated if the problem does not respond to conservative therapy within 24 hours

(3) Perforation can occur secondary to Oglivie's syndrome, CMV disease, or PTLD; mortality is higher than 30%.

(4) *Clostridium difficile* colitis: may present with abdominal pain and colonic distention without diarrhea

e. Cholecystitis

(1) Serious complication in immunosuppressed patient

(2) Cholecystectomy is sometimes performed prior to transplant in patients with cholelithiasis.

4. Neurologic

a. Immunosuppressive agents, notably tacrolimus, can cause CNS side effects including tremor, encephalopathy, central pontine myelinolysis, and seizures.

b. Infections

(1) Encephalitis: herpes simplex virus

(2) Meningitis: *Listeria, Cryptococcus*

(3) Abscess: bacterial or fungal

Key Prognosis (for Graft Survival)

- For organs from living related donors, graft survival is 94% at 1 year, with an estimated half-life of 22 years (36 years if deaths are censored).

- For organs from cadaveric donors, graft survival is 88% at 1 year with an estimated half-life of 14 years (20 years if deaths are censored).

Bibliography

Hariharan S, Johnson CP, Bresnahan BA, et al. Improved graft survival after renal transplantation in the United States, 1998 to 1996. N Engl J Med 2000;342:605–612.

Kusne S, Shapiro R. Surgical infections in immunocompromised patients—prevention and treatment. Adv Surg 1997; 31:299–331.

Rao VK. Posttransplant medical complications. Surg Clin North Am 1998;78:113–132.

Sadaghdar H, Chelluri L, Bowles SA, et al. Outcome of renal transplant recipients in the ICU. Chest 1995;107:1402–1405.

Suthanthiran M, Strom TB. Renal transplantation. N Engl J Med 1994;331:365–376.

148 Hypothermia

Nicola A. Hanania

Key Definitions

- *Hypothermia:* unintentional decline in core body temperature to less than 35°C (95°F)

- *Primary (accidental) hypothermia:* spontaneous reduction of core body temperature from exposure to a cold environment without adequate protection

- *Secondary hypothermia:* hypothermia complicating an underlying medical disorder

Etiology and Risk Factors

A. Decreased heat production
   1. Endocrine failure
      a. Hypothyroidism
      b. Hypoadrenalism
      c. Hypopituitarism
   2. Insufficient substrate
      a. Hypoglycemia
      b. Malnutrition
   3. Neuromuscular inefficiency
      a. Extremes of age
      b. Impaired shivering
      c. Inactivity
B. Increased heat loss
   1. Environmental exposure
   2. Induced vasodilation
      a. Alcohol
      b. Drugs and toxins
   3. Skin disorders
      a. Burns
      b. Psoriasis
      c. Exfoliative dermatitis
   4. Iatrogenic
      a. Infusion of cold IV fluids
      b. Emergent (out of hospital) parturition
C. Impaired thermoregulation
   1. Central nervous system (CNS) failure
      a. Metabolic derangements
      b. Drugs: barbiturates, cyclic antidepressants, sedatives, ethanol
      c. Primary CNS causes: trauma, cerebrovascu-

lar accidents, subarachnoid hemorrhage, Parkinsonism, hypothalamic dysfunction, multiple sclerosis
      d. Anorexia nervosa
   2. Peripheral failure
      a. Neuropathy
      b. Spinal cord transection
      c. Diabetes mellitus
D. Miscellaneous
   1. Sepsis
   2. Pancreatitis
   3. Carcinomatosis
   4. Uremia
   5. Vascular insufficiency

Key Epidemiology

- Annual U.S. death rate is 0.3 per 100,000.

- 50% of deaths are in patients over 65 years old.

- The male : female fatality rate is 3 : 1.

- At highest risk are the homeless, the mentally ill, trauma victims, outdoor workers, and individuals at the extremes of age and with serious underlying medical conditions or ethanol or drug intoxication.

Clinical Features

A. Diagnosis
   1. Straightforward with cold exposure history
   2. Measure core body temperature.
   3. Use a rectal probe thermometer capable of registering temperatures as low as 25°C.
B. Grading
   1. Mild hypothermia: 32.2° to 35°C (90° to 95°F)
   2. Moderate hypothermia: 28° to 32.2°C (82.4° to 90°F)
   3. Severe hypothermia: <28°C (<82.4°F)
C. Manifestations
   1. Onset is insidious.
   2. Initial symptoms are vague: hunger, nausea, dizziness, chills, pruritus, or dyspnea
   3. Manifestations correlate with temperature re-

TABLE 148-1. CLINICAL MANIFESTATIONS OF HYPOTHERMIA

System	Mild Hypothermia	Moderate Hypothermia	Severe Hypothermia
Central nervous system	Confusion, slurred speech, impaired judgment, amnesia	Lethargy, hallucinations, loss of pupillary reflex, EEG abnormalities	Loss of cerebrovascular regulation, decline in EEG activity, coma, loss of ocular reflexes
Cardiovascular	Tachycardia, increased cardiac output and systemic vascular resistance	Progressive bradycardia (unresponsive to atropine), decreased cardiac output and blood pressure, atrial and ventricular dysrhythmias, Osborn waves	Decline in blood pressure and cardiac output, ventricular fibrillation ($<28°C$) and asystole ($<20°C$)
Respiratory	Tachypnea, bronchorrhea	Hypoventilation, decreased O_2 consumption and CO_2 production, loss of cough reflex	Pulmonary edema, apnea
Renal	Cold diuresis	Cold diuresis	Decreased renal perfusion, oliguria
Hematologic	Increased hematocrit, decreased platelet, white blood cell count, coagulopathy and disseminated intravascular coagulation		
Gastrointestinal	Ileus, pancreatitis, gastric stress ulcers, hepatic dysfunction		
Metabolic and endocrine	Increased metabolic rate, hyperglycemia	Decreased metabolic rate, hyperglycemia or hypoglycemia	
Musculoskeletal	Increased shivering	Decreased shivering ($<32°C$), muscle rigidity	Patient appears dead ("pseudo-rigor mortis")

duction and pre-morbid condition (see Table 148–1).

Key Tests

- Basic panel: blood glucose concentration, serum electrolyte concentrations, renal and hepatic function tests, complete blood cell and platelet counts, coagulation profile, electrocardiogram, chest x-ray

- Arterial blood gases (correction for temperature not necessary)

- Serial tests during rewarming: serum electrolyte concentrations, hematocrit, coagulation panel

- Selective tests: thyroid function studies, serum creatine phosphokinase (CK) activity (including MB isoenzymes) and troponin levels, serum ethanol concentration and toxicology screen, microbiologic cultures, other imaging studies as indicated

Laboratory Findings

A. Arterial blood gases
1. PaO_2 and $PaCO_2$ decrease with decrease in temperature.
2. Respiratory acidosis and metabolic acidosis are common.

B. Complete blood cell count
1. Increased hematocrit
2. Decreased white blood cell and platelet counts

C. Coagulation profile
1. Disseminated intravascular coagulation
2. Prolonged prothrombin and partial thromboplastin times

D. Serum biochemical tests
1. Hypokalemia or hyperkalemia
2. Elevated serum urea nitrogen and creatinine concentrations
3. Hyperglycemia (initially) or hypoglycemia (subsequently)
4. Elevated serum amylase and CK activities

E. Electrocardiogram
1. Prolonged PR, QRS, and QT intervals
2. J (Osborn) waves
   a. Positive deflection in left ventricular leads at junction of QRS interval and ST segment
   b. Not always present and not pathognomonic for hypothermia

CAUTION

Use of an esophageal probe is an alternative to rectal temperature monitoring, but readings may be falsely elevated in an intubated patient receiving heated gases by inhalation.

Treatment

A. Initial stabilization

1. Confirm and quantify hypothermia with accurate measurement of core temperature (use hypothermia thermometer).

2. Perform continuous core temperature monitoring.

3. Confirm spontaneous pulse or blood pressure; use of Doppler ultrasound may be necessary.

4. Caution: pulse oximetry may be inaccurate in hypothermia because of poor peripheral perfusion

5. Give supplemental oxygen pending assessment of oxygenation.

6. Intubate trachea (exception: alert patients with intact airway reflexes).

7. In moderate to severe hypothermia, place nasogastric or orogastric tube to relieve gastric distention.

8. Place urinary catheter.

   a. Monitor urine output as an indicator of the adequacy of volume resuscitation.

   b. Caution: cold-induced tubular dysfunction may induce a "cold diuresis," which may interfere with the use of urine output as an indicator of volume status

9. Peripheral (or femoral) venous catheters are preferred over central venous catheters to minimize precipitating cardiac dysrhythmias.

10. Similarly, avoid pulmonary artery catheterization.

11. Avoid rough movement and excess activity; maintain horizontal position.

12. Search for associated conditions requiring urgent intervention: e.g., trauma, hypoglycemia, adrenal, pituitary, or thyroid insufficiency

B. Volume resuscitation

1. Volume depletion is common with moderate to severe hypothermia; assess volume status and give fluids.

2. Begin with rapid infusion of 250 to 500 mL 5% dextrose in normal saline.

3. Additional fluid is needed during rewarming to manage hypotension.

4. Avoid lactated Ringer's solution (impaired hepatic lactate metabolism).

5. Warm fluids to 40° to 42°C before IV infusion, if possible.

6. Monitor closely for fluid overload during rewarming.

7. Consider red cell transfusion if there is a baseline low hematocrit, which may be due to preexisting anemia or hemorrhage.

C. Circulatory support

1. Nonperfusing rhythm (e.g., ventricular fibrillation or asystole) or absence of pulse: perform cardiopulmonary resuscitation

2. Bradycardia: no pharmacologic manipulation of rate required

3. Chest wall compressions require more force in hypothermic patient because of decreased chest wall elasticity and decreased pulmonary compliance.

4. Attempt initial defibrillation for ventricular fibrillation or ventricular tachycardia without pulse: attempts may be unsuccessful if temperature is lower than 30° to 32°C

5. If unsuccessful, continue rewarming, reattempt defibrillation after each 1° to 2°C increase in temperature, or when a core temperature of 30° to 32°C is achieved.

6. Antidysrhythmic and vasoactive drugs are usually ineffective at temperature lower than 30°C (excess administration may lead to toxicity after rewarming due to altered metabolism).

7. Hypothermia-induced dysrhythmias usually convert spontaneously with rewarming.

8. Bretylium tosylate may be more effective than lidocaine; procainamide may increase the risk of ventricular fibrillation.

9. Manage hypotension initially with fluid loading; vasopressor agents are less effective in moderate to severe hypothermia and increase the risk of dysrhythmia.

D. Rewarming

1. Passive external rewarming

   a. Definition: insulating material applied over patient to prevent further heat loss

   b. Method of choice for mild hypothermia; use as an adjunct in moderate or severe hypothermia.

2. Active rewarming

   a. Definition: transfer of exogenous heat to patient via internal or external devices

   b. Indications

      (1) Cardiovascular instability

      (2) Poikilothermia (<32°C)

      (3) Inadequate rewarming with other methods

      (4) Endocrinologic insufficiency

(5) Traumatic peripheral vasodilation (i.e., spinal cord injury)

c. Active external rewarming

(1) Techniques

(a) Forced-air rewarming

(b) Warming blankets, heating pads

(c) Radiant heat

(d) Immersion in a 40°C water bath

(2) Disadvantages

(a) Peripheral vasodilation may worsen hypotension.

(b) Vasodilation in extremities and transport of colder peripheral blood to warmer core can result in decrease in core temperature ("after-drop").

(c) Immersion in warm water bath can impede monitoring and active resuscitation, including defibrillation.

(d) Thermal injury can occur with heating pads, warming blankets, and radiant heat sources.

d. Active core rewarming

(1) Airway rewarming using heated humidified oxygen

(a) Easily implemented

(b) Indicated for most patients with moderate or severe hypothermia

(2) Heated irrigation to transfer heat from fluids to internal areas using a variety of techniques

(a) Peritoneal dialysis or lavage (with potassium-free dialysate): not routinely advocated for stable patients, but can consider in combination with other rewarming methods for patient with poor or undetectable perfusion

(b) Closed thoracic (mediastinal irrigation and myocardial) lavage: warms the heart and great vessels; may consider in severe hypothermia without spontaneous perfusion

(c) Irrigation of the stomach, bladder, or colon: limited utility due to minimal surface area for heat transfer

(d) Extracorporeal blood rewarming: using hemodialysis, continuous arteriovenous rewarming, continuous venovenous rewarming, or cardiopulmonary bypass

E. Supportive care

1. Intensive care unit admission is required for all cases of moderate and severe hypothermia.

2. Anticipate complications.

a. Rhabdomyolysis

(1) Electrolyte disturbances

(2) Renal dysfunction

(3) Compartment syndromes (may not be detected during initial resuscitation)

b. Acute respiratory distress syndrome

c. Acute tubular necrosis

d. Disseminated intravascular coagulation

e. Sepsis

3. Do not aggressively treat hyperglycemia.

a. Hypothermia decreases sensitivity to insulin.

b. Hypoglycemia may result on rewarming.

Key Treatment

- Prompt removal of wet clothing and protection against continued heat loss

- Continuous monitoring of cardiac status

- Fluid resuscitation and circulatory support

- Rewarming measures

- Treatment of underlying cause

- Supportive care

Prognosis

A. Prognosis improved by prompt recognition

B. Risk of death is related to age, preexisting illnesses or trauma, nutritional status, and alcohol or drug intoxication.

C. Resuscitation is often successful if cardiac arrest is due to hypothermia, and not a consequence of anoxia or other injuries.

D. Rapid rewarming is not proven to improve outcome in severe hypothermia.

E. Temper the dictum "no one is dead until warm and dead," with clinical judgment regarding therapy and termination of efforts.

F. There are no validated indicators of survival in severe hypothermia, but poor prognostic signs on admission may include venous pH lower than 6.5; severe coagulopathy; severe hyperkalemia (>10 mmol/L), reflecting death prior to hypothermia.

> **PEARL**
>
> Careful monitoring and frequent reassessments of metabolic, neurologic, and hemodynamic parameters are essential for successful outcome.

Bibliography

Braun R, Krishel S. Environmental emergencies. Emerg Med Clin North Am 1997;15:451–476.

Brunette DD, McVaney K. Hypothermic cardiac arrest: an 11 year review of ED management and outcome. Am J Emerg Med 2000;18:418–422.

Danzl DF, Pozos RS. Accidental hypothermia. N Engl J Med 1994;331:1756–1760.

Danzl DF, Pozos RS, Hamlet MP. Accidental hypothermia. In: Auerbach PS (ed). Wilderness Medicine: Management of Wilderness and Environmental Emergencies, 3rd ed. St. Louis: Mosby, 1995; p 51.

Eddy VA, Morris JA Jr, Cullinane DC. Hypothermia, coagulopathy and acidosis. Surg Clin North Am 2000;80: 845–854.

Greif R, Rajek A, Laciny S, et al. Resistive heating is more effective than metallic-foil insulation in an experimental model of accidental hypothermia: a randomized controlled trial. Ann Emerg Med 2000;35:337–345.

Hanania NA, Zimmerman JL. Accidental hypothermia. Crit Care Clin 1999;15:235–249.

Larach MG. Accidental hypothermia. Lancet 1995;345: 493–498.

Lee-Chiong TL Jr, Stitt JT. Accidental hypothermia. When thermoregulation is overwhelmed. Postgrad Med 1996; 99:77–88.

Thomas R, Cahill CJ. Successful defibrillation in profound hypothermia (core body temperature 25.6°C). Resuscitation 2000;47:317–320.

149 Heat Stroke

Adriana H. Wechsler

This hyperthermic disorder is associated with central nervous system (CNS) depression and core temperatures that may exceed 41°C. It is a life-threatening condition associated with profound physiologic and biochemical abnormalities, and a high mortality rate.

Definitions

A. Heat exhaustion
1. Mild pyrexia with reversible end-organ signs and symptoms primarily due to dehydration
2. May be difficult to distinguish from exertional heat stroke
3. May progress to classic heat stroke if inadequately treated

B. Exertional heat stroke
1. External heat load with endogenous heat production (exercise) overwhelming thermoregulatory mechanisms
2. Otherwise healthy subject
3. Cardinal feature is CNS dysfunction.

C. Classic heat stroke (non-exertional)
1. Failure of endogenous thermoregulatory mechanisms due to overwhelming environmental heat stress
2. Cardinal features include extreme hyperthermia, CNS dysfunction, and diffuse end-organ damage.

Etiology

A. Increased heat production
1. Exercise
2. Thyrotoxicosis
3. Fever

B. Impaired dissipation of heat
1. High ambient temperature or humidity
2. Advanced age
3. Lack of acclimatization
4. Dehydration
5. Impaired cardiovascular performance, decreased cutaneous blood flow for evaporation of heat
6. Debilitation due to physical or psychiatric conditions
7. Alcoholism or drug intoxication: amphetamines, barbiturates, cocaine, lysergic acid diethylamide

8. Drugs
a. Anticholinergics: e.g., benztropine, antihistamines, scopolamine, anti-Parkinsonian agents
b. Antidepressants: e.g., cyclic antidepressants, monoamine oxidase inhibitors
c. Barbiturates
d. β-Adrenergic blockers
e. Diuretics
f. Haloperidol
g. Lithium
h. Phenothiazines: prochlorperazine, chlorpromazine, promethazine
9. Skin diseases
10. Inappropriate clothing
11. Lack of air-conditioning, ventilation, or means of transport to cool environments

Pathophysiology

A. Heat dissipation is normally mediated by circulation (blood is shunted from core to cutaneous vasculature) plus conductive and evaporative heat loss (sweating).
B. Conductive and evaporative heat loss are overwhelmed by high ambient temperature and humidity.
C. Hyperthermia can lead to cerebral edema and multiple organ failure.
D. At temperatures higher than 42°C, hyperthermia causes direct cellular toxicity with uncoupling of oxidative phosphorylation.

Key Epidemiology

- 200 heat stroke deaths/year in the United States; mortality increases during heat waves
- Occupational heat stress affects more than 6 million U.S. workers.
- Desert or tropical climates have the highest incidence of heat stroke.

Risk Factors

A. Extremes of age: neonates and the elderly (80% of heat stroke victims are older than 65 years old)

530

B. Hot, humid, or tropical climates; heat waves in temperate climates

C. Debilitation and poor judgment: physical, mental handicaps impairing access to cooler environments and protective maneuvers

   1. Alcohol intoxication and drug abuse

   2. Psychiatric disorders

   3. Dementia

D. Increased heat production: vigorous exercise (e.g., military recruits, marathon runners)

E. Lack of acclimatization or proper hydration

F. Underlying cardiovascular disease

Key Clinical Findings

- History of environmental exposure or vigorous exercise

- Pyrexia, often higher than 41°C or 106°F

- Confusion, coma, stupor

- Anhydrosis

Clinical Findings

A. Heat exhaustion

   1. Pyrexia less than 40°C (104°F)

   2. Tachycardia, orthostasis

   3. Central nervous system depression

     a. Headache

     b. Dizziness

     c. Irritability

     d. Confusion (mild)

   4. Nausea, vomiting

   5. Fatigue, weakness

   6. Muscle cramps, myalgias

   7. Peripheral edema

B. Heat stroke

   1. Findings of heat exhaustion plus severe CNS dysfunction and multiorgan failure

   2. Pyrexia greater than 41°C or 106°F

   3. Central nervous system dysfunction

     a. Coma

     b. Bizarre behavior

     c. Hallucinations

     d. Confusion

     e. Seizures (1/3 of patients)

     f. Cerebral thrombosis or hemorrhage

   4. Anhydrosis

     a. Late finding

     b. Present in only 50% of cases

   5. Coagulopathy

     a. Disseminated intravascular coagulation

     b. Thrombocytopenia

     c. Consumption coagulopathy

     d. Bleeding: melena, hemoptysis, hematuria

   6. Renal

     a. Azotemia

     b. Acute tubular necrosis

     c. Anuria or oliguria

     d. Myoglobinuria

   7. Musculoskeletal: rhabdomyolysis

   8. Hepatic (a later finding: effects typically peak at 48 to 72 hours)

     a. Hepatocellular necrosis

     b. Jaundice

   9. Respiratory

     a. Tachypnea leading to respiratory alkalosis

     b. Mild hypoxemia

     c. Pulmonary edema

     d. Acute respiratory distress syndrome

   10. Cardiovascular

     a. Hyperdynamic or hypodynamic state

     b. Circulatory failure: due to either direct thermal injury to muscle or decreased coronary blood flow

> **PEARL**
>
> The classic heat stroke triad (i.e., coma, hot dry skin, and hyperthermia) is not uniformly present. Neurologic dysfunction, plus renal, muscle, hematologic, cardiovascular, and hepatic alterations are common.

Differential Diagnosis

A. Delirium tremens

B. Drug toxicity (see earlier list under Etiology)

C. Drug withdrawal

D. Encephalitis, meningitis

E. Hypothalamic infarction or hemorrhage

F. Malaria

G. Malignant hyperthermia

H. Neuroleptic malignant syndrome

I. Serotonin syndrome

J. Septic shock

K. Thyrotoxicosis

L. Pheochromocytoma storm

M. Typhoid fever

Diagnosis

A. History of heat exposure/vigorous exercise

B. Pyrexia greater than 40°C (use a thermometer that registers above 41°C)

C. Altered mentation

D. Assess fluid status and end-organ damage

E. Evidence of rhabdomyolysis

Laboratory and Other Tests

A. Hematology
   1. Complete blood cell count
   2. Platelet count

B. Coagulation
   1. Prothrombin time and international normalized ratio
   2. Partial thromboplastin time
   3. Fibrinogen level
   4. Fibrin(ogen) split products

C. Serum biochemical tests
   1. Electrolyte concentrations, including magnesium and phosphorus
   2. Urea nitrogen and creatinine concentrations
   3. Glucose concentrations
   4. Creatine phosphokinase activity and troponin levels
   5. Liver function tests

D. Arterial blood gas

E. Urinalysis

F. Chest radiography

G. Computed tomography scan of head

Key Monitoring

- Continuous core temperature (rectal or esophageal probe)
- Urine output (Foley catheter)
- Consider pulmonary artery catheterization in selected patients.

Treatment

A. Stabilize airway; ensure ventilation and oxygenation.

B. Crystalloid fluid resuscitation

C. Cooling measures: institute rapidly to minimize end-organ damage
   1. Remove from hot environment immediately.
   2. Lower core temperature by 0.2°C/minute to 39°C.
      a. Facilitate evaporation: undress patient, spray with tepid water or cover with wet sheet; expose to breeze from electric fans
      b. Accelerate cooling: place ice packs at neck, axilla, groin
      c. Consider ice water gastric, rectal, or peritoneal lavage in refractory cases—although this treatment has been associated with complications.
      d. Cardiopulmonary bypass as last resort, if available

WARNING

Cold water immersion impairs evaporative cooling, restricts access to patient, and prohibits defibrillation.

D. Pharmacologic measures
   1. Antipyretics
      a. Are of no benefit because of impaired hypothalamic function
      b. Contraindicated: may exacerbate hepatic or hematologic abnormalities
   2. Avoid anticholinergic and adrenergic agents: they impair evaporation.
   3. Neuroleptic drugs may be used to suppress shivering: e.g., thorazine 25 to 50 mg intravenously.
   4. Mannitol has been used for osmotic diuresis and renal protection: 0.5 to 1 g/kg, followed by 0.25 to 0.5 g/kg every 4 to 6 hours to a maximum dose of 200 g in 24 hours; ensure adequate fluid balance

E. Hydration
   1. Most patients with heat stroke are euvolemic initially.
   2. Hypotension is due primarily to vasodilatation and redistribution of volume.
   3. Cautious fluid loading is indicated with central venous pressure monitoring.

F. Additional maneuvers
   1. Early mechanical ventilation and positive end-expiratory pressure for acute respiratory distress syndrome (ARDS); see Chapter 8, Acute Respiratory Distress Syndrome, Chapter 223, Conventional Mechanical Ventilation, and Chapter 225, Positive End-Expiratory Pressure.
   2. Fluid loading, alkalinization of urine, and diuretics for rhabdomyolysis and renal failure (see Chapter 153, Rhabdomyolysis)
   3. Benzodiazepines for seizures
   4. Reserve calcium repletion for patients with elec-

trocardiographic or CNS manifestations of hypocalcemia (risk of rebound hypercalcemia).

5. Bicarbonate for refractory acidosis

Key Treatment

- Stabilize airway, ensure adequate ventilation.

- Institute rapid cooling: undress patient, use tepid water spray, wet sheets, fanning.

- Assess intravascular volume and replete if hypovolemic.

- Give benzodiazepines for seizures.

- Consider other etiologies of fever and confusion.

Complications

A. Pulmonary
  1. Pulmonary edema (ARDS)
  2. Aspiration pneumonia
  3. Respiratory alkalosis
B. Neurologic
  1. Coma
  2. Motor deficits, hemiplegia
  3. Cerebellar dysfunction
  4. Dysarthria, aphasia
  5. Seizures
  6. Dementia
C. Cardiac
  1. High-output cardiac failure
  2. Decompensation of underlying compensated cardiac failure
  3. Subendocardial hemorrhage, myocardial necrosis
  4. Cardiac muscle rupture
D. Renal and metabolic
  1. Rhabdomyolysis
  2. Acute renal failure
    a. In exertional heat stroke incidence is 35%.
    b. Mechanisms
      (1) Dehydration
      (2) Acute tubular necrosis
      (3) Myoglobinuric renal failure
  3. Electrolyte imbalance
    a. Hypokalemia from excessive sweating
    b. Hyperkalemia from severe cellular injury (especially in exertional heat stroke)
    c. Hypocalcemia 2 to 3 days post-injury, with potential for rebound hypercalcemia 2 to 3 weeks later
    d. Hypernatremia
    e. Hypoglycemia
    f. Mild hypophosphatemia
    g. Hyperuricemia
  4. Lactic acidosis
E. Hematologic
  1. Coagulopathy
  2. Disseminated intravascular coagulation
F. Hepatic: hepatocellular necrosis peaks 2 to 3 days after insult

Prognosis

A. Mortality: 10% to 70%; highest if treatment delayed more than 2 hours
B. Survival affected by premorbid condition, age, and level of core temperature
C. Poor prognostic signs
  1. Coagulopathy, disseminated intravascular coagulation
  2. Lactic acidosis
  3. Rectal temperature higher than 42.2°C (108°F)
  4. Acute renal failure
  5. Prolonged coma longer than 4 hours
  6. Hyperkalemia
  7. Serum alanine aminotransferase activity higher than 1000 units/L
  8. Prolonged hyperthermia
D. Rapid body cooling is key to survival.

 Bibliography

Bouchama A, Hammami MM, Haq A, et al. Evidence for endothelial cell activation/injury in heatstroke. Crit Care Med 1996;24:1173–1178.

Bouchama A, Hammami MM, al Shail E, et al. Differential effects of in vitro and in vivo hyperthermia on the production of interleukin-10. Intensive Care Med 2000;26: 1646–1651.

Curley FJ, Irwin RS. Disorders of temperature control: hyperthermia. In: Irwin RS, Cerra FB, Rippe JM (eds). Intensive Care Medicine, 4th ed. Philadelphia: Lippincott-Raven, 1999; pp 844–858.

Dematte JE, O'Mara K, Buescher J, et al. Near-fatal heat stroke during the 1995 heat wave in Chicago. Ann Intern Med 1998;129:173–181.

Duthie DJR. Heat-related illness. Lancet 1998;352:1329–1330.

Hubbard RW, Gaffin SL, Squire DL. Heat-related illnesses. In: Auerbach PS (ed). Wilderness Medicine: Management of Wilderness and Environment Emergencies, 3rd ed. St. Louis: Mosby, 1995; pp 167–212.

Khosla R, Guntupalli KK. Heat-related illnesses. Crit Care Clin 1999;15:251–263.

Lin MT. Heatstroke-induced cerebral ischemia and neuronal damage: involvement of cytokines and monoamines. Ann NY Acad Sci 1997;813:572–580.

Simon HB. Hyperthermia. N Engl J Med 1993;329:483–487.

Tek D, Olshaker JS. Heat Illness. Emerg Med Clin North Am 1992;10:299–310.

150 Anaphylaxis

Marilyn T. Haupt

Anaphylactic reactions are life-threatening events that are allergic in nature. They are generally mediated by immunoglobulin (Ig) E and involve the activation of mast cells, basophils, and various biochemical mediators. Anaphylactoid reactions are clinically identical events in which a chemical or physical stimulus leads to the release of cellular mediators without the involvement of IgE. Anaphylactic and anaphylactoid reactions are usually explosive in onset and are typically observed in individuals with a history of atopy.

Etiology

A. Antibiotics
  1. β-Lactam antibiotics (e.g., penicillins and cephalosporins)
  2. Tetracyclines
  3. Macrolides
B. Nonsteroidal anti-inflammatory agents
  1. Aspirin
  2. Ibuprofen
  3. Indomethacin
C. Local anesthetics
  1. Lidocaine
  2. Cocaine
D. General anesthetics
  1. Thiopental
  2. Etomidate
  3. Ketamine
E. Neuromuscular blocking agents
  1. D-Tubocurarine
  2. Pancuronium
  3. Succinylcholine
  4. Atracurium
  5. Vecuronium
F. Blood products and antisera
  1. Red cell, white cell, and platelet transfusions
  2. Gamma globulin preparations
  3. Rabies, tetanus, and diphtheria antitoxins
  4. Snake and spider antivenom
G. Allergenic extracts
H. Radiographic contrast agents

I. Foods
  1. Peanuts and other legumes (e.g., soybeans, kidney beans)
  2. True nuts (e.g., walnuts, pecans)
  3. Shellfish
  4. Fish
  5. Dairy products (e.g., milk, eggs)
J. Venoms
  1. Hymenoptera (e.g., bee, wasp, hornet, fire ant)
  2. Snake
  3. Spider
  4. Scorpion
K. Latex rubber products
L. Chemotherapeutic agents
  1. Cisplatin
  2. Daunorubicin
  3. Cyclophosphamide
  4. Methotrexate
M. Other drugs
  1. Acetylcysteine
  2. Pancreatic enzyme supplements
  3. Protamine
  4. Insulin
  5. Parenteral iron
  6. Iodine compounds
  7. Thiazide diuretics
  8. Morphine
  9. Meprobamate

Symptoms

A. Constitutional
  1. Feeling of impending doom
  2. Anxiety
  3. Lightheadedness
B. Respiratory
  1. Dyspnea
  2. Stridor
  3. Wheezing
C. Cardiac
  1. Chest tightness
  2. Palpitations

534

D. Gastrointestinal

　1. Nausea and vomiting

　2. Diarrhea

　3. Abdominal cramping

E. Skin and mucous membranes

　1. Pruritus: skin, eyes, palate, nasal areas

　2. Hoarseness

　3. Dysphagia

F. Central nervous system

　1. Loss of consciousness

　2. Seizures

　3. Dizziness

PEARL

Recurrence of symptoms can occur 6 to 12 hours after anaphylaxis (late-phase reaction) due to new release of cell-derived mediators.

Physical Examination

A. Vital signs: fever, tachycardia, hypotension, tachypnea

B. Head and neck: periorbital or perioral edema, tongue swelling and protrusion

C. Cardiovascular: flat neck veins, bounding pulses, irregular heart rhythm

D. Respiratory: prolonged inspiration or stridor from laryngeal edema and obstruction; prolonged expiration from wheezes; rales; respiratory arrest

E. Skin: hives, erythema, urticaria, angioedema; identifiable site of toxin exposure or envenomation may be apparent when etiologic

F. Gastrointestinal: diffuse abdominal tenderness, hyperactive bowel sounds

Laboratory Findings

A. Elevated hematocrit (hemoconcentration)

B. Metabolic acidosis and increased anion gap (lactic acidosis)

C. Hypoxemia

D. Respiratory alkalosis

E. Eosinophilia

F. Neutrophilia

G. Elevated tryptase levels (from mast cells) are helpful to distinguish anaphylaxis from other acute events.

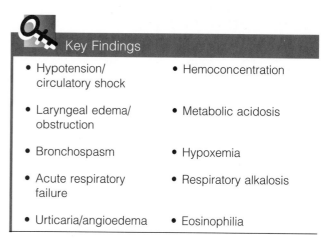

Key Findings

- Hypotension/circulatory shock
- Laryngeal edema/obstruction
- Bronchospasm
- Acute respiratory failure
- Urticaria/angioedema
- Hemoconcentration
- Metabolic acidosis
- Hypoxemia
- Respiratory alkalosis
- Eosinophilia

Differential Diagnosis

A. Vasovagal episode

B. Acute asthmatic attack

C. Acute pulmonary edema

D. Pulmonary embolism

E. Spontaneous pneumothorax

F. Myocardial ischemia or infarction

G. Paroxysmal cardiac dysrhythmia

H. Drug overdose or poisoning

I. Insulin shock

J. Carcinoid attack

Treatment

A. Assure a patent airway; endotracheal intubation or emergency cricothyroidotomy may be necessary.

B. Maintain adequate cardiopulmonary function.

　1. Cardiopulmonary resuscitation may be required.

　2. Mechanical ventilation may be necessary.

C. Establish IV access.

D. Epinephrine

　1. For severe cases: 3 to 5 mL of a 1:10,000 solution intravenously over 5 to 10 minutes with continuous electrocardiographic monitoring

　2. For mild cases: 0.3 to 0.5 mL of a 1:1000 solution subcutaneously

E. Intravenous fluid therapy with isotonic crystalloids or colloids to reverse hemoconcentration or to optimize hemodynamic parameters, guided by hemodynamic monitoring

F. Hydrocortisone: 100 to 200 mg intravenously (to prevent late phase reactions)

G. Histamine receptor blocking drugs

　1. H_1 receptor blocker: diphenhydramine 25 to 50 mg intravenously or orally

2. H$_2$ receptor blocker: cimetidine 300 mg in 50 mL normal saline intravenously may also be tried if no contraindications

H. Treat ongoing hypotension with inotropic/vasoactive sympathomimetic drugs, as appropriate.

I. Treat continued bronchospasm with inhaled β-adrenergic agonist and, if necessary, anticholinergic drugs.

J. Remove ongoing toxin exposure.

1. Washing of exposed skin or removal of a retained stinger may be necessary.

2. Absorption of toxin into the circulation can be slowed by placing a constricting band on the extremity at a point proximal to the toxin exposure; the band should be tight enough to occlude venous flow without occluding arterial flow.

K. Monitor for late-phase reactions.

L. After acute management, attention should be directed to methods for preventing repeat occurrences.

Bibliography

Binkley K, Cheema A, Sussman G, et al. Generalized allergic reactions during anaesthesia. J Allergy Clin Immunol 1992;89:768–774.

Kemp SF, Lieberman P. Inhibitors of angiotensin II: potential hazards for patients at risk for anaphylaxis. Ann Allergy Asthma Immunol 1997;78:527–529.

Nicklas RA, Bernstein IL, Li JT (eds). The diagnosis and management of anaphylaxis. J Allergy Clin Immunol 1998;101(Suppl Part 2):S465–S528.

Sampson HA, Metcalfe DD. Food allergies. JAMA 1992; 268:2840–2844.

Sussman GL, Beezhold DH. Allergy to latex rubber. Ann Intern Med 1995;122:43–46.

Valentine MD. Anaphylaxis and stinging insect hypersensitivity. JAMA 1992;268:2830–2833.

151 Near Drowning

Syed K. Shahryar
Richard W. Carlson

Key Definitions

- *Near-drowning:* survival following a drowning episode

- *Drowning:* death from suffocation in a liquid medium

- *Wet drowning:* drowning associated with aspiration of fluids (occurs in >80% of instances)

- *Dry drowning:* asphyxia secondary to laryngospasm

Pathophysiology

A. Drowning process: panic, air hunger, breath-holding, ultimately followed by reflexive inspiratory efforts with aspiration or laryngospasm

B. Pulmonary injury is highly variable.
1. Minor to diffuse infiltrates (acute respiratory distress syndrome)
2. Modest ventilation–perfusion mismatch disturbances to severe intrapulmonary shunting
3. Surfactant loss

C. Similar clinical features are seen in most cases of sea water or fresh water immersion.

D. Cardiac dysrhythmias or arrest

E. Central nervous system (CNS) hypoxia

F. Hypothermia

G. Head and spinal cord injuries are common.

> ### PEARL
>
> Hypoxia, aspiration, and asphyxia are leading causes of morbidity and mortality.

Epidemiology

A. More than 6,000 drowning fatalities occur in the United States annually.

B. Males have more drowning episodes.

C. Bimodal age distribution: younger than 4 years and 15 to 24 years

D. Alcohol, other drugs, trauma, hypothermia, myocardial or central nervous system events may precede or lead to the drowning episode.

Clinical Findings

A. History
1. Consider trauma, such as diving injury.
2. Duration of submersion
3. Water temperature
4. Alcohol or drug involvement

B. Physical examination
1. Rectal temperature
2. Emphasize cardiovascular, pulmonary, and neurologic assessments.
3. Document level of consciousness.

C. Imaging
1. Chest x-ray
2. Cervical spine x-ray
3. Computed tomography (head, spine)

D. Laboratory and other tests
1. Complete blood count
2. Serum biochemical tests
3. Arterial blood gas analysis
4. Toxicologic studies
5. Creatine phosphokinase activity
6. Electrocardiogram

Key Prognosis

Clinical assessment after initial resuscitation and admission is predictive of survival and neurologic outcome.

Category	Description	Outcome
A	Awake	Good survival with few sequelae
B	Blunted	Increased morbidity
C	Coma	Highest morbidity and mortality

Treatment

A. Prehospital management
1. Begin immediate cardiopulmonary resuscitation at scene.
2. Full aggressive efforts should be provided unless rigor mortis is present.
3. Sinus bradycardia or atrial fibrillation induced by hypothermia requires no initial treatment.

4. Rewarm all hypothermic (<33°C) patients as soon as possible.

B. Emergency department management

1. Hospitalize all victims submerged for longer than 1 minute, those with cyanosis or apnea, and those resuscitated in the field.

2. Admit to the intensive care unit if chest x-ray, arterial blood gases, or neurologic examination is abnormal.

3. Continue resuscitation and rewarming.

   a. Avoid declaring death in the presence of hypothermia.

   b. The minimal resuscitation effort should always exceed 20 minutes.

4. Body temperature lower than 28°C impairs spontaneous cardiac activity and ability to defibrillate.

5. Rewarming

   a. Heated IV fluids (36 to 40°C)

   b. Heated humidified oxygen (40 to 44°C) via endotracheal tube

   c. Warmed gastric, bladder or peritoneal lavage

   d. Hemodialysis and extracorporeal circulation, if available

6. Observe for cardiac dysrhythmias, acid-base, rhabdomyolysis, and coagulation and renal-electrolyte derangements.

C. Intensive care unit management

1. Neurologic

   a. Goal: prevent or reduce secondary CNS damage from hypoxia acidosis, hypotension, hypothermia, hyperglycemia, seizures, or fluid overload

   b. Intracranial pressure (ICP) monitoring is not routinely employed.

      (1) If high ICP is suspected or documented, sedate the patient and elevate the head of bed.

      (2) No confirmed benefit from hyperventilation, dehydration, induced coma, sedation, neuromuscular blockade, or hypothermia

   c. Correct acid-base and electrolyte defects and ensure euglycemia.

2. Cardiovascular

   a. Attempt to achieve a core temperature higher than 32°C.

   b. Assess volume status; hypothermia may induce diuresis.

   c. Inotropic support may be required.

   d. Consider pulmonary artery catheterization for unstable patients.

3. Pulmonary

   a. Indications for intubation

      (1) Coma or near-coma

      (2) Inability to maintain PaO_2 higher than 60 to 90 torr by high-flow oxygen using a non-rebreathing mask

      (3) Progressive hypercapnia

   b. See Chapter 8, Acute Respiratory Distress Syndrome.

   c. Permissive hypercapnia may not be suitable if there is CNS injury and elevated ICP.

   d. Treat bronchospasm with aerosolized β-adrenergic agents.

   e. Monitor tracheal aspirate as an indicator for antibiotic therapy.

   f. Fungi isolated from sputum may indicate a fungal bronchopulmonary infection requiring treatment.

   g. Underwater diving incidents may be associated with dysbaric injuries that necessitate hyperbaric (decompression) treatment.

CAUTION

Corticosteroids, prophylactic antibiotics, intracranial pressure monitoring, and deep sedation with neuromuscular blockade are no longer recommended for routine use.

B | **Bibliography**

Bonnor R, Siddiqui M, Ahuja TS. Rhabdomyolysis associated with near-drowning. Am J Med Sci 1999;318:201–202.

DeNicola LK, Falk JL, Swanson ME, et al. Submersion injuries in children and adults. Crit Care Clin 1997;13:477–502.

Ender PT, Dolan MJ. Pneumonia associated with near-drowning. Clin Infect Dis 1997;25:896–907.

Modell JH. Drowning. N Engl J Med 1993;328:253–256.

Sachdeva RC. Near Drowning. Crit Care Clin 1999;15:281–296.

Spicer ST, Quinn D, Nyi Nyi NN, et al. Acute renal impairment after immersion and near-drowning. J Am Soc Nephrol 1999; 10:382–386.

Van Berkel M, Bierens JJL, Lie RLK, et al. Pulmonary oedema, pneumonia and mortality in submersion victims; a retrospective study in 125 patients. Intensive Care Med 1996;22:101–107.

Zuckerman GB, Gregory PM, Santos-Damiani SM. Predictors of death and neurologic impairment in pediatric submersion injuries: the Pediatric Risk of Mortality Score. Arch Pediatr Adolesc Med 1998;152:134–140.

152 Fat Embolism

Remzi Bag

Fat embolism syndrome (FES) is a triad of respiratory dysfunction, neurologic manifestations, and petechiae that is caused by the entry of fat particles into the microcirculation.

Etiology

A. Traumatic
1. Long bone fractures
2. Other fractures
3. Orthopedic surgery
4. Liposuction
5. Bone marrow biopsy
6. Blunt trauma to fatty organs
7. Median sternotomy

B. Nontraumatic
1. Pancreatitis
2. Diabetes mellitus
3. Lipid infusions
4. Sickle cell crisis and acute chest syndrome
5. Burn injury
6. Cardiopulmonary bypass
7. Decompression sickness
8. Corticosteroid therapy
9. Osteomyelitis
10. Alcoholic fatty liver
11. Acute fatty liver of pregnancy
12. Lymphangiography
13. Cyclosporine infusion
14. Severe infections
15. Inhalation anesthesia
16. Renal infarction, renal transplantation
17. Blood transfusion
18. Acute decompression sickness

Pathophysiology

A. Traumatic
1. Release of neutral fat from the bone or adipose tissue
2. Fat droplets enter the veins and are transported to the pulmonary vascular bed.
3. Particles larger than 8 μm can embolize.
4. Lung lipases hydrolyze fat and toxic free fatty acids (FFA) are released.
5. Pulmonary endothelial injury is due to toxic FFA.
6. Elevated right heart pressures may cause transient opening of foramen ovale.
7. Fat particles and FFA pass to the systemic circulation causing endothelial injury in brain, kidney, retina, or skin.

B. Nontraumatic
1. Controversial
2. C-reactive protein or other mediators agglutinate blood lipids with subsequent embolization.
3. Liberation of FFA from fat stores due to catecholamines

> ### PEARL
>
> In many conditions, especially long bone fractures, small amounts of fat enter the circulation, but without significant clinical findings. Fat embolism syndrome is the occurrence of clinical manifestations that occur in some patients in which fat embolism is more severe or protracted.

Epidemiology

A. Fat embolism is common after blunt trauma (80% of cases).
B. Fat embolism syndrome occurs in a minority of patients with fat embolism.
1. Occurs in 0.5% to 2% of patients with isolated long bone fractures
2. Occurs in 5% to 10% of patients with multiple long bone fractures or concomitant pelvic fractures
C. Risk of FES with closed bone fractures versus open bone fractures is controversial.
D. Most commonly seen in second and third decades of life
E. No sex predilection
F. There is a latent period of FES, which occurs 12 to 72 hours after trauma (occasionally up to 1 week).
G. Fat embolism syndrome without pulmonary involvement is uncommon.

539

Clinical Findings

A. Constitutional: fever

B. Pulmonary

  1. Dyspnea

  2. Tachypnea

  3. Hypoxemia

  4. Rales and rhonchi

  5. Pleural friction rub (rare)

  6. Findings of permeability (low pressure) pulmonary edema and the acute respiratory distress syndrome (ARDS; see Chapter 8)

C. Neurologic

  1. Mental status changes: confusion, delirium, obtundation, coma

  2. Headache, irritability

  3. Convulsions

  4. Hemiparesis, hemiplegia, cerebral edema due to fat microemboli or petechial hemorrhagic infarcts

D. Cutaneous: petechiae on upper chest, axilla, neck, face

E. Ocular

  1. Intravascular fat emboli on funduscopic exam (Purtscher's retinopathy)

  2. Exudates, edematous patches, cotton wool spots

  3. Perivascular or petechial hemorrhage

  4. Subconjunctival petechia

F. Cardiovascular

  1. Tachycardia

  2. Electrocardiogram

    a. Usually normal

    b. Right heart strain or nonspecific T wave changes may be seen.

Key Differential Diagnosis

- Multi-organ trauma
- Neurologic trauma
- Severe infections
- Sepsis syndrome
- Thrombocytic thrombocytopenic purpura

Diagnosis (Gurd Criteria)

A. Major criteria (most patients have more than 1)

  1. Axillary or subconjunctival petechiae

  2. Hypoxemia (PaO$_2$ <60 torr at FIO$_2$ ≤0.40)

  3. Central nervous system depression disproportionate to hypoxemia

  4. Pulmonary edema

B. Minor criteria (should have 4 or more)

  1. Tachycardia

  2. Fever (body temperature 38.5°C or higher)

  3. Retinal emboli

  4. Fat in urine

  5. Fat globules in sputum

  6. Fall of hematocrit or platelet count; rise of sedimentation rate

Laboratory and Other Tests

A. Blood

  1. Sensitivity and specificity of blood tests are poor.

  2. Cytologic examination of blood drawn from pulmonary artery catheter may reveal fat globules.

  3. Anemia

  4. Thrombocytopenia

  5. Hypofibrinogenemia

  6. Elevated serum lipase activity

  7. Elevated serum lipid levels

B. Bronchoalveolar lavage

  1. More than 30% of lavage cells contain neutral fat.

  2. Most useful in patient with overt pulmonary and neurologic abnormalities that cannot be ascribed to FES (confirmatory test)

Imaging Studies

A. Chest x-ray

  1. Normal in mild cases

  2. In severe cases, x-ray is initially normal but infiltrates develop over the next 48 to 72 hours.

  3. Diffuse bilateral alveolar or interstitial infiltrates ("snowstorm" pattern)

  4. May progress to diffuse capillary permeability type edema; i.e., acute respiratory distress syndrome (ARDS)

  5. May reveal complications of ARDS (e.g., pneumothorax or fibrosis)

B. Transcranial Doppler detection of fat emboli is a research tool.

C. Transesophageal echocardiography

  1. May be useful in monitoring during orthopedic surgery (nailing procedures of long bones)

  2. Fat emboli are seen as echogenic material.

3. Only some of the patients with echocardiographic evidence of emboli develop FES.

D. Ventilation–perfusion scanning is not helpful.

Key Diagnostic Points

- High index of suspicion
- Hypoxemia
- Pulmonary edema
- Central nervous system depression
- ARDS pattern on chest x-ray

Monitoring

A. Hemodynamic
   1. Noninvasive blood pressure monitoring
   2. Tissue perfusion; urine output
   3. Consider pulmonary artery catheter in selected patients.

B. Pulmonary
   1. Oxygenation: arterial blood gases, pulse oximetry
   2. Pulmonary mechanics

Key Treatment

- Supportive pulmonary care
- Treatment of respiratory failure and ARDS
- Hemodynamic monitoring and support
- Corticosteroid use is controversial.

Complications

A. Neurologic complications (often resolve)
B. Respiratory failure and complications of ARDS
   1. Hypoxemia
   2. Pneumothorax

3. Oxygen toxicity
4. Pulmonary fibrosis
5. Pulmonary infections

Key Prevention

- Early fixation of long bone fractures
- Prophylactic corticosteroids are controversial.

Prognosis

A. Mortality rate is approximately 10%.
B. Most neurologic dysfunction is reversible.
C. Grave prognostic signs include
   1. Coma
   2. Severe ARDS
   3. Pneumonia
   4. Superimposed congestive heart failure
   5. Sepsis

Bibliography

Bulger EM, Smith DG, Maier RV, Jurkovick GJ. Fat embolism syndrome: a 10-year review. Arch Surg 1997;132:435–439.

Fabian TC. Unravelling the fat embolism syndrome. N Engl J Med 1993;329:961–963.

Fabian TC, Hoots AV, Stanford DS, et al. Fat embolism syndrome: prospective evaluation in 92 fracture patients. Crit Care Med 1990;18:42–46.

Godeau B, Schaeffer B, Bachir D, et al. Bronchoalveolar lavage in adult sickle cell patients with acute chest syndrome: value for diagnostic assessment of fat embolism. Am J Respir Crit Care Med 1996;153:1691–1696.

Gurd AR. Fat embolism: an aid to diagnosis. J Bone Joint Surg Br 1970;52:732–737.

Mellor A, Soni N. Fat embolism. Anaesthesia 2001;56:145–154.

Pell AC, Hughes D, Keating J, et al. Brief report: fulminating fat embolism syndrome caused by paradoxical embolism through a patent foramen ovale. N Engl J Med 1993;329:926–929.

Pitto RP, Koessler M, Draenert K. Prophylaxis of fat and bone marrow embolism in cemented total hip arthroplasty. Clin Orthop 1998;355:23–34.

Stanley JD, Hanson RR, Hicklin GA, et al. Specificity of bronchoalveolar lavage for the diagnosis of fat embolism syndrome. Am Surgeon 1994;60:537–541.

153 Rhabdomyolysis

James A. Kruse

Rhabdomyolysis is a syndrome characterized by skeletal muscle injury and necrosis that results in characteristic laboratory findings and a variety of potential complications, most notably acute renal failure and compartment syndrome.

Etiology

A. Physical muscle injury
  1. Trauma, especially crush injuries
  2. Thermal (burn) injury
  3. Electrical shock
  4. Lightning injury
  5. Pressure necrosis
  6. Other: jackhammer use, mechanical bull rides, bongo drum playing

B. Extreme exertion
  1. Extreme exercise, contact sports, noncontact sports (e.g., marathon running)
  2. Seizures
  3. Status asthmaticus
  4. Delirium tremens
  5. Fighting against physical restraints

C. Ischemic/hypoxic muscle injury
  1. Postural arterial compression due to coma, incapacitation, anesthesia
  2. Arterial thrombosis, clot embolism, or surgical occlusion
  3. Compartment syndrome
  4. Prolonged tourniquet application
  5. Sickle cell hemoglobinopathy
  6. Arterial air embolism
  7. Vasculitis
  8. Carbon monoxide poisoning

D. Infection
  1. Bacterial infections: e.g., *Clostridium perfringens* (gas gangrene), *Clostridium tetani* (tetanus), *Streptococcus, Staphylococcus, Legionella, Salmonella, Vibrio, Escherichia coli, Listeria,* leptospirosis, tularemia, brucellosis, shigellosis
  2. Mycoplasmal infection: *Mycoplasma pneumoniae*
  3. Viruses: e.g., Epstein-Barr virus, herpesviruses, adenovirus, influenza, echovirus, coxsackievirus, cytomegalovirus, hantavirus
  4. Rickettsial infections: Rocky Mountain spotted fever
  5. Parasitic causes: trichinosis

E. Chemical toxins
  1. Carbon monoxide poisoning
  2. Alcohols, glycols, hydrocarbons: ethanol, methanol, isopropanol, ethylene glycol, toluene, gasoline
  3. Other organic toxins: strychnine, iodoacetate, sodium fluoroacetate, chlorphenoxy herbicides
  4. Heavy metals: mercury, $HgCl_2$, tetraethyl lead, copper, selenium
  5. Other inorganic toxins: cyanide, hydrogen sulfide, phosphine, phosphorus

F. Nonbacterial biotoxins
  1. Arthropod envenomations: hymenopteran stings, brown recluse spider bite, centipede bite
  2. Various snake bites
  3. Quail meat or water hemlock (?)

G. Drug associations
  1. Sedative, hypnotic, narcotic drug overdoses: e.g., benzodiazepines, glutethimide, ethchlorvynol, doxylamine, heroin, methadone, propoxyphene, propofol
  2. Other illicit drugs: cocaine, amphetamines, phencyclidine, lysergic acid diethylamide
  3. Other drug overdoses: salicylates, isoniazid, cyclic antidepressants (e.g., amitriptyline, amoxapine, doxepin), theophylline, lithium, neuroleptics (e.g., butyrophenones, phenothiazines)
  4. 3-Hydroxy-3-methylglutaryl coenzyme A reductase inhibitors: e.g., lovastatin, simvastatin, pravastatin, fluvastatin
  5. Miscellaneous drugs: succinylcholine, clofibrate, quinine, quinidine, epsilon aminocaproic acid, corticosteroids

H. Metabolic associations
  1. Hypokalemia
  2. Hypophosphatemia
  3. Diabetic ketoacidosis
  4. Hyperosmolar nonketotic syndrome
  5. Hyponatremia and hypernatremia
  6. Hypothyroidism
  7. Thyroid storm
  8. Pheochromocytoma

I. Temperature-related disorders
  1. Exposure hypothermia
  2. Heat stroke
  3. Malignant hyperthermia
  4. Neuroleptic malignant syndrome

J. Genetic disorders
  1. Abnormal carbohydrate metabolism
    a. Various muscle enzyme deficiencies: e.g., myophosphorylase (McArdle's syndrome), phosphofructokinase (Tarui's disease), α-glucosidase deficiency (Pompe's disease), phosphohexomerase, amylo-1,6-glucosidase, lactate dehydrogenase (LDH) M-subunit transferase
  2. Abnormal lipid metabolism: e.g., carnitine palmityltransferase deficiency, carnitine deficiency
  3. Muscular dystrophies
K. Psychiatric disorders
  1. Psychosis, catatonia
  2. Neuroleptic malignant syndrome
  3. Neuroleptic agent-induced dystonic reactions
  4. Strait jacket restraint
L. Miscellaneous
  1. Polymyositis, dermatomyositis
  2. Systemic lupus erythematosus
  3. Idiopathic recurrent rhabdomyolysis

Key Etiologies

- Severe trauma and crush injuries
- Drug overdose or alcohol intoxication
- Compression injury from any cause of coma
- Status epilepticus
- Systemic viral infections such as influenza
- Locally invasive bacterial soft-tissue infection
- Various inborn errors of metabolism

Clinical Manifestations

A. History
  1. Consistent with etiology
  2. Local myalgias, weakness
  3. Local or distal pain, paresthesias, hypesthesia
  4. Brown-colored urine, oliguria
B. Physical findings
  1. Consistent with etiology
  2. Muscle tenderness, muscle compartment tenseness or swelling
  3. Muscle weakness
  4. Peripheral neuropathy
  5. Skin bullae (due to pressure necrosis of skin)

Key Complications

- Acute myoglobinuric renal failure
- Compartment syndrome with neuropathy or nonviable extremity
- Hypocalcemia (early) and hypercalcemia (late)
- Iatrogenic fluid overload, hypokalemia, or severe alkalemia

Laboratory Findings

A. Increased serum creatine phosphokinase (CK) activity
  1. Due to CK release (mainly CK-MM isoenzyme) from skeletal muscle
  2. Mild to extreme elevations are possible (just over upper normal limit to >1,000,000 units/L).
B. Increased serum aldolase, LDH, LDH-5 isoenzyme, aspartate aminotransferase, alanine aminotransferase activity
C. Myoglobinemia: may be transient
D. Elevated serum urea nitrogen and creatinine
  1. Elevated serum urea nitrogen may be due to hypovolemia or myoglobinuric renal failure.
  2. Serum creatinine may rise more rapidly than typical of acute renal failure, due to high creatine load from infarcted muscle.
E. Alterations in serum potassium
  1. Severe hypokalemia may be present as a causative or contributory factor.
  2. Severe hyperkalemia can occur as a result of release of potassium from infarcted muscle tissue (~100 mmol potassium/kg muscle), development of acute renal failure, or both.
F. Alterations in serum calcium
  1. Hypocalcemia may occur early in course due to sequestration of calcium in infarcted muscle tissue.
  2. Hypercalcemia can occur later in course, typically within 2 days to 2 weeks after entering diuretic phase of acute renal failure.
    a. May be secondary to mobilization of sequestered calcium, alterations in parathormone or vitamin D, and physical immobilization
    b. Particularly likely if calcium supplementation was given for hypocalcemia early in course
G. Alterations in serum phosphorus
  1. Hypophosphatemia may be present as a causative or contributory factor.
  2. Hyperphosphatemia may occur from intracellular phosphate release, acute renal failure, or both.

H. Acid-base disturbances are common.

1. Metabolic acidosis secondary to myoglobinuric renal failure or lactic acidosis due to associated hypovolemic or septic shock

2. Increased anion gap

   a. From acute renal failure and possibly release of intracellular anions

   b. Increase may be more severe than expected for the degree or duration of renal failure.

3. Metabolic alkalosis resulting from $NaHCO_3$ administration

4. Respiratory acid-base disturbances may occur related to underlying cause

I. Hyperuricemia: breakdown product of myocyte-derived nucleic acids

J. Evidence of disseminated intravascular coagulation: e.g., increased prothrombin time, increased partial thromboplastin time, thrombocytopenia, increased D-dimer or fibrin monomer levels

K. Urine abnormalities

1. Myoglobinuria

   a. If severe (>100 mg/dL): grossly visible, dark-brown urine

   b. May be transient and missed by biochemical analysis

2. Urinalysis showing positive dipstick test for blood, but few or no red blood cells (RBCs)

   a. Can be indicative of myoglobinuria

      (1) Myoglobin cross–reacts with dipstick test for hemoglobin.

      (2) Paucity of RBCs suggests lack of hemoglobin in specimen.

   b. Pattern can also be seen in hematuria with hypotonic urine due to osmotic hemolysis.

3. Proteinuria

4. Signs of acute tubular necrosis: e.g., presence of renal tubular cells

---

Key Treatment

- Maintain adequate hydration.

- Maintain high urine output, if possible.

- Alkalinize urine with sodium bicarbonate, if possible.

- Correct hypokalemia and hypophosphatemia.

- Hemodialysis may be necessary.

- Monitor for development of compartment syndrome.

- Fasciotomy may be necessary to preserve threatened limb.

Treatment

A. General measures

1. Ensure adequate hydration using IV fluids.

   a. Use isotonic fluid initially if hypovolemic (common unless established renal failure).

   b. Consider central venous pressure monitoring to aid in ensuring adequate hydration and avoiding hypovolemia.

   c. Consider pulmonary artery catheterization in patients with circulatory shock or serious underlying cardiac disease.

2. Consider specific diagnostic tests if etiology is not obvious: e.g., toxicologic screening tests, thyroid function tests, body fluid cultures, carboxyhemoglobin levels, etc.

3. Correct hypoxemia or impaired tissue oxygen delivery.

4. Control seizures or severe agitation.

5. Correct hypothermic or hyperthermia.

6. Provide specific treatment for underlying cause.

B. Maintain adequate diuresis: e.g., urine output 200 to 300 mL/hour, if possible

1. May minimize risk of acute myoglobinuric renal failure

2. Generally accomplished using hydration with IV fluid

3. Intravenous mannitol has also been used in conjunction with IV fluid loading.

   a. Mannitol: 1 g/kg of 20% solution IV over 30 minutes, may repeat every 6 hours

   b. Alternative is 10 to 25 g mannitol added to each liter of titrated IV fluid.

   c. Monitor serum osmolality.

   d. Do not use if established renal failure.

4. In patients with established renal insufficiency, fluid overload, or impending fluid overload, a loop diuretic may be tried (avoid hypovolemia).

C. Alkalinize urine.

1. Aim is for urine pH >7, to minimize separation of the nephrotoxic heme moiety from myoglobin within renal tubules.

2. Accomplished using IV sodium bicarbonate

   a. Typical starting dose: 100 mmol in 1 L 5% dextrose, or 50 mmol in 1 L 5% dextrose in 0.45% saline, at 250 mL/hour

   b. Monitor volume status, acid-base status, potassium, glucose, and sodium levels frequently.

   c. Titrate infusion rate to achieve alkaline urine while avoiding excessive alkalemia, or to maintain arterial blood pH ~7.50.

d. Helpful to use two different IV access routes and two separate IV solutions: one IV solution containing $NaHCO_3$ with rate titrated for desired acid-base effect, and a second IV solution containing isotonic or hypotonic saline titrated to achieve additional hydration and diuresis as necessary

3. If urine pH not alkaline despite arterial pH ≥7.48, consider use of acetazolamide.

4. Urinary alkalinization is unlikely to be meaningful if patient is oliguric or has severe impairment in glomerular filtration rate.

D. Monitor for electrolyte imbalance.

1. Serial serum assays of sodium, potassium, ionized calcium, magnesium, phosphorus, urate

2. Treat hyperkalemia if present (e.g., insulin + glucose, sodium polystyrene sulfonate, hemodialysis).

3. Hypokalemia is particularly likely to occur during $NaHCO_3$ administration.

4. Administer potassium and phosphate supplements if necessary.

5. Avoid giving calcium for hypocalcemia, unless symptomatic.

6. Monitor throughout course for hypercalcemia, which may develop during recovery phase.

E. Monitor acid-base balance.

1. Monitor arterial blood gases and serum CO_2 content.

2. Use results to titrate $NaHCO_3$ to maintain mild alkalemia.

3. Avoid excessive alkalemia (pHa >7.53) during $NaHCO_3$ infusion.

F. Consider hemodialysis early in course if acute renal failure develops.

G. Monitor for signs of compartment syndrome.

1. Perform serial assessments.

a. Assess for subjective neurologic symptoms indicative of peripheral nerve compression, e.g., peripheral paresthesias or pain.

b. Assess for objective signs of peripheral neurovascular compression, e.g., peripheral pulse deficits, hypesthesia, decreased motor strength, and loss of deep tendon reflexes.

c. Assess for physical signs of increased compartment pressure, e.g., tense swelling of compartment (significant false negative rate).

2. Consider compartment pressure measurement.

a. Indicated if suspected compartment syndrome, especially in unconscious patients

b. Normal resting, passive compartment pressure is lower than 10 mm Hg (postural compression, e.g., lying on hard surface with torso compressing limb, can result in increases to more than 100 mm Hg).

3. Most patients are at highest risk for compartment syndrome during first few days after presentation.

H. Decompressive fasciotomy

1. Sustained compartment pressure greater than 20 to 30 mm Hg may indicate need for fasciotomy.

2. Performed to avoid vascular compromise, compressive peripheral nerve injury, worsening muscle necrosis, and potential loss of limb

I. Amputation necessary for nonviable limb

Key Prognostic Points

- Prognosis for survival varies with underlying cause and its severity.

- Most survivors recover some or all renal function.

- Permanent renal failure requiring life-long dialysis may occur.

- Peripheral neuropathies may be reversible or permanent.

Bibliography

Guglielminotti J, Guidet B. Acute renal failure in rhabdomyolysis. Minerva Anesthesiol 1999;65:250–255.

Mars M, Hadley GP. Raised intracompartmental pressure and compartment syndrome. Injury 1998;29:403–411.

Ruttenber AJ, McAnally HB, Wetli CV. Cocaine-associated rhabdomyolysis and excited delirium: different stages of the same syndrome. Am J Forensic Med Pathol 1999;20:120–127.

Visweswaran P, Guntupalli J. Rhabdomyolysis. Crit Care Clin 1999;15:415–428.

154 Tumor Lysis Syndrome

Lisa Mueller

Tumor lysis syndrome is a metabolic emergency that can occur in patients with neoplastic disease. It occurs chiefly after cytotoxic therapy in patients with large tumor burdens, but it can also occur without cytotoxic therapy in bulky disease.

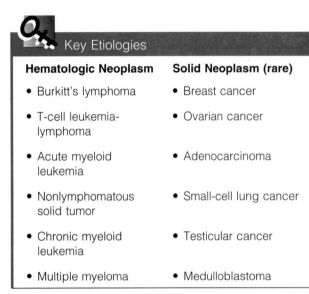

Key Etiologies

Hematologic Neoplasm	Solid Neoplasm (rare)
• Burkitt's lymphoma	• Breast cancer
• T-cell leukemia-lymphoma	• Ovarian cancer
• Acute myeloid leukemia	• Adenocarcinoma
• Nonlymphomatous solid tumor	• Small-cell lung cancer
• Chronic myeloid leukemia	• Testicular cancer
• Multiple myeloma	• Medulloblastoma

Pathophysiology

A. Mechanism is tumor degradation, development of inadequate renal function, and accumulation of toxic metabolites.

B. Occurrence
   1. Usually occurs 1 to 2 (but up to 5 or more) days after start of chemotherapy or radiation therapy
   2. Particularly likely to occur with rapidly growing tumors that are very chemosensitive
   3. Rarely, can occur spontaneously (i.e., without cytotoxic therapy); mostly in Burkitt's lymphoma

C. Specific metabolite accumulation
   1. Uric acid
      a. Derived from breakdown of nucleic acids
      b. Precipitates in an acidic environment causing urate nephropathy and nephrolithiasis
   2. Phosphate
      a. Released from lysed tumor cells
      b. Precipitates as calcium phosphate if the calcium-phosphate product is greater than 60 mg^2/dL^2

   c. Precipitation within the microvasculature can lead to renal failure, hypocalcemia, and seizures.
   3. Potassium
      a. Released from lysed tumor cells promoting development of hyperkalemia
      b. Hyperkalemia also develops as a result of renal failure occurring as a complication of tumor lysis.
      c. Hyperkalemia can lead to ventricular dysrhythmias and death.

Key Risk Factors

- Bulky, rapidly proliferating, chemosensitive tumors
- Chemotherapy administration
- Older age
- Elevated serum uric acid level
- Increased serum lactate dehydrogenase activity
- Poor urine output
- Renal parenchymal involvement (azotemia)
- Dehydration

Clinical Findings

A. Symptoms
   1. Anorexia
   2. Vomiting
   3. Abdominal pain or fullness
   4. Back or flank pain
   5. Change in urine volume
   6. Muscle cramps, spasms, or tetany
   7. Confusion
   8. Seizures

B. Physical examination
   1. Hypertension
   2. Cardiac rhythm disturbances
   3. Oliguria or polyuria
   4. Hematuria
   5. Pleural effusion
   6. Ascites
   7. Alterations in consciousness

Laboratory and Other Tests

A. Serum biochemical tests
   1. Sodium
   2. Potassium
      a. Pseudohyperkalemia may be seen with hyperleukocytosis.
      b. If serum level is elevated and pseudohyperkalemia is a possibility, check the plasma potassium level.
   3. Chloride
   4. Total CO_2 content
   5. Calcium (total and ionized)
   6. Phosphorus
   7. Urea nitrogen
   8. Creatinine
   9. Uric acid
   10. Lactate dehydrogenase
B. Complete blood cell count
C. Urinalysis with urine pH and microscopic examination
D. Electrocardiogram (ECG): to assess for dysrhythmias and ECG signs of hyperkalemia
E. Abdominal ultrasonography or computed tomography (avoid IV contrast) to exclude obstructive uropathy (uncommon)

Key Laboratory Findings

- Hyperuricemia
- Hyperkalemia
- Hyperphosphatemia
- Azotemia

Treatment

A. Major goals
   1. Prevent or minimize risk of developing renal failure.
   2. Promote excretion of uric acid and phosphorus.
   3. Restore metabolic stability.
B. Hydration and alkalinization
   1. Adequate hydration is the most important measure.
   2. Infuse 5% dextrose in 0.25 normal saline at 2 to 4 times maintenance to maintain urine specific gravity below 1.010.
   3. Add $NaHCO_3$ to IV solution (50 to 100 mmol/L) to target a urine pH of 7.0 to 7.5.

C. Allopurinol
   1. Inhibits xanthine oxidase, blocking purine degradation of hypoxanthine and xanthine to uric acid and increasing their excretion
   2. Dose: 10 mg/kg per day or 300 mg/m² (300 to 900 mg) per day orally every 12 hours
   3. Consider initiating 48 hours before cytoxic therapy in patients with high urate levels or those at high risk.
   4. Avoid urine pH higher than 8 as hypoxanthine stones and calcium phosphate crystals may form in the urinary tract.
D. Monitor laboratory tests (see above) every 4 to 6 hours.
E. Stop all potassium administration until hyperkalemia is excluded.
F. Treat hyperkalemia, if present (see Chapter 40, Hyperkalemia).
G. Dialysis
   1. For impending or overt renal failure and
      a. Hyperkalemia (potassium >6 mmol/L)
      b. Serum uric acid level higher than 10 mg/dL
      c. Serum creatinine level more than 10× normal
      d. Serum phosphorus level higher than 10 mg/dL
      e. Symptomatic hypocalcemia
   2. Hemodialysis is preferable to peritoneal dialysis.
H. Chemotherapy
   1. Purpose is to decrease tumor burden.
   2. Begun once uric acid level is decreasing, urine specific gravity is lower than 1.010, urine pH is 7.0 to 7.5, or the patient is stabilized on dialysis
I. Avoid drugs that inhibit tubular reabsorption of urate.
   1. Salicylates
   2. Probenecid
   3. Ethambutol
   4. Thiazide diuretics
   5. Radiocontrast agents
J. Other (?)
   1. Leukapheresis or exchange transfusion, in the setting of marked leukocytosis
   2. Low-dose corticosteroids (however, have been reported to induce acute uric acid nephropathy)

Monitoring

A. Frequent vital signs
B. Continuous electrocardiographic monitoring
C. Chest examination and chest x-ray for pleural effusions
D. Abdominopelvic examination (for evidence of renal mass, distended bladder, ascites)

E. Foley catheterization and strict monitoring of fluid intake and output

F. Serial biochemical tests
   1. See above.
   2. Monitor serum CO_2 content or arterial blood gases during alkali therapy to obviate excessive alkalemia (avoid pHa >7.5).

Key Complications

- Secondary renal failure

- Hypocalcemia

- Fluid overload

- Metabolic alkalosis (iatrogenic) or acidosis

- Cardiac dysrhythmias, cardiac arrest

Bibliography

Castro MP, VanAuken J, Spencer-Cisek P, et al. Acute tumor lysis syndrome associated with concurrent biochemotherapy of metastatic melanoma: a case report and review of the literature. Cancer 1999;85:1055–1059.

Cohen LF, Balow JE, Magrath IT, et al. Acute tumor lysis syndrome. Am J Med 1980;68:486–491.

Fassas AB, Desikan KR, Siegel D, et al. Tumour lysis syndrome complicating high-dose treatment in patients with multiple myeloma. Br J Haematol 1999;105:938–941.

Kalemkerian GP, Darwish B, Varterasian ML. Tumor lysis syndrome in small cell carcinoma and other solid tumors. Am J Med 1997;103:363–367.

O'Regan S, Carson S, Chesney RW, et al. Electrolyte and acid-base disturbances in the management of leukemia. Blood 1977;49:345–353.

Schelling JR, Ghandour FZ, Strickland TJ, et al. Management of tumor lysis syndrome with standard continuous arteriovenous hemodialysis: case report and a review of the literature. Ren Fail 1998;20:635–644.

155 Superior Vena Cava Syndrome
Lisa Mueller

Superior vena cava (SVC) syndrome is a thoracic emergency resulting from compression or obstruction of the superior vena cava. If left untreated this disorder can lead to respiratory compromise and death.

Pathophysiology

A. The SVC is thin walled and easily compressed by abnormally expanding adjacent structures (e.g., lymph nodes, thymus, adjacent pericardium, coronary vessels), due to infiltrative, infectious, or other pathologic process.

B. The SVC can also become obstructed by intraluminal processes, most commonly thrombosis or invading tumor.

C. Superior vena cava thrombosis can occur as a secondary process, once external compression or non-thrombotic intraluminal obstruction decreases flow sufficiently to induce it.

D. Effects of compression or obstruction
   1. Upstream venous hypertension resulting in plethora and edema
   2. Decreased venous blood return from the head, neck, upper extremities, and upper thorax
   3. Cerebral edema and compromised brain perfusion with resulting central nervous system dysfunction
   4. Concomitant potential for compression and air flow through trachea and major bronchi

E. If due to malignant tumor, the onset of clinical manifestations in adults is often insidious.

Etiology

A. Mediastinal tumors
   1. Malignant tumors
      a. Bronchogenic carcinoma, especially the small-cell variety (the most common malignant cause)
      b. Non-Hodgkin's lymphoma
      c. Metastases (breast cancer, germ cell and gastrointestinal malignancies, etc.)
      d. Hodgkin's lymphoma
      e. Leukemia
      f. Neuroblastoma
      g. Ewing's sarcoma
      h. Thymoma
      i. Thyroid cancer
   2. Benign tumors
      a. Lymphoid hyperplasia
      b. Benign thymoma
      c. Benign teratoma
      d. Neuroma
      e. Hygroma
      f. Atrial myxoma

B. Mediastinal fibrosis
   1. Histoplasmosis
   2. Sarcoidosis
   3. Other granulomatous diseases
   4. Post-radiation
   5. Pyogenic
   6. Idiopathic

C. Cardiovascular
   1. Aortic aneurysm
   2. Congenital heart disease
   3. Complications of cardiovascular surgery
   4. Pericarditis
   5. Pericardial cyst
   6. Mitral stenosis

D. Superior vena cava thrombosis
   1. Central venous catheterization
   2. Transvenous pacemaker insertion
   3. Secondary thrombosis (i.e., secondary to another cause of SVC syndrome)

E. Hydrocephalus

F. Infections
   1. Tuberculosis
   2. Syphilis

G. Goiter

H. Behçet's syndrome

I. Tracheal or bronchial cysts

Key Etiologies

- Malignancy is the most common etiology.

- Among cancers, the most common is bronchogenic carcinoma.

- Among bronchogenic neoplasms, the most common is small-cell cancer.

Symptoms

A. Early
1. Dyspnea
2. Cough
3. Hoarseness
4. Dysphagia
5. Orthopnea
6. Chest pain

B. Late
1. Lethargy
2. Headache
3. Distorted vision
4. Sense of ear fullness
5. Syncope
6. Symptoms of spinal cord compression (rare)

Key History

- Symptoms are often aggravated in supine or flexed positions.

- There may be a history of cancer, cardiac disease, exposure to infections or pertinent past operations.

Physical Examination

A. General
1. Anxiety
2. Diaphoresis
3. Tachypnea

B. Cutaneous (head, neck, upper thorax, upper extremities)
1. Ruddy facial complexion
2. Plethora, facial edema
3. Telangiectases
4. Cyanosis

C. Head
1. Chemosis
2. Glossal edema
3. Findings of Horner's syndrome

D. Neck
1. Laryngeal paralysis
2. Dilated neck veins
3. Neck edema

E. Chest
1. Dilated veins of upper thorax
2. Upper chest edema

3. Stridor
4. Wheezing

F. Extremities
1. Upper extremity edema
2. Notable lack of lower extremity edema

G. Neurological
1. Confusion, alterations in mentation
2. Alterations in sensorium, coma
3. Focal cerebral signs
4. Signs of spinal cord compression (rare)

Imaging Studies

A. Chest x-ray
1. Usually abnormal
2. Frequently shows evidence of a superior mediastinal mass

B. Computed tomography
1. May reveal an extrinsic mass lesion compressing the SVC
2. Intravenous contrast will delineate intraluminal obstruction and show dilated collateral vessels.

C. Magnetic resonance imaging

D. Doppler ultrasound

E. Echocardiography

F. Conventional venography (usually unnecessary)

Laboratory and Other Tests

A. Blood tests
1. Routine biochemical tests (to screen for underlying etiology)
2. Complete blood cell and differential white blood cell count
3. Tumor markers
   a. Carcinoembryonic antigen
   b. α-Fetoprotein
   c. Lactate dehydrogenase
   d. Human chorionic gonadotropin
   e. Neuron-specific enolase

B. Sputum cytology

C. Microbiological smears and cultures

D. Bronchoscopic washings, brushing, lavage

E. Biopsy of pertinent site(s)
1. Bronchoscopic biopsy (increased risk of bleeding complication)
2. Mediastinoscopy
3. Bone marrow biopsy
4. Lymph node biopsy
5. Other (depends on suspicion for specific underlying tumor)

Key Diagnostic Points

- Rapid diagnosis is essential.

- Diagnosis should be made by the least invasive means.

- Consider biopsy only in low-risk patients when the diagnosis is otherwise not clear.

- Avoid sedation or general anesthesia in high-risk patients because of potential for inducing circulatory or respiratory compromise.

Treatment

A. Uncover and treat underlying etiology.

B. Monitor closely for the possibility of impending cardiovascular or respiratory compromise.

C. Elevate head of bed.

D. Diuretics may be palliative if hemodynamic status allows.

E. Treatment for malignant processes

   1. Diagnosis known

      a. Treat with appropriate chemotherapy, radiation therapy, or both, based on clinical picture and radiosensitivity of tumor.

      b. Radiation therapy is employed in most cases; doses as low as 200 cGy can shrink tumor rapidly if radiosensitive.

      c. Small-cell lung cancer may respond well initially to chemotherapy.

   2. Diagnosis not known

      a. Controversy exists over the circumstances in which radiation or chemotherapy should be employed when a tissue diagnosis is lacking.

      b. Empiric therapy offers the advantage of expeditious and potentially life-prolonging treatment.

      c. The disadvantage is the possibility of exposure to radiation or chemotherapy for a nonmalignant process, including attendant risks of this treatment and the risks of delaying diagnosis and definitive treatment.

   3. Anticoagulation not used routinely in malignant etiologies because of risk of bleeding, especially during antineoplastic therapy

   4. Steroids may be of value in lymphoma and some other malignancies.

   5. Rarely, post-radiation therapy airway edema and respiratory compromise occur, requiring a short course of prednisone (e.g., 40 mg/m^2 per day every 6 hours).

F. Central venous catheter thrombosis

   1. Medical emergency

   2. Thrombolytic therapy (see Chapter 174, Thrombolytic Agents)

      a. Streptokinase: 250,000 U bolus followed by 100,000 U per hour intravenously for 24 to 72 hours

      b. Monitor thrombin time (2 to 3 times normal recommended).

      c. Remove catheter if thrombus is not lysed.

   3. Heparin

      a. Used to prevent clot propagation, but ineffective for clot lysis

      b. Recommended following thrombolysis with streptokinase

      c. Dose: 5,000 to 10,000 U bolus followed by continuous infusion at 1,300 U per hour; titrate for partial thromboplastin time of 1.5× normal

G. Percutaneous endovascular stent placement

H. Surgical intervention

   1. May be indicated in some refractory cases with progressive symptoms

   2. Examples

      a. Malignant tumor unresponsive to radiation or chemotherapy

      b. Benign tumor

      c. Thrombosis

      d. Chylous effusion

   3. High risk of bleeding

Bibliography

Adelstein DJ, Hines JD, Carter SG, et al. Thromboembolic events in patients with malignant superior vena cava syndrome and the role of anticoagulation. Cancer 1988;62:2258–2262.

Mineo TC, Ambrogi V, Nofroni I, et al. Mediastinoscopy in superior vena cava obstruction: analysis of 80 consecutive cases. Ann Thorac Surg 1999;68:223–226.

Neuman GC, Weingarten AE, Abramowitz RM, et al. The anesthetic management of the patient with an anterior mediastinal mass. Anesthesiology 1984;60:144–147.

Qanadli SD, El Hajjam M, Bruckert F, et al. Helical CT phlebography of the superior vena cava: diagnosis and evaluation of venous obstruction. AJR Am J Roentgenol 1999;172:1327–1333.

Thony F, Moro D, Witmeyer P, et al. Endovascular treatment of superior vena cava obstruction in patients with malignancies. Eur Radiol 1999;9:965–971.

Yahalom J. Superior vena cave syndrome. In: DeVita VT Jr, Hellman S, Rosenberg SA (eds). Cancer: Principles and Practice of Oncology, 5th ed. Philadelphia: Lippincott, 1997; pp 2469–2476.

156 Obstetric Crises

Brian A. Mason

Pregnancy may complicate or exacerbate any number of catastrophic conditions. Any condition that may occur in a nonpregnant reproductive aged woman can generally occur in the gravida as well. There are, however, certain maladies unique to pregnancy. Several of the more acute and potentially disastrous of these are outlined here.

Peripartum Cardiomyopathy

Key Definition and Epidemiology

- Idiopathic heart failure about the time of pregnancy
- Most commonly manifests during labor or shortly after delivery
- Affects approximately 1 in 15,000 deliveries

Clinical Findings

A. Symptoms
   1. Fatigue
   2. Dyspnea
   3. Orthopnea
   4. Cough
   5. Palpitations
   6. Chest and abdominal pain
B. Physical signs
   1. Elevated jugular venous pressure
   2. Pulmonary rales
   3. S_3 gallop
   4. Peripheral edema
   5. Normotension (usually); may be hypertensive due to vasoconstriction
   6. Reduced pulse pressure secondary to low cardiac output

Tests

A. Chest x-ray
   1. Cardiomegaly
   2. Pulmonic infiltrates and pulmonary vascular congestion
B. Electrocardiogram (usually nondiagnostic)

   1. Sinus tachycardia
   2. Dysrhythmias common
C. Echocardiogram
   1. Increased internal end-diastolic dimensions
   2. Decreased ventricular wall motion

Treatment

A. Treat as with other forms of heart failure.
B. Digoxin (use cautiously as many of these patients have complex ventricular dysrhythmias)
C. Diuretics
D. Limit sodium intake.
E. Avoid hypokalemia.
F. Afterload reduction
   1. Frequently associated with superimposed preeclampsia (see Chapter 26, Pregnancy-Induced Hypertension)
   2. Angiotensin converting enzyme inhibitors if patient has delivered
   3. Hydralazine if patient undelivered
G. Consider anticoagulation with heparin.
   1. High incidence of mural thrombi and pulmonary embolism
   2. Warfarin contraindicated
H. Treat anemia and infection aggressively.

> **WARNING**
>
> **Angiotensin converting enzyme inhibitors are contraindicated during pregnancy.**

Prognosis

A. Important to distinguish from reversible causes
B. Prognosis for true peripartum cardiomyopathy is very poor.
C. Persistent cardiomyopathy and development of ventricular dysrhythmias suggest poor outcome.
D. Up to 50% of patients with true peripartum cardiomyopathy die within 1 year.
E. Heart transplantation is the only definitive treatment if end-stage heart failure ensues.

Anaphylactoid Syndrome of Pregnancy

Key Definition and Pathophysiology

- A catastrophic anaphylactoid reaction occurring in pregnancy; formerly known as amniotic fluid embolism

- Pathophysiology remains unclear; may be an anaphylactic reaction to thromboplastin-rich amniotic fluid.

Diagnosis

A. Sudden onset of agitation, dyspnea, and respiratory arrest, often occurring during labor, delivery, or the immediate postpartum period
B. Differential diagnosis
   1. Acute pulmonary edema (cardiogenic or noncardiogenic)
   2. Pulmonary thromboembolism
   3. Cardiac dysrhythmia
   4. Classic anaphylactic reaction to drug or environmental agent
   5. Sepsis

Treatment

A. Primarily supportive
B. Endotracheal intubation and mechanical ventilation
C. Cardiac resuscitative measures
D. Left ventricular failure may necessitate inotropic therapy.
E. Pulmonary artery catheterization
   1. Survivors of the initial event require meticulous cardiac and renal management.
   2. Obtain blood sample from distal pulmonary artery catheter lumen during balloon inflation for histological staining to detect fetal squamous cells and mucin.
F. Perform platelet count and coagulation studies including prothrombin time, partial thromboplastin time, fibrin(ogen) degradation products, fibrinogen, fibrin monomer, and D-dimer assays.
G. Consider component therapy if disseminated intravascular coagulation (DIC) is present.
H. Survivors of initial cardiopulmonary event typically have a 2 to 5 day course of respiratory failure due to acute respiratory distress syndrome.

Prognosis

A. Accounts for over 10% of maternal mortality in the United States

B. Mortality rate during the initial resuscitative effort is 50%; overall mortality rate approaches 80%.
C. Survivors may develop left ventricular failure, acute respiratory distress syndrome or DIC.

Septic Abortion

Key Definition

- Aborted pregnancy with intrauterine infection resulting in secondary generalized sepsis

- Often associated with instrumentation of uterine cavity: e.g., illegal abortion attempt or pregnancy occurring with intrauterine device (IUD) in situ

Clinical Findings

A. Fever
B. Pelvic pain
C. Uterine cramping
D. Vaginal bleeding
E. History of uterine instrumentation
F. IUD in situ
G. Altered mental status
H. Signs of circulatory shock

Tests

A. Pregnancy test to confirm gravid state
B. Complete blood count with differential white blood cell and platelet count
C. Blood, cervical, and urine cultures
D. Coagulation studies
E. Type and cross match
F. Abdominal x-ray studies (observe for air under diaphragm, because bowel perforation may occur from instrumentation of the uterus)
G. Pelvic ultrasonography

Complications and Prognostic Risk Factors

A. Evidence of circulatory shock or cardiovascular instability
B. Coagulopathy
C. Acute respiratory distress syndrome
D. Uterine or bowel perforation
E. Intra-abdominal bleeding
F. Oliguria
G. Advanced (second trimester or beyond) pregnancy

Treatment

A. Low-risk patient
1. Intravenous antibiotics: aminoglycoside plus cephalosporin or penicillinase-resistant β-lactam agent
2. Uterine evacuation (suction, dilation and curettage)
B. High-risk patient
1. Intravenous antibiotics as above
2. Aggressive management of circulatory shock
3. Expedite surgical intervention.
4. If no bowel or uterine injury, peritoneal signs, or active bleeding, then evacuate uterus under direct laparoscopic visual control.
5. If uterine or bowel perforation, peritonitis, or intra-abdominal bleeding present, proceed to exploratory laparotomy.
   a. Evacuate uterine cavity.
   b. Drain abdomen.
   c. Repair or resect injured tissue.

Uterine Rupture

Definition and Risk Factors

A. Catastrophic separation of uterine musculature
B. Usually at site of previous surgical scarring (from cesarean section, myomectomy, etc.)
C. Predisposing factors include
1. History of uterine surgery
2. Intrauterine instrumentation
3. Oxytocin-induced hyperstimulation
4. Obstructed labor
5. Abdominal trauma
6. Cocaine use

Clinical Findings

A. Acute abdominal pain
B. Evidence of fetal distress (perform ultrasound or electronic fetal monitoring)
C. Vaginal bleeding
D. Tachycardia (maternal and fetal)
E. Hematuria
F. Circulatory collapse (out of proportion to apparent vaginal blood loss)

Key Laboratory Tests in Uterine Rupture

- Serial hematocrit assays
- Coagulation studies
- Type and cross match for packed red cells

Treatment

A. Assess cardiovascular status and treat as with any hemorrhagic event.
1. Crystalloid volume resuscitation
2. Blood and component therapy as needed
3. Treat other complications of shock.
B. Immediate delivery of fetus via cesarean section if undelivered and fetal distress present
C. Repair versus remove uterus during cesarean delivery.

Abruptio Placentae

Definition

A. Premature separation of placenta from uterine wall
B. Often catastrophic with potentially disastrous consequences for mother and fetus
C. Predisposing risk factors:
1. Pregnancy-induced hypertension
2. High parity
3. Direct abdominal trauma
4. Uterine anomalies
5. Cocaine use
6. Cigarette smoking
7. Sudden uterine decompression

Clinical Findings

A. Uterine tenderness
B. Increased uterine tone
C. Fetal distress
D. Cardiovascular decompensation
E. Vaginal bleeding

Key Tests in Abruptio Placentae

- Complete blood cell and platelet counts
- Serial hematocrit assays
- Serial coagulation studies
- Obstetrical ultrasound
- Continuous electronic fetal heart rate monitoring
- Assessment of cardiovascular stability and blood loss

Differential Diagnosis

A. Placenta previa
B. Acute surgical abdomen
C. Degeneration of myoma
D. Uterine rupture

Treatment

A. Assess degree of severity
   1. Mild separation, stable maternal and fetal conditions, minimal bleeding
   2. Severe separation, unstable mother, fetal distress, heavy bleeding
B. Mild separation with preterm (< 36 weeks gestation) fetus
   1. Bed rest
   2. Fetal monitoring
   3. Serial ultrasonography
   4. Await onset of labor unless change in status, then proceed to delivery.
C. Mild separation with term gestation
   1. Proceed to delivery room with "double setup" (immediate capability for cesarean or vaginal birth).
D. Severe separation with viable fetus in no distress
   1. Provide fluid, blood, and cardiovascular support as needed.
   2. Proceed to immediate cesarean delivery.

Postpartum Hemorrhage

Definition and Classification

A. Largely a clinical judgement
B. Classic definition is greater than 500 mL of blood loss after delivery but hemodynamic stability in pregnant women usually maintained with up to 2 L of blood loss.
C. Classified as early if it occurs within first 24 hours of delivery
D. Classified as late if more than 24 hours but less than 6 weeks after delivery
E. Accounts for up to 11% of maternal deaths in the United States

Etiology

A. Uterine atony (most common etiology)
   1. Uterine overdistension
   2. Rapid or prolonged labor
   3. High parity
   4. Oxytocic agents
   5. Chorioamnionitis
   6. Uterine relaxing agents
B. Trauma
   1. Forceps delivery
   2. Precipitous delivery
   3. Large birth weight
C. Retained placenta
   1. Prior cesarean delivery
   2. Placenta accreta
   3. High parity
D. Uterine rupture
E. Coagulopathy
   1. Pregnancy-induced hypertension
   2. Abruptio placentae
   3. Anaphylactoid syndrome of pregnancy
   4. Sepsis
   5. Retained dead fetus
   6. Inherited coagulopathy

Treatment

A. The most important aspect of management is preparation based on recognition of risk factors.
   1. All pregnant women should have blood type and rh factors determined.
   2. If risk factors are present, place a large-bore (16 g) IV access, keep patient well hydrated, and have uterotonic agents immediately available.
B. If postpartum hemorrhage does occur
   1. Determine cause.
      a. Inspect for lacerations.
      b. Perform bimanual examination for uterine atony, uterine rupture, or retained products of conception.
   2. Perform laboratory studies.
      a. Complete blood cell and platelet count
      b. Prothrombin and partial thromboplastin times
      c. Fibrin(ogen) degradation products, fibrinogen, D-dimer, and fibrin monomer assays
      d. Bedside clot retraction test
   3. Correct identified cause.
      a. Lacerations packed or sutured
      b. Atony treated as needed with uterotonic agents
      c. Treat hemorrhagic shock aggressively.
      d. Avoid uterine packing.
   4. Uterotonic agents
      a. Oxytocin, prepared to 20 U/L crystalloid, and given by continuous IV infusion titrated to effect
      b. Methylergonovine 0.2 mg intramuscularly
      c. 15-Methylprostaglandin F 0.25 mg intramuscularly or intramyometrially
   5. If bleeding persists from uterine source despite uterotonic agents consider surgical intervention.
      a. Uterine artery ligation
      b. Hypogastric artery ligation

c. Selective arterial embolization

d. Hysterectomy

Key Treatment for Postpartum Hemorrhage

- Ensure adequate IV access.
- Initiate resuscitation with crystalloid fluids.
- Blood product transfusion
- Administer uterotonic agent.
- Determine cause and address.
- Serial hematocrit, platelet, and coagulation studies
- Consider surgical intervention.

 Bibliography

Case records of the Massachusetts General Hospital. Weekly clinicopathological exercises. Case 9–1998. Cardiovascular collapse after vaginal delivery in a patient with a history of cesarean section. N Engl J Med 1998; 338:821–826.

Heider AL, Kuller JA, Strauss RA, et al. Peripartum cardiomyopathy: a review of the literature. Obstet Gynecol Surv 1999;54:526–531.

Locksmith GJ. Amniotic fluid embolism. Obstet Gynecol Clin North Am 1999;26:435–444.

Pelage JP, Soyer P, Repiquet D, et al. Secondary postpartum hemorrhage: treatment with selective arterial embolization. Radiology 1999;212:385–389.

Pridmore BR, Chambers DG. Uterine perforation during surgical abortion: a review of diagnosis, management and prevention. Aust NZ J Obstet Gynaecol 1999;39: 349–353.

157 Pressure Ulcers

Jai K. Prasad

Epidemiology

A. More than 2 million people afflicted annually in the United States

B. Significant prevalence in intensive care unit (ICU) patients

C. Approximately 60% of patients with decubitus ulcers are more than 70 years old

D. Approximately 20% incidence in paraplegic patients

E. Approximately 25% incidence in quadriplegic patients

Pathophysiology and Etiology

A. Pathophysiology

1. Pressure is transmitted from cutaneous surface to underlying bone, compressing all the intervening tissues.

2. Unrelieved external compression exceeding capillary blood pressure results in ischemia and necrosis.

3. The greatest extent of ischemia and necrosis takes place at the bony interface and not on the skin surface.

B. Factors contributing to pressure sore formation

1. Altered activity and mobility

2. Friction and shear force

3. Lack of sensory perception

4. Accumulation of moisture

5. Secondary wound infection

C. High-risk patients

1. Traumatic brain injury

2. Spinal cord injury

3. Encephalopathic or comatose condition

4. Dementia or chronic brain syndromes

5. Age more than 70 years

6. Poor nutritional status

7. Morbidly obese

D. Most common sites affected

1. Sacral area

2. Heel

3. Ischial tuberosity

4. Trochanteric area

Key Clinical Findings

- *Stage I:* nonblanchable erythema of intact skin, reddened for more than 1 hour after relief of pressure

- *Stage II:* partial-thickness skin loss involving epidermis and, in some cases, dermis; may manifest as cracked, blistered, abraded, or broken skin, or a shallow crater

- *Stage III:* full-thickness skin loss with subcutaneous destruction that may extend down to, but not through, fascia

- *Stage IV:* full thickness skin loss with extensive tissue necrosis or destruction involving muscle, tendon, bone, or joint capsule; there may be undermining or sinus tract formation

Treatment

A. Integrate prevention with treatment: routine periodic inspection for pressure ulceration allows diagnosis in stage I or II of the disease process, making treatment simpler

B. Nutritional therapy

1. Perform nutritional assessment (see Chapter 213, Nutritional Assessment).

2. Ensure diet or nutritional support with adequate calorie and protein intake.

3. Provide vitamin and mineral supplements, as indicated.

C. Pain management

1. Assess patient for pain related to ulcer and treatment.

2. Provide adequate analgesia.

3. Analgesia may be necessary during dressing changes and debridement.

D. Incontinence management

E. Infection management

1. Swab wound culture: not useful because only detects organisms at surface, which is normally colonized with bacteria

2. Needle aspiration or tissue biopsy: can be useful to diagnose soft tissue infection

3. Bone biopsy: criterion standard for diagnosis of osteomyelitis

4. Topical antibiotic therapy

a. Not routinely recommended

b. May be considered (e.g., silver sulfadiazine) as a 2-week trial for ulcers that are not healing or continue to produce exudate after 2 to 4 weeks of optimal care

5. Systemic antibiotic therapy: necessary if there are signs of cellulitis, osteomyelitis, bacteremia, or sepsis

6. Debridement: see below

F. Positioning techniques

1. Avoid positioning immobile patients so that pressure is applied to an existing ulcer or to areas at high risk of developing pressure sores (e.g., trochanters).

2. Regular turning (minimum every 2 hours) of immobile patients is prophylactic and therapeutic.

3. Avoid sitting position for patients with pressure ulcer on sitting surface; if used, reposition every hour.

4. Avoid use of doughnut-type cushion devices.

a. Lead to edema formation, local venous congestion, and circumferential ischemia

b. More likely to cause than prevent or treat pressure ulcers

5. Use positioning devices (e.g., pillows, foam wedges, sheepskin) to prevent direct contact between bony eminences (e.g., knees or ankles).

6. Consider foam wedges or other devices to suspend ankles and totally relieve pressure on heels.

7. Limit duration of head of bed elevation, and maintain at lowest elevation possible, consistent with other therapeutic considerations.

G. Special support surfaces

1. Static support surfaces

a. Standard mattress

b. Foam overlay

(1) Reduces pressure by increasing support area

(2) Low cost

c. Flotation (air or water)

(1) Increases support area and reduces shear

(2) Low cost

2. Dynamic support surfaces: consider if patient cannot assume a variety of positions without bearing weight on pressure ulcer, patient fully compresses static support surface, or ulcer does not show signs of healing after 2 to 4 weeks

a. Alternating-pressure air mattress

(1) Increases support area, reduces shear, provides dynamic pressure reduction

(2) Moderate cost

b. Low air loss bed (KinAir)

(1) Consists of multiple, inflatable cushions attached to a modified hospital bed frame; allows elevation of head and foot of bed

(2) Increases support area, reduces heat accumulation, has low moisture retention, provides dynamic pressure reduction

(3) Consider for patients with stage III or IV ulcers on multiple turning surfaces, or if patient "bottoms out" or fails to heal on dynamic overlay or mattress.

(4) Lightweight, similar to regular hospital bed, high cost

c. Air-fluidized bed (Clinitron)

(1) Glass beads fluidized by pressurized air and contained under a polyester sheet

(2) Increases support area, reduces shear, provides dynamic pressure reduction, has low moisture retention

(3) Consider for bed-bound patients with stage III or IV ulcers on multiple turning surfaces, who "bottom out," fail to heal on dynamic overlay or mattress, and are incontinent.

(4) Heavy, generates heat, noisy, very high cost

H. Relief of spasticity

1. Spasticity frequently seen in patients with spinal cord injuries, especially proximal cord lesions

2. Incidence of spasm is 100% in cervical region, 75% in thoracic region, and 50% in thoracolumbar region.

3. Spasms in these patients are believed to be from loss of supraspinal inhibitory pathways.

4. Treatment options for reducing spasticity include pharmacotherapy (e.g., benzodiazepines), peripheral nerve block, epidural stimulators, and rhizotomy.

5. Spasms must be eliminated before surgical procedures; otherwise, pressure sores will recur.

I. Becaplermin (Regranex) gel 0.01%

1. Recombinant platelet derived growth factor

2. Accelerates ulcer healing by promoting chemotactic recruitment and proliferation of cells involved in formation of granulation tissue and wound healing

3. Approved for use in lower extremity ulcers due to diabetic neuropathy

4. Efficacy in pressure ulcer treatment demonstrated in preliminary investigations

J. Wound cleansing

1. Removal of necrotic tissue, exudate, and metabolic wastes optimizes wound healing.

2. Routinely cleanse wounds initially and with each dressing change, using a minimum of chemical and mechanical trauma.

3. Selection of cleansing agent

   a. Normal saline is recommended for routine use.

   b. Avoid use of cytotoxic skin cleansers or antiseptic agents (e.g., iodophor, povidone iodine, hydrogen peroxide, sodium hypochlorite).

4. Mechanical methods

   a. Gauze, cloth, or sponges

   b. Moderate irrigation pressure (4 to 15 psi) enhances cleansing without trauma.

      (1) Water Pik at low setting (~6 psi)

      (2) 35-mL syringe with 19 gauge needle or angiocatheter (~8 psi)

      (3) 250 mL squeeze bottle with irrigation cap (~4.5 psi)

      (4) Bulb syringes may have limited efficacy due to low pressures (typically ~2 psi).

   c. Whirlpool hydrotherapy: consider for stable patients with thick exudate, slough, or necrotic tissue

K. Debridement (removal of devitalized tissue)

1. Sharp debridement

   a. Limited surgical debridement (e.g., unroofing eschar) may be performed at bedside.

   b. Debridement of large or extensive ulcers

      (1) Definitive surgical debridement may need to be performed in the operating room.

      (2) Bone biopsy should be considered to detect osteomyelitis.

   c. Debridement may be facilitated by instilling methylene blue solution inside the cavity to delineate the extent of excision necessary.

   d. Use dry dressings for 8 to 24 hours after sharp debridement associated with bleeding, then resume moist dressings.

2. Mechanical and chemical debridement

   a. Saline wet-to-dry dressings: should not be used on clean, granulating wounds

   b. Povidone iodine wet-to-dry dressings: not recommended, because it is cytotoxic to fibroblasts and macrophages and it delays healing

   c. Buffered Dakin's solution (0.025%) may be used.

      (1) Bacteriocidal, but nontoxic to fibroblasts and macrophages

      (2) Dressings should be changed every 8 hours to eliminate exudate and effect debridement.

   d. Wound irrigation and hydrotherapy: see section J. Wound cleansing

3. Enzymatic debridement (topical application of enzymes to devitalized tissue on wound surface)

   a. Trypsin (e.g., Granulex aerosol)

   b. Papain-urea (e.g., Accuzyme)

   c. Collagenase (e.g., Santyl ointment)

   d. Fibrinolysin + desoxyribonuclease (e.g., Elase ointment)

   e. Streptokinase + streptodornase (e.g., Veridase)

4. Autolytic debridement

   a. Use of synthetic dressings to cover wound and allow self-digestion of devitalized tissue by enzymes naturally present in wound fluids

   b. Should not be used in the presence of wound infection

L. Other surgical options

1. Simple debridement and nonoperative measures should be tried first.

2. Ostectomy procedures

   a. Surgical excision of bony eminence

   b. May be partial or complete

3. Pressure ulcer closure procedures

   a. Skin graftings may be possible in case of superficial ulceration, but the success rate is only around 30%; therefore, wound closure is usually accomplished by rotation of local skin, fasciocutaneous flaps, or musculocutaneous flaps.

   b. Musculocutaneous flap is superior to other alternatives in the closure of infected wounds.

      (1) Advantages: has excellent blood supply and provides a bulky padding

      (2) Disadvantages: sensitivity of muscle to external pressure and atrophic muscles in spinal cord patients

   c. Fasciocutaneous flap

      (1) Offers additional advantages: adequate blood supply, durable coverage, and anatomic padding over boney eminence

      (2) Disadvantage: limited bulk

M. Dressings

1. Purpose

   a. Protects the wound

   b. Controls exudate

   c. Maintains hydration within the ulcer bed

   d. Maintains surrounding, intact skin dry

2. Specific types of dressings

a. Dry gauze dressing

(1) Used temporarily after sharp debridement to absorb blood

(2) Used if heavy exudate

b. Continuously moist saline dressing

(1) Routine dressing

(2) Maintains hydration of ulcer tissue

(3) Minimally absorptive, inexpensive, versatile

(4) Requires frequent dressing changes

c. Saline wet-to-dry dressings

(1) Used only for debridement

(2) Not used to maintain moisture

d. Transparent polymer film dressings (e.g., Tegaderm, Opsite)

(1) Gas-permeable, self-adhesive polyurethane film

(2) Moisture-retaining properties, nonabsorptive

(3) Requires less nursing time than continuously moist saline gauze dressing

(4) Useful for stage I and II sores

e. Hydrocolloid dressing (e.g., DuoDerm, Tegasorb)

(1) Nontransparent, self-adhesive, semipermeable or occlusive

(2) Moisture-retaining properties

(3) Hydrocolloid material forms a gel at dressing-wound interface; promotes autolysis.

(4) Requires less nursing time than continuously moist saline gauze dressing

(5) Potentially useful for all stages, especially stages II and III

f. Calcium alginate dressing (e.g., Sorbsan, Kaltostat)

(1) Highly absorptive dressing material derived from seaweed

(2) Potential utility in stage II through IV lesions with moderate to heavy exudate, and as cavity filler

(3) Not for use on dry wounds

g. Loose packing: used if there is a cavity, to prevent abscess formation

N. Other therapeutic modalities

1. Electrotherapy: shown to have efficacy in stage III and IV ulcers unresponsive to conventional therapy

2. Hyperbaric oxygen therapy: insufficient data to recommend

3. Ultraviolet or infrared radiation: insufficient data to recommend

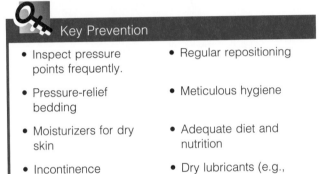

Key Prevention

- Inspect pressure points frequently.

- Pressure-relief bedding

- Moisturizers for dry skin

- Incontinence management

- Regular repositioning

- Meticulous hygiene

- Adequate diet and nutrition

- Dry lubricants (e.g., cornstarch) to reduce friction injury

Bibliography

Bergstrom N, Bennett MA, Carlson CE, et al. Pressure Ulcer Treatment. Clinical Practice Guideline. Quick Reference Guide for Clinicians, No. 15. Rockville, MD: U.S. Department of Health and Human Services, Public Health Service, Agency for Health Care Policy and Research, AHCPR Pub. No. 95-06532. Dec. 1994.

Evans JM, Andrews KL, Chutka DS, et al. Pressure ulcers: prevention and management. Mayo Clin Proc 1995;70: 789–799.

Pierce GF, Tarpley JE, Allman RM, et al. Tissue repair processes in healing chronic pressure ulcers treated with recombinant platelet-derived growth factor BB. Am J Pathol 1994;145:1399–1410.

Pompeo M, Baxter C. Sacral and ischial pressure ulcers: evaluation, treatment, and differentiation. Ostomy Wound Manage 2000;46:18–23.

Rees RS, Robson MC, Smiell JM, et al. Becaplermin gel in the treatment of pressure ulcers: a phase II randomized, double-blind, placebo-controlled study. Wound Rep Reg 1999;7:141–147.

Thomson JS, Brooks RG. The economics of preventing and treating pressure ulcers: a pilot study. J Wound Care 1999;8:312–316.

158 Air Embolism

Elizabeth S. Guy

Air embolism is a potentially fatal condition that occurs when air is entrained into blood vessels as a complication of certain invasive procedures or trauma. Two types of gas embolism are recognized, related to the portal of entry: venous (VAE) or arterial air embolism. Paradoxical arterial embolism (PAE) occurs when there is right-to-left shunting, as may occur in atrial septal defect, patent foramen ovale, or when the filtering function of the lung is overwhelmed. This chapter reviews venous and paradoxical air embolism.

Etiology

A. Requirements for air entry into the venous system
   1. Breach in venous integrity with atmospheric communication
   2. Positive atmospheric-to-venous pressure gradient
      a. A gradient of 5 cm H_2O or more between atmosphere and right atrium
      b. Experimentally, 100 mL of air can enter 14-gauge needle in 1 second in the presence of a 5 cm H_2O gradient.
B. Procedures associated with VAE
   1. Central or peripheral venous catheters: during insertion, removal or disconnect (open to atmosphere)
   2. Surgical procedures
      a. Neurosurgery in the sitting position
      b. Head and neck surgery
      c. Gas insufflation during laparoscopic surgery
      d. Transurethral resection of the prostate
      e. Liver transplantation
      f. Total hip replacement
      g. Cesarean section
      h. Intraoperative use of hydrogen peroxide
   3. Gastrointestinal endoscopy
   4. Nd:YAG laser bronchoscopy
   5. Intrauterine gas insufflation during pregnancy
C. Trauma
   1. Chest trauma, blunt or penetrating
   2. Blast injury

Pathophysiology

A. Gas in the right ventricle and pulmonary outflow tract obstructs blood flow from the right ventricle, resulting in rapid cardiopulmonary decompensation.
   1. Volume of gas that can be tolerated in humans is unknown.
   2. Animal studies suggest that 100 to 300 mL may be fatal in adults.
B. Large bolus of gas can lead to paradoxical air embolism via patent foramen ovale.
   1. Foramen ovale is probe-patent in 30% of the population.
   2. Acute rise of right atrial pressure by air lock promotes right-to-left shunting.
C. Effects of air bubbles in pulmonary arterioles and capillaries
   1. Ventilation–perfusion mismatching with increased dead space
      a. Hypoxemia
      b. Hypercarbia
      c. Low end-tidal P_{CO_2} (PetCO$_2$) and increased end-tidal P_{N_2}
   2. Increased airway resistance occurs.
   3. Noncardiogenic pulmonary edema is a common result of endothelial injury and increased capillary permeability.
D. Air lodged in the pulmonary arterioles is dissipated into alveolar space.
E. Pulmonary filtering capacity can be overwhelmed by a large bolus of gas, resulting in air passing to pulmonary veins.

Clinical Findings

A. Symptoms
   1. Dyspnea
   2. Chest pain
   3. Sense of impending death
B. Physical findings
   1. Respiratory
      a. Tachypnea
      b. Wheezing
      c. Reflex gasping respiration in spontaneously breathing patients
   2. Cardiovascular
      a. Hypotension
      b. Tachycardia or bradycardia
      c. Cardiac dysrhythmias
      d. Mill-wheel murmur may be heard late and transiently; caused by agitation of blood and air in the right ventricle.

e. Angina pectoris

f. Livedo reticularis

3. Neurologic

a. Confusion, altered mentation, seizures, or focal neurologic deficit

b. Caused by hypoxia and hypotension, or by paradoxical brain embolism

C. Laboratory findings

1. Hypoxemia

2. Hypercarbia

D. Hemodynamic findings

1. Elevated central venous and pulmonary artery pressures

2. Decreased cardiac output

E. Electrocardiogram may show right heart strain.

Key Diagnostic Features

- Dyspnea, chest pain, sense of impending death

- Hypotension

- Signs of paradoxical arterial embolism

- Decreased $PetCO_2$

- Detection of air by Doppler ultrasound or echocardiography

Diagnosis

A. Requires knowledge of risks for air embolism during invasive procedures, and a high index of clinical suspicion

B. Transesophageal echocardiography

1. The most sensitive method to detect VAE (as little as 0.02 mL/kg)

2. Position the probe at level of aortic valve to visualize right ventricular outflow tract or to display right and left atria or four chambers.

3. May detect patent foramen ovale or paradoxical air embolus

4. Drawbacks include invasive nature, expense, and requirement for trained personnel.

C. Precordial Doppler ultrasound

1. Can detect 0.25 mL air

2. Place along right parasternal border between intercostal spaces 3 to 6.

3. Turbulent noise generated by the air–blood interface and alterations of heart tones are associated with intracardiac air.

4. Consider intraoperative monitoring with precordial Doppler ultrasound when incision is made above the level of the heart.

D. End-tidal PCO_2 monitoring

1. Sensitive to detect VAE

2. Practical and convenient

3. Useful in conjunction with Doppler ultrasound to assess hemodynamic significance of intravascular air

4. Decrease in $PetCO_2$ identifies significant embolus with ventilation–perfusion mismatching.

5. Drawback: decreased $PetCO_2$ alone is not specific; consider other causes

E. Increased pulmonary artery pressures

1. May be suggestive in appropriate setting; e.g., high-risk surgical procedure

2. Correlates with volume and rate of entry of air into pulmonary circuit

F. Direct observation of surgical field

1. Venous bleeding indicates that venous pressure exceeds atmospheric pressure.

2. Observation of air entrainment during catheter placement warrants immediate evaluation and assessment of cardiopulmonary status.

Key Differential Diagnosis

- Other causes of pulmonary edema, cardiogenic and noncardiogenic

- Venous thromboembolism

- Acute ischemic event

Treatment

A. Identify source of air entry and stop air entrainment.

B. Initiate cardiopulmonary support, including cardiopulmonary resuscitation and vasopressors.

C. Give 100% oxygen to reduce the size of air bubbles by increasing the gradient for nitrogen to diffuse from emboli.

D. Consider positioning a multi-orifice catheter at the junction of the superior vena cava and right atrium to retrieve the embolus.

1. May remove up to 50% of embolus and prevent death

2. Drawback: not suited to most situations except high-risk posterior fossa cranial surgery and similar conditions

E. Increase central venous pressure by fluid loading to reduce gradient for air entry into venous circuit.

F. Positioning (Trendelenburg, left lateral decubitus) advocated but of little effectiveness because the buoyancy of air bubbles is exceeded by the force of blood flow

G. Consider hyperbaric therapy for paradoxical arterial embolism and clinical deterioration (hyperbaric therapy is not indicated in VAE).

H. Heparin administration is controversial; complications may exceed potential benefit.

I. Corticosteroids: controversial, but generally not recommended

J. Lidocaine: may be considered for arterial gas embolism in therapeutic doses; avoid overdose

Key Treatment

- Stop additional air entry immediately.

- Support cardiopulmonary function.

- Administer 100% oxygen.

- Provide volume expansion.

- Institute hyperbaric treatment in PAE.

Bibliography

Albin MS. Air embolism. In: Albin MA (ed). Textbook of Neuroanesthesia with Neurosurgical and Neuroscience Perspectives. New York: McGraw-Hill, 1997, pp 1009–1025.

Annane D, Troche G, Delisle F, et al. Effects of mechanical ventilation with normobaric oxygen therapy on the rate of air removal from cerebral arteries. Crit Care Med 1994;22:851–857.

Muth CM, Shank ES. Gas embolism. N Engl J Med 2000; 342:476–482.

Palmon SC, Moore LE, Lundberg J, Toung T. Venous air embolism: a review. J Clin Anesth 1997;9:251–257.

Porter JM, Pidgeon C, Cunningham AJ. The sitting position in neurosurgery: a critical appraisal. Br J Anaesth 1999;82:117–128.

Toung TJ, Rossberg MI, Hutchins GM. Volume of air in a lethal venous air embolism. Anesthesiology 2001;94:360–361.

Weaver LK, Morris A. Venous and arterial gas embolism associated with positive pressure ventilation. Chest 1998; 113:1132–1134.

159 Intravenous Fluids

James A. Kruse

Indications

A. Maintenance fluid replacement (e.g., in patients who are n.p.o.)

B. Maintaining patent IV access (e.g., for potential emergency use in unstable patients)

C. Correction of fluid deficits (e.g., for treating dehydration or hypovolemia)

D. Replacement of on-going fluid losses (e.g., treatment of polyuria or diarrhea)

E. Resuscitation (e.g., treatment of hypovolemic or septic shock)

F. Correction of electrolyte derangements (e.g., use of potassium-containing IV solutions to treat hypokalemia)

G. Correction of acid-base disorders (e.g., saline treatment of metabolic alkalosis)

H. Correction of abnormal osmolality (e.g., treatment of hyperosmolar coma)

I. Caloric supplementation (e.g., dextrose infusions, partial or total parenteral nutrition)

J. Forced diuresis (e.g., for treatment of rhabdomyolysis, salicylate intoxication, or hypercalcemia)

K. Vehicle for IV drug infusions (e.g., to administer dopamine infusions)

PEARL

Do not administer blood transfusions through Ringer's or Ringer's lactate solution; the calcium-containing IV fluid can neutralize the citrate anticoagulant.

Formulations (Table 159–1)

A. Isotonic crystalloids

1. Include fluids that are approximately iso-osmolar to plasma

2. Expand the extracellular space; i.e., the interstitial and intravascular compartments

3. Are second to colloid preparations in ability to rapidly expand intravascular volume

4. Are commonly available with and without added 5% (5 g/dL) dextrose

5. Common formulations

a. Normal saline (NS)

(1) Contains only NaCl (0.9 g/dL)

(2) Tends to cause non-anion gap metabolic acidosis (dilutional acidosis) when large volumes are administered

b. Ringer's lactate

(1) More physiologic than normal saline because it contains potassium, calcium, and buffer at near-physiologic concentrations

(2) Contains lactate as a buffer, which tends to alkalinize body fluids once metabolized

(3) Has a greater number of IV drug incompatibilities compared to saline

(4) Cannot be used as diluent for blood transfusions

(5) Avoid in patients with renal dysfunction or hyperkalemia (contains potassium), or hypercalcemia (contains calcium).

c. Proprietary physiologic preparations

(1) Various formulations are commercially available; e.g., Normosol R, Plasma-Lyte A

(2) Contain Na^+, Cl^-, other electrolytes

(3) Many preparations include stable buffer anions (e.g., acetate), which counter the tendency to develop dilutional acidosis seen with large volumes of NS.

B. Hypotonic fluids

1. Not useful for rapid intravascular volume expansion

2. Useful for treating hyperosmolar states (once intravascular volume is replete) and administering parenteral fluid without excessive sodium loading

3. Dextrose-containing formulations can have an osmolarity in excess of physiologic plasma osmolality, but they are considered hypotonic because the dextrose component is ultimately metabolized.

4. Formulations

a. Hypotonic saline

(1) 0.45 g/dL saline (half-strength NS), with or without 5% dextrose; useful for maintenance parenteral fluid

TABLE 159–1. COMPOSITION OF REPRESENTATIVE CRYSTALLOID AND COLLOID-BASED IV FLUIDS*

SOLUTION	Na^+	K^+	Cl^-	Ca^{2+}	Mg^{2+}	LAC-TATE	ACE-TATE	GLUC-ONATE	DEX-TROSE (g/dL)	~pH (RANGE)	OSMO-LARITY (mOsm/L)	~ONCOTIC PRESSURE (torr)
			(mEq/L)									
0.9% (normal) saline	154	—	154	—	—	—	—	—	—	5.0 (4.5–7.0)	308	—
0.9% saline + D5	154	—	154	—	—	—	—	—	5	4.0 (3.2–6.5)	560	—
0.45% (1/2-normal) saline	77	—	77	—	—	—	—	—	—	5.0 (4.5–7.0)	154	—
0.45% saline + 2.5% dextrose	77	—	77	—	—	—	—	—	2.5	4.5 (3.2–6.5)	280	—
0.45% saline + D5	77	—	77	—	—	—	—	—	5	4.0 (3.2–6.5)	406	—
0.33% saline + D5	56	—	56	—	—	—	—	—	5	4.0 (3.2–6.5)	365	—
0.3% saline + D5	51	—	51	—	—	—	—	—	5	4.0 (3.2–6.5)	355	—
0.3% saline + 3.3% dextrose	51	—	51	—	—	—	—	—	3.3	4.5 (3.5–6.5)	270	—
0.225% saline + D5	38.5	—	38.5	—	—	—	—	—	5	4.3 (3.5–6.5)	329	—
0.2% saline + D5	34	—	34	—	—	—	—	—	5	4.0 (3.2–6.5)	321	—
3% (hypertonic) saline	513	—	513	—	—	—	—	—	—	5.0 (4.5–7.0)	1027	—
5% (hypertonic) saline	856	—	856	—	—	—	—	—	—	5.0 (4.5–7.0)	1712	—
7.5% (hypertonic) saline†	1283	—	1283	—	—	—	—	—	—	5.0 (4.5–7.0)	2566	—
5% dextrose	—	—	—	—	—	—	—	—	5	4.0 (3.2–6.5)	252	—
10% dextrose	—	—	—	—	—	—	—	—	10	4.0 (3.2–6.5)	505	—
20% dextrose	—	—	—	—	—	—	—	—	20	4.0 (3.2–6.5)	1010	—
Ringer's	148	4	156	4.5	—	—	—	—	—	5.5 (5.0–7.5)	309	—
Ringer's lactate	130	4	109	2.7	—	28	—	—	—	6.5 (6.0–7.5)	273	—
D5 + Ringer's lactate	130	4	109	2.7	—	28	—	—	5	6.0 (4.0–6.5)	525	—
D2.5 +1/2-Ringer's lactate	65	2	55	1.4	—	14	—	—	2.5	5.0 (4.0–6.5)	263	—
Normosol R + D5	140	5	98	—	3.0	—	27	23	5	5.2 (4.0–6.0)	547	—
Plasma-Lyte A pH 7.4	140	5	98	—	3.0	—	27	23	—	7.4 (6.5–8.0)	294	—
Plasma-Lyte R	140	10	103	5.0	3.0	8	47	—	—	5.5 (4.0–8.0)	312	—
Plasma-Lyte M + D5	40	16	40	5.0	3.0	12	12	—	5	5.0 (4.0–6.5)	377	—
5% albumin	145 ± 15	<2.5	145 ± 15	—	—	—	—	—	—	6.9 (6.4–7.4)	~290	20
25% albumin	145 ± 15	<2.5	145 ± 15	—	—	—	—	—	—	6.9 (6.4–7.4)	~290	100
10% dextran-40 in NS	154	—	154	—	—	—	—	—	—	5.0 (3.5–7.0)	311	68
10% dextran-40 in D5	—	—	—	—	—	—	—	—	5	4.0 (3.0–7.0)	255	68
6% dextran-70 in NS	154	—	154	—	—	—	—	—	—	5.0 (4.0–6.5)	309	60
4% modified fluid gelatin‡	154	—	120	—	—	—	—	—	—	7.4 (7.1–7.7)	274	33
6% hetastarch	154	—	154	—	—	—	—	—	—	5.5 (3.5–7.5)	310	30
Lactated 6% hetastarch	143	3	124	5	0.9	28	—	—	0.1	5.9 (5.8–6.1)	307	30
10% pentastarch§	154	—	154	—	—	—	—	—	—	4.8 (3.5–7.0)	326	40

* Exact values of some components of preparations may vary depending on specific proprietary formulation; D5 = 5% dextrose; D2.5 = 2.5% dextrose; NS = normal saline; 1/2 = half-strength.

† Used investigationally for resuscitation from hemorrhagic shock.

‡ Not available in the United States.

§ Current U.S. labeling restricted to use as an adjunct for leukapheresis.

(2) 0.33 g/dL saline with 5% dextrose

(3) 0.3 g/dL saline with 5% dextrose

(4) 0.225 g/dL saline (quarter-strength NS) with 5% dextrose

(5) 0.2 g/dL saline with 5% dextrose

b. Pure dextrose solutions

  (1) Pure dextrose preparations have no electrolytes and represent free water administration.

  (2) Use cautiously in patients with hyperglycemia or glucose intolerance.

  (3) Have negligible impact on intravascular volume

  (4) Most efficient solutions for expanding the intracellular compartment

  (5) Caloric content is 3.4 kcal/g dextrose; however, not a substitute for enteral or parenteral nutrition formulas.

  (6) Formulations

    (a) 5% (5 g/dL) dextrose in water: isotonic in vitro and during infusion

    (b) 10% (10 g/dL) dextrose in water: used for treatment or prevention of hypoglycemia, especially in patients prone to fluid overload (may be given via peripheral IV catheter)

    (c) 20% (20 g/dL) dextrose in water: used for refractory hypoglycemia or as caloric source (must be given by central venous catheter)

    (d) 50% (50 g/dL) dextrose in water: widely available in 50 mL ampules for emergency IV bolus treatment of hypoglycemia

C. Hypertonic saline

  1. Mainly used clinically for treatment of severe, symptomatic hyponatremia (see Chapter 37, Hyponatremia)

  2. Requires careful dosing to avoid excessive in-

creases in plasma sodium concentration and precipitation of osmotic demyelination

3. Available formulations include 3%, 5%, and 7.5% NaCl.

4. Has also been used experimentally for initial volume resuscitation in traumatic hypovolemic shock because it increases intravascular volume in excess of the infused volume, at the expense of intracellular volume

D. Colloidal fluids

1. Expand intravascular space exclusively and provide the most rapid intravascular volume expansion

2. Generally expand intravascular volume to at least 3 times that of equal volumes of isotonic crystalloid fluids, depending on the colloid oncotic pressure of the preparation

3. Substantially more expensive than crystalloids

4. Clinically used colloids

a. Albumin

(1) Prepared from human plasma; therefore, potentially limited availability

(2) Pasteurized; no known reported cases of viral transmission

(3) Molecular weight (MW) is between 66,300 and 69,000 daltons.

(4) Not indicated as intravenous nutrition

(5) 5% formulation in NS contains 50 g/L and has approximately 3 times the volume expansion effect of NS.

(6) 25% formulation contains 25 g/dL and has been used to increase intravascular volume in patients with hypovolemia in the face of interstitial edema; e.g., hypotension following excessive hemodialysis in patients with renal failure.

b. Starch preparations

(1) 6% hetastarch

(a) A synthetic polysaccharide colloid (hydroxyethyl starch)

(b) Contains a mixture of various length polymers of MW ranging from 10,000 to more than 1 million (number average approximately 70,000, weight average approximately 450,000) daltons

(c) Hydroxyethyl substitutions bestow reduced degradation by amylase.

(d) Has somewhat greater volume-expanding properties than 5% albumin, approximately equal to volume infused

(e) Less expensive than albumin

(f) Usual maximum daily dose is 20 mL/kg or 1500 mL.

(g) Large doses can affect coagulation parameters.

(h) Allergic reactions are extremely rare.

(2) 10% pentastarch

(a) A synthetic polysaccharide analog of hetastarch with lower MW and lower molar substitution ratio (fewer hydroxyethyl side groups)

(b) Shorter half-life than hetastarch; essentially cleared within 24 hours

(c) Expands intravascular volume by a factor of approximately 1.5 the volume infused

c. Dextran preparations

(1) Glucose-based polysaccharides produced by the bacterium *Leuconostoc mesenteroides*

(2) Expand intravascular volume in excess of infused volume, at the expense of interstitial volume

(3) Anaphylactic reactions are more common than with other colloids.

(4) Cause dose-related coagulation defects, especially at doses higher than 20 mL/kg per day

(5) Acute renal failure has been described rarely (more so with dextran-40).

(6) 6% dextran-70 in NS or 5% dextrose

(a) Weight average MW of 70,000 (90% range from 25,000 to 125,000) daltons

(b) Longer half-life than dextran-40

(7) 10% dextran-40 in normal saline or 5% dextrose

(a) Weight average MW of 40,000 (90% range from 10,000 to 80,000) daltons

(b) More rapid volume-expanding effect than with dextran-70, but the effect is transient because of the shorter half-life

(c) Has rheological properties that decrease coagulation tendency and improve microcirculatory flow

d. Gelatin preparations

(1) Bovine gelatin polymers (weight average MW approximately 35,000 daltons)

(2) Formulations (none available in the United States) include 3.5% urea-bridged gelatin (polygeline) and 4% succinyl-linked, modified fluid gelatin, both in NS.

Key Complications

- Phlebitis and other complications of IV access

- Electrolyte or acid-base disorders

- Fluid overload, with systemic or pulmonary edema

- Hyperglycemia (from glucose-containing fluids)

- Hyponatremia (from excess hypotonic fluids)

- Coagulation abnormalities (from certain colloids)

Bibliography

AuBuchon JP. Blood-volume expanders: current issues and trends in selection and use. Formulary 1997;32(Suppl 3): S2–S28.

Electrolyte Solutions. In: McEvoy GK, Welsh OH Jr, Snow EK, et al (eds). AHFS Drug Information. Bethesda, MD: American Society of Health-System Pharmacists, 1999, pp 2271–2274.

Rainey TC, Read CA. Pharmacology of colloids and crystalloids. In: Chernow B (ed). The Pharmacologic Approach to the Critically Ill Patient, 3rd ed. Baltimore: Williams & Wilkins, 1994, pp 272–290.

Vermeulen LC, Ratko TA, Erstad BL, et al. A paradigm for consensus. The University Hospital Consortium guidelines for the use of albumin, nonprotein colloid, and crystalloid solutions. Arch Intern Med 1995;155:373–379.

160 Amrinone and Milrinone

Allison L. Somerville
James A. Kruse

Amrinone and milrinone are bipyridine phosphodiesterase (PDE) inhibitors that exhibit positive inotropic effects as well as vasodilating properties. They differ from other inotropes (e.g., dopamine, dobutamine, and digoxin) in that they do not stimulate α- or β-adrenergic receptors, inhibit Na^+-K^+-ATPase, or cause histamine or prostaglandin release. Amrinone and milrinone exert their effects by inhibiting the enzyme PDE III, which breaks down cAMP in cardiac and vascular smooth muscle. Phosphodiesterase inhibitors increase cardiac performance without increasing myocardial oxygen demand because they also act as direct vasodilators, causing decreases in preload and afterload with a reduction in myocardial oxygen consumption (MvO_2). Amrinone and milrinone are FDA approved for short-term therapy of acute episodes of congestive heart failure; however, their use in the intensive care unit (ICU) is limited by their potential for adverse effects, inability to titrate easily because of their long elimination half-life, and lack of studies showing positive effects on morbidity and mortality.

Mechanisms and Effects

A. Inhibition of PDE III in cardiac and vascular smooth muscle
1. Increases cAMP levels and thereby increases peak developed tension and rate of tension development
2. Promotes Ca^{2+} influx
   a. Increases flow through the slow inward Ca^{2+} channel
   b. Possible activation of the Na^+-Ca^{2+} exchange mechanism, further increasing intracellular Ca^{2+}

B. Vasodilatory effect
1. Exerts a direct vasodilatory action on vascular smooth muscle and coronary arteries, reducing coronary artery resistance by 30% to 40%
   a. Arterial dilation leads to increased stroke volume by reducing ventricular afterload.
   b. Venodilation leads to decreased filling pressures by reducing ventricular preload.
   c. Unpredictable effect on renal blood flow
2. Indirectly decreases sympathetic tone by improving cardiac contractility

C. May reestablish mechanical activity in K^+-depolarized tissues in which the fast inward current was previously inactivated

D. Hemodynamic effects
1. Increases stroke volume, cardiac output, and ventricular dP/dt
   a. Increases in cardiac output, typically of 25% to 50% or more, can be observed within 5 minutes of a bolus dose.
   b. Most prominent effects are seen in patients with high filling pressures.
   c. Effects are due to both vasodilation and inotropic action.
2. Lowers central venous and pulmonary artery occlusion pressures
3. Increases heart rate (effect is dose dependent and may not appear until there is a plateau in dose-response effect on cardiac output)
4. Lowers systemic vascular resistance
5. Variable effect on blood pressure
   a. Blood pressure may decrease, especially at high doses and in patients with limited inotropic reserve.
   b. Blood pressure may be maintained by inotropic action balanced against vasodilation.
   c. Risk of inducing hypotension is high in patients with low filling pressures or hypovolemia.
6. Little effect on MvO_2, due to a balance between inotropic and vasodilatory effects
   a. Inotropic effect: increases myocardial oxygen demand, but may also improve myocardial oxygen supply by increasing stroke volume and decreasing filling pressures, thus improving coronary perfusion
   b. Vasodilatory effect: decreases myocardial oxygen demand by decreasing ventricular wall tension via lowering preload and afterload

Indications

A. Short-term therapy of acute congestive heart failure that has failed conventional therapy (FDA approved)

B. Patients not responding to inotropic therapy (e.g., dopamine, dobutamine) secondary to downregulation of β-adrenergic receptors

C. "Pharmacologic bridge" to cardiac transplantation

D. Treatment of low cardiac output states following open-heart surgery

E. Treatment of circulatory shock (once hypotension is controlled)

Contraindications

A. Absolute

1. Severe aortic or pulmonic valvular disease

2. Sulfite hypersensitivity (amrinone contains sodium metabisulfite)

B. Relative

1. Hypotension

a. Risk of worsening hypotension

b. Dobutamine may be reconsidered once blood pressure is controlled with fluids or vasopressor agents.

2. Low cardiac filling pressures (hypovolemia)

3. Supraventricular and ventricular dysrhythmias

4. Post–myocardial infarction without signs of heart failure

5. Renal impairment

6. Pregnancy (category C)

Drug Interactions

A. Concomitant disopyramide administration can cause severe hypotension.

B. Loop and thiazide diuretics potentiate potassium excretion and may predispose the patient to hypokalemia.

Typical Dosing

A. Amrinone

1. Loading dose: 0.75 mg/kg IV over 3 minutes

2. Maintenance dose: 5 μg/kg per minute IV; may titrate up to 15 μg/kg per minute

3. Dosing in renal insufficiency

a. 40% of amrinone is excreted in the urine unchanged.

b. May need dosage adjustment in renal insufficiency, although no specific guidelines

B. Milrinone

1. Loading dose: 50 μg/kg IV over 10 minutes

2. Maintenance IV dose: 0.375 to 0.75 μg/kg per minute

3. Dosing in renal insufficiency is based on creatinine clearance (Ccr) since 80% to 85% of milrinone is excreted in the urine unchanged.

a. Ccr <50 mL/minute: 0.43 μg/kg per minute

b. Ccr <40 mL/minute: 0.38 μg/kg per minute

c. Ccr <30 mL/minute: 0.33 μg/kg per minute

d. Ccr <20 mL/minute: 0.28 μg/kg per minute

e. Ccr <10 mL/minute: 0.23 μg/kg per minute

f. Ccr <5 mL/minute: 0.20 μg/kg per minute

Adverse Effects

A. Amrinone

1. Ventricular dysrhythmias (3%)

2. Dose-dependent reversible thrombocytopenia

a. 2.4% incidence with IV use

b. 10% to 20% incidence with PO use

c. Platelets usually return to baseline within 4 days after discontinuance of the drug.

3. Gastrointestinal (GI) intolerance (<2%)

a. Nausea, emesis

b. Anorexia

c. Abdominal pain

d. Diarrhea

4. Hypotension (1.3%)

5. Fever (1%)

6. Liver function abnormalities (0.2%)

a. Jaundice

b. Elevation of plasma liver enzyme activities and bilirubin concentration

7. Myocardial ischemia (0.2%)

B. Milrinone

1. Ventricular dysrhythmias (12.1%)

a. Premature ventricular contractions (8.5%)

b. Ventricular tachycardia (2.8%)

c. Sustained ventricular tachycardia (1%)

d. Ventricular fibrillation (0.2%)

2. Diarrhea (11.9%)

3. Blurred vision (7.7%)

4. Syncope (4.5%)

5. Headache (2.9%)

6. Thrombocytopenia (0.4%)

Key Monitoring

- Follow hemodynamic parameters to assess clinical benefit of drug (e.g., cardiac output, pulmonary artery occlusion pressure, heart rate, blood pressure).

- Continuously monitor electrocardiogram to detect tachydysrhythmias.

- Monitor for electrolyte disturbances secondary to diuretic actions.

Special Considerations

A. Amrinone vs milrinone
   1. Amrinone exerts its major effect through vasodilation, with little inotropic effect.
   2. Milrinone may be advantageous because of its greater inotropic effect.
   3. Intravenous milrinone use is not associated with dose-dependent thrombocytopenia, fever, or GI intolerance.

B. Long-term therapy with PDE inhibitors
   1. Associated with accelerated progression of left ventricular dysfunction and increased risk of ventricular dysrhythmias
   2. The PROMISE Trial showed a 28% increase in total mortality associated with milrinone treatment in 1088 patients with chronic New York Heart Association (NYHA) class III to class IV heart failure; 53% if analysis restricted to NYHA class IV.

C. Use of PDE inhibitors in combination with other inotropic agents having different mechanisms of action
   1. Pretreatment with β-adrenergic agonists increases the levels of cAMP and provides more substrate for the PDE inhibitors.
   2. Dobutamine and dopamine have complementary and synergistic effect with PDE inhibitors.
   3. Amrinone + dobutamine increases stroke volume index significantly and decreases left ventricular end-diastolic pressure and systemic vascular resistance.
   4. Digoxin effects are additive.

5. Because of the increased potential for side effects, combination therapy is indicated only when the effects of single-agent therapy are inadequate.

PEARLS

- PDE inhibitors may provoke the development of serious ventricular dysrhythmias.

- Long-term therapy with oral milrinone increases morbidity and mortality of patients with advanced heart failure.

- Amrinone and milrinone have prolonged elimination half-lives that complicate titration.

 Bibliography

Alousi AA, Johnson DC. Pharmacology of the bipyridines: Amrinone and milrinone. Circulation 1986;73(Suppl III):10–23.

Colucci WS. Positive inotropic/vasodilator agents. Cardiol Clin 1989;7:131–144.

Colucci WS, Richard WF, Braunwald E. New positive inotropic agents in the treatment of congestive heart failure. Mechanisms of action and recent clinical developments. N Engl J Med 1986;314:349–358.

Cuffe MS, Califf RM, Adams Jr KF, et al. Short-term intravenous milrinone for acute exacerbation of chronic heart failure. A randomized controlled trial. JAMA 2002;287:1541–1547.

Hatzizacharias A, Makris T, Krespi P, et al. Intermittent milrinone effect on long-term hemodynamic profile in patients with severe congestive heart failure. Am Heart J 1999;138:241–246.

Packer M, Carver JR, Rodeheffer RJ, et al. Effect of milrinone on mortality in severe chronic heart failure. N Engl J Med 1991;325:1468–1475.

161 Vasoactive Catecholamines

James A. Kruse

The vasoactive catecholamines considered in this chapter are clinically important sympathomimetic drugs that can be administered by IV infusion to induce hemodynamic effects. These effects are mediated either by direct or indirect action of these agents on adrenergic or dopaminergic (DA) receptors, or both, located in blood vessels, the myocardium, and other tissues. Indirect action refers to stimulation of endogenous catecholamine release from neurons. These drugs have a rapid onset of action (seconds to minutes) and a short duration of action (minutes), which allows them to be titrated to achieve desired therapeutic effects. Their IV use requires continuous electrocardiographic monitoring and frequent or continuous blood pressure monitoring.

Key Pharmacology

- α_1-Adrenergic receptors: mediate arteriolar vasoconstriction and glycogenolysis

- α_2-Adrenergic receptors: presynaptic receptors mediate inhibition of synaptic norepinephrine release; smooth muscle receptors mediate arteriolar vasoconstriction

- β_1-Adrenergic myocardial receptors: mediate inotropic and chronotropic effects, and increase atrioventricular conduction velocity

- β_2-Adrenergic receptors: mediate arteriolar vasodilation, bronchodilation, glycogenolysis, and insulin secretion

- DA_1 receptors: mediate vasodilation, especially in the mesenteric, renal, and coronary vasculature

Mechanisms and Effects (see Table 161–1)

A. Norepinephrine
1. A direct-acting endogenous catecholamine with α_1, α_2, β_1, and (weak) β_2-adrenergic actions
2. Inotropic and vasoconstrictor effects
3. Little or no chronotropic effect

B. Epinephrine
1. A direct-acting endogenous catecholamine with moderate β_2- and potent α- and β_1-adrenergic properties
2. Vasoconstrictor, inotropic, and chronotropic effects

3. β-Adrenergic effects predominate at lower doses; α-adrenergic effects predominate at higher doses.

C. Dopamine
1. An endogenous catecholamine with direct and indirect actions
2. Acts on dopaminergic receptors throughout clinical dose range
   a. Acts on vascular DA_1 receptors, located mainly in mesenteric, renal, and coronary vessels, causing vasodilation
   b. Acts on DA_1 receptors on proximal renal tubular cells and causes natriuresis and diuresis
   c. Acts on DA_2 receptors in autonomic nervous system, resulting in inhibition of norepinephrine release
3. At moderate doses, acts on cardiac β_1-adrenergic receptors
   a. Inotropic effect
   b. Chronotropic effect, which can be marked, especially if there is hypovolemia
4. At high doses, acts on vascular α-adrenergic receptors
   a. Produces systemic vasoconstriction
   b. Can override the vasodilatory effects of DA_1 receptor stimulation

D. Dobutamine
1. A racemic mixture of a synthetic, direct-acting catecholamine
   a. d (+) stereoisomer has strong β_1- and some β_2-adrenergic action, but little or no α-adrenergic action.
   b. l (−) stereoisomer has some β-adrenergic actions, but only weak α_1-adrenergic effects.
2. Inotropic and mild chronotropic effects on heart (occasionally chronotropic effects are marked, especially in hypovolemia)
3. Net effect on blood pressure is variable: may have little or no effect, mild increase, or mild to marked decrease

E. Isoproterenol
1. A direct-acting pure β_1-adrenergic agonist
2. Inotropic and vasodilating effects
3. Potent chronotrope

TABLE 161–1. KEY EFFECTS OF VASOACTIVE CATECHOLAMINES AND SELECTED NON-CATECHOLAMINE VASOACTIVE AGENTS

DRUG	VASODILATION	VASOCONSTRICTION	INOTROPIC EFFECT	CHRONOTROPIC EFFECT	RENAL BLOOD FLOW AND DIURESIS	DYSRHYTHMO-GENICITY
Epinephrine	++	+++	++++	+++	0	+++
Norepinephrine	0	++++	++	0	0	+
Phenylephrine	0	+++	0	−	0	0
Isoproterenol	+++	0	++++	++++	0	++++
Dopamine	+	0 to +++	++	+++	+	++
Dobutamine	++	0 to +	++++	++	0	+
Dopexamine	++	0	++	++	+	++
Fenoldopam	+++	0	0	+	+	0
Amrinone	++	0	++++	+	0	+
Nitroprusside	++++	0	0	0	0	0
Nitroglycerin	++	0	0	0	0	0

See respective chapters for details on non-catecholamine vasoactive drugs.
0 = little or no effect; + to ++++ = relative extent of positive effect; − = baroreceptor reflex-mediated decrease in heart rate.

a. Main clinical utility has been as a pharmacologic means of urgently treating bradycardia, usually as a prelude to emergency cardiac pacing.

b. Because of the drug's marked vasodilator properties and propensity for causing dysrhythmias, its use as an emergency chronotrope has been largely supplanted by dopamine.

F. Phenylephrine

1. A direct-acting pure α-adrenergic agonist

2. Potent vasoconstrictor

3. No direct cardiac effects

4. Resulting increases in systemic vascular resistance and blood pressure increase left ventricular afterload, which can potentially decrease cardiac output in patients with impaired myocardial reserve.

5. May decrease atrioventricular conduction and decrease heart rate by baroreceptor reflex

6. May be a useful vasoconstrictor if tachycardia limits use of other vasopressors, or in patients with hypotension and underlying hypertrophic obstructive cardiomyopathy

G. Dopexamine

1. A synthetic DA$_1$, DA$_2$, and β_2-adrenergic agonist

2. Has systemic and renomesenteric vasodilating actions

3. Increases cardiac output by afterload reduction and possibly by direct inotropic action (mechanism unclear)

4. Can cause reflex tachycardia

5. Not currently available in the United States

 Key Indications

- Hypotension: norepinephrine, dopamine, phenylephrine

- Cardiogenic or septic shock: norepinephrine, dopamine

- Left ventricular failure: dobutamine

- Oliguria: dopamine (?)

Typical Dosing

A. Norepinephrine

1. Typical dilution for infusion (final concentration): 4 mg in 250 mL 5% dextrose in water, or other dextrose-containing fluid (16 μg/mL)

2. Starting dose (typical range) for hypotension: 1 (0.5 to 20+) μg/minute; titrate to desired mean arterial blood pressure

B. Epinephrine

1. For circulatory shock

a. Typical dilution for infusion (final concentration): 1 mg in 250 mL normal saline (4 μg/mL)

b. Starting infusion dose (typical range): 0.5 to 1 (0.5 to 10+) μg/minute

2. For cardiac arrest: 1.0 mg (10 mL of 1:10,000 solution) every 3 to 5 minutes by IV bolus or (if no IV access) through endotracheal tube

3. For anaphylaxis

a. Mild to moderate: 0.3 to 0.5 mg (0.3 to 0.5 mL of a 1:1000 solution) subcutaneously; may repeat every 20 minutes

b. Severe shock: 0.1 to 0.5 mg (1 to 5 mL of a 1:10,000 solution) IV over 5 to 10 minutes

c. Cardiac arrest: 1 to 3 mg IV, then (after 3 minutes) 3 to 5 mg, then (after 3 minutes) start an infusion at 1 to 10 μg/minute

4. For laryngeal edema: 0.5 mL of 2.25% racemic epinephrine in 3 to 4 mL normal saline (nebulized) by inhalation

C. Dopamine

1. Typical dilution for infusion (final concentration): 800 mg in 500 mL (1.6 mg/mL) in normal saline or 5% dextrose in water

2. Starting dose (typical range)

a. For augmenting renal and mesenteric perfusion: 3 (0.5 to 5) μg/kg per minute (questionable efficacy)

b. For inotropic effect: 5 (5 to 10) μg/kg per minute

c. For vasoconstrictor effect: 10 (8 to 20+) μg/kg per minute, titrated to desired mean arterial blood pressure

3. There is wide person-to-person variation in the above dose–response ranges.

D. Dobutamine

1. Typical dilution for infusion (final concentration): 500 mg in 250 mL (2 mg/mL) in normal saline or 5% dextrose in water

2. Starting dose (typical range): 5 (2.5 to 20) μg/kg per minute

E. Isoproterenol

1. Typical dilution for infusion (final concentration): 1 mg in 250 mL of 5% dextrose in water (4 μg/mL)

2. Starting dose (typical range): 2 (0.5 to 20+) μg/minute; titrate to desired heart rate, when used for chronotropic effect

F. Phenylephrine

1. Typical dilution for infusion (final concentration): 20 mg in 250 mL 5% dextrose in water (80 μg/mL)

2. Starting dose (typical range): 20 (20 to 200) μg/minute; titrate to desired mean arterial blood pressure

Key Contraindications

- Vasoactive catecholamines are contraindicated in hypovolemia, except as a temporizing measure.

- β-Adrenergic catecholamines are contraindicated in hypertrophic obstructive cardiomyopathy.

Adverse Effects

A. Hypertension: can occur with vasoconstrictive catecholamines (e.g., norepinephrine, dopamine, phenylephrine)

B. Hypotension

1. Can occur with vasodilatory catecholamines (e.g., isoproterenol; sometimes with dobutamine)

2. Use of these drugs may be considered (e.g., for their inotropic or chronotropic effects) once hypotension is reversed using fluids, vasoconstrictor agents, or other means.

C. Marked tachycardia, particularly with isoproterenol, dobutamine, epinephrine, dopamine

D. Tachydysrhythmias

1. Mediated by β-adrenergic action

2. Relative propensity: isoproterenol > epinephrine > dopamine > dobutamine > norepinephrine

3. Sinus tachycardia is most common, but other supraventricular and ventricular dysrhythmias (including ventricular tachycardia) can occur.

E. Ischemia

1. Due to vasoconstriction-induced decreases in perfusion

2. Higher risk in patients with low-flow states, preexisting arteriosclerotic vascular disease, or receiving high doses of vasopressor

3. Distal extremities at high risk, but ischemia can develop in any organ

4. Risk can be minimized by avoiding excessive vasopressor doses, i.e., unnecessarily high elevations of blood pressure.

F. Drug extravasation

1. Avoid infusion of vasoconstrictive drugs via peripheral IV catheter.

a. Dislodgement from vessel and subcutaneous infiltration of drug can cause local tissue necrosis and skin sloughing.

b. Extravasation can be severe enough to require wide debridement and skin grafting.

2. Provide prompt local treatment.

a. Immediately stop the infiltrating drug infusion.

b. Dilute 5 to 10 mg of phentolamine mesylate, an α-adrenergic antagonist, in 10 to 15 mL normal saline and use a fine ($\geq$25 gauge) needle and multiple injections to liberally infiltrate the entire volume throughout the affected area.

c. The extremity may be elevated, but avoid warm compresses, ice, or other local temperature manipulation.

Key Monitoring

- Infuse vasoconstrictive catecholamines through a central venous catheter to minimize risk of extravasation.

- Employ continuous electrocardiographic monitoring to detect induced tachydysrhythmias.

- Follow hemodynamic parameters to assess clinical benefit of drug (blood pressure, heart rate, cardiac output, pulmonary artery occlusion pressure, etc.).

- Titrate vasoactive drug dosage to hemodynamic or other physiologic endpoints (e.g., reversal of oliguria or hyperlactatemia).

Bibliography

Bellomo R, Cole L, Ronco C. Hemodynamic support and the role of dopamine. Kidney Int 1998;53(Suppl 66): S71–S74.

Chen JL, O'Shea M. Extravasation injury associated with low-dose dopamine. Ann Pharmacother 1998;32:545–548.

Flancbaum L, Dick M, Dasta J, et al. A dose-response study of phenylephrine in critically ill, septic surgical patients. Eur J Clin Pharmacol 1997;51:461–465.

Meier-Hallmann A, Reinhart K, Bredle DL, et al. Epinephrine impairs splanchnic perfusion in septic shock. Crit Care Med 1997;25:399–404.

Task Force of the American College of Critical Care Medicine, Society of Critical Care Medicine. Practice parameters for hemodynamic support of sepsis in adult patients in sepsis. Crit Care Med 1999;27:639–660.

Velasco M, Luchsinger A. Dopamine: pharmacologic and therapeutic aspects. Am J Therapeut 1998;5:37:43.

162 Antihypertensives

Allison L. Somerville

Hypertension is prevalent among critically ill patients. The goal of treating hypertension in the acute setting is to decrease blood pressure and thereby prevent or halt acute progression of end organ damage. There are many antihypertensive agents available and the choice is often dependent on the etiology, concomitant disease states, severity of hypertension, and the desired timeframe to normalize the blood pressure. This chapter focuses on those antihypertensive agents that are preferred for various causes of hypertension in the ICU and that do not have their own chapter in this book.

Mechanisms and Effects

A. Vasodilators

   1. Hydralazine

      a. Direct arteriolar vasodilator

      b. Reflex sympathetic stimulation occurs through activation of baroreceptor mechanisms and results in increased heart rate.

      c. May be combined with a β-adrenergic blocking agent to counter reflex tachycardia

      d. Does not decrease blood flow to vital organs, and so is useful in hypertension complicated by renal failure or vascular insufficiency

      e. Potential for increased myocardial oxygen demand limits use in coronary artery disease

   2. Minoxidil

      a. Direct arteriolar vasodilating effect

      b. Can increase pulmonary artery pressure

      c. Reflex tachycardia occurs

      d. May be combined with a β-adrenergic blocking agent to counter reflex tachycardia

      e. Fluid retention may necessitate the addition of a diuretic.

   3. Diazoxide

      a. Opens adenosine triphosphate (ATP)-sensitive potassium channels on arteriolar smooth muscle to reduce vascular resistance

      b. No effect on venous resistance beds

      c. Reflex tachycardia occurs.

      d. Increases velocity of left ventricular ejection

   4. Nitroglycerin (see Chapter 164, Nitroglycerin)

   5. Nitroprusside (see Chapter 165, Nitroprusside)

   6. Fenoldopam (see Chapter 163, Fenoldopam)

B. Central-acting α_2-adrenergic receptor agonists

   1. Specific agents: clonidine, methyldopa, guanabenz, guanfacine

   2. Act within the central nervous system to decrease sympathetic neuronal stimulation to the heart, kidneys, and peripheral vasculature

   3. Indirectly reduce renin release by decreasing adrenergic tone to the juxtaglomerular apparatus via renal innervation

   4. Do not induce reflex tachycardia

C. Peripheral α_1-adrenergic receptor blockers

   1. Specific agents: prazosin, terazosin, doxazosin

   2. Provide balanced vasodilation (i.e., both arterial and venous dilation) mediated by peripheral α_1-adrenergic blockade

   3. No reflex tachycardia

D. Angiotensin converting enzyme (ACE) inhibitors

   1. Specific agents: captopril, enalapril, lisinopril, quinapril, ramipril, benazepril, moexipril, trandolapril, and fosinopril

   2. Peripheral vasodilation mediated by decreased formation of the vasoconstrictor angiotensin II, secondary to ACE inhibition

   3. Pronounced effect in patients with high plasma renin activity

   4. Decreases aldosterone secretion and inactivation of vasodilatory bradykinins

E. Trimethaphan camsylate (a ganglionic blocker)

   1. Interferes with the action of acetylcholine on ganglionic cells in the autonomic nervous system

   2. Inhibits venous capacitance vessels from constricting and thus reduces venous return

   3. Decreases blood pressure and cardiac output because sympathetic reflexes are blocked

   4. Rate of rise of arterial pressure during systole (dP/dt) is reduced.

5. No reflex tachycardia

F. Phentolamine mesylate

1. Blocks α_1- and α_2-adrenergic receptors

2. Rapid onset and short duration of action

3. Drug of choice for hypertensive crises associated with pheochromocytoma, tyramine–monoamine oxidase inhibitor (MAOI) interactions, and clonidine withdrawal

G. β-Adrenergic receptor antagonists (also see Chapter 66, Calcium Channel and β-Blocker Drug Overdoses)

1. Nonselective agents

a. Specific agents: propranolol, nadolol, sotalol, and pindolol

b. Block β_1-adrenergic receptors (on myocardium) with β_2-adrenergic receptors (on bronchial and vascular smooth muscle)

c. Inhibit chronotropic, inotropic, vasodilator, and bronchodilator responses to β-adrenergic stimulation

2. β_1-Selective antagonists

a. Specific agents: metoprolol, acebutolol, esmolol, and atenolol

b. Preferentially inhibit β_1-adrenergic receptors (dose-dependent cardioselectivity)

c. Safer for patients with asthma, chronic obstructive pulmonary disease, peripheral vascular disease, and diabetes

3. Intrinsic sympathomimetic activity (ISA)

a. Specific agents: pindolol and acebutolol

b. Have partial sympathomimetic agonist activity, which manifests as a smaller reduction in resting cardiac output and heart

H. Calcium channel antagonists (also see Chapter 66, Calcium Channel and β-Blocker Drug Overdoses)

1. Act on slow calcium channels with varying degrees of selectivity in their effects on vascular smooth muscle, myocardium, and cardiac conduction tissue

2. Dihydropyridines

a. Specific agents: nifedipine, amlodipine, felodipine, israpidine, and nicardipine

b. Decrease in systemic vascular resistance with minimal to no effect on myocardial conduction and heart rate

c. May result in reflex tachycardia

3. Non-dihydropyridines

a. Specific agents: diltiazem and verapamil

b. Decrease heart rate, slow atrioventricular conduction, and produce a negative inotropic effect (verapamil > diltiazem)

c. Dilate the corony arteries and arterioles

d. Reduce systemic blood pressure, afterload and myocardial oxygen demand

Indications

A. Aortic dissection

1. Nitroprusside + β-adrenergic blocker

a. Standard regimen

b. β-Blocker must be used in conjunction with nitroprusside to avoid worsening dissection due to increased dP/dt induced by nitroprusside.

2. Trimethaphan camsylate

a. Reduces blood pressure, left ventricular afterload, and dP/dt

b. An alternative to the use of combined therapy using a β-blocker and nitroprusside when one of those agents is contraindicated

3. Labetalol

a. Has been used as monotherapy

b. Limited experience

4. Also see Chapter 31, Aortic Dissection, Chapter 25, Hypertensive Crisis, and Chapter 165, Nitroprusside.

B. Hypertensive nephropathy

1. ACE inhibitors: may decrease proteinuria associated with some forms of renal disease

2. Loop diuretics may be a useful adjunct in patients with underlying renal disease and fluid overload, if they can mount a diuresis.

C. Cerebral infarction

1. Labetalol: does not raise intracranial pressure

2. Hydralazine: does not reduce cardiac output or cerebral perfusion

3. ACE inhibitors: limited effects on cerebral vessels; less titratable than above agents

D. Eclampsia and preeclampsia (see Chapter 26, Pregnancy-Induced Hypertension)

1. Hydralazine

2. Labetalol

3. Nicardipine

E. Pheochromocytoma (see Chapter 57, Pheochromocytoma)

1. Phentolamine mesylate: first-line agent

2. Substitute sodium nitroprusside if phentolamine is ineffective.

3. Patients may be maintained on oral phenoxybenzamine or prazosin.

F. Drug and ethanol withdrawal syndromes

1. Clonidine: effective for sympathetic overactivity in mild cases

2. Phentolamine mesylate: consider when other agents fail or for severe cases

G. Monoamine oxidase inhibitor interaction with tyramines

1. Phentolamine mesylate

2. Important to add a β-adrenergic antagonist to mitigate risk of cardiac dysrhythmias

H. Autonomic hyperreflexia

1. Trimethaphan camsylate

2. Phentolamine mesylate

Contraindications

A. Hydralazine

1. Ischemic heart disease

2. Aortic dissection

B. Minoxidil

1. Pheochromocytoma

2. Ischemic heart disease

3. Aortic dissection

4. Cerebrovascular disease

C. Diazoxide

1. Aortic dissection

2. Intracranial hemorrhage

3. Pulmonary edema

4. Ischemic heart disease

D. Clonidine

1. Noncompliant patients, because of rebound hypertension

2. Ischemic stroke

3. Breast-feeding

E. Angiotensin converting enzyme inhibitors

1. History of angioedema

2. Use caution with impaired renal function.

3. Bilateral renovascular disease (or unilateral renal artery stenosis if only one functioning kidney)

4. Pregnancy

F. Trimethaphan camsylate

1. Pregnancy toxemia

2. Stroke

3. Respiratory insufficiency

4. Glaucoma

G. Phentolamine mesylate

1. Coronary artery disease

2. History of gastric or peptic ulcer

H. β-Adrenergic receptor antagonists

1. Hypotension or cardiogenic shock

2. Severe sinus bradycardia

3. Second or third degree heart block

4. Severe bronchial asthma or chronic obstructive lung disease

I. Calcium channel antagonists

1. Dihydropyridines

a. Aortic stenosis (nicardipine, nifedipine)

b. Heart failure (if used in conjunction with a β-adrenergic blocker)

2. Non-dihydropyridines

a. Aortic stenosis

b. Heart failure

c. Second and third degree heart block

Key Contraindications

- Ischemic heart disease: hydralazine, minoxidil, diazoxide, phentolamine

- Aortic dissection: hydralazine, minoxidil, diazoxide

- Cerebrovascular disease: minoxidil, diazoxide, clonidine

- Pregnancy: ACE inhibitors

- Second and third degree heart block: β-adrenergic blockers, diltiazem, verapamil

Drug Interactions

A. Hydralazine

1. Drugs that potentiate its antihypertensive effect

a. Monoamine oxidase inhibtors

b. Diuretics

2. Drugs that lessen its antihypertensive effect

a. Sympathomimetic drugs

b. Estrogens

c. Nonsteroidal anti-inflammatory drugs (NSAIDs)

B. Minoxidil

1. Diuretics can potentiate its antihypertensive effect.

2. Drugs that lessen its antihypertensive effect

a. Sympathomimetic drugs

b. Estrogens

c. NSAIDs

C. Diazoxide: can increase or decrease plasma phenytoin levels

D. Clonidine

1. Diuretics can potentiate its antihypertensive effect.

2. Drugs that lessen its antihypertensive effect

a. Tricyclic antidepressant drugs

b. Sympathomimetic drugs

c. NSAIDs

3. May potentiate the action of other CNS depressants

4. May increase cyclosporin blood levels

E. Prazosin

1. Diuretics potentiate antihypertensive effect.

2. α-Adrenergic agonists can lessen its antihypertensive effect.

F. ACE inhibitors

1. Diuretics potentiate antihypertensive effect.

2. NSAIDs lessen antihypertensive effect.

3. ACE inhibitors enhance the effects of oral hypoglycemic agents.

4. ACE inhibitors can increase plasma lithium concentration.

5. ACE inhibitors have additive effect on risk of hyperkalemia when combined with potassium-sparing diuretics or potassium supplements.

G. Trimethaphan camsylate

1. Bethanechol and diuretics can potentiate its antihypertensive effect.

2. Enhances succinylcholine-induced neuromuscular blockade

H. β-adrenergic receptor antagonists

1. Drugs that increase β-adrenergic blocker concentration: H_2-receptor antagonists, propafenone, quinidine, quinolones

2. Propranolol may increase the effects of warfarin.

I. Calcium channel blockers

1. Increase effects of digoxin

2. Bioavailability is increased by H_2-receptor antagonists.

3. Increase concentrations of carbamazepine, cyclosporin, and theophylline (non-dihydropyridines and nicardipine)

Typical Dosing

A. Intravenous administration for hypertensive emergency

1. Nitroprusside (see Chapter 165, Nitroprusside)

2. Nitroglycerin (see Chapter 164, Nitroglycerin)

3. Fenoldopam (see Chapter 163, Fenoldopam)

4. Hydralazine

a. Initial dose: 5 to 20 mg by IV injection

b. Maintenance dose: 5 to 40 mg every 4 to 6 hours by IV injection

c. Onset of action: 10 to 30 minutes

d. Duration of action: 2 to 8 hours

e. May also be used orally at same doses

5. Diazoxide

a. Initial dose: 50 to 100 mg single IV injection and may repeat initial dose every 10 to 15 minutes until blood pressure is controlled or 600 mg given, or

b. Has been given as a 10 to 30 mg/minute infusion up to a total of 5 mg/kg

c. Onset of action: less than 5 minutes

d. Duration of action: 3 to 12 hours

e. Generally not recommended due to unpredictable effect

6. Enalaprilat

a. Initial dose: 0.625 mg by IV injection

b. Maintenance dose: titrate up to 5 mg every 6 hours intravenously

c. Onset of action: 30 to 60 minutes

d. Duration of action: up to 6 hours

7. Esmolol

   a. Initial dose: 500 μg/kg over 1 minute

   b. Maintenace dose: 25 to 50 μg/kg per minute

   c. Titration: increase by 25 μg/kg per minute every 10 to 20 minutes (maximum 300 μg/kg per minute)

   d. Onset of action: almost immediate

   e. Duration of action: 2 to 15 minutes

8. Labetalol

   a. Initial dose: 20 mg IV bolus

   b. Maintenance dose: 20 to 80 mg boluses, or an infusion

   c. Titration: start at 1 mg/minute and titrate to goal blood pressure

   d. Onset of action: 5 to 20 minutes

   e. Duration of action: 3 to 6 hours

9. Nicardipine

   a. Initial dose: 5 mg/hour

   b. Titration: increase by 2.5 mg/hour every 5 minutes (maximum 15 mg/hour)

   c. Onset of action: 5 to 10 minutes

   d. Duration of action: 3 hours

10. Trimethaphan camsylate

    a. Initial dose: 0.5 mg/minute by IV infusion

    b. Maintenance dose: titrate up to 5.0 mg/minute

    c. Onset of action: immediate, peak within 5 minutes

    d. Duration of action: 10 to 20 minutes

11. Phentolamine mesylate

    a. Initial dose: 2 to 15 mg by IV injection

    b. Acute titration: can be repeated every 5 to 15 minutes

    c. Onset of action: 1 to 5 minutes

    d. Duration of action: 3 to 15 minutes

B. Oral administration for hypertensive urgency

   1. Minoxidil

      a. Initial dose: 5 mg

      b. Acute titration: double dose every 6 hours until desired effect or 20 mg

      c. Maintenance dose: 5 to 50 mg every 12 to 24 hours

      d. Onset of action: 30 to 60 minutes, peak effect in 2 to 4 hours

      e. Duration of action: 1 to 5 days

   2. Clonidine

      a. Initial dose: 0.1 to 0.2 mg

      b. Acute titration: repeat every 1 to 6 hours, up to a total of 0.6 mg

      c. Maintenance dose: 0.2 to 1 mg every 8 to 12 hours

      d. Onset of action: 30 minutes, peak effect 2 to 4 hours

      e. Duration of action: 6 to 18 hours

   3. Prazosin

      a. Initial dose: 1 to 2 mg

      b. Maintenance dose: 2 to 10 mg every 6 to 12 hours

      c. Onset of action: 2 hours, peak effect 2 to 4 hours

      d. Duration of action: 6 to 12 hours

   4. Captopril

      a. Initial dose: 12.5 to 25 mg

      b. Acute titration: repeat dose every 4 to 6 hours

      c. Maintenance dose: 12.5 to 50 every 6 to 12 hours

      d. Onset of action: 15 to 60 minutes

      e. Duration of action: 2 to 12 hours, dependent on renal function

TABLE 162-1. SELECTED ORAL AGENTS FOR NON-URGENT TREATMENT OF HYPERTENSION

Drug	Initial Dose	Maintenance Dose (mg/day)	Onset of Action (hours)	Duration of Action (hours)	Time to Steady-State (weeks)
Verapamil (immediate release)	80 mg every 8 hours	↑ to 480	1 to 2	6 to 8	1
Diltiazem	60 to 240 mg/day	↑ to 360 to 540	1	3 to 6	2
Nifedipine (extended release)	30 to 60 mg/day	↑ to 90 to 120	0.5	4 to 8	<1
Metoprolol	50 to 100 mg/day	↑ to 450	1	3 to 6	1
Atenolol	50 mg/day	↑ to 100	3	24	1 to 2

5. Labetalol
   a. Initial dose: 200 to 400 mg every 6 to 8 hours
   b. Maintenance does: double the dose if blood pressure response not adequate after 24 hours (maximum dose is 2400 mg/day)
   c. Onset of action: 1 to 2 hours
   d. Duration of action: 3 hours

C. Oral administration for non-urgent treatment of hypertension: see Table 162–1

D. Also see Chapter 166, Diuretics

Adverse Effects

A. Hydralazine
   1. Severe hypotension
   2. Tachycardia
   3. Cardiac ischemia (due to tachycardia)
   4. Headache
   5. Nausea, vomiting
   6. Long-term side effects: drug fever, skin rash, peripheral neuropathy and reversible lupus-like syndrome

B. Minoxidil
   1. Sodium and fluid retention
   2. Hypotension
   3. Reflex tachycardia
   4. Angina or myocardial infarction
   5. Hirsutism with chronic use
   6. Pericardial effusion with chronic use

C. Diazoxide
   1. Severe hypotension
   2. Tachycardia
   3. Hyperglycemia, hyperuricemia
   4. Renal sodium retention
   5. Nausea and vomiting
   6. Pain and cellulitis with drug extravasation
   7. Exacerbation of aortic dissection

D. Clonidine
   1. Hypotension, frank or orthostatic
   2. Depressed sensorium
   3. Dry mouth
   4. Impotence
   5. Bradycardia or heart block

E. Prazosin
   1. Hypotension, frank or orthostatic (especially after first dose)
   2. Syncope (especially after first dose)
   3. Tachycardia
   4. Drowsiness
   5. Anticholinergic effects

F. ACE inhibitors
   1. Hyperkalemia
   2. Azotemia and increased serum creatinine concentration
   3. Angioedema
   4. Leukopenia
   5. Rash
   6. Fever
   7. Chronic cough
   8. Proteinuria
   9. Ageusia or dysgeusia

G. Trimethaphan camsylate
   1. Hypotension, frank and orthostatic
   2. Dry mouth
   3. Mydriasis or blurred vision
   4. Constipation, paralytic ileus
   5. Urinary retention
   6. Weakness
   7. Impotence
   8. Respiratory arrest

H. Phentolamine mesylate
   1. Hypotension
   2. Tachycardia
   3. Headache

I. β-adrenergic receptor antagonists (also see Chapter 66, Calcium Channel and β-Blocker Drug Overdoses)
   1. Atrioventricular block, bradydysrhythmias
   2. Bronchoconstriction
   3. Cold extremities
   4. Glucose intolerance

J. Calcium channel antagonists (also see Chapter 66, Calcium Channel and β-Blocker Drug Overdoses)
   1. Dihydropyridines
      a. Peripheral edema
      b. Palpitations

c. Gastrointestinal complaints

d. Dizziness, headache, flushing

2. Non-dihydropyridines

a. Atrioventricular block, bradydysrhythmias

b. Hypotension

c. Constipation (verapamil), anorexia, nausea

Special Considerations

A. Hydralazine

1. Tolerance may develop in patients receiving the drug for extended periods.

2. Tachycardia may be attenuated by concomitant administration of a β-blocker.

3. Increased heart rate is less likely to occur in patients with chronic, advanced heart failure.

4. Dose reductions may be necessary if creatinine clearance less than 50 ml/minute.

B. Minoxidil

1. Tachycardia may be attenuated by concomitant administration of a β-blocker.

2. Concomitant diuretic improves efficacy.

C. Diazoxide

1. May be advantagous in patients with renal insufficiency, as it may enhance renal blood flow

2. Tachycardia may be attenuated by concomitant administration of a β-blocker.

D. Clonidine

1. Doses should be tapered over 2 to 4 days to avoid withdrawal (rebound) symptoms.

2. Dose reduction may be needed in patients with renal impairment.

E. Prazosin

1. Use associated with less reflex tachycardia than nonselective α-adrenergic receptor antagonists (e.g., phentolamine mesylate)

2. Hypotension and syncope may follow first dose.

F. ACE inhibitors

1. Decreases blood pressure with little or no change in heart rate

2. Slows the progression of nephropathy in diabetic patients

3. Useful in congestive heart failure and in patients at risk for cerebral hypoperfusion

4. Dose reductions may be necessary in patients with creatinine clearance less than 50 mL/minute.

G. Trimethaphan camsylate

1. Intravenous bolus dosing leads to more histamine release and adverse effects; continuous IV infusion is preferred.

2. Blood pressure can fluctuate rapidly, so continuous monitoring is necessary.

3. Reverse Trendelenburg position increases hypotensive effect.

H. Phentolamine mesylate

1. Hemodynamic effects are dose dependent.

2. β-Adrenergic blockers may be used to attenuate associated tachycardia.

I. β-adrenergic receptor antagonists

1. Abrupt cessation can precipitate unstable angina or myocardial infarction.

2. Induce glucose intolerance, increase triglycerides, and decrease high density lipoproteins (except labetalol and agents with ISA)

J. Calcium channel antagonists

1. Diltiazem may worsen congestive heart failure in patients with impaired ventricular function secondary to negative inotropic effects.

2. No effect on lipid profiles or glucose tolerance

PEARLS

- Agents that can induce reflex tachycardia: hydralazine, minoxidil, diazoxide, and dihydropyridine calcium channel blockers (except amlodipine)

- Agents that do not induce reflex tachycardia: clonidine, prazosin, trimethaphan, and β-adrenergic blockers

---

Bibliography

Grossman E, Ironi AN, Messerli FH. Comparative tolerability profile of hypertensive crisis treatments. Drug Safety 1998;19;99–122.

Harrison BA, Murray MJ. Care of the hypertensive patient

in the intensive care unit. In: Murray MJ, Coursin DB, Pearl RG, et al (eds). Critical Care Medicine: Perioperative Management. Philadelphia: Lippincott-Raven, 1997, pp 341–354.

Hirschl MM, Binder M, Bur A, et al. Clinical evaluation of different doses of intravenous enalaprilat in patients with hypertensive crisis. Arch Intern Med 1995;155:2217–2223.

Joint National Committee on Prevention, Detection, Evaluation, and Treatment of High Blood Pressure (JNC). The Sixth Report of the JNC. Arch Intern Med 1997;157: 2413–2446.

163 Fenoldopam

Jorge A. Guzman

Pharmacology

A. Fenoldopam mesylate is an arteriolar vasodilator.

B. Mechanism
1. Selective postsynaptic dopamine (DA)-1 receptor agonist
2. Its DA$_1$-receptor activity is 6 to 9 times as potent as dopamine.
3. Unlike dopamine, it has no affinity for the DA$_2$-receptor or α_1- or β-adrenergic receptors.

C. Pharmacokinetics
1. Volume of distribution is approximately 0.50 L/kg.
2. Onset of action occurs within 5 minutes.
3. Elimination half-life is 5 to 10 minutes; duration of action is 15 to 30 minutes.

D. Metabolism
1. Does not involve the cytochrome P-450 system.
2. Metabolized mainly to inactive conjugates by sulfation, methylation, and glucuronidation
3. Conjugates are excreted in urine (90%) and feces (10%); 4% is excreted unchanged.

Actions

A. Dose dependent decrease in systolic and diastolic blood pressure comparable to nitroprusside

B. Systemic, renal, and mesenteric vasodilation mediated by vascular DA$_1$-receptors

C. Increases renal blood flow and decreases renal vascular resistance

D. Decreases renal tubular sodium and water reabsorption, thereby increasing sodium and water excretion

E. Does not cross the blood–brain barrier

Indications

A. Hypertensive crisis

B. Management of perioperative and intraoperative hypertension

Contraindications

A. Contraindicated if known hypersensitivity to metabisulfite

B. Avoid in patients with known open-angle glaucoma or intraocular hypertension.

C. Avoid in patients with uncorrected hypokalemia.

Typical Dosing and Administration

A. Standard preparation: 10 mg added to 250 mL 5% dextrose in water or normal saline (40 μg/mL)

B. Administered by continuous IV infusion using an infusion pump; do not administer by bolus injection

C. Initiate infusion at 0.1 μg/kg per minute and titrate upward by 0.05 to 0.10 μg/kg per minute, at increments no more frequently than every 15 minutes, to a maximum of 1.6 μg/kg per minute.

D. Intra-arterial blood pressure monitoring is not always needed; however, blood pressure should be assessed at frequent (e.g., every 15 minutes) intervals.

PEARLS

- Potent arteriolar vasodilator with rapid onset of action

- Consider as an alternative to nitroprusside for management of hypertensive crisis, especially in the presence of hepatic or renal failure.

- May exert protective effects on the renal circulation during mechanical ventilation with high levels of end-expiratory pressure

---

Side Effects

A. Cardiovascular
1. Hypotension: orthostatic or frank; asymptomatic or symptomatic
2. Dose-related tachycardia secondary to baroreceptor-mediated reflex mechanisms
3. Ventricular extrasystoles
4. Cardiac ischemia
5. Electrocardiographic T wave flattening or inversion

B. Metabolic: hypokalemia

C. Gastrointestinal
1. Nausea

2. Emesis

3. Abdominal pain

D. Central nervous system

1. Headache

2. Nervousness

3. Dizziness

E. Other effects

1. Cutaneous flushing

2. Increased intraocular pressure

3. Allergic reactions to sodium metabisulfite, including anaphylaxis

Bibliography

Brogden RN, Markham A. Fenoldopam. A review of its pharmacodynamic and pharmacokinetic properties and intravenous clinical potential in the management of hypertensive urgencies and emergencies. Drugs 1997;54:634–650.

Murphy MB, Murray C, Shorten GD. Fenoldopam—a selective peripheral dopamine-receptor agonist for the treatment of severe hypertension. N Engl J Med 2001;345:1548–1557.

O'Connell DP, Ragsdale NV, Boyd DG, et al. Differential human renal tubular responses to dopamine type 1 receptor stimulation are determined by blood pressure status. Hypertension 1997;29:115–122.

Oparil S, Aronson S, Deeb GM, et al. Fenoldopam: a new parenteral antihypertensive. Am J Hypertension 1999;12:653–664.

Panacek EA, Bednarczyk EM, Dunbar LM, et al. Randomized prospective trial of fenoldopam vs sodium nitroprusside in the treatment of acute severe hypertension. Acad Emerg Med 1995;2:959–965.

Post IV JB, Frishman WH. Fenoldopam: a new dopamine agonist for the treatment of hypertensive urgencies and emergencies. J Clin Pharmacol 1998;38:2–13.

Tumlin JA, Dunbar LM, Oparil S, et al. Fenoldopam, a dopamine agonist, for hypertensive emergency: a multicenter randomized trial. Acad Emerg Med 2000;7:653–662.

164 Nitroglycerin

Jorge A. Guzman

Pharmacology

A. Nitroglycerin causes relaxation of vascular smooth muscle, resulting in generalized vasodilation.
   1. Predominantly affects the venous vasculature
   2. Higher doses are also capable of producing arterial vasodilation, including coronary artery vasodilation.
B. Mechanism of action
   1. Nitroglycerin is metabolized to nitric oxide (NO) at or near the plasma membrane of vascular smooth cells.
   2. Nitric oxide activates guanylate cyclase, resulting in an increase in cyclic guanosine-3′,5′-monophosphate, which leads to the dephosphorylation of myosin light chains, resulting in smooth muscle relaxation.
C. Pharmacokinetics
   1. Rapid onset of action (1 to 2 min) when given by IV or sublingual route
   2. Metabolized to mono- and dinitrates, predominantly by liver
   3. Short plasma half-life of 2 to 3 minutes
   4. Short duration of action (<10 minutes), making it easily titratable by IV route
D. Tolerance develops as a function of dosage and duration or frequency of administration.

Actions

A. Arterial blood pressure
   1. Low doses affect predominantly venous vasodilation, and usually have little effect on blood pressure.
   2. Hypotension more likely at high doses or in the face of hypovolemia or compromised compensatory mechanisms
B. Cardiac effects
   1. Decreases ventricular preload
      a. Venous vasodilation results in decreased venous return, which decreases central venous pressure, pulmonary artery occlusion pressure, and left and right ventricular diastolic pressure and volume.
      b. Occurs at low and high doses
   2. Decreases ventricular afterload
      a. Arterial vasodilation results in decreased systemic vascular resistance, decreased left ventricular volume during systole, and decreased left ventricular wall tension during systole.
      b. Occurs mainly at higher doses
   3. Variable effect on cardiac output
   4. Heart rate usually increases slightly, probably mediated by baroreceptor reflex.
   5. Dilates epicardial coronary arteries

Indications

A. Oral and topical uses
   1. Stable ischemic heart disease
   2. Chronic angina pectoris
   3. Congestive heart failure
B. Intravenous uses
   1. Unstable angina
   2. Acute myocardial infarction
   3. Congestive heart failure
   4. Hypertension associated with myocardial ischemia
   5. Intraoperative controlled hypotension
   6. Perioperative hypertension

Key Contraindications

- Uncontrolled hypotension
- Hypovolemia
- Severe aortic or subaortic stenosis
- Increased intracranial pressure

Typical Dosing and Administration

A. Nitroglycerin
   1. Intravenous use
      a. Standard IV preparation: 100 mg/500 mL of 5% dextrose in water (200 μg/mL)
      b. Initiate at a dose of 5 μg/min and increase by 5 to 10 μg/min at 3- to 10-minute intervals, while monitoring blood pressure and symptoms.
      c. Titrated to affect (blood pressure or angina)
      d. Usual maximum dose is 400 μg/min.

585

e. Substantial absorption by some polyvinyl-chloride IV tubing

2. Sublingual route (Nitrostat and others)

a. For relief of acute angina pectoris

b. One 0.3 or 0.4 mg tablet sublingually; generally may repeat up to 3 times, 5 minutes apart

3. Lingual aerosol spray (Nitrolingual)

a. For relief of acute angina pectoris

b. 1 to 2 metered dose sprays (0.4 to 0.8 mg) onto or under tongue; generally may repeat up to 3 times, 5 minutes apart

4. Buccal transmucosal tablet (e.g., Nitrogard)

a. For relief of acute angina pectoris

b. 1 mg every 3 to 5 hours during waking hours

5. Topical use

a. Ointment (e.g., Nitrol, Nitro-bid ointment)

(1) Not for acute relief of angina attacks

(2) Applied topically to a 1- by 3-inch area

(3) 1/2 to 2 inches (7.5 to 30 mg) of 2% ointment every 4 to 8 hours

b. Transdermal delivery system (e.g., Nitro-Dur, Deponit)

(1) Not for acute relief of angina attacks

(2) Provides continuous controlled release of the drug through intact skin

(3) Delivered dose is proportional to area of device in contact with skin: approximately 0.2 mg/hour per cm²

(4) Usual dose is 0.2 to 0.8 mg/hour during a 12- to 14-hour patch-on period followed by a 10- to 12-hour patch-off period, daily.

6. Extended-release oral capsule or tablet (e.g., Nitrong)

a. For prophylactic use only

b. Typical dose: 2.5 to 10 mg, 2 to 3 times daily

B. Related nitrates

1. Isosorbide dinitrate (e.g., Isordil, Sorbitrate)

a. Sublingual, chewable, oral tablets or capsules

b. Slower onset than nitroglycerine, so not usually used to abort acute angina

c. Usual oral dose range: 20 to 40 mg, 2 to 3 times daily

d. Sublingual form: 2.5 to 5 mg

2. Isosorbide mononitrate (e.g., Imdur, Monoket)

a. For prophylactic use only

b. 10 to 40 mg, twice daily (sustained-release form: 30 to 120 mg, once daily)

3. Erythrityl tetranitrate (Cardilate)

a. For chronic prophylaxis

b. Usual dose: 5 to 10 mg up to 3 times daily

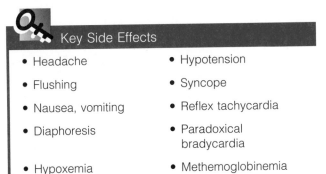

Key Side Effects

- Headache
- Flushing
- Nausea, vomiting
- Diaphoresis
- Hypoxemia
- Hypotension
- Syncope
- Reflex tachycardia
- Paradoxical bradycardia
- Methemoglobinemia

Bibliography

Buckley R, Roberts R. Symptomatic bradycardia following the administration of sublingual nitroglycerin. Am J Emerg Med 1993;11:253–255.

Jugdutt BI. Nitrates in myocardial infarction. Cardiovasc Drug Ther 1994;8:635–646.

Milicevic G, Goldner V, Vrhovac B, et al. How long can escalation of dose override tolerance to the hypotensive efficacy of nitroglycerin infusion in coronary care patients? Cardiovasc Drug Ther 1999;13:531–536.

Robertson RM, Robertson D. Drugs used for the treatment of myocardial ischemia. In: Hardman JG, Limbird LE, Molinoff PB, et al (eds). Goodman & Gilman's The Pharmacological Basis of Therapeutics, 9th ed. New York: McGraw-Hill, 1996, pp 759–779.

165 Nitroprusside

Jorge A. Guzman

Pharmacology

A. Sodium nitroprusside (SNP) is a potent parenteral antihypertensive agent.
1. It is an inorganic compound: $Na_2[Fe(CN)_5NO] \cdot 2H_2O$
2. Solutions of SNP are sensitive to light and must be protected from exposure to light.

B. Metabolism
1. Metabolized by reaction with hemoglobin to form cyanide (CN^-) and cyanmethemoglobin
2. CN^- is eliminated by several routes.
   a. Forming hydrogen cyanide, which is expired via the lungs, but only to a limited extent
   b. Combining with methemoglobin to form cyanmethemoglobin
   c. Reacting with thiosulfate and mitochondrial rhodenase to form thiocyanate, which is excreted by the kidney

C. Mechanism of action
1. Nitric oxide, the active metabolite, activates intracellular guanylate cyclase to form cyclic guanosine monophosphate (cGMP).
2. Cyclic GMP directly mediates vascular smooth muscle cell relaxation and vasodilation.

D. Pharmacokinetics
1. Sodium nitroprusside rapidly distributes throughout the extracellular space.
2. Rapid onset of action ($\sim$1 minute)
3. Half-life is approximately 2 minutes.

Key Actions
- Potent antihypertensive effect
- Dilates both arterial and venous vessels
- Reduces cardiac preload and afterload
- Decreases myocardial oxygen demand

Indications

A. Hypertensive emergencies
B. Acute congestive heart failure
C. Management of arterial hypertension during acute aortic dissection (in conjunction with pharmacologic β-adrenergic blockade)
D. Controlled hypotension during anesthesia to reduce intraoperative bleeding
E. Perioperative management of pheochromocytoma crisis
F. Perioperative hypertension

Contraindications

A. Certain rare disorders associated with abnormal cyanide metabolism
1. Leber's congenital optic atrophy
2. Tobacco amblyopia
B. Hepatic and renal failure are relative contraindications because of the increased risk of cyanide and thiocyanate toxicity.
C. Inability to monitor blood pressure closely

Key Side Effects
- Hypotension
- Cyanide intoxication
- Thiocyanate intoxication
- Intracranial hypertension
- Methemoglobinemia (rare)

Typical Dosing and Administration

A. Preparation
1. 50 mg SNP in at least 250 mL of 5% dextrose and water
2. Protect infusate container from light using aluminum foil or other opaque material.

B. Dosing
1. Initiate administration using 0.1 μg/kg per minute by continuous IV infusion.
2. Administer using a volumetric infusion pump.
3. Titrate dose upward in increments of 0.1 to 0.5 μg/kg per minute, every few minutes, to effect.
4. Maximum recommended infusion rate is 10 μg/kg per minute.
5. Avoid doses greater than 2 μg/kg per minute for prolonged periods (>48 hours).

PEARLS

- Sodium nitroprusside is a predictable and effective IV vasodilator with rapid onset of action and short half-life.

- Risk of cyanide toxicity is reduced by addition of sodium thiosulfate to SNP solution.

- To lower toxicity risk, minimize duration of use by substituting alternative antihypertensive agents as soon as possible.

- Especially avoid infusions of more than 2 μg/kg per minute and use that exceeds 48 hours

C. Closely monitor blood pressure.
  1. Automated, noninvasive sphygmomanometry devices may be considered in some circumstances.
  2. Intra-arterial pressure monitoring is preferred.
D. Initiate alternative antihypertensive agent(s) as soon as possible to allow timely discontinuation of SNP.
E. Addition of 1 g sodium thiosulfate per 100 mg of SNP in the IV solution decreases the risk of cyanide toxicity.
F. A high index of suspicion in the presence of suggestive clinical findings is key to recognizing cyanide or thiocyanate toxicity (see Chapter 70, Cyanide Poisoning).

Bibliography

Capomolla S, Pozzoli M, Opasich C, et al. Dobutamine and nitroprusside infusion in patients with severe congestive heart failure: hemodynamic improvement by discordant effects on mitral regurgitation, left atrial function, and ventricular function. Am Heart J 1997;134:1089–1098.

Curry SC, Arnold-Capell P. Nitroprusside, nitroglycerin, and angiotensin-converting enzyme inhibitors. Crit Care Clin 1991;7:555–581.

Friederich JA, Butterworth JF IV. Sodium nitroprusside: twenty years and counting. Anesth Analg 1995;81:152–162.

Kieback AG, Iven H, Stolzenburg K, et al. Saterinone, dobutamine, and nitroprusside: comparison of cardiovascular profiles in patients with congestive heart failure. J Cardiovasc Pharmacol 1998;32:629–636.

166 Diuretics

Mary M. Meyer

Diuretics are pharmacologic agents that are used chiefly in the treatment of edema by causing natriuresis and diuresis. Urgency of treatment is related to the location and cause of the expanded interstitial fluid. The only emergent condition is pulmonary edema, although massive fluid collections, such as large-volume ascites or pleural effusion, may necessitate urgent treatment. In addition, anasarca may contribute to skin breakdown, ulceration, and infection. Despite massive edema, diuretics may not be tolerated in the presence of hemodynamic instability. In such situations, continuous renal replacement techniques may be employed.

Pharmacology

A. Acetazolamide
   1. Inhibits carbonic anhydrase in the proximal convoluted tubule, in effect, preventing reabsorption of sodium bicarbonate
   2. Causes metabolic acidosis
   3. Weak diuretic effect

B. Furosemide, bumetanide, torsemide, ethacrynic acid ("loop diuretics")
   1. Block sodium-potassium-chloride co-transport in the renal medulla at the level of the ascending limb of the loop of Henle, impairing the urinary concentration mechanism
   2. Decreases renal vascular resistance and increases renal blood flow
   3. Potent diuretic effect

C. Thiazides, metolazone, indapamide
   1. Block sodium-chloride co-transport at the distal convoluted tubule (the "distal diluting segment") impairing the urinary dilution mechanism
   2. Block calcium entry into the cell and can lead to hypercalciuria

D. Spironolactone, amiloride, triamterene ("potassium-sparing diuretics")
   1. Spironolactone: blocks aldosterone at the collecting duct
      a. Decreases sodium absorption, which leads to natriuresis and diuresis
      b. Decreases potassium ion secretion, which can lead to hyperkalemia

   2. Amiloride and triamterene: block sodium channels

E. Mannitol ("osmotic diuretic")
   1. A non-reabsorbable sugar-alcohol that increases intravascular and intratubular osmotic pressure and inhibits sodium and water reabsorption in the proximal tubule and the loop of Henle, producing a water diuresis
   2. Must reach the renal tubule to act as a diuretic; thus, in renal insufficiency it increases intravascular volume but may not induce diuresis.

F. Dopamine
   1. Increases renal blood flow when used at low doses (typically, 0.5 to 2.0 μg/kg per minute), inducing natriuresis and diuresis
   2. Plasma dopamine clearance is reduced in critically ill patients such that the "renal dose" may be within what is typically the β- or α-adrenergic range.

Indications

A. Acetazolamide
   1. Metabolic alkalosis, including metabolic alkalosis generated by loop diuretic use
   2. Used to treat metabolic alkalosis-driven hypoventilation in patients with severe chronic obstructive lung disease and chronic hypercapnia
   3. Prophylaxis and treatment of acute mountain sickness and high-altitude pulmonary and cerebral edema
   4. Glaucoma

B. Furosemide, bumetanide, torsemide, ethacrynic acid
   1. Edematous disorders, e.g., cirrhosis, congestive heart failure (CHF), and nephrotic syndrome
   2. Sodium and water retention in renal insufficiency
   3. Hypercalcemia
   4. Hypertension associated with renal insufficiency
   5. Acute tubular necrosis (ATN)
      a. Experimentally, to reduce metabolic demand of tubular cells by blocking active ion

589

transport and to decrease tubular obstruction from cell debris by increasing tubular flow

    b. Practically, to increase urine output and simplify fluid management

  6. Some forms of hyponatremia

C. Thiazides, metolazone, indapamide

  1. Edema

  2. Hypertension

  3. Synergism in conjunction with loop diuretic

D. Spironolactone, amiloride, triamterene

  1. Used in conjunction with other diuretics to counteract their hypokalemic effect

  2. Spironolactone

    a. First-line diuretic for ascites associated with cirrhosis

    b. Congestive heart failure

    c. Primary hyperaldosteronism

  3. Amiloride

    a. Primary hyperaldosteronism

    b. Lithium-induced nephrogenic diabetes insipidus

    c. Used in lieu of spironolactone if gynecomastia occurs

  4. Triamterene: also may be used in lieu of spironolactone if gynecomastia occurs

E. Mannitol

  1. Cardiovascular surgery (efficacy debated)

  2. Rhabdomyolysis, to mitigate myoglobinuric renal failure (efficacy debated)

  3. Hemolytic transfusion reaction

  4. Elevated intraocular or intracranial pressure

  5. Irrigating solution during transurethral resection of prostate

  6. Prevention of disequilibrium syndrome during initiation of dialysis

  7. Early stages of post-ischemic, acute oliguric renal failure, in attempt to prevent progression to ATN (efficacy unproven)

F. Dopamine

  1. No benefit of prophylactic renal-dose dopamine

  2. May observe mild tubular diuretic and saluretic effect of low-dose dopamine and saline in some patients, but no proven renal protective effect

Key Contraindications

- Acetazolamide: hyperchloremic acidosis, hypersensitivity to sulfonamides

- Furosemide, bumetanide, torsemide, ethacrynic acid: sulfonamide hypersensitivity

- Thiazides, metolazone, indapamide: diabetes mellitus and hypercholesterolemia (relative contraindication), hypersensitivity to sulfonamides; ineffective when glomerular filtration rate is <50 mL/minute

- Spironolactone, amiloride, triamterene: hyperkalemia, anuria

- Mannitol: anuria, diuretic unresponsive renal failure, pulmonary edema, CHF

Typical Dosing

A. Acetazolamide: 250 mg one to three times daily, intravenously or orally

B. Furosemide, bumetanide, torsemide, ethacrynic acid

  1. Effective dose is based on the glomerular filtration rate (Tables 166–1 and 166–2).

  2. The threshold dose is that below which no natriuresis occurs; determined empirically by escalating the dose until natriuresis occurs.

  3. The effective oral dose may exceed the effective IV dose, depending on bioavailability.

C. Hydrochlorothiazide: edema: 25 to 200 mg/day in divided oral doses (12.5 to 25 mg/day for hypertension)

TABLE 166–1. SELECTION OF LOOP DIURETIC DOSE (mg) USING IV BOLUS ADMINISTRATION ACCORDING TO LEVEL OF RENAL DYSFUNCTION

DIURETIC	BIOAVAILABILITY	LEVEL OF RENAL IMPAIRMENT		
		NONE	MODERATE	SEVERE
Furosemide	50%	10 to 20	80 to 160	160 to 200
Bumetanide	80% to 100%	0.5 to 2	4 to 8	8 to 10

TABLE 166–2. SELECTION OF LOOP DIURETIC DOSE (mg/hr) USING CONTINUOUS IV INFUSION ACCORDING TO GLOMERULAR FILTRATION RATE

DIURETIC	IV LOADING DOSE (MG)	GLOMERULAR FILTRATION RATE (ML/MIN)		
		<25	25 TO 75	>75
Furosemide	40	20 to 40	10 to 20	1 to 10
Bumetanide	1	1 to 2	0.5 to 1	0.5

D. Metolazone

  1. For edema: 5 to 20 mg/day orally for edema

  2. For synergistic effect with loop diuretic: 2.5 to 5 mg orally 30 minutes before the loop diuretic

E. Chlorothiazide: 250 to 1000 mg/day in one or two IV doses

F. Spironolactone

  1. For edema: 25 to 200 mg/day in divided oral doses

  2. For hypertension or cirrhosis: 25 to 100 mg/day orally

  3. For CHF: 25 mg/day PO

  4. For primary aldosteronism: 100 to 400 mg/day in divided oral doses

G. Amiloride: 5 to 20 mg/day

H. Triamterene: 100 mg twice daily

I. Mannitol

  1. Acute renal failure: test dose 12.5 g intravenously; if no diuresis, repeat test dose

  2. If diuretic responsive, give 50 to 100 g intravenously over 90 minutes.

  3. For increased intracranial pressure: 250 mg/kg intravenously over 30 to 60 minutes

---

PEARL

Metolazone is inconsistently absorbed from the gastrointestinal tract, and its long half-life can lead to drug accumulation. When used in combination diuretic therapy, this can result in a late excessive response, leading to volume depletion.

Side Effects and Precautions

A. Acetazolamide

  1. Severe hypokalemia, agranulocytosis, aplastic anemia

  2. Decreased urinary excretion of amphetamines, ephedrine, and antidysrhythmic and cyclic antidepressant drugs

  3. Increased urinary excretion of lithium

B. Furosemide, bumetanide, torsemide, ethacrynic acid

  1. Hypokalemia, hypomagnesemia, hypocalcemia, hypovolemia

  2. Hyperuricemia

  3. Allergic interstitial nephritis

  4. Ototoxicity, tinnitus (higher risk with large IV bolus dosing)

C. Thiazides, metolazone, indapamide

  1. Hypokalemia, hyponatremia, hypercalcemia

  2. Hyperglycemia

  3. Hyperuricemia

  4. Hypercholesterolemia

  5. Enhanced urinary stone formation

D. Amiloride

  1. Hyperkalemia, hyponatremia

  2. Headache

  3. Aplastic anemia, positive Coombs' test

E. Triamterene

  1. Hyperkalemia

  2. Hyperuricemia

  3. Megaloblastic anemia, granulocytopenia

F. Spironolactone

  1. Hyperkalemia

  2. Gynecomastia, erectile dysfunction, androgenic effects (hirsutism, low voice, irregular menses)

  3. Rash

G. Mannitol

  1. Hyponatremia, hypertonicity

  2. Intravascular volume expansion leading to pulmonary edema or CHF

3. Renal medullary wash-out and impaired renal concentrating ability

H. Dopamine

  1. Tachycardia

  2. Hypokalemia, hypophosphatemia

Key Causes of Diuretic Resistance

- Insufficient diuretic dose

- Decreased bioavailability of diuretic

- Excess dietary or IV sodium administration

- Intravascular volume depletion

- Hypoalbuminemia

- Concurrent administration of angiotensin converting enzyme inhibitor, angiotensin receptor blocker, or nonsteroidal antiinflammatory drugs

Bibliography

Australian and New Zealand Intensive Care Society Clinical Trials Group. Low-dose dopamine in patients with early renal dysfunction: a placebo-controlled randomized trial. Lancet 2000;356:2139–2143.

Brater DC. Diuretic therapy. N Engl J Med 1998;339:387–395.

Dormans TPJ, van Meyel JJM, Gerlag PGG, et al. Diuretic efficacy of high dose furosemide in severe heart failure: bolus injection versus continuous infusion. J Am Coll Cardiol 1996;28:376–382.

Ellison DH. Diuretic drugs and the treatment of edema: from clinic to bench and back again. Am J Kidney Dis 1994;23:623–643.

Ichai C, Soubielle J, Carles M, et al. Comparison of the renal effects of low to high doses of dopamine and dobutamine in critically ill patients: a single-blind randomized study. Crit Care Med 2000;28:921–928.

Kellum JA. Use of diuretics in the acute care setting. Kidney Int 1998;53(Suppl 66):S67–S70.

Mazur JE, Devlin JW, Peters MJ, et al. Single versus multiple doses of acetazolamide for metabolic alkalosis in critically ill medical patients: a randomized double-blind trial. Crit Care Med 1999;27:1257–1261.

Rudy DW, Voelker JR, Greene PK, et al. Loop diuretics for chronic renal insufficiency: a continuous infusion is more efficacious than bolus therapy. Ann Intern Med 1991;115:360–366.

167 Acid-Inhibiting Agents and Sucralfate

John W. Devlin
James A. Kruse

The gastric cytoprotective agent sucralfate, or a gastric acid inhibiting agent (i.e., histamine-2 receptor antagonist [H2RA] or proton-pump inhibitors [PPI]) are routinely used in the intensive care unit (ICU) to prevent stress ulcer-related gastrointestinal bleeding or as empiric treatment for patients experiencing an acute upper gastrointestinal (GI) hemorrhage. Newer literature suggests that stress ulcer prophylaxis may not be cost-effective in ICU patients at low risk for developing GI bleeding. In addition, H2RAs, as compared to sucralfate for stress ulcer prophylaxis, may prevent more bleeding without increasing the risk of nosocomial pneumonia. The specific role for PPIs in the ICU remains to be elucidated. The benefits of treating acute upper GI hemorrhage with acid-inhibiting therapy has not been well documented in the literature. Any of these agents may induce undesired side effects, and thus therapy should be carefully monitored, particularly in critically ill patients.

Actions

A. H2RAs: reduce gastric acid output
B. PPIs
 1. Reduce gastric acid output
 2. Decrease pepsin activity
 3. Increase gastrin level
C. Sucralfate: protects areas of gastrointestinal mucosal ulceration

Pharmacology

A. H2RAs: competitively inhibit the action of histamine on H_2 receptors of parietal cells under basal conditions and when stimulated by food, gastrin, or muscarinic agonists
B. PPIs
 1. Suppress gastric acid secretion by specific inhibition of the H^+/K^+-ATPase enzyme system (the proton pump) at the secretory surface of the gastric parietal cell (the final step in acid production)
 2. Decrease blood flow in the antrum, pylorus, and duodenal bulb
 3. Decrease conversion of pepsinogen to pepsin, resulting in decreased pepsin secretion and activity

 4. Increase serum gastrin levels in relation to inhibition of acid secretion
C. Sucralfate
 1. A basic aluminum salt of sulfated sucrose
 2. Dissociates in acidic gastric juice to an anion that binds to areas of gastric ulceration
 3. This ulcer-adherent complex covers the ulcer site and protects it against acid, pepsin, and bile salts.
 4. Minimal, if any, acid neutralizing capacity

Indications

A. Specific indications
 1. H2RA
  a. Prevention of stress ulcer–related upper GI bleeding
  b. Acute treatment of upper GI bleeding
  c. Acute and maintenance therapy for gastric or duodenal ulcers, or GI reflux disease
  d. *Helicobacter pylori* eradication (as part of a multi-drug regimen)
  e. Treatment of allergic manifestations in anaphylaxis and contact dermatitis
 2. PPIs
  a. Prevention of stress ulcer–related upper GI bleeding
  b. Acute treatment of upper GI bleeding
  c. Acute and maintenance therapy for gastric or duodenal ulcers, or GI reflux disease
  d. *Helicobacter pylori* eradication (as part of a multi-drug regimen)
  e. Pathological hypersecretory conditions, such as Zollinger-Ellison syndrome
 3. Sucralfate
  a. Prevention of stress ulcer–related upper GI bleeding
  b. Acute and maintenance therapy for duodenal ulcers
  c. Maintenance therapy for gastric ulcers
B. Intensive care unit patients in whom stress ulcer prophylaxis should be considered

1. Bleeding diathesis (e.g., platelets <50,000/mm³, baseline prothrombin time >16 seconds)
2. Acute respiratory failure requiring mechanical ventilation for longer than 24 hours
3. Circulatory shock requiring vasopressor therapy
4. Burns involving more than 30% of body surface area
5. Significant intracranial trauma or hemorrhage
6. Spinal injury requiring immobilization for longer than 24 hours
7. Bone marrow transplantation
8. High-dose corticosteroid therapy (>250 mg/day hydrocortisone or equivalent)
9. Gastrointestinal bleeding within 12 weeks of admission

PEARLS

- Antacids, to effectively neutralize gastric acid, must be administered frequently (every 3 to 4 hours) and in high doses (>30 mL/dose); however, intensity of therapy is both cumbersome for the nurse and associated with a higher incidence of adverse events (e.g., electrolyte abnormalities) than the agents described in this chapter.

- H2RAs, when compared to sucralfate as stress ulcer prophylaxis therapy, have been shown to be more efficacious (less GI hemorrhage) without increasing the incidence of nosocomial pneumonia.

- No specific H2RA has been shown to be more efficacious than other agents in its class when equipotent doses are compared; ranitidine and famotidine are generally associated with fewer adverse effects than cimetidine, but may have higher acquisition costs.

- Combined therapy using sucralfate and either H2RA or PPI is unlikely to be of greater benefit than the use of either agent alone, because sucralfate is dependent on an acid pH for its binding action to areas of gastrointestinal mucosal ulceration.

Contraindications

A. All agents: previous hypersensitivity reactions to respective drug
B. Sucralfate: should be avoided in patients with end-stage renal disease, including those patients undergoing peritoneal dialysis or hemodialysis, because aluminum toxicity can occur

Precautions

A. H2RAs
  1. Reversible central nervous system (CNS) effects (e.g., mental confusion, psychosis) reported predominantly with cimetidine in critically ill patients; advanced age and preexisting renal or liver failure are predisposing factors.
  2. Each agent has rarely been associated with thrombocytopenia, although causality, in each case, has not been well established, particularly in critically ill patients, who frequently have a host of reasons for becoming thrombocytopenic.
  3. Rapid IV administration of cimetidine and ranitidine has been associated, in rare instances, with cardiac dysrhythmias and hypotension.
B. PPIs: although evidence to date has not suggested that humans exposed to PPI therapy are at risk, a dose-related increase in gastric carcinoid tumors has been observed during long-term exposure in animals
C. Sucralfate (and most PPIs), unlike H2RAs, require gastroenteral administration; use of nasogastric tubes has been associated with an increased incidence of nosocomial pneumonia in mechanically ventilated patients.

Side Effects

A. H2RAs
  1. Central nervous system: headache, confusional states
  2. Hematologic: thrombocytopenia (rare)
  3. Other: gynecomastia (cimetidine, rare)
B. PPIs: adverse reactions are generally rare and usually are limited to GI symptoms (e.g., diarrhea) or minor CNS effects (e.g., headache)
C. Sucralfate: adverse reactions are rare; usually limited to GI complaints (e.g., diarrhea, nausea, vomiting)

Interactions

A. H2RAs
  1. All agents: oral absorption of iron salts, ketoconazole, and tetracycline may be decreased
  2. Cimetidine: may block the metabolism and thus increase the activity of the following agents: calcium channel blockers, carbamazepine, metoprolol, phenytoin, quinidine, theophylline, valproic acid, warfarin
B. PPIs: omeprazole may prolong the elimination of diazepam, warfarin, phenytoin and other agents that are metabolized by cytochrome P450–medi-

TABLE 167-1. DOSING OF HISTAMINE-2 RECEPTOR ANTAGONISTS*

FORM OF TREATMENT	CIMETIDINE (TAGAMET)	FAMOTIDINE (PEPCID)	RANITIDINE (ZANTAC)
Oral treatment and stress ulcer prophylaxis	300 to 400 mg PO q 4–6 hr	20 mg PO q 12 hr	150 mg PO q 12 hr
Intermittent IV dosing	300 mg q 6–8 hr (maximum of 2400 mg/day)	20 mg q 12 hr (maximum of 160 mg/day)	50 mg q 8 hr (maximum of 400 mg/day)
Continuous IV infusion	50 mg/hr to a maximum of 100 mg/hr	1.6 mg/hr to a maximum of 3.2 mg/hr	6.3 mg/hr to a maximum of 12.5 mg/hr
Dose adjustment in renal failure	If Ccr <30 mL/min, decrease dose by 50%	If Ccr <10 mL/min, decrease dose by 50%	If Ccr <50 mL/min, 150 mg PO q 24 hr or 50 mg IV q 18–24 hr

*Ccr = creatinine clearance rate; PO signifies per os or by GI tract feeding tube.

ated oxidation in the liver (clinical significance of these interactions is unclear)

C. Sucralfate: may bind to phenytoin, fluoroquinolones (e.g., ciprofloxacin), quinidine, digoxin, and ketoconazole if administered concomitantly; should separate dosing by at least 2 hours with any of these agents

Typical Dosing

A. Histamine-2 receptor antagonists

1. Dosing: see Table 167–1

2. Gastroenteral administration

   a. Generally well absorbed and may be administered by the GI tract (using the less expensive oral liquid formulation) rather than IV

3. IV administration

   a. May be given by intermittent or continuous IV infusion

   b. Continuous IV infusions may be more cost-effective than intermittent IV dosing, particularly at high doses.

   c. Compatible with total parenteral nutrition solutions

B. PPIs

1. See Table 167–2.

2. Capsules (i.e., lansoprazole, omeprazole) contain enteric-coated drug granules, which must be protected from destruction during administration via feeding tubes by mixing contents with 10 mL of 8.4% sodium bicarbonate solution.

3. Pantoprazole is available as an intravenous formulation, administered as 40 mg once daily by IV injection at less than 3 mg/min.

C. Sucralfate (Carafate)

1. For stress ulcer prophylaxis or active treatment: 1 g orally every 6 hours

2. For maintenance therapy: 1 g orally every 12 hours

3. Tablets may be easily dissolvable in 10 to 15 mL sterile water and can be administered through a feeding tube.

Use in Renal or Hepatic Dysfunction

A. H2RAs: see Table 169–1

B. Proton-pump inhibitors

1. Renal: none

2. Hepatic: lansoprazole dosing adjustment should be considered in patients with severe hepatic disease

C. Sucralfate

1. Renal: aluminum may accumulate with prolonged use in patients with end-stage renal disease; alternative agents should be considered

2. Hepatic: none

TABLE 167-2. DOSING (ORAL OR BY GI TRACT FEEDING TUBE) OF PROTON PUMP INHIBITORS

DRUG	ACUTE THERAPY	MAINTENANCE THERAPY
Lansoprazole (Prevacid)	30 mg daily (maximum of 120 mg/day in hypersecretors)	15 mg daily
Omeprazole (Prilosec)	40 mg daily (maximum of 360 mg/day in hypersecretors)	20 mg daily
Esomeprazole (Nexium)	20 or 40 mg daily	20 mg daily
Pantoprazole (Panto)*	40 or 80 mg daily (maximum of 480 mg/day in hypersecretors)	40 mg daily
Rabeprazole (Aciphex)*	20 mg daily (maximum of 120 mg/day in hypersecretors)	20 mg daily

*Enteric coated tablet, do not crush.

Monitoring

A. Stress ulcer prophylaxis therapy (all agents): monitor for signs and symptoms of gastrointestinal bleeding
B. Acid-Inhibiting agents (H2RA, PPI)
   1. Gastric pH monitoring may be employed for titrating therapy between the usual dose and the maximum recommended dose, to achieve gastric $pH \geq 4$ (stress ulcer prophylaxis) and gastric ≥ 6 (acute upper GI hemorrhage).
   2. Evidence supporting the clinical utility of this as routine practice is scant.

 Bibliography

Cook DJ, Guyatt G, Marshall J, et al. A comparison of sucralfate and ranitidine for the prevention of upper gastrointestinal bleeding in patients requiring mechanical ventilation. N Engl J Med 1998;338:791–797.

Cook DJ, Heyland D, Griffith L, et al. Risk factors for clinically important upper gastrointestinal bleeding in patients requiring mechanical ventilation. Crit Care Med 1999;27:2812–2817.

Devlin JW, Ben-Menachem T, Ulep SK, et al. Stress ulcer prophylaxis in medical ICU patients: annual utilization in relation to the incidence of endoscopically proven stress ulceration. Ann Pharmacother 1998;32:869–874.

Khuroo MS, Yattoo GN, Javid G, et al. A comparison of omeprazole and placebo for bleeding peptic ulcer N Engl J Med 1997;336:1054–1058.

Richardson P, Hawkey CJ, Stack WA. Proton pump inhibitors: pharmacology and rationale for use in gastrointestinal disorders. Drugs 1998;56:307–335.

Robertson JA, Salusky IB, Goodman WG, et al. Sucralfate intestinal absorption and aluminum toxicity in a patient on dialysis. Ann Intern Med 1989;111:179–181.

168 Neuromuscular Blocking Drugs

John W. Devlin
James A. Kruse

Pharmacology

A. Actions
1. Neuromuscular blocking drugs (NBDs) chemically interrupt neuromuscular transmission by reacting with the nicotinic cholinergic receptors on skeletal muscle.
2. The NBDs thus prevent the normal action of acetylcholine, and result in weakness or paralysis.

B. Muscles affected by neuromuscular blockade
1. First affected are muscles producing fine, rapid movements such as those of the eyes, face, and neck.
2. Next affected are muscles of the limbs, abdomen, and chest.
3. Last affected is the diaphragm.
4. Recovery of muscle function generally occurs in the reverse order.

C. Classification
1. Succinylcholine
   a. A depolarizing NBD
   b. Has a high affinity for acetylcholine receptors at the neuromuscular junction
   c. Highly resistant to acetylcholinesterase
2. Nondepolarizing NBDs
   a. Competitively antagonize acetylcholine binding at nicotinic pre- and postsynaptic membrane receptors at the neuromuscular junction
   b. Structurally categorized as aminosteroids or benzylisoquinolines
   c. Functionally categorized by duration of action: short, intermediate, or long

Indications

A. The depolarizing NBD succinylcholine is used to induce complete skeletal muscle relaxation of short duration.
1. Endotracheal intubation
2. Endoscopic examination
3. Electroconvulsive therapy
B. Nondepolarizing NBDs
1. Rapid-sequence intubation

2. Optimization of mechanical ventilation, particularly when using advanced ventilation strategies to minimize lung injury (the most common reason for using NBDs in the intensive care unit [ICU] setting)
   a. Ventilator asynchrony
   b. Excessive peak or plateau airway pressures
   c. Excessive intrinsic positive end-expiratory pressure (i.e., resulting in hemodynamic compromise)
   d. Pressure control mode ventilation
   e. Permissive hypercapnic ventilation
   f. Inverse ratio or independent lung ventilation
3. Lowering systemic oxygen demand in the face of inadequate oxygen delivery
4. Intracranial hypertension unresponsive to first-line therapies
5. Tetanus

Key Indications

- Succinylcholine is the drug of choice to facilitate endotracheal intubation in patients not having contraindications for its use.

- Sedation (e.g., benzodiazepines, opioids, propofol) and mechanical ventilation settings should be optimized before considering continuous neuromuscular blocker therapy in the ICU.

- Aminosteroid nondepolaring NBDs (e.g., pancuronium) are generally more cost-effective than benzylisoquinoline class agents (e.g., cisatracurium), and are recommended as first-line therapy unless there are contraindications.

- Shorter half-life agents (e.g., cisatracurium) are more conveniently administered by continuous infusion than by intermittent injection.

Contraindications

A. Depolarizing NBDs
1. Known hypersensitivity to the drug
2. Genetically determined disorders of plasma pseudocholinesterase
3. Personal or family history of malignant hyperthermia

4. Skeletal muscle myopathies

5. Angle-closure glaucoma or penetrating eye injury

6. Acute phase of extensive burn injury

7. Acute phase of multiple trauma

8. Upper motor neuron injury

9. Extensive denervation of skeletal muscle

B. Nondepolarizing NBDs: known hypersensitivity to the drug

Precautions

A. Depolarizing NBDs
1. Patients with electrolyte imbalance, particularly potassium and magnesium
2. Patients with suspected digoxin toxicity
3. Hyperkalemia
4. Risk factors for developing hyperkalemia
   a. Neuromuscular disease or paralysis, including paraplegia, hemiplegia, myopathy, muscular dystrophy, spinal cord injury, or other upper motor neuron or central nervous system injury
   b. Multiple trauma
   c. Extensive or severe burns

B. Nondepolarizing NBDs
1. Should be used only in facilities where the personnel for endotracheal intubation, administration of oxygen, and mechanical ventilation are readily available
2. Factors that may inhibit or potentiate effects of NBDs (see Interactions, later in this chapter)
3. Prolonged persistence of neuromuscular blockade following discontinuation of NBD
   a. A temporal and anecdotal association with prolonged skeletal muscle weakness or paralysis is well documented.
   b. These effects are often challenging to differentiate from myopathies and axonal polyneuropathies associated with critical illness.
4. If there is a need for long-term mechanical ventilation, the benefits of continued neuromuscular blockade therapy should be weighed against the risks.
5. All patients receiving continuous NBDs should
   a. Receive standard eye care
   b. Receive decubitus precautions according to nursing standards
   c. Be properly positioned or splinted to prevent peroneal and brachial plexus palsies during paralysis

d. Receive prophylaxis for deep-vein thrombosis

> ## WARNING
> NBDs will cause apnea and death if administered to patients not receiving controlled mechanical ventilation.

Interactions

A. Factors inhibiting the effects of NBDs
1. Drugs
   a. Halogenated anesthetics
   b. Local anesthetics
   c. Antibiotics
      (1) Aminoglycosides
      (2) Clindamycin
      (3) Vancomycin
   d. Antiarrhythmic drugs
      (1) Procainamide
      (2) Quinidine
      (3) Bretylium
   e. β-Adrenergic blocking drugs
   f. Calcium channel blockers
   g. Corticosteroids
   h. Cyclophosphamide
   i. Cyclosporin A
   j. Dantrolene
   k. Lithium
2. Clinical factors
   a. Acidosis
   b. Electrolyte abnormalities
      (1) Hypermagnesemia
      (2) Severe hypocalcemia
      (3) Severe hypokalemia
      (4) Severe hyponatremia
   c. Neuromuscular diseases
      (1) Myasthenia gravis
      (2) Muscular dystrophy
      (3) Poliomyelitis
      (4) Multiple sclerosis
      (5) Eaton-Lambert syndrome
   d. Hypothermia
   e. Acute intermittent porphyria

TABLE 168–1. TYPICAL PROPERTIES AND IV DOSING OF NONDEPOLARIZING NBDS

Drug	Chemical Class	Loading Dose (μG/KG)	Intermittent Dose (μG/KG)	Continuous Infusion (μG/KG per min)	Onset (min)	Duration (min)	Dosage Adjustment Required in Organ Failure
Atracurium (Tracrium)	Benzylisoquinoline	300–500	80–100 q 30–60 min	5–15	2–4	30–40	None
Cisatracurium (Nimbex)	Benzylisoquinoline	150–200	30 q 30 to 60 min	0.5–10	2–6	60–120	None
Pancuronium (Pavulon)	Aminosteroid	40–150	40–150 q 1–3 hr	1.0–1.7	4–6	120–180	Renal failure
Rocuronium (Zemuron)	Aminosteroid	600	300–600 q 1 hr	3–15	1–2	30–40	Hepatic failure
Vecuronium (Norcuron)	Aminosteroid	60–130	10–15 q 1–2 hr	0.8–1.2	2–4	30–40	Hepatic failure
Mivacurium (Mivacron)	Benzylisoquinoline	150–200	100 q 15 min	4–12	2–4	12–18	Hepatic and renal failure
Doxacurium (Nuromax)	Benzylisoquinoline	25–50	5–10 q 30–45 min	Not recommended	4–6	80–130	Renal failure
Pipecuronium (Arduan)	Aminosteroid	70–85	10–15 q 30 to 45 min	Not recommended	3–5	80–100	Renal failure
Rapacuronium (Raplon)	Aminosteroid	1500	500 q 15 min	Not recommended	1.5	15	Renal failure

f. Renal failure

g. Hepatic failure

B. Factors potentiating the effects of NBDs

  1. Drugs

    a. Phenytoin

    b. Carbamazepine

    c. Anticholinesterase agents

      (1) Edrophonium

      (2) Neostigmine

      (3) Pyridostigmine

    d. Theophylline

    e. Azathioprine

    f. Ranitidine

  2. Clinical factors

    a. Alkalemia

    b. Hypercalcemia

    c. Demyelinating lesions

    d. Peripheral neuropathies

    e. Diabetes mellitus

Typical Dosing

A. Depolarizing NBDs

  1. Succinylcholine (Anectine, Quelicin) 0.6 mg/kg (range 0.3 to 1.1 mg/kg) intravenously over 10 to 30 seconds

  2. Continuous infusion of succinylcholine generally not recommended

B. Nondepolarizing NBDs (see Table 168–1)

  1. Loading dose: usually administered to initiate therapeutic paralysis

  2. Maintenance dose

    a. Medium and long half-life agents (e.g., pancuronium, rocuronium, vecuronium) may be administered either as intermittent bolus injections or as a continuous IV infusion.

    b. Short half-life agents (e.g., atracurium, cisatracurium) should be administered as a continuous infusion.

Patients with Renal or Hepatic Dysfunction

A. Renal dysfunction (creatinine clearance <30 mL/min)

  1. Cisatracurium is the drug of choice.

  2. Pancuronium is nearly 100% renally excreted and thus should be avoided in patients with renal failure.

B. Hepatic dysfunction

  1. Pancuronium and cisatracurium are the drugs of choice.

  2. Vecuronium is hepatically metabolized to an active metabolite (3-desacetyl-vecuronium) and should not be used in patients with hepatic failure.

Adverse Effects

A. All NBDs

  1. Extensions of the pharmacologic action: dose-related prolonged apnea and residual muscle weakness

  2. Complications of therapeutic paralysis

  3. Prolonged muscle weakness

4. Cutaneous pressure ulcers

5. Corneal ulcers

6. Nerve compression syndromes

7. Hypoventilation or apnea

8. Allergic or idiosyncratic hypersensitivity reactions

9. Malignant hyperthermia

10. Unrecognized anxiety (conscious patients receiving inadequate sedation)

B. Adverse effects that may be associated with only one or some of the available NBDs

1. Histamine release

a. This dose-related effect is associated more commonly with benzylisoquinoline class agents, particularly atracurium, than with the aminosteroids.

b. Manifestations: flushing, erythema, urticaria, bronchospasm, hypotension

2. Cardiovascular effects

a. Transient changes in blood pressure and heart rate can occur with all agents.

b. Pronounced vagolytic effect (tachycardia, hypertension) can be seen with pancuronium.

3. Seizures

a. Atracurium and cisatracurium are metabolized to laudanosine by Hoffman elimination (rate independent of renal or hepatic function).

b. Laudanosine has been shown to have cerebral excitatory effects, including seizures, in animal models.

c. Seizures have been reported anecdotally in patients receiving atracurium; however, virtually all of these patients had other concomitant risk factors for seizure development (e.g., cranial trauma).

C. Reversal of nondepolarizing NBDs

1. Not routinely performed when using NBDs in the ICU setting

2. In situations where reversal is desired, a cholinesterase inhibitor (e.g., neostigmine, pyridostigmine, or edrophonium) is used.

3. An antimuscarinic drug (e.g., atropine or glycopyrrolate) is sometimes given in conjunction with the cholinesterase inhibitor to block any adverse muscarinic effects.

Monitoring

A. Patients should undergo a baseline neurologic evaluation consisting of an assessment of reflexes, muscle atrophy, mental status, motor strength, and sensory perception before initiation of therapy with a neuromuscular blocking agent.

B. Patients receiving continuous therapy should have heart rate, blood pressure, and respiratory rate monitored continuously.

C. Patients receiving continuous therapy should be regularly assessed via peripheral nerve stimulation with train-of-four (TOF) monitoring.

1. The TOF stimulation should be performed 15 minutes after each dose adjustment and every 4 hours for patients receiving continuous IV NBD infusions.

2. The goal of monitoring is to maintain 75% to 90% neuromuscular blockade (1-of-4 to 3-of-4 twitches), although the minimum amount of NBD to achieve the desired clinical end point should always be used.

3. Procedure

a. Apply two small electrocardiograph-type adhesive electrode pads, approximately 1/2 inch apart, to the ulnar surface of the wrist, 2 inches proximal to the wrist crease.

b. Apply positive and negative electrode leads to the pads (polarity not important).

c. Using 20 mA current setting, deliver TOF electrical stimuli at 0.5-second increments and note (visually and by tactile assessment) the number of twitch responses.

d. If no twitches are detected, repeat the TOF assessment at 60-second intervals using esca-

Key Monitoring

- Dose and duration of neuromuscular therapy should not exceed that needed to achieve the desired clinical outcome.

- Interrupt neuromuscular blocker therapy on a daily basis to assess the need for continued administration.

- If train-of-four testing reveals no twitches, hold neuromuscular blocker therapy until a twitch response is observed.

- Unrecognized wakefulness is known to occur in paralyzed patients; patients receiving NBDs should always receive concomitant sedation.

- To minimize the risks associated with these drugs, always employ all ventilator alarms, periodic patient repositioning, deep-vein thrombosis prophylaxis, ocular lubrication, and foot splinting.

lating currents of 40, 60, and then 80 mA until a response is obtained.

4. If no twitch is detected with the TOF test at 80 mA, check to ensure batteries are charged and there is adequate contact between electrodes and patient.

5. Alternative monitoring sites (e.g., facial nerve) can be used in patients with excessive peripheral edema.

6. If no twitches are observed with properly performed TOF testing, discontinue NBD until a response returns.

D. NBD therapy should be interrupted on a daily basis to reevaluate neurologic status, need for further therapeutic paralysis, and adequacy of sedation and pain management.

E. After discontinuation of NBD, the patient should be monitored for return of spontaneous respiration and movement.

 Bibliography

Hunter JM. New neuromuscular blocking drugs. N Engl J Med 1995;332:1691–1699.

Rudis MI, Sikora CA, Angus E, et al. A prospective, randomized, controlled evaluation of peripheral nerve stimulation versus standard clinical dosing of neuromuscular blocking drugs in critically ill patients. Crit Care Med 1997;25:575–583.

Segredo V, Caldwell JE, Matthay MA, et al. Persistent paralysis in critically ill patients after long-term administration of vecuronium. N Engl J Med 1992;327:524–528.

Shapiro BA, Warren J, Egol AB, et al. Practice parameters for sustained neuromuscular blockade in the adult critically ill patient: an executive summary. Crit Care Med 1995;23:1601–1605.

169 Narcotic Agonists and Naloxone

John W. Devlin

Narcotic agonists such as morphine and fentanyl are commonly used in the intensive care unit (ICU) to control pain and to facilitate mechanical ventilation. Morphine is generally the narcotic of choice because of its potency, side-effect profile, and low cost. Synthetic opiates (opioids) such as fentanyl may be used in patients requiring rapid-onset analgesia of short duration (e.g., during dressing changes), having a history of morphine allergy, having renal failure, or in whom the potential for histamine release associated with morphine use may be deleterious (e.g., asthmatics). Meperidine use should generally be avoided in the ICU setting because of its relatively short duration of action, its higher incidence of adverse effects compared to morphine (e.g., nausea, confusion), and the risk for accumulation of its active metabolite, normeperidine, in patients with renal insufficiency. The ultra-short-acting opioid, remifentanil, is frequently used for sedation and to lower intracranial pressure in neurosurgery patients. Naloxone, a competitive narcotic antagonist, may be used to rapidly reverse the effects of opioids. Its use in the ICU is limited, however, as many patients have a protected airway and are receiving mechanical ventilation, and the acute withdrawal reaction that may result from naloxone administration can be deleterious. Any of these agents may induce unwanted effects and thus therapy should be carefully monitored, particularly in critically ill patients.

Actions

A. Narcotic agonists
   1. Mechanism: by interaction with specific receptors at several sites within the central nervous system
   2. Potentially therapeutic effects
      a. Sedation, narcosis
      b. Analgesia
      c. Cough suppression
      d. Relief of dyspnea
B. Narcotic antagonists
   1. Antagonize effects of opioids by competing for the same receptor sites
   2. Classification
      a. Partial agonists (e.g., burprenorphine)
      b. Agonist/antagonists (e.g., pentazocine, nalbuphine)
      c. Pure antagonist: naloxone (has no narcotic agonist effects)

Indications

A. Narcotic agonists
   1. Temporary analgesia in the symptomatic treatment of moderate to severe pain
   2. Acute cardiogenic pulmonary edema
   3. Sedation in mechanically ventilated patients
B. Naloxone
   1. Complete or partial reversal of opiate effects (e.g., respiratory depression)
   2. For the diagnosis of a suspected opioid overdose
   3. Investigational treatment of refractory septic shock
   4. Treatment of pruritus in biliary cholestasis

Contraindications

A. Narcotic agonists
   1. Previous hypersensitivity reaction to the drug
   2. Respiratory depression (not applicable to patients with a protected airway receiving mechanical ventilation)
   3. Paralytic ileus
B. Naloxone: previous hypersensitivity reactions to naloxone

Precautions

A. Narcotic agonists
   1. May cause significant respiratory or circulatory depression (rapid IV administration may increase the severity of this reaction)
   2. Employ close monitoring of vital signs and oxygenation when used parenterally.
   3. Patients with hypovolemia are more sensitive to the hypotensive effects of opiate agonists.
   4. May interfere with the neurologic assessment, particularly assessment of level of consciousness and pupillary changes
   5. Patients with cranial trauma or increased intracranial pressure

6. May cause urinary retention and oliguria, particularly in patients with an inadequate circulating volume

7. Decreases gastrointestinal (GI) motility, which may decrease drug absorption and cause constipation

8. Can increase biliary tract pressure resulting in biliary spasm or colic

9. Some agents may have a prolonged duration and accumulate in patients with hepatic or renal failure.

B. Naloxone

1. Administer cautiously to persons who are known or suspected to be physically dependent on opioids, because naloxone can precipitate acute withdrawal.

2. Patients who have a satisfactory clinical response to naloxone may require repeat dosing because the duration of action of some opioids is longer than that of naloxone.

3. Use with caution in patients with preexisting cardiac disease or anyone who have received potentially cardiotoxic drugs.

Side Effects

A. Narcotic agonists

1. Central nervous system: dizziness, sedation, euphoria, mood changes, coma, tremor, convulsion, increased intracranial pressure, withdrawal reactions

2. Respiratory: respiratory depression, decreased sensitivity and responsiveness to increases in $PaCO_2$, apnea, suppression of cough reflex, chest wall rigidity (fentanyl and some other high-potency opioids), bronchoconstriction, laryngeal edema

3. Cardiovascular: flushing, hypotension, syncope, tachycardia, tachydysrhythmias, heart block, cardiac arrest

4. Gastrointestinal: nausea, vomiting, abdominal pain or cramps, constipation, biliary tract spasm, ileus, decreased drug absorption

5. Renal: urinary retention, oliguria, antidiuretic effect

6. Muscular: muscle rigidity, including thoracic muscle rigidity leading to decreased pulmonary compliance or apnea (fentanyl and some other high-potency opioids)

7. Miscellaneous: miosis, pruritus, urticaria, anaphylaxis

B. Naloxone

1. Patients with acute or chronic opiate use: abrupt reversal of narcotic depression can cause nausea, vomiting, sweating, tachycardia, hypertension, tremulousness, anxiety

2. Postoperative patients: excessive dosage may result in excitement and significant reversal of analgesia, hypotension or hypertension, pulmonary edema, cardiac dysrhythmias including sinus tachycardia, ventricular tachycardia, and ventricular fibrillation

3. Seizures

PEARLS

• Morphine is generally the opiate of choice in the ICU because of its potency, duration of action, side-effect profile, and cost.

• Fentanyl is a useful opioid for use in patients who have a history of morphine or codeine allergy, those with renal insufficiency, those requiring rapid onset and short duration analgesia (e.g., dressing change), and those in whom the potential for morphine-induced histamine release may be deleterious.

• Hydromorphone (Dilaudid), because of its high potency, is a useful alternative in patients requiring high doses of morphine.

• Meperidine (Demerol), should not be used as a first-line analgesic in the ICU because of its low potency, short duration of action, greater frequency of side effects, and the risk for accumulation of its active metabolite in patients with renal insufficiency.

Typical Dosing

A. Narcotic agonists (Table 169–1)

B. Naloxone

1. Intermittent IV dosing

a. Postoperative opiate depression: 0.1 to 0.2 mg IV push every 1 to 2 hours, as needed

b. Known or suspected opiate overdosage

(1) 0.4 to 2.0 mg IV push every 2 to 3 minutes until a response is observed

(2) No response after 10 mg suggests the depressive condition is due to a drug or disease process not responsive to naloxone.

2. Continuous IV infusion

a. Known or suspected opiate overdose

b. In situations where repeated IV bolus doses of naloxone have been required, or when it is anticipated that the duration of effect of the opioid being reversed is longer than that

TABLE 169-1. EQUIANALGESIC POTENCY AND DOSING OF OPIATE AND OPIOID ANALGESICS*

DRUG	APPROXIMATE EQUIANALGESIC ORAL DOSE	APPROXIMATE EQUIANALGESIC PARENTERAL DOSE	RECOMMENDEDS ORAL STARTING DOSE (TYPICAL DOSING RANGE)	RECOMMENDED PARENTERAL STARTING DOSE (TYPICAL DOSING RANGE)
Morphine, immediate release	30 mg q 3–4 hr	10 mg q 3–4 hr	10 mg q 3–4 hr (10–40 mg)	5 mg q 3–4 hr (2–15 mg)
Morphine, controlled release	100 mg q 12–hr	—	30 mg q 12 hr (15–200 mg)	—
Codeine†	130 mg q 3–4 hr	75 mg q 3–4 hr	30 mg q 4–6 hr (15–60 mg)	30 mg q 3 hr (IM/SQ) (max. 360 mg/day)
Methadone (Dolophine)‡	20 mg q 6–8 hr	10 mg q 6–8 hr	10 mg q 6–8 hr (5–20 mg)	5 mg q 6–8 hr (2.5–10 mg)
Fentanyl‡ (Sublimaze)	—	100 μg q 30 min–2 hr	—	50 μg q 1 hr (0.5–2 μg/kg/hr)
Sufentanil (Sufenta)	—	10–25 μg q 1 hr	—	15 μg q 30–60 min (10–30 μg)
Remifentanil (Ultiva)	—	0.05 μg/kg per min	—	0.1 μg/kg per min (0.05–0.2 μg/kg per min)
Alfentanil (Alfenta)	—	250–500 μg	—	(8–50 μg/kg loading then 3–15 μg/kg q 5–20 min or 0.5–5 μg/kg per min)
Hydromorphone (Dilaudid)	7.5 mg q 3–4 hr	1.5 mg q 3–4 hr	4 mg q 3–4 hr (3–10 mg)	1 mg q 2–4 hr (1–3 mg)
Meperidine§ (Demerol)	300 mg q 2–3 hr	100 mg q 3 hr	Not recommended	75 mg q 3 hr (50–100 mg)
Oxycodone (Percocet, others)	20 mg q 3–4 hr	—	10 mg q 3–4 hr (5–30 mg)	—
Pentazocine (Talwin)	150 mg q 3–4 hr	60 mg q 3–4 hr	50 mg q 4–6 hr (50–100 mg)	Not recommended
Levorphanol (Levo-Dromoran)	4 mg q 6–8 hr	2 mg q 6–8 hr	4 mg q 6–8 hr (4–8 mg)	2 mg q 6–8 hr (2–4 mg)
Buprenorphine (Buprenex)	—	0.2–0.5 mg q 6–8 hr	—	0.4 mg q 6–8 hr (0.2–0.5 mg)
Butorphanol (Stadol)	—	2 mg q 3–4 hr	—	2 mg q 3–4 hr (1–3 mg)
Nalbuphine (Nubain)	—	10 mg q 3–4 hr	—	10 mg q 3 to 4 hr (5–20 mg)
Hydrocodone (Vicodin, others)	30 mg q 3–4 hr	—	10 mg q 3–4 hr (5–20 mg)	—

*Adapted from Acute Pain Management Guideline Panel. Acute Pain Management in Adults: Operative Procedures. Quick Reference Guide for Clinicians. AHCPR Pub. No. 92-0019. Rockville, MD: Agency for Health Care Policy and Research, Public Health Service, U.S. Department of Health and Human Services, 1992. Recommended doses may not apply to patients with hepatic or renal insufficiency; some proprietary formulations contain other drugs in combination. IM = intramuscular injection; SQ = subcutaneous injection.
†Codeine doses greater than 65 mg are associated with diminishing efficacy and increased side effects.
‡Equivalent transdermal dose is 50 μg every 72 hours.
§Limit use of meperidine to brief courses (i.e., <72 hr) and 600 mg/day; avoid in renal insufficiency and seizure disorders.

of naloxone, continuous IV infusions of naloxone may be considered.

c. Starting dose is 0.0025 mg/kg per hour or 0.4 mg/hour.

Key Dosing Factors

- An objective pain scale (e.g., a visual analog scale) should be used to regularly assess adequacy of analgesia.

- Erroneous substitution of high-potency morphine for regular strength injectable morphine can result in overdosage (e.g., respiratory depression, seizures).

- Morphine is highly water soluble and thus can be concentrated in up to an 8:1 ratio for patients requiring fluid restriction.

- Oral morphine solution may be administered via gastric or enteric feeding tube; sustained-release morphine preparations should not be crushed.

- Most IV drugs are compatible (at least via Y-site) with IV morphine infusions.

Monitoring

A. Vital signs

B. Adequacy of ventilation and oxygenation

C. Level of sensorium

D. Airway control

E. Gastrointestinal signs and symptoms (e.g., nausea, vomiting, constipation)

 Bibliography

Ayres J, Rees J, Lee T, et al. Intravenous naloxone in acute respiratory failure. BMJ 1982;284:927–928.

Chamberlain KL, Klein BL. A comprehensive review of naloxone for the emergency physician. Am J Emerg Med 1994;12:650–660.

Cherny NI. Opioid analgesics: comparative features and prescribing guidelines. Drugs 1996;51:713–737.

Davies G, Kingswood C, Street M. Pharmacokinetics of opioids in renal dysfunction. Clin Pharmacokinet 1996;6: 410–422.

Duthie DJ, Nimmo WS. Adverse effects of opioid analgesic drugs. Br J Anaesth 1987;59:61–77.

Main A. Remifentanil as an analgesic in the critically ill. Anaesthesia 1998;53:823–824.

Ostermann ME, Keenan SP, Seiferling RA, et al. Sedation in the intensive care unit: a systematic review. JAMA 2000;283:1451–1459.

170 Benzodiazepines and Flumazenil

Michael J. Ruffing
James A. Kruse

Benzodiazepines (BZDs) are the most commonly used agents for anxiolysis and sedation in the critical care setting. As a class these agents possess anxiolytic, amnestic, sedative, anticonvulsant, and skeletal muscle relaxant properties. Although chlordiazepoxide and diazepam were the first agents to be approved and used in the intensive care unit (ICU), at this time, lorazepam and midazolam are by far the most frequently used benzodiazepines in the ICU. Lorazepam and midazolam more closely maintain the properties of an ideal sedative than other agents in this class. They are relatively short-acting, can be given by IV infusion, have a low adverse effect profile, and may be more cost effective.

Flumazenil is the only FDA approved benzodiazepine antagonist at this time. Appropriate dosing with flumazenil promptly reverses the anxiolytic, sedative, amnestic, and anticonvulsant effects of benzodiazepines. It has a variable response in reversing benzodiazepine-induced respiratory depression.

Pharmacology

A. Mechanism of action of BZD agonists
   1. Benzodiazepines bind to a specific receptor on the γ-aminobutyric acid (GABA) receptor complex in the central nervous system (CNS).
   2. An allosteric interaction with GABA receptors opens chloride channels, allowing influx of chloride ions, which causes hyperpolarization of the cell membrane making it less excitable.
   3. Benzodiazepines also influence the action of glycine, which acts as a CNS inhibitory neurotransmitter in the spinal cord to produce muscle relaxation.
   4. Benzodiazepine receptor occupancy determines CNS effect.
      a. Lower BZD concentrations and occupancy result in anxiolysis.
      b. Increasing concentrations and occupancy result in sedation, anticonvulsant activity, and hypnosis.
   5. The major differences among BZDs in clinical practice is based on potency, pharmacokinetics, and patient-specific factors.
B. Mechanism of action of flumazenil
   1. Acts as a competitive antagonist at the BZD receptor
   2. Effectively reverses the CNS effects, and to a variable degree, the respiratory effects of BZDs

C. Pharmacokinetics of BZDs and flumazenil
   1. Absorption
      a. Healthy subjects: BZDs are readily absorbed orally
      b. Intensive care unit patients: gut absorption may be impaired because of decreased gastric emptying, diminished intestinal blood flow, gut edema, and concomitant enteral feedings or medications
      c. Intramuscular absorption of chlordiazepoxide and diazepam is slow and erratic.
      d. Intramuscular absorption of midazolam and lorazepam is relatively rapid and complete.
   2. Distribution
      a. Widely distribute throughout body tissues and readily cross the blood–brain barrier
      b. High volume of distribution (Vd) of BZDs is increased in the ICU population as a result of a relative increase in extracellular volume and a decrease in protein binding.
      c. Benzodiazepines and their metabolites cross the placenta and are distributed into milk.
   3. Metabolism
      a. Their high protein binding ($>70\%$) and effects on certain metabolic pathways make BZDs susceptible to drug interactions.
      b. Chlordiazepoxide, diazepam, and midazolam undergo oxidative metabolism in the liver to active metabolites.
      c. Lorazepam is conjugated by glucuronidases to inactive metabolites excreted by the kidneys.
   4. Half-life
      a. Chlordiazepoxide: 5 to 30 hours
      b. Desmethylchlordiazepoxide (metabolite of chlordiazepoxide): approximately 18 hours
      c. Demoxepam (metabolite of desmethylchlordiazepoxide): 14 to 95 hours
      d. Desmethyldiazepam (metabolite of diazepam and demoxepam): 30 to 200 hours
      e. Oxazepam (metabolite of desmethyldiazepam): 3 to 21 hours
      f. Diazepam: 20 to 50 hours (20 to 120 hours in ICU patients)
      g. Lorazepam: 10 to 20 hours
      h. Midazolam: 3 to 4 hours (7 to 11 hours or more in ICU patients)
      i. Flumazenil: 40 to 80 minutes

5. The terminal half-life of the BZDs and their metabolites is highly variable, particularly in ICU patients; dependent on age, hepatic function, renal function, disease pathology, and interacting drug therapy.

Indications

A. Clordiazepoxide
   1. FDA-approved indications
      a. Anxiety, including preoperative anxiety
      b. Alcohol withdrawal
   2. Also has been used effectively in opiate withdrawal

B. Diazepam (FDA-approved indications)
   1. Anxiety, including as premedication for procedures and surgery
   2. Alcohol withdrawal
   3. Reflex skeletal muscle spasm secondary to local pathology and spasticity due to upper motor neuron diseases
   4. Initial management of status epilepticus and as adjunct therapy in other convulsive disorders

C. Lorazepam
   1. FDA-approved indications
      a. Anxiety, including as preanesthetic medication
      b. Status epilepticus
   2. Other common uses
      a. Alcohol withdrawal
      b. Mania and psychotic agitation
      c. Benzodiazepine of choice for long-term sedation in the ICU

D. Midazolam
   1. FDA-approved indications
      a. Sedation in critically ill patients
      b. Preoperative anxiety
      c. Postoperative sedation
      d. Anesthesia induction
   2. Other common uses
      a. Delirium tremens
      b. Psychosis
      c. Status epilepticus and other convulsive disorders
      d. Benzodiazepine of choice for short-term (<24 hours) sedation in ICU patients

E. Flumazenil
   1. Complete or partial reversal of the sedative effects of BZDs used for diagnostic or therapeutic purposes
   2. Diagnostic assessment of depressed sensorium to attribute or exclude BZD administration as etiologic
   3. Management of BZD overdose

Key Indications

- Chlordiazepoxide: alcohol withdrawal
- Diazepam: status epilepticus
- Midazolam: premedication for procedures and short-term (<24 hours) ICU sedation
- Lorazepam: alcohol withdrawal, status epilepticus, and long-term (>24 hours) ICU sedation
- Flumazenil: reversal of sedative effects of BZDs

Contraindications

A. Benzodiazepine agonists
   1. Known hypersensitivity to the drug
   2. Acute angle-closure glaucoma
   3. Avoid in patients with acute alcohol intoxication with depressed vital signs.

B. Flumazenil
   1. Known hypersensitivity to BZDs or flumazenil
   2. Avoid in patients where BZDs are used to treat a life-threatening condition.
      a. Status epilepticus
      b. Elevated intracranial pressure
      c. Serious cyclic antidepressant overdose (may precipitate seizures)

Side Effects and Precautions (BZD agonists)

A. Cardiopulmonary effects
   1. Hypotension
   2. Bradycardia or tachycardia
   3. Respiratory depression (decreased tidal volume; variable effect on respiratory rate)

B. Although generally mild, these effects can be significant when the agents are given by rapid IV injection, particularly in the elderly, those with hypovolemia, and those given concomitant opiates.

C. Tolerance with subsequent withdrawal reactions
   1. May occur if taking BZDs (particularly the short-acting ones) in high doses or for prolonged periods
   2. Manifestations: agitation, dysphoria, insomnia, sweating, tremors, psychosis, and seizures
   3. Patients receiving continuous infusions in the ICU for at least 2 weeks may require a tapering regimen of 7 to 10 days.

D. Uncommon side effects: rash, nausea, constipation, diarrhea, urinary retention, psychosis, hepatic dysfunction, and blood dyscrasias (leukopenia, agranulocytosis, thrombocytopenia, eosinophilia, and anemia), burning and redness following IM injection

Typical Dosing

A. Chlordiazepoxide
  1. Anxiety
     a. Oral: 5 to 25 mg every 6 to 8 hours
     b. Parenteral: 50 to 100 mg initially, IM or IV; then 25 to 50 mg IM every 6 to 8 hours
  2. Acute alcohol withdrawal: 50 to 100 mg (oral, IM or IV); repeat, if necessary, up to 300 mg/day
  3. Intensive care unit sedation: 25 to 50 mg intramuscularly or intravenously every 2 to 4 hours as needed
  4. Special precautions for parenteral use
     a. Use special diluent for IM administration.
     b. Use 5 ml sterile water for injection or normal saline for IV use; give IV over 1 minute.

B. Diazepam
  1. Anxiety
     a. Oral: 2 to 10 mg every 6 to 12 hours; or 15 to 30 mg sustained-release daily
     b. Parenteral: 2 to 10 mg intravenously or intramuscularly every 3 to 4 hours, as needed
  2. Acute alcohol withdrawal
     a. Oral: 10 mg 3 to 4 times daily initially; reduce to 5 mg 3 to 4 times daily as appropriate
     b. Parenteral: 10 mg intravenously or intramuscularly; then 5 to 10 mg every 3 to 4 hours, if necessary
  3. Adjunct in muscle spasm
     a. Oral: 2 to 10 mg every 6 to 8 hours
     b. Parenteral: 5 to 10 mg intravenously or intramuscularly; repeat in 3 to 4 hours, if necessary; tetanus may require higher doses (e.g., 20 mg)
  4. Endoscopic procedures
     a. Intravenous: approximately 10 mg administered slowly just prior to procedure to sedative response
     b. Intramuscular: 5 to 10 mg 30 minutes prior to procedure
  5. Seizures: 5 to 10 mg IV initially; then 5 to 10 mg every 15 to 30 minutes up to 30 mg
  6. ICU sedation
     a. Preferred parenteral route: IV
     b. 1 to 15 mg intravenously every 2 to 4 hours; titrate to sedative effect
     c. Continuous IV infusion is not recommended because of potential incompatibilities with solutions, IV bag, and IV tubing.

C. Lorazepam
  1. Anxiety
     a. Oral: 2 to 6 mg/day, in 2 or 3 divided doses
     b. Parenteral: same
  2. Preoperative sedation
     a. IM: 0.05 mg/kg IM 2 hours before procedure
     b. IV: 0.044 mg/kg IV 15 to 30 minutes before procedure
  3. ICU sedation
     a. IM/IV: 1 to 4 mg every 2 to 4 hours as needed for appropriate sedation
     b. IV infusion
        (1) 1 to 10 mg/hour adjusted every 4 hours to sedation
        (2) Best stability is attained in glass bottles at concentrations of 8 mg/dL in 5% dextrose in water or in normal saline.
        (3) Also may be diluted in equal volumes of sterile water for injection, normal saline, or 5% dextrose in water, to deliver a 1 mg/mL solution

D. Midazolam
  1. Preoperative sedation, anxiolysis, or amnesia: 0.07 to 0.08 mg/kg intramuscularly, 1 hour before surgery
  2. Sedation, anxiolysis, amnesia
     a. 1 to 2.5 mg intravenously over 2 minutes
     b. Wait at least 2 minutes and administer additional small increments.
     c. Use 30% less if given with concomitant narcotic or other CNS depressant.
  3. Induction of anesthesia
     a. 0.30 to 0.35 mg/kg over 20 to 30 seconds, if not premedicated
     b. Premedicated: 0.15 to 0.35 mg/kg (usually 0.25 mg/kg) intravenously over 20 to 30 seconds
     c. Maintenance infusion is 0.02 to 0.1 mg/kg per hour.
  4. ICU sedation
     a. 0.07 mg/kg intramuscularly every 2 to 4 hours, titrated to effect
     b. 0.02 to 0.1 mg/kg intravenously every 2 to 4 hours, titrated to effect
     c. 0.02 to 0.25 mg/kg per hour, titrated to effect
  5. Patients that are elderly, receiving concomitant CNS depressants, or are hemodynamically compromised should be initiated at doses 25% to 50% lower than normal.

E. Flumazenil
  1. Reversal of sedation
     a. 0.2 mg intravenously over 15 seconds
     b. Repeat every 60 seconds, up to 1 mg.
     c. May need additional doses after a few hours depending on the BZD used
  2. BZD overdose
     a. 0.2 mg intravenously over 30 seconds
     b. If no response, repeat in 30 seconds with 0.3 mg.

TABLE 170-1. PARTIAL LIST OF POTENTIAL DRUG INTERACTIONS WITH BENZODIAZEPINES (BZDs)

DRUG	BZD	EFFECT	COMMENT
Ethanol	All	Enhances sedative effects	Additive effects; may inhibit BZD metabolism; ethanol-induced hepatic dysfunction may impair BZD metabolism
Barbiturates	All	Enhance sedative effects	—
Carbamazepine	Diazepam, lorazepam	Decreases BZD effect	Induces metabolism in gut and liver
Cimetidine	Chlordiazepoxide, diazepam, lorazepam	Enhances BZD effect	Inhibits metabolism of BZDs
Macrolides (clarithromycin, erythromycin, troleandomycin)	Diazepam, midazolam	Enhance BZD effect	Inhibit metabolism of BZDs (azithromycin and erythromycin less likely to interact)
Calcium channel blockers (diltiazem, verapamil)	Midazolam	Enhance BZD effect	Inhibit metabolism of BZDs
Opioids	All	Enhance BZD and opioid effects	Possibly decrease cardiovascular and respiratory effects
Azole antibiotics (ketoconazole, itraconazole, fluconazole)	Chlordiazepoxide, diazepam, midazolam	Enhance BZD effect	Inhibit metabolism of BZDs; less likely with fluconazole than with other azoles antibiotics
Fluvoxamine	Diazepam, midazolam	Enhances BZD effect	Inhibits metabolism of BZD
Phenytoin, fosphenytoin	Midazolam, diazepam, chlordiazepoxide	Decrease BZD effect; may increase or decrease phenytoin levels	Induce metabolism of BZD
Indinavir, saquinavir, nelfinavir, amprenavir, ritonavir, delaviridine, efavirenz	Midazolam (possibly diazepam)	Increase effect of midazolam	Inhibit metabolism of midazolam
Omeprazole	Midazolam	Enhances effect of midazolam	Inhibits metabolism of midazolam
Probenecid	Midazolam	Enhances effect of midazolam	Inhibits metabolism of midazolam
Theophylline	All	Antagonizes effects of BZDs	Blocks adenosine receptors, causing CNS stimulation; may increase metabolism of BZDs

c. May give additional doses of 0.5 mg at 1-minute intervals, up to 3 mg total

Key Dosing Considerations

- Benzodiazepine dosing is highly variable within and between patients.
- Dosing for sedation or agitation should be based on a standardized sedation or anxiety scale.
- Patients should be allowed to awaken daily; this has been shown to shorten ventilator days and length of ICU days.
- Many drugs interfere with the hepatic cytochrome P450 system, thereby potentially altering the metabolism and effects of BZDs metabolized by this system (see Table 170-1).

Bibliography

Barr J, Donner A. Optimal intravenous dosing strategies for sedatives and analgesics in the intensive care unit. Crit Care Clin 1995;11:827–847.

McCollam JS, O'Neil MG, Norcross ED, et al. Continuous infusions of lorazepam, midazolam, and propofol for sedation of the critically ill surgery trauma patient: a prospective, randomized comparison. Crit Care Med 1999; 27:2454–2458.

Shapiro BA, Warren J, Egol AB, et al. Practice parameters for intravenous analgesia and sedation for adult patients in the intensive care unit: an executive summary. Crit Care Med 1995;23:1596–1600.

Wagner BK, O'Hara DA. Pharmacokinetics and pharmacodynamics of sedatives and analgesics in the treatment of agitated critically ill patients. Clin Pharmacokinet 1997; 33:426–453.

Young C, Knudsen N, Hilton A, et al. Sedation in the intensive care unit. Crit Care Med 2000;28:854–866.

171 Propofol

Michael J. Ruffing

Adequate sedation is necessary for the appropriate management of patients in the intensive care unit (ICU). Until recently ICU sedation was commonly induced with the use of benzodiazepine, antipsychotic, and narcotic analgesic drugs. Propofol, a relatively newer agent, produces dose-dependent sedation and hypnosis of rapid onset and short duration. It also has analgesic, amnestic, and anticonvulsant properties. In patients with head trauma, propofol decreases intracranial and mean arterial pressure, but generally maintains cerebral perfusion pressure. The pharmacokinetic and pharmacodynamic characteristics of propofol make it an attractive agent for short-term ICU sedation, particularly in neurosurgery patients.

Pharmacology

A. Description: propofol is an alkyl phenol derivative that is formulated as a 1% oil-in-water emulsion of propofol, soybean oil, glycerol, and egg phosphatide

B. Actions
1. Produces dose-dependent sedation and amnesia
2. Effects are synergistic with barbiturates, benzodiazepines, and opioids.
3. Has some analgesic and anticonvulsant activity
4. Decreases cerebral blood flow, intracranial pressure, and cerebral metabolic oxygen requirements
5. Can cause hypotension, secondary to decreased systemic vascular resistance, with decreased cardiac output

C. Mechanism of action
1. Binds to a γ-aminobutyric acid receptor that is different from the benzodiazepine receptor
2. Receptor interaction results in global central nervous system (CNS) depression.

D. Pharmacokinetics
1. Highly lipophilic and distributes rapidly into the CNS and other well-perfused tissues
2. Subsequently distributes into lean muscle, and then fat
3. Propofol is 96% bound to plasma proteins.

E. Metabolism and elimination
1. Eliminated primarily by hepatic conjugation to inactive metabolites that are excreted by the kidney

2. Extrahepatic elimination is also apparent as propofol clearance exceeds typical hepatic clearance.
3. The vehicle provides 1 kcal/mL in the form of fat.

Key Pharmacologic Points

- Propofol is highly lipophilic, and thus has a rapid onset of activity in the CNS.

- Propofol has a short initial half-life (2 to 4 minutes), responsible for its very short duration of action.

- Hepatic and renal dysfunction have little effect on the pharmacokinetics of propofol.

Indications

A. Induction or maintenance of anesthesia as part of balanced anesthesia

B. Initiation and maintenance of monitored anesthesia care (MAC) sedation during diagnostic procedures

C. Continuous sedation and control of stress responses in mechanically ventilated patients in the ICU

D. Status epilepticus refractory to conventional treatment

Drug Interactions

A. Central nervous system depressants such as benzodiazepines, narcotics, and inhalational anesthetics enhance the CNS effects and cardiovascular effects of propofol.

B. Lower doses of propofol may be necessary if used in combination.

Contraindications

A. Hypersensitivity to propofol or ingredients of the emulsion

B. Situations where general anesthesia or sedation are contraindicated

Side Effects

A. Pain at injection site
1. Especially if given into a small peripheral vein
2. Minimized by

a. Use of larger peripheral veins of the forearm or antecubital fossa

b. Central venous administration

c. Injection of 1 mL of 1% lidocaine intravenously prior to propofol infusion

B. Respiratory depression

1. Can cause apnea

2. Necessitates close monitoring

C. Hypotension

1. Dose dependent and infusion rate related

2. More likely in hemodynamically unstable patients

D. Central nervous system effects

1. Neuroexcitatory effects: e.g., tremor, twitching, opisthotonos

2. Hallucinations

E. Metabolic effects

1. Hypertriglyceridemia with prolonged infusions (>3 days)

2. Increased CO_2 production, secondary to metabolism of fat contained in the emulsion

F. Other

1. Pancreatitis

2. Green urine

3. Sepsis (secondary to contamination of product)

Typical Dosing

A. Indication

1. Anesthesia

a. Induction: 20 to 40 mg every 10 seconds until induction

b. Maintenance

(1) Intermittent IV injection: 25 to 50 mg, as needed.

(2) Continuous IV infusion: 100 to 200 μg/kg per minute; titrate to clinical effect

2. MAC sedation

a. Initiate with 100 to 150 μg/kg per minute over 3 to 5 minutes.

b. Maintenance

(1) Intermittent IV injection: 10 to 20 mg, as needed

(2) Continuous IV infusion: 25 to 75 μg/kg per minute

3. ICU sedation

a. Initiate with 5 μg/kg per minute.

b. Increase at 5 to 10 μg/kg per minute increments at 5- to 10-minute intervals.

c. Usual maintenance rates are 5 to 50 μg/kg per minute.

d. Discontinue daily to assess patient's condition.

4. Refractory status epilepticus

a. Initiate with 1 to 2 mg/kg.

b. Titrate to clinical effect or burst suppression on electroencephalography.

c. May require more than 50 to 100 μg/kg per minute

B. Administration

1. Do not mix with other agents prior to administration.

2. Propofol may be diluted with 5% dextrose in water to concentrations no less than 2 mg/mL.

3. Propofol can promote microbial growth.

4. Propofol is stable for 12 hours if administered from its original vial, but it should be discarded after 6 hours if transferred to a different container prior to administration.

5. Intravenous lines should be changed every 12 hours, along with a new bottle of propofol.

PEARLS

- Patients receiving propofol may develop a green tint in the urine.

- Generic propofol may show a slight yellow discoloration after being spiked (i.e., exposed to air); however, the efficacy should still be intact.

- Patients receiving total parenteral nutrition with lipids should have the lipid portion of their caloric regimen decreased in proportion to the lipid administered via propofol (1 kcal/10 mg propofol).

Bibliography

Barrientos-Vega R, Sanchez-Soria MM, Morales-Garcia C, et al. Prolonged sedation of critically ill patients with midazolam or propofol: impact on weaning and costs. Crit Care Med 1997;25:33–40.

Fulton B, Sorkin EM. Propofol: an overview of its pharmacology and a review of its clinical efficacy in intensive care sedation. Drugs 1995;50:636–657.

Lund N, Papadakos PJ. Barbiturates, neuroleptics, and propofol for sedation. Crit Care Clin 1995;11:875–886.

Marinella MA. Propofol for sedation in the intensive care unit: essentials for the clinician. Respir Med 1997;91:505–510.

172 Anticonvulsants

Michael J. Ruffing

Pharmacology

A. Phenytoin
1. Gastrointestinal (GI) absorption
   a. 70% to 100% with capsules
   b. Peak level: 8 to 12 hours with extended-release product, 1.5 to 3 hours with prompt release product
2. Volume of distribution (Vd): 0.6 L/kg
3. Protein binding: 90%
4. Metabolism
   a. Hepatic (capacity limited)
   b. Half-life is 20 to 24 hours with levels lower than 10 μg/mL.
   c. At higher concentrations (>10 μg/mL), metabolic saturation occurs and small increases in dose may lead to disproportionate increases in plasma concentrations.
   d. Therapeutic range: 10 to 20 μg/mL (total) or 1 to 2 μg/mL (free)
5. Carbamazepine (CBZ)
   a. Gastrointestinal absorption: slowly absorbed; peak level achieved in 1.5 hours with suspension, 4 to 8 hours with tablets and capsules
   b. Distribution: widely distributed
   c. Protein binding: 75% to 90%
   d. Metabolism
      (1) Hepatic metabolism via cytochrome P-450 to CBZ epoxide (active), and then to trans-CBZ-diol and excreted in urine
      (2) Half-life 25 to 65 hours, initially; then 12 to 17 hours with chronic dosing
   e. Therapeutic range: 4 to 12 μg/mL
6. Valproic acid
   a. Gastrointestinal absorption: rapid and complete absorption
   b. Peak levels achieved in 15 minutes to 2 hours (sodium valproate syrup), 1 to 4 hours (valproic acid capsules), and 3 to 5 hours (delayed-release divalproex sodium)
   c. Protein binding
      (1) 90% protein bound
      (2) Concentration-dependent: free drug increases to 15% to 20% at levels higher than 100 μg/mL
      (3) Decreased in renal insufficiency and hepatic disease

   d. Metabolism: hepatic; half-life 6 to 16 hours
   e. Therapeutic range: 50 to 100 μg/mL
7. Phenobarbital
   a. Gastrointestinal absorption: 70% to 90% (slow); peak level achieved in 8 to 12 hours
   b. Distribution: 20% to 45% protein bound
   c. Metabolism: 75% hepatic, 25% renal; half-life is 2 to 6 days
   d. Therapeutic range: 15 to 40 μg/mL
8. Pentobarbital
   a. Absorption: nearly complete by oral and rectal routes; peak levels achieved in 30 to 60 minutes
   b. Distribution: 35% to 45% protein bound
   c. Metabolism: hepatic; half-life is 15 to 50 hours
   d. Therapeutic range: 2 to 4 mg/dL for status epilepticus and induced coma
9. Lorazepam
   a. Absorption: nearly complete, orally and intramuscularly; peak level achieved in 2 to 4 hours
   b. Protein binding: 85% to 90%
   c. Metabolism: hepatic glucuronidation; half-life is 10 to 20 hours
   d. Therapeutic range: titrated to effect
10. Diazepam
    a. Absorption is nearly complete, orally; peak level achieved in 30 minutes to 2 hours (IM absorption is erratic).
    b. Protein binding: 98%
    c. Metabolism: hepatic, to active and inactive metabolites; half-life: 20 to 80 hours
    d. Therapeutic range: titrated to effect

Key Pharmacology Points

- Plasma levels of phenytoin can be substantially affected by changes in dose, extent of protein binding, and concurrent use of drugs that alter hepatic enzyme activity.

- Carbamazepine induces its own metabolism, resulting in marked changes in serum levels several weeks after initiation of therapy.

- Valproic acid levels may vary by approximately 100% between doses; they should be measured at the same time of day (and just prior to a dose).

Action and Effects

A. Phenytoin: limits seizure propagation by reducing the passive influx of sodium ions at voltage-sensitive sodium channels, leading to a reduction in postetanic potentiation; also has antidysrhythmic properties

B. Benzodiazepines: limit the spread of seizure activity by enhancing γ-aminobutyric acid (GABA) inhibition

C. Barbiturates: modulate the GABA receptor to enhance inhibitory transmission; can enhance spike-wave discharges and potentially be proconvulsant

D. Carbamazepine: mechanism is similar to phenytoin

E. Valproic acid: reduces the sodium-mediated effects at voltage-sensitive sodium channels, inhibits the metabolism of GABA, and reduces calcium currents in afferent neurons

F. Other, newer anticonvulsant drugs
1. Felbamate, gabapentin, lamotrigine, oxcarbazepine, tiagabine, topiramate, vigabatrin, zonisamide
2. Mechanisms: prevent sustained repetitive firing by activity at the voltage-dependent sodium channel, enhance GABA inhibitory effect, reduce voltage-dependent calcium currents, and reduce glutamate-mediated excitation

Indications

A. Phenytoin
1. Generalized tonic-clonic seizures
2. Partial seizures with complex symptomatology
3. Post-traumatic and perineurosurgical seizures
4. Status epilepticus

B. Fosphenytoin
1. Status epilepticus
2. Lack of IV access in phenytoin-treatable seizures

C. Carbamazepine
1. Generalized tonic-clonic seizures
2. Partial seizures with complex symptomatology
3. Post-traumatic seizures
4. Also used for chronic pain syndromes (e.g., trigeminal neuralgia)

D. Phenobarbital
1. Generalized tonic-clonic seizures
2. Partial seizures
3. Status epilepticus

E. Valproic acid

1. Generalized tonic-clonic seizures
2. Partial seizures
3. Absence seizures

F. Lorazepam, diazepam: status epilepticus

G. Pentobarbital: status epilepticus

Contraindications

A. Phenytoin and fosphenytoin
1. Sinus bradycardia, sino-atrial block, second- or third-degree atrioventricular block, or Adam-Stokes syndrome (because phenytoin can decrease ventricular automaticity)
2. Known hypersensitivity to phenytoin
3. Avoid IV administration in patients with severely compromised myocardial function.

B. Carbamazepine
1. History of bone marrow depression
2. Use of monoamine oxidase inhibitors within 14 days
3. Hypersensitivity to CBZ or tricyclic antidepressants

C. Phenobarbital and pentobarbital
1. Hypersensitivity to barbiturates
2. Porphyria

D. Valproic acid
1. Hypersensitivity to valproic acid
2. Significant hepatic dysfunction

Drug Interactions

A. Phenytoin
1. Decrease absorption of phenytoin: antacids, charcoal, sucralfate
2. Inhibit metabolism of phenytoin (and thereby increase the effects of phenytoin): allopurinol, amiodarone, cimetidine, ethanol (acute use), fluconazole, isoniazid, metronidazole, omeprazole, sulfonamides, trimethoprim, valproic acid
3. Increase metabolism of phenytoin (and thereby decrease effects of phenytoin): barbiturates, CBZ, ethanol (chronic use), rifampin, theophylline
4. Displace phenytoin from binding sites (lowering total phenytoin concentration and thereby increasing the free fraction of phenytoin): salicylates, tricyclic antidepressants, valproic acid
5. Metabolism increased by phenytoin (effects of these drugs may thereby be reduced): acetamin-

ophen, amiodarone, CBZ, corticosteroids, digoxin, disopyramide, doxycycline, haloperidol, meperidine (increased formation of normeperidine, a toxic metabolite), methadone, mexiletine, quinidine, theophylline, valproic acid

6. Displaced from binding sites by phenytoin: warfarin (may thereby increase its anticoagulant effects)

7. Neuromuscular blocking agent interactions: resistance possible with chronic phenytoin treatment (related to duration of phenytoin use); not observed with atracurium

B. Carbamazepine

1. Decreases the absorption of CBZ: charcoal

2. Inhibit metabolism of CBZ (and thereby increases the effects of CBZ): barbiturates, cimetidine, diltiazem, isoniazid, lamotrigine, macrolides, propoxyphene, valproic acid

3. Increase the metabolism of CBZ (effects of decreased CBZ levels may be minimized by an increased ratio of CBZ-epoxide/CBZ levels): felbamate, phenytoin

4. Increases degradation of isoniazid to hepatotoxic metabolite

5. Metabolism increased by CBZ (and effects of these drugs may thereby be reduced): acetaminophen, cyclosporin A, doxycycline, felbamate, haloperidol, lamotrigine, tricyclic antidepressants, warfarin

6. Decrease duration of neuromuscular blocking effect: neuromuscular blocking drugs (not observed with atracurium)

C. Valproic acid

1. Decreases absorption of valproic acid: charcoal

2. Inhibit metabolism of valproic acid: cimetidine, erythromycin, felbamate

3. Increase metabolism of valproic acid: CBZ, lamotrigine, phenobarbital, phenytoin, rifampin

4. Metabolism inhibited by valproic acid: CBZ, diazepam, lamotrigine, phenobarbital, zidovudine

5. Valproic acid displaces drug from protein binding (thereby increasing effect of these drugs): diazepam, warfarin

D. Barbiturates

1. Decreases absorption of barbiturates: charcoal

2. Increases metabolism of barbiturates: rifampin

3. Inhibits metabolism of barbiturates: valproic acid

4. Metabolism increased by barbiturates: metoprolol, propranolol, corticosteroids, doxorubicin, doxycycline, metronidazole, quinidine, theophylline, verapamil, warfarin

E. Benzodiazepines

1. Decrease the metabolism of benzodiazepines that undergo oxidative metabolism (e.g., diazepam): cimetidine, fluoxetine, isoniazid, ketoconazole, metoprolol, propoxyphene, propranolol, valproic acid

2. Increases the metabolism of benzodiazepines that undergo oxidative metabolism (e.g., diazepam): rifampin

3. May increase digoxin levels

Typical Dosing

A. Phenytoin

1. Loading dose

   a. IV: 15 to 20 mg/kg intravenously at 50 mg/minute or less

   b. Oral: 15 to 20 mg/kg given in three divided doses 2 to 4 hours apart (may be administered at one time, if necessary, with caution)

2. Maintenance dose

   a. 5 to 7 mg/kg per day

   b. Should be increased slowly; ideally, not to increase by more than 25 to 50 mg/day every 2 to 4 weeks

   c. In critically ill patients it is more practical to adjust the dose by 50 to 100 mg/day every 3 to 5 days.

   d. Phenytoin levels should be monitored closely.

   e. Oral doses of up to 300 mg/day may be given once daily in some patients if using extended phenytoin sodium capsules.

   f. All other oral dosage forms should be administered 2 to 3 times daily.

3. Precautions during IV administration

   a. Phenytoin is poorly soluble and is formulated with sodium hydroxide, propylene glycol, and alcohol.

   b. The vehicle can cause serious adverse effects, including cardiac arrest, if given overly rapidly.

   c. The loading dose infusion rate should be limited to 20 mg/minute in patients with cardiovascular disease.

   d. Do not administer through isotonic saline or dextrose-free solutions.

   e. Best practice is to flush IV tubing before and after administration of IV phenytoin.

4. Precautions for maintenance administration with enteral feedings

   a. The suspension is erratically absorbed when administered with enteral feedings.

b. Phenytoin suspension may adhere to vinyl tubing of enteral feeding tubes and should be diluted (e.g., in sterile water, normal saline, or 5% dextrose in water) prior to administration.

c. Subsequent flushing (approximately 20 mL) should be performed.

d. When feasible, hold feedings 1 to 2 hours before and after administration of phenytoin suspension.

e. In the intensive care unit setting it is often more practical to administer phenytoin by the IV route until the patient is no longer critically ill.

5. Intramuscular administration

a. Should not be used due to erratic absorption, pain, necrosis, and abscess formation

b. Fosphenytoin can be used intramuscularly, in place of phenytoin.

6. Therapeutic range

a. Total phenytoin: 10 to 20 μg/mL

b. Free phenytoin: 1 to 2 μg/mL

B. Fosphenytoin

1. Doses are expressed in phenytoin equivalents (PE).

2. When expressed as PEs, fosphenytoin dosing is the same as phenytoin dosing.

3. Intravenous administration should not exceed 100 mg (PE)/min.

4. Elderly and hemodynamically unstable patients should receive fosphenytoin at no more than 50 mg (PE)/min.

5. Intramuscular administration may be given in 1 to 4 separate injections.

6. 1 g PE = 20 mL

C. Carbamazepine

1. Initiate at 400 mg/day in 2 divided doses (or 4 divided doses if using suspension).

2. Increase by 200 mg/day per week in 3 to 4 divided doses/day until response is achieved.

3. Most adults require 800 to 1200 mg/day.

4. Extended-release tablets may be given twice a day.

5. Carbamazepine can induce its own metabolism.

6. As a result of its enzyme-inducing properties and the potential inhibition of other agents on CBZ metabolism, combined use with other anticonvulsants often requires dose adjustment for one or both agents.

D. Valproic acid

1. Initiate at 10 to 15 mg/kg per day and increase by 5 to 10 mg/kg each week until response is achieved.

2. Rapid IV loading with 15 to 30 mg/kg has been used.

3. Intravenous administration should be given over 60 minutes (or ≤20 mg/min).

4. The maximum recommended dosage is 60 mg/kg per day.

5. If more than 250 mg/day is needed, give in divided doses.

6. Most patients require dosing every 6 to 8 hours.

7. Divalproex sodium can be given every 12 hours at an equivalent daily dose.

8. Rectal administration (oral syrup with 30 mL water) has been successful, given every 6 or 8 hours.

E. Phenobarbital

1. Loading dose: 15 mg/kg intravenously at 60 mg/minute or less

2. Maintenance dose: 2 to 4 mg/kg per day in single or divided doses

3. Administration of IM phenobarbital should be deep into a large muscle; avoid areas where injection into arteries or nerves is a significant risk.

F. Pentobarbital

1. Loading dose: 5 to 10 mg/kg intravenously

2. Maintenance dose: 2 to 3 mg/kg per hour titrated to burst suppression by electroencephalogram

3. Intramuscular injection should be made deeply into a large muscle mass.

4. Do not give more than 250 mg (in 5 mL) at one site to avoid tissue irritation.

G. Lorazepam

1. Intravenous: 0.1 mg/kg at a rate of 2 mg/minute

2. Prior to administration, dilute with an equal volume of sterile water for injection, normal saline, or 5% dextrose in water.

3. Intramuscular route is not recommended for status epilepticus.

4. If necessary, inject undiluted at maximum doses of 4 mg.

H. Diazepam

1. Intravenous administration

a. 0.15 to 0.3 mg/kg at a rate of 5 mg/minute in status epilepticus

b. May repeat in 2 to 4 hours up to a maximum dose of 30 mg total

2. Oral administration: 2 to 10 mg two to four times a day.

3. Intramuscular administration

a. Not recommended because of low and erratic absorption

b. Use only if not able to give intravenously.

4. Rectal administration

a. Diazepam rectal gel has been used for intermittent seizures in patients already on stable antiepileptic regimens.

b. Dose is 0.2 mg/kg rounded to the nearest 5 mg.

Side Effects and Precautions

A. Phenytoin or fosphenytoin

1. Cardiovascular: hypotension and heart block following rapid IV administration

2. Central nervous system: nystagmus (at ~20 to 30 μg/mL), ataxia (~30 to 40 μg/mL), sensorial and mental status changes (>40 μg/mL), respiratory depression (high concentrations)

3. Dermatologic

a. Morbilliform or scarlatiniform rash; bullous, exfoliative, or purpuric dermatitis; lupus erythematosus; Stevens-Johnson syndrome; or toxic epidermal necrolysis

b. Some rashes may occur with fever, lymphadenopathy, arthralgias, and hepatic dysfunction. Stop phenytoin immediately.

c. May restart if morbilliform or scarlatiniform in nature and has completely resolved

4. Hematologic: thrombocytopenia, leukopenia, pancytopenia, megaloblastic anemia

B. Carbamazepine

1. Cardiovascular: congestive heart failure, hypotension, thromboembolism, aggravation of coronary artery disease, dysrhythmias, conduction disturbances

2. Central nervous system: dizziness, drowsiness, sedation, confusion, nystagmus, blurred vision, oculomotor disturbances, abnormal involuntary movements, peripheral neuritis and paresthesias, tinnitus, muscle relaxation, anticholinergic and antidepressant effects

3. Dermatologic: pruritic and erythematous rashes; urticaria; photosensitivity reactions; erythema multiforme; lupus erythematosus; hypersensitivity reactions with fever, rash, eosinophilia; and reversible aseptic meningitis

4. Gastrointestinal: nausea, vomiting, diarrhea, dry mouth

5. Genitourinary: acute urinary retention

6. Hematologic

a. Rarely, aplastic anemia and agranulocytosis can occur.

b. Transient decreases in platelets or white blood cell counts are not uncommon, but rarely progress to aplastic anemia or agranulocytosis.

c. Monitor hematologic profile at baseline and during therapy.

d. Watch for early signs and symptoms such as fever, sore throat, bruising.

7. Metabolic: hyponatremia from syndrome of inappropriate antidiuresis or water intoxication

C. Valproic acid

1. Central nervous system: sedation, tremor, hallucinations, headache, nystagmus, visual disturbances, vertigo, incoordination, confusion

2. Dermatologic: skin rash, dry skin, seborrhea, Stevens-Johnson syndrome, erythema multiforme, toxic epidermal necrolysis (rare)

3. Gastrointestinal:

a. Nausea, vomiting, diarrhea, anorexia

b. Fewer GI effects with divalproex

4. Hematologic

a. Inhibits secondary phase of platelet aggregation, potentially prolonging bleeding time

b. Thrombocytopenia: more likely with higher levels

c. Bone marrow suppression

5. Hepatic

a. Idiopathic hepatotoxicity can occur (uncommon in adults).

b. Monitor activity of serum aminotransferases and lactate dehydrogenase, and serum bilirubinemia and ammonia concentrations.

D. Phenobarbital and pentobarbital

1. Cardiovascular: hypotension, bradycardia

2. Respiratory: respiratory depression, apnea

3. Central nervous system: sedation, hypnosis, agitation, confusion, nightmares

4. Gastrointestinal: nausea, vomiting, constipation

5. Hypersensitivity reactions

a. Rashes: angioedema, exfoliative dermatitis

b. More likely in those with asthma, urticaria, and angioedema

E. Lorazepam and diazepam

1. Cardiovascular: bradycardia, tachycardia, hypotension

2. Respiratory: respiratory depression, apnea

3. Central nervous system: anxiolysis, amnesia, sedation, hypnosis, confusion, agitation, skeletal muscle relaxation

4. Dermatologic: rash

Key Precautions

- Intravenous injection of phenytoin at more than 50 mg/min can cause hypotension and heart block.

- Carbamazepine can cause bone marrow suppression.

- High IV doses of phenobarbital and pentobarbital can cause hypotension.

- Intravenous lorazepam and diazepam are more likely to induce apnea in elderly patients.

Bibliography

Arroyo S, Sander WA. Carbamazepine in comparative trials. Pharmacokinetic characteristics too often forgotten. Neurology 1999;53:1170–1174.

Browne TR. Pharmacokinetics of antiepileptic drugs. Neurology 1998;51(Suppl. 4):S2–S7.

Meek PD, Davis SN, Collins DM, et al. Guidelines for nonemergency use of parenteral phenytoin products. Proceedings of an expert panel consensus process. Arch Intern Med 1999;159:2639–2644.

Schachter SC. Antiepileptic drug therapy: general treatment principles and application for special patient populations. Epilepsia 1999;40(Suppl. 9):S20–S25.

173 Anticoagulants

Mark A. Douglass
James A. Kruse

Anticoagulants are commonly used in the intensive care unit (ICU) for prevention and treatment of venous thromboembolism (VTE). Current literature suggests that, compared to low molecular weight heparin (LMWH), unfractionated heparin (UFH) is equally efficacious for the treatment of VTE. Therefore, most ICU patients with deep venous thrombosis (DVT) or pulmonary embolism (PE) are treated routinely with IV UFH. For VTE prophylaxis, UFH remains the drug of choice for most medical ICU patients; however, LMWH has been shown to be superior in subgroups of patients such as orthopedic surgery patients. Warfarin, an oral anticoagulant with a long half-life, is uncommonly used in the ICU because critically ill patients are unstable, subject to invasive procedures, and at increased risk of bleeding. Due to its limited application in the ICU, warfarin use is not addressed in this chapter. The thrombin inhibitors and danaparoid have been used in patients with heparin-induced thrombocytopenia (HIT).

Mechanisms and Effects

A. Unfractionated heparin
  1. Low (prophylactic) doses prevent new clot formation but do not arrest propagation of existing thrombus.
  2. Higher (therapeutic) doses prevent clot formation and propagation.
  3. Effect is mediated by inactivation of coagulation factors primarily by heparin-antithrombin III complex.
B. Low molecular weight heparin
  1. Anticoagulant effect is similar to UFH, but LMWHs are more potent at inactivating factor Xa than they are at inactivating thrombin.
  2. Longer plasma half-life compared to UFH
C. Thrombin inhibitors
  1. Inhibition of free and clot-bound thrombin through formation of a tight 1:1 complex with thrombin
  2. Currently approved agents are bivalirudin, lepirudin (hirudin) and argatroban
D. Danaparoid
  1. A glycosaminoglycan (heparinoid)
  2. Similar to LMWH, its anticoagulant effect is primarily mediated by inactivation of factor Xa

Indications

A. Unfractionated heparin
  1. Prevention of VTE: evidence supports use for patients with acute myocardial infarction (AMI), ischemic stroke, lower extremity paralysis, and in general surgery and general medical patients with clinical risk factors for VTE
  2. Treatment of DVT and PE
  3. Treatment of unstable angina and AMI
  4. Prevention or treatment of thromboembolism associated with valvular heart disease (including prosthetic valves), atrial fibrillation, atrial flutter, or intracardiac thrombus
  5. Vascular and cardiac (bypass) surgery
  6. Percutaneous coronary interventions
  7. Disseminated intravascular coagulation with clinical evidence of thromboembolism
B. LMWH (FDA-approved indications vary with particular drug)
  1. Prevention of VTE
    a. Medical patients
    b. Abdominal surgery and joint (knee and hip) replacement surgery
    c. Orthopedic and spinal trauma (not currently FDA-approved indications)
  2. Treatment of DVT and PE
  3. Unstable angina and non-ST-segment elevation AMI
C. Thrombin inhibitors
  1. Argatroban and lepirudin: prophylaxis and treatment for thromboembolism in patients with HIT or heparin-induced thrombocytopenia and thrombosis syndrome (HITTS)
  2. Bivalirudin: unstable angina in patients undergoing coronary angioplasty
D. Danaparoid
  1. Prevention of postoperative DVT in patients undergoing hip replacement surgery
  2. Has been used off-label for anticoagulation in patients with HIT; however, see later under Side Effects and Precautions.

Contraindications

A. All therapeutic anticoagulation
  1. Previous hypersensitivity reaction to the drug

617

2. Hemorrhagic diathesis (e.g., hemophilia, idiopathic thrombocytopenic purpura)

3. Active, major bleeding

4. Use (at full dose) during invasive procedures with risk of critical bleeding, e.g., lumbar puncture, spinal anesthesia, central venous catheterization, most surgical procedures

B. Heparin (UFH and LMWH)

1. Heparin-induced thrombocytopenia, HITTS, or a history of either disorder

2. Known hypersensitivity reaction to pork products (for porcine-derived formulations)

C. Danaparoid: known hypersensitivity reaction to pork products

Side Effects and Precautions

A. Unfractionated heparin

1. Bleeding

    a. Most common side effect (incidence 5% to 10%)

    b. Can occur from any site, varies from minor local ecchymosis to major hemorrhagic complication

    c. Increased risk with elderly patients, full-dose therapy, concurrent use of antiplatelet agents, recent surgery or trauma, and patients with underlying coagulopathy

    d. An unexplained drop in hematocrit, blood pressure, or other signs consistent with hemorrhage should be closely monitored while patients are receiving heparin.

2. Heparin-induced thrombocytopenia

    a. Type I

        (1) Variable incidence (10% to 20%)

        (2) Minor drop in platelet count

        (3) Does not necessarily require interruption of anticoagulation therapy

    b. Type II

        (1) Lower incidence (3% to 5%) than HIT I

        (2) Associated with a larger drop in platelet count (30% to 50% decrease, or to < 100,000 platelets/mm^3) than HIT I

        (3) May also manifest as skin lesions at injection sites

        (4) Higher risk (30% to 80%) of thromboembolic sequelae without treatment, compared to HIT I

3. Skin reactions

    a. Typically occur at the site of injection (~5 days after subcutaneous heparin administration)

    b. Develop as urticarial lesions, erythematous papules, or skin necrosis (most serious)

4. Hypersensitivity reactions

    a. Well documented to occur, but rare

    b. Common manifestations include chills, fever, and urticaria.

5. Hyperkalemia

    a. Although uncommon, may occur as a result of inhibition of aldosterone production by heparin

    b. Patients at risk include those with renal failure and those receiving concomitant agents that cause hyperkalemia.

B. Low molecular weight heparin

1. Bleeding

    a. The most common side effect

    b. Current evidence suggests the risk of bleeding with LMWH in the treatment of VTE is not higher compared with UFH.

    c. Patients undergoing spinal anesthesia, epidural or lumbar puncture, and those with indwelling epidural catheters are at risk for the development of epidural or spinal hematomas and possible paralysis with concomitant use of LMWH.

    d. Protamine can also be used for the treatment of major hemorrhage or overdose attributable to LMWH.

2. Heparin-induced thrombocytopenia

    a. Risk of developing HIT from LMWH is lower than from UFH, but not zero.

    b. Therefore, LMWH is not recommended for the treatment of patients with suspected HIT.

3. Elevated serum transaminase activity

    a. Benign elevations (>3 times upper limit of normal) in serum aspartate and alanine aminotransferase levels have been reported in patients receiving LMWH and UFH.

    b. Resolves upon discontinuation of LMWH

C. Thrombin inhibitors

1. Bleeding

    a. Most common adverse event

    b. Can occur from multiple sites but most frequently reported from wounds and puncture sites

    c. Intracranial bleeding, although rare, occurred most frequently in non-HIT patients who received concomitant thrombolytic therapy.

2. Hepatic disease: the anticoagulant effect of lepirudin may be prolonged

3. Hypersensitivity reactions have been reported with lepirudin, although most reactions (cough,

bronchospasm, stridor, dyspnea) occurred in patients also receiving thrombolytic agents.

D. Danaparoid

1. Bleeding: 0 to 6% frequency of major hemorrhagic events

2. Neurological bleeding complications: similar risk as with LMWH in patients with epidural catheters, those undergoing spinal anesthesia, repeated or traumatic spinal puncture

3. Heparin-induced thrombocytopenia: low incidence (0 to 5%) of in vivo cross-reactivity with HIT antibodies (lower than LMWH); however, this finite incidence represents potential risk for causing thrombosis

4. Injection site reactions: moderate to severe pain at the injection site reported in 14% of patients in clinical trials

Key Treatment of Patients with Heparin-Induced Bleeding

- Discontinue heparin for minor hemorrhagic episodes and closely monitor.

- Administer protamine sulfate for serious hemorrhage or heparin overdose.

- 1 mg of protamine neutralizes approximately 100 U of heparin.

- Administer protamine slowly (over 10 minutes) to avoid hypotension.

- Severe hemorrhage may require stat fluid resuscitation, blood transfusion, and surgical intervention.

Interactions

A. Concomitant use of anticoagulants and other drugs that may induce a bleeding diathesis increases the risk of hemorrhage.

B. Drugs having this potential include

1. Platelet active agents: e.g., aspirin, nonsteroidal antiinflammatory drugs, glycoprotein IIb/IIIa antagonists

2. Warfarin

3. Cephalosporins (e.g., moxalactam, cefamandole, and cefoperazone): can result in depletion of vitamin K dependant clotting factors and subsequent prolongation of prothrombin time (PT)

4. Thrombolytic agents

Typical Dosing

A. Unfractionated heparin

1. Prevention of VTE: 5,000 U subcutaneously every 8 to 12 hours

2. Acute treatment of DVT, PE, coronary syndromes, atrial fibrillation: see Table 173–1

3. Although continuous IV infusion therapy is preferred and more convenient, subcutaneous adjusted-dose therapy can also be used.

B. Low molecular weight heparin: see Table 173–2

C. Thrombin inhibitors

1. Lepirudin

a. Normal renal function: 0.4 mg/kg IV bolus over 15 to 20 seconds followed by 0.15 mg/kg per hour continuous IV infusion

b. Do not exceed 44 mg for bolus or 16.5 mg/hour for IV infusion.

c. Also see later under Dosing in Renal or Hepatic Dysfunction.

2. Argatroban

a. Initiate at 2 μg/kg per minute by continuous IV infusion.

b. Titrate dosage to achieve activated partial thromboplastin time (aPTT) of 1.5 to 3.0 times baseline.

c. Do not exceed 10 μg/kg per minute.

3. Bivalrudin

a. Initiate with 0.75 to 1 mg/kg bolus, followed by 1.75 to 2.5 mg/kg per hour for 4 hours.

b. Decrease infusion to 0.2 mg/kg per hour for an additional 14 to 20 hours, if needed.

TABLE 173–1. WEIGHT-BASED DOSING NOMOGRAM FOR TITRATING INTRAVENOUS UNFRACTIONATED HEPARIN*

1. Bolus dose: 80 U/kg
2. Initial continuous infusion dose: 18 U/kg per hour
3. Titrate infusion on the basis of aPTT results:

APTT (SEC)	RECOMMENDED CHANGE IN DOSING
<37	Rebolus with 80 U/kg, then increase infusion by 4 U/kg per hour
37 to 47	Rebolus with 40 U/kg, then increase infusion by 2 U/kg per hour
48 to 71	No change
72 to 93	Decrease infusion rate by 2 U/kg per hour
>93	Hold infusion for 1 hour; then decrease infusion rate by 3 U/kg per hour

*Based on total body weight; maximum initial bolus is 10,000 U and maximum continuous infusion rate is 2,300 U/hour. For use in cerebral infarction delete bolus and target a PTT of 1.5 to 2.0 × baseline (45 to 60 seconds).

TABLE 173–2. SUBCUTANEOUSLY ADMINISTERED LOW MOLECULAR WEIGHT HEPARIN DOSING

	DEEP VENOUS THROMBOSIS PROPHYLAXIS	DEEP VENOUS THROMBOSIS AND PULMONARY EMBOLISM TREATMENT	UNSTABLE ANGINA OR NON-ST-SEGMENT ELEVATION ACUTE MYOCARDIAL INFARCTION
Ardeparin (Normiflo)	50 U/kg q 12 hr	No data currently	No data currently
Dalteparin (Fragmin)	2,500 to 5,000 U daily*	100 U/kg q 12 hr or 200 U/kg daily†	120 U/kg q 12 hr (unstable angina)
Enoxaparin (Lovenox)	30 mg q 12 hr or 40 mg daily	1 mg/kg q 12 hr or 1.5 mg/kg q 24 hr	1 mg/kg q 12 hr
Tinzaparin (Innohep)	2,500 to 4,500 U daily†	175 U/kg q 24 hr	3,500 U q 12 hr × 5 days† (pilot study)

*Post hip replacement and abdominal surgery
†Not currently approved indications by U.S. Food and Drug Administration

E. Danaparoid: 750 U every 8 to every 12 hours subcutaneously (postoperative prophylactic dose)

Key Considerations for the Initiation of IV UFH Therapy

- Ensure no contraindications (e.g., active bleeding, thrombocytopenia).

- Obtain baseline aPTT, PT, platelet, and complete blood cell counts (CBC).

- When indicated, administer UFH bolus using a weight-based nomogram (Table 135–1).

- Start continuous IV infusion of UFH (Table 135–1).

- Order next aPTT to be drawn 6 hours after initiating UFH.

Dosing in Renal or Hepatic Dysfunction

A. Renal failure
  1. Unfractionated heparin: a small proportion is cleared by the kidneys, but there are no specific recommendations for dose reduction in patients with renal dysfunction
  2. Low molecular weight heparin: use with caution and consider dosage reduction in patients with severe renal dysfunction (creatinine clearance [Ccr] less than 30 mL/minute); consider monitoring anti–factor Xa levels for drug accumulation
  3. Lepirudin
     a. Ccr 45 to 60 mL/minute (or serum creatinine concentration [Cr$_s$] 1.6 to 2.0 mg/dL): 0.2 mg/kg IV bolus, followed by 0.075 mg/kg per hour
     b. Ccr 30 to 44 mL/minute (or Cr$_s$ 2.1 to 3.0 mg/dL): 0.2 mg/kg IV bolus, followed by 0.045 mg/kg per hour
     c. Ccr 15 to 29 mL/minute (or Cr$_s$ 3.1 to 6.0 mg/dL): 0.2 mg/kg IV bolus, followed by 0.225 mg/kg per hour

     d. Ccr less than 15 mL/minute (or Cr$_s$ >6.0 mg/dL) or receiving dialysis: avoid if possible; if not, consider intermittent bolus dose of 0.1 mg/kg every other day (if aPTT <1.5 times control)
  4. Danaparoid: half-life and clearance may be prolonged in patients with severe renal dysfunction, but there are no specific dosing recommendations; monitoring of anti–factor Xa levels is recommended
  5. Argatroban: no dose adjustment is necessary for renal dysfunction
  6. Bivalirudin: dose reduction is necessary in renal dysfunction (up to 90% decrease in dosage for patients on hemodialysis)

B. Hepatic dysfunction
  1. Anticoagulant effect of lepirudin and argatroban may be prolonged because of slowed elimination in patients with hepatic disease.
  2. Argatroban initiation dose should be decreased to 0.5 µg/kg per minute in patients with moderate hepatic dysfunction.
  3. Patients with liver disease should be monitored closely for signs of bleeding when using these agents.

Special Considerations

A. Pregnancy
  1. Low molecular weight heparin (enoxaparin, dalteparin), and lepirudin are FDA Category B.
  2. Unfractionated heparin, LMWH (ardeparin), and danaparoid are Category C.
  3. Based on the available studies, UFH is still recommended for the prevention and treatment of VTE in the pregnant patient.
  4. Warfarin (Category X) is contraindicated in pregnancy.

B. Obesity
  1. Dosing based on actual body weight (kg) is preferred.

2. Consider 5,000 units UFH subcutaneously every 8 hours (compared to every 12 hours) for VTE prophylaxis in the obese patient.

3. Enoxaparin dosing studied up to 150 kg in clinical trials

4. See Table 173–1 for maximum IV UFH dosing.

5. Weight-based dosing for lepirudin and argatroban is given earlier, under "C, Thrombin inhibitors."

6. Many studies excluded patients with morbid obesity, and so limited empiric data exists.

C. Conversion between low molecular weight heparin and UFH

1. Low molecular weight heparins have a longer half-life (3 to 5 hours) compared to UFH (60 minutes).

2. Upon converting a patient from LMWH to UFH, it is advisable to hold the first dose of UFH at least 12 hours (longer if there is significant renal dysfunction).

3. Since the half-life of UFH is relatively short, LMWH can be started within 60 minutes of UFH discontinuation.

Monitoring

A. Unfractionated heparin

1. Treatment: order aPTT every 6 hours after therapy initiation or change until stable (two therapeutic aPTT results), then once daily

2. Complete blood count and platelet count at least every other day

B. Low molecular weight heparin

1. Complete blood count and platelet count monitoring (baseline and periodically)

2. Serum creatinine concentration (baseline and as needed for patients with declining renal function)

3. Routine aPTT monitoring not useful

C. Thrombin inhibitors

1. Lepirudin

a. Baseline aPTT, PT, and CBC, then daily CBC

b. Target aPTT for lepirudin is 1.5 to 2.5 times patient baseline or mean of normal range.

c. Repeat aPTT 4 hours after initiation or dosage adjustment.

d. Stop infusion for 2 hours if aPTT is high; decrease infusion rate by 50% when restarted.

e. If aPTT is low, increase infusion rate by 20%; avoid exceeding infusion rate of 0.2 mg/kg per hour.

f. After two consecutive therapeutic aPTT values, obtain aPTTs once daily.

g. Watch for elevated aPTT due to anti-hirudin antibodies or vitamin K deficiency.

2. Argatroban

a. Baseline aPTT, PT, and CBC, then daily CBC

b. Target aPTT for argatroban is 1.5 to 3 times initial baseline (not to exceed 100 seconds).

c. Obtain aPTT 2 hours after initiation of therapy or dosage adjustment.

D. Danaparoid

1. Baseline aPTT, PT, and CBC, then daily CBC

2. aPTT levels are not useful for danaparoid.

E. All therapeutic anticoagulants: routinely monitor for signs and symptoms of bleeding

B Bibliography

Clagett GP, Anderson FA, Geerts WH, et al. Prevention of venous thromboembolism. Chest 1998;114:S531–S560.

Hirsh J, Warkentin TE, Raschke R, et al. Heparin and low molecular weight heparin: mechanisms of action, pharmacokinetics, dosing considerations, monitoring, efficacy, and safety. Chest 1998;114:S489–S510.

Hyers TM, Agnelli G, Hull RD, et al. Antithrombotic therapy for venous thromboembolic disease. Chest 1998;114:S561–S578.

Legere BM, Dweik RA, Arroliga AC. Venous thromboembolism in the intensive care unit. Clin Chest Med 1999;20:367–384.

Matthai WH Jr, Siegel JE. Heparin-induced thrombocytopenia: diagnostic and therapeutic considerations. JCOM 2000;7:47–53.

174 Thrombolytic Agents

Robert I. Parker

Pharmacology

A. Specific agents
1. Streptokinase
2. Urokinase, urokinase plasminogen activator (u-PA), tissue complex u-PA
3. Recombinant tissue plasminogen activator (alteplase, rt-PA)
4. Derivatives of rt-PA: reteplase (rPA), lanoteplase (nPA), tenecteplase (TNK-rt-PA)
5. Anisoylated plasminogen-streptokinase activator complex (anistreplase, APSAC)
6. Recombinant single chain u-PA (prourokinase, saruplase, or pro-u-PA)
7. Recombinant staphylokinase (investigational)

B. Mechanism of action
1. All agents generate plasmin, the active fibrinolytic enzyme, by cleavage of plasminogen.
2. Action requires the presence of plasminogen.
3. All agents cause degradation of both plasma fibrinogen and clot-bound fibrin.
4. Streptokinase and staphylokinase bind with a molecule of plasminogen, creating a complex that cleaves a second molecule of plasminogen to form plasmin.
5. Urokinase, rt-PA, and their derivatives, and APSAC act directly on a plasminogen molecule to form plasmin.

C. Pharmacokinetics: the in vivo half-life of these agents is measured in minutes.

Key Indications

- Acute myocardial infarction (within 12 hours)
- Thrombotic cerebrovascular accident (within 3 hours)
- (Massive) pulmonary embolism
- Deep vein thrombosis (best if treated within 72 hours; benefit possible beyond 72 hours)
- Peripheral arterial thromboembolic occlusion (within 14 days)
- Vascular graft thrombosis

Contraindications

A. Absolute contraindications:
1. Hemorrhagic stroke
2. Intracranial neoplasm
3. Recent cranial, spinal, or intraocular surgery or trauma (within 3 months)
4. Active or recent (within 10 days) severe internal bleeding (e.g., gastrointestinal hemorrhage)
5. (For streptokinase only) history of prior administration of streptokinase

B. Relative contraindications
1. Uncontrolled, severe hypertension
   a. Systolic blood pressure higher than 180 mm Hg
   b. Diastolic blood pressure higher than 110 mm Hg
2. Major surgery of the thorax or abdomen (within 10 days)
3. Prolonged cardiopulmonary resuscitation
4. Thrombocytopenia
5. Preexisting coagulopathy
6. Intracardiac thrombus
7. Advanced age (≥70 years)
8. Diabetic retinopathy

Key Contraindications

- Active bleeding
- Intracranial pathology
- Recent major surgery
- Recent major trauma

Dosing

A. Recombinant t-PA
1. Acute myocardial infarction (MI)
   a. 100 mg intravenously over 90 minutes (15 mg bolus then 0.75 mg/kg, not to exceed 50 mg over 30 minutes, and 0.5 mg/kg not to exceed 35 mg over the next 1 hour)
   b. Combined with 160 to 325 mg aspirin and IV heparin (5,000 U bolus then 1,000 U/

hour infusion monitored by activated partial thromboplastin time [PTT])

2. For peripheral artery occlusion

a. 0.05 to 0.1 mg/kg per hour by local intraarterial infusion (rt-PA is the agent of choice)

B. Urokinase

1. For pulmonary emboli: 2,200 or 4,400 U/kg bolus intravenously followed by 2,200 or 4,400 U/kg per hour by IV infusion for 24 to 72 hours

2. For peripheral artery occlusion

a. 37,500 U/hour by IV infusion or 4,000 U/minute (for 2 to 4 hours) followed by 1,000 U/minute by IV infusion

b. Once arterial flow has been reestablished, follow with IV infusion of heparin.

C. Streptokinase

1. For acute MI: 1.5 million units intravenously over 30 to 60 minutes, combined with aspirin 160 to 325 mg daily

2. For peripheral arterial occlusion: 2,500 U over 5 minutes intraarterially

3. For pulmonary embolism: 250,000 U by IV bolus, then 100,000 U/hour by IV infusion for 24 to 72 hours

D. APSAC for acute MI: 30 U by IV bolus over 2 to 5 minutes

E. Staphylokinase for acute MI: 20 to 30 mg by IV bolus; may repeat after 30 to 60 minutes

Monitoring

A. Establishment of a thrombolytic state can be demonstrated by showing the following.

1. Decreased plasma fibrinogen level

2. Decreased plasminogen level

3. Increased fibrin(ogen) degradation product level

4. Shortened euglobulin clot lysis time

B. The magnitude of these changes is not entirely predictive of the intensity of fibrinolysis, and these values do not need to be driven to a specific target level.

C. Profound hypofibrinogenemia ($\leq$50 g/dL) increases the risk of bleeding.

D. Monitor during therapy

1. Daily complete blood cell and platelet count

a. Thrombolytic therapy may be associated

with thrombocytopenia and can produce a qualitative platelet defect.

b. May need to provide platelet transfusion if count is lower than 40,000 to 50,000 platelets/mm^3

2. Measure prothrombin time and PTT every 6 to 12 hours while on therapy.

3. Fibrinogen every 6 to 12 hours while on therapy (transfuse with cryoprecipitate to maintain a fibrinogen level greater than 50 mg/dL)

4. Thrombin time while on therapy (optional); may be prolonged as a consequence of fibrin(ogen) degradation products or hypofibrinogenemia

5. Monitor for occult or overt bleeding.

Special Considerations

A. Embolism secondary to thrombolytic therapy

1. Risk of embolism occurring from a dissolving clot is small, but it must be considered in a patient with new pulmonary findings or ischemic manifestations who is receiving thrombolytic therapy.

2. The incidence of peripheral arterial emboli resulting from arterial thrombolytic therapy may be as high as 10%.

B. Many thrombolytic regimens employ either aspirin or heparin in conjunction with the thrombolytic agent, which increases both the efficacy of the therapy and the risk of bleeding.

B Bibliography

Collen D. The plasminogen (fibrinolytic) system. Thromb Haemost 1999;82:259–270.

Hacke W, Ringleb P, Stingele R. Thrombolysis in acute cerebrovascular disease: indications and limitations. Thromb Haemost 1999;82:983–986.

Kandarpa K. Catheter-directed thrombolysis of peripheral arterial occlusions and deep vein thrombosis. Thromb Haemost 1999;82:987–996.

Marder VJ, Hirsh J, Bell WR. Rationale and practical basis of thrombolytic therapy. In: Colman RW, Hirsh J, Marder VJ, et al (eds). Hemostasis and Thrombosis: Basic Principles and Clinical Practice, 3rd ed. Philadelphia: JB Lippincott, 1994; pp 1514–1541

Schlandt RC (chairman), International Society and Federation of Cardiology and World Health Organization Task Force on Myocardial Reperfusion. Reperfusion in acute myocardial infarction. Circulation 1994;90:2091–2102.

Weitz JI, Stewart RJ, Fredenburgh JC. Mechanism of action of plasminogen activators. Thromb Haemost 1999; 82:974–982.

175 Glycoprotein IIb/IIIa Receptor Antagonists

Vivian L. Clark

Definition

Drugs that block the glycoprotein (GP) IIb/IIIa platelet receptor, which mediates platelet aggregation via fibrinogen, von Willebrand factor, and fibronectin, thereby interrupting the final common pathway of platelet aggregation

Indications

A. During percutaneous coronary intervention (PCI), particularly in high-risk patients (i.e., patients with acute coronary syndromes—see below—, thrombus, complex coronary artery lesions, or coronary artery dissection)

B. Pretreatment of patients with unstable angina prior to percutaneous coronary intervention

C. High-risk patients with acute coronary syndromes (ACS)
   1. Ischemic chest pain at rest with electrocardiographic (ECG) changes and positive troponin
   2. Complicated by hemodynamic instability or heart failure

D. As an adjunct to thrombolytic therapy for treatment of acute myocardial infarction (MI) (under investigation)

Contraindications

A. Bleeding diathesis

B. Active hemorrhage

C. Thrombocytopenia (<100,000 platelets/mm^3) is a relative contraindication even in the absence of bleeding.

D. Major surgery within the past 6 weeks

E. History of intracranial hemorrhage or nonhemorrhagic stroke within the past 2 years

F. Intracranial neoplasm, aneurysm, or arteriovenous fistula

G. Severe uncontrolled hypertension

H. History of documented vasculitis

I. Significant gastrointestinal or genitourinary bleeding within the past 6 weeks

J. History of sensitivity to the drug

K. Oral anticoagulant and thrombolytic drug administration are relative contraindications; the use of GP IIb/IIIa inhibitors with low-dose thrombolytics is under investigation.

L. Eptifibatide should be avoided in patients with chronic renal insufficiency; tirofiban should be administered at a reduced dose.

Side Effects

A. Bleeding
   1. Some trials have shown a significantly increased risk of major bleeding with GP IIb/IIIa inhibitors.
   2. Risk can be minimized by weight-adjusted dosing of concomitant unfractionated heparin.
   3. Treatment of bleeding complications includes discontinuation of the drug; platelet transfusions may be effective in bleeding related to abciximab.

B. Thrombocytopenia
   1. Higher incidence with abciximab compared to small molecule GP IIb/IIIa inhibitors
   2. Generally abates with discontinuation of the drug
   3. Treatment for severe thrombocytopenia (<50,000 platelets/mm^3) includes platelet transfusions and blood transfusions if complicated by bleeding.
   4. Platelet counts should be monitored while a patient is receiving these agents.

C. Readministration
   1. Antibodies to abciximab develop in about 5% of patients.
   2. No reported cases of hypersensitivity reactions have occurred.
   3. Incidence of thrombocytopenia may be higher with readministration.

Key Side Effects

• Bleeding

• Thrombocytopenia

Specific GP IIb/IIIa Inhibitors

A. Abciximab (ReoPro)
   1. A chimeric human-murine monoclonal antibody

2. High affinity for GP IIb/IIIa receptors and a slow dissociation rate

3. Half-life is 10 to 30 minutes; antiplatelet activity can last up to a week or more.

4. Reduces platelet aggregation up to 80%

5. Has additional activity against vitronectin receptor resulting in antithrombin action

6. Approved in the United States for PCI, and for ACS when an intervention is planned within 24 hours

7. May be used in renal dysfunction without dose adjustment

B. Eptifibatide (Integrelin)

1. A small molecule synthetic peptide inhibitor of GP IIb/IIIa

2. Half-life is 2.5 hours.

3. Approved in the United States for use in ACS and PCI

4. May be used at reduced dosage in patients with a serum creatinine level of 2.0 to 3.9 mg/dL; not recommended if creatinine level is 4.0 mg/dL or higher

C. Tirofiban (Aggrastat)

1. A non-peptide, small molecule inhibitor of GP IIb/IIIa

2. Half-life is 2 hours.

3. Approved in the United States for ACS, but not for PCI

4. May be administered at reduced dose for patients with renal insufficiency (1/2 dose for creatinine clearance lower than 30 ml/min)

D. Lamifiban (Lamistat)

1. A non-peptide, small molecule inhibitor of GP IIb/IIIa

2. Half-life is 2 hours.

3. Not approved in the United States

Clinical Trials

A. Glycoprotein IIb/IIIa inhibitors have been shown to reduce incidence of death, MI, and short term need for revascularization after percutaneous re-vascularization in both low-risk and high-risk patients. Most of the available data is with abciximab, although recent trials also show efficacy for eptifibatide and tirofiban.

B. Small molecule GP IIb/IIIa inhibitors have been shown to reduce the risk of death and MI at 30 days among patients with acute coronary syndromes. A recent trial also confirms improved outcome with eptifibatide during percutaneous coronary intervention.

Key Dosing

- Abciximab for PCI: 0.25 mg/kg bolus, then 0.125 μg/kg per min (up to 10 μg/min), for 12 hours

- Abciximab for ACS: same as above except drug is initiated 18 to 24 hours before PCI and continued for 12 hours after

- Eptifibatide for PCI (with normal renal function): 180 μg/kg bolus, repeated in 10 minutes, and 2.0 μg/kg per minute infusion for 20 to 24 hours

- Eptifibatide for ACS (with normal renal function): same as above except no second bolus and the infusion may be continued for up to 96 hours

- Tirofiban for ACS (with normal renal function): 0.4 μg/kg for 30 minutes, then 0.1 μg/kg per minute infusion for 48 to 108 hours

Bibliography

Bhatt DL, Topol EJ. Current role of platelet glycoprotein IIb/IIIa inhibitors in acute coronary syndromes. JAMA 2000;284:1549–1558.

Kong DF, Califf RM. Glycoprotein IIb/IIIa receptor antagonists in non-ST elevation acute coronary syndromes and percutaneous revascularization: a review of trial reports. Drugs 1999;58:609–620.

Lincoff M, Califf RM, Topol EJ. Platelet glycoprotein IIb/IIIa receptor blockade in coronary artery disease. J Am Coll Cardiol 2000;35:1103–1115.

Pitts WR, Lange RA. Platelet glycoprotein IIb/IIIa receptor blockade: lessening the risk of coronary interventions. Thromb Haemost 1999;82(Suppl I):136–138.

Weitz JI, Bates SM. Beyond heparin and aspirin: new treatments for unstable angina and non-Q wave myocardial infarction. Arch Intern Med 2000;160:749–758.

176 Digoxin

Salmaan Kanji
John W. Devlin

Actions

A. Vagomimetic actions
   1. Negative chronotropic effect
   2. Decrease in sinoatrial node and atrioventricular (AV) nodal conduction
B. Positive inotropic effect
   1. Inhibits Na-K-ATPase in myocardial cells causing an increase in intracellular Na
   2. Increased intracellular Na activates a Na–Ca active transport system, which then pumps Na out of the cell in exchange for Ca.
   3. The resulting increase in intracellular Ca improves cardiac muscle excitation–contraction coupling, resulting in increased myocardial contractility.

Indications

A. Supraventricular dysrhythmias
   1. Atrial fibrillation and flutter
      a. Effective for rate control but not for conversion to sinus rhythm
      b. May be ineffective for ventricular rate control in patients with high sympathetic drives; in these cases, β-adrenergic antagonists or calcium channel blockers may be required to control ventricular rate
   2. Chronic suppression of paroxysmal atrial tachycardia
B. Congestive heart failure (CHF)
   1. Effective for improving cardiac output, quality of life, exercise tolerance, and functional class
   2. Digoxin has not been shown to reduce mortality associated with CHF, but it has been shown to reduce the frequency of hospitalization, both overall and for worsening heart failure.
   3. Digoxin is the drug of choice for patients with concomitant atrial fibrillation.
   4. Digoxin has not been shown to benefit diastolic dysfunction.

Precautions

A. Hypertrophic obstructive cardiomyopathy
B. Suspected digitalis intoxication
C. Second- or third-degree heart block (in the absence of permanent pacemaker)
D. Atrial fibrillation with accessory AV pathway (e.g., Wolff-Parkinson-White syndrome)
E. Atrioventricular block
F. Recent myocardial infarction
G. Electrolyte imbalance (e.g., hyperkalemia, hypokalemia, hypomagnesemia, hypercalcemia)
H. Renal dysfunction
I. Elderly patients

Interactions

A. Drugs that can decrease plasma digoxin concentration
   1. Acarbose
   2. Penicillamine
   3. Antacids (aluminum and magnesium salts)
   4. Rifampin
   5. Cholestyramine
   6. Sucralfate
   7. Colestipol
   8. Metoclopramide
B. Drugs that can increase plasma digoxin concentration
   1. Amiodarone
   2. Propafenone
   3. Cyclosporin A
   4. Quinidine and quinine
   5. Diltiazem and verapamil
   6. Fluoxetine
   7. Spironolactone
   8. Itraconazole
   9. Clarithromycin, erythromycin, tetracycline
C. Other drug interactions
   1. β-Adrenergic antagonists, calcium channel blockers
      a. β-Adrenergic antagonists and non-dihydropyridine calcium channel blockers (verapamil, diltiazem) may potentiate digoxin's effect on redirecting AV node conduction.
      b. Verapamil and diltiazem increase serum concentrations of digoxin by blocking its renal excretion.
   2. Loop diuretics (furosemide, bumetanide), thia-

zide diuretics (hydrochlorothiazide, metolazone), amphotericin B: drug-induced electrolyte imbalances (e.g., hypokalemia, hypomagnesemia) may predispose to digitalis-induced dysrhythmias

3. Pancuronium, succinylcholine, Vaughn-Williams class I and III antidysrhythmic drugs: concurrent use with digoxin increases the risk of digoxin-related cardiac dysrhythmias

D. Drug–food interactions: rate of absorption of oral digitalis preparations is slowed when taken with food, but the total extent of absorption is unchanged

E. Drug–laboratory test interactions

1. Spironolactone may interfere with some digoxin assays (radioimmunoassay-based tests do not seem to be affected).

2. Digoxin may interfere with some urine glucose tests (e.g., Clinistix, Diastix) leading to spuriously low results.

Typical Dosing

A. Loading

1. 10 μg/kg orally or intravenously, based on ideal body weight

2. Must be given in divided doses: usually, half the loading dose is given initially, followed by two divided doses given at 6- to 8-hour intervals or until clinical response is achieved

B. Maintenance

1. Usually 125 to 500 μg orally or intravenously each day

2. Maintenance doses should be based on both clinical indication and renal function.

C. Intravenous versus oral dosing

1. Intravenous dosing is often necessary in intensive care unit patients with an acute indication.

2. Each IV dose is usually administered as an IV piggyback over 15 minutes.

3. Tablets and elixir have a bioavailability of approximately 80%.

D. Serum digoxin levels

1. In patients not receiving a loading dose, steady-state plasma digoxin concentrations will not be reached for approximately 5 to 7 days.

2. In patients with end-stage renal disease the half-life of the drug may exceed 5 days.

3. Blood samples for digoxin concentrations should be drawn at least 6 to 8 hours after a dose to allow for tissue redistribution.

4. Therapeutic plasma concentrations for adults are generally 0.5 to 2.0 ng/mL (higher plasma digoxin concentrations have been associated with better control of rapid atrial fibrillation).

5. The likelihood for toxicity increases at concentrations above 2.0 ng/mL.

Dosing in Renal Failure

A. The dose of digoxin must be reduced in renal insufficiency.

B. Volume of distribution and total body clearance are decreased in end-stage renal disease (ESRD).

C. Loading doses in ESRD should be reduced by 50%.

D. Adjustment of the dose and dosing interval are required when the creatinine clearance (Cl_{Cr}) is less than 50 mL/minute.

1. Cl_{Cr} can be determined by 24-hour urine collection, or estimated by:

a. For males: $Cl_{Cr} = [Wt \times (140 - Age)] / [72 \times S_{Cr}]$

b. For females: $Cl_{Cr} = 0.85 \times [Wt \times (140 - Age)] / [72 \times S_{Cr}]$
where S_{Cr} is serum creatinine (mg/dL), Wt is adjusted body weight (kg), and Age is chronological age (years)

2. Typical maintenance dosing in renal insufficiency

a. Cl_{Cr} greater than 50 mL/minute: 100% of standard dose, every 24 hours

b. Cl_{Cr} 10 to 50 mL/min: 25% to 75% of standard dose, every 36 hours

c. Cl_{Cr} less than 10 mL/minute: 10% to 25% of usual standard, every 48 hours

E. No supplemental doses are required after hemodialysis.

Key Monitoring

- Maintain normal plasma electrolyte concentrations, including K, Mg, and Ca.

- Use serum creatinine and urea nitrogen assays to assess renal function.

- Electrocardiographic monitoring is necessary when toxicity is suspected.

- Serum digoxin concentrations are indicated when toxicity is suspected (see Chapter 67, Digoxin Overdose).

- Digoxin serum concentration should be measured at least 6 to 8 hours after the last dose.

Side Effects

A. Cardiovascular
   1. Dysrhythmias
      a. Unifocal or multiform ventricular premature contractions
      b. Bigeminal or trigeminal rhythms
      c. Atrioventricular re-entry tachycardia
      d. Ventricular tachycardia
      e. Atrioventricular block (all degrees)
      f. Electrolyte imbalances, specifically hypokalemia and hypomagnesemia, increase the risk of toxic dysrhythmias.
      g. Virtually any dysrhythmia or conduction disturbance can be seen with digitalis toxicity.
   2. Electrocardiographic changes
      a. Inverted T waves or decrease in T wave amplitude
      b. ST segment depression
      c. Prolonged PR interval
      d. QT interval shortening
B. Gastrointestinal
   1. Anorexia
   2. Nausea
   3. Vomiting
   4. Diarrhea
C. Central nervous system
   1. Visual disturbances (blurred or yellow vision)
   2. Headache
   3. Weakness
   4. Apathy
   5. Psychosis
D. Other
   1. Gynecomastia
   2. Maculopapular rash

Key Side Effects

- Bigeminal or trigeminal rhythms
- Atrioventricular block (all degrees)
- Paroxysmal atrial tachycardia with heart block
- Accelerated junctional rhythm
- Ventricular tachycardia

Precautions

A. Atrial fibrillation: discontinuation of digoxin may result in undesirable increases in heart rate
B. Electrical cardioversion: risk of dysrhythmias is increased if cardioversion is attempted in the face of a toxic serum digoxin concentration
C. Cardiogenic shock
   1. Digoxin is probably not useful in circulatory shock unless there is concomitant atrial fibrillation.
   2. Rapid IV administration may increase peripheral vascular resistance and worsen hypoperfusion.
D. Acute myocardial infarction: digoxin may worsen myocardial ischemia
E. Elderly patients: often require dose reductions due to reduced lean body mass and reduced renal clearance

Bibliography

The Digitalis Investigation Group. The effect of digoxin on mortality and morbidity in patients with heart failure. N Engl J Med 1997;336:525–533.

Hauptman PJ, Rekha G, Kelly RA. Cardiac glycosides in the next millennium. Progr Cardiovasc Dis 1999;41:247–254.

Lewis RP. Digitalis: a drug that refuses to die. Crit Care Med 1990;18:S5–S13.

Riaz K, Forker AD. Digoxin use in congestive heart failure: current status. Drugs 1998;55:747–758.

177 Antidysrhythmic Agents

Michael J. Ruffing
Vivian L. Clark

Actions

A. Class I

1. Class IA: significant depression of phase 0; prolongation of the action potential duration, slowed conduction velocity, increased refractoriness, decreased automaticity

2. Class IB: minimal depression of phase 0, shortening of the action potential duration, minimal effect on conduction velocity and refractoriness, decrease in automaticity

3. Class IC: significant depression of phase 0, slight effect on action potential duration, significant decrease in conduction velocity, mild increase in refractoriness, decrease in automaticity

B. Class II: depression of phase 4 of action potential; decrease in automaticity; decrease in conduction velocity and increase in refractoriness of atrioventricular (A-V) node

C. Class III: prolongation of phase 3 of the action potential, decrease automaticity, slow conduction velocity, increase in refractoriness

D. Class IV: depression of phase 4 of the action potential; prolongation of phases 1 and 2, decrease in automaticity and conduction velocity; increase in refractoriness of A-V node

Contraindications

A. Procainamide: second- or third-degree heart block (unless pacemaker in place), systemic lupus erythematosus, torsade de pointes, hypersensitivity to procainamide

B. Quinidine: myasthenia gravis, complete or second- or third-degree heart block, torsade de pointes, long QT syndrome, hypersensitivity or thrombocytopenic purpura associated with quinidine administration

C. Lidocaine: Wolff-Parkinson-White syndrome, Adams-Stokes syndrome, significant sinoatrial, A-V nodal, or intraventricular block without an appropriate pacemaker, hypersensitivity to lidocaine or amide anesthetics

D. Flecainide: second- or third-degree A-V block or right bundle branch block without a pacemaker, cardiogenic shock, recent myocardial infarction, hypersensitivity to flecainide

E. Propafenone: congestive heart failure (CHF); conduction abnormalities (heart block, sick sinus syndrome, etc.) without a pacemaker; hypotension; bronchospasm; hypersensitivity to propafenone

F. Bretylium: significant hypotension, fixed cardiac output, hypersensitivity to bretylium

G. Amiodarone: marked sinus node dysfunction with bradycardia and second- or third-degree block without an appropriate pacemaker; hypersensitivity to amiodarone

H. Adenosine: second- or third-degree A-V block or sick sinus syndrome without an appropriate pacemaker; hypersensitivity to adenosine

I. Ibutilide: hypersensitivity to ibutilide

J. Sotalol: second- or third-degree A-V block, sick sinus syndrome, cardiogenic shock, congenital or acquired long QT syndrome, hypersensitivity to sotalol

K. Dofetilide: congenital or acquired long QT syndrome (avoid in patients with a baseline QTc >440 msec); concomitant use of verapamil or renal cationic transport inhibitors (cimetidine, trimethoprim, ketoconazole, prochlorperazine, megestrol); severe renal impairment (creatinine clearance [Cl_{cr}] <20 mL/min); hypersensitivity to dofetilide

Precautions

A. Procainamide: heart block, prolonged QT interval, CHF, renal impairment, lupus erythematosus (long-term use), myasthenia gravis, embolization during conversion of atrial fibrillation, agranulocytosis

B. Quinidine: hepatic and renal impairment, heart block, prolonged QT interval, severe CHF, asthma, fever, muscle weakness

C. Lidocaine: malignant hyperthermia; hepatic and renal impairment; bradycardia or conduction disturbances (risk of suppressing ventricular escape rhythm)

D. Propafenone: lupus erythematosus, hepatic impairment, pulmonary disease

E. Bretylium: renal impairment, aortic stenosis, pulmonary hypertension

F. Amiodarone: pulmonary, thyroid, and ophthalmologic disorders; photosensitivity

G. Adenosine: asthma, heart block

H. Ibutilide: heart block

I. Sotalol: heart block, bradycardia, bronchospasm, renal impairment, CHF

J. Dofetilide: conduction abnormalities, hypokalemia, hypomagnesemia, renal impairment

Key Precaution: Noncardiac Drugs that Can Prolong QT Interval

(Potentially Causing Torsade De Pointes)

- Antihistamines: astemizole, terfenadine

- Antimicrobials: azithromycin, cotrimoxazole, chloroquine, clarithromycin, erythromycin, fluconazole, ketoconazole, itraconazole, pentamidine, quinine

- Psychotropics: haloperidol, tricyclic antidepressants, phenothiazines, risperidone

- Miscellaneous: cisapride, probucol, most diuretics (via hypokalemia)

Pharmacokinetics

A. Procainamide
   1. Therapeutic level
      a. Procainamide: 4 to 10 μg/mL (some ventricular dysrhythmias may require higher levels)
      b. N-acetylprocainamide (NAPA): 10 to 30 μg/mL
   2. Metabolism and excretion: 15% to 35% of procainamide (half-life 2 to 5 hours with normal renal function, 6 to 13 hours with renal impairment) is metabolized to NAPA (half-life 6 to 10 hours with normal renal function, 10 to 40 hours with renal impairment)

B. Quinidine
   1. Therapeutic level: 2 to 6 μg/mL
   2. Metabolism and excretion: 60% to 80% metabolized by liver, less than 50% unchanged in the urine (half-life 4 to 10 hours; may be prolonged in cirrhosis)

C. Lidocaine
   1. Therapeutic level: 1.5 to 5 μg/mL
   2. Metabolism and excretion
      a. 90% metabolized in liver to monoethylglycinexylidide and glycinexylidide; both have antidysrhythmic activity
      b. Metabolites eliminated by kidneys (half-life 1 to 2 hours)
      c. Heart failure or shock may impair hepatic metabolism.

D. Propafenone
   1. Therapeutic level: 60 to 1,100 ng/mL
   2. Metabolism and excretion
      a. Rapid nonlinear hepatic metabolism in 90% of population (half-life 2 to 10 hours)
      b. Slow linear hepatic metabolism in 10% of population (half-life 10 to 30 hours)

c. Active metabolites: 5-hydroxypropafenone and N-depropylpropafenone (<20% of parent compound)

E. Bretylium metabolism: more than 80% renal elimination (half-life 5 to 10 hours with normal renal function, 16 to 32 hours with Cl_{cr} <20 mL/minute)

F. Amiodarone metabolism: hepatic, with excretion in bile

G. Adenosine metabolism: by erythrocytes and endothelial cells to inosine and adenosine monophosphate (half-life 10 seconds)

H. Ibutilide metabolism and excretion: more than 80% renal elimination (half-life 6 hours)

I. Sotalol metabolism and excretion: renal (half-life 12 hours)

J. Dofetilide metabolism and excretion: 80% excreted unchanged by kidney (half-life 10 hours)

Drug Interactions

A. Procainamide
1. Cimetidine, ranitidine, trimethoprim, ofloxacin, and amiodarone may increase plasma procainamide concentrations.
2. Class III agents and diuretics may increase likelihood of torsade de pointes.

B. Quinidine
1. Amiodarone, cimetidine, verapamil, and urinary alkalinizers may increase plasma quinidine concentration.
2. Phenytoin, rifampin, barbiturates, and carbamazepine may decrease plasma quinidine concentration.
3. Plasma digoxin levels increase (decrease digoxin dose by 50%).
4. Increased effect of warfarin

C. Lidocaine
1. Amiodarone, β-adrenergic blockers, cimetidine, and protease inhibitors may increase plasma lidocaine concentration.
2. Rifampin and phenytoin may decrease plasma lidocaine concentration.
3. Prolonged neuromuscular blockade is possible with succinylcholine use.
4. Increased cardiodepressant effect and enhanced electrophysiologic activity with other type I antidysrhythmic drugs

D. Propafenone
1. Cimetidine and quinidine may increase plasma propafenone concentration.
2. Rifampin may decrease plasma propafenone concentration.

3. May accentuate effects of drugs that depress nodal function, intraventricular conduction, or inotropic state

E. Bretylium
1. Effects of catecholamines may be enhanced by bretylium.
2. Digoxin toxicity may be exacerbated.

F. Amiodarone
1. Cimetidine and ritonavir may increase the plasma concentration of amiodarone.
2. Warfarin effect increased
3. Plasma digoxin, theophylline, cyclosporine, methotrexate, lidocaine, procainamide, and quinidine levels may be increased.
4. Effects of many interactions can last for several weeks after discontinuation of amiodarone (secondary to long half-life of amiodarone).
5. Additive prodysrhythmic effect when combined with drugs that prolong QT interval

G. Adenosine
1. Carbamazepine and dipyridamole may augment the effects of adenosine.
2. Theophylline may antagonize the effects of adenosine.

H. Ibutilide: drugs with the potential to prolong the QT interval may increase the risk of prodysrhythmia

I. Sotalol: may augment effect of drugs that prolong QT interval

J. Dofetilide
1. Drugs that may increase the concentration of dofetilide: cimetidine, verapamil, inhibitors of cationic renal transport secretion (amiloride, metformin, megestrol, prochlorperazine, triamterene, ketoconazole)
2. Class I or III antidysrhythmic drugs may enhance potential for torsade de pointes.
3. Cisapride, phenothiazines, tricyclic antidepressants, and some macrolides may cause QT prolongation and increase the risk of torsade de pointes.

Typical Dosing

A. Procainamide
1. IV: 14 to 17 mg/kg (or up to 1 g) at 20 mg/minute; then 1 to 4 mg/minute by continuous infusion (lower doses with renal impairment)
2. PO: 40 to 50 mg/kg per day in 6 to 8 divided doses for immediate release and 4 doses for extended-release formulations
3. IM: 40 to 50 mg/kg per day in 4 to 8 divided doses

B. Lidocaine

1. Initial dose: 1.0 to 1.5 mg/kg by slow IV injection; may repeat at 0.5 to 0.75 mg/kg every 5 to 10 minutes up to 3 mg/kg

2. Continuous maintenance infusion: 1 to 4 mg/minute intravenously; reduce dose if heart failure or liver disease

C. Propafenone: 150 to 300 mg PO every 8 hours (increase dose minimally every 3 to 4 days until effect)

D. Bretylium

1. Ventricular fibrillation or pulseless ventricular tachycardia: 5 mg/kg by IV injection; may repeat at 10 mg/kg for 2 doses if persists

2. Ventricular tachycardia: 5 to 10 mg/kg, diluted and given over 8 minutes

3. Continuous infusion rate: 1 to 2 mg/minute

E. Amiodarone

1. Oral

a. Life-threatening ventricular dysrhythmias: 800 to 1600 mg/day in divided doses for 1 to 3 weeks, then 400 to 600 mg/day

b. Supraventricular dysrhythmias: 600 to 800 mg/day for 7 to 10 days, then 200 to 400 mg/day

2. Parenteral

a. Ventricular fibrillation or pulseless ventricular tachycardia: 300 mg by IV injection, then 150 mg repeated in 3 to 5 minutes until effect

b. Stable ventricular tachycardia

(1) 150 mg in 100 mL 5% dextrose in water over 10 minutes (15 mg/minute); may be repeated at 10-minute intervals if needed

(2) 360 mg (900 mg in 500 mL 5% dextrose in water) over 6 hours (1 mg/minute)

(3) Then 540 mg over 18 hours (0.5 mg/minute); may continue 0.5 mg/minute infusion for a limited period beyond 24 hours

F. Adenosine

1. Initially 6 mg by IV injection over 1 to 2 seconds (follow injection with rapid saline flush)

2. If no response after 1 to 2 minutes, give 12 mg intravenously; may repeat this dose once if no response.

G. Ibutilide

1. >60 kg: 1 mg over 10 minutes

2. <60 kg: 0.01 mg/kg over 10 minutes

3. May repeat dose in 10 minutes if no effect

4. Observe or continue ECG monitoring for at least 4 hours after infused.

H. Sotalol

1. Initiate at 80 mg every 12 hours and titrate upward every 2 to 3 days to effect.

2. Usual dose is 160 to 320 mg/day in divided doses.

3. Renal impairment: initiate at 80 mg at the following dosing intervals

a. Cl_{cr} 30 to 59 mL/minute: every 24 hours

b. Cl_{cr} 10 to 30 mL/minute: every 36 to 48 hours

c. Cl_{cr} <10 mL/minute: individualize

I. Dofetilide

1. Only available to prescribers and hospitals that have undergone dofetilide education from the manufacturer

2. Must initiate in setting where continuous ECG monitoring with trained personnel is present for a minimum of 3 days.

3. Patient must not be discharged within 12 hours of conversion to normal sinus rhythm.

4. Initiating dosing

a. Obtain baseline ECG; if QTc is greater than 440 msec or heart rate is lower than 60 beats/minute, do not initiate.

b. Obtain Cl_{cr} for initial dose.

(1) Cl_{cr} >60 mL/minute: 500 μg every 12 hours

(2) Cl_{cr} 40 to 60 mL/minute: 250 μg every 12 hours

(3) Cl_{cr} 20 to 40 mL/minute: 125 μg every 12 hours

(4) Cl_{cr} <20 mL/minute: avoid dofetilide

c. Determine QTc 2 to 3 hours after first dose. If QTc increased by 15% or is greater than 500 msec, dose as follows based on starting dose.

(1) Starting dose of 500 μg every 12 hours: 250 μg every 12 hours

(2) Starting dose of 250 μg every 24 hours: 125 μg every 12 hours

(3) 125 μg every 12 hours: 125 μg once daily

5. Discontinue if QTc is greater than 500 msec at any time after the second dose has been given.

Electrocardiographic and Side Effects

A. Procainamide: widening of QRS complex, prolongation of QT and JT intervals, hypotension, heart block, dizziness, nausea, vomiting, agranulocytosis, leukopenia, thrombocytopenia, lupus erythematosus

B. Quinidine: widening of QRS complex; prolongation of QT and JT intervals, prodysrhythmic effect, hypotension (particularly after rapid IV administration), paradoxical tachycardia, heart block, headache, confusion, ataxia, rash, nausea, vomiting, diarrhea, acute hemolytic anemia, thrombocytopenic purpura, cinchonism

C. Lidocaine: possible shortening of QT interval, hypotension, bradycardia, drowsiness, blurred vision, tremors, twitching, convulsions

D. Propafenone: prolonged PR, QRS, or QT interval; A-V block; intraventricular conduction delay; CHF; dizziness; nausea; vomiting; constipation; dysgeusia

E. Bretylium: prolonged JT interval, hypotension, dizziness, nausea, vomiting (especially with rapid IV push in awake patients)

F. Amiodarone: increased PR or QT interval, visual disturbances, optic neuritis, corneal microdeposits, photophobia, bradycardia, hypotension (high daily doses), ventricular tachycardia or fibrillation, A-V block, pulmonary fibrosis, hypersensitivity pneumonitis, interstitial or alveolar pneumonitis, malaise, ataxia, nausea, vomiting, anorexia, dysgeusia, hepatitis, photosensitivity, blue discoloration of skin, solar dermatitis, hyperthyroidism, hypothyroidism

G. Adenosine: increased PR interval, facial flushing, prolonged asystole, dyspnea, dizziness, headache, nausea

H. Ibutilide: prolonged QT interval, polymorphic ventricular tachycardia, hypotension, A-V block

I. Sotalol: QT prolongation, CHF, bradycardia, heart block, dizziness, fatigue, headache, sleep disturbances, nausea, vomiting

J. Dofetilide: QT prolongation, torsade de pointes, hypotension, lightheadedness, nausea

Bibliography

Chaudhry GM, Haffajee CI. Antiarrhythmic agents and prodysrhythmia. Crit Care Med 2000;28(Suppl.):N158–N164.

Chung MK. Cardiac surgery: postoperative dysrhythmias. Crit Care Med 2000;28(Suppl):N136–N144.

Kowey PR, Marinchak RA, Rials SJ, et al. Intravenous antiarrhythmic therapy in the acute control of in-hospital destabilizing ventricular tachycardia and fibrillation. Am J Cardiol 1999;84:46R–51R.

Levy S. Pharmacologic management of atrial fibrillation: current therapeutic strategies. Am Heart J 2001;141:S15–S21.

Pollak PT. Clinical organ toxicity of antiarrhythmic compounds: ocular and pulmonary manifestations. Am J Cardiol 1999;84:37R–45R.

Trujillo TC, Nolan PE. Antiarrhythmic agents. Drug interactions of clinical significance. Drug Safety 2000;23:509–532.

178 Dantrolene

Jeff D. Huntress

Pharmacology

A. Indications: useful in the management of muscle spasticity and injury from environmental, drug-induced, or other neuromuscular insults

B. Mechanism of action
1. Induces skeletal muscle relaxation by reducing the release of calcium from the sarcoplasmic reticulum by the muscle action potential
2. Leads to decreased muscle contraction caused by direct stimulation as well as contractions mediated through monosynaptic and polysynaptic reflexes
3. Reduces the release of calcium from the sarcoplasmic reticulum in anesthesia-induced malignant hyperthermia, which may prevent the increase in myoplasmic calcium with activation of acute skeletal muscle cell catabolism
4. Does not affect electrical activity at myoneuronal junction or rate of acetylcholine synthesis or release
5. Has minimal effect on contraction of cardiac or intestinal smooth muscle, except at high concentrations

C. Pharmacokinetics
1. Oral absorption is approximately 35%.
2. Extensively bound to plasma proteins, especially albumin
3. Plasma half-life is approximately 9 hours.
4. Metabolized primarily by the liver to less active 5-hydroxy derivatives, which are excreted in the urine

Key Indications

- Malignant hyperthermia
- Neuroleptic malignant syndrome
- Spasticity resulting from upper neuron disorders (e.g., multiple sclerosis, cerebral palsy, spinal cord injury)

Side Effects and Precautions

A. Dantrolene has a narrow therapeutic window.

B. Side effects occur primarily with long-term oral therapy.

C. Adverse signs and symptoms
1. Muscle weakness
2. Dizziness, lightheadedness
3. Drowsiness
4. Malaise
5. Fatigue
6. Nausea
7. Diarrhea

D. Liver function abnormalities
1. Elevated serum aspartate aminotransferase, alanine aminotransferase, alkaline phosphatase, and lactate dehydrogenase activity
2. Elevated serum total bilirubin concentration
3. Fatal or nonfatal hepatitis may occur, most frequently after taking over 300 mg daily for over 2 months or after intermittent short courses of 800 mg or more daily.

Key Side Effects Associated with Acute IV Therapy

- Thrombophlebitis
- Pulmonary edema (uncommon)
- Urticaria and erythema (rare)

Interactions

A. There are no clinically significant drug–drug interactions.

B. Metabolism is not affected by concurrent administration of phenobarbital or diazepam.

Typical Dosing

A. Malignant hyperthermia
1. Prevention in at-risk patients
   a. Oral: 4 to 8 mg/kg per day in 3 or 4 divided doses, for 1 to 2 days preoperatively, with the last dose administered 3 to 4 hours before surgery
   b. Intravenous: 2.5 mg/kg given over 1 hour beginning 1.25 hours before anticipated anesthesia induction
2. Hyperthermic crisis
   a. Give 1 mg/kg or more intravenously rapidly.

b. Repeat dose as necessary until physiologic abnormalities subside or a maximum dose of 10 mg/kg is reached.

c. Prevention of recurrence following initial IV therapy: oral dantrolene 4 to 8 mg/kg/day in four divided doses for up to 3 days after the crisis. May be given intravenously if necessary, initiating therapy with 1 mg/kg or more as clinically indicated.

B. Neuroleptic malignant syndrome

1. Intravenous dose can range from 0.37 to 2.8 mg/kg per day, with duration of treatment from 2 to 16 days; typical dosage is 2 to 3 mg/kg per day in divided doses.

2. Oral dose is 2 to 4 mg/kg per day.

3. Dosing and route of administration have not been well studied, and other regimens for management of malignant hyperthermia treatment have been used.

4. One case report describes 400 mg/day continuous infusion of IV dantrolene supplemented with boluses of 60 to 100 mg for a total daily dose of 6 mg/kg for the initial 72 hours.

5. Fever and rigidity should respond within a few hours of the initial dose.

WARNING

Use of IV dantrolene in hyperthermic crises must be accompanied by emergency supportive measures. See Chapter 86, Neuroleptic Malignant Syndrome and Malignant Hyperthermia.

Bibliography

Heiman-Patterson TD. Neuroleptic malignant syndrome and malignant hyperthermia. Important issues for the medical consultant. Med Clin North Am 1993;77:477–492.

McEvoy GK, Welsh OH, Snow EK, et al (eds). Dantrolene sodium. In: American Hospital Formulary Service. Drug Information 2000. Bethesda: American Society of Health-System Pharmacists, 2000, pp 1274–1276.

Sakkas P, Davis JM, Hua J, et al. Pharmacotherapy of neuroleptic malignant syndrome. Psychiatric Ann 1991; 21:157–164.

Tsujimoto S, Maeda K, Sugiyama T, et al. Efficacy of prolonged large-dose dantrolene for severe neuroleptic malignant syndrome. Anesth Analg 1998;86:1143–1144.

179 Inhaled Bronchodilators

Jeff D. Huntress

Drugs with potent bronchodilator activity are highly effective for the treatment of reversible airway obstruction. In the critical care environment, the bronchodilator drugs most commonly employed are inhaled β_2-adrenergic receptor agonists and the inhaled anticholinergic agent ipratropium. Their potency and more favorable side effect profiles are responsible for their more frequent use compared to the methylxanthine drugs aminophylline and theophylline, and β_2-agonists administered by other routes.

Key Indication

Treatment of acute bronchospasm in patients with reversible, obstructive airway disease

Pharmacology

A. β_2-Adrenergic receptor agonists
  1. Increase intracellular cyclic adenosine monophosphate concentration by β-adrenergic receptor stimulation, causing
     a. Smooth muscle relaxation
     b. Mast-cell membrane stabilization
     c. Skeletal muscle stimulation
  2. Activation of Na–K-ATPase, resulting in
     a. Gluconeogenesis
     b. Enhanced insulin secretion
     c. Mild to moderate decreases in serum potassium due to an intracellular shift
  3. Positive chronotropic response mediated by
     a. Baroreceptor reflex mechanism
     b. Direct stimulation of cardiac β_1- and β_2-adrenergic receptors
  4. Relative potency, selectivity, and pharmacokinetics: see Table 179–1

B. Ipratropium bromide
  1. A synthetic quaternary anticholinergic ammonium compound chemically related to atropine
  2. Inhibits vagal reflexes by blocking acetylcholine-induced stimulation of guanyl cyclase, with reduction of cyclic guanosine monophosphate, a mediator of bronchoconstriction
  3. A greater antimuscarinic effect generally occurs on bronchial smooth muscle than on secretory glands.

4. Has no substantial effect on sputum viscosity or mucociliary clearance
5. The extent of bronchodilation produced by ipratropium is related to the level of cholinergic parasympathetic bronchomotor tone.
6. Pharmacokinetics
   a. Onset of action is at least 15 minutes.
   b. Duration of action is 3 to 6 hours.

Contraindications

A. β_2-Adrenergic agonists: no absolute contraindications for the use of β_2-agonists in the acute management of bronchospasm
B. Ipratropium: hypersensitivity to ipratropium, atropine or its derivatives, or to soya lecithin or related food products such as soy bean or peanut (inhalation aerosol)

CAUTION

Consider the potential for inducing or exacerbating hypokalemia and cardiac dysrhythmias when administering high doses of β-adrenergic agonists to critically ill patients.

Precautions

A. β_2-Adrenergic receptor agonists
  1. β_2-Adrenergic receptor agonists administered via the inhaled route cause fewer systemic adverse effects than those administered orally, subcutaneously, or intravenously.
  2. Administer with caution to patients with diabetes mellitus, hyperthyroidism, prostatic hypertrophy, or history of seizures.
  3. Use with caution in patients with cardiovascular disorders including ischemic heart disease, cardiac dysrhythmias, congestive heart failure, and hypertension.
  4. Electrocardiographic changes include sinus tachycardia, atrial and ventricular tachydysrhythmias, T wave flattening, QT interval prolongation, and ST segment depression.
  5. Prolonged sympathomimetic amine aerosol use can lead to tolerance, possibly due to desensitization of β_2-adrenergic receptors.

TABLE 179–1. RELATIVE SELECTIVITY AND POTENCY OF β_2-ADRENERGIC AGONISTS USED AS INHALED BRONCHODILATORS

AGENT	β-SELECTIVITY		β_2-POTENCY*	DURATION OF ACTION	
	β_1	β_2		ONSET (MIN)	DURATION (HR)
Metaproterenol	+++	+++	15	5 to 30	1 to ≥6
Isoetharine	++	+++	6	0.5 to 2.0	2 to 3
Albuterol	+	++++	2	≤5	3 to 6
Levalbuterol	+	++++	4	≤15	5 to 8
Bitolterol	+	++++	2 to 4	4 to 8	2 to 4
Pirbuterol	+	++++	5	5	2 to 4
Terbutaline	+	++++	4	5 to 30	3 to 6
Formoterol	+	++++	0.24	1 to 3	>12
Salmeterol	+	++++	0.50	≤20	>12

*Relative molar potency (lower is more potent)

B. Ipratropium bromide
1. Use as a single agent for relief of bronchospasm in acute exacerbations of chronic obstructive lung disease has not been adequately studied.
2. Pregnancy category B
   a. Adequate controlled studies have not been conducted in pregnant women.
   b. Use during pregnancy only if clearly indicated.

Key Side Effects

β_2-Adrenergic Agonists	Ipratropium Bromide
• Tremor	• Tremor
• Tachycardia	• Blurred vision
• Palpitations	• Palpitations
• Cardiac dysrhythmias	• Cough
• Hyperactivity	• Dry oropharynx
• Insomnia	• Rash
• Nervousness	• Nervousness
• Dizziness	• Dizziness
• Headache	• Headache
• Hypokalemia	• Fatigue
• Nausea, vomiting	• Nausea
• Gastrointestinal distress	• Gastrointestinal distress
• Paradoxical bronchospasm	• Urinary difficulty

Interactions

A. β_2-Adrenergic agonists
1. Digoxin
   a. Decrease in digoxin concentrations may occur following administration of albuterol.
   b. Monitor digoxin level in patients receiving concomitant therapy.
2. Medications that can lower serum potassium concentration: monitor for additive effects.
3. Nonspecific β-adrenergic receptor antagonists (e.g., propranolol, nadolol)
   a. May antagonize the action of β_2-adrenergic agonists
   b. Can precipitate severe bronchospasm in asthmatic patients taking albuterol or salmeterol
   c. If β-adrenergic antagonist use is necessary, consider a cardioselective agent.
B. Ipratropium
1. Unlikely to interact with systematically administered drugs due to limited systemic absorption and low plasma concentrations with oral inhalation
2. Some potential for additive effects to occur with concomitantly used antimuscarinic agents

Typical Dosing

A. When administered in equipotent doses, all short-acting β-adrenergic agonists produce the same intensity of response; the only differences lie in duration of action and cardiac toxicity.
B. Intensity and duration of the bronchodilator response is dose dependent and related to the intensity of bronchoconstriction. With increasing levels of bronchoconstriction, duration of bronchodilation may be decreased with need for higher, more frequent doses.
C. Either nebulization or metered dose inhalers (MDIs) may be used for mechanically ventilated patients. MDIs are generally considered easier to administer, involve less personnel time, and can

possibly result in significant cost savings while providing reliable drug administration.

D. Specific agents

1. Metaproterenol (Alupent)

   a. Available as a 5% (50 mg/mL) solution for nebulization: administer 0.3 mL (15 mg) diluted with 2.5 mL normal saline every 2 to 4 hours

   b. Available as a 0.4% (10 mg in 2.5 mL) solution for nebulization: administer 2.5 mL (10 mg) every 2 to 4 hours

   c. Available as a 0.6% (15 mg in 2.5 mL) solution for nebulization: administer 2.5 mL (15 mg) every 2 to 4 hours

   d. Available as an MDI containing 0.65 mg per metered actuation: administer 2 to 3 puffs every 3 to 4 hours

2. Isoetharine (Bronkometer)

   a. Available as a 1% inhalation solution: dilute 1:3 with normal saline and administer 1 to 4 mL every 4 hours

   b. Available as an MDI (340 μg per puff): administer 1 to 2 puffs every 4 hours

3. Albuterol (Ventolin, Proventil)

   a. Available as a 0.5% (2.5 mg/mL) solution or a 0.083% solution for inhalation: administer 2.5 to 5 mg diluted to 3 mL in normal saline every 4 to 6 hours

   b. Available as an MDI (90 μg per puff): administer 1 to 2 puffs every 4 to 6 hours

4. Levalbuterol (Xopenex)

   a. Available as a 0.21 mg/mL solution for nebulization: administer 0.63 to 1.25 mg (3 to 6 mL) every 8 hours

   b. Available as a 0.417 mg/mL solution for nebulization: administer 0.63 to 1.25 mg (1.5 to 3 mL) every 8 hours

5. Bitolterol (Tornalate)

   a. Available as a 0.2% solution: administer 1 to 2 mg every 8 hours

   b. Available as an MDI (370 μg per puff): administer 1 to 3 puffs every 4 to 6 hours

6. Pirbuterol (Maxair): available as an MDI (0.2 mg per puff): administer 1 to 2 puffs every 4 to 6 hours

7. Terbutaline (Brethaire, Brethine)

   a. Available as an aerosol (0.2 mg per actuation): administer 1 to 2 puffs every 4 to 6 hours

   b. Available as a 1 mg/mL solution for nebulization: administer 0.01 to 0.03 mg/kg per dose

8. Formoterol (Foradil): available as capsules containing 12 μg of inhalation powder for use in an aerosolizer inhaler: administer 12 μg every 12 hours

9. Salmeterol (Serevent): available as an MDI (25 μg per puff): administer 2 puffs every 12 hours

10. Ipratropium (Atrovent)

    a. Available as an MDI (18 μg per puff): administer 2 puffs every 6 hours

    b. Available as a 0.02% solution for nebulization: administer 500 μg every 6 to 8 hours by nebulization

11. Ipratropium–albuterol combination MDI (Combivent): formulated as 18 μg ipratropium plus 103 μg albuterol per actuation: administer 2 puffs every 6 hours

Bibliography

Burnham TH, Short RM, Bell WL, et al (eds). Drug Facts and Comparisons. St. Louis: Facts and Comparisons 2001, pp 643–653, 660–661.

Dhand R, Tobin MJ. Inhaled bronchodilator therapy in mechanically ventilated patients. Am J Respir Crit Care Med 1997;156:3–10.

Duarte AG, Momii K, Bidani A. Bronchodilator therapy with metered-dose inhaler and spacer versus nebulizer in mechanically ventilated patients: comparison of magnitude and duration of response. Respir Care 2000;45: 817–823.

Kelly HW, Kamada AK. Asthma. In: Dipiro JT, Talbert RL, Yee GC, et al (eds). Pharmacotherapy. Stamford, CT: Appleton & Lange, 1999, pp 430–459.

McEvoy GK (ed). Ipratropium bromide. In: American Hospital Formulary Service. Drug Information 2001. Bethesda: American Society of Health-System Pharmacists, 2001, pp 1199–1205.

McEvoy GK (ed). Albuterol, albuterol sulfate, levalbuterol hydrochloride. In: American Hospital Formulary Service. Drug Information 2001. Bethesda, MD: American Society of Health-System Pharmacists, 2001, pp 1211–1221.

NHLBI, National Asthma Education and Prevention Program. Expert Panel Report 2. Guidelines for the Diagnosis and Management of Asthma. NIH Publication No. 98-4051. Bethesda, MD: US Department of Health and Human Services, 1997.

Seligman M. Bronchodilators. In: Chernow B (ed). The Pharmacologic Approach to the Critically Ill Patient. Baltimore: Williams & Wilkins, 1994, pp 567–578.

180 Filgrastim

Mitchell P. Fink

Filgrastim is recombinant human granulocyte colony-stimulating factor (G-CSF). The native protein contains 174 amino acids and is extensively glycosylated. The recombinant version, which has a molecular weight of 18,800 daltons, contains an added *N*-terminal methionine residue and is nonglycosylated.

Key Effects

- Increases absolute neutrophil count (ANC) in peripheral blood

- Increases the number of immature neutrophils in peripheral blood (i.e., causes a "left shift" of the differential white blood cell count)

- Increases bone marrow cellularity

- Increases production of superoxide ("oxidant burst") by neutrophils stimulated with the bacterial peptide, formyl-methionyl-leucyl-phenylalanine

Indications

A. Filgrastim is indicated to decrease the incidence of infection, as manifested by febrile neutropenia, in patients with nonmyeloid malignancies who are receiving myelosuppressive and cancer drugs associated with a significant incidence of severe neutropenia with fever.

B. Filgrastim is indicated for reducing the time to neutrophil recovery and the duration of fever after induction or consolidation chemotherapy treatment of adults with acute myelogenous leukemia.

C. Filgrastim is indicated to reduce the duration of neutropenia and neutropenia-related clinical sequelae (e.g., febrile neutropenia) in patients with nonmyeloid malignancies who are undergoing myeloablative chemotherapy followed by marrow transplantation.

D. Filgrastim is indicated for the mobilization of hematopoietic progenitor cells into the peripheral blood for collection by leukapheresis. Mobilization allows for the collection of increased numbers of progenitor cells capable of engraftment compared with collection by leukapheresis without mobilization or bone marrow harvest.

E. Filgrastim is indicated for chronic administration to reduce the incidence and duration of sequelae of neutropenia (e.g., fever, infections, oropharyngeal ulcers) in symptomatic patients with congeni-

tal neutropenia, cyclic neutropenia, or idiopathic neutropenia.

F. In pre-clinical studies, treatment of non-neutropenic animals with G-CSF has been shown to improve outcome in a variety of models of sepsis and infection. Unfortunately, clinical trials to date have not shown that similar beneficial effects occur in humans with serious infectious diseases.

Contraindications and Adverse Effects

A. Filgrastim is contraindicated in patients with known hypersensitivity to *Escherichia coli*–derived proteins, filgrastim, or any component of the product.

B. Transient mild bone pain occurs in 20% to 25% of patients.

C. Minor changes in some serum biochemical markers are common. These changes can include increased activities of lactate dehydrogenase and alkaline phosphate, and increased concentration of uric acid.

D. Filgrastim is remarkably safe. In phase I testing, even massive doses (>100 μg/kg per day) were well tolerated.

E. Allergic-type reactions occurring on initial or subsequent treatment have been reported in fewer than one in 4000 patients treated with filgrastim. These have generally been characterized by systemic symptoms such as rash, urticaria, facial edema, wheezing, dyspnea, hypotension, and tachycardia.

Dosage and Administration

A. The recommended starting dose of filgrastim is 5 μg/kg per day, administered as a single daily injection by subcutaneous bolus injection, by short IV infusion (15 to 30 minutes), or by continuous IV infusion.

1. A complete blood cell count and platelet count should be obtained before instituting filgrastim therapy, and monitored twice weekly during therapy.

2. Doses may be increased in increments of 5 μg/kg for each chemotherapy cycle, according to the duration and severity of the ANC nadir.

B. Filgrastim should be administered no earlier than 24 hours after the administration of cytotoxic chemotherapy.

C. Filgrastim should not be administered in the period 24 hours before the administration of chemotherapy.

D. Filgrastim should be administered daily for up to 2 weeks, until the ANC has reached 10,000 cells/mm³ after the expected chemotherapy-induced neutrophil nadir.

E. Filgrastim therapy should be discontinued if the ANC surpasses 10,000 cells/mm³ after the expected chemotherapy-induced neutrophil nadir.

Bibliography

Heard SO, Fink MP, Gamelli RL, et al. Effect of prophylactic administration of recombinant human granulocyte colony-stimulating factor (filgrastim) on the frequency of nosocomial infections in patients with acute traumatic brain injury or cerebral hemorrhage. Crit Care Med 1998;26:748–754.

Nelson S, Belknap SM, Carlson RW, et al. A randomized controlled trial of filgrastim as an adjunct to antibiotics for treatment of hospitalized patients with community-acquired pneumonia. J Infect Dis 1998;178:1075–1080.

181 Complications of Chemotherapeutic Agents

Lisa Mueller

The side effects of chemotherapy are numerous and varied, involving many organ systems. Fortunately, life-threatening complications are rare, but when they do occur are dramatic and require rapid intervention. It is important to distinguish the cause of severe organ dysfunction that occurs during cancer therapy. The cause potentially involves the tumor itself, or can be due to infection, other underlying illnesses, paraneoplastic syndromes, effects of other prior therapy including surgery, radiation, and drugs. The latter includes chemotherapy, complications of which are the subject of this chapter. Often the cause of severe organ dysfunction in cancer patients is multifactorial. This chapter summarizes some of the most severe forms of chemotherapy complications that require intervention in the intensive care unit.

Pulmonary Toxicity

Etiology and Side Effects

A. Chronic pneumonitis and pulmonary fibrosis: bleomycin, carmustine, mitomycin C, cyclophosphamide, methotrexate, azathioprine, busulfan, melphalan, chlorambucil

B. Hypersensitivity pneumonitis: bleomycin, methotrexate, procarbazine

C. Acute respiratory distress syndrome: cytarabine, cyclophosphamide, methotrexate, mitomycin, teniposide, *all-trans*-retinoic acid, interleukin-2

D. Acute chest syndrome: bleomycin, methotrexate

E. Bronchiolitis obliterans: bone marrow transplant (BMT)

F. Radiation-induced lung toxicity

Clinical Findings

A. Chronic pneumonitis and pulmonary fibrosis
 1. History: insidious onset of dyspnea, nonproductive cough, malaise, fatigue, weight loss
 2. Examination: fever and bibasilar "Velcro-like" rales
 3. Arterial blood gases: hypoxemia, respiratory alkalosis
 4. Chest x-ray: bibasilar reticulonodular infiltrates
 5. Pulmonary function tests: restrictive process with decreased CO diffusion
 6. Lung biopsy: interstitial inflammation and thickening, cellular atypia, fibrosis

B. Hypersensitivity pneumonitis
 1. History: subacute onset of dyspnea, nonproductive cough, chills, headaches, rash
 2. Examination: fever, pulmonary crackles, skin rash
 3. Chest x-ray: diffuse interstitial infiltrates, often in an acinar pattern
 4. Lung biopsy: interstitial eosinophilic infiltrates with histiocytic cells

C. Acute respiratory distress syndrome
 1. History: acute onset of respiratory distress
 2. Examination: rales, respiratory failure
 3. Chest x-ray: pulmonary edema (due to increased permeability of the pulmonary capillary endothelium)
 4. Arterial blood gases: hypoxemia
 5. Pulmonary artery occlusion pressure: not elevated
 6. Lung biopsy: pulmonary edema, some focal hemorrhages and thrombi, hyaline membranes

D. Acute chest syndrome
 1. Pleuritic or retrosternal chest pain
 2. Pleural friction rub: uncommon
 3. Chest x-ray: normal

E. Bronchiolitis obliterans
 1. History: insidious onset of cough, exertional dyspnea, with or without wheezing
 2. Examination: similar to emphysema
 3. Chest x-ray: patchy infiltrates
 4. Pulmonary function tests: obstructive pattern
 5. Lung biopsy: lymphocytic or mixed inflammatory infiltrates with granulation tissue or fibrosis obstructing bronchiolar lumina

F. Radiation-induced lung toxicity
 1. Dose-related toxicity
 2. Signs and symptoms: dyspnea, cough, fever
 3. Typically occurs 2 to 3 months after irradiation

Treatment

A. Chronic pneumonitis and pulmonary fibrosis
 1. Stop the offending drug.

2. Administer corticosteroids (1 mg/kg per day prednisone equivalent).

3. Avoid excessive or unregulated supplemental oxygen (bleomycin).

B. Hypersensitivity pneumonitis
1. Stop the offending agent.
2. Administer corticosteroids
3. Outcome is generally good (better than with chronic pneumonitis).

C. Noncardiogenic pulmonary edema
1. Discontinue the offending agent.
2. Administer corticosteroids
3. Provide supportive care

D. Acute chest syndrome: analgesia

E. Bronchiolitis obliterans
1. Give high-dose corticosteroids
2. Administer bronchodilators
3. Immunosuppression (?)

F. Radiation-induced lung toxicity
1. Corticosteroids for acute toxicity
2. Corticosteroids not indicated for fibrosis

Circulatory Shock

Etiology and Side Effects

A. Hypovolemic shock
1. Sepsis
a. Due to severe prolonged myelosuppression from high-dose chemotherapy
b. Specific agents: busulfan, carboplatin, carmustine (BCNU), cyclophosphamide, cytarabine, doxorubicin, etoposide, fludarabine, idarubicin, ifosfamide, melphalan, mercaptopurine, methotrexate, mitomycin, procarbazine, thiotepa, topotecan
2. Hemorrhagic shock from hemorrhagic cystitis: cyclophosphamide, ifosfamide
3. Pancreatitis: L-asparaginase, glucocorticoids
4. Addisonian crisis: glucocorticoid withdrawal
5. Uncontrolled diabetes mellitus: glucocorticoid administration

B. Distributive shock
1. Septic shock: see 1. Sepsis, above
2. Anaphylaxis: etoposide, teniposide, carboplatin, L-asparaginase, cytarabine, cisplatin, melphalan, methotrexate, mitomycin C, procarbazine, pentostatin

C. Cardiogenic shock
1. Anthracycline toxicity: see next section
2. High dose cyclophosphamide in BMT
3. Radiation therapy

Treatment (see respective chapters for each disorder)

Cardiac Toxicity

Etiology and Side Effects

A. Congestive heart failure
1. Anthracyclines: doxorubicin, daunorubicin, idarubicin, epirubicin, mitoxantrone
a. Cumulative dose effect leading to cardiomyopathy
b. Acute myocarditis is uncommon.
c. Early ST segment and T wave electrocardiographic changes (do not require drug discontinuation)
2. Cyclophosphamide: hemorrhagic myocarditis

B. Myocardial ischemia or necrosis
1. Cyclophosphamide
a. Occurs after high doses used in preparation for BMT
b. Electrocardiographic abnormalities, heart failure, and pericardial effusion can occur within days to weeks after dosing.
2. 5-Fluorouracil
a. May induce coronary artery spasm
b. Can occur within minutes to hours after dosing
3. Other agents: cisplatin, vinblastine, vincristine

C. Pericarditis
1. Anthracyclines (rarely)
2. Radiation
a. Develops in approximately 50% of cases of thoracic irradiation
b. Typically occurs 6 months to 2 years after irradiation
c. Cardiac ischemia, fibrosis, or tamponade can occur.

D. Cardiac dysrhythmias
1. Cyclophosphamide, 5-fluorouracil, ifosfamide, amsacrine, taxol, doxorubicin, interleukin-2
2. Atrial or ventricular dysrhythmias, heart block

Key Risk Factors for Anthracycline Cardiotoxicity

- High cumulative dose
- History of mediastinal radiation
- Preexisting cardiac disease
- Age
- Malnutrition

Treatment

A. Discontinue anthracycline if left ventricular ejection fraction is less than 35% or absolute decrease is greater than 10%.

B. Consider endocardial biopsy.

C. Appropriate pharmacotherapy for heart failure

Renal Toxicity (Rare)

Etiology and Side Effects

A. Most common

  1. Cisplatin

    a. Dose-related, cumulative proximal and distal renal tubular injury

    b. Renal tubular acidosis, hypomagnesemia, hypocalcemia

  2. Methotrexate: precipitates in renal tubules with high doses

  3. Streptozotocin

    a. Dose-related, cumulative nephrotoxicity

    b. Interstitial nephritis, proteinuria

B. Carmustine

  1. Cumulative dose nephrotoxicity

  2. Glomerular sclerosis, interstitial fibrosis, tubular atrophy

C. Mitomycin C

  1. Renal insufficiency

  2. Hemolytic uremic syndrome

D. Cyclophosphamide and ifosfamide

  1. Tubular injury

  2. Hemorrhagic cystitis

E. Others: asparaginase, cisplatin, cyclosporin A, lomustine, pentostatin, plicamycin, suramin, radiation

Key Risk Factors

- Older age
- Poor nutritional status
- Concurrent use of other nephrotoxic drugs
- Preexisting renal dysfunction

Treatment

A. Discontinue the agent.

B. Provide dialysis.

C. Adjust doses of other nephrotoxic drugs.

Neurotoxicity

Etiology and Side Effects

A. Ifosfamide

  1. Clinical manifestations

    a. Confusion

    b. Cerebellar deficits

    c. Cranial nerve paralysis

    d. Seizures

    e. Stupor or coma

  2. Risk factors

    a. Rapid infusion

    b. High cumulative dose cisplatin

    c. Renal or hepatic dysfunction

  3. Recovery is usual.

B. Cytarabine

  1. Manifestations

    a. Cerebellar deficits

    b. Acute necrotizing leukoencephalopathy

    c. Seizures

  2. Risk factors

    a. Renal or hepatic dysfunction

    b. High cumulative dose

    c. Underlying neurologic disease

    d. Advanced age

  3. Recovery is usual.

C. Fludarabine

  1. Peripheral neuropathy

  2. Cortical blindness

  3. Coma

D. L-Asparaginase

  1. Cerebral hemorrhage or infarction

  2. Metabolic encephalopathy with lethargy and confusion

E. Methotrexate

  1. Clinical manifestations

    a. Chronic necrotizing leukoencephalopathy

    b. Paraplegia

    c. Arachnoiditis

  2. Risk factors

    a. Intrathecal dosing

    b. High-dose or long-term systemic dosing

    c. Younger age

    d. Prior cranial radiation therapy

  3. Complete recovery is uncommon (except for arachnoiditis).

F. Pentostatin

  1. Seizures

  2. Coma

Key Risk Factors

- High-dose chemotherapy
- Intrathecal chemotherapy
- Age
- Renal or hepatic impairment
- Concomitant use of other neurotoxic agents
- Prior cranial irradiation

Treatment

A. Discontinue the offending agent.

B. Supportive care until symptoms resolve

Gastrointestinal and Hepatic Toxicity

Etiology and Side Effects

A. Nausea and vomiting: cisplatin, nitrosourea, hydroxyurea, methotrexate, cytarabine, cyclophosphamide, doxorubicin, 5-fluorouracil, others

B. Mucositis

  1. Etiology

    a. Methotrexate, 5-fluorouracil, doxorubicin, hydroxyurea, cytarabine

    b. Head and neck irradiation

  2. Clinical grading

    a. Grade 0: none

    b. Grade 1: mild soreness, erythema, or painless ulcers

    c. Grade 2: painful erythema, edema, or ulcers; able to eat

    d. Grade 3: same as grade 2, but unable to eat

    e. Grade 4: requires enteral or parenteral nutritional support

C. Diarrhea: 5-fluorouracil, cyclophosphamide, cytarabine

D. Veno-occlusive disease

  1. Etiology

    a. Mitomycin C, carmustine, busulfan, cyclophosphamide, dactinomycin

    b. Bone marrow transplant (~20% incidence); chronic graft-versus-host disease

    c. Radiotherapy

  2. History: acute onset upper abdominal pain, weight gain

  3. Examination: jaundice, hepatomegaly, ascites, oliguria

  4. Laboratory studies: hyperbilirubinemia, elevated serum transaminase activities

  5. Biopsy: centrilobular cholestasis, hemorrhagic necrosis or fibrosis, central venule luminal obliteration

E. Hepatic toxicity

  1. Cytarabine, methotrexate, 6-mercaptopurine, nitrosoureas, hydroxyurea, pentostatin, L-asparaginase, plicamycin: increased serum transaminase activity, alkaline phosphatase activity, and bilirubin concentration

  2. Methotrexate: cirrhosis (cumulative dose >1.5 g)

  3. Decarbazine: hepatic vein thrombosis

  4. L-Asparaginase, plicamycin: coagulopathy (decreased factor II, V, VII, X)

Treatment

A. Mucositis

  1. Mouth care

  2. Intravenous hydration

  3. Sucralfate (direct cytoprotectant)

  4. Chlorhexidine gluconate oral rinse to reduce microbial colonization

  5. Dyclonine hydrochloride oral rinse for topical anesthesia

  6. Nutritional support, if necessary

B. Veno-occlusive disease

  1. Supportive therapy

  2. Mortality in BMT is approximately 35% (lower in autologous BMT).

C. Hepatic toxicity: supportive care, treatment of hepatic failure

Bibliography

Jain D. Cardiotoxicity of doxorubicin and other anthracycline derivatives. J Nucl Cardiol 2000;7:53–62.

Komblau S, Benson AB, Catalano R, et al. Management of cancer treatment-related diarrhea. Issues and therapeutic strategies. J Pain Symptom Manage 2000;19:118–129.

Plevova P. Prevention and treatment of chemotherapy- and radiotherapy-induced oral mucositis: a review. Oral Oncol 1999;35:453–470.

Wadler S, Benson AB III, Engelking C, et al. Recommended guidelines for the treatment of chemotherapy-induced diarrhea. J Clin Oncol 1998;16:3169–3178.

Weiss RB. Miscellaneous toxicities. In: DeVita VT Jr, Hellman S, Rosenberg SA (eds). Cancer: Principles and Practice of Oncology, 5th ed. Philadelphia: Lippincott, 1997; pp 2796–2806.

Wesselius LJ. Pulmonary complications of cancer therapy. Compr Ther 1999;25:272–277.

Windebank AJ. Chemotherapeutic neuropathy. Curr Opin Neurol 1999;12:565–571.

182 Penicillins and Cephalosporins

Geneen M. Gibson

All penicillins contain a β-lactam ring structure conveying antibacterial activity. Variable side chains on the molecule result in derivatives that allow for differences in spectrum of activity, stability against β-lactamases, acid stability, gastrointestinal absorption, and protein binding. Penicillins, in particular the extended-spectrum and β-lactam/β-lactamase combinations, are frequently used in the intensive care unit (ICU) because of their rapid bactericidal action, spectrum of activity, low toxicity profile, and tissue penetration.

Cephalosporins are β-lactam antibiotics structurally and pharmacologically similar to the penicillins. The cephalosporin nucleus consists of a β-lactam ring fused to a six-membered dihydrothiazine ring instead of the five-membered thiazolidine ring of penicillin. Molecular modifications alter antibacterial activity and pharmacokinetic properties. Like the penicillins, the cephalosporins are bactericidal, with excellent penetration into most tissues and body fluids. Because of the broad spectrum of activity, low toxicity profile, and good tissue penetration, the third- and fourth-generation cephalosporins see most use in the ICU setting.

Classification

A. Penicillins

1. Natural penicillins: benzylpenicillin (IV), procaine penicillin G (IM), benzathine penicillin G (IM), penicillin V (phenoxymethyl penicillin, PO)

2. Penicillinase-resistant penicillins: methicillin (no longer available in the U.S.), oxacillin (IV, IM, PO), nafcillin (IV, IM, PO), cloxacillin (PO), dicloxacillin (PO)

3. Extended-spectrum penicillins

   a. Aminopenicillins: ampicillin (IV, IM, PO), amoxicillin (PO)

   b. Anti-pseudomonal carboxypenicillins: carbenicillin (PO), ticarcillin (IV)

   c. Anti-pseudomonal ureidopenicillins: mezlocillin (IV), piperacillin (IV)

4. β-Lactam/β-lactamase combinations: amoxicillin/clavulanate (PO), ampicillin-sulbactam (IV), ticarcillin/clavulanate (IV), piperacillin/tazobactam (IV)

B. Cephalosporins

1. First generation: cefazolin (IV, IM), cephalexin (PO), cephadroxil (PO)

2. Second generation: cefuroxime (IV, IM), cefuroxime axetil (PO), cefotetan (IV, IM), cefoxitin (IV, IM), cefprozil (PO), cefaclor (PO), loracarbef (PO)

3. Third generation: cefotaxime (IV, IM), ceftizoxime (IV, IM), ceftriaxone (IV, IM), cefixime (PO), ceftibuten (PO), cefpodoxime proxetil (PO), cefdinir (PO)

4. Third generation with anti-pseudomonal activity: ceftazidime (IV, IM), cefoperazone (IV, IM)

5. Fourth generation: cefepime (IV, IM)

PEARL

Cephalosporins are ineffective against enterococci and methicillin-resistant staphylococci.

Pharmacology

A. Penicillins

1. Mechanisms of action

   a. Bind to and inhibit high-molecular-weight penicillin-binding proteins

   b. Interfere with synthesis of bacterial cell walls

   c. Require actively replicating bacteria

   d. Promote autolysis of bacterial cell wall and therefore cell death

2. Mechanisms of resistance

   a. Inactivation of antibiotic by β-lactamases

   b. Failure of antibiotic to reach its penicillin-binding protein target

   c. Alteration of target site on penicillin-binding protein, thus altering affinity of antibiotic to target site

3. Pharmacokinetics

   a. Widely distributed into most tissues and fluids, except that cerebrospinal fluid (CSF) penetration is poor unless meninges are inflamed

645

b. Half-life of most penicillins is approximately 1 hour.

c. Primary route of elimination for most penicillins is renal.

d. Primary route of elimination for the penicillinase-resistant penicillins is hepatic (to varying degrees), ± renal.

e. Most agents are moderately (20% to 50%) removed by hemodialysis (exceptions: penicillinase-resistant penicillins).

4. Spectrum of activity is narrow to broad depending on the penicillin side chain and presence or absence of a β-lactamase inhibitor. Antibiograms for the ICU should be reviewed.

a. Penicillin G: *Streptococcus* (group A, B, C, G), *Streptococcus pneumoniae*, viridans streptococci, *Listeria monocytogenes* (high dose Penicillin G), *Neisseria meningitidis*, *Pasteurella multocida*, *Actinomyces* spp., *Clostridium* spp. (not *C. difficile*), peptostreptococci, *Enterococcus faecalis* (± *Enterococcus faecium*)

b. Nafcillin, oxacillin, cloxacillin, dicloxacillin: methicillin-susceptible *Staphylococcus aureus*, *Streptococcus* (group A, B C, G), *Streptococcus pneumoniae*, viridans streptococci, peptostreptococci (± coagulase-negative staphylococci)

c. Ampicillin, amoxicillin: *Streptococcus* (group A, B, C, G), *Streptococcus pneumoniae*, viridans streptococci, *Listeria monocytogenes*, *Neisseria meningitidis*, *Pasturella multocida*, *Enterococcus faecalis*, *Enterococcus faecium*, *Actinomyces* spp., *Clostridium* spp. (not *C. difficile*), peptostreptococci (± coagulase-negative staphylococci, *Haemophilus influenzae*, *Escherichia coli*)

d. Amoxicillin/clavulanate, ampicillin/sulbactam: *Streptococcus* (group A, B, C, G), *Streptococcus pneumoniae*, viridans streptococci, *Haemophilus influenzae*, *Listeria monocytogenes*, *Moraxella catarrhalis*, *Neisseria meningitidis*, *Neisseria gonorrhoeae*, *Escherichia coli*, *Klebsiella* spp., *Pasturella multocida*, *Enterococcus faecalis*, *Enterococcus faecium*, methicillin-susceptible *Staphylococcus aureus*, coagulase-negative staphylococci, *Actinomyces* spp., *Clostridium* spp. (not *C. difficile*), peptostreptococci

e. Ticarcillin: *Streptococcus* (group A, B, C, G), *Streptococcus pneumoniae*, viridans streptococci, *Listeria monocytogenes*, *Neisseria meningitidis*, *Serratia* spp., *Citrobacter* spp., *Pseudomonas aeruginosa* (± *Enterococcus faecalis*, *Enterococcus faecium*, *Haemophilus influenzae*, *Escherichia coli*, and coagulase-negative staphylococci), *Clostridium* spp. (not *C. difficile*), peptostreptococci

f. Ticarcillin-clavulanate: as for ticarcillin, plus *Moraxella catarrhalis*, methicillin-susceptible *Staphylococcus aureus*, *Haemophilus influenzae*, *Escherichia coli*, *Klebsiella* spp., *Acinetobacter* spp., *Bacteroides fragilis*

g. Piperacillin: *Streptococcus* (group A, B, C, G), *Streptococcus pneumoniae*, viridans streptococci, *Enterococcus faecalis* (± *Enterococcus faecium*), *Listeria monocytogenes*, *Neisseria meningitidis* (± *Moraxella catarrhalis*, *Haemophilus influenzae*), *Escherichia coli*, *Klebsiella* spp., *Citrobacter* spp., *Pseudomonas aeruginosa*, *Clostridium* (not *C. difficile*), peptostreptococci

h. Piperacillin-tazobactam: as for piperacillin, plus methicillin-susceptible *Staphylococcus aureus*, coagulase-negative staphylococci, *Moraxella catarrhalis*, *Haemophilus influenzae*, *Serratia* spp., *Acinetobacter* spp., *Bacteroides fragilis*

i. Mezlocillin: *Streptococcus* (group A, B, C, G), *Streptococcus pneumoniae*, viridans streptococci, *Listeria monocytogenes*, *Neisseria meningitidis*, *Enterococcus faecalis* (± *Enterococcus faecium*, *Haemophilus influenzae*), *Escherichia coli*, *Klebsiella* spp., *Serratia* spp., *Citrobacter* spp., *Pseudomonas aeruginosa*, *Clostridium* (not *C. difficile*), peptostreptococci

B. Cephalosporins

1. Mechanisms of action

a. Cephalosporins bind to and inhibit penicillin-binding proteins.

b. Interfere with synthesis of bacterial cell walls

c. Require actively replicating bacteria

d. Promote autolysis of bacterial cell walls and therefore cell death

2. Mechanisms of resistance

a. Inactivation of antibiotic by β-lactamases

b. Failure of antibiotic to reach its penicillin-binding protein target

c. Alteration of target site on penicillin-binding protein thus altering affinity of antibiotic to target site

3. Pharmacokinetics

a. Widely distributed into most tissues; cerebrospinal fluid penetration for cefotaxime, ceftriaxone, and ceftazidime is good in the presence of inflamed meninges

b. Half-life is less than 2.5 hours for most agents, 3 to 4 hours for cefixime, and 5 to 9 hours for ceftriaxone.

c. Primary route of elimination is renal (exception: ceftriaxone 50% renal and 40% biliary); dose adjustment required in renal failure for most agents (exception: ceftriaxone).

4. Spectrum of activity by generation

a. First generation: active against Gram-positive cocci and limited number of Gram-negative bacilli (e.g., *Escherichia coli, Proteus mirabilis*)

b. Second generation: variable activity against Gram-positive cocci, improved activity against select Gram-negative bacilli, anaerobic activity (cefoxitin and cefotetan only)

c. Third generation: active against Gram-positive cocci, plus enhanced activity against Gram-negative bacilli

d. Anti-pseudomonal third generation: active against *Pseudomonas aeruginosa*, but poor activity against Gram-positive cocci

e. Fourth generation: active against Gram-positive cocci, Gram-negative cocci and bacilli, *Pseudomonas aeruginosa*, and many Enterobacteriaceae that possess inducible chromosomal β-lactamases

5. Spectrum of activity against specific organisms

a. Cefazolin: *Streptococcus* (group A, B, C, G), *Streptococcus pneumoniae*, viridans streptococci, methicillin-susceptible *Staphylococcus aureus* (± coagulase-negative staphylococci), *Neisseria gonorrhoeae, Moraxella catarrhalis, Haemophilus influenzae, Escherichia coli, Klebsiella* spp., *Proteus mirabilis*

b. Cefuroxime: *Streptococcus* (group A, B, C, G), *Streptococcus pneumoniae*, viridans streptococci, methicillin-susceptible *Staphylococcus aureus* (± coagulase-negative staphylococci), (± *Neisseria gonorrhoeae*), (± *Citrobacter* spp.), *Neisseria meningitidis, Moraxella catarrhalis, Haemophilus influenzae, Escherichia coli, Klebsiella* spp., *Proteus mirabilis, Clostridium* (not *C. difficile*), peptostreptococci

c. Cefotaxime and ceftriaxone: *Streptococcus* (group A, B, C, G), *Streptococcus pneumoniae*, viridans streptococci, methicillin-susceptible *Staphylococcus aureus* (± coagulase-negative staphylococci), *Acinetobacter* spp., *Neisseria gonorrhoeae* (± for cefotaxime), *Neisseria meningitidis, Moraxella catarrhalis, Haemophilus influenzae, Escherichia coli, Klebsiella* spp., *Serratia* spp., *Proteus mirabi-*

lis, *Citrobacter* spp., *Clostridium* (not *C. difficile*), peptostreptococci

d. Ceftazidime: *Streptococcus* (group A, B, C, G) (± methicillin-susceptible *Staphylococcus aureus, Neisseria gonorrhoeae, Neisseria meningitidis*), *Acinetobacter* spp., *Moraxella catarrhalis, Haemophilus influenzae, Escherichia coli, Klebsiella* spp., *Serratia* spp., *Proteus mirabilis, Citrobacter* spp., *Pseudomonas aeruginosa, Clostridium* (not *C. difficile*), peptostreptococci

e. Cefepime: *Streptococcus* (group A, B, C, G), *Streptococcus pneumoniae*, viridans streptococci, methicillin-susceptible *Staphylococcus aureus* (± coagulase-negative staphylococci), *Neisseria meningitidis*, (± *Acinetobacter* spp.), *Neisseria gonorrhoeae, Moraxella catarrhalis, Haemophilus influenzae, Escherichia coli, Klebsiella* spp., *Serratia* spp., *Proteus mirabilis, Citrobacter* spp., *Pseudomonas aeruginosa*, peptostreptococci

Key Indications

Penicillins	Cephalosporins
• Bacterial meningitis	• Bacterial meningitis (ceftriaxone)
	• Nosocomial meningitis
• Pneumonia	• Community-acquired pneumonia, severe community-acquired pneumonia third-generation cephalosporin (second- or third-generation drugs)
• Skin and soft-tissue infections	• Surgical prophylaxis (e.g., cefazolin)
• Polymicrobial infections	• Pseudomonas infections (cefepime, ceftazidime)

Typical Dosing

A. Penicillins

1. Penicillin G: 2 to 24 million units/day intravenously in divided doses every 4 hours, depending on susceptibility of organism and severity of infection

2. Penicillin V: 125 to 500 mg PO every 6 to 8 hours

3. Oxacillin and nafcillin: 1 to 2 g intravenously every 4 to 6 hours

4. Cloxacillin: 250 to 500 mg PO every 6 hours

5. Dicloxacillin: 125 to 250 mg PO every 6 hours

6. Ampicillin: 1 to 3 g intravenously every 4 to 6 hours (maximum dose is 12 g/day)

7. Amoxicillin and amoxicillin-clavulanate: 500 mg PO every 8 hours or 875 mg every 12 hours

8. Ampicillin-sulbactam: 1.5 to 3 g intravenously every 6 hours

9. Ticarcillin: 3 g intravenously every 4 to 6 hours

10. Ticarcillin-clavulanate: 3.1 g intravenously every 4 to 6 hours

11. Piperacillin or mezlocillin: 3 to 4 g intravenously every 4 to 6 hours

12. Piperacillin-tazobactam: 3.375 to 4.5 g intravenously every 6 hours (4.5 g dose may be needed for *Pseudomonas* infections causing pneumonia)

B. Cephalosporins

1. Cefazolin: 1 to 2 g intravenously every 8 hours

2. Cephalexin: 500 mg to 1 g PO every 6 hours

3. Cefuroxime: 750 mg to 1.5 g intravenously every 8 hours

4. Cefotaxime and ceftazidime: 2 g intravenously every 8 hours

5. Ceftriaxone: 1 g intravenously every 24 hours (2 g every 12 hours for meningitis)

6. Cefepime: 1 to 2 g intravenously every 8 to 12 hours

Dosing with Renal Dysfunction

A. Penicillins

1. Penicillin G
   a. Creatinine clearance (C_{cr}) 10 to 50 mL/minute: normal dose, but decrease dosing frequency to every 6 to 8 hours; or use 75% of normal dose
   b. C_{cr} <10 mL/minute: normal dose every 12 hours dosing, or 20% to 50% of normal dose

2. Ampicillin
   a. C_{cr} 10 to 50 mL/minute: normal dose every 6 to 12 hours
   b. C_{cr} <10 mL/minute: normal dose every 12 hours

3. Ampicillin-sulbactam
   a. C_{cr} 10 to 50 mL/minute: normal dose every 8 to 12 hours
   b. C_{cr} <10 mL/minute: normal dose every 24 hours

4. Ticarcillin
   a. C_{cr} 10 to 50 mL/minute: 1 to 2 g every 8 hours
   b. C_{cr} <10 mL/minute: 1 to 2 g every 12 hours

5. Ticarcillin-clavulanate
   a. C_{cr} 10 to 50 mL/minute: 2 g every 4 to 8 hours
   b. C_{cr} <10 mL/minute: 2 g every 12 hours

6. Piperacillin
   a. C_{cr} 10 to 50 mL/minute: normal dose every 6 to 8 hours
   b. C_{cr} <10 mL/minute: normal dose every 8 hours

7. Piperacillin-tazobactam
   a. C_{cr} 10 to 50 mL/minute: 2.25 g every 6 hours
   b. C_{cr} <10 mL/minute: 2.25 g every 8 hours

B. Cephalosporins

1. Cefazolin
   a. C_{cr} 10 to 50 mL/minute: normal dose every 12 hours
   b. C_{cr} <10 mL/minute: normal dose every 24 to 48 hours

2. Cefuroxime
   a. C_{cr} 10 to 50 mL/minute: normal dose every 8 to 12 hours

Key Side Effects

Penicillins	Cephalosporins
• Allergic reactions	• Allergic reactions
• Diarrhea	• Nausea, emesis, diarrhea
• Drug-related fever	• Biliary sludge (ceftriaxone)
• Platelet dysfunction (ticarcillin, carbenicillin)	• Phlebitis
• Neutropenia	• Thrombocytopenia, thrombocytosis
• Elevated serum aspartate transaminase activity (oxacillin, nafcillin)	

b. C_{cr} <10 mL/minute: normal dose every 24 hours

3. Cefotaxime and ceftazidime

a. C_{cr} 50 to 90 mL/minute: normal dose every 8 to 12 hours

b. C_{cr} 10 to 50 mL/minute: normal dose every 12 to 24 hours (cefotaxime) or 24 hours (ceftazidime)

c. C_{cr} <10 mL/minute: normal dose every 24 hours (cefotaxime) or 48 hours (ceftazidime)

4. Ceftriaxone: no change in renal failure

5. Cefepime

a. C_{cr} 10 to 50 mL/minute: normal dose every 12 to 24 hours

b. C_{cr} <10 mL/minute: 1 g every 24 hours

Bibliography

American Hospital Formulary Service. Drug Information 2001. Bethesda, MD: American Society of Health-System Pharmacists, 2001.

Asbel LE, Levison ME. Cephalosporins, carbapenems, and monobactams. Infect Dis Clin North Am 2000;14:435–447.

Gilbert DN, Moellering RC Jr, Sande MA (eds). The Sanford Guide to Antimicrobial Therapy, 32st ed. Hyde Park, VT: Antimicrobial Therapy, 2002.

Marshall WF, Blair JE. The cephalosporins. Mayo Clin Proc 1999;74:187–195.

Wright AJ. The penicillins. Mayo Clin Proc 1999;74:290–307.

183 Aminoglycosides

Robert DiCenzo

For the past several decades, aminoglycosides have been a mainstay in the therapy of severe Gram-negative infections in the intensive care unit (ICU). Dosing remains complex because of unpredictable changes in aminoglycoside disposition. Interpatient and intrapatient variability in the ICU is a consequence of critical pathophysiologic alterations, such as changes in fluid and hemodynamic status. Accordingly, it may be difficult to achieve adequate drug exposure, and this can lead to treatment failure. Understanding alterations in aminoglycoside disposition and the need for aggressive and individualized therapy will facilitate dosing of aminoglycosides to maximize their effectiveness.

Key Actions

- Bactericidal with a rapid induction of lethal effect

- Concentration-dependent killing: increased rate of in vitro bacterial killing at higher concentrations

- Postantibiotic effect: ability to suppress bacterial growth when levels are below the minimum inhibitory concentration; related to the infecting organism and the aminoglycoside concentration achieved

Pharmacology

A. Serum concentrations and outcome
1. Peak serum concentration and area under the concentration versus time curve (AUC) provide estimates of overall exposure during the dosing interval.
2. Factors affecting drug exposure and the desired exposure target include the patient's clinical condition, the infecting organism, and the site of infection.
3. There is a higher risk of ototoxicity and nephrotoxicity for gentamicin, tobramycin, and netilmicin troughs greater than 2 μg/mL, and for amikacin troughs greater than 8 to 10 μg/mL.

B. Desired concentrations
1. Reported relationships between peak concentrations and outcome may be limited by such methodological problems as small sample size, differing definitions of peak concentrations, and lack of randomization.

a. Targeted daily AUC: 75 to 100 mg · hr/L; for serious or life-threatening infections, aim for an AUC at the upper end of this range
b. Targeted peak concentration varies with the seriousness and site of the infection.
   (1) For serious infections: 6 to 8 μg/mL for gentamicin, tobramycin, and netilmicin; 20 to 25 μg/mL for amikacin
   (2) For life-threatening infections: 8 to 10 μg/mL for gentamicin, tobramycin, and netilmicin; 25 to 30 μg/mL for amikacin
   (3) For urinary tract infections: 4 to 5 μg/mL for gentamicin, and 4 to 5 μg/mL for tobramycin
   (4) For synergy against Gram-positive organisms: 3 to 4 μg/mL for gentamicin
c. Targeted trough concentration
   (1) For serious infections: 0.5 to 1.0 μg/mL for gentamicin, tobramycin, and netilmicin; 1 to 4 μg/mL for amikacin
   (2) For life-threatening infections: 1 to 2 μg/mL for gentamicin, tobramycin, and netilmicin; 4 to 8 μg/mL for amikacin

C. Factors that alter the disposition of aminoglycosides in critically ill patients
1. Altered volume of distribution: typically larger for critically ill patients, necessitating larger doses
   a. Cachexia, ascites, congestive heart failure, fluid overload, capillary leak secondary to sepsis
   b. Protein malnutrition, cancer, mechanical ventilation
2. Unpredictable changes in glomerular filtration, frequently occurring in burn injury, septic shock, trauma, and other conditions necessitating dosing based on observed drug levels

Key Indications

- Primary use is against aerobic Gram-negative bacilli, e.g., *Escherichia coli* and *Proteus, Enterobacter, Pseudomonas, Klebsiella, Acinetobacter, Serratia,* and *Providencia* species.

- Also used for synergistic effect against certain Gram-positive organisms, e.g., *Enterococcus*

Typical Dosing

A. Initial dosing for gentamicin and tobramycin and timing of measurements of serum concentrations
1. Initial dose: 3 mg/kg ideal body weight (IBW)
   a. Men: IBW (kg) = 48.2 + (2.3 × height in inches >5 feet)
   b. Women: IBW (kg) = 45.5 + (2.3 × height in inches >5 feet)
   c. If actual body weight (ABW) exceeds 125% of IBW, use the following adjustment for dosing weight:
   Adjusted body weight = IBW + 0.4 × (ABW − IBW)
2. Subsequent serum measurements
   a. Obtain 2 serum concentrations: one sampled 30 minutes to 1 hour after initiation of the 30-minute infusion, and one sampled approximately 1.5 half-lives later
   b. $t_{1/2} = 0.693 / (0.0026 × Cl_{cr} + 0.014)$
   c. Definitions: $t_{1/2}$ = half-life (hr); Cl_{cr} = creatinine clearance (mL/min)

B. Estimate pharmacokinetic parameters after first dose.
1. $Vd = \dfrac{dose × (1 − e^{-k × IT}) × (e^{-k × T_1})}{k × IT × C_1}$
2. $k = \dfrac{\ln (C_1/C_2)}{\Delta t}$
3. $t_{1/2} = 0.693/k$
4. Definitions: IT = infusion time (hr); T_1 = time (hr) since the end of infusion; C_1 = concentration (mg/L) obtained 30 minutes to 1 hour after the initial dose; C_2 = concentration (mg/L) obtained 1.5 half-lives after the first dose; k = elimination rate constant (hr^{-1}); Vd = volume of distribution (L); Δt = time elapsed (hr) between drawing C_1 and C_2

C. Individualizing dosing regimens
1. Select a dosing interval of at least 2 half-lives, but no more frequent than every 12 hours.
2. If 12 hours is too frequent, increase to 24 hours.
3. If 24 hours is too frequent, increase by 24-hour increments.
4. For gentamicin and tobramycin, determine a regimen that produces AUC of 75 to 100 mg · hr/L.
5. For serious or life-threatening Gram-negative infections, select AUC at the higher end of the range.
6. 24-hour dose = total dose (mg) to be given in a 24-hour interval, determined by: 24-hour dose = AUC × k × Vd
7. If dosing interval is not 24 hours, divide the 24-hour dose by the number of doses given per day to determine the dose per dosing interval.

D. Predicting peak and trough
1. Unnecessary to predict the peak and trough when dosing per AUC
2. If predicted true peak and trough at steady state are desired, use:
   a. True peak = $\dfrac{dose × (1 − e^{-k × IT})}{k × Vd × IT × (1 − e^{-k × \tau})}$
   b. Trough = true peak × $e^{-k × (\tau − IT)}$
   c. Definitions: true peak = concentration (mg/L) at the end of infusion; trough = drug concentration (mg/L) just before the next dose; τ = dosing interval (hr)

E. Subsequent monitoring
1. Frequency of subsequent serum measurements is based on clinical response, physiologic changes, and risks for toxicity.
2. Repeat above steps to determine the 24-hour dose; adjust as needed.

Key Dosing Points

- Traditional starting doses are often inadequate in ICU patients because of higher volumes of distribution and the potential for increased clearance.

- Use 3 mg/kg as initial dose.

- Regardless of the method used to estimate the initial dose, interpatient variability necessitates monitoring aminoglycoside concentrations.

Dosing in Renal Failure

A. Aminoglycoside elimination rate depends on type of dialysis and rate of extra-renal elimination; may necessitate dosing based on random serum concentrations.

B. May require a dose (~1 mg/kg) after each dialysis

C. Chronic renal replacement therapy requires more frequent administration.

Key Monitoring Points

- Aminoglycoside efficacy and toxicity are related to serum concentrations.

- It is not appropriate to wait to achieve a steady state before monitoring aminoglycoside concentrations in ICU patients.

- Monitoring after the first dose will allow more rapid achievement of therapeutic concentrations.

Side Effects and Precautions

A. Toxicities of concern are nephrotoxicity and ototoxicity.

B. Aminoglycoside clearance is slower from renal, cochlear, and vestibular tissue.

C. Because basement membrane binding is saturable, high concentrations may not result in increased binding.

D. Higher doses with prolonged dosing intervals provide more time for clearance from these tissues and may result in decreased toxicity.

E. Nephrotoxicity occurs at least 5 days after the onset of therapy; it is reversible in most patients.

F. Ototoxicity can occur during treatment or up to 4 to 6 weeks after treatment.

G. Hearing deficits are less likely to be reversible; vestibular damage is usually permanent.

PEARL

In the ICU, interpatient variability necessitates individualized dosing based on aminoglycoside concentrations whether using "pulse" or "traditional" dosing methods.

 Bibliography

Barclay ML, Begg EJ, Duffull SB, et al. Experience of once-daily aminoglycoside dosing using a target area under the concentration-time curve. Aust NZ J Med 1995;25:230–235.

Edson RS, Terrell CL. The aminoglycosides. Mayo Clin Proc 1999;74:519–528.

Tholl DA, Shikuma LR, Miller TQ, et al. Physiologic response of stress and aminoglycoside clearance in critically ill patients. Crit Care Med 1993;21:248–251.

Watling SM, Dasta JF. Aminoglycoside dosing considerations in intensive care unit patients. Ann Pharmacother 1993;27:351–357.

Zaske DE. Aminoglycosides. In: Evans WE, Schentag JJ, Jusko WJ, et al (eds). Applied Pharmacokinetics: Principles of Therapeutic Drug Monitoring, 3rd ed. Vancouver, WA: Applied Therapeutics, 1992;14:1–14:47.

184 Fluoroquinolone Antibiotics

Mitchell P. Fink

The fluoroquinolone antibiotics are synthetic molecules based on a basic chemical structure (4-oxo-6-fluoro-1,4-dihydroquinolone). The biochemical mechanism responsible for the antibacterial activity of these compounds is thought to be inhibition of bacterial DNA topoisomerases, including topoisomerase IV and DNA gyrase. Inhibition of these enzymes by the antibiotic interferes with bacterial DNA replication. The fluoroquinolones currently approved for IV administration in the United States are ciprofloxacin, ofloxacin, and levofloxacin. All three of these agents are also available for oral administration.

In Vitro Spectrum of Activity

A. Ciprofloxacin
  1. All organisms (except *Neisseria gonorrhoeae*) with a minimal inhibitor concentration (MIC) of 1 μg/mL or less are considered susceptible to ciprofloxacin.
  2. The following organisms are typically susceptible to ciprofloxacin.
     a. Gram-negative facultative aerobes, including *Escherichia coli, Klebsiella pneumoniae, Enterobacter* spp., *Citrobacter* spp., *Proteus mirabilis*, indole positive *Proteus* spp., *Serratia marcesens*, and *Acinetobacter calcoaceticus*
     b. *Haemophilus influenzae* (both β-lactamase–positive and –negative strains)
     c. *Moraxella catarrhalis* (both β-lactamase–positive and –negative strains)
     d. *Neisseria meningitidis*
     e. *Pseudomonas aeruginosa* (resistance occurs rapidly with monotherapy)
     f. *Stenotrophomonas maltophilia*
     g. *Staphylococcus aureus* (both methicillin-susceptible and methicillin-resistant strains; resistance is increasingly common)
B. Ofloxacin
  1. Organisms with an MIC of 2 μg/mL or less are considered susceptible.
  2. The in vitro spectrum of activity for ofloxacin is similar to that for ciprofloxacin; however, ofloxacin is less active than ciprofloxacin against *P. aeruginosa*.
C. Levofloxacin
  1. Organisms with an MIC of 2 μg/mL or less are considered susceptible.
  2. The in vitro spectrum of activity for levofloxacin is similar to that for ciprofloxacin; however, levofloxacin is more active against *Streptococcus pneumoniae* than ciprofloxacin and less active against *P. aeruginosa* than ciprofloxacin.

PEARL

None of the available parenteral fluoroquinolones are active against obligate Gram-negative anaerobes (e.g., *Bacteroides fragilis*) or enterococcal species.

Pharmacology

A. Ciprofloxacin
  1. Absorption is rapid and essentially complete following oral administration.
  2. Distribution
     a. Volume of distribution is very large (~250 L), indicating that the antibiotic penetrates extensively into tissues and body fluids.
     b. Ciprofloxacin penetrates well into bronchial secretions; the bronchial fluid to plasma area under the curve ratio is approximately 0.1 : 0.5.
  3. Metabolism and excretion
     a. Approximately 40% to 50% of administered ciprofloxacin is excreted in the urine as the unchanged drug.
     b. The drug is cleared by the kidney by both glomerular filtration and active tubular secretion.
     c. The serum elimination half-life is approximately 5 to 6 hours.
B. Ofloxacin
  1. Absorption
     a. Rapid and essentially complete following oral administration
     b. Bioavailability is approximately 98%.
     c. Maximum plasma concentrations are achieved 1 to 2 hours after oral administration.
  2. The volume of distribution is large (~120 L).
  3. Metabolism and excretion
     a. Elimination of ofloxacin is primarily by renal excretion; approximately 4% to 8% of the drug is excreted in the feces.

b. Most of the drug is cleared without metabolism.

c. The plasma elimination half-life is approximately 6 hours.

C. Levofloxacin

1. Absorption

a. Rapid and essentially complete following oral administration

b. Bioavailability is approximately 99%.

c. Maximum plasma concentrations are achieved 1 to 2 hours after oral administration.

2. Distribution

a. The volume of distribution is large (~90 to 110 L).

b. Lung tissue concentrations are typically two- to five-fold higher than plasma concentrations.

3. Metabolism and excretion

a. Elimination of levofloxacin is primarily by

renal excretion; less than 4% of the drug is recovered in feces.

b. Most of the drug is cleared without metabolism.

c. The plasma elimination half-life is approximately 6 to 8 hours.

Precautions and Adverse Reactions

A. The parenteral fluoroquinolones are contraindicated in persons with a history of hypersensitivity to either the agent in question or any member of the fluoroquinolone class of antimicrobial agents.

B. Serious and fatal reactions have been reported in patients receiving concurrent administration of ciprofloxacin and theophylline.

1. These reactions have included cardiac arrest, seizure, status epilepticus, and respiratory failure.

2. Although theophylline alone can cause similar adverse reactions, the possibility exists of potentiation by ciprofloxacin.

3. Accordingly, if concurrent therapy with these two agents cannot be avoided, then theophylline serum levels should be closely monitored.

C. Parenteral doses of ciprofloxacin and ofloxacin should be administered by slow IV infusion over 60 minutes.

D. Antibiotic-associated colitis (pseudomembranous colitis) has been reported after treatment with most antibacterial agents, including the parenteral fluoroquinolones.

Key Indications

- The available parenteral fluoroquinolones are indicated for the treatment of a wide range of infections relevant to critical care medicine, including urinary tract infections, lower respiratory tract infections (including ventilator-associated pneumonia), and intra-abdominal infections (in combination with an agent active against obligate anaerobes).

- When parenteral fluoroquinolones are used for empiric treatment of patients with severe late-onset hospital-acquired pneumonia (i.e., onset after 4 days of hospitalization), then the antibiotic regimen should include an additional agent active against *P. aeruginosa* and *Acinetobacter* spp. (e.g., an antipseudomonal penicillin, piperacillin-tazobactam, ceftazidime, cefepime, cefoperazone, imipenem).

- Parenteral fluoroquinolones can be used as monotherapy for patients with early-onset hospital-acquired pneumonia (i.e., onset within 5 days of hospitalization).

Bibliography

Culley CM, Lacy MK, Klutman N, et al. Moxifloxacin: clinical efficacy and safety. Am J Health Pharm 2001:58:379–388.

Fink MP, Snydman DR, Niederman MS, et al. Treatment of severe pneumonia in hospitalized patients: results of a multicenter, randomized, double-blind trial comparing intravenous ciprofloxacin with imipenem-cilastatin. The Severe Pneumonia Study Group. Antimicrob Agents Chemother 1994;38:547–557.

Saravolatz L, Manzor O, Check C, et al. Antimicrobial activity of moxifloxacin, gatifloxacin and six fluoroquinolones against *Streptococcus pneumoniae*. J Antimicrob Chemother 2001;47:875–877.

Solomkin JS, Wilson SE, Christou NV, et al. Results of a clinical trial of clinafloxacin versus imipenem/cilastatin for intra-abdominal infections. Ann Surg 2001;233:79–87.

Talan DA. Clinical perspectives on new antimicrobials: focus on fluoroquinolones. Clin Infect Dis 2001;32(Suppl 1):S64–S71.

185 Macrolides

Rebecca L. Corey

Pharmacology

A. Spectrum of activity

1. All of the following three macrolides are effective for pulmonary infections caused by *Mycoplasma pneumoniae*, *Chlamydia pneumoniae* and *Legionella* spp., but some differences exist regarding in vitro spectra of activity and potency against various microorganisms.

   a. Azithromycin: more active against Gram-negative bacteria (e.g., *Haemophilus influenzae* and *Moraxella catarrhalis*)

   b. Clarithromycin: most active against *Mycobacterium avium* complex (MAC); less active than azithromycin against *H. influenzae*, but 14-OH metabolite augments the activity of the parent compound

   c. Erythromycin: relatively inactive against *H. influenzae*

2. Resistance patterns vary with geographic location and prior antibiotic exposure; in vitro susceptibility testing is recommended.

3. Microorganisms generally susceptible to azithromycin, clarithromycin, and erythromycin in vitro are listed in Table 185–1 (macrolides may also have some activity against organisms not listed).

B. Pharmacokinetics

1. Oral bioavailability

   a. Erythromycin: 18% to 45%

   b. Clarithromycin: approximately 50%

   c. Azithromycin: approximately 37%

2. Protein binding

   a. Erythromycin: 73% to 81% (estolate 96%)

   b. Clarithromycin: 42% to 72%

   c. Azithromycin: 7% to 51%

3. Distribution

   a. All three agents are widely distributed into most body fluids and tissues.

   b. Minimal distribution into cerebrospinal fluid

   c. Tissue concentrations are higher than serum concentrations.

4. Metabolism

   a. Erythromycin: partial hepatic metabolism to inactive metabolites

   b. Clarithromycin

   (1) Extensive hepatic metabolism to multiple metabolites

   (2) Principal active metabolite, 14-OH clarithromycin, is thought to have additive or synergistic action with the parent compound against various microorganisms (e.g., *H. influenzae*).

   c. Azithromycin: partial hepatic (35%) to inactive metabolites

5. Elimination half-life

   a. Erythromycin: 1.5 to 2 hours (range is 0.8 to 3 hours; may be prolonged to 5 to 6 hours in anuric patients, but not considered clinically important)

   b. Clarithromycin: 3 to 7 hours in patients with normal renal function (5 to 9 hours for the 14-OH clarithromycin metabolite); prolonged in patients with renal impairment

   c. Azithromycin: terminal $t_{1/2}$ 68 hours; tissue $t_{1/2}$ 24 to 96 hours (prolonged tissue levels and long $t_{1/2}$ allow for shorter duration of therapy)

6. Excretion

   a. Erythromycin: primarily by biliary excretion of unchanged drug; 2.5% to 15% excreted unchanged in urine

   b. Clarithromycin: 20% to 40% renal elimination (rate approximates normal glomerular filtration rate); only small amounts excreted in bile

   c. Azithromycin: primarily (50%) by biliary excretion of unchanged drug; 6% to 14% excreted unchanged in urine

Key Pharmacology

- Inhibit RNA-dependent protein synthesis by reversibly binding to 50S ribosomal subunits of susceptible microorganisms

- Generally bacteriostatic, but may be bactericidal in high concentrations or against highly susceptible microorganisms

- Activity increases in alkaline pH, possibly due to greater bacterial cell wall penetration of un-ionized drug.

- Erythromycin enhances gastrointestinal motility by mimicking the effects of the stimulatory peptide motilin.

TABLE 185–1.   MICROORGANISMS GENERALLY SUSCEPTIBLE TO MACROLIDES IN VITRO*

Microorganism	Azithromycin	Clarithromycin	Erythromycin
Gram-positive aerobes			
Group A, B, C, G *Streptococcus*	√	√	√
Streptococcus pneumoniae	√	√	√
Staphylococcus aureus	√	√	±
Corynebacterium diphtheriae			√
Gram-negative aerobes			
Haemophilus influenzae	√	√	±
Haemophilus ducreyi	√		
Moraxella catarrhalis	√	√	√
Bordatella pertussis	√		√
Legionella spp.	√	√	√
Neisseria gonorrhoeae	±	±	±
Anaerobes			
Actinomyces israeli	√		√
Other			
Chlamydia spp.	√	√	√
Mycoplasma pneumoniae	√	√	√
Campylobacter jejuni	√	√	√
Mycobacterium avium complex	√	√	√
Ureaplasma urealyticum	√		√
Helicobacter pylori		√	
Bartonella henselae, B. quintana	√	√	√

* √ = usually effective clinically or >60% susceptible; ± = clinical trials lacking or 30% to 60% susceptible; blank = data not available

Indications and Clinical Uses

A. Erythromycin (oral, IV)

1. Pneumonia: *M. pneumoniae, Legionella* spp., *Chlamydia* spp.

2. Pertussis (whooping cough): *Bordatella pertussis*

3. Gastroenteritis:* *Campylobacter jejuni*

   a. Shortens the duration of illness, prevents relapse when initiated early

   b. Therapy initiated 4 or more days after onset of symptoms hastens the eradication of organism from feces but does not appear to alter clinical course.

4. Bacillary angiomatosis* in patients with advanced human immunodeficiency (HIV) virus infection or acquired immunodeficiency syndrome (AIDS): *Bartonella henselae* and *B. quintana*

5. Diphtheria (adjunct to antitoxin): *Corynebacterium diphtheriae*

6. Pharyngitis or tonsillitis: alternative to first-line therapy against *Streptococcus pyogenes*

7. *Coxiella burnetii* (Q fever):* alternative to first-line therapy in acute disease

8. Urogenital infections: alternative to first-line therapy

   a. *Haemophilus ducreyi* (chancroid)*

   b. *Chlamydia trachomatis,* including lymphogranuloma venereum* serotypes L1, L2, L3

   c. Granuloma inguinale (donovanosis):* *Calymmatobacterium granulomatis*

   d. *Ureaplasma urealyticum*

9. Uncomplicated, superficial skin and skin structure infections: *Strep. pyogenes, Staphylococcus aureus, Corynebacterium minutissimum (erythrasma)*

10. Preoperative gastrointestinal (GI) prophylaxis:* oral erythromycin base + oral neomycin

11. Diabetic gastroparesis*

B. Clarithromycin (oral)

1. Pharyngitis or tonsillitis: *Strep. pyogenes* (alternative to first-line therapy)

2. Acute maxillary sinusitis: *H. influenzae, Moraxella catarrhalis, Strep. pneumoniae*

3. Acute bacterial exacerbation of chronic bronchitis: *H. influenzae, H. parainfluenzae, M. catarrhalis, Strep. pneumoniae*

4. Community-acquired pneumonia: *M. pneumoniae, Strep. pneumoniae, C. pneumoniae* (TWAR)

5. Uncomplicated, superficial skin and skin structure infections: *Staph. aureus, Strep. pyogenes*

6. Disseminated MAC infection: prophylaxis in patients with advanced HIV infection or AIDS; or treatment in combination with other agents (e.g., ethambutol ± rifabutin)

7. Eradication of *Helicobacter pylori* infection in patients with peptic ulcer disease (additional

---

* Use is not currently approved by the U.S. Food and Drug Administration.

combination regimens, i.e., with metronidazole or tetracycline have also been used)

    a. Clarithromycin, amoxicillin, and either lansoprazole or omeprazole

    b. Clarithromycin, ranitidine bismuth citrate (Tritec)

    c. Clarithromycin and omeprazole

    d. Regimens with clarithromycin as single antimicrobial agent are more likely to be associated with clarithromycin resistance among patients who fail therapy.

    8. *Coxiella burnetii* (Q fever): potential alternative to first-line therapy

C. Azithromycin (oral, IV)

    1. Community-acquired pneumonia: *C. pneumoniae, H. influenzae, Legionella pneumophila, M. catarrhalis, M. pneumoniae, Staph. aureus* (susceptible strains), *Strep. pneumoniae* (susceptible strains)

    2. Mild to moderate acute bacterial exacerbation of chronic obstructive pulmonary disease: *H. influenzae, M. catarrhalis, Strep. pneumoniae*

    3. Pharyngitis or tonsillitis: *Strep. pyogenes* (alternative to first-line therapy)

    4. Uncomplicated, superficial skin or skin structure infections: *Staph. aureus, Strep. pyogenes, S. agalactiae*

    5. Urogenital infections: *C. trachomatis, H. ducreyi* (chancroid), *Neisseria gonorrhoeae, Mycoplasma hominis*

    6. Disseminated MAC infection* prophylaxis in patients with advanced HIV infection or AIDS; alternative for treatment in combination with other agents (e.g., ethambutol ± rifabutin)

    7. Gastroenteritis:* alternate to first-line therapy: *Campylobacter jejuni, Salmonella typhi* and *Shigella* spp.

PEARL

Resistance to macrolides may develop; methicillin and oxacillin-resistant strains of *Staph. aureus* are almost always resistant to macrolides.

Interactions

A. Macrolide antibiotics (erythromycin, clarithromycin) inhibit cytochrome P-450 (CYP450) microsomal enzyme systems and can reduce hepatic metabolism of certain drugs, thereby decreasing elimination and increasing serum concentrations.

B. Azithromycin appears to have little or no effect on the CYP450 enzyme system. Interactions would not be expected to occur; however, the possibility that drug interactions may occur cannot be ruled out.

C. Potential clinically significant drug interactions produced by macrolide antibiotics; interactions generally lead to increased levels of the drugs listed below due to inhibition of CYP450 metabolism (except digoxin) by macrolide antibiotics (azithromycin does not appear to significantly inhibit CYP450 metabolism)

D. Specific interactions

    1. Anticonvulsants: carbamazepine, valproic acid

    2. Antihistamines: astemizole (see Contraindications), terfenadine (see Contraindications)

    3. Psychiatric drugs: clozapine, pimozide (see Contraindications)

    4. Cardiac drugs: disopyramide, digoxin (in approximately 10% of patients serum digoxin concentrations may be elevated due to the effect of the antibiotic on gut flora that metabolize digoxin), felodipine, quinidine, dofetilide

    5. Sedative-hypnotic and narcotic drugs: alfentanil, benzodiazepines (alprazolam, triazolam, midazolam, diazepam), buspirone, hexobarbital

    6. Miscellaneous: bromocriptine, cilostazol, cisapride (see Contraindications), cyclosporine, dolasetron, ergot alkaloids, HMG-CoA reductase inhibitors, protease inhibitors, sildenafil, sirolimus, tacrolimus, theophylline, vinblastine, warfarin, itraconazole

    7. Erythromycin may have additive effects on QT prolongation when used with other drugs that may also prolong the QT interval (i.e., dolasetron, fluoroquinolones, IV haloperidol, antiarrhythmics, ziprasidone, etc.).

Key Contraindications

- History of hypersensitivity to macrolide antibiotics

- Concomitant therapy with pimozide: combination may result in life-threatening cardiac dysrhythmias

- When terfenadine, astemizole, and cisapride were commercially available in the United States, these drugs were also contraindicated with macrolide antibiotics due to development of life-threatening cardiac dysrhythmias.

- Pre-existing liver disease (erythromycin estolate)

Typical Dosing (Adult)

A. Respiratory tract infections

    1. Erythromycin

---

* Use is not currently approved by the U.S. Food and Drug Administration.

a. *M. pneumoniae* pneumonia: 500 mg every 6 hr for 14 to 21 days

b. *Legionella* spp pneumonia: 500 mg to 1 g every 6 hours (± rifampin) for 10 to 21 days

c. *Chlamydia* spp. pneumonia: 10 mg/kg every 6 hours

d. Pertussis: 500 mg every 6 hours for 10 to 14 days

e. Diphtheria: 2 to 4 g/day intravenously, followed by 500 mg orally every 6 hours for 10 days, as adjunct to antitoxin; 500 mg every 6 hours for 10 days for carrier state

f. Pharyngitis or tonsillitis: 250 to 500 mg every 6 hours for 10 days

2. Clarithromycin

a. Community-acquired pneumonia: 250 mg every 12 hours for 7 to 14 days

b. Sinusitis: 500 mg every 12 hours for 14 days

c. Pharyngitis or tonsillitis: 250 mg every 12 hours for 10 days

d. Acute exacerbations of chronic bronchitis: 250 to 500 mg every 12 hours for 7 to 14 days.

3. Azithromycin

a. 500 mg IV once daily for at least 2 days, then follow with 500 mg orally once daily to complete 7 to 10 day course of therapy, for community-acquired pneumonia

b. Mild to moderate exacerbation of chronic obstructive pulmonary disease: 500 mg as single dose on first day, then 250 mg daily on days 2 to 5

c. Pharyngitis or tonsillitis: 500 mg as single dose on first day, then 250 mg daily on days 2 to 5

B. GI indications

1. Erythromycin

a. Preoperative GI prophylaxis, 1 g each of erythromycin base and oral neomycin at 1, 2, and 11 PM on the day before 8 AM surgery

b. Gastroenteritis: 250 mg every 6 hours for 7 days

c. Diabetic gastroparesis: 125 to 500 mg two to four times daily before meals and/or at bedtime (dosage not well-defined)

2. Azithromycin

a. *Salmonella* spp.: (severe illness): 1 g on first day, then 500 mg daily for 6 days

b. *Shigella* spp.: 500 mg on first day, then 250 mg daily for 4 days

c. *C. jejuni* gastroenteritis: 500 mg once a day for 3 days

3. Clarithromycin for *H. pylori* treatment

a. As part of triple combination therapy: 500 mg every 12 hours for 10 to 14 days

b. As part of dual combination therapy: 500 mg every 8 to 12 hours for 14 days

C. Urogenital infections

1. Erythromycin

a. *H. ducreyi*: 500 mg every 6 hours for 7 days

b. *C. trachomatis*: 500 mg every 6 hours for 7 days

c. *C. trachomatis* (lymphogranuloma venereum serotypes): 500 mg every 6 hours for 21 days

d. *C. granulomatis* (donovanosis): 500 mg every 6 hours for at least 21 days

e. *Ureaplasma urealyticum*: 500 mg every 6 hours for 7 days

2. Azithromycin

a. Nongonococcal urethritis (e.g., *C. trachomatis*): single 1 g dose

b. *Neisseria gonorrhoeae* urethritis or cervicitis: single 2 g dose

c. Genital ulcer disease (chancroid): single 1 g dose

D. Skin or skin structure infections

1. Erythromycin

a. Uncomplicated skin infections: 250 to 500 mg every 6 hours for 10 days

b. Bacillary angiomatosis: 500 mg every 6 hours for 8 to 12 weeks (longer if indicated)

2. Clarithromycin: 250 mg every 12 hours for 7 to 14 days

3. Azithromycin: 500 mg as single dose on first day, then 250 mg daily for 4 days (for uncomplicated, superficial skin infections)

E. MAC infections

1. Prevention: 500 mg clarithromycin every 12 hours or 1200 mg azithromycin once weekly

2. Treatment: 500 mg clarithromycin every 12 hours (or, alternatively, azithromycin 600 mg daily) with ethambutol ± rifabutin

Key Dosing Points

- Dosing varies with indication, renal and hepatic function, and severity of infection.

- Erythromycin and azithromycin are available for oral or IV use; clarithromycin is available for oral use only.

- Erythromycin dosages listed herein are oral doses stated as erythromycin base (250 mg base = 250 mg stearate = 400 mg ethylsuccinate salt).

- Erythromycin: use IV therapy (2 to 4 g/day) for serious illness or when oral therapy is not possible or reliable

Dosing in Renal or Hepatic Dysfunction

A. Hepatic impairment

1. Erythromycin: exercise caution when administering to patients with impaired hepatic function (see also Contraindications)

2. Clarithromycin: no dosage adjustment necessary in patients with hepatic impairment if renal function is normal

3. Azithromycin: no data available; use caution because the drug is eliminated principally by the liver

B. Renal impairment

1. Erythromycin: no dosage adjustment necessary in mild to moderate renal impairment

2. Clarithromycin: in severe renal impairment (creatinine clearance less than 30 mL/min), with or without coexisting hepatic impairment, decrease dose by 50% or double-dosing interval

3. Azithromycin: no data available; small amount excreted in urine

---

PEARL

The role of macrolides in the intensive care unit relates primarily to their excellent activity against atypical respiratory pathogens (*C. pneumoniae* and *M. pneumoniae*) and *Legionella* spp.

Adverse Effects

A. Gastrointestinal irritation (dose-related and more common with erythromycin): abdominal cramps, nausea, vomiting, diarrhea

B. Prolongation of QT interval and development of ventricular dysrhythmias including torsade de pointes (erythromycin). Use caution when administering with other drugs that prolong the QT interval.

C. Dysgeusia (clarithromycin)

D. Thrombophlebitis (IV use): particularly problematic with erythromycin, but minimized by appropriate dilution of dose and avoidance of rapid infusions

E. Allergic reactions, including skin rash, fever, and eosinophilia are uncommon.

F. Cholestatic hepatitis

1. Rare and almost always associated with the erythromycin estolate preparation

2. Occurs mainly in adults, usually after repeated courses or prolonged therapy (exceeding 10 days)

G. Reversible hearing loss (erythromycin)

1. May occur in patients with impaired hepatic or renal function or high doses of erythromycin (≥4 g/day)

2. Usually reverses 6 to 14 days after discontinuing or decreasing the dose of erythromycin

H. Use in pregnancy

1. Erythromycin and azithromycin: category B

2. Clarithromycin: category C

Bibliography

Alvarez-Elcoro S, Enzler MJ. The macrolides: erythromycin, clarithromycin, and azithromycin. Mayo Clin Proc 1999;74:613–634.

Bartlett JG, Dowell SF, Mandell LA, et al. Practice guidelines for the management of community-acquired pneumonia in adults. Infectious Diseases Society of America. Clin Infect Dis 2000;31:347–382.

Burnham TH, Short RM, Bell WL, et al (eds). Drug Facts and Comparisons. St. Louis: Facts and Comparisons 2001, pp 1300–1312.

Gikas A, Kofteridis DP, Manios A, et al. Newer macrolides as empiric treatment for acute Q fever infection. Antimicrob Agents Chemother 2001;45:3644–3646.

Gilbert DN, Moellering RC, Sande MA (eds). The Sanford Guide to Antimicrobial Therapy, 32st ed. Hyde Park, Vermont: Antimicrobial Therapy, Inc., 2002.

McEvoy GK (ed). Macrolides. In: American Hospital Formulary Service. Drug Information 2001. Bethesda, MD: American Society of Health-System Pharmacists, 2001, pp 271–314.

Steigbigel NH. Macrolides and clindamycin. In: Mandell GL, Bennett JE, Dolin R (eds). Principles and Practice of Infectious Diseases, 5th ed. Philadelphia: Churchill Livingstone, 2000, pp 366–382.

186 Antituberculosis Drugs

Dana G. Kissner

Overview

A. Goals and principles of treatment
1. Rapid sterilization of sputum: most effective method of preventing tissue damage and further spread of tuberculosis (TB)
   a. Suspect, diagnose, and treat disease quickly and efficiently.
   b. Select appropriate and most effective drugs.
   c. Assure adherence to treatment.
   d. Medications should be administered parenterally if adequate gastrointestinal (GI) absorption cannot be assured.
2. Prevention of drug resistance
   a. Approximately 1 of every 10^4 to 10^8 bacilli will spontaneously mutate and develop resistance to one drug. The more organisms there are, as in cavitary TB, the more likely it is that resistant organisms will emerge. Therefore,
   b. Treat with at least two drugs to which the organism is susceptible, so that each prevents emergence of tubercle bacilli resistant to the other.
   c. Obtain in vitro drug susceptibility studies on all first isolates, those obtained after three months of therapy, and when there is clinical evidence of poor response to treatment.
   d. However, because treatment needs to be initiated before results of in vitro susceptibility studies are available, resistance should be suspected when there is
      (1) A history of previously treated TB
      (2) A history of exposure to a drug-resistant case
      (3) Residence in, or origination from, an area where drug resistance is common: Asia, Central and South America, Africa, Russia
      (4) There is greater than 4% primary resistance to isoniazid in the community. Primary resistance is that which occurs in patients not previously treated with anti-TB medications. Secondary resistance refers to that which occurs in previously treated persons.
   e. If resistance is suspected, begin treatment with four drugs, at least two of which the patient (or the patient's drug-resistant contact) has not been exposed to.
   f. Never add a single agent to a failing regimen.
   g. Never use a single agent (isoniazid) preventively until active disease has been excluded.
3. Prevention of relapse, sterilization of disease sites
   a. Treat for a long enough time to achieve a cure.
   b. Treat with appropriate medications at sufficient doses: isoniazid, rifampin, or both are necessary for 6- to 9-month regimens; pyrazinamide for the first 2 months allows shortening of treatment duration of smear-positive TB to 6 months if rifampin can be administered.
   c. Assure that the patient continues to take medications. Directly observed therapy (DOT) should be available.
4. Control the transmission of TB within institutions.
   a. Isolation of TB suspects patients with known communicable TB
   b. Prompt initiation of appropriate chemotherapy
   c. Adequate ventilation to dilute the infectious droplet nuclei: 6 air exchanges/hour recommended by Centers for Disease Control and Prevention (CDC)
   d. Ultraviolet germicidal irradiation
   e. High-efficiency particulate aerosol (HEPA) filtration units
   f. Personal respiratory protective devices

Actions and Dosing

A. Isoniazid (INH)
1. Action: bactericidal against actively growing bacilli; inhibits the synthesis of cell wall components; most potent of the anti-TB drugs
2. Forms: parenteral (IM), tablets (100 and 300 mg), syrup (50 mg/5 mL)
3. Once daily dose: 5 mg/kg; maximum and usual adult dose 300 mg
4. Twice weekly dose: 15 mg/kg; maximum and usual adult dose 900 mg

5. Metabolized in the liver: acetylation rate genetically determined

6. Effect of renal failure: none, except perhaps in slow acetylators with creatinine clearance lower than 10 mL/min

7. Diffuses into fluids such as cerebrospinal fluid (CSF)

B. Rifampin (RIF)

1. Action: bactericidal against slow and intermittently growing bacilli; inhibits DNA-dependent RNA polymerase in mycobacteria; allows shortened duration of therapy (6 months)

2. Forms: parenteral (IV), capsules (150 and 300 mg), syrup (10 mg/mL)

3. Once daily dose: 10 mg/kg, maximum and usual adult dose 600 mg

4. Twice weekly dose: same as once daily

5. Significant liver dysfunction: reduce dose to 150 to 200 mg/day and monitor serum levels

6. No dose adjustment in renal failure

7. Diffuses into CSF when meninges are inflamed

C. Pyrazinamide (PZA)

1. Action: not active at pH >6

2. Forms: 500 mg tablets

3. Daily dose: 15 to 30 mg/kg, maximum 2 g; may be given in divided doses

4. Twice weekly dose: 50 to 70 mg/kg

5. Dosing in end-stage renal failure: 25 to 30 mg/kg 3 times a week, postdialysis (significant clearance by hemodialysis)

6. Diffuses into CSF

D. Combination tablets

1. Rifamate: INH 150 mg + RIF 300 mg; dose is twice daily

2. Rifater: INH 50 mg + RIF 120 mg + PZA 300 mg; dose is 4 times daily if less than 45 kg; 5 times daily if 45 to 54 kg; 6 times daily if 55 kg or more

E. Ethambutol (EMB)

1. Action: bactericidal at higher doses, bacteriostatic at lower doses; inhibits synthesis of metabolites; effective at preventing emergence of resistance when combined with INH

2. Forms: 100 and 400 mg tablets

3. Once daily dose: 25 mg/kg during initial phase of treatment (first 1 to 2 months), 15 mg/kg for continuation phase

4. Twice weekly dose: 50 mg/kg

5. Requires dose adjustment in renal insufficiency; 15 to 25 mg/kg 3 times a week in end-stage renal failure

6. Does not produce high levels in CSF, even with inflamed meninges

F. Streptomycin (SM)

1. Action: bactericidal in alkaline environment; interferes with protein synthesis

2. Forms: parenteral (IM; not FDA approved for IV use)

3. Once daily dose: 15 mg/kg (maximum 1000 mg) if age 60 years or less; 10 mg/kg if older than 60 years (maximum 750 mg)

4. Twice weekly dose: 25 to 30 mg/kg

5. Total cumulative dose 120 g, unless no other options exist

6. Dosing in renal insufficiency: loading dose of 5 to 7.5 mg/kg followed by usual daily dose (mg) × creatinine clearance (mL/min)/100; avoidance of SM or pharmacokinetic monitoring is advisable (can cause renal failure)

7. Does not enter CSF

G. Capreomycin (CA)

1. Once daily dose: 15 to 30 mg/kg, maximum 1 g (750 mg if age >60 years) IM

2. Dose should be reduced in the presence of renal insufficiency; renal toxicity more common than with SM.

H. Kanamycin: same form, dose, and renal effects as CA, but is FDA approved for IV use

I. Ethionamide (ETA)

1. Action: bacteriostatic derivative of isonicotinic acid

2. Form: 250 mg tablets

3. Daily dose: 15 to 20 mg/kg; maximum 1 g per day

4. No dose adjustment in renal failure

J. Para-aminosalicylic acid (PAS)

1. Action: bacteriostatic

2. Form: 500 mg and 1 g tablets, bulk powder, and delayed-release granules

3. Daily dose: 150 mg/kg, maximum 12 g per day

4. No dose adjustment in renal failure

K. Cycloserine (CS)

1. Action: bacteriostatic

2. Form: 250 mg capsules

3. Daily dose: 15 to 20 mg/kg, maximum 1 g per day

4. Renally excreted and cleared by dialysis; reduce dose in renal insufficiency (250 to 500 mg 3 times a week postdialysis in end-stage renal failure)

L. Amikacin (A)

1. Action: bactericidal

2. Forms: parenteral (IM or IV)

3. Once daily dose: 15 mg/kg
4. Dose adjustment required in renal insufficiency; nephrotoxic

M. Quinolones

1. Action: bactericidal; inhibit DNA gyrase; not FDA approved for TB treatment
2. Forms:
   a. Ciprofloxacin: parenteral (IV); 100, 250, 500, and 750 mg tablets; 5% and 10% oral suspension
   b. Ofloxacin: parenteral (IV); 200, 300, and 400 mg tablets
   c. Levofloxacin: parenteral (IV); 250, 500, and 750 mg tablets
3. Daily dose
   a. Few data available for TB treatment
   b. One approach is to adjust dose to achieve serum concentration several times higher than the minimum inhibitory concentration.
   c. Another approach is to use the dose recommended for treatment of other respiratory infections.
   d. Suggestions for initiation of treatment in ICU setting
      (1) Ciprofloxacin: 500 to 750 mg PO, or 400 mg IV every 12 hours
      (2) Ofloxacin: 200 to 400 mg PO or IV every 12 hours
      (3) Levofloxacin: 500 to 750 mg PO or IV daily
4. Reduce dose if creatinine clearance is less than 50 mL/min.

N. Rifabutin

1. Action: similar to rifampin
2. Form: 150 mg capsules
3. Dose: 300 mg PO daily

PEARLS

- Suspect drug resistance if there is more than 4% primary resistance to INH in community.
- HIV⁺ individuals may be exogenously reinfected during or after treatment.
- Never use a single drug to treat disease.
- Never add a single drug to a failing regimen.
- It is not the number of drugs used that determines treatment duration, but rather the specific ones.
- Anti-TB drugs available in parenteral form: INH, RIF, SM, CA, kanamycin, amikacin, ciprofloxacin, levofloxacin

---

Indications

A. First-line agents for the treatment of TB are INH, RIF, PZA, EMB, and SM. The following recommendations include HIV-infected persons if clinical and bacteriologic response is adequate.

1. Preferred: initiate with INH, RIF, PZA daily for 8 weeks. If drug resistance is suspected, add EMB or SM until susceptibility studies are available. Continue therapy with INH, RIF daily or 2 to 3 times/week for 4 months for drug-susceptible TB; RIF and EMB or SM may be continued when INH resistance alone is present. For smear and culture-negative TB, a total of 4 months of treatment may be adequate.

2. Administer isoniazid and RIF for 9 months. Where drug resistance is suspected, add PZA and EMB or SM until susceptibility studies are available. If INH resistance is present, continue RIF and EMB for at least 12 months.

B. Second-line agents for the treatment of active TB are CA, ETA, kanamycin, PAS, and CS. These medications are indicated when there is resistance or intolerance to first-line agents, or if there are contraindications. They are most useful in cases of multiple–drug-resistant TB (MDR-TB), defined as resistance to at least INH and RIF. They are less effective and more toxic than first-line drugs. For MDR-TB, five or more drugs may be necessary; chosen on the basis of susceptibility studies, if available. If unavailable, select drugs to which the patient (or contact) has not been previously exposed.

C. Newer agents have in vitro activity against *M. tuberculosis*, but they have been less vigorously studied for the treatment of TB, and are not approved by the FDA for this purpose. Amikacin, and the quinolones have in vitro activity against *M. tuberculosis*, but there is less clinical evidence regarding their efficacy and dosing. These may be used for MDR-TB, or when multiple other preferable agents are not tolerated.

D. Treatment of latent TB (also called preventive therapy): INH, RIF, and PZA have been shown to be useful in preventing disease in those at high risk for TB. High-risk groups include those who have been infected recently, or who have clinical conditions that are associated with an increased risk for progression from latent TB infection to active disease.

1. Indications for treatment of latent TB infection (preventive therapy)

   a. Positive skin test and no clinical, radiologic, or microbiological evidence of active disease

b. For those considered to have a positive skin test when reaction size is greater than 14 mm induration, the decision to treat should be individualized.

c. Note that age is not a factor in the decision to treat latent TB infection except for those in category b, above.

2. Treatment of latent TB infection (preventive therapy)

a. INH 300 mg/day for 9 months (preferred regimen for HIV-positive and HIV-negative individuals)

b. RIF 600 mg/day and PZA 1 to 2 g/day for 2 months (preferred for HIV positive individuals, acceptable in HIV-negative persons)

c. RIF 600 mg/day for 4 months is acceptable for HIV-positive and HIV-negative individuals.

E. Rifabutin may be substituted for RIF.

Major Side Effects and Interactions

A. Isoniazid

1. Hepatitis: may be life-threatening; risk increases with age and probably with co-infection with hepatitis C and co-administration of RIF. Asymptomatic elevation of liver function tests occurs in 10% to 20% of patients taking INH and do not require stopping the drug. Caution should be exercised in the presence of preexisting liver disease. Isoniazid should be avoided in the presence of acute serious liver disease.

2. Peripheral neuropathy (stocking and glove): may be caused by INH's ability to increase urinary excretion of pyridoxine. Supplementation with 10 mg per day of pyridoxine is advisable for chronically undernourished persons, alcoholics, adolescent girls, the elderly, pregnant women, uremic individuals, and those with cancer.

3. Other side effects: mild central nervous system effects; hypersensitivity reactions with fever, rash and a lupus-like syndrome; a variety of hematologic abnormalities

4. Interactions: phenytoin (increased serum concentrations of phenytoin and INH), disulfiram (unsteady gait, mental status changes)

B. Rifampin

1. Gastrointestinal upset (may subside with further treatment), hepatitis, cholestatic jaundice

2. Skin eruptions

3. Turns body fluids orange

4. Acute renal failure, thrombocytopenia, influenza-like syndrome, and hemolytic uremia when used at a dose greater than 10 mg/kg intermittently or when therapy is interrupted

5. Interactions

a. Rifampin induces hepatic cytochrome P450 system (CYP450) activity, and thus can accelerate degradation or elimination of protease inhibitors and nonnucleoside reverse transcriptase inhibitors (NNRTIs), azol antifungal agents, corticosteroids (including endogenous cortisol), warfarin, methadone and other opiates, anticonvulsants, antidysrhythmics, β-blockers, calcium channel blockers, benzodiazepines, and cyclosporine; rifabutin is a less active inducer of CYP450.

b. Other drugs that inhibit CYP450 can decrease elimination of RIF and other rifamycins, e.g., protease inhibitors and NNRTIs, azol antifungal agents, ciprofloxacin.

c. Co-administration of RIF (or rifabutin) and other drugs, such as ciprofloxacin or clarithromycin, may cause a lupus-like syndrome.

C. Pyrazinamide

1. Arthralgias associated with elevated serum uric acid levels

2. Erythematous pruritic rash (rarely requires discontinuation of the drug)

3. Gastrointestinal upset (usually resolves over time)

4. Hepatitis rare (resolves over 4 to 6 weeks)

D. Ethambutol: optic neuritis and vision impairments (occurs most commonly in doses higher than 25 mg/kg per day); hyperuricemia; GI upset

E. Streptomycin, CA, kanamycin, amikacin

1. Irreversible vestibular dysfunction or ataxia (especially with SM)

2. High-frequency hearing loss (irreversible, especially with amikacin or kanamycin)

3. Nephrotoxicity and electrolyte abnormalities (least common with SM)

4. Rash and fever

F. Ethionamide: dysgeusia, GI distress, diarrhea, hepatitis, arthralgias

G. Para-aminosalicylic acid: GI distress, nausea, bloating, diarrhea, rash, edema

H. Cycloserine: cognitive impairment, mood changes, psychosis, seizures

I. Quinolones: GI distress, headache, anxiety, tremulousness

Key Precautions

- Isoniazid: hepatitis, neuropathy

- Streptomycin: irreversible damage to eighth cranial nerve

- Rifampin: turns body fluids orange; induces CYP450; reduces serum levels of methadone, corticosteroids, warfarin; interacts in a complex way with protease inhibitors and nonnucleoside reverse-transcriptase inhibitors

Special Considerations

A. Surgical adjuncts to chemotherapy
   1. Resectional surgery: consider for
      a. Local resectable destructive cavitary disease likely to be a source of relapse and
      b. Persistence of MDR-TB by culture, despite prolonged (3 to 4 months) drug therapy
      c. Patterns of drug resistance unlikely to be cured with drugs
   2. Open drainage with Eloesser flap procedure for bronchopleural fistula (BPF); tube thoracostomy is contraindicated in tuberculous effusions without BPF
   3. Thoracoplasty for space problems
   4. Adjunctive surgery may be necessary for some forms of extrapulmonary TB.

B. Corticosteroids (to suppress aspects of the immune response that cause injury or severe symptoms)
   1. Pulmonary TB: symptoms and x-ray findings may improve more rapidly, but rebound occurs with discontinuation; dose is 40 to 60 mg prednisone per day, tapered over 4 to 8 weeks
   2. TB meningitis: not useful in early or late (coma) disease. In intermediate disease there may be benefit for survival, frequency of sequelae, and time to resolution of elevated CSF pressures. Dose is 8 to 12 mg per day dexamethasone, tapered over 6 to 8 weeks.
   3. TB pericarditis: may be useful in acute effusive stage to decrease amount and reaccumulation of fluid as well as mortality. Does not seem to decrease incidence of progression to constrictive disease. Dose is 60 mg prednisone, tapered over 6 to 12 weeks.

Bibliography

American Thoracic Society. Treatment of tuberculosis and tuberculosis infection in adults and children. Am J Respir Crit Care Med 1994;149:1359–1374.

American Thoracic Society. Targeted tuberculin testing and treatment of latent tuberculosis infection. Am J Respir Crit Care Med 2000;161:S221–S247.

Bradford WZ, Daley CL. Multiple drug-resistant tuberculosis. Infect Dis Clin North Am 1998;12:157–172.

Burman BJ, Jones BE. Treatment of HIV-related tuberculosis in the era of effective antiretroviral therapy. Am J Respir Crit Care Med 2001;164:7–12.

CDC. Notice to readers: Updated guidelines for the treatment and prevention of tuberculosis among HIV-infected patients taking protease inhibitors or nonnuclioside reverse transcriptase inhibitors. MMWR 2000;49:185–189.

Dooley DP, Carpenter JL, Rademacher S. Adjunctive corticosteroid therapy for tuberculosis: a critical reappraisal of the literature. Clin Infect Dis 1997;25:872–887.

Yew WW, Chan CK, Chau CH et al. Outcomes of patients with multidrug-resistant pulmonary tuberculosis treated with ofloxacin/levofloxacin-containing regimens. Chest 2000;117:744–751.

187 Miscellaneous Antibiotics

Jeff D. Huntress

Pharmacology

A. Vancomycin
1. Poorly absorbed from the gastrointestinal (GI) tract
2. Widely distributed in body tissues following IV administration, but does not readily distribute into cerebrospinal fluid (CSF) in the absence of inflammation
3. Elimination half-life with normal renal function averages 4 to 6 hours.
4. Only minimally removed by intermittent hemodialysis or peritoneal dialysis, but increasingly removed by continuous venovenous hemodialysis (CVVHD)

B. Carbapenems (imipenem cilistatin and meropenem)
1. Cilistatin inhibits the renal brush border enzyme dehydropeptidase I, which would otherwise hydrolyze and thus inactivate imipenem.
2. Widely distributed into most tissues
   a. Only low concentrations of imipenem (1% to 10% of concurrent serum concentration) appear in CSF.
   b. Meropenem penetrates into CSF, matching or exceeding concentrations required to inhibit most susceptible bacteria.
3. The elimination half-life of imipenem and meropenem averages 1 hour with normal renal function.

C. Quinupristin-dalfopristin (Synercid)
1. Combination of two streptogramins (30% quinupristin, 70% dalfopristin)
2. The elimination half-life of each component is less than 1 hour.
3. Biliary (fecal) excretion is the main elimination route for both parent drugs and their metabolites; urinary excretion accounts for less than 20%.

D. Linezolid
1. A synthetic oxazolidinone that may be administered orally or intravenously without dose adjustment
2. Rapidly and extensively absorbed after oral dosing, with 100% bioavailability
3. Readily distributes into well-perfused tissue and is primarily metabolized by oxidation to two inactive metabolites

4. Non-renal clearance accounts for about 65% of the total clearance; renal clearance is low, suggesting net tubular reabsorption.

E. Clindamycin
1. Oral bioavailability is about 90% for clindamycin HCl.
2. Distributes into many body tissues and fluids, but does not penetrate well into CSF (even in the presence of inflamed meninges)
3. About 10% of an oral dose of clindamycin is excreted in the urine, and 4% is excreted in feces as active drug and metabolites.
4. Plasma half-life is 2 to 3 hours with normal renal function; slightly longer with markedly reduced renal or hepatic function.

F. Metronidazole
1. Well absorbed from the GI tract; plasma levels are similar following equivalent oral and IV doses.
2. Widely distributed into most body tissues and fluids, including CSF
3. Readily crosses the placenta and is excreted into breast milk
4. 30% to 60% is metabolized by hepatic hydroxylation, side-chain oxidation, and glucuronide conjugation.
   a. Plasma half-life is 6 to 8 hours with normal renal and hepatic function.
   b. Half-life is not affected by changes in renal function, but may be prolonged in patients with impaired hepatic function.

Indications

A. Vancomycin
1. Serious infections caused by β-lactam-resistant Gram-positive organisms
2. Infections caused by Gram-positive organisms in patients who have serious allergies to β-lactam antimicrobials
3. Antibiotic-associated colitis that fails to respond to metronidazole or is severe and potentially life-threatening
4. Prophylaxis against endocarditis after certain procedures in patients at high risk
5. Prophylaxis for major surgical procedures involving implantation of prosthetic materials or

665

devices at institutions with a high prevalence of methicillin-resistant *Staphylococcus aureus* (MRSA) or methicillin-resistant *Staphylococcus epidermidis* (MRSE)

B. Imipenem and meropenem

1. Urinary tract infections, intra-abdominal infections, gynecologic infections, bacterial sepsis, bone and joint infections, skin and skin structure infections, endocarditis, polymicrobial infections, lower respiratory tract infections, febrile neutropenia, bacterial meningitis

2. Should not be used for the treatment of monobacterial infections when an agent with a narrower spectrum of activity would be effective

C. Quinupristin-dalfopristin

1. Infections caused by susceptible strains of vancomycin-resistant *Enterococcus faecium* (VREF) infections, including serious or life-threatening infections associated with concurrent VREF bacteremia

2. Complicated skin and skin structure infections caused by *Streptococcus pyogenes* or methicillin-susceptible *Staphylococcus aureus* (MSSA)

D. Linezolid

1. Treatment of VREF infections, including those associated with concurrent bacteremia

2. Community-acquired or nosocomial pneumonia caused by susceptible strains of *Streptococcus pneumoniae* (penicillin-susceptible strains only), MSSA, MRSA

3. Uncomplicated skin and skin structure infections caused by MSSA or *Streptococcus pyogenes,* and for complicated skin and skin structure caused by MSSA, MRSA, *Streptococcus pyogenes,* or *Streptococcus agalactiae*

E. Clindamycin

1. Useful alternative in penicillin-allergic patients where other less toxic antibiotics are contraindicated

2. Most often used as part of combination therapy (e.g., in combination with an aminoglycoside)

   a. Anaerobic bacterial infections: serious lower respiratory tract infections, serious skin and skin structure infections, sepsis, intra-abdominal infections, gynecologic infections, acute pelvic inflammatory disease

   b. Gram-positive aerobic bacterial infections: bone and joint infections caused by susceptible strains of *Staphylococcus aureus,* serious respiratory tract infections, skin and skin structure infections, sepsis, invasive group A streptococci, perioperative prophylaxis

   c. Intra-abdominal procedures

3. Other indications include bacterial vaginosis, alternative agent for endocarditis prophylaxis, post-traumatic endophthalmitis, malaria (in conjunction with oral quinine), toxoplasmosis (in combination with pyrimethamine), *Pneumocystis carinii* pneumonia (with primaquine, when standard therapy has failed).

F. Metronidazole

1. Anaerobic and (in combination with other agents) mixed aerobic-anaerobic bacterial infections

2. *Clostridium difficile* diarrhea

3. Other: trichomoniasis, amebiasis, giardiasis, bacterial vaginosis, pelvic inflammatory disease, *Helicobacter pylori* infections, perioperative prophylaxis

Key Indications

- Vancomycin: methicillin-resistant staphylococci

- Imipenem or meropenem: broad-spectrum Gram-negative, Gram-positive, and anaerobic coverage

- Quinupristin-dalfopristin or linezolid: Gram-positive aerobe coverage, including vancomycin-resistant *Enterococcus faecium*

- Clindamycin: anaerobic and Gram-positive aerobic bacterial infections

- Metronidazole: anaerobic infections

Actions and Spectrum of Activity

A. Vancomycin

1. Inhibits cell wall synthesis, impairs RNA synthesis, injures protoplasts

2. Bactericidal against most Gram-positive organisms except enterococci

3. Spectrum is largely limited to aerobic and anaerobic Gram-positive organisms, including staphylococci, *Streptococcus pneumoniae*, *Streptococcus pyogenes* (group A β-hemolytic streptococci), enterococci, *Corynebacterium* spp., *Clostridium* spp. (including *C. difficile*).

4. Vancomycin-resistant enterococci (*E. faecalis, E. faecium, and E. gallinarum*) have been reported with increasing frequency.

   a. Strains with high-level resistance generally require vancomycin concentrations of 128 μg/mL or more, whereas strains with low-level resistance generally require concentrations of 16 to 64 μg/mL for in vitro inhibition.

b. Some strains of VREF may be susceptible in vitro to linezolid or quinupristin-dalfopristin.

c. Strains of *Enterococcus faecalis* may be susceptible to linezolid in vitro, but these strains are resistant to quinupristin-dalfopristin.

5. Vancomycin-resistant staphylococci (*S. haemolyticus and S. epidermidis*) have been reported rarely; strains of MRSA with reduced susceptibility to vancomycin have been reported.

B. Imipenem and meropenem

1. Inhibit mucopeptide synthesis in the bacterial cell wall

2. Have a high degree of stability against hydrolysis by bacterial β-lactamases

3. Gram-positive spectrum

a. Usually covered: Group A, B, C, G streptococci, *Streptococcus pneumoniae*, viridans streptococci, MSSA, *Staphylococcus epidermidis*, *Listeria monocytogenes*, *Enterococcus faecalis* (imipenem)

b. Sometimes covered: *Enterococcus faecalis* (meropenem), *Enterococcus faecium* (imipenem)

c. Not covered: MRSA, *Enterococcus faecium* (meropenem)

4. Gram-negative spectrum

a. Usually covered: *Escherichia coli*, *Klebsiella* spp., *Enterobacter* spp., *Proteus mirabilis*, *Citrobacter* spp., *Serratia* spp., *Pseudomonas aeruginosa*, *Pseudomonas cepacia*, *Acinetobacter* spp., *Salmonella* spp., *Shigella* spp., *Haemophilus influenzae*, *Moraxella catarrhalis*, *Neisseria gonorrhoeae*, *Neisseria meningitidis*

b. Not covered: *Stenotrophomonas maltophilia*, *Legionella*

5. Anaerobic spectrum: *Peptostreptococcus* spp., *Bacteroides fragilis*

C. Quinupristin-dalfopristin

1. Inhibit bacteria protein synthesis: quinupristin inhibits peptide chain elongation, whereas dalfopristin directly interferes with peptidyl transferase

2. When resistance to only one of the streptogramin components occurs, the organism may continue to be inhibited but not killed.

3. Active only against Gram-positive organisms

a. Bacteriostatic against *Enterococcus faecium* and bactericidal against methicillin-susceptible and -resistant staphylococci

b. Active both in vitro and clinically against most strains of *Enterococcus faecium*, MSSA, and *Streptococcus pyogenes*, and in vitro (limited clinical experience) against most strains of *Corynebacterium jeikeium*, MRSA, *Staphylococcus epidermidis* (including MRSE), and *Streptococcus agalactiae*

4. Not active against *Enterococcus faecalis*

D. Linezolid

1. Interferes with bacterial protein synthesis

2. Bacteriostatic against enterococci and staphylococci, and bactericidal against most strains of streptococci

3. Clinically active against *Enterococcus faecium*, *Staphylococcus aureus* (including MRSA), *Streptococcus agalactiae*, *Streptococcus pneumoniae* (penicillin-susceptible strains only), *Streptococcus pyogenes*

4. Activity shown in vitro but clinical significance is unknown against *Enterococcus faecalis* (including vancomycin-resistant strains), *Enterococcus faecium* (vancomycin-susceptible strains), *Staphylococcus epidermidis* (including MRSE), *Staphylococcus haemolyticus*, *Streptococcus pneumoniae* (penicillin-resistant strains), viridans streptococci, *Pasteurella multocida*.

E. Clindamycin

1. Inhibits protein synthesis

2. Can be bacteriostatic or bactericidal in action, depending on the concentration of drug attained at the site of infection and the susceptibility of the infecting organism

3. Gram-positive aerobic activity: *Streptococcus pneumoniae* and other streptococci; methicillin-susceptible staphylococci

4. Anaerobic and microaerophilic Gram-negative and Gram-positive activity: microaerophilic streptococci, *Peptococcus* spp., *Peptostreptococcus* spp., *Bacteroides* spp., *Eubacterium* spp., *Fusobacterium* spp., *Propionibacterium* spp.

5. Active against *Actinomyces*

6. Not effective against *Enterococcus faecalis*

F. Metronidazole

1. Disrupts DNA and inhibits nucleic acid synthesis

2. Active against most obligatory anaerobic bacteria and many protozoa

a. Gram-negative anaerobic bacteria: *Fusobacterium* spp., *Bacteroides fragilis*, other *Bacteroides* spp.

b. Gram-positive anaerobic bacteria: *Clostridium* spp. (including *C. perfringens* and *C. difficile*), *Peptococcus* spp., *Peptostreptococcus* spp., *Eubacterium* spp.

c. Other organisms: *Helicobacter pylori, Trichomonas vaginalis, Entamoeba histolytica, Giardia lamblia*

3. *Actinomyces; Lactobacillus* spp.; *Propionibacterium acnes, Propionibacterium avidum,* and *Propionibacterium granulosum* are generally resistant to metronidazole.

Side Effects and Precautions

A. Vancomycin

1. Ototoxicity and nephrotoxicity occur rarely and are most likely to occur in patients who are receiving other ototoxic or nephrotoxic agents.

2. Very irritating to tissue; care must be taken to avoid extravasation.

3. Hypersensitivity reactions, including urticaria, exfoliative dermatitis, macular rashes, occur in 5% to 10% of patients.

4. Red man syndrome
   a. Possibly caused in part by release of histamine
   b. Characterized by a sudden drop in blood pressure, which can be accompanied by flushing, an erythematous rash of the face, neck, chest and upper extremities, wheezing, dyspnea, angioedema, urticaria, or pruritus
   c. Minimized by infusing over 1 or 2 hours

5. Hematologic: leukopenia, neutropenia, eosinophilia, and rarely thrombocytopenia

B. Imipenem and meropenem

1. Gastrointestinal: nausea, vomiting, diarrhea; *Clostridium difficile*-associated diarrhea and colitis have occurred during administration or after discontinuation of carbapenems

2. Hematologic: eosinophilia, transient leukopenia, neutropenia, agranulocytosis, pancytopenia, bone marrow depression, hemolytic anemia, thrombocytopenia

3. Neurologic: seizures (imipenem)

4. Miscellaneous: phlebitis, thrombophlebitis, rash, drug fever, transient increases in serum activity of aspartate aminotransferase, alanine aminotransferase, or alkaline phosphatase

C. Quinupristin-dalfopristin: venous irritation, arthralgias, myalgias, pseudomembranous colitis, hyperbilirubinemia

D. Linezolid

1. Myelosuppression: anemia, leukopenia, pancytopenia, thrombocytopenia
   a. Complete blood counts should be monitored weekly in patients who receive linezolid, particularly those who receive it for longer than 14 days, those with preexisting myelosuppression, and those receiving concomitant drugs that produce bone marrow suppression.
   b. Consider discontinuation in patients who develop or have worsening myelosuppression.

2. Gastrointestinal: nausea, dyspepsia, abdominal pain, diarrhea, pseudomembranous colitis

3. Miscellaneous: headache, oral and vaginal moniliasis, hypertension

E. Clindamycin

1. Gastrointestinal: anorexia, nausea, vomiting, esophagitis, bloating, abdominal pain, antibiotic-associated diarrhea, tenesmus, flatulence, colitis, weight loss

2. Hematologic: neutropenia, eosinophilia, thrombocytopenia, agranulocytosis

3. Miscellaneous: morbilliform rash, thrombophlebitis, transient hyperbilirubinemia, transient increases in serum alkaline phosphatase or aspartate aminotransferase activity

F. Metronidazole

1. Gastrointestinal: unpleasant metallic taste, nausea, abdominal discomfort, diarrhea

2. Neurologic: headache, peripheral neuropathy (use with caution in patients with central nervous system diseases)

3. Hematologic: mild, transient leukopenia and thrombocytopenia reported rarely

4. Hypersensitivity reactions: urticaria, pruritus, erythematous rash, flushing, fever

5. Use with caution and with reduced dosage in patients with severe hepatic impairment.

Key Dosing of Vancomycin in Renal Dysfunction

- Creatine clearance (C_{cr}) >65 mL/minute: dose every 12 hours
- C_{cr} 35 to 65 mL/minute: dose every 24 hours
- C_{cr} 20 to 34 mL/minute: dose every 48 hours
- C_{cr} <20 mL/minute should have individualized dosing based on serum concentration monitoring.

Typical Dosing

A. Vancomycin

1. Usual IV dose with normal renal function: 1 g (12 to 15 mg/kg actual body weight) every 12 hours

a. Hemodialysis patients typically require maintenance dosing every 4 to 7 days. Re-dosing should be guided by serum concentrations that fall into the 5 to 15 μg/mL range, depending on the severity of the infection.

b. Patients receiving CVVHD usually require dosing every 24 hours.

2. Bacterial endocarditis: typical dose is 1 g intravenously every 12 hours

3. Prophylaxis of enterococcal endocarditis in penicillin-allergic patients at high or moderate risk: a single 1 g dose given over 1 to 2 hours with the infusion completed within 30 minutes of the start of the procedure

4. Perioperative prophylaxis when a cephalosporin cannot be used or when use of vancomycin is considered necessary because of a high incidence of methicillin-resistant staphylococci: a single 1 g dose of vancomycin may be given just prior to the procedure

5. Oral dosage for *Clostridium difficile*–associated diarrhea and colitis that fails to respond to metronidazole: 125 mg four times daily for 7 to 10 days

B. Imipenem and meropenem

1. Imipenem: usual dose is 250 to 500 mg every 6 to 12 hours, not to exceed 50 mg/kg per day or 4.0 g/day, whichever is lower

a. Dose adjustment required in renal dysfunction

b. Moderately dialyzable (20% to 50%); administer dose post-dialysis

2. Meropenem: usual dose is 1 g intravenously every 8 hours

a. Dose adjustment is required in renal dysfunction.

b. Should be re-dosed after dialysis

C. Quinupristin-dalfopristin

1. Administered by IV infusion in 5% dextrose in water only (incompatible with saline) over 60 minutes

2. Central venous route is preferred, but peripheral administration is possible as long as the patient is monitored for venous irritation.

3. Treatment of VREF: 7.5 mg/kg every 8 hours

4. Treatment of complicated skin and skin structure infections: 7.5 mg/kg every 12 hours

5. No dosage adjustment is required for use in patients with renal insufficiency.

6. Pharmacokinetic data in patients with hepatic cirrhosis suggest that a dosage reduction may be necessary in these patients, but exact recommendations are currently unavailable.

D. Linezolid

1. Vancomycin-resistant *Enterococcus faecium* infections, including concurrent bacteremia: 600 mg intravenously or orally every 12 hours for 14 to 28 days

2. Uncomplicated skin and skin structure infections: 400 mg oral every 12 hours for 10 to 14 days

3. Community-acquired pneumonia (including concurrent bacteremia), nosocomial pneumonia, complicated skin and skin structure infections: 600 mg intravenously or orally every 12 hours for 10 to 14 days

4. Methicillin-resistant *Staphylococcus aureus* infections: 600 mg every 12 hours

E. Clindamycin

1. 600 mg intravenously every 8 hours is usually recommended; 900 mg intravenously every 8 hours is preferred for some gynecologic infections and morbidly obese patients.

2. Duration of therapy depends on the type and severity of infection.

3. Dosage adjustment may be required in patients with severe renal or hepatic impairment.

F. Metronidazole

1. Anaerobic bacterial infections

a. Loading dose is 15 mg/kg intravenously followed by a maintenance dose of 7.5 mg/kg intravenously every 6 to 8 hours; typical dosing for a 70 kg adult is 500 mg intravenously or orally every 6 or 8 hours.

b. Because of the long half-life, doses can be

Key Dosing of Carbapenems in Renal Dysfunction

Imipenem ciliastatin

- C_{cr} >70 mL/minute per 1.73 m²: 500 mg every 6 hours

- C_{cr} 30 to 70 mL/minute per 1.73 m²: 500 mg every 8 hours

- C_{cr} 20 to 29 mL/minute per 1.73 m² (or CVVHD use): 500 mg every 12 hours

- C_{cr} 5 to 19 mL/minute per 1.73 m²: 250 mg every 12 hours

Meropenem

- C_{cr} 26 to 50 mL/minute: 1 g every 12 hours

- C_{cr} 10 to 25 mL/minute: 500 mg every 12 hours

- C_{cr} <10 mL/minute: 500 mg every 24 hours

given at 6-, 8-, or 12-hour intervals; higher doses given at one time may cause more GI side effects.

c. The maximum recommended daily dose (IV or PO) is 4 g.

2. *Clostridium difficile*–associated diarrhea

a. 250 mg PO every 6 hours, or 500 mg intravenously every 6 to 8 hours, for 10 to 14 days

b. Oral therapy is preferred but intravenous therapy is appropriate for patients unable to receive enteral therapy.

B Bibliography

Cantú TG, Yamanaka-Yuen NA, Lietman PS. Serum vancomycin concentrations: reappraisal of their clinical value. Clin Infect Dis 1994;18:533–543.

Clemett D, Markham A. Linezolid. Drugs 2000;59:815–827.

Hellinger WC, Brewer NS. Carbapenems and monobactams: imipenem, meropenem, and aztreonam. Mayo Clin Proc 1999;74:420–434.

McEvoy GK (ed). American Hospital Formulary Service. Drug Information 2001. Bethesda: American Society of Health-System Pharmacists, 2001.

Reese RE, Betts RF, Gumustop B. Handbook of Antibiotics, 3rd ed. Philadelphia: Lippincott Williams & Wilkins, 2000.

188 Antifungal Therapy

Peter K. Linden

The decision to initiate antifungal therapy optimally is based on laboratory (mycologic and serologic) studies or histopathological evidence of fungal infection. Obtaining these results, however, takes time. Accordingly, in rapidly deteriorating or critically ill patients, empiric antifungal therapy is often prescribed in an effort to decrease morbidity and risk of death. Superficial (dermatophyte) infections are not addressed in this chapter

Classification and Pharmacology

A. Polyene class

  1. Polyenes are naturally occurring compounds.

    a. These agents exert antifungal activity by binding to the sterol component (ergosterol) of fungal membranes.

    b. This action increases the permeability of fungal cells, leading to the leakage of cytosolic contents and cell death on this basis.

  2. Amphotericin B

    a. Produced by *Streptomyces nodosus*

    b. Available as a colloidal suspension in a solution containing sodium desoxycholate and sodium phosphate (amphotericin B desoxycholate)

    c. Pharmacokinetics

      (1) 95% bound to serum proteins

      (2) Rapid uptake from intravascular space to multiple viscera

      (3) Blood levels not affected by either hepatic or renal failure

      (4) Concentration in inflamed tissue is less than 70% of serum concentration.

      (5) Penetrates poorly into normal or inflamed meninges

    d. Antifungal spectrum of activity

      (1) Amphotericin B has the broadest spectrum of all available antifungal agents.

      (2) In vitro susceptibility testing does not provide dependable prediction of clinical outcome.

      (3) Almost all *Candida* spp. are susceptible to amphotericin B, although many strains of *C. lusitaniae* are resistant.

      (4) *Cryptococcus neoformans*

      (5) Dimorphic fungi, including *Histoplasmosis encapsulatum, Coccidioides immitis, Blastomyces dermatiditis*

      (6) *Aspergillus, Fusaria,* and most other mycelial pathogens

      (7) Zygomycetes (*Mucor, Rhizomucor, Rhizopus,* others)

      (8) Pigmented molds (*Dactylaria*)

    e. Amphotericin B lipid formulations

      (1) The three marketed lipid amphotericin B products are amphotericin B lipid complex, amphotericin B colloidal dispersion, and liposomal amphotericin B.

      (2) These formulations differ with respect to the type of lipid complexed with amphotericin B, physical structure, pharmacokinetics, approved antifungal spectrum, infusion-related toxicity, and cost.

      (3) All appear to be less nephrotoxic than amphotericin B based upon comparative data, but all are significantly more expensive than amphotericin B (Table 188–1).

  3. Nystatin

    a. Polyene produced by *Streptomyces noursei*

    b. Available as an oral suspension (100,000 U/mL), lozenges, tablets and powder for topical mucosal therapy against oral/esophageal candidiasis or selective bowel decontamination

    c. Fungal spectrum includes *Candida* spp. and other yeasts.

B. Azole class

  1. The azoles class includes an imidazole (ketoconazole) and two triazoles (fluconazole and itraconazole). Their antifungal activity is based on interference with a fungal cytochrome P-450 enzyme, which converts lanosterol to ergosterol (the major steroid of most fungal membranes).

  2. Ketoconazole

    a. Second-line agent for itraconazole-intolerant patients

    b. Limited spectrum of activity

    c. Requires gastric acidity for absorption after enteric administration

    d. Plagued by adverse side effects and numerous drug interactions

    e. Pharmacology

TABLE 188–1. CLINICAL DIFFERENCES BETWEEN THREE LIPID AMPHOTERICIN PRODUCTS

	AMPHOTERICIN B LIPID COMPLEX (ABLC)	AMPHOTERICIN B COLLOIDAL DISPERSION (ABCD)	LIPOSOMAL AMPHOTERICIN B
Proprietary name	Abelcet	Amphotec	(AmBisome)
Infusion-toxicity*	Lower	Higher	Lower
Nephrotoxicity*	Lower	Lower	Lower
Approved indications†	All mycoses	*Aspergillus*	*Aspergillus, Candida, Cryptococcus*, febrile neutropenia
Daily dose (mg/kg per day)			
Yeast	3	3 to 6	3
Mycelia	5	—	5
Cost‡	$300 to $350	$200 to $250	$600 to $1,000

*Compared to amphotericin B
†All three agents are second-line therapy for amphotericin-refractory or amphotericin-intolerance
‡Pharmacy-acquisition costs ($US) for 70 kg patient at 5 mg/kg per day

(1) Available as 200 mg and 400 mg tablets

(2) Serum protein binding exceeds 99%.

(3) Penetrates well into most tissues except cerebrospinal fluid (CSF), eye, and urinary tract

(4) Excreted in bile as inactive metabolites

  f. Antifungal spectrum

    (1) *H. capsulatum*

    (2) *B. dermatiditis*

    (3) *C. immitis*

    (4) Paracoccidioidomycosis

    (5) *Pseudallescheria boydii*

    (6) *Candida* spp.

3. Fluconazole

  a. This agent is the mainstay of azole therapy due to its favorable pharmacological and safety profile and its activity against a broad spectrum of fungal pathogens.

  b. Pharmacology

    (1) Available as oral (50, 100, 150, and 200 mg tablets) and parenteral formulations (10 to 40 mg/mL)

    (2) Oral formulation does not require gastric acidity for absorption and is 85% to 90% bioavailable.

    (3) Penetrates most important body tissues and fluid compartments

    (4) Metabolized in liver, but 80% is excreted unchanged in the urine

  c. Fungal spectrum

    (1) *Candida* spp. (except *C. glabrata* and *C. krusei*)

    (2) *Cryptococcus neoformans*

    (3) *H. capsulatum*

    (4) *C. immitis*

    (5) *Blastomyses dermatitidis*

    (6) *Sporothrix schenkii*

4. Itraconazole

  a. This agent is a broad-spectrum triazole with enhanced activity in aspergillosis, sporotrichosis, cryptococcosis, and coccidioidomycosis, but pharmacological and toxicological characteristics are less favorable than those for fluconazole.

  b. Pharmacology

    (1) Available in 100 mg oral capsules, but the oral suspension (10 mg/mL) achieves more predictable serum levels and is pH-insensitive

    (2) Parenteral formulation approved in year 2000

  c. Antifungal spectrum

    (1) *S. schenkii*

    (2) *H. capsulatum*

    (3) *B. dermatitidis*

    (4) *Aspergillus* spp.

    (5) *C. neoformans*

    (6) *C. immitis*

    (7) *Candida* spp.

    (8) Paracoccidioidomycosis

    (9) Chromomycosis

5. 5-Flucytosine (5-FC)

  a. This agent is a competitive inhibitor of fungal DNA synthesis. It is useful as a therapeutic adjunct in combination with either amphotericin B or fluconazole in the therapy of candidiasis or cryptococcosis. It is rarely used alone.

  b. Pharmacology

    (1) Available only as an oral formulation (250 and 500 mg capsules)

    (2) Undergoes rapid and complete absorption

    (3) Little protein binding

(4) 90% of dose is excreted unchanged in the urine.

(5) Urinary levels greater than plasma levels

c. Antifungal spectrum

(1) *Candida* spp.

(2) *C. neoformans*

(3) Chromomycosis

6. Other systemic antifungals for critically ill patients

a. Miconazole: indicated for infections caused by *Pseudallescheria boydii* and other unusual mycelial infections

b. Voriconazole

(1) Investigational agent currently in phase 3 trials for treatment of infections caused by *Candida* and *Aspergillus* spp.

(2) Parenteral azole with a broad spectrum of antifungal activity

c. Caspofungin

(1) Recently approved as second line therapy for invasive aspergillosis

(2) Chitin-synthesis inhibitor with broad activity against yeast and mycelia

Typical Dosing

A. Amphotericin B (Fungizone)

1. A test dose of 1 mg should only be employed in patients suspected to be at risk for anaphylaxis.

2. Immediate escalation to the intended daily therapeutic dose is both safe and important for clinical efficacy.

3. General daily dose ranges are 0.3 to 1.5 mg/kg per day (depending on the specific fungal infection).

4. The drug should be administered as a daily single 2- to 4-hour infusion.

B. Nystatin

1. 100,000 units every 4 to 6 hours

2. Higher doses (2 to 8 million U/day) are used in selective bowel decontamination.

C. Ketoconazole (Nizoral)

1. 200 to 800 mg/day

2. Serum levels should be monitored in liver failure.

3. No dosage adjustment for dialysis

D. Fluconazole (Diflucan).

1. Recommended dose is 200 to 800 mg/day.

2. Avoid doses lower than 400 mg/day in serious infections.

3. Reduce dose by 50% for creatinine clearance (C_{Cr}) 11 to 50 mL/min.

4. Administer after dialysis.

5. Monitoring of drug levels is suggested in patients with renal failure to keep the plasma level in the 6 to 20 μg/mL range.

6. Consider fungal mean inhibitory concentration (MIC) testing in candidal infections that fail to respond to therapy.

E. Itraconazole (Sporanox)

1. 200 mg/day for oral candidiasis

2. Higher doses (400 to 600 mg/day) for aspergillosis and endemic mycoses

3. No adjustment of oral dosing is required for patients with renal failure or receiving dialysis.

4. Because of accumulation of cyclodextran, use of the parenteral formulation is contraindicated when C_{Cr} is lower than 30 mL/minute.

F. 5-FC (Ancobon)

1. 150 mg/kg per day administered orally in 4 divided doses every 6 hours

2. Total daily doses decreased to 75 mg/kg with C_{Cr} 26 to 50 mL/min and to 37 mg/kg with C_{Cr} 13 to 25 mL/minute

3. Peak 5-FC levels (drawn 2 hours after dosing) should be 50 to 100 μg/mL to avoid toxicity.

G. Miconazole: 800 mg intravenously every 8 hours

Side Effects

A. Amphotericin B

1. Adverse reactions include both acute "infusion-related" events and subacute or chronic effects from the cumulative actions of the drug.

2. Shaking, chills, fever, tachypnea, and dyspnea may occur during infusion and last for several hours.

3. Patients with underlying cardiac or respiratory disease are at higher risk for significant morbidity from cardiac ischemia or respiratory fatigue.

4. Acetaminophen (650 mg oral dose) and diphenhydramine (25 to 50 mg oral dose) prior to infusion may reduce the severity of these effects.

5. Meperidine (25 to 50 mg intravenously) is the treatment of choice for severe rigors.

6. Administering hydrocortisone (25 to 100 mg intravenously) prior to infusing amphotericin B is of doubtful benefit.

7. Anaphylactoid reactions (urticaria, bronchospasm, hypotension) are extremely rare.

8. Nephrotoxicity

a. Dose-dependent; due to renal afferent arteriolar vasoconstriction and tubular damage

b. Findings include a transient or permanent

Key Indications and Dosing

Fungal Infection	First-Line Therapy	Alternative(s)
• Invasive candidiasis†	Amphotericin B (0.6 mg/kg per day) ± 5-FC	Fluconazole (400 to 800 mg/day) ± 5-FC (excluding *C. krusei* and *C. glabrata*)
• Invasive aspergillosis‡	Amphotericin B (1.0 to 1.5 mg/kg per day), surgical excision of isolated lesions (lung, brain)	Amphotericin lipid formulations or itraconazole (400 mg/day)
• Cryptococcosis	Amphotericin B (0.4 to 0.6 mg/kg per day) + 5-FC (150 mg/kg per day)	Fluconazole (400 mg/day) ± 5-FC
• Mucorales (*Mucor, Rhizomucor, Rhizopus*, others)	Amphotericin B (1.0 to 1.5 mg/kg per day), early surgical debridement	Amphotericin lipid formulations
• Histoplasmosis (disseminated)	Amphotericin B (0.6 to 1.0 mg/kg per day) or itraconazole (400 mg/day)	Itraconazole (400 mg/day); first-line therapy for mild disease
• Coccidioidomycosis§	Fluconazole (400 to 800 mg/day) for pulmonary, extrapulmonary, or meningitis	Itraconazole (400 mg/day) or amphotericin B (0.6 to 1.0 mg/kg per day)

*5-FC = flucytosine.

†Amphotericin B and fluconazole have shown therapeutic equivalency in neutropenic and non-neutropenic candidemia. Amphotericin B + 5-FC has shown better response rates in candidal peritonitis. Optimal cumulative amphotericin B dose is not established, but usually is at least 7 to 15 mg/kg. Usual duration of fluconazole is a minimum of 14 days.

‡Benefits of concomitant amphotericin B and itraconazole not known. Optimal cumulative dose of amphotericin B is not established, but usually is a minimum of 2.0 to 2.5 g.

§Duration of fluconazole therapy for pulmonary and nonmeningeal extrapulmonary disease is a minimum of 12 to 18 months. Meningeal disease requires treatment indefinitely.

decrease in glomerular filtration rate and electrolyte (K^+, Mg^{2+}) wasting.

    c. Hypovolemia, age, concomitant administration of other nephrotoxins, preexisting renal insufficiency, daily and cumulative dose, all correlate with nephrotoxicity.

  9. Other important but less common toxicities include bone marrow suppression (usually normocytic anemia and less frequently leukopenia or thrombocytopenia), gastrointestinal disturbances, and phlebitis.

B. Nystatin: toxicity consists of gastrointestinal disturbances

C. Ketoconazole

  1. Gastrointestinal (decreased with food intake)

  2. Rash

  3. Elevated serum transaminase activity (2% to 10%)

  4. Symptomatic hepatitis (1 per 10,000)

  5. Hypoadrenalism

  6. Hypogonadism (decreased libido, gynecomastia)

D. Fluconazole

  1. Gastrointestinal (1% to 4%)

  2. Headache

  3. Rash

  4. Transient increase in serum transaminase activity (1%)

  5. Reversible alopecia

E. Itraconazole

  1. Gastrointestinal

  2. Headache

  3. Rash

  4. Pruritus

  5. Dizziness

  6. Mild, reversible elevations of serum transaminase activity (1% to 7%)

  7. Hypokalemia

  8. Hypertension with long-term therapy

  9. Causes significant inhibition of cytochrome P-450 enzymes, leading to potentiation of the effects of numerous concomitantly administered drugs (e.g., cyclosporine, tacrolimus, digoxin, terfenadine, astemizole, oral hypoglycemics, and cholesterol-lowering agents, among others)

F. 5-flucytosine

  1. Rash

2. Diarrhea

3. Hepatic dysfunction

4. Bone marrow suppression (leukopenia, thrombocytopenia) is more common in patients with renal insufficiency caused by drug accumulation.

G. Miconazole: significant toxicity effects (e.g., cardiac dysrhythmias) can occur if the drug is infused too rapidly

Special Considerations

A. Fungal pathogens

1. Definitive identification of the fungal pathogen responsible for the infection usually narrows the choice to only one or two potential antifungal agents.

2. Presumptive identification is based on body fluid or tissue stains showing yeast or mycelia.

   a. Pseudohyphae: *C. albicans*

   b. 45-degree dichotomous branching forms: most likely *Aspergillus* spp., but other mycelia, such as *Fusaria* and *Dactylaria*, are possible.

   c. 90-degree broad-branching forms: probably *Mucor* or other *Zygomycetes* spp.

3. Empiric therapy before culture results are available is warranted in certain clinical situations.

   a. Neutropenia and persistent fever of longer than 5 to 7 days in duration despite empiric antibacterial chemotherapy

   b. Patients at high risk for developing candidemia, candidal peritonitis, or disseminated candidiasis, with clinical findings suggestive of fungal infection

   c. Cavitating or noncavitating pulmonary nodule(s) and a clinical picture consistent with aspergillosis

   d. Enhancing mass lesion evident in the brain by computed tomography (CT) or magnetic resonance imaging (MRI) in a patient felt to be at high risk for cerebral aspergillosis

B. Documented or suspected antifungal resistance

1. *C. krusei* and most strains of *C. glabrata* are resistant to fluconazole.

2. Consider fluconazole resistance in any candidal infection that fails to respond to fluconazole.

3. Mean inhibitory concentration testing for susceptibility to fluconazole can be performed.

4. Consider in vitro testing for non-albicans *Candida* spp to ensure susceptibility to 5-FC.

5. *C. lusitaniae* is usually resistant to amphotericin B.

6. Mycelial organisms may have variable susceptibility to both amphotericin B and the azoles.

7. Consider reference laboratory susceptibility testing for these organisms.

   a. *Fusaria* spp.

   b. *Pseudallescheria boydii*

   c. *Trichosporon beigelii*

   d. *Curvularia*

   e. *Dactylaria*

   f. Mucorales and related species

C. Special anatomic site(s) of fungal infection

1. Central nervous system

   a. Lower amphotericin B concentrations in the meninges and CSF may compromise efficacy.

   b. Consider supplementing systemic amphotericin B with intrathecal amphotericin B (0.1 to 0.3 mg/day via intrathecal or intraventricular route) for meningitis due to *C. immitis* or *Candida*, and for refractory cryptococcal meningitis.

2. Lower urinary tract

   a. Except for cases caused by fluconazole-resistant strains, efficacy for the treatment of candidal cystitis is similar for a 5-day course of systemic fluconazole or a 2-day course of bladder irrigation with amphotericin B (50 mg/day).

   b. Consider presence of a "fungus ball" or renal candidiasis if there is no response to treatment or relapse.

3. Candidal endocarditis almost always requires valve replacement and a minimum of 6 to 10 weeks of amphotericin B (0.6 mg/kg per day) + 5-FC.

4. Candidal peritonitis associated with peritoneal dialysis

   a. Treated with fluconazole (200 mg/day) + 5-FC (1 to 2 g/day), or continuous intraperitoneal amphotericin (1.5 mg amphotericin/L dialysis fluid) for 4 to 6 weeks

   b. Consider removal of the peritoneal dialysis catheter for infections failing to respond to treatment.

5. Rhinocerebral mucormycosis mandates early surgical debridement to achieve "clean" surgical margins, since this infection responds poorly to antifungal therapy alone.

D. Severity of illness

1. Use the parenteral route in septic patients and patients with disturbances of gastrointestinal motility or absorption.

2. Document the adequacy of serum levels if the oral route is used.

E. Organ toxicity

1. Strategies to limit renal toxicity of amphotericin B
   a. Infuse 500 mL of normal saline 30 minutes before giving the drug.
   b. Avoid concomitant administration of other nephrotoxins.
   c. Avoid intravascular volume depletion.
   d. Use lipid-based formulations of amphotericin B.
   e. Use triazole therapy if evidence for comparable efficacy is available.
   f. Avoid unnecessarily high daily or cumulative doses of amphotericin B.
2. Strategies to minimize bone marrow suppression
   a. Consider administration of erythropoietin.
   b. Consider administration of filgrastim.
F. Antifungal–antifungal synergism
   1. Amphotericin B + 5-FC
      a. Cryptococcal meningitis
      b. Candidal infection
   2. Fluconazole + 5-FC for cryptococcal meningitis
G. Antifungal–antifungal antagonism
   1. Sterol synthesis inhibitors (azoles) and the sterol degrader (amphotericin B) are antagonistic in some in vitro and animal models of infection with yeast and *Aspergillus* infections.
   2. However, the clinical significance of this finding is unknown.
H. Antifungal-drug interactions
   1. Potentiation of nephrotoxicity can occur when amphotericin B is used along with other nephrotoxins (e.g., cyclosporine A, tacrolimus, IV contrast agents, cis-platinum).
   2. Azole + drugs metabolized by cytochrome P-450 3A4
      a. This interaction should not influence the decision to use an azole.
      b. It is critical, however, to monitor the potential interaction, which can have serious or even fatal sequelae.
I. Cost should be only one of several issues considered when choosing among antifungal agents.
   1. Amphotericin lipid formulations are the most expensive (see Table 188–1).
   2. Amphotericin B (0.3 to 1.0 mg/kg per day) costs $8 to $25 per day.
   3. Nystatin (500,000 to 2,000,000 U/day) costs $2 to $8 per day.
   4. Fluconazole (400 mg/day)
      a. Parenteral formulation costs $120 per day.
      b. Oral formulation costs $22 per day.
   5. Itraconazole (400 mg/day)
      a. Oral tablet costs $25 per day.
      b. Oral suspension costs $26 per day.
   6. 5-FC (150 mg/kg per day) costs $90 per day to treat a 70 kg patient.

Key Treatment Points

- Empiric therapy before culture results are available is warranted in certain clinical situations (e.g., persistent fever for longer than 5 to 7 days despite adequate empiric antibacterial chemotherapy in a neutropenic patient, cavitating or noncavitating pulmonary nodules with a clinical picture consistent with aspergillosis, presence of an enhancing mass lesion on brain by CT or MRI in a patient at high risk for cerebral aspergillosis).

- Definitive identification of the fungal pathogens responsible for the infection usually narrows the choice to only one or two potential antifungal agents.

- Use the parenteral route in septic patients and in patients with disturbances of gastrointestinal motility or absorption.

- Consider supplementing systemic amphotericin B with intrathecal amphotericin B (0.1 to 0.3 mg/day via intrathecal or intraventricular route) for meningitis due to *C. immitis, Candida,* and for refractory cryptococcal meningitis.

- Except for cases caused by fluconazole-resistant strains, efficacy for the treatment of candidal cystitis is similar for a 5-day course of systemic fluconazole or a 2-day course of bladder irrigation with amphotericin B (50 mg/day).

- Potentiation of nephrotoxicity can occur when amphotericin B is used along with other nephrotoxins (e.g., cyclosporine A, tacrolimus, IV contrast agents, cis-platinum).

Bibliography

Kauffman CA, Carver PL. Antifungal agents in the 1990s. Current status and future developments. Drugs 1997;53: 539–549.

Patel R. Antifungal agents. Part I. Amphotericin B preparations and flucytosine. Mayo Clin Proc 1998;73:1205–1225.

Rex JH, Pfaller MA, Galgiani JN, et al. Development of interpretive breakpoints for antifungal susceptibility testing: conceptual framework and analysis of in vitro-in vivo correlation data for fluconazole, itraconazole and Candida infections. Subcommittee on Antifungal Susceptibility Testing of the National Committee for Clinical Laboratory Standards. Clin Infect Dis 1997;24:235–247.

Robinson RF, Nahata MC. A comparative review of conventional and lipid formulations of amphotericin B. J Clin Pharm Ther 1999;24:249–257.

Summers KK, Hardin TC, Gore SJ, et al. Therapeutic drug monitoring of systemic antifungal therapy. J Antimicrob Chemother 1997;40:753–764.

Terrell CL. Antifungal agents. Part II. The azoles. Mayo Clin Proc 1999;74:78–100.

189 Endotracheal Intubation

James A. Kruse

Key Indications

- Airway control in the unconscious patient

- Upper airway obstruction, trauma, bleeding, or edema

- Delivery of high concentrations of supplemental oxygen

- Use of mechanical ventilation

- Bronchoscopy in unstable patient

- Tracheobronchial suctioning

Procedure

A. Identify anatomic factors heralding potentially difficult intubation.

1. Short neck: thyromental distance less than 6 cm or 3 to 4 finger breadths during extension

2. Limited gape: interdental gap less than 5 cm or 2 to 3 finger breadths

3. Protruding incisors, poor dentition, high arched palate, or macroglossia

4. Limitation in neck extension, e.g., cervical arthritis

5. Decreased mobility of temporomandibular joint

6. Receding mandible or inability to protrude mandible beyond upper incisors

7. Marked obesity

8. Facial trauma

9. Inability of conscious patient to flex neck and touch chin to chest

10. History of difficult intubation, rheumatoid arthritis, ankylosing spondylitis, or congenital deformities of face or neck

11. Modified Mallampati classification (assess ability to visualize faucial pillars, soft palate, and uvula while patient is seated with tongue fully protruded)

    a. Class I (complete visualization of all three structures): near 100% chance of visualizing glottis; easy intubation

    b. Class II (only uvula is not visualized): much less likely to visualize glottis, but probably can intubate without problem

    c. Class III (only soft palate is visualized): unlikely to visualize glottis; difficult intubation

    d. Class IV (none of the above structures visualized): unlikely to visualize glottis; very difficult intubation

12. Possible cervical spine injury (necessitates use of blind nasotracheal intubation, application of continuous cervical traction during orotracheal intubation, or establishment of surgical airway)

B. Preparation

1. Explain procedure to patient and obtain informed consent, if possible.

2. If not urgent, make patient n.p.o., stop enteral feeding, and delay procedure (ideally, at least 6 hours after solid food or tube feeding and 3 hours after clear liquids).

3. For conscious patients at risk for aspiration, decide on method.

    a. Awake intubation (with topical anesthesia and conscious sedation) is preferred if any difficulty is anticipated.

    b. Rapid-sequence procedure employs induction dose sedative drug (e.g., 3 mg/kg thiopental) followed by paralytic dose (1.5 mg/kg) of succinylcholine; should be used only by experienced operators.

4. Ensure adequate intravenous access.

5. Employ pulse oximetry and continuous electrocardiographic monitoring, if available.

6. Have all equipment and supplies readily available, including

    a. Rigid-tipped suction catheter and working vacuum source

    b. Resuscitation cart (defibrillator, advanced cardiac life-support drugs, etc.)

    c. Appropriate size of resuscitation bag, valve, and mask

7. Select endotracheal tube.

    a. Average-sized adult woman: 7.5 or 8.0 mm

    b. Average-sized adult man: 8.0 or 8.5 mm

c. Larger-diameter tubes offer less airway resistance and facilitate pulmonary toilet.

d. For nasal approach, only use tubes 8.0 mm or smaller.

e. Tubes smaller than 8.0 mm generally do not allow passage of a bronchoscope.

8. Prepare tube.

a. Attach syringe and inflate balloon to full volume to test competence.

b. Insert malleable stylet, if desired (not used for nasotracheal approach).

(1) End of stylet should not protrude from distal end of endotracheal tube.

(2) Form distal end of endotracheal tube into hockey stick shape.

c. Lubricate distal end of endotracheal tube with sterile lubricant (which may contain topical anesthetic).

9. Test laryngoscope light to ensure lamp operates (do not allow blade to remain in working position during preparation lest batteries become depleted).

10. Adjust bed to height that is comfortable for operator.

11. Remove patient's dentures, if any.

12. Administer 100% oxygen by bag-valve mask device.

13. Ensure that ventilation can be achieved using bag-valve mask device, and provide as required.

14. Periodically assess heart rate, blood pressure, and SpO_2 throughout procedure.

15. Inspect oral cavity and suction any secretions.

16. If nasal approach is contemplated

a. Have patient sniff while separately occluding each naris to determine which is the more patent.

b. If either can be used, the right side is preferred because most endotracheal tubes have a left-facing bevel.

C. Drugs

1. Topical anesthesia (for awake intubations)

a. Topical benzocaine or other local anesthetic may be sprayed onto posterior pharynx, if desired.

b. Alternatively, lidocaine (1 mg/kg) may be administered topically once vocal cords are visualized.

2. Lidocaine (1.0 to 1.5 mg/kg) may be administered intravenously to blunt sympathetic response to procedure.

3. Local vasoconstrictor (e.g., phenylephrine

spray) is administered intranasally if preparing for awake nasotracheal intubation.

4. Intravenous sedative-hypnotic agents

a. Can be used to produce conscious sedation using incremental dosing, or used in induction dose for rapid-sequence intubation

b. Commonly used agents include benzodiazepines (e.g., midazolam, lorazepam, diazepam), narcotics (e.g., morphine, fentanyl), short-acting barbiturates (e.g., thiopental sodium), propofol, ketamine, and etomidate.

c. Seldom required in unconscious patients

5. Paralytic agents (see Chapter 168, Neuromuscular Blocking Drugs)

a. Used in rapid-sequence intubation procedure

b. Should be used by experienced operators only

c. Can result in death if unable to establish airway

d. Succinylcholine

(1) Rapidly acting, depolarizing neuromuscular blocker

(2) Used along with induction dose sedative drug as part of rapid-sequence intubation in patients at risk for aspiration

(3) Can cause hyperkalemia in patients with trauma, burn injury, and neurologic disorders

e. Nondepolarizing agents

(1) Including, for example, pancuronium, vecuronium, atricurium, cis-atricurium

(2) Sometimes given to prevent fasciculations from succinylcholine

(3) Longer acting, used postintubation if prolonged therapeutic paralysis is indicated

D. Optimize upper airway configuration and establish noncannulating airway.

1. Tilt head back to "sniffing" position to optimize alignment of oral, pharyngeal, and laryngeal axes for oral intubation.

a. Flex neck at lower cervical spine (facilitated by placing a few layers of toweling under the head).

b. Extend head at the atlanto-occipital joint.

2. Lift chin upward.

3. Place fingers of one hand under mandible and lift up and back.

4. Remove debris from oral cavity, if necessary.

5. Suction secretions from oral cavity.

6. Apply bag-valve mask and provide ventilation.

7. Ensure that chest excursions occur with provided ventilation.

8. Maximize oxyhemoglobin saturation prior to attempting intubation.

9. Insert temporary oral airway if there is difficulty achieving adequate oxygenation or ventilation.

E. Endotracheal tube insertion

1. Oral intubation

a. Advantages compared to nasal approach

(1) Can be accomplished more rapidly

(2) Generally has a higher success rate

(3) Allows larger-diameter endotracheal tube

(4) Low incidence of sinusitis

b. Operator takes a position at the head of the bed.

c. Operator always holds the laryngoscope in the left hand and inserts blade into patient's mouth from right side.

d. For patients at risk for aspiration, an assistant performs the Sellick maneuver.

(1) Assistant applies pressure to the cricoid cartilage using thumb and forefinger.

(2) This maneuver occludes the esophagus and minimizes the risk of regurgitation of stomach contents and entry of air into the stomach while bagging.

(3) Pressure is maintained until the endotracheal tube is in place and the cuff is inflated.

e. Sweep the patient's tongue toward left side of the oral cavity as the blade is advanced toward the base of the tongue.

f. If using a curved blade (e.g., MacIntosh), insert the tip of the blade anterior to the epiglottis into the vallecula, and exert upward traction on the laryngoscope handle to indirectly displace the epiglottis anteriorly to expose the glottis (Fig. 189–1, top).

g. If using a straight blade (e.g., Miller), insert the tip of the blade under the epiglottis and exert upward traction on the laryngoscope handle to directly displace epiglottis and base of tongue anteriorly to expose the glottis (Fig. 189–1, middle).

h. Be attentive to preventing dental trauma. Always lift the entire laryngoscope to afford visualization of the glottis. Do not use a prying or levering motion, which can easily lead to dental fracture or avulsion when the teeth are inadvertently used as fulcrum.

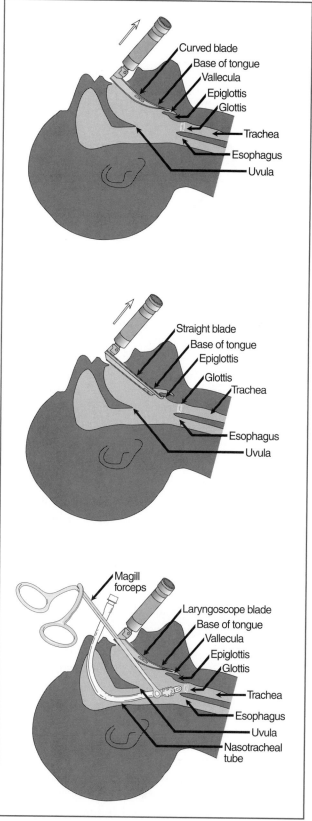

Figure 189–1 Laryngoscopic endotracheal intubation. Open arrow denotes lifting action applied to laryngoscope handle to facilitate visualization of glottis. *Top:* Orotracheal intubation using curved (MacIntosh) blade. Note tip of blade lies in vallecula and epiglottis is indirectly displaced anteriorly. *Middle:* Orotracheal intubation using straight (Miller) blade. Note tip of blade is positioned under epiglottis, allowing direct anterior displacement of epiglottis. *Bottom:* Nasotracheal intubation using direct laryngoscopy and Magill forceps.

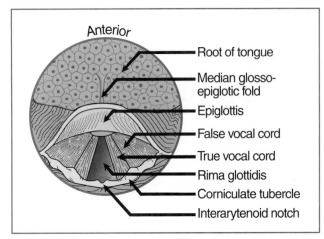

Anterior

Root of tongue

Median glosso-epiglotic fold

Epiglottis

False vocal cord

True vocal cord

Rima glottidis

Corniculate tubercle

Interarytenoid notch

Figure 189–2 Normal anatomy of the structures visible during direct laryngoscopy. Vocal cords are depicted in the open (non-phonating) position.

    i. Suction secretions while the laryngoscope is in place, if necessary to facilitate visualization of the glottis.

    j. Once the glottic opening is visualized (Fig. 189–2), use the right hand to insert the endotracheal tube into the oral cavity from the right corner of the mouth.

    k. Advance the tip of the tube through the vocal cords.

  2. Nasal intubation

    a. Advantages

      (1) More comfortable for the patient

      (2) May be performed without visualizing the vocal cords

      (3) Endotracheal tube is more easily stabilized

      (4) Easier to perform in an awake patient

      (5) Facilitates mouth care

    b. Contraindications

      (1) Patient apneic or in extremis

      (2) Coagulopathy or thrombocytopenia

      (3) Nasal polyps or obstruction

      (4) Facial or basal skull fracture

    c. Blind, awake, nasotracheal approach

      (1) Posterior pharynx should already be well anesthetized with topical anesthetic spray, and a topical nasal decongestant spray should be applied.

      (2) Insert a soft nasal trumpet (Guedel airway) after lubricating liberally with anesthetic jelly (may use smaller airway first, followed by larger size).

      (3) After testing the balloon and lubricat-

ing the tip, insert an appropriately sized nasotracheal tube (usually one French size smaller than appropriate oral tube, up to 8.0 Fr) into the selected naris.

      (4) Direct tube straight back (posterior, not cephalad) along the floor of the nasal cavity using steady, even, light pressure.

      (5) Pause when the tip of the tube is in vicinity of the glottis, often indicated by appearance of condensation within tube synchronous with expiration (best seen if opposite naris is manually occluded).

      (6) Anticipate inspiration by noting phasic changes in tube fogging and air flow from tube, and advance the tube quickly during inspiration.

      (7) Tracheal placement is usually signaled by coughing, continued expiratory condensation within the tube, increased expired air flow from the tube, and the patient's inability to phonate.

      (8) Esophageal entry is usually indicated by loss of phasic condensation, absence of cough and air flow from tube, and ability of patient to phonate.

    d. Nasotracheal intubation using direct laryngoscopy

      (1) Tube is inserted through naris as in the blind method, to the supraglottic level.

      (2) The laryngoscope blade is inserted and the vocal cords are visualized as in orotracheal intubation.

      (3) The tube is advanced between the vocal cords and through the glottis.

      (4) If the tube is directed to one side of the glottic opening, rotate it to redirect toward glottis.

      (5) If the tube still does not enter the glottis, insert Magill forceps through the mouth to grasp the end of the tube and direct it into the glottis while an assistant advances the tube at naris on operator's command (Fig. 189–1, bottom).

F. Remove the stylet (if used) and inflate the cuff with air.

G. Institute ventilation using 100% oxygen with the bag-valve attached to the endotracheal tube.

H. Confirm tube placement within the trachea and at the proper level (no method is foolproof).

  1. Directly visualize tube passage between the

vocal cords (best method, but the tube can become displaced from the trachea after procedure).

2. Auscultate to confirm bilaterally equal breath sounds during bagging (however, sounds can sometimes be transmitted from the abdomen to the chest).

3. Auscultate over the epigastrium to confirm absence of gastric insufflation during bagging.

4. Observe chest expansion during bag-valve insufflation through the endotracheal tube (sometimes it is difficult to distinguish chest from abdominal movements).

5. Note high compliance of the resuscitation bag during bagging (low bag compliance can be due to esophageal intubation, high airway resistance, or low lung or chest wall compliance).

6. Note high or increasing oxyhemoglobin saturation by pulse oximetry (desaturation may take up to several minutes in some cases of esophageal intubation).

7. Note inability of conscious patient to phonate if the tube lies between the vocal cords.

8. Detect end-tidal CO_2 using a disposable chemical detector, capnometry or capnography (high levels of CO_2 may emanate from the stomach during initial bagging if the tube is in the esophagus).

9. Check the position of the tube on chest x-ray: tube should be below the larynx and above the carina (confirms level of placement if within trachea, but does not exclude esophageal placement).

10. Note phasic appearance of water vapor condensation within the endotracheal tube during expiration (can occur with esophageal placement).

11. Palpate the trachea at the suprasternal notch while rapidly inflating and deflating the cuff, either using a syringe, or by squeezing the pilot balloon.

12. The ability to freely and rapidly aspirate gas using a 60 mL syringe securely attached to the end of the endotracheal tube suggests intratracheal placement; resistance suggests esophageal intubation.

13. Visualize the trachea using a fiberoptic bronchoscope through endotracheal tube (reliable but expensive and can be logistically difficult).

14. Perform arterial blood gas measurement (takes time to obtain sample, perform assay, and obtain results).

I. Insert an oral airway or bite block, if necessary.
   1. Prevents kinking of tube by biting
   2. Uncomfortable for conscious patients

J. Secure the tube at the proper position.
   1. In average sized adult, optimal orotracheal tube position is approximately 23 cm at the lip for men and approximately 21 cm for women.
   2. Unequal breath sounds may signify excessive tube insertion and right mainstem bronchus intubation.
   3. A variety of devices are in common use for securing tube in place, including
      a. Twill umbilical tape (nonadhesive)
      b. Intravenous tubing
      c. Various proprietary devices

Common Pitfalls in Orotracheal Intubation

- Head positioned improperly
- Mouth not open wide enough
- Blade not inserted to right side of tongue
- Laryngoscope levered against incisors
- Tube inserted without visualizing vocal cords

Complications

A. Failure to intubate

B. Malpositioned tube
   1. Esophageal intubation
   2. Inadvertent displacement of the tube from the trachea (early or late)
   3. Right main stem bronchus intubation with left lung atelectasis
   4. Tube too high, cuff impinges on vocal cords (can cause coughing and agitation)

C. Aspiration of gastric contents leading to pneumonitis, pneumonia, acute lung injury

D. Hypoxemia

E. Tissue injury
   1. Trauma with bleeding from oral cavity, pharynx, larynx, trachea
   2. Epistaxis (nasotracheal intubation)
   3. Traumatic laryngeal dysfunction
   4. Glottic edema (late)
   5. Tracheoesophageal fistula (late)
   6. Tracheoinnominate artery fistula (late)

7. Late cutaneous injury due to tube ties (e.g., at corners of mouth, cheeks, or ears)

8. Late injury to lips or tongue (oral tubes) or ala nasi (nasal tubes)

9. Esophageal perforation

10. Spinal cord injury (caused by hyperextension of neck in patients with cervical spine injury)

F. Endotracheal tube obstruction

   1. Mucus plug or inspissated secretions

   2. Blood clot

   3. Cuff herniation around end of tube

G. Endotracheal tube cuff problems

   1. Inadequate cuff inflation with inadequate seal

   2. Cuff rupture

   3. Cuff overinflation

     a. Cuff herniation

     b. Tracheal mucosal necrosis leading to tracheal malacia or tracheal stenosis (late)

H. Mechanical problems with tube

   1. Kinking of tube, resulting in airway obstruction

   2. Incompetent cuff inflation valve

   3. Inadvertent cutting of cuff inflation tubing

I. Dental trauma including tooth avulsion or fracture, or breakage of dental prosthesis

J. Foreign body aspiration

K. Barotrauma

   1. Pneumothorax

   2. Pneumomediastinum

   3. Subcutaneous emphysema

   4. Gastric rupture (from esophageal intubation)

   5. Pneumoperitoneum

L. Nosocomial infection (late effects)

   1. Pneumonia

   2. Tracheobronchitis

   3. Sinusitis

   4. Infected labial or ala nasi ulceration

   5. Facial cellulitis

M. Sympathetic stimulation

   1. Hypertension

   2. Tachycardia

   3. Dysrhythmias

   4. Increased intracranial pressure

 Bibliography

Bergen JM, Smith DC. A review of etomidate for rapid sequence intubation in the emergency department. J Emerg Med 1997;15:221–230.

Hamilton PH, Kang JJ. Emergency airway management. Mt Sinai J Med 1997;64:292–301.

Knapp S, Kofler J, Stoiser B, et al. The assessment of four different methods to verify tracheal tube placement in the critical care setting. Anesth Analg 1999;88:766–770.

Orebaugh SL. Succinylcholine: adverse effects and alternatives in emergency medicine. Am J Emerg Med 1999;17:715–721.

Reed DB, Clinton JE. Proper depth of placement of nasotracheal tubes in adults prior to radiographic confirmation. Acad Emerg Med 1997;4:1111–1114.

Walls RM. Management of the difficult airway in the trauma patient. Emerg Med Clin North Am 1998;16:45–61.

190 Central Venous Catheterization
James A. Kruse

Central venous catheterization is performed frequently in the intensive care unit (ICU). Although other insertion methods are in current use, the method reviewed below is based on the Seldinger (guide wire) technique.

Indications

A. Need for IV access and lack of accessible peripheral veins
B. Use of potentially sclerosing, irritating or vasoconstricting IV solutions
 1. Vasopressor agents: e.g., dopamine, norepinephrine
 2. Hypertonic solutions: e.g., total parenteral nutrition formula, 3% saline, dextrose concentrations higher than 10%
 3. Certain parenteral chemotherapy agents
 4. Other irritant infusates: e.g., concentrated potassium solutions
C. Access for pulmonary artery catheterization
D. Access for temporary transvenous cardiac pacing
E. Access for acute hemodialysis
F. Cardiopulmonary resuscitation and lack of IV access
G. Fluid resuscitation
H. Central venous pressure monitoring
 I. Frequent venous blood sampling

Contraindications (all are relative)

A. Significant coagulopathy or thrombocytopenia
 1. Especially at internal jugular (IJ) and subclavian sites because bleeding cannot be controlled by manual pressure
 2. Femoral and peripheral sites relatively safer
B. Infection at access site
C. Morbid obesity
D. Ipsilateral arteriovenous fistula or shunt graft for hemodialysis (IJ, subclavian)
E. Prior surgery at selected site
F. Venous thrombosis at or near intended site
G. Presence of inferior vena cava filter

Procedure

A. Preparation
 1. Explain procedure to patient and obtain informed consent.

2. Select site and side of body.
 a. Consider patient factors; examples:
 (1) Avoid subclavian approach in patient with large apical emphysematous blebs and receiving positive pressure ventilation.
 (2) Avoid subclavian approach in patient with severe thrombocytopenia.
 (3) If unilateral chest tube is in place, the ipsilateral subclavian vein is preferable to the contralateral vein.
 b. Consider operator experience and preference.
3. Have all needed supplies readily available.
4. Position patient.
 a. For IJ or subclavian approaches: supine 10° to 20° Trendelenburg position with ipsilateral arm retracted inferiorly and close to the patient's side
 b. For femoral approach: supine position, bed flat, ipsilateral knee extended, ipsilateral leg externally rotated and abducted 30°
5. Don mask, eye protection, hat, sterile gown and gloves.
6. Prepare site with suitable antiseptic scrub, e.g., povidone-iodine solution.
7. Apply sterile drapes to create an ample sterile field.
8. Infiltrate site with local anesthetic.
 a. 1% lidocaine without epinephrine is suitable.
 b. First use a small (e.g., 25-gauge) needle to infiltrate superficial dermis.
 c. Then use a somewhat larger (e.g., 21- or 22-gauge × ~3.8 cm) needle to infiltrate deeper subcutaneous tissue.
 d. Aspirate before each injection to avoid intravascular injection.
 e. At completion of infiltration, operator may optionally locate vein using anesthesia needle and syringe, noting angle and depth of needle entry.
9. Nick intended entry site with #11 scalpel blade.
10. Fit a 5- or 10-mL non-Luer lock syringe onto a thin-walled insertion needle of appropriate length (depends on site selected) and internal

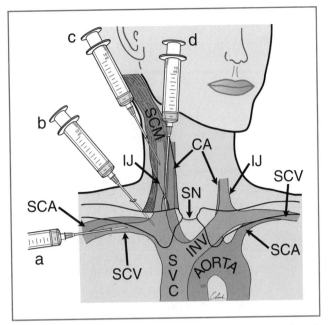

Figure 190–1 Sites of needle entry for central venous catheterization using (a) infraclavicular subclavian approach, (b) supraclavicular subclavian approach, (c) posterior internal jugular approach, and (d) middle internal jugular approach. CA = carotid artery, IJ = internal jugular vein, INV = innominate vein, SCA = subclavian artery, SCM = sternocleidomastoid muscle, SCV = subclavian vein, SN = suprasternal notch, SVC = superior vena cava.

caliber (depends on guidewire used; typically 18 gauge).

11. Make needle puncture through skin nick, with bevel of needle directed upward.

B. Site-specific technique

1. IJ approaches (see Fig. 190–1)

a. Anterior IJ approach

(1) Make needle puncture along the anterior (medial) edge of the sternocleidomastoid muscle (SCM).

(2) Advance the needle at 30° to 45° to skin, toward the ipsilateral nipple, lateral to and away from the carotid pulse.

(3) This approach is not recommended because of the increased risk of carotid artery puncture.

b. Middle (central) IJ approach

(1) Position the patient's head in neutral position or turned only slightly from the side of insertion.

(2) Make needle puncture at the apex of a triangle formed by the superior surface of the clavicle, the sternal head of SCM, and the clavicular head of SCM.

(3) Advance the needle at a 30° to 60° an-

gle to frontal plane toward ipsilateral nipple, away from the carotid pulse.

(4) The vein is usually reached at 2 to 4 cm depth in an average-sized adult.

c. Posterior IJ approach

(1) Rotate the patient's head away from the side of insertion.

(2) Make puncture at the posterior (lateral) edge of SCM approximately midway between its origin at the mastoid process and its insertion at the clavicle.

(3) Avoid striking the external jugular vein.

(4) Advance the needle toward the suprasternal notch, just under the belly of SCM at an angle approximately 45° to the transverse plane and 15° to 45° (negative) angle to the frontal plane

(5) The vein is usually reached by a depth of 7 cm in an average-sized adult.

2. Subclavian vein approach (see Fig. 190–1)

a. Infraclavicular approach

(1) Make a puncture 1 to 2 cm caudal to the juncture of the medial and middle thirds of the clavicle.

(2) Once superficial tissue has been penetrated, rotate the needle to orient the bevel inferiorly.

(3) Advance the needle toward the suprasternal notch at less than a 30° angle, under the clavicle and over the first rib into the subclavian vein.

(4) The vein is usually reached at 1 to 3 cm depth in an average-sized adult.

b. Supraclavicular approach

(1) Make needle puncture at the superior edge of the clavicle, 0 to 3 cm lateral to the lateral edge of SCM.

(2) Advance the needle at a −15° to +20° angle to the frontal plane toward the contralateral nipple at a 45° angle to the sagittal plane.

(3) The subclavian vein is usually reached at 2 cm depth (or less) in an average-sized adult.

3. Femoral vein approach (see anatomic depiction in Chapter 191, Arterial Catheterization).

a. Make needle puncture 2 to 3 cm below the inguinal ligament, 1 to 2 cm medial to the femoral pulse.

b. Advance the needle toward the umbilicus at an angle approximately 45° to the frontal plane.

c. The vein is usually reached at 3 to 5 cm

depth in an average–sized, nonobese, non-cachectic adult.

   d. Do not allow the needle to enter tissue cephalad to the inguinal ligament.

C. Seldinger catheterization technique

1. Ensure that venous blood is freely aspirated into the syringe.

2. Remove the syringe from the needle and immediately place a gloved digit over the needle hub to prevent air embolism.

3. When the guidewire is in position at the needle hub, remove digit from the hub to momentarily expose hub orifice, and quickly insert the J-end of the guidewire into the needle.

4. Advance the guidewire into the vessel, as long as there is no resistance, to the desired depth (approximately 1 cm further than the intended dilator-sheath assembly or catheter insertion distance).

5. Do not allow the guidewire to extend into the right atrium; average distances from the insertion site to the junction of the superior vena cava and the right atrium are
   a. Right IJ: 16 ± 2 cm
   b. Left IJ: 19 ± 2 cm
   c. Right subclavian: 18 ± 3 cm
   d. Left subclavian: 21 ± 2 cm

6. Remove the needle over the guidewire.

7. Enlarge the skin nick, if necessary, using a #11 scalpel blade.

8. Device placement (ensure any side ports or auxiliary lumen hubs are capped)
   a. For central venous catheter or hemodialysis catheter
      (1) Insert tapered vessel dilator over wire, advance into vessel using a twisting motion as long as there is no undue resistance.
      (2) Remove the vessel dilator over the wire.
      (3) Insert the desired catheter over the wire and advance it the appropriate distance, but not beyond the tip of the guidewire or into the right atrium.
      (4) Remove the guidewire and cover the hub of the catheter immediately to prevent air embolism.
   b. For introducer sheath with hemostasis valve (e.g., for pulmonary artery catheterization)
      (1) Insert vessel dilator–sheath assembly into the vein over the guidewire.
      (2) Use twisting motion during advancement.

   (3) When fully advanced, remove the wire and dilator simultaneously.

9. Flush catheter lumen (each lumen if multilumen catheter) and side-port (if any).
   a. Ensure that venous blood can be freely aspirated.
   b. Aspirate all air from lumen and hub.
   c. Flush lumen with sterile saline solution.
   d. Cap lumen or connect to IV fluid source.

10. Ensure that all connections are tightened.

11. Suture the catheter into place.

Key Precautions

- Weigh benefits versus risks before performing catheterization.

- Wear mask, cap, and gown; meticulously maintain sterile field.

- Make skin nick wide enough for cannula, but not excessively deep.

- Do not expose cannula hubs to air for more than 1 second lest air embolism occur.

- Do not allow guidewire or catheter to enter the right atrium.

- The tip of the dilator or catheter should not extend deeper than the tip of the guidewire.

Complications

A. Arterial puncture
B. Other inadvertent tissue penetration (subclavian, IJ sites)
   1. Pneumothorax
   2. Hemothorax
   3. Hydrothorax
   4. Perforation of cardiac chamber, with cardiac tamponade
C. Hemorrhage: venous or arterial
D. Infection
   1. Local site infection, cellulitis
   2. Catheter-related blood stream infection
E. Catheter malposition (e.g., tip of catheter in right atrium)
F. Cardiac dysrhythmias
G. Venous thromboembolism
H. Air embolism
I. Thoracic duct injury (subclavian, IJ sites)
J. Nerve injury (e.g., phrenic nerve, brachial plexus, femoral nerve)
K. Catheter fragmentation or guidewire embolism

Key Follow-up Measures

- Ensure proper disposal of all sharps.

- Dress site using minimal occlusive dressing.

- Document procedure in the medical record.

- Obtain and review chest x-ray (IJ, subclavian sites).

- Provide periodic dressing changes according to institutional protocol.

- Periodically inspect site according to institutional protocol.

Bibliography

Andrews RT, Bova DA, Venbrux AC. How much guidewire is too much? Direct measurement of the distance from subclavian and internal jugular vein access sites to the superior vena cava–atrial junction during central venous catheter placement. Crit Care Med 2000;28:138–142.

CVC Working Group, Office of Training and Assistance, Food and Drug Administration. Central venous catheter complications [videotape series]. Rockville, MD: FDA; Capitol Heights, MD: National Audio-visual Center; 1994.

Miller JA, Singireddy S, Maldjian P, et al. A re-evaluation of the radiographically detectable complications of percutaneous venous access lines inserted by four subcutaneous approaches. Am Surg 1999;65:125–130.

Tan BK, Hong SW, Huang MH, et al. Anatomic basis of safe percutaneous subclavian venous catheterization. J Trauma Injury Infect Crit Care 2000;48:82–86.

191 Arterial Catheterization

James A. Kruse

Indications

A. Continuous arterial blood pressure monitoring
   1. Hypotension or high likelihood of developing hypotension
   2. Hypertensive emergencies
   3. Continuous vasoactive drug infusion (e.g., norepinephrine, nitroprusside)
   4. Inability to obtain blood pressure by sphygmomanometry
   5. High-risk surgical procedures
B. Frequent arterial blood sampling (e.g., for arterial blood gases)

Key Contraindications

- Significant coagulopathy or thrombocytopenia
- Infection at access site
- Prior vascular surgery at selected site
- Lack of collateral circulation (radial artery site)
- Severe peripheral arterial disease
- Downstream ischemia or arterial thromboembolism

Technique

A. Have all needed supplies readily available, including catheter (typically 20 g).
B. Select site.
   1. Evaluate adequacy of distal pulses.
   2. Check for other signs of arterial insufficiency.
   3. If radial artery site selected, collateral circulation may be evaluated using Allen test or modified Allen test.
      a. Allen test
         (1) Patient forms tight fist with wrist in neutral position.
         (2) Clinician occludes radial artery by applying pressure with thumb for approximately 1 minute.
         (3) Patient opens fist (thumb pressure maintained).
         (4) Ulnar circulation is adequate if blanching abates within approximately 5 seconds, inadequate if hand remains pale for longer than 10 seconds.
      b. Modified Allen test
         (1) Patient forms tight fist with wrist in neutral position.
         (2) Clinician occludes radial and ulnar arteries by applying pressure with thumbs for approximately 1 minute.
         (3) Patient opens fist, revealing blanched palm.
         (4) Clinician releases pressure on ulnar artery, but maintains pressure on radial artery.
         (5) Ulnar circulation is adequate if blanching abates within approximately 5 seconds, inadequate if hand remains pale for more than 10 seconds.
C. Don mask, eye protection, hat, sterile gown and gloves.
D. Radial artery catheterization
   1. Supinate and immobilize the hand and forearm, using an armboard if necessary.
   2. Place a folded towel under the wrist to maintain extension.
   3. Scrub site with suitable antiseptic (e.g., povidone-iodine).
   4. Apply sterile drapes to create an ample sterile field.
   5. Locate radial artery 1 to 2 cm proximal to wrist crease by palpation of pulse.
   6. Infiltrate site with 2% lidocaine without epinephrine.
      a. Use a small (e.g., ≥25 gauge) needle and infiltrate on each side of vessel.
      b. Do not raise an intradermal wheal or infiltrate directly over artery.
      c. Use minimal volume of anesthetic (i.e., approximately 1 mL total).
   7. Carefully nick skin with a #11 scalpel blade at intended site.
   8. Insert thin-wall needle or catheter-over-needle.
      a. Do not use an attached syringe.
      b. Insert the needle parallel to vessel at an approximately 30° to 45° angle.
      c. Direct the needle bevel upward, and advance slowly until pulsatile arterial blood is visible at the hub.
   9. Device-specific techniques
      a. Simple catheter-over-needle device

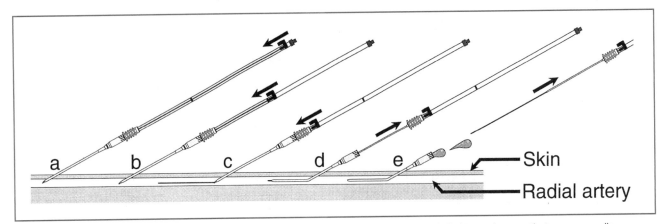

Figure 191–1 Percutaneous cannulation of radial artery by a modified Seldinger technique using a catheter-over-needle device with integral guidewire. *(a)* Tab is used to advance guidewire into needle after artery is punctured. *(b)* Tip of guidewire is at the level of the needle orifice once tab reaches marker. *(c)* Guidewire is advanced into artery. *(d)* Catheter is advanced over needle and guidewire into artery. *(e)* Needle and guidewire are removed.

(1) Once blood return is obtained, advance the entire device an additional 1/8 inch into the artery so that the distal end of the catheter is within the lumen of the vessel.

(2) After ensuring that blood return is still present, slide the catheter over the needle using a twisting motion.

(3) Advance the catheter fully into the artery as long as no resistance is encountered.

(4) Remove the needle.

b. Seldinger technique

(1) Once blood return is obtained from the thin-wall needle, insert an appropriate sized, J-tipped guidewire through the needle.

(2) Advance the wire to a depth beyond the anticipated catheter insertion distance, as long as no resistance is encountered.

(3) Remove the needle over the wire (wire remains in place).

(4) Advance the catheter over the wire.

(5) Remove the guidewire.

c. Modified Seldinger technique using catheter-over-needle device with integral guidewire (Fig. 191–1)

(1) Once blood return is visible from the device hub, fully advance the integral guidewire through the catheter-over-needle device, as long as no resistance is encountered.

(2) Using a rotating or twisting motion, fully advance the catheter over the needle and wire into the artery.

(3) Remove the needle and guidewire assembly from the catheter.

E. Femoral artery technique (Fig. 191–2)

1. Ensure that the bed is flat.

2. Position the patient supine with the ipsilateral knee extended and the ipsilateral ankle externally rotated.

3. Scrub the site with suitable antiseptic (e.g., povidone-iodine).

4. Apply sterile drapes to create an ample sterile field.

5. Locate the femoral artery inferior to the inguinal ligament and inguinal crease by palpation of pulse.

6. Infiltrate the superficial and subcutaneous site with several mL of 1% lidocaine without epinephrine using a small (≥21 gauge) needle.

7. Carefully nick the skin with a #11 scalpel blade at the intended site.

8. Catheter-over-needle devices are not recommended at this site.

9. Insert a thin-wall needle directly over the femoral pulse below the inguinal ligament.

   a. Do not use an attached syringe.

   b. Needle should enter at an angle approximately 45° to the skin.

   c. Orient the needle parallel to the vessel with the needle bevel directed upward.

   d. Advance the needle slowly toward the umbilicus until pulsatile arterial blood is visible at the needle hub.

10. Complete the procedure using needle-and-guidewire method, as described under D. Radial artery catheterization, Seldinger technique, above.

F. After momentarily allowing pulsatile arterial blood to emerge from the catheter hub, connect the hub to fluid-flushed, low-compliance tubing connected to a pressure transducer, flush device, and electronic monitor.

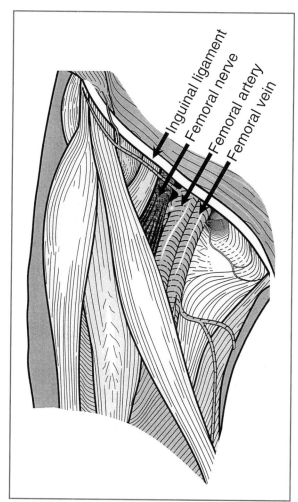

Figure 191-2 Anatomic relationships of femoral artery, femoral vein, femoral nerve, inguinal ligament, and adjacent muscles of the upper anterior thigh.

G. Flush the catheter briefly.
H. Confirm typical arterial pressure waveform on the monitor.
I. Ensure that all connections are tightened.
J. Suture the catheter hub to the skin.
K. Level and zero system (see Chapter 215, Fast Flush Test)
L. Document the procedure in the medical record.
M. Postcatheterization care
   1. Dress the site with minimal occlusive dressing, as with venous catheterization.
   2. Immobilize the involved limb to prevent flexion at the insertion site.
   3. Maintain connection to the pressure transducer and the continuous flush device, and monitor at all times.
   4. Regularly check limb appearance, temperature, and pulses distal to the insertion site.
   5. Periodically inspect the insertion site and change the dressing, per institutional protocol.
N. Remove the catheter when no longer required or if there are signs of ischemia (e.g., diminished or

absent pulses, coolness or mottling of skin, or paresthesias) or if infection develops.

Complications

A. Catheter clotted or kinked
   1. Waveform damped or unobtainable
   2. Unable to aspirate blood
B. Hemorrhage
   1. Visible bleeding at site
   2. Hematoma
C. Infection
   1. Local site infection, cellulitis, abscess
   2. Catheter-related blood stream infection
D. Distal ischemia
   1. Causes
      a. Thrombosis
      b. Embolism
      c. Arterial spasm
      d. Intimal dissection
      e. Cholesterol emboli
   2. Risk factors
      a. Hypotension or low flow states
      b. Vasopressor infusion
      c. Underlying atherosclerotic disease
E. Pseudoaneurysm
F. Arteriovenous fistula
G. Peripheral neuropathy
H. Catheter fragmentation or guidewire embolism
I. Cerebral air embolism

Key Risk Factors for Complications

- Coagulopathy or therapeutic anticoagulation
- Thrombocytopenia
- Hypotension or vasopressor infusion
- Low flow state
- Prior vascular surgery at insertion site
- Peripheral arterial disease
- Bacteremia, sepsis, local site infection
- Duration of catheterization

Bibliography

Clark VL, Kruse JA. Arterial catheterization. Crit Care Clin 1992;8:687–697.

Frezza EE. Indications and complications of arterial catheter use in surgical or medical intensive care units: analysis of 4932 patients. Am Surg 1998;64:127–131.

Mangar D, Thrush DN, Connell GR, et al. Direct or modified Seldinger guide wire–directed technique for arterial catheter insertion. Anesth Analg 1993;76:714–717.

Sfeir R, Khoury S, Khoury G, et al. Ischaemia of the hand after radial artery monitoring. Cardiovasc Surg 1996;4:456–458.

192 Pulmonary Artery Catheterization

James A. Kruse

The balloon-tipped pulmonary artery (PA) catheter is flow-directed, allowing bedside insertion guided by pressure monitoring without need for fluoroscopic visualization. Basic catheters allow pressure measurements and thermodilution cardiac output measurement. More advanced catheters are available that can be used for automated and near-continuous cardiac output determinations; continuous fiberoptic mixed venous oxyhemoglobin saturation monitoring; right ventricular (RV) end-diastolic volume, end-systolic volume, and ejection fraction measurements; and right ventricular cardiac pacing.

Indications

A. Circulatory shock
B. Acute myocardial infarction (MI)
  1. Right ventricular MI
  2. Mechanical complications of MI
  3. Cardiogenic shock
C. Severe heart failure
D. Cardiac tamponade
E. Acute oliguric renal failure
F. Acute respiratory distress syndrome
G. Perioperative monitoring in high-risk patients

Key Precautions

- Once distal catheter is outside introducer sheath, never advance catheter unless balloon is fully inflated.

- Continuously monitor electrocardiogram (ECG) for cardiac dysrhythmias during insertion.

- Never retract catheter with the balloon inflated.

- Never rapidly inflate balloon to full volume while it is in PA, lest PA rupture occur.

- Ensure that an undamped PA pressure waveform is visible during routine monitoring.

- Promptly retract catheter if waveform assumes a "permanent wedge" configuration.

- Avoid unnecessary or routine balloon inflation in patients with severe pulmonary hypertension.

Contraindications

A. Contraindication to venous access procedure (see Chapter 190, Central Venous Catheterization)
B. High risk for ventricular dysrhythmia or complete heart block
C. Marked hypothermia
D. Prosthetic tricuspid or pulmonic valve
E. Central venous or right heart thrombus

Procedure

A. Patient preparation
  1. Explain procedure to patient and obtain informed consent.
  2. Select access route: internal jugular and subclavian vein are most commonly employed for bedside insertion
    a. For internal jugular route, right side preferred because of more direct route to heart
    b. For subclavian route, left side preferred because of single curvature route to heart
  3. Ensure large sterile field; e.g., 3/4 length sterile drape.
  4. Obtain central venous access and insert introducer sheath with hemostasis valve (see Chapter 190, Central Venous Catheterization).
  5. If introducer sheath has a side-arm port, aspirate blood from the port, connect to sterile, fluid-filled IV connection tubing, and flush the lumen.
B. Prepare the PA catheter for insertion.
  1. Connect the syringe to the balloon lumen and test balloon inflation.
  2. Connect fluid-filled connection tubing to all pressure monitoring and infusion lumen hubs.
    a. Specific configurations may vary per institutional practice; a representative arrangement is shown in Figure 192–1.
    b. Low-compliance (high pressure) tubing must be used to connect distal lumen to transducer.
    c. Low-compliance tubing must also be used for connection path between right atrial pressure monitoring lumen and transducer.

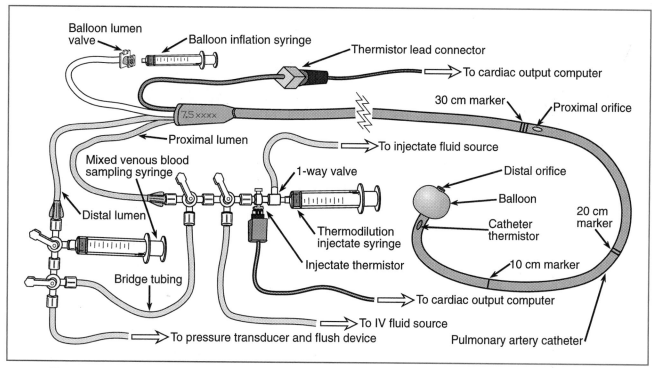

Figure 192-1 Typical configuration of pulmonary artery (PA) catheter and associated connections. Adjustment of stopcocks allows either PA (and PA occlusion) pressure monitoring, right atrial (central venous) pressure measurement, aspiration of mixed venous blood samples from distal orifice, or thermodilution injections into proximal (right atrial) orifice for cardiac output measurements.

d. Interpose the minimum number of stopcocks needed to allow

   (1) Right atrial port injections for thermodilution cardiac output determination

   (2) Mixed venous blood sampling from distal lumen port

   (3) Choice of pressure measurement from distal (PA) orifice or right atrial orifice (if a one-transducer configuration is employed)

e. Flush all pressure monitoring and infusion lumens and their associated connection tubing with sterile saline.

f. Ensure that no air bubbles remain in the catheter, connection tubing, stopcocks, or transducer(s).

3. Insert distal end of the PA catheter into the correct end of a compressed sterility sleeve and slide the compressed sleeve onto the proximal portion of the catheter.

C. Ensure electrical connection between pressure transducer and electronic monitor.

1. Flat tracing should be visible on display screen of electronic monitor.

2. Adjust scale to either 0 to 30 or 0 to 60 mm Hg.

D. Test the system for pressure measuring capability.

1. Ensure that all PA catheter lumens are properly connected and that connections are tight.

2. Adjust stopcocks so there is a continuous, open luminal path between the distal catheter orifice and the transducer.

3. Ensure that no intravascular ports are exposed to the atmosphere, directly or via stopcocks, and that all connections are tight.

4. Observe the pressure tracing while moving the catheter ex vivo.

   a. Sharply shaking or accelerating the distal catheter should produce pressure deflections on the electronic display.

   b. Slowly raising and lowering the distal catheter (and thus the hydrostatic pressure level) should raise and lower the pressure tracing and digital pressure readings on the electronic display.

E. Catheter insertion

1. Insert the PA catheter through the hemostasis valve of the introducer sheath and advance until the catheter tip extends just beyond the end of the sheath (typically 20 cm, depending on the length of the sheath).

2. Confirm the appearance of a central venous pressure waveform, which is characterized by

   a. Atrial pressure wave configuration, usually with a, v, and possibly c waves visible

b. Slower pressure fluctuations corresponding to respiration-induced intrathoracic pressure changes

3. Inflate the PA catheter balloon to the full recommended volume (typically 1.5 mL on a 7.5 French catheter).

4. Advance the catheter while continuously observing the pressure waveform (Figure 192–2) and ECG.

5. Observe the transition from a central venous or right atrial pressure waveform to a right ventricular waveform, which is characterized by

a. An increase in systolic pressure compared to right atrial pressure

b. Wide pulse pressure

c. Diastolic pressure similar to right atrial or central venous pressure

d. Positive slope to diastolic portion of waveform

6. Continue advancing the catheter and observe transition to a PA pressure waveform, which is characterized by

a. Usually the same systolic pressure as right ventricular pressure

b. Narrower pulse pressure compared to right ventricular waveform

c. Dicrotic notch

d. Diastolic pressure higher than right atrial or central venous pressure

e. Negative slope to diastolic portion of waveform

7. Continue advancing the catheter and observe transition to a PA occlusion pressure (PAOP) waveform, which is characterized by

a. Change in waveform configuration, normally with a substantial decrease in pulse pressure

b. Atrial-type a and v waves (may be visible)

c. Average PAOP less than mean PA pressure

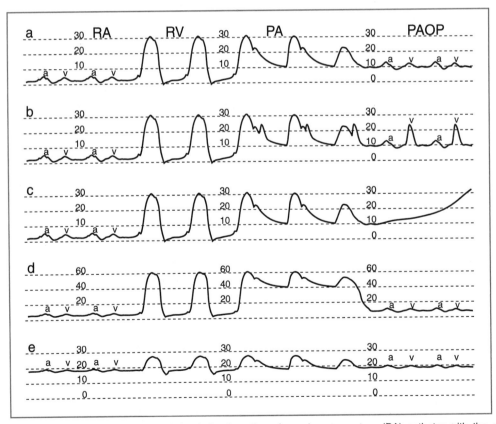

Figure 192–2 Sweep pressure–time tracings during insertion of a pulmonary artery (PA) catheter with the catheter balloon inflated. (a) Normal sweep showing typical waveforms, including atrial a and v waves. Note positive slope to diastolic portion of right ventricular (RV) waveform, negative slope to diastolic portion of PA waveform, dicrotic notch in PA waveform, and transition from PA to PAOP. (b) Mitral insufficiency showing large pathological v wave visible in PA and PAOP waveforms. (c) So called "over-wedge," due to occlusion of the distal catheter orifice by the PA wall. (d) Pulmonary arterial hypertension, showing elevated RV and PA systolic and PA diastolic pressure, and a wide gradient between PA diastolic pressure and PAOP. (e) Cardiac tamponade, showing high diastolic pressures, narrow RV and PA pulse pressure, and diastolic equalization. RA = right atrial pressure; PAOP = pulmonary artery occlusion pressure. Numbers indicate pressure scale (mm Hg).

d. PAOP only slightly less than PA diastolic pressure, unless there is pulmonary arterial hypertension (Fig. 192–2d)

e. Rise in oxyhemoglobin saturation (fiberoptic oximetry catheters)

8. Deflate the balloon.

a. Waveform should revert to PA pressure tracing.

b. If PAOP remains visible, or if a damped PA tracing appears, the catheter tip is too distal and should be retracted somewhat.

9. Test for reproducibility of the PAOP waveform.

a. Inflate the balloon slowly (e.g., over 15 seconds) or incrementally (e.g., 0.5 mL every 5 seconds) while observing the monitor.

b. If the PAOP waveform appears before full balloon inflation is achieved, the catheter is too far distal and should be retracted somewhat (after fully deflating balloon).

10. Repeat steps 8 and 9 until the optimal position is reached, in which

a. Undamped PA waveform is visible when balloon is deflated.

b. PAOP waveform does not appear with partial balloon inflation.

c. PAOP waveform is apparent when balloon is fully inflated.

F. Postprocedure

1. Fully extend the sterility sleeve, affix one end securely to the sheath hub (typically employing an integral locking mechanism) and the opposite end to the catheter (with tape, if necessary).

2. Suture the introducer sheath to skin using 3-0 silk.

3. Ensure proper disposal of all sharps.

4. Dress the site using minimal occlusive dressing.

5. Document the procedure in the medical record.

6. Obtain and review the chest x-ray.

7. Obtain and review the full hemodynamic profile.

a. PA, PAOP, and RA pressures at end–expiration

b. Thermodilution cardiac output

c. Mixed venous blood and arterial blood gases and oxyhemoglobin saturations

d. Systemic arterial blood pressures (systolic, diastolic, and mean)

e. Derived hemodynamic and oxygen transport parameters (see Chapter 214, Hemodynamic Monitoring; and Chapter 216, Monitoring Oxygen Transport)

f. Arterial blood lactate concentration

8. Provide periodic dressing changes per institutional protocol.

9. Periodically inspect site per institutional protocol.

PITFALLS

- Do not attempt insertion without visible continuous ECG and pressure waveforms.

- If an "over-wedge" waveform appears (Fig. 192–2c), deflate the balloon, retract the catheter partially, and reattempt insertion.

- If seemingly unable to obtain typical PAOP waveform, consider the possibility of mitral regurgitation (Fig. 192–2b).

- Mean PAOP should not exceed mean PA pressure.

- Measure all pressures at end-expiration.

Complications

A. Complications related to venous access procedure (see Chapter 190, Central Venous Catheterization)

B. Cardiac dysrhythmias and conduction defects
1. Ectopy
2. Ventricular tachycardia or cardiac arrest
3. Right bundle branch block
4. Complete heart block (if preexisting left bundle branch block)

C. Balloon rupture

D. Endocarditis

E. Thrombocytopenia (heparin-induced, due to use of heparin-coated catheter)

F. Pulmonary infarction

G. Valvular injury

H. Thromboembolism

I. Catheter knotting or entrapment

J. Pulmonary artery rupture

K. Cardiac perforation

Bibliography

Brandstetter RD, Grant GR, Estilo M, et al. Swan-Ganz catheter: misconceptions, pitfalls, and incomplete user knowledge—an identified trilogy in need of correction. Heart Lung 1998;27:218–222.

Nelson LD. The new pulmonary artery catheters: continuous venous oximetry, right ventricular ejection fraction, and continuous cardiac output. New Horizons 1997;5: 251–258.

Perret C, Tagan D, Feihl F, Marini JJ. The Pulmonary Artery Catheter in Critical Care. A Concise Handbook. Cambridge, MA: Blackwell Science, 1996.

Pulmonary Artery Catheter Consensus Conference Participants. Pulmonary artery catheter consensus conference: Consensus statement. New Horizons 1997;5:175–194.

193 Temporary Transvenous Pacemaker

James A. Kruse

This chapter describes the procedure of temporary transvenous ventricular pacing using balloon-tipped, bipolar electrode pacing catheters inserted via internal jugular or subclavian vein access.

Key Indications

- Indications require that the patient is either symptomatic, unstable, or at high risk for progressing to complete heart block.

- High degree atrioventricular block: e.g., complete heart block or Mobitz type II second-degree heart block

- Severe or symptomatic bradycardia

- New onset of bundle branch block (BBB) in setting of acute myocardial infarction

- Prophylactic use in patients with bifascicular or second-degree block who are undergoing high-risk surgery

- Overdrive suppression of tachydysrhythmias

Supplies and Equipment

A. Supplies for central venous access
B. Pacing catheter
   1. Typically, 5 French, 110 cm bipolar electrode catheter
   2. Balloon-tipped catheter recommended
C. Introducer sheath and mating dilator
   1. Introducer sheath with hemostasis valve preferred
   2. Sheath caliber must be large enough to allow passage of pacing catheter.
   3. Hemostasis valve must be either
      a. Matched in caliber to the diameter of the pacing catheter to allow its passage without air or blood leakage around the catheter, or
      b. Adjustable (Tuohy-Borst), set to the appropriate size before insertion, and lightly tightened after insertion
D. Pacemaker generator
   1. Ensure that the battery is fresh.
   2. Test the generator to ensure operation.

3. Configure for desired mode and settings, typically:
   a. Mode: VVI (some models allow only this mode)
   b. Rate: initially set to at least 10 beats/minute higher than the patient's intrinsic rate
   c. Output (current): initially set at 5 to 10 mA
   d. Sensitivity: initially set to asynchronous mode
E. Standard intensive care unit electrocardiograph (ICU ECG) monitor (needed for all insertion methods)
F. A separate 12-lead ECG (needed for internal electrographic guidance method)
G. Sterile lead wire or connection adaptor (needed for internal electrographic guidance method)
   1. Allows connection between distal catheter electrode and V-lead connector of 12-lead ECG
   2. One end of the lead wire or adaptor may have either a connector that fits the standard ECG lead connector or an alligator clip.
   3. The other end of the lead wire or adaptor may have either a connector that fits the distal pacing catheter electrode lead connector or an alligator clip.

Preparation

A. Explain the procedure to the patient and obtain informed consent.
B. Ensure adequate ECG monitoring.
   1. Ensure that chest leads are connected to standard ICU ECG monitor.
   2. Configure the ECG monitor so that signals from two different leads are simultaneously visible.
C. If an internal electrographic guidance technique is to be used, ensure patient connection to standard 12-lead ECG.
   1. Attach four limb leads to the patient and connect to a standard 12-lead ECG.
   2. Do not connect precordial leads, but ensure that they are accessible to the operator.
   3. For single-channel ECGs, configure the device

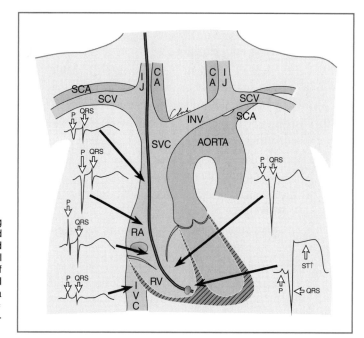

Figure 193–1 Insertion of temporary transvenous pacing catheter using intracardiac electrographic guidance. Closed arrows show representative positions within great veins and right-sided cardiac chambers and corresponding internal electrograms. Open arrows delineate P and QRS waves of internal electrograms. CA = carotid artery; IJ = internal jugular vein; INV = innominate vein; IVC = inferior vena cava; RA = right atrium; RV = right ventricle; SCA = subclavian artery; SCV = subclavian vein; ST↑ = ST segment elevations; SVC = superior vena cava.

so that one V-lead is visible on the screen or paper recording.

4. For multichannel ECGs, configure the device so that one V-lead and two limb lead signals are visible on the screen or paper recording.

D. Wear mask, cap, eye protection, sterile gown and gloves.

E. Employ large sterile field; e.g., 3/4 length sterile drape.

F. Obtain central venous access and insert introducer sheath (see Chapter 190, Central Venous Catheterization).

G. If the introducer sheath has a side-arm port, aspirate blood from the port, connect to sterile, fluid-filled IV connection tubing, and flush the lumen.

H. Insert the distal end of the pacing catheter into the correct end of the compressed sterility sleeve and slide the compressed sleeve onto the proximal portion of the catheter.

I. For balloon-tipped pacing catheters, connect the syringe to the balloon lumen and test balloon inflation using recommended volume.

Insertion Techniques (using bipolar electrode catheter)

A. Internal electrographic guidance technique

1. Using a sterile adaptor or lead wire, connect the distal pacing electrode lead to the monitored V-lead of the 12-lead ECG.

2. Insert the catheter through the hemostasis valve of the introducer sheath with the curvature directed so as to facilitate passage through the tricuspid valve.

3. Advance the catheter an appropriate distance until the tip is just beyond the end of the sheath.

4. Observe the internal electrogram signal on the V-lead of the 12-lead ECG (Fig. 193–1).

5. Inflate the pacing catheter balloon to the full recommended volume.

6. Advance the catheter while continuously observing the monitored V-lead signal on the 12-lead ECG.

   a. Advance until the right atrial intracavitary electrogram is visualized, which is characterized by

      (1) Large P wave and small QRS complex

      (2) P wave deflection negative in the superior right atrium and positive in the inferior right atrium

      (3) PR segment elevation indicates contact with the atrial wall.

   b. Advance further and observe the transition from the right atrial to the right ventricular (RV) electrogram, which is characterized by

      (1) P wave becoming smaller

      (2) QRS complex becoming larger

   c. Stop advancing when the catheter tip contacts the RV endocardium, which may be signaled by

      (1) Appearance of ST segment elevation on internal electrogram (Fig. 193–1)

      (2) Ventricular ectopy visible on the standard ECG monitor

      (3) Any physical resistance to advancement

7. Deflate the balloon.

8. Retract the catheter slightly if ST segment elevation exceeds 2 mV (may signify excessive pressure on endocardium).

9. Verify that ST segment elevation is still visible (if not, it may be necessary to cautiously advance catheter slightly).

10. Disconnect the adaptor or lead wire from the distal catheter electrode.

11. Connect the pacing catheter electrode lead wires to the pacemaker generator.

    a. Proximal catheter electrode connects to positive pole of generator.

    b. Distal catheter electrode connects to negative pole of generator.

12. Ensure that the generator is turned on, with desired settings (see D.3. under Supplies and Equipment, above), and that the pulse firing indicator is flashing.

13. Verify pacing spikes on the ECG monitor with 1:1 capture.

B. Fluoroscopic guidance technique

1. Unless bedside fluoroscopy is available, the patient must be moved to the cardiac catheterization laboratory or other location where fluoroscopy is available.

2. Insert the catheter through the hemostasis valve of the introducer sheath with the curvature directed so as to facilitate passage through the tricuspid valve.

3. Advance the catheter until its tip is just beyond the end of the sheath.

4. If a balloon-tipped catheter is used, inflate the balloon to the full recommended volume.

5. Advance the catheter into the right atrium while continuously monitoring its course under fluoroscopy.

6. Advance the catheter through the right atrium and into the right ventricle.

    a. Direct advancement is usually simple with flow-directed (balloon-tipped) catheters.

    b. For non-flow-directed catheters it may be necessary to position the catheter tip against the free wall of the right atrium and form a loop that allows the tip to enter the right ventricle as the catheter is rotated.

7. Connect pacing catheter electrode lead wires to the pacemaker generator.

    a. Proximal catheter electrode to positive pole of generator

    b. Distal catheter electrode to negative pole of generator

8. Turn the pacemaker generator on and ensure appropriate settings (see D.3. in Supplies and Equipment above), and that the pulse firing indicator is flashing.

9. Advance the catheter tip toward the right ventricular apex.

10. Stop advancing the catheter when

    a. Electrical capture is obtained.

    b. Ectopy or dysrhythmia occurs.

    c. Any degree of resistance is encountered.

    d. The catheter tip reaches the right ventricular apex.

    e. The catheter tip is misdirected into the outflow tract or any other undesired direction.

11. If necessary, deflate the balloon, retract and redirect the catheter as required to achieve position in right ventricular apex.

12. Once capture is obtained, deflate the balloon.

13. Verify pacing spikes on the ECG monitor with 1:1 capture.

C. Blind insertion technique

1. Not recommended except in an emergency; e.g., insertion during cardiac resuscitation

2. Connect the pacing catheter electrode lead wires to the pacemaker generator.

    a. Proximal catheter electrode to positive pole of generator

    b. Distal catheter electrode to negative pole of generator

3. Insert the catheter through the hemostasis valve of the introducer sheath with the curvature directed so as to facilitate passage through the tricuspid valve.

4. Advance the catheter until its tip is just beyond the end of the sheath.

5. Turn pacemaker generator on and ensure appropriate settings (see D.3. under Supplies and Equipment, above).

6. Inflate the pacing catheter balloon to the full recommended volume.

7. Advance the catheter while continuously monitoring:

    a. Physical depth of insertion, indicated by markers along the length of the catheter

    b. Surface ECG monitor, noting

       (1) Patient's intrinsic rhythm

       (2) Pacemaker spikes (initially will be asynchronous with patient's intrinsic rhythm)

       (3) Presence of electrical capture, signaled

by wide-complex synchronous beats immediately following a pacing spike

    (4) Any ectopy or dysrhythmia, which may signal contact of the catheter with the endocardium

8. Stop advancing the catheter when

  a. Electrical capture is obtained.

  b. Ectopy or dysrhythmia occurs.

  c. Any degree of resistance is encountered.

  d. The insertion distance exceeds the expected distance to the right ventricular apex.

    (1) Distance depends on access site.

    (2) Excessive distance indicates catheter is entering the inferior vena cava, coiling in the right atrium, or is otherwise misdirected.

    (3) Retract the catheter to sheath and reattempt.

9. Once capture is obtained, deflate the balloon.

Threshold Testing

A. Determine pacing threshold (also known as capture or stimulation threshold).

1. First ensure consistent 1:1 capture by the pacemaker.

  a. Generator set to VVI mode

  b. Generator set to a rate higher than the patient's intrinsic rate (e.g., by ~10 beats/minute and at ≥50 beats/minute)

  c. Observe the ECG monitor for pacing spikes consistently followed by captured beats.

  d. If capture is not occurring, increase output current or reposition the catheter.

2. Then slowly or incrementally decrease the generator output current until capture no longer occurs or no longer occurs reliably (i.e., <1:1 capture).

3. Increase current to minimum value that results in reliable 1:1 capture, which is designated as the pacing threshold.

  a. Values lower than 1 mA are ideal.

  b. Values 1 to 2 mA are acceptable

  c. Values above 2 mA

    (1) Indicate suboptimal electrode position

    (2) May be acceptable in emergencies

    (3) Should prompt an attempt at electrode repositioning

4. Increase current 3 to 5 mA above threshold value as a safety margin.

B. Determine the sensing threshold

1. Principle

  a. Represents the amplitude of spontaneous QRS voltage required at the pacing electrode to inhibit firing of a current spike by the pacemaker generator

  b. The higher the sensitivity, the lower the QRS voltage level required to inhibit firing

  c. Important if pacemaker is to be used in demand mode

  d. May not be able to safely test if patient lacks an intrinsic rhythm of sufficient rate

2. Method

  a. Ensure that the generator is configured appropriately.

    (1) Set to VVI mode.

    (2) Set rate to approximately 10 beats/minute lower than the patient's intrinsic rate (assuming it is safe to do so).

    (3) Set sensitivity to approximately 3 mV.

  b. Slowly or incrementally increase the sensing voltage level (thus, decreasing the sensitivity) until intrinsic beats are no longer reliably sensed and the pacemaker fires.

  c. Decrease the sensing voltage level to the highest value that results in reliable sensing; this is designated the *sensing threshold*.

  d. Decrease the sensing voltage level well below threshold to ensure an adequate margin of safety for reliable sensing.

  e. Setting sensing voltage to an unnecessarily low value (maximum sensitivity) risks spurious pacemaker inhibition; e.g., inhibition caused by sensing atrial depolarization or extraneous electrical activity.

Post-Procedure

A. Fully extend the sterility sleeve, affix one end securely to the sheath hub (typically employing an integral locking mechanism), and affix the opposite end to the catheter (with tape, if necessary).

B. Suture the introducer sheath to the skin using 3-0 silk.

C. Ensure proper disposal of all sharps.

D. Dress the site using minimal occlusive dressing.

E. Enter the desired settings for mode, rate, output current, and sensitivity in orders section of patient's medical record.

F. Document the procedure in the medical record, including pacing and sensing thresholds.

G. Obtain and review a chest x-ray.

H. Provide for periodic dressing changes and site inspections per institutional protocol.

Complications

A. Complications related to venous access procedure (see Chapter 190, Central Venous Catheterization)

B. Cardiac dysrhythmias

  1. Atrial or ventricular ectopy

  2. Ventricular tachycardia, ventricular fibrillation, or cardiac arrest

  3. Bradycardia or asystole due to pacemaker failure

C. Pacing failure

  1. Catheter electrode dislodgement

  2. Exit block

  3. Cardiac perforation

  4. Lead disconnection or fracture

  5. Generator malfunction

  6. Expended battery

D. Infection or sepsis

  1. Local access site infection

  2. Catheter-related blood stream infection

  3. Endocarditis

E. Hemodynamic decompensation due to loss of atrial contribution to ventricular function

F. Thromboembolism

G. Balloon rupture (flow-directed pacing catheters)

H. Catheter knotting or entrapment

I. Cardiac perforation

J. Pericardial effusion or hemopericardium

K. Cardiac tamponade

Key Findings Implicating Cardiac Perforation by Pacing Catheter

- Pacing evokes synchronous contractions of diaphragm.

- Pacing evokes synchronous contractions of intercostal muscles.

- Tip of pacing catheter extends beyond right ventricular apex on chest x-ray.

- Paced beat morphology changes from left BBB to right BBB pattern.

- New pericardial friction rub develops.

- Hemodynamic decompensation or signs of cardiac tamponade occur.

Bibliography

Anonymous. Choice of route for insertion of temporary pacing wires: recommendations of the Medical Practice Committee and Council of the British Cardiac Society. Br Heart J 1993;70:592.

Francis GS. Clinical compentence in insertion of a temporary transvenous ventricular pacemaker. A statement for physicians from the ACP/ACC/AHA Task Force on Clinical Privileges in Cardiology. Circulation 1994;89:1913–1916.

Goldberger J, Kruse J, Ehlert FA, et al. Temporary transvenous cardiac pacemaker placement: what constitutes an adequate pacing site? Am Heart J 1993;126:488–493.

Jafri SM, Kruse JA. Temporary transvenous cardiac pacing. Crit Care Clin 1992;8:713–725.

194 Transcutaneous Pacing

Steven Borzak

Definition

A method to provide ventricular cardiac pacing using electrode pads applied to the surface of the chest

Indications

A. Therapeutic indications
1. Symptomatic severe bradycardia
2. Symptomatic high-grade atrioventricular block
3. Asystole or sinus node arrest
4. Bradycardia-dependent ventricular tachycardia (e.g., torsade de pointes)
5. Indication for temporary transvenous pacing, but inability to place transvenous pacemaker catheter

B. Prophylactic indications
1. Transient dysrhythmias described above, with a risk of recurrence (pacer is placed in a "standby" or demand mode)
2. Used in situations where bradycardia is anticipated (e.g., following elective cardioversion)

C. Transcutaneous versus transvenous pacing
1. In general, transcutaneous pacing is less consistently reliable than transvenous pacing, and more prone to cause discomfort to the patient.
2. Transvenous pacing is preferred when patients are pacemaker dependent, or the demand for intermittent pacing is frequent or not likely reversible (e.g., after washout of a drug causing bradycardia or heart block).

Supplies and Equipment

A. Transcutaneous pacing device (usually a cardioverter–defibrillator with transcutaneous pacing capability)

B. Adhesive pacing electrodes
1. Pacing electrode pads must be compatible with the particular device; they are not necessarily interchangeable.
2. Some pads have dual transcutaneous pacing and cardioversion function; others do not.
3. Electrode pads are attached to the pacing device via cables.

Procedure

A. Turn on the device.
B. Attach skin electrodes to the patient by applying adhesive backing to the chest.
1. Anterior-posterior position is preferred.
   a. Anterior pad: left of sternum anteriorly and centered over point of maximum cardiac impulse
   b. Posterior pad: left of spine at same craniocaudal level as anterior pad
2. Avoid covering monitor leads and female breast with electrode pads.
3. Avoid covering implanted permanent pacemakers or defibrillators, if present.
4. If excessive hair is present, trimming with scissors may be required.
C. Identify the patient's intrinsic rhythm (if present).
D. Set the pacing rate (generally 60 beats per minute for bradycardia).
E. Turn on the pacing function.
F. Increase electrical current output (in milliamperes) until capture occurs.
1. Capture is identified by a pacing spike followed immediately by a wide QRS complex.
2. Determine the minimum current threshold for pacing.
3. Electrical capture should be confirmed by palpation of carotid pulsations associated with captured beats.
G. Set pacing energy at 10% to 20% above threshold.

Key Procedure Steps

- Apply pads: center anterior pads over point of maximum impulse
- Increase pacing energy (milliamperes) until capture is verified on electrocardiograph display and by carotid pulse palpation
- Set pacing energy at 10% to 20% above threshold value.

Post-Procedure Management

A. Periodically reassess the need for pacing.
B. Assess patient comfort; if the patient is pacemaker dependent and experiencing distress, transvenous pacing should be considered.

CAUTION

- Every pacemaker–defibrillator device is different, and some familiarity is required prior to use of a new device.

- The location of usual controls on the operation console can differ among devices.

- Not all devices have both cardioversion and defibrillation capabilities.

- Different types of skin adhesive electrodes are available.

- Skin irritation under electrode pads is common if they are used for long periods (>24 hours) or if extensive pacing is required.

C. If the pacemaker is in predominantly "standby" mode, assess pacing energy threshold periodically (i.e., each nursing shift).

 Bibliography

American Heart Association. AMA guidelines 2000 for CPR and ECC: international consensus on science. Circulation 2000;102(Suppl I):I1-I384.

Barold SS, Zipes DP. Cardiac pacemakers and antiarrhythmic devices. In: Braunwald E (ed). Heart Disease, 5th ed. Philadelphia: WB Saunders, 1997; pp 705–706.

Cummins RO, Graves JR, Larsen MP, et al. Out-of-hospital transcutaneous pacing by emergency medical technicians in patients with asystolic cardiac arrest. N Engl J Med 1993;328:1377–1382.

Robinson ES. How to set up and use a transcutaneous pacemaker. Nursing 1995;25:32FF–32HH.

Zoll PM. Noninvasive temporary pacing. In: Bartecchi CE, Mann DE (eds). Temporary Cardiac Pacing. Chicago: Precept Press, 1990; pp 124–136.

195 Cardioversion and Defibrillation

Steven Borzak

Cardioversion and defibrillation are similar but distinct maneuvers to restore normal sinus rhythm in the setting of atrial or ventricular tachydysrhythmias. These procedures can be elective or emergent, are generally performed with the same device (a cardioverter-defibrillator), and are likely to be successful when proper technique is employed.

Definitions

A. Cardioversion: a synchronized electrical countershock applied concurrent with the electrocardiographic QRS complex
B. Defibrillation: a nonsynchronized electrical countershock
C. Synchronization: a function performed by the cardioversion device, in which the device identifies the patient's QRS complex and ensures that any electrical countershock is delivered concurrent with the QRS complex

Indications

A. Cardioversion
   1. Stable patients (no hemodynamic compromise attributable to the dysrhythmia)
      a. Atrial tachycardia, atrial fibrillation, or atrial flutter with rapid ventricular response
      b. Atrioventricular nodal re-entrant tachycardia
      c. Ventricular tachycardia
   2. Unstable patients (i.e., circulatory shock, symptomatic hypotension, angina or heart failure attributable to the dysrhythmia)
      a. Atrial tachycardia, atrial fibrillation, or atrial flutter with rapid ventricular response
      b. Atrioventricular nodal re-entrant tachycardia
   3. Ventricular tachycardia
B. Defibrillation
   1. Ventricular fibrillation
   2. Ventricular flutter

Supplies and Equipment

A. Cardioverter-defibrillator device
B. Electrodes and leads
   1. Hand-held paddles are applied manually to the chest wall with a conductive gel between surface of paddle and skin.
      a. Apply electrode gel to each of the pads in a thin continuous layer that fully covers the paddle surface.
      b. Only specific electrode gel should be used; do not use echocardiography gel, water-based or petroleum-based lubricants, or other substances.
      c. Saline-soaked gauze pads may be used, provided excess liquid is squeezed from the gauze before applying it to the chest.
      d. Do not use petroleum-impregnated gauze.
      e. While paddles are applied to the chest, the device can function in "quick look" mode to display cardiac rhythm.
   2. Skin adhesive pads can be applied to the chest wall as an alternative to hand-held paddles.
      a. Adhesive defibrillator pads can serve doubly as monitor leads on some devices.
      b. Pads come with electrical connections that are specific to the defibrillator device and are not interchangeable.
      c. Some pads have dual transcutaneous pacing function; others do not.
C. Anesthesia or sedation, and associated equipment, is required in conscious patients.
   1. Elective procedures
      a. General anesthesia or conscious sedation (e.g., using methohexital or propofol) is generally preferred over lower levels of sedation (e.g., using benzodiazepines) or narcotics (e.g., morphine).
      b. Administration of anesthesia should be by a practitioner experienced in the use of these pharmacologic agents and airway management.
      c. Supplemental oxygen is administered.
      d. Resuscitation bag-valve mask, laryngoscope, endotracheal tube, and related supplies should be immediately available for use if necessary.
      e. Pulse oximeter
      f. Suction catheter and vacuum source
      g. Automated cycling blood pressure cuff

2. For emergency procedures: the above provisions are desirable, but urgency (based on the clinical situation of the patient) may preclude some of these measures

Key Preparation

- Obtain informed consent.

- Correct hypoxemia, hypokalemia, and digoxin excess.

- Consider adequate anticoagulation.

- Ensure the presence of an experienced individual to administer anesthesia and control airway.

- Prepare monitoring equipment: pulse oximeter, automatic sphygmomanometer, bag-valve and mask, and cardioverter–defibrillator

Procedure

A. Elective cardioversion (Table 195–1)
  1. Obtain informed consent.
  2. Ensure absence of hypokalemia or signs of digoxin toxicity.
  3. For atrial fibrillation (and probably flutter), consider use of adequate anticoagulation.
  4. Ensure equipment (see earlier under Supplies and Equipment) is present.
  5. Turn on device and identify acceptable electrocardiograph (ECG) signal and rhythm on monitor; confirmation of rhythm by 12-lead ECG is desirable.
  6. Set synchronization mode on the device, and confirm the presence of the synchronization indicator over QRS complex on monitor.
  7. Select initial energy setting (suggested initial energy is 200 J for all procedures).
  8. Plan paddle position (i.e., hand-held paddles or skin adhesive pads).
    a. Anterior-posterior: left of sternum anteriorly, and left of spine at same cranial-caudal level posteriorly

    b. Right of sternum, apex of left ventricle
  9. Administer anesthesia.
  10. Deliver countershock.
    a. Establish unconsciousness of patient.
    b. Assure that other personnel are not touching the patient or the bed.
    c. Deliver synchronized shock.
      (1) Energy delivery may take several seconds due to synchronization.
      (2) For hand-held paddles, apply continuous, constant and even pressure.
  11. Re-assess rhythm.
    a. Repeat above if sinus rhythm is not restored.
    b. Note that most devices require resynchronization.
    c. Use increasing energy delivery.

B. Emergency cardioversion
  1. Perform steps for elective cardioversion as above, as the stability of the patient permits.
  2. Obtaining informed consent and pre-procedure laboratory studies may not be possible.
  3. If the patient is conscious, use of some sedation with minimal hemodynamic effects (e.g., midazolam) is recommended.

C. Defibrillation
  1. Perform steps as for emergency cardioversion.
  2. Do not use synchronization.
  3. Anesthesia or sedation not required because patient is unconscious.

Key Procedure Points

- Assure proper paddle position and avoid the sternum.

- If using paddles, apply firm and even pressure.

- Check for synchronization before each shock (for cardioversion).

- Keep pressure on paddles after discharging energy, as synchronization may introduce a delay in energy delivery.

TABLE 195–1. DISTINGUISHING FEATURES OF CARDIOVERSION AND DEFIBRILLATION

FEATURE	ELECTIVE CARDIOVERSION	EMERGENCY CARDIOVERSION	DEFIBRILLATION
Dysrhythmia indication	Atrial or supraventricular rhythm	Unstable patient with atrial or supraventricular rhythm	Pulseless ventricular tachycardia
	Ventricular tachycardia with pulse	Ventricular tachycardia with pulse	Ventricular fibrillation
Synchronization	Always	Always, except for pulseless ventricular tachycardia	Never
Anesthesia or sedation	Always	As stability of patient permits	Not required (patient is unconscious)

Postprocedure Management

A. Observe for dysrhythmic complications of cardioversion.

   1. Bradycardia

      a. If sinus node or conduction system disease is present, return of sinus rhythm may be delayed, with a bradycardic escape.

      b. In some circumstances, atropine or temporary transcutaneous pacing may be required (see Chapter 194, Transcutaneous Pacing).

   2. Ventricular tachycardia or fibrillation may result, particularly if a nonsynchronized countershock is delivered; immediate cardioversion (ventricular tachycardia) or defibrillation (ventricular fibrillation) is then required.

B. Observe patient for return of consciousness and spontaneous respiration; monitor oxyhemoglobin saturation and provide ventilation with resuscitation bag as necessary.

C. Be alert for embolic complications (atrial fibrillation and flutter), which manifest as new neurologic deficits.

D. Inspect skin at site of electrode contact; erythema can be treated with a weak steroid (e.g., 1% hydrocortisone) cream.

Special Considertaions

A. Every cardioverter-defibrillator device is different, and some familiarity is required; machines may differ, particularly regarding

   1. Presence or absence of transcutaneous pacing through machine

   2. Type of skin adhesive electrodes employed

   3. Location of controls on operation console

B. Unsuccessful cardioversion

   1. Repeated attempts are warranted.

   2. Increase to maximum energy.

   3. Change electrode position.

   4. For atrial fibrillation and flutter, consider ibutilide infusion, which can decrease the defibrillation threshold and energy requirements and increase the success rate of cardioversion.

Bibliography

American Heart Association. AMA guidelines 2000 for CPR and ECC: international consensus on science. Circulation 2000;102(Suppl I):I1–I384.

Bossaert LL. Fibrillation and defibrillation of the heart. Br J Anaesth 1997;79:203–213.

Fotuhi PC, Epstein AE, Ideker RE. Energy levels for defibrillation: what is of real clinical importance? Am J Cardiol 1999;83:24D–33D.

Main ML, Klein AL. Cardioversion in atrial fibrillation: Indications, thromboembolic prophylaxis, and role of transesophageal echocardiography. J Thromb Thrombolysis 1999;7:53–60.

Truong JH, Rosen P. Current concepts in electrical defibrillation. J Emerg Med 1997;15:331–338.

196 Pericardiocentesis

Vivian L. Clark

Key Indications

- Treatment of pericardial tamponade; pericardiocentesis may be used to stabilize a patient until a more definitive procedure can be performed

- Determination of the etiology of a pericardial effusion

Key Contraindications (relative)

- Bleeding diathesis

- Small or loculated effusions, because of the risk of cardiac perforation

- Surgical pericardiotomy is preferable for treating some effusions, particularly those due to penetrating trauma, free wall rupture, bacterial infections, or malignancy.

Procedure

A. Patient preparation

1. The procedure should be done in an ICU setting, catheterization laboratory, or operating room.

2. The patient should be in a semirecumbant position.

3. Establish continuous electrocardiographic, intra-arterial, and central venous pressure monitoring.

4. Limb leads from a second electrocardiograph (ECG) are connected to the patient; the V_1 lead wire is not connected to a skin electrode, but it is positioned for ready availability during the procedure (see below).

5. Pulmonary artery catheterization is useful to confirm the presence of tamponade, to document improvement with fluid removal, and to aid in the management of potential complications.

B. Site selection

1. The subxiphoid approach is the most frequently used and has a low risk of complications.

2. An apical (transthoracic) approach may be used in effusions that are primarily localized to the apex, but the risk of pleural or coronary artery perforation may be higher.

C. Subxiphoid approach (Fig. 196–1)

1. The patient's chest is cleansed with a suitable antiseptic solution (e.g., povidone-iodine).

2. Local anesthetic (e.g., 1% lidocaine without epinephrine) is infiltrated intradermally and then subcutaneously just below and to the right of the xiphoid process.

3. An alligator clip lead wire is used to establish an electrical connection between a spinal needle and lead V_1 of the secondary electrocardiograph to signal contact with the epicardium.

4. Simultaneous transthoracic echocardiography should be performed, if available.

5. The pericardial (spinal) needle with its inner stylet in place is inserted just inferior to and to the right of the xiphoid process and directed toward the left nipple at an angle to allow the needle to pass just below the xiphoid process.

6. The needle is incrementally advanced and the stylet intermittently removed to assess for the presence of pericardial fluid; a slight degree of give is often felt as the needle enters the pericardial space.

7. ST segment elevation observed on the monitored ECG V-lead signifies contact with the epicardium and indicates that the needle should be withdrawn slightly.

8. After fluid is obtained a small amount is withdrawn using a syringe.

   a. If the fluid is bloody, a hematocrit is obtained to exclude cardiac perforation.

   b. If fluoroscopy is available, a small amount of contrast can be injected to verify needle position.

9. 50 to 100 ml of fluid is collected in syringes, transferred to appropriate tubes, and sent for biochemical, hematologic, microbiologic, and cytologic studies, including blood cell counts, pH, protein, glucose, lactate dehydrogenase, cytology, Gram stain, acid-fast stain, and bacterial, fungal and mycobacterial cultures.

10. A guidewire is advanced through the needle into the pericardial space several centimeters beyond the tip of the needle.

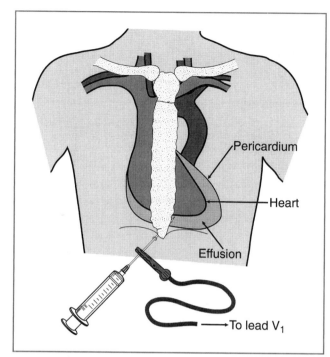

Figure 196-1 Needle-electrocardiography guided pericardiocentesis by the subxiphoid approach.

11. Withdraw the needle, leaving the guidewire in place, and advance a pig-tail catheter over the wire into the pericardial space.

12. Remove the guidewire and attach the pig-tail catheter to a vacuum bottle using low-compliance connection tubing.

13. If necessary, adjust the catheter position to allow fluid to flow into the vacuum bottle.

D. Apical approach
   1. After cleansing and anesthetizing the site, insert the needle at the 4th or 5th intercostal space about two finger breadths medial to the outer limit of cardiac dullness and at an angle nearly perpendicular to the chest wall.
   2. Follow steps C3 through C13 above.
   3. Both needle-electrocardiographic and echocardiographic monitoring are recommended with this approach.

E. Post-catheterization care
   1. When satisfactory catheter position is achieved, the catheter should be anchored to the skin with a suture and covered with a sterile dressing.
   2. Confirm catheter position with a chest x-ray.

3. Serial echocardiography can be used to determine whether residual effusion remains and can identify loculated effusions.

4. When drainage from the catheter is minimal and there is no significant residual fluid by echocardiography, the catheter should be removed.

Complications

A. Right atrial or ventricular free wall perforation
   1. The most frequent complication
   2. Should be considered if grossly bloody fluid is obtained
   3. ST segment elevation (if needle-electrocardiographic monitoring is used) or ectopy signals needle contact with the epicardium.
   4. Can be confirmed fluoroscopically by injecting a small amount of contrast through the needle; rapid clearance suggests it is intraventricular.
   5. Treatment includes removal of the needle; if the catheter is already in place it should be removed in the operating room.
   6. Open pericardiotomy and repair of the perforation are usually required.

B. Cardiac dysrhythmias including supraventricular and ventricular ectopy, and marked bradycardia

C. Coronary artery perforation

D. Hollow viscus perforation: more common with the subxiphoid approach

E. Pneumothorax: more common with the apical approach

B Bibliography

Atar S, Chiu J, Forrester JS, et al. Blood pericardial effusion in patients with cardiac tamponade: is the cause cancerous, tuberculous, or iatrogenic in the 1990s? Chest 1999;16:1564–1569.

Kirkland LL, Taylor RW. Pericardiocentesis. Crit Care Clin 1992;8:699–712.

Meyers DG, Meyers RE, Prendergast TW. The usefulness of diagnostic tests on pericardial fluid. Chest 1997;111:1213–1221.

Sagrista-Sauleda J, Angel J, Permanyer-Miraldo G, et al. Long-term follow-up of idiopathic chronic pericardial effusion. N Engl J Med 1999;341:2054–2059.

Tsang TSM, Enriquez-Sarano M, Freeman WK, et al. Consecutive 1127 therapeutic echocardiographically guided pericardiocenteses: clinical profile, practice patterns, and outcomes spanning 21 years. Mayo Clin Proc 2002;77:429–436.

Tsang TS, Freeman WK, Sinak LJ, et al. Echocardiographically guided pericardiocentesis: evolution and state-of-the-art technique. Mayo Clin Proc 1998;73:647–652.

197 Intra-Aortic Balloon Counterpulsation

Vivian L. Clark

Indications

A. Unstable angina pectoris unresponsive to standard medical therapy

B. Cardiogenic shock; in patients with acute myocardial infarction (MI) this is usually combined with revascularization

C. Congestive heart failure, as a bridge to left ventricular assist device or transplant

D. Mechanical complications of acute MI; i.e., severe mitral insufficiency or ventricular septal defect

E. High-risk patient undergoing percutaneous coronary intervention

F. High-risk patient undergoing coronary artery bypass surgery; e.g., significant left main coronary artery disease

Key Contraindications

- Aortic insufficiency (even mild degrees of aortic insufficiency can be worsened by diastolic balloon inflation)

- Aortic dissection

- Abdominal aortic aneurysm

- Peripheral vascular occlusive disease

- Severe bleeding diathesis

- Certain dysrhythmias, e.g., atrial fibrillation with a rapid ventricular response

Catheter Insertion

A. Usually the catheter is inserted percutaneously via the femoral artery; peripheral circulation must be assessed prior to catheter insertion by checking peripheral pulses, listening for bruits, and looking for signs of arterial insufficiency.

B. Most devices are 8 to 10 French.

C. Bedside insertion is feasible, but fluoroscopic guidance should be used if readily available.

D. Percutaneous femoral artery insertion technique using a sheath introducer

  1. Femoral arterial access is obtained using the Seldinger technique.

2. A predilator may be used prior to insertion of the sheath–dilator assembly.

3. The sheath–dilator assembly is inserted over the guidewire and the dilator is removed.

4. The catheter should be prepared prior to insertion by flushing the lumen with heparinized saline; depending upon the size and design of the balloon catheter, a one-way valve may be placed on the balloon port and suction applied with a syringe.

5. Under fluoroscopic guidance, the catheter is then advanced over the wire and the distal radiopaque marker on the catheter is positioned just caudal to the origin of the left subclavian artery; if the catheter is inserted without fluoroscopic control, the insertion distance should be roughly estimated by first laying the catheter on the sterile drape over the patient.

6. Blood is aspirated from the hub of the intravascular lumen, which is then connected to a pressure transducer and heparinized saline flush; after flushing the intravascular lumen, a pressure waveform should be observed on the drive-unit monitor.

7. The balloon lumen is then connected to the helium supply in the device console, after removal of the one-way valve.

8. After catheter placement and confirmation of adequate counterpulsation (Fig. 197–1) the catheter position (Fig. 197–2) should be confirmed on chest x-ray.

Key Effects of Intra-aortic Balloon Counterpulsation

- Increases diastolic coronary perfusion

- Reduces left ventricular afterload

- May increase cardiac output by up to 20%

Pitfalls of Intra-aortic Balloon Counterpulsation

A. Poor diastolic augmentation may be due to incomplete balloon filling, malposition of the catheter, incorrect timing during the cardiac cycle, and tachydysrhythmias.

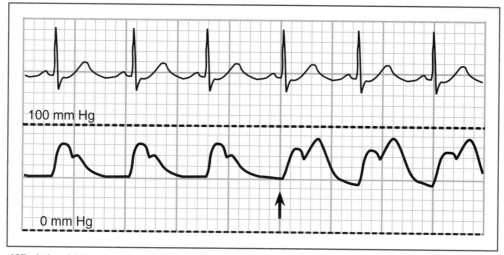

Figure 197–1 Arterial blood pressure waveform before and after (arrow) initiation of intra-aortic balloon counterpulsation

1. Catheter malposition
   a. Balloon positioned in the aortic arch or subclavian orifice
   b. Balloon not fully exited from the introducer sheath; this may be a problem in patients of short stature and may require partial withdrawal of the introducer sheath
   c. Position of the balloon within a false lumen should be considered if blood cannot be aspirated from the balloon lumen and no pressure waveform is visualized upon connecting the intravascular lumen to the pressure transducer; balloon inflation must not be initiated until appropriate catheter position is confirmed.
2. Insufficient augmentation due to tachydysrhythmia
   a. May be managed by changing the pumping ratio to 2 : 1
   b. Treatment of the dysrhythmia is critical.

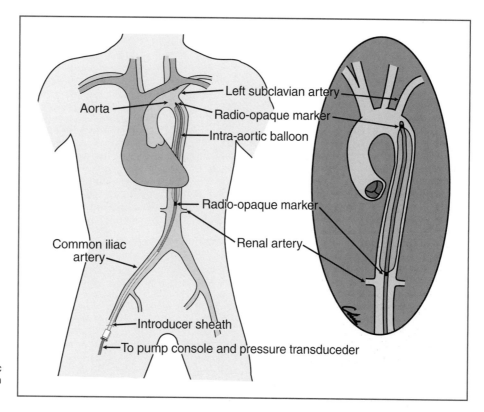

Figure 197–2 Inflated intra-aortic balloon catheter in correct position within aorta

c. Dysrhythmias related to ischemia may improve after initiation of balloon counterpulsation.

3. Incomplete balloon filling due to failure of the balloon to unwrap completely is usually confirmed by visualizing the balloon fluoroscopically; this can sometimes be corrected by rapid manual inflation and deflation of the balloon.

B. Thrombosis of catheter lumen with loss of pressure waveform is more frequent with smaller catheters; it can be minimized by frequent flushing with heparinized saline.

C. Intra-aortic balloon pumping may be ineffective in patients with certain dysrhythmias, e.g., atrial fibrillation with a rapid ventricular response.

Complications

A. Vascular complications are the most common and range from mild arterial insufficiency to gangrene with limb loss.

1. Usually manifest initially by loss or significant decrease in peripheral pulse; other findings include extremity pain and cool, pale extremities.

2. Risk is increased in women and patients with diabetes.

3. Management includes removal of the device, anticoagulation, thrombolytic therapy, surgical thrombectomy and surgical limb revascularization.

B. Device-related blood stream infection or local infection at the insertion site

C. Bleeding complications occur more commonly in patients who have received thrombolytic therapy or glycoprotein IIb/IIIa inhibitors.

D. Insertion failure

E. Rare complications include balloon entrapment, aortic dissection or perforation, paraplegia, mesenteric ischemia, and renal insufficiency.

Bibliography

Arafa OE, Pedersen TH, Svennevig JL, et al. Vascular complications of the intra-aortic balloon pump in patients undergoing open heart operations: 15 year experience. Ann Thorac Surg 1999;67:645–651.

Bates ER, Stomel JR, Hochman JS, et al. The use of intra-aortic balloon counterpulsation as an adjunct to reperfusion therapy for cardiogenic shock. Int J Cardiol 1998; 65(Suppl 1):S37–S42.

Cohen M, Dawson MS, Kopistansky C, et al. Sex and other predictors of intra-aortic balloon counterpulsation-related complications: prospective study of 1119 consecutive patients. Am Heart J 2000;139:282–287.

Kantrowitz A, Cardona RR, Freed P. Percutaneous intra-aortic balloon counterpulsation. Crit Care Clin 1992;8: 819–837.

198 Fiberoptic Bronchoscopy

Willane S. Krell

Flexible fiberoptic bronchoscopy serves diagnostic and therapeutic roles in the intensive care unit (ICU). It is essential that any physician performing bronchoscopy in the critical care setting know the bronchial anatomy and the mechanics of performing the procedure. A certain amount of athletic ability and good hand–eye coordination is necessary to wield the bronchoscope from the side, from the front, or from behind the patient, overcoming catheters, ventilator circuitry, and other life-support equipment surrounding the bed. The physician should also be aware of expected yields, potential benefits, and possible complications in determining the utility of bronchoscopy for a given patient.

Indications

A. Diagnostic indications

1. Suspected infection

2. New or nonresolving chest x-ray findings

3. Assessment of airway injury

   a. Inhalation injury

   b. Thermal injury

   c. Aspiration

4. Evaluation of hemoptysis

5. Suspected malignancy

B. Therapeutic indications

1. Difficult endotracheal intubation

   a. Cervical injury

   b. Craniofacial injury or abnormality

   c. Reintubation

2. Endotracheal tube placement issues

   a. Assure correct placement (>2 cm above carina).

   b. Evaluate for and remove obstructions (blood clots, mucus plugs, foreign bodies).

   c. Bronchoscopy is required for correct placement of double-lumen endotracheal tubes for differential lung ventilation.

3. Foreign body removal

4. Persistent mucus plugging, retained secretions

5. Hemostasis

Key Contraindications

- Inexperienced bronchoscopist

- Intractable hypoxemia

- Malignant dysrhythmias

- Bleeding diathesis

Monitoring

A. Pre-procedure

1. Assess factors that signify increased risk.

   a. Uncooperative or combative patient

   b. Hypoxemia

   c. Debilitation

   d. Unstable angina or recent myocardial infarction

   e. Ventricular dysrhythmia

   f. Partial airway obstruction

   g. Mechanical ventilation and positive end-expiratory pressure (PEEP)

   h. Lung abscess

   i. Bleeding diathesis

   j. Elevated vascular pressures

      (1) Pulmonary hypertension

      (2) Superior vena cava obstruction

2. Obtain platelet count.

   a. Platelet count is more important than prothrombin or partial thromboplastin time in predicting the risk of bleeding.

   b. More than 60,000 platelets/mm³ are required for transbronchial biopsy.

3. Obtain blood urea nitrogen (BUN) and creatinine concentrations to assess for functional platelet defect from uremia.

4. Consider airway size for intubated patients undergoing bronchoscopy.

   a. Minimum practical tube diameter is 8 mm

   b. Options for patients intubated with smaller size endotracheal tubes

      (1) Fiberoptic reintubation with a larger tube

    (2) Ventilating the patient with heliox during bronchoscopy

    (3) Bypass endotracheal tube (only if PEEP is not used).

B. During procedure

  1. Use continuous pulse oximetry.

    a. Decrease in oxygen saturation is expected.

    b. Greater decreases are expected in patients with respiratory compromise.

    c. Greater decreases are expected with increasing procedure duration.

    d. Titrate supplemental oxygen to patient's requirements.

  2. Use continuous electrocardiography.

    a. Cardiac dysrhythmias can occur due to vagal stimulation in airways.

      (1) Atrial dysrhythmias: usually minor

      (2) Ventricular dysrhythmias: can be life threatening

    b. Both hypoxemia and unstable angina create a high risk for dysrhythmias.

  3. Frequently reassess the comfort level of the patient.

C. Post-procedure

  1. Use continuous pulse oximetry.

    a. Desaturation may persist several hours.

    b. Desaturation may signal other complications.

  2. Monitor respiratory rate, pulse, blood pressure, and physical examination.

    a. Pneumothorax

    b. Bleeding

    c. Bronchospasm

  3. Perform chest x-ray.

    a. Displacement of endotracheal tube

    b. Pneumothorax

Key Monitoring

- Platelet count
- Blood urea nitrogen and creatinine level
- Continuous pulse oximetry
- Continuous electrocardiography

Preparation (pharmacologic)

A. Local anesthetics

  1. Watch for allergic reactions.

    a. More common with ester-type "caines" (e.g., procaine)

    b. Amide-type agents (e.g., lidocaine) are generally safer.

  2. Watch for toxicity.

    a. Track dosing; assume 30% to 50% is absorbed systemically.

    b. Watch for central nervous system toxicity; e.g., tremors, seizures.

    c. Watch for cardiac toxicity; e.g., dysrhythmias, cardiovascular collapse.

  3. Lidocaine is a good choice.

    a. Good cough suppression

    b. Less respiratory depression

B. Opiates

  1. Role: antitussive, mild sedation

  2. Avoid long-acting narcotics.

  3. No clear advantage or disadvantage for any short-acting drug

  4. Can cause respiratory depression

C. Sedative-hypnotic drugs

  1. Important role, even in ICU setting

    a. Patient comfort

    b. Decreases complications

  2. Choose short-acting agents.

  3. Can cause respiratory depression

D. Anticholinergic drugs

  1. Decrease upper airway secretions in non-intubated patients

  2. Reduce watery lower airway secretions

  3. May prevent vagally induced cardiac dysrhythmias

Procedure

A. General principles

  1. Minimize total procedure time.

    a. Less than 10 minutes is ideal.

    b. If longer than 30 minutes, significant oxygen desaturation is more likely.

  2. Assure adequate local anesthesia for comfort and to minimize cough.

  3. Assure adequate sedation; will help minimize airway trauma.

B. Washings

  1. Instill 5 to 10 mL nonbacteriostatic sterile saline into a major airway and aspirate.

  2. Yield approximates good endotracheal tube specimens.

  3. Helpful for excluding acid-fast bacteria (AFB) and fungi

  4. Not useful for identifying bacterial infection

  5. Minimal added risk over bronchoscopy itself

C. Brushings

1. Endobronchial lesions are brushed under direct vision to obtain specimens for cytologic analysis.

    a. Slide preparation at bedside is crucial.

    b. Yield is 30% to 40% positive for cancer.

2. Protected brushing of visible or beyond-visible areas of suspected infection

    a. Uses

        (1) Only way to deliver an anaerobic specimen

        (2) Quantitative cultures for aerobic bacteria

        (3) Identification of AFB, fungi, *Legionella*, and in some cases *Pneumocystis carinii* pneumonia (PCP)

        (4) Modest increase in bleeding over bronchoscopy alone

    b. Use caution in brushing beyond visible airways.

D. Bronchoalveolar lavage (BAL)

1. Wedge bronchoscope in a subsegmental bronchus.

    a. Look for mucosal blanching.

    b. Do not overwedge.

2. Instill nonbacteriostatic sterile saline into the subsegment.

    a. Instill serial aliquots of 20 to 100 mL each.

    b. Total volume instilled is 100 to 300 mL.

    c. Do not push fluid with excessive force.

3. Remove fluid by low continuous suction (<80 mm Hg).

    a. Suction serially after each aliquot is instilled.

    b. Minimum return volume for analysis is 40 mL of BAL fluid.

    c. If poor return volume

        (1) Increase instilled volume.

        (2) Reposition bronchoscope tip.

        (3) Lower or raise suction pressure.

4. Results in greater oxygen desaturation at 4 to 6 hours than bronchoscopy alone

E. Biopsy

1. Endobronchial

    a. For visible airway lesions

    b. Uses large-jawed forceps

    c. Increased risk of bleeding

2. Transbronchial

    a. For peripheral pulmonary processes

    b. Has the highest yield of bronchoscopic procedures

        (1) Malignancy, especially if localized process

        (2) Infection, especially if diffuse process

    c. Has the highest complication rate of routine bronchoscopic procedures

        (1) Bleeding

            (a) In ICU patients, significant bleeding occurs in up to 30%.

            (b) Increases with increasing risk factors

        (2) Pneumothorax

            (a) Risk reported from 5% to 20%

            (b) Increased risk with coughing and with combative patients

            (c) Increased risk with use of positive pressure ventilation

            (d) Further increased risk with PEEP

3. Needle aspiration/biopsy

    a. Central/mediastinal extraluminal disease (lymph nodes)

    b. Cellular aspirate or core biopsy

    c. Good yield for malignancy; poor yield for infections

    d. Increased risk of bleeding and pneumothorax

F. Therapeutic tools

1. Basket forceps to retrieve foreign bodies

2. Balloon catheter

    a. To tamponade bleeding pulmonary segment

    b. To isolate a subsegment of lung for lavage

3. Airway stents

    a. Silicone stents require rigid bronchoscopy (generally impractical in ICU).

    b. Metal stents

        (1) Useful for stenotic or highly compliant airway segments

        (2) Problematic with progressive lesions (e.g., malignancies, granulation tissue)

        (3) Risk of misplacement, distal migration, and perforation

4. Endobronchial irradiation (brachytherapy) for endobronchial tumors

5. Laser therapy for benign and malignant airway obstruction

Laboratory Studies

A. Washings

1. AFB stain and culture

2. Fungal stains and cultures

3. Less useful for bacteria (upper airway contamination common)

B. Protected catheter brushings

1. Gram stain

2. Quantitative cultures for aerobic bacteria

3. Anaerobic culture

4. Acid-fast bacteria stain and culture

5. Fungi

6. *Legionella*

7. *Pneumocystis carinii* stain

C. Bronchoalveolar lavage fluid analysis

1. Same tests as brushings, plus cytology

2. Microbiology: 40% to 95% yield

   a. Better for PCP, AFB, fungi, *Legionella,* and viruses than brushings

   b. Yield in patients with AIDS is much greater than in other immunocompromised hosts.

3. Cytology: 40% to 70% yield

4. Cell counts

   a. High lymphocyte counts

     (1) Sarcoidosis

     (2) Tuberculosis

     (3) Hypersensitivity pneumonitis

     (4) Lymphoid malignancy

   b. High polymorphonuclear cell counts

     (1) Bacterial infection

     (2) Radiation injury

     (3) Acute inflammatory response

       (a) Bronchiolitis

       (b) Parenchymal inflammation

   c. High eosinophil counts

     (1) Eosinophilic pneumonias

     (2) Acute inflammation

D. Biopsy

1. Histologic analysis

   a. Inflammation

   b. Granulomas

   c. Malignancy

   d. Fibrosis

2. Special stains for organisms

   a. Silver stain for PCP, fungi

   b. Fluorescent antibody stain for *Legionella*

   c. Acid-fast or flourescent stains for *Mycobacteria*

Bibliography

Dasgupta A, Mehta AC. Transbronchial needle aspiration. An underused technique. Clin Chest Med 1999;20:39–51.

Davies L, Mister R, Spence DP, et al. Cardiovascular consequences of fiberoptic bronchoscopy. Eur Respir J 1997;10:695–698.

O'Brien JD, Ettinger NA, Shevlin D, et al. Safety and yield of transbronchial biopsy in mechanically ventilated patients. Crit Care Med 1997;25:440–446.

Prakash UBS. Bronchoscopy. New York: Raven Press, 1994.

White P, Bonacum JT, Miller CB. Utility of fiberoptic bronchoscopy in bone marrow transplant patients. Bone Marrow Transpl 1997;20:681–687.

199 Lumbar Puncture

James A. Kruse

Lumbar puncture allows laboratory examination of the cerebrospinal fluid (CSF). In the ICU setting, it is most often performed when meningitis is suspected.

Indications

A. Diagnosis of meningitis and encephalitis: e.g., bacterial, viral, mycobacterial, fungal

B. Diagnosis of subarachnoid hemorrhage, if suspected despite negative brain imaging studies

C. Other potential diagnostic indications: e.g., aseptic meningitis, neurosyphilis, demyelinating disease, meningeal carcinomatosis, vasculitis, pseudotumor cerebri

D. Therapeutic indications: e.g., intrathecal antibiotic or chemotherapy administration

Key Contraindications

- Increased intracranial pressure with mass lesion or obstruction of ventricular system

- Thrombocytopenia, coagulopathy, or therapeutic anticoagulation

- Focal infection at intended site of puncture, including paraspinal abscess or osteomyelitis

Procedure

A. Preparation

1. Ensure no contraindications; consider necessity of preprocedural computed tomography.

2. Explain procedure to patient and obtain informed consent.

3. Have all needed supplies readily available.

4. Position patient (Fig. 199–1).

   a. Lateral decubitus position with back perpendicular to bed surface

   b. Neck, hips, and knees fully flexed

   c. For acutely ill patients, have one or more assistants maintain patient in position.

5. Determine and mark the intended point of needle entry, usually at the midline of the L4–L5 interspace (Fig. 199–1); L3–L4 and L5–S1 are alternative sites.

6. Don mask, eye protection, hat, sterile gown and gloves.

7. Prepare site with suitable antiseptic scrub, e.g., povidone-iodine solution.

8. Apply sterile drapes to create an ample sterile field.

9. Wipe residual antiseptic from intended puncture site with alcohol gauze.

10. Assemble sterile manometer apparatus.

    a. Connect the manometer extension column, if included.

    b. Connect a sterile 3-way stopcock to the manometer, either directly or using a short length of sterile extension tubing.

    c. Adjust the stopcock so that when it is connected to the spinal needle hub CSF will flow from the needle into the manometer column.

    d. Place the apparatus on a sterile field within easy reach of the operator.

11. Arrange prelabeled (as #1 through #4 to indicate order of sampling), sterile CSF collection tubes within easy reach of operator with caps removed.

B. Procedure for lumbar dural puncture

1. Using a ≥25 gauge needle, raise a skin wheal and infiltrate the underlying soft tissue with 1% or 2% lidocaine, aspirating before each injection to avoid intravascular injection.

2. Select the desired size of spinal needle, typically 20 to 22 gauge.

3. With the stylet fully inserted within the needle lumen and the needle bevel directed upward, puncture the skin at midline of selected interspace.

4. Maintain the needle parallel with the floor throughout the procedure.

5. Advance the needle, aiming toward the umbilicus (Fig. 199–2).

6. Once the depth of penetration is into the soft tissue overlying the vertebrae and conceivably close to the posterior spinal canal, halt needle advancement.

7. Remove stylet and observe for possible CSF escape.

8. If no CSF droplets are visible at the hub after a few seconds, replace the stylet and advance needle 1 to 2 mm.

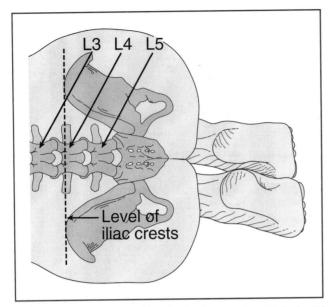

Figure 199-1 Patient position for lumbar puncture. Note frontal plane of back from shoulders to hips is perpendicular to bed, thoracolumbar spine is parallel with bed, hips and knees are flexed in knee-chest position, and head rests on pillow with neck flexed. Line segment connecting the left and right iliac crests usually crosses L3–L4 interspace or L4 spinous process. Recommended level of needle entry is L4–L5 interspace.

9. Repeat steps 7 and 8 until CSF appears or bone is encountered.

10. If the needle strikes bone, keep the stylet in place, retract the needle to superficial soft tissue, redirect angle slightly more cephalad or

caudad, and re-advance (repeating steps 6 through 9).

11. If bone is again encountered, consider that the needle may not be optimally centered at the midline of the interspace and restart with puncture slightly lateral to the original puncture site.

C. Procedure for measuring CSF pressure and collecting CSF

1. Once the stylet is removed from needle and CSF freely flows from hub, quickly connect the manometer to the spinal needle hub using a stopcock.

2. Allow CSF to rise into manometer column (held vertically) until it reaches equilibrium hydrostatic height.

3. After noting peak intrathecal pressure, hold collection tube #1 under the open stopcock port and adjust the stopcock valve to allow CSF in the manometer to drain into the collection tube.

4. Remove the manometer apparatus and continue collecting CSF into tube #1 by holding tube directly beneath needle hub until desired CSF volume is obtained; never aspirate fluid with a syringe.

5. Sequentially collect the desired volume of CSF into tubes #2 through 4 (typically 2 to 4 mL/ tube).

6. If closing pressure is desired, reconnect the

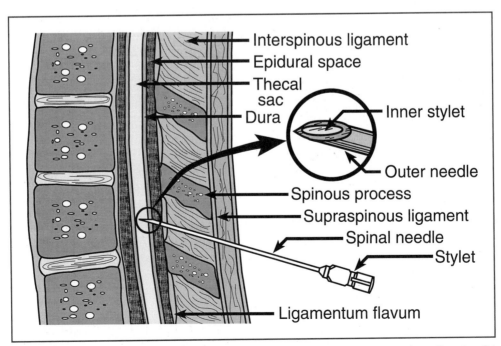

Figure 199-2 Sagittal section depicting lumbar puncture at L4–L5 interspace. Note angle of needle entry. Orientation of needle bevel should be toward patient's side.

manometer apparatus to the spinal needle hub with the stopcock appropriately positioned; note the pressure, then remove the manometer apparatus.

7. Replace the stylet fully into the spinal needle.

8. Remove the needle, apply digital pressure, and rub the site briefly.

9. Apply a bandage to the site.

10. Ensure that all CSF collection tubes are tightly capped.

D. Postprocedure

1. Order that the patient remain supine for at least 3 hours.

2. Note the gross appearance (color and clarity) of the first and last collected specimens.

3. Label all specimen tubes with patient identification.

4. Order all indicated (routine and any specific) laboratory tests to be performed on CSF; typical routine tests include:

a. Tube #1: RBC count

b. Tube #2: Gram stain, bacterial culture and susceptibility testing; acid-fast stain and culture; fungal culture, if indicated

c. Tube #3: cytologic analysis (>5 mL desirable if malignancy specifically suspected)

d. Tube #4: second RBC count, WBC count, and differential; assessment for xanthochromia, total protein, glucose; serologic test for syphilis, fungal and cryptococcal antigen tests; polymerase chain reaction test for herpes encephalitis, if indicated

5. Consider other specific tests when indicated: e.g., oligoclonal bands and myelin basic protein in suspected multiple sclerosis.

6. Review critical CSF test results as soon as available.

7. Order any necessary treatment or further testing prompted by CSF examination findings.

Key Complications

- Brain herniation
- Nerve root irritation
- Radicular nerve laceration
- Infection
- Hemorrhage at puncture site
- Epidural or intraspinal hematoma
- Retroperitoneal hemorrhage
- Post–lumbar puncture positional headache

Bibliography

Gopal AK, Whitehouse JD, Simel DL, et al. Cranial computed tomography before lumbar puncture: a prospective clinical evaluation. Arch Intern Med 1999;159:2681–2685.

Lederman RJ. Lumbar puncture: essential steps to a safe and valid procedure. Geriatrics 1996;51:51–58.

Quality Standards Committee of the American Academy of Neurology. Practice parameters: lumbar puncture. Summary statement. Neurology 1993;43:625–627.

200 Paracentesis

James A. Kruse

Abdominal paracentesis is the removal of fluid from the peritoneal space using a needle or catheter for purposes of diagnosis or therapy.

Key Indications

- Determination of etiology of ascites

- Diagnosis of peritonitis

- Diagnosis of hemoperitoneum

- Assessment of etiology of acute abdomen

- Therapeutic removal of ascites

Key Contraindications

- Pregnancy

- Significant stomach, bowel, or bladder distention

- Organomegaly in vicinity of intended site

- Prior surgery or adhesions at intended site

- Skin or soft tissue infection at intended site

Procedure

A. Site selection
1. Confirm presence of peritoneal fluid using one or more of the following methods.
   a. Physical examination, i.e., percussion and palpation (low sensitivity for detecting small volumes)
   b. Abdominal x-ray (low sensitivity for detecting small volumes)
   c. Ultrasonography
   d. Computed tomography
2. Select intended puncture site.
   a. Midline infraumbilical approach (~5 cm inferior to umbilicus between rectus abdominus muscles)
   b. Just lateral to rectus sheath at or near level of umbilicus
   c. Left or right lower quadrant, approximately midway between anterior superior iliac spine and umbilicus, lateral to rectus sheath
3. Mark intended puncture site.

B. Patient preparation
1. Explain procedure to patient and, if possible, obtain informed consent.
2. Have all needed supplies readily available.
3. Insert a nasogastric tube to decompress the stomach.
4. Insert a Foley catheter to decompress the urinary bladder.
5. Position the patient supine or with the head of the bed at an angle less than 30°, or slight reverse Trendelenburg; knees may be slightly bent above the level of the bed.
6. Prepare the site with a suitable antiseptic scrub, e.g., povidone-iodine solution.
7. Don mask, eye protection, hat, sterile gown and gloves.
8. Apply sterile drape(s) to create an ample sterile field and work space.

C. Local anesthetic infiltration
1. Use 1% lidocaine with epinephrine.
2. First use a 25-gauge needle to infiltrate the superficial dermis.
3. A 22-gauge needle may be substituted to infiltrate deeper subcutaneous tissue if necessary.
4. During superficial infiltration, aspirate before each injection to avoid intravascular injection.
5. During superficial infiltration, maintain negative pressure within the syringe barrel as the needle is advanced.
6. Aspiration of ascitic fluid into the syringe as needle is advanced signals penetration of the peritoneum; if this occurs, note the depth of penetration but do not advance needle further.

D. Device insertion
1. Diagnostic paracentesis
   a. Attach a 50 mL sterile syringe to an 18- or 20-gauge needle (a smaller syringe may be used initially and then changed to a larger syringe once fluid is obtained).
   b. Insert the needle into the skin at or near the intended site.
   c. Displace the skin 2 to 3 cm in relation to deeper tissue and advance the needle perpendicular to the skin into soft tissue (to create a Z-track).
   d. Continue slow and incremental advancement through the soft tissue with the needle per-

pendicular to the skin while intermittently attempting to aspirate with the syringe.

(1) Slow advancement allows detection of inadvertent blood vessel entry as well as immediate recognition of entry into the peritoneal space.

(2) Intermittent aspiration minimizes the chance of needle occlusion by omentum or bowel once the peritoneum is entered.

e. When ascitic fluid is obtained, aspirate the desired volume (50 mL is typically sufficient for diagnostic tests).

f. Optionally, a catheter-over-needle device may be used in place of the simple needle (see 2. Therapeutic paracentesis, below).

Key Laboratory Tests on Ascitic Fluid

- Total and differential cell counts
- Total protein and albumin concentrations
- Lactate dehydrogenase activity
- Gram stain, bacterial culture, and susceptibility
- Cytology, if malignancy is suspected
- Optional microbiological tests: acid-fast bacillus stain and culture; fungal culture
- Optional biochemical tests: glucose, amylase, triglyceride, bilirubin levels

2. Therapeutic paracentesis

a. Attach a 20 mL sterile syringe to a 16- to 20-gauge catheter-over-needle device (commonly used for intravenous access), length in excess of abdominal wall thickness.

b. Insert and advance the device toward the peritoneal space (as above), maintaining negative pressure on the syringe, until ascitic fluid is aspirated.

c. Advance the assembly an additional 1/8″ or so and ensure that fluid can still be aspirated.

d. Hold the needle portion of the assembly stationary and slide the catheter over the needle and into the peritoneal space, using a twisting motion if necessary.

e. Hold the catheter hub in position during the remainder of the procedure so that the catheter tip does not retract out of the peritoneal space.

f. Remove the needle, attach a syringe to the catheter hub, and aspirate to ensure that free-flowing peritoneal fluid is obtained.

g. Remove the desired volume of fluid using one of the following methods.

(1) Attach a length of sterile extension tubing between the catheter hub and a large vacuum collection bottle.

(2) Attach a sterile 3-way stopcock to the catheter hub, with the second hub of the stopcock connected to a 50-mL syringe, and the third hub connected to a length of sterile extension tubing leading to a large collection bag or other container. By repetitively manipulating the stopcock and syringe, 50-mL aliquots of fluid can be aspirated into the syringe and expelled into the collection container.

(3) If flow stops before the desired volume of fluid has been obtained, several maneuvers may result in resumption of flow.

(a) Rotation of cannula (needle or catheter)

(b) If a plastic catheter has been used, rotation or slight advancement or retraction of the device

(c) Intermittently ceasing application of negative pressure during manipulation of the cannula

(d) Allowing fluid to flow from the hub of the cannula without application of negative pressure

Key Complications

- Bloody (traumatic) tap
- Bleeding or hematoma at puncture site
- Persistent ascitic fluid leakage at puncture site
- Site infection or peritonitis
- Hemoperitoneum
- Bowel or bladder perforation
- Large vessel (e.g., aorta) puncture
- Hepatorenal syndrome (due to large-volume ascites removal)
- Hypotension (due to hemorrhage or large-volume ascites removal)

TABLE 200–1. TYPICAL LABORATORY FINDINGS IN ASCITES OF VARIOUS ETIOLOGIES*

	TOTALS PROTEINS (G/DL)	LDH (IU/L)	LDH A:S	ALB S–A GRADIENT (G/DL)	GRAM STAIN C/S	WBC COUNT (MM⁻³)	GLUCOSE (MG/DL)	CYTOLOGY	AMYLASE (IU/L)
Cirrhosis	<2.5	<400	<0.6	>1.1	−	<500†	−	−	−
Congestive heart failure	>2.5	−	<0.6	>1.1	−	<500†	−	−	−
Nephrosis	<2.5	−	<0.6	<1.1	−	<250†	−	−	−
Secondary bacterial peritonitis	>1.0	>225	>0.6	<1.1	+	>5000‡	<50	−	−
Spontaneous bacterial peritonitis	<1.0	<225	>0.6	>1.1	+	>250‡	>50	−	−
Tuberculous peritonitis	>2.5	>300	>0.6	<1.1	§	>1000†	nl- ↓	−	>100
Pancreatitic ascites	>2.5	>300	>0.6	<1.1	−	>250‡	−	−	−
Peritoneal carcinomatosis	>2.5	>300	>0.6	<1.1	−	>500†	nl- ↓	+	−
Massive hepatic metastases	<3.0	<400	<0.6	>1.1	−	>500†	−	±	−

*LDH = lactate dehydrogenase; Alb = albumin; s = serum concentration or activity; a = ascites concentration or activity; c/s = culture/susceptibility testing; WBC = white blood cell; + = positive; nl = normal; ↓ = decreased.
†Fewer than 50% polymorphonuclear cells.
‡More than 50% polymorphonuclear cells.
§Acid-fast bacillus stain and culture positive.

h. Alternatives to the catheter-over-needle method (see Chapter 201, Thoracentesis, for detailed description of devices and techniques)

   (1) Seldinger procedure: using an 18-gauge thin-walled needle with mating guidewire and catheter

   (2) Catheter-through-needle device

   (3) Safety needle or catheter-over-safety needle

E. Remove needle or catheter.

F. Postprocedure

   1. Apply bandage to site.

   2. Order tests to be performed on collected fluid (Table 200–1).

3. Document procedure in the medical record.

4. Monitor patient for signs of bleeding or other complications.

Bibliography

Arnold C, Haag K, Blum HE, et al. Acute hemoperitoneum after large-volume paracentesis. Gatroenterology 1997; 113:978–982.

Habeeb KS, Herrera JL. Management of ascites. Paracentesis as a guide. Postgraduate Med 1997;101:195–200.

Kravetz D, Romero G, Argonz J, et al. Total volume paracentesis decreases variceal pressure, size, and variceal wall tension in cirrhotic patients. Hepatology 1997;25: 59–62.

Runyon BA, Montano AA, Akriviadis EA, et al. The serum–ascites albumin gradient is superior to the exudate–transudate concept in the differential diagnosis of ascites. Ann Intern Med 1992;117:215–220.

201 Thoracentesis

James A. Kruse

Thoracentesis is the removal of air or fluid from the pleural space using a needle or catheter. A variety of methods are in use for performing this procedure, several of which are described.

Key Indications

- Determination of etiology of pleural effusion
- Diagnosis of empyema, hydrothorax, hemothorax, or chylothorax
- Therapeutic removal of fluid from pleural space
- Treatment of minor pneumothorax
- Pleurodesis

Key Contraindications

- Thrombocytopenia
- Coagulopathy
- Bullous disease near site
- Known pleural malignancy
- Adhesions at intended site
- Prior surgery at intended site

Procedure

A. Site selection
   1. Confirm presence of effusion.
      a. By percussion and auscultation
      b. By chest x-ray (preferably lateral decubitus views)
      c. By ultrasonography or computed tomography
   2. Select point of entry.
      a. Locate level of effusion by percussion. Intended entry point is usually 2 interspaces below superior margin of dullness at posterolateral chest.
      b. Alternatively, employ ultrasonographic imaging.
   3. Mark intended puncture site.

B. Preparation
   1. Explain the procedure to the patient and obtain informed consent, if possible.
   2. Coach the patient regarding the necessity of remaining still and avoiding coughing during the critical portion of procedure.
   3. Consider the need for supplemental oxygen.
   4. Have all needed supplies readily available.
   5. Position the patient seated erect at the edge of bed with arms folded and resting on a bedside table adjusted to a suitable height so arms are horizontal to floor.
   6. Prepare the site with a suitable antiseptic scrub, e.g., povidone-iodine solution.
   7. Don mask, eye protection, hat, sterile gown and gloves.
   8. Tape a fenestrated sterile drape to the patient's back, and place a sterile drape on the bed or an adjacent table to create a work area for sterile supplies.

C. Local anesthetic infiltration
   1. Use 1% lidocaine.
   2. First use a 25 gauge needle to infiltrate superficial dermis.
   3. Next use a 21 or 22 gauge needle to infiltrate deeper subcutaneous tissue.
   4. During anesthetic infiltration
      a. Aspirate before each injection to avoid intravascular injection.
      b. Maintain negative pressure within the syringe barrel as the needle is advanced.
      c. When infiltrating deep tissue, direct the needle over the superior edge of the rib to avoid contact with the neurovascular bundle at inferior rib edge.
   5. Aspiration of fluid into the syringe as the needle is advanced signals penetration of parietal pleura (aspiration of air signifies either the presence of pneumothorax or penetration of lung parenchyma).
   6. Upon aspirating pleural fluid, clamp a small hemostat onto the needle flush with the skin before withdrawing needle (allows assessment of depth of penetration needed to reach pleural space).

D. Device insertion (description is for aspiration of pleural fluid)
   1. Simple needle method (Fig. 201–1)
      a. Attach a sterile syringe (e.g., 20 to 50 mL) to a sterile 3-way stopcock and an appropri-

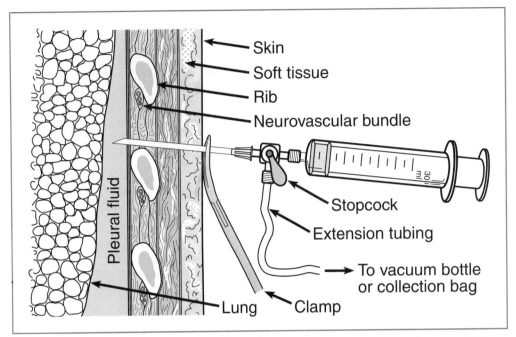

Figure 201–1 Thoracentesis using a simple needle, syringe, 3-way stopcock, and clamp (see text).

ately sized sterile needle (e.g., 14 to 18 gauge by approximately 4 cm).

b. Optionally, a length of sterile extension tubing may be interposed between the needle hub and the stopcock–syringe assembly.

c. Attach a length of sterile extension tubing between the exposed port of the stopcock and a suitable specimen collection container, e.g.:

(1) Sterile vacuum bottle

(2) Sterile specimen collection bag

(3) One or more sterile open collection tubes or containers

d. Ensure that the stopcock position is adjusted so there is continuity only between the syringe and the needle.

e. Using the anesthesia needle and attached clamp as a guide, clamp the thoracentesis needle at same distance from its tip.

f. Puncture the skin at intended site with the needle and advance the needle while maintaining negative pressure in syringe barrel.

g. Direct the needle over the superior aspect of the rib to avoid contact with the neurovascular bundle at the inferior edge of rib.

h. Aspiration of pleural fluid should occur when the needle is advanced to the depth marked by the clamp.

i. After filling syringe with pleural fluid, turn the stopcock handle to allow fluid to be ex-

pelled from the syringe into the specimen collection container.

j. If a vacuum collection bottle is used, adjust the stopcock position for fluid path between bottle and needle.

k. If a vacuum bottle is not employed, alternately adjust the stopcock, first to allow aspiration into the syringe and then to allow fluid to be expelled into the container, repeating until the desired volume of fluid is removed.

2. Safety needle method

a. Device description

(1) Consists of an outer, sharp-tipped, beveled needle (e.g., 14 gauge) and a longer inner cannula with a closed, blunt tip and a side hole near the tip

(2) Inner cannula is spring-loaded so it only protrudes from the outer needle tip when there is no resistance at the tip to advancement.

(3) Proximal end has a Luer hub for connection to a stopcock and syringe.

b. Employed as with the simple needle method

c. Blunt, inner cannula is automatically pressed into outer needle during advancement through skin and soft tissue, but it extends from the end of the needle once the pleural space is entered.

d. Avoids puncture or laceration of visceral pleura while the device is in the pleural space

3. Conventional catheter-over-needle method

   a. Device consists of a plastic catheter over a hollow needle (same as used commonly for peripheral vein cannulation).

   b. Syringe is connected to the device and it is advanced through the skin to the pleural space with constant negative pressure applied.

   c. Once pleural fluid is aspirated, the assembly is advanced an additional 1/8 inch and then the plastic cannula is advanced over the stationary needle.

   d. Syringe and inner needle are removed and the catheter hub is immediately occluded with a gloved finger.

   e. Syringe and stopcock are applied to the catheter hub and the desired volume of fluid is repetitively aspirated or allowed to flow to a vacuum bottle.

   f. Alternatively, sterile connection tubing can be used to directly connect catheter hub to vacuum bottle (with no syringe or stopcock).

4. Catheter-over-safety-needle method (Fig. 201-2)

   a. Device is the same as safety needle described above, except that it has a plastic catheter over the needle.

   b. Syringe is connected to the device and it is advanced through the skin to the pleural space with constant negative pressure applied.

   c. Once the needle is within the pleural space and pleural fluid aspirated, the catheter is advanced over the needle into the pleural space, and the needle portion is removed.

   d. Catheter portion of device incorporates a one-way valve mechanism that prevents entry of atmospheric air into the catheter lumen through the hub (and prevents the needle from being re-inserted once it has been removed from the catheter).

   e. Catheter portion of device has an integral side port for connection to a syringe or vacuum bottle.

5. Catheter-through-needle method

   a. Device consists of (1) a large-bore needle (e.g., 14 gauge) and, (2) a plastic catheter designed to fit through the needle bore (e.g., 16 gauge), with an inner stiffening wire.

   b. Attach syringe to the needle hub and ad-

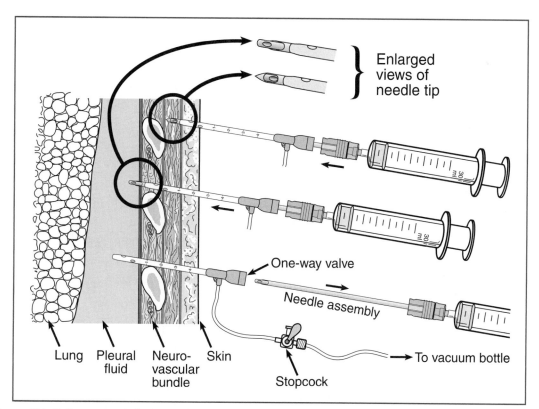

Figure 201-2 Sequence of thoracentesis using a catheter-over-safety-needle device. Upper enlarged view shows spring-loaded, blunt-tipped, inner cannula with side-hole, in normal passive position, i.e., extruding from end of sharp outer needle. Lower enlarged view shows same end of device with inner cannula depressed (as when pressure is applied to tip during penetration of soft tissue), thereby exposing sharp tip of outer needle. One-way valve on catheter hub prevents escape of pleural fluid or entry of atmospheric air via hub.

vance the needle to the pleural space while maintaining negative pressure in the syringe.

c. When pleural fluid is aspirated, remove the syringe and quickly insert the catheter (with inner stiffening wire in place) through the needle hub.

d. Once the catheter has been advanced past the end of the needle it must not be retracted through the needle (the needle bevel could shear off the distal portion of the catheter).

e. Once the catheter is advanced into the pleural space, retract the needle out of the body and cover it with the included safety guard.

f. Remove the inner stiffening wire from the catheter and immediately connect the catheter hub to the syringe and stopcock.

g. Proceed as above.

6. Seldinger method

a. Device consists of a thin-walled needle and mating spring guidewire and catheter.

b. Attach a syringe to the needle hub and advance the needle to the pleural space while maintaining negative pressure in the syringe.

c. When pleural fluid is aspirated, remove the syringe and quickly insert the guidewire through the needle hub.

d. Once the wire is advanced well into the pleural space, remove the needle.

e. If necessary, nick the skin with a #11 scalpel.

f. Advance the catheter over the guidewire.

g. Before advancing the catheter through the cutaneous entry point, ensure that the guidewire is visible at the hub end of the catheter.

h. Advance the catheter into the pleural space.

i. Remove the guidewire and immediately connect the catheter hub to a syringe and stopcock.

j. Proceed as above.

7. Catheter-through-sheath method

a. Device consists of a thin-walled needle and a mating spring guidewire, tissue dilator, introducer sheath, and catheter.

(1) Components are specially designed for large-bore (e.g., up to 28 French) chest catheter insertion (differs from introducer sheaths commonly used for vascular access).

(2) Generally used as an alternative to surgical placement of an indwelling chest tube rather than for thoracentesis

b. Attach syringe to needle hub and advance needle to pleural space while maintaining negative pressure in syringe.

c. When pleural fluid is aspirated, remove the syringe and quickly insert the guidewire through the needle hub.

d. Once the wire is advanced well into the pleural space, remove the needle.

e. Enlarge the skin incision with a #11 scalpel.

f. Bluntly dissect soft tissue using a Kelly clamp, as necessary.

g. Advance the dilator-sheath assembly over the guidewire; ensure that the guidewire is visible at the hub end of the assembly before the dilator tip enters skin.

h. Advance the dilator-sheath assembly into the pleural space.

i. Remove the guidewire and dilator, and immediately occlude the sheath hub.

j. Advance the chest catheter through the introducer sheath and into the pleural space.

k. Remove the sheath over the chest catheter.

l. Proceed as above.

Key Laboratory Tests Performed on Pleural Fluid

- Complete and differential cell count
- Total protein, glucose, and lactate dehydrogenase (and simultaneous serum tests for comparison)
- Amylase (if suspect pancreatitis, esophageal rupture, neoplasm)
- Gram stain, culture, and susceptibility testing
- Acid fast smear and culture (if suspect tuberculosis)
- Cytology (if suspect neoplasm)
- Anaerobic pH (if suspect parapneumonic effusion or empyema)
- Cholesterol and triglycerides (if suspect chylothorax)
- Hematocrit (if hemothorax)
- Rheumatoid factor and antinuclear antibody (if suspect collagen vascular disease)

E. Post-procedure

1. Apply a bandage to the site.

2. Write orders for the desired laboratory tests to be performed on pleural fluid.

3. Document the procedure in the medical record.

4. Obtain and review stat portable upright chest x-ray for signs of pneumothorax, effusion, or hemothorax.

5. Monitor the patient for pneumothorax or other complications.

Key Complications

- Pneumothorax

- Site infection or empyema

- Bronchopleural fistula

- Diaphragm injury

- Bleeding at puncture site or hemothorax

- Re-expansion pulmonary edema (>1 L drainage)

- Intercostal nerve injury

- Visceral puncture (liver or spleen)

Bibliography

Grogan DR, Irwin RS, Channick R, et al. Complications associated with thoracentesis. A prospective, randomized study comparing three different methods. Arch Intern Med 1990;150:873–877.

Heffner JE, Brown LK, Barbieri CA. Diagnostic value of tests that discriminate between exudative and transudative pleural effusions. Chest 1997;111:970–980.

Lichtenstein D, Hulot JS, Rabiller A, et al. Feasibility and safety of ultrasound-aided thoracentesis in mechanically ventilated patients. Intensive Care Med 1999;25:955–958.

Light RW, Rodriguez RM. Management of parapneumonic effusions. Clin Chest Med 1998:19:373–382.

Sasse S, Nguyen T, Teixeira LR, et al. The utility of daily therapeutic thoracentesis for the treatment of early empyema. Chest 1999;116:1703–1708.

202 Chest Tube Thoracostomy

James A. Kruse

Chest tube thoracostomy is the placement of an indwelling drainage tube through the chest wall and into the pleural space, usually for the purpose of removing air, fluid, or blood. A variety of methods and devices are available for performing the procedure, including the use of large-bore, catheter-over-needle devices; Foley catheters; Seldinger techniques using needle, guidewire, dilator, sheath-introducer, and catheter; the McSwain dart; the Heimlich valve; and trochar devices. The method described here is the conventional surgical approach.

Key Indications

- Pneumothorax
- Hemothorax
- Chylothorax
- Pleurodesis
- Thoracotomy
- Chest trauma
- Empyema
- Complicated parapneumonic effusion

Key Contraindications (relative)

- Thrombocytopenia
- Coagulopathy
- Bullous disease at site
- Pleural malignancy
- Adhesions at insertion site
- Prior surgery at insertion site

Procedures

A. Preparation

1. Explain procedure to the patient and, if possible, obtain informed consent.
2. Consider the need for supplemental oxygen, sedation, and systemic analgesia.
3. Have all needed supplies readily available.
4. Select the chest tube size.
   a. 20 to 28 French for pneumothorax
   b. 28 to 34 French for serous effusions
   c. 34 to 42 French for viscous effusions, empyema, or hemothorax
5. Select the insertion site.

   a. Anterior site (for pneumothorax): second intercostal space at the midclavicular line
   b. Lateral site (for pneumothorax, hemothorax, or effusion): cutaneous entry at fifth, sixth, or seventh intercostal space at the midaxillary line and pleural entry one intercostal space cephalad to the cutaneous entry site

6. Position the patient.

   a. For anterior insertion: 30° upright position with arms at side (the following description of technique details the more common lateral approach)
   b. For lateral insertion: 30° upright position with ipsilateral arm above head, with patient rolled slightly toward the contralateral side to expose the lateral chest; a pillow or folded towels may be placed under the ipsilateral back for support

7. Prepare the site with a suitable antiseptic scrub, e.g., povidone-iodine solution.
8. Don mask, eye protection, hat, sterile gown and gloves.
9. Apply sterile drape(s) to create an ample sterile field and work space.
10. Infiltrate the site with local anesthetic.

    a. Use ample 1% lidocaine (10 to 30 mL total).
    b. First use a 25-gauge needle to infiltrate the superficial dermis.
    c. Next use a 21- or 22-gauge needle to infiltrate deeper subcutaneous tissue (of both involved intercostal spaces for lateral approach).
    d. Aspirate before each injection to avoid intravascular injection.
    e. Anesthetize the parietal pleura.
    f. If pneumothorax or effusion is present, it may be useful to aspirate air or fluid with the anesthesia syringe to demonstrate that infiltration is to the level of the parietal pleura.

B. Special consideration for tension pneumothorax

1. Tension pneumothorax is a life-threatening emergency requiring immediate intervention; do not delay treatment awaiting x-ray confirmation.

Key Manifestations of Pneumothorax

Any Pneumothorax	Tension Pneumothorax
• Dyspnea	• Increased ipsilateral hemithoracic size
• Tachypnea	• Decreased ipsilateral respiratory movements
• Respiratory distress	• Contralateral tracheal deviation
• Apprehension	• High resistance to positive pressure ventilation
• Ipsilateral hyperresonance to percussion	• High airway pressure while on positive pressure ventilation
• Ipsilateral decreased breath sounds	• Hyperexpanded ipsilateral hemithorax on x-ray
• Pleuritic chest pain	• Contralateral shift of mediastinum on x-ray
• Subcutaneous emphysema	• Flattened ipsilateral diaphragm on x-ray
• Cyanosis	• Widened intercostal spaces on x-ray
• Tachycardia	• Hypotension, circulatory shock
• Hypoxemia	• Pulseless electrical activity (cardiac arrest)

2. The above-described preparation is abbreviated, and a needle or cannula-over-needle device (12- to 16-gauge) is inserted into the pleural space at the second intercostal space, midclavicular line, or the fourth or fifth intercostal space at the midaxillary line.

3. Exposure of the needle or cannula hub to the atmosphere converts tension pneumothorax to simple, open pneumothorax, relieving hemodynamic embarrassment.

4. Provide hemodynamic and respiratory stabilization.

5. Complete preparation for tube thoracostomy and proceed with chest tube insertion in a controlled manner as described next.

C. Dissection

1. Use a #10 scalpel to make a 2- to 4-cm skin incision parallel with the ribs, one intercostal space inferior to the intended level of pleural entry.

2. Use a large, curved Kelly clamp to bluntly dissect a tract through the soft tissue to the immediately superior intercostal space, creating a subcutaneous tunnel outside the rib cage.

3. Direct the dissection between the ribs (at the interspace just cephalad to the interspace at which the skin incision was made) to the parietal pleura (Fig. 202–1, left).

4. Focus the intercostal dissection at the caudal portion of the intercostal space to avoid trauma to the intercostal neurovascular bundle at the inferior rib edge.

5. When the dissection is to the level of the parietal pleura, use the tips of the clamp to bluntly dissect the pleural membrane part-way through.

6. Close the clamp jaws, apply controlled pressure, and puncture the parietal pleura with the tip of the clamp.

7. Pleural entry is signaled by an audible pop or palpable give, often followed by noise of air entry or egress from the incision or appearance of pleural fluid from the site.

8. Before removing the clamp, enlarge the pleural defect by opening and closing the jaws, rotating the clamp, and repeating this several times while the jaw tips are within the defect.

D. Digital probing (Fig. 202–1, middle)

1. Insert a gloved finger into the wound and advance it to the pleural defect.

2. Probe the pleural defect to ensure that the pleural cavity has been entered and that the opening is sufficient to allow digital insertion.

3. Advance the fingertip through the pleural defect, rotate it 360° and ensure that the lung is not adherent to the parietal pleura.

E. Tube insertion

1. Grasp the tip of the chest tube with the clamp and insert it into the wound with the curve of the clamp oriented to facilitate pleural entry (Fig. 202–1, right).

2. Advance the tip of the clamp and tube through the pleural opening.

3. Use the clamp to direct the tube in the desired direction.

   a. If a basal tube position is desired, relax the clamp jaws and advance the tube.

   b. If a superior tube position is desired, rotate the clamp 180° to direct the tube superiorly,

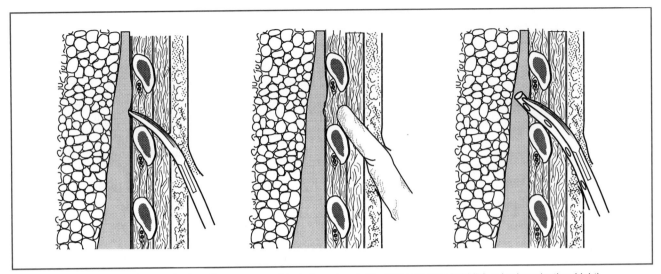

Figure 202–1 Chest tube insertion sequence: blunt dissection (left), digital probing (middle), tube introduction (right).

and then relax the jaws and advance the tube.

   c. Aim the tube posteriorly to drain fluid.

   d. Aim the tube anteriorly to relieve pneumothorax.

4. Remove the clamp and advance the tube the desired distance.

5. Ensure that the most proximal side hole of the chest tube is within the pleural space. Position of the proximal side hole may be indicated by distance markers printed on the tube.

6. Immediately connect the external end of the chest tube to the drainage apparatus (Fig. 202–2).

7. Close the skin incision tightly around the tube using one or two knotted 0 or 00 silk sutures, wrap the free ends tightly around the tube several times and tie securely in place.

F. Postprocedure

1. Apply sterile petrolatum gauze to the incision site, if desired.

2. Apply a minimal sterile occlusive dressing to the incision site.

3. At a distance from the bandage, secure the tube to skin using adhesive tape, with or without tincture of benzoin.

4. Ensure that all fittings between the chest tube and the drainage device are securely tightened and taped.

5. Ensure proper functioning of the drainage device.

6. Document the procedure in the medical record.

7. Obtain and review stat portable chest x-ray for

   a. Radiographic signs of new or residual pneumothorax

   b. Chest tube position

   c. Presence of effusion or hemothorax

   d. Complications

8. Monitor the patient for pneumothorax or other complications.

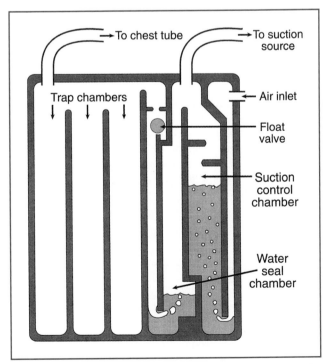

Figure 202–2 Schematic sectional view of a one-piece chest tube drainage apparatus.

9. Provide analgesia, if necessary.

G. Removal

1. Remove the tube when its use is no longer indicated, generally signaled by

   a. Sustained resolution of pneumothorax on chest x-ray

   b. No pleural air leak for more than 24 hours (without suction or clamping)

   c. Fluid drainage of less than 100 mL/day

   d. No need for positive pressure ventilation

2. Technique

   a. Explain procedure to the patient.

   b. Remove tape and dressing.

   c. Cut the suture knots securing the tube.

   d. To avoid creating a pneumothorax, withdraw the tube quickly.

   (1) If the patient is breathing spontaneously, withdraw the tube during expiration, or at the peak of maximal inspiration, or while patient performs the Valsalva maneuver.

   (2) If the patient is receiving positive pressure ventilation, withdraw the tube during inspiration.

   e. If original sutures were not knotted to skin the released free ends may be tied together to further close wound (and fully removed at a later date).

   f. Apply sterile petrolatum gauze and occlusive dressing.

3. Obtain chest x-ray to exclude pneumothorax.

4. Monitor the patient for pneumothorax or other complications.

Key Aspects of Drainage Apparatus

- Trap chambers: allow collection and quantification of pleural fluid drainage

- Water seal chamber: provides one-way passage for air to exit the pleural space

- Float valve: prevents siphoning of fluid from the water seal chamber into the trap chamber

- Hydrostatic level of water seal: determines the pleural pressure needed to expel gas from the pleural space

- Suction control chamber: limits the degree of applied suction

- Hydrostatic water level in control chamber: determines maximum applied suction

Complications

A. Pain

B. Cough

C. Tube malposition

   1. Suboptimal positioning within the pleural space (e.g., superiorly or anteriorly in cases of effusion)

   2. Chest tube fenestration located outside pleural space

   3. Interfissural placement

   4. Drainage holes not in proximity to loculated pleural air or fluid collection

   5. Impinging on mediastinal structures

   6. Subcutaneous placement (outside of chest cavity)

   7. Intra-abdominal placement

D. Mechanical problems with tube

   1. Tube occluded with viscous fluid or clotted blood

   2. Tube kinked

   3. Leak in tube, connecting tubing, or fittings

E. Inadvertent removal of tube (fully or partially)

F. Hemorrhage

   1. From surgical wound, including soft tissue and intercostal vessels

   2. From vascular adhesions

   3. From pulmonary vessel

   4. Hemothorax

   5. Intra-abdominal bleeding

   6. Hemorrhagic shock

G. Pneumothorax

H. Subcutaneous emphysema

I. Infection

   1. Surgical site infection

   2. Empyema

   3. Pneumonia

   4. Sepsis

J. Reexpansion pulmonary edema

   1. After drainage of large (>1 L) effusion

   2. After relief of tension pneumothorax

K. Lung entrapment

L. Lung laceration

M. Bronchopleural fistula

N. Diaphragm injury

O. Cardiac injury or perforation

P. Visceral injury, laceration, or perforation

   1. Esophageal injury or perforation

   2. Liver or spleen laceration

Q. Nerve injury

1. To intercostal nerve, resulting in pain or hypesthesia at site

2. To long thoracic nerve, resulting in winged scapula

3. To phrenic nerve, resulting in diaphragmatic weakness or paralysis

4. To upper thoracic sympathetic nerves, resulting in Horner's syndrome

B Bibliography

Baumann MH, Strange C. The clinician's perspective on pneumothorax management. Chest 1997;112:822–828.

Iberti TJ, Stern PM. Chest tube thoracostomy. Crit Care Clin 1992;8:879–895.

Luketich JD, Kiss M, Hershey J, et al. Chest tube insertion: A prospective evaluation of pain management. Clin J Pain 1998;14:152–154.

Martino K, Merrit S, Boyakye K, et al. Prospective randomized trial of thoracostomy removal algorithms. J Trauma Injury Infection Crit Care 1999;46:369–371.

203 Hemodialysis

Fayyaz H. Sagarwala
Richard W. Carlson

Acute hemodialysis is performed for complications of uremia and for certain drug overdoses. There are considerable differences in opinion and practice patterns regarding indications for dialysis in the intensive care unit (ICU) setting. No definite level of serum urea nitrogen (BUN) or creatinine concentration are agreed on as absolute indicators to initiate dialysis.

Indications

A. Uremic signs, symptoms, and complications
1. Nausea, vomiting, anorexia
2. Encephalopathy, including lethargy, somnolence, stupor, asterixis, myoclonus, coma
3. Volume overload refractory to diuretic therapy
4. Serositis: pericarditis, pleuritis; uremic pulmonary edema
5. Hyperkalemia resistant to other therapy
6. Bleeding diathesis from uremia
7. Severe hypermagnesemia
8. Hyperuricemia
9. Severe metabolic acidosis or complex acid-base disturbances uncontrolled by other measures

B. Drug overdoses and poisonings
1. Salicylates
2. Lithium
3. Methanol, ethylene glycol, isopropanol
4. Theophylline
5. Bromide
6. Chloral hydrate
7. Paraquat
8. Phenobarbital

Key Contraindications and Barriers to Dialysis

- Hemodynamic: hypotension, shock

- Hemostatic: uncontrolled bleeding diathesis or inability to tolerate anticoagulation

- Access-related: inability to establish vascular access

- Ethical: patient's or surrogate's decision to withhold dialysis

Overview

A. Biophysical principles
1. Solute removal
    a. Passive diffusion
        (1) Primary mechanism of metabolic waste product removal; diffusion down the concentration gradient from blood to dialysate
        (2) Solute transport by blood flow interacting with dialysis solution at high surface area dialysis membrane
        (3) Blood and dialysate flow in opposite directions, maintaining concentration gradient for diffusion across membrane.
    b. Convective transport: solute drag with fluid movement across membrane
    c. Solute features that facilitate removal by hemodialysis: water-soluble, low molecular weight, low protein binding, low volume of distribution (<250 L or <3 L/kg)
2. The fluid-removal mechanism is the hydrostatic pressure gradient across the dialysis membrane, causing fluid movement from a high-pressure compartment (blood) to a low-pressure compartment (dialysate).

B. Types of hemodialysis membranes
1. Cellulose
    a. Manufactured from processed cotton; contains many hydroxy groups
    b. May be associated with more type B reactions by complement activation at hydroxyl groups
2. Modified cellulose
    a. Improved biocompatibility or improved diffusive and ultrafiltration properties
    b. Examples: cuprammonium cellulose, cellulose acetate
3. Synthetic polymers
    a. High absorptive capacity; generally more biocompatible
    b. Occasionally associated with type A anaphylactoid reactions
    c. Examples: polysulfone, polymethylmethacrylate, polyacrylonitrile (PAN), polyamide

C. Membrane–blood interactions (physiology of bioincompatibility)

TABLE 203–1.   COMPARISON OF HEMODIALYSIS, HEMOFILTRATION, HEMOPERFUSION, AND PERITONEAL DIALYSIS IN THE ACUTE CARE SETTING

	HEMODIALYSIS	HEMOFILTRATION AND CRRT	HEMOPERFUSION	PERITONEAL DIALYSIS
Indication	Uremia, volume control, intoxications	Uremia, volume control	Intoxications, hepatic failure	Uremia (limited use in ICU setting)
Access	AV, VV	AV, VV	AV, VV	Peritoneal
Interval	Intermittent	Continuous	As needed	>12 hr or auto-exchange
Duration	Daily or less frequently	Many hours	Hours	Auto-exchange
Anticoagulation	Regional or systemic	Systemic (most cases)	Systemic	Not required
Skill level required	High skill, but less labor intensive	Low skill, but labor intensive	Moderate skill and labor intensive	Low skill; bedside procedure; moderately labor intensive
Biophysics	Convective and diffusive	Convective; high-flux membrane; clearance is related to diffusion	Adsorption to charcoal membrane	Less efficient clearance except for high molecular weight substances
Advantages	Standard of care; available; excellent for hyperkalemia and acidosis; effective for many drugs and toxins	Little hemodynamic perturbation; efficient for volume control in ICU patients; cytokine removal (?)	Very effective for some toxins	Little hemodynamic perturbation; good clearance of high molecular weight substances
Disadvantages	Hypotension	Immobilization	Limited availability	Less efficient
Complications	Hypoxemia, dysrhythmias, allergic reactions, infection, disequilibrium syndrome, spallation, dialysis-induced electrolyte and acid-base disorders	Hypothermia, bleeding, infection, thrombosis	Hypocalcemia, thrombocytopenia	Peritonitis, limitation in use in patients with abdominal pathology

CRRT = continuous renal replacement therapies, AV = arteriovenous, VV = venovenous.

1. Complement activation can occur and result in vascular smooth muscle contraction, increased vascular permeability (including acute respiratory distress syndrome), formation of membrane attack complex (C5-C9), and activation of neutrophils with release of free radicals and intracellular enzymes.

2. Activation of coagulation, contact pathway, and cellular components can occur.

3. Inflammatory response is affected by dialysate composition and temperature, clearance process (diffusion or convection), and bioincompatibilty.

D. Comparison of hemodialysis, hemofiltration, plasmapheresis hemoperfusion and peritoneal dialysis (Table 203–1)

Procedures

A. Vascular access devices

1. Temporary multilumen hemodialysis catheters

    a. Two- and three-lumen devices available (third lumen useful for non-dialysis-related access in many ICU patients)

    b. Preferred access for temporary, acute dialysis

    c. Can be inserted at bedside at femoral, subclavian, or internal jugular sites

    d. Ultrasound visualization may assist in vessel location and detection of thrombosis and distorted anatomy.

    e. X-ray required after jugular or subclavian vein cannulation to ensure position and to detect complications

    f. Vessel thrombosis and stenosis are potential risks.

2. Scribner shunt

    a. External plastic arteriovenous fistulas

    b. Common application: two silicone elastomer tubes connect radial artery to cephalic vein

    c. Advantage: useful for both hemodialysis and continuous hemofiltration

    d. Disadvantages: requires surgical insertion; higher infection rate; risk of dislodgement with major bleeding

3. Cuffed tunneled silicone elastomer catheters

    a. Double-lumen silicone catheters with felt cuffs or two separate single-lumen catheters with cuffs

    b. Can be used for longer duration

    c. Silicone reduces risk of thrombosis and perforation.

B. Vascular insertion sites

1. Femoral vein

    a. Advantages: easily placed at bedside, less skill required, relatively low risk, reverse

Trendelenburg position can be used for patients who cannot tolerate horizontal position during procedure

b. Disadvantages: possible increased risk of infection and thrombosis, catheter must be larger than 18 cm to minimize recirculation and increase dialysis efficiency; sitting position to be avoided when catheter in place; limited duration of use

2. Subclavian vein

a. Advantages: high blood flow rates achievable; patient can sit up or walk after the procedure; nursing care is facilitated; can be used with tracheostomy

b. Disadvantages: greater operator skill for insertion; patient must be supine or in Trendelenburg position during insertion; risk of pneumothorax; risk of superior vena cava or subclavian thrombosis or stenosis, especially after repeated cannulations; limited duration of use (2 to 3 weeks)

3. Internal jugular

a. Advantages: bedside insertion, less operator skill required, good flow rates

b. Disadvantages: risk of bleeding and injury to neck structures during insertion; patient must be supine or in Trendelenburg position during insertion; not preferred if tracheostomy; risk of vena cava thrombosis; limited duration (2 to 3 weeks)

CAUTION

Patients <7 days after major surgery (14 days for intracranial surgery), or those with pericarditis, should undergo hemodialysis without heparin.

Dosing and Monitoring

A. Dosing

1. In the acute care setting, dialysis dose requirements are highly variable and affected by several factors.

a. Indication: e.g., hyperkalemia, volume control, uremia, toxin management

b. Technical issues: e.g., availability of dialysis personnel, equipment, vascular access, time on dialysis, membrane

c. Patient variables: hemodynamic and coagulation status

B. Factors affecting the effectiveness of dialysis

1. Blood and dialysate flow rates

2. Duration of treatment

C. Monitoring the effectiveness of dialysis

1. Clinical assessment of uremic symptoms

2. Intake-output; dry weight assessment at estimated euvolemia

3. Pre- and post-dialysis blood concentrations of BUN, creatinine, toxin, drug, electrolytes

a. For example, can calculate the urea nitrogen ratio (R) as post-dialysis BUN/pre-dialysis

b. Low R values signify high clearance.

4. Urea reduction ratio

a. Calculated as 1-R

b. High urea reduction ratio values signify high urea clearance.

5. Fractional reduction of urea for urea distribution volume

a. Calculated as $K \times t / V$; where K = hemodialyzer clearance (L/hr), t = duration of dialysis (hr), and V = volume of distribution of urea (equal to total body water or approximately 60% of body weight, in liters)

b. Does not account for convective clearance

c. Varies inversely with R

d. Goal is >1.2.

Post-Procedure Management

A. Obtain post-dialysis laboratory studies.

1. Serum electrolytes, BUN, and creatinine concentrations

2. Caution: white blood cell and platelet counts may be dramatically altered immediately after dialysis

3. Toxin levels as appropriate

4. Techniques of pre- or post-dialysis blood sampling are crucial for consistent results.

B. Evaluate clinical status.

1. Hemodynamics

2. Uremic symptoms

3. Bleeding

CAUTION

Low serum potassium levels obtained within a few hours of hemodialysis do not indicate a need for potassium supplementation, as a 30% rebound increase in potassium concentration can occur up to 5 hours after hemodialysis.

Complications

A. Cardiovascular
   1. Hypotension
      a. Hypovolemia due to excessive ultrafiltration
      b. Vasodilation due to eating, drug effects, or autonomic neuropathy
      c. Cardiac dysfunction
      d. Air embolism
   2. Angina or acute myocardial infarction
   3. Cardiac dysrhythmias
   4. Steal syndrome (decreased blood flow distal to access)

B. Respiratory: hypoxemia, air embolism, white blood cell or complement-induced pulmonary reactions

C. Neurologic: disequilibrium syndrome (mental confusion, delirium, coma, seizures), muscle cramps

D. Hematologic: bleeding, leukopenia, thrombocytopenia, hemolysis

E. Metabolic: electrolyte and acid-base disturbances

F. Dialyzer related: dialyzer rupture or clotting, dialysate contamination (fluoride), mechanical complications, spallation (roller pump–induced release of plasticizer from tubing)

G. Access-related: thrombosis, infection

H. Allergic and bioincompatibilily reactions
   1. Type A ("first use syndrome")
      a. Uncommon (4 per 100,000)
      b. Related to ethylene oxide sterilization and leachable material from dialysis membrane
      c. Manifestations: hypotension, urticaria, and angioedema occur within minutes
      d. Treatment: stop dialysis, do not return blood, give antihistamines, steroids, epinephrine, bronchodilators, vasopressors as needed
   2. Type B
      a. Common (3% to 5%)
      b. Occurs after 15 to 30 minutes; related to complement–cellulose interaction and white blood cell effects
      c. Manifestations: chest-back pain, shortness of breath, nausea, vomiting, hypotension
      d. Treatment: symptomatic; often improves with ongoing dialysis
   3. Anaphylactoid reactions: occur in patients taking angiotensin converting enzyme (ACE) inhibitors and use of some high-flux PAN dialysis membranes
   4. Other clinical effects of bioincompatibilily
      a. Reduced survival rate and recovery from acute renal failure
      b. Loss of residual renal function
      c. Increased incidence of infection
      d. Increased catabolism
      e. Adverse nutritional effects

PEARL

Anaphylactoid reactions can occur during dialysis with some PAN membranes in patients treated with ACE inhibitors.

B Bibliography

Arieff AI. Dialysis disequilibrium syndrome: current concepts on pathogenesis and prevention. Kidney Int 1994;45:629–635.

Caruana RJ, Raja RM, Zeit RM, et al. Thrombotic complications of indwelling central catheters used for chronic hemodialysis. Am J Kidney Dis 1987;9:497–501.

Cruz DN, Mahnensmith RL, Brickel HM, Perazella MA. Midodrine and cool dialysate are effective therapies for symptomatic intradialytic hypotension. Am J Kidney Dis 1999;33:920–926.

Daugirdas JT. Dialysis hypotension: a hemodynamic analysis. Kidney Int 1991;39:233–346.

Hamel MB, Phillips RS, Davis RB, et al. Outcomes and cost-effectiveness of initiating dialysis and continuing aggressive care in seriously ill hospitalized adults. Ann Intern Med 1997;127:195–202.

Schwab SJ, Quarles LD, Middleton JP, et al. Hemodialysis-associated subclavian vein stenosis. Kidney Int 1988;33:1156–1159.

Van Bommel E, Bouvy ND, So KL, et al. Acute dialytic support for the critically ill: intermittent hemodialysis versus continuous arteriovenous hemodiafiltration. Am J Nephrol 1995;15:192–200.

Vanholder R, Van Biesen W, Lameire N. What is the renal replacement method of first choice for intensive care patients? J Am Soc Nephrol 2001;12(Suppl 17):S40–S43.

204 Continuous Renal Replacement Therapy

Ali H. Al-Khafaji
Howard L. Corwin

Nomenclature

A. Continuous renal replacement therapy (CRRT)

1. A wide variety of methods applied over a 24-hour period to support patients with acute renal failure

2. Encompasses each of the following techniques

B. Continuous arteriovenous hemofiltration (CAVH)

1. Blood is driven by the patient's own blood pressure through a filter containing a permeable membrane.

2. The extracorporeal circuit flows from the patient's artery and returns to a vein.

3. The ultrafiltrate produced is replaced (partly or completely) to achieve solute clearance and to adjust fluid balance.

4. Clearance of solutes occurs by convection.

5. This simple technique has been largely superseded by a variety of more complicated pump-driven systems.

C. Continuous veno-venous hemofiltration (CVVH)

1. Blood is driven by a pump through a filter containing a permeable membrane.

2. The extracorporeal circuit flows from a vein and returns to a vein.

3. The ultrafiltrate produced is replaced (partly or completely) to achieve solute clearance and to adjust fluid balance.

4. Clearance of solutes occurs by convection.

5. Offers higher efficiency than CAVH both because of the pump and because there is no need for arterial access

D. Slow continuous ultrafiltration (SCUF)

1. A form of CAVH or CVVH in which fluid is not replaced

2. This modality provides continuous isosmotic fluid removal.

3. Minimal solute clearance is obtained.

E. Continuous arteriovenous hemodialysis (CAVHD) or continuous venovenous hemodialysis (CVVHD)

1. Either CAVH or CVVH modified by addition of a slow countercurrent dialysate flow through the filtrate compartment of the filter

2. Fluid is not replaced and clearance is predominantly by diffusion.

F. Continuous arteriovenous hemodiafiltration (CAVHDF) or continuous venovenous hemodiafiltration (CVVHDF)

1. Either CAVH or CVVH modified by addition of a slow countercurrent dialysate flow through the filtrate compartment of the filter

2. Ultrafiltration is maximized and fluid is replaced.

3. Clearance of solutes occurs by diffusion and convection.

4. Both large and small solutes are effectively removed.

Indications

A. Classic indications for renal replacement therapy

1. Severe volume overload and oliguric renal failure

2. Metabolic acidosis

3. Azotemia with uremic manifestations

B. Expanded indications

1. Congestive heart failure

   a. Application of CRRT is effective for fluid removal in patients resistant to conventional therapy.

   b. The SCUF alternative may be employed for this indication.

2. Liver failure

   a. The use of CAVH may be preferable to "pump-driven" CRRT (e.g., CVVH) in patients with fulminant hepatic failure.

   b. Various forms of CRRT have been used in chronic liver disease.

      (1) Hepatorenal syndrome, as a "bridge" to liver transplantation

      (2) Perioperative period in liver transplant recipients

3. Sepsis and multiple organ failure

   a. This indication is predicated on the ability of CRRT to remove circulating cytokines.

   b. Impact on outcome is still uncertain.

   c. This indication must be regarded as experimental.

4. Intoxications

a. For acute indications, CRRT is not routinely used.

b. Major role is for the treatment of intoxications with certain drugs with these characteristics.

    (1) Circulating levels tend to rebound due to release from tissue stores

    (2) Higher molecular weight

C. Comparison of CRRT versus intermittent hemodialysis (IHD)

1. The control of azotemia is as good if not better with CRRT (especially CVVH or CVVHD) as with IHD.

2. Hemodynamic stability is better with CRRT.

3. Fluid balance can be controlled more tightly with CRRT.

4. Use of CRRT avoids disequilibrium syndrome.

5. The IHD alternative is preferable if very rapid metabolic control is necessary (e.g., hyperkalemia).

6. Also, IHD is easier to manage without anticoagulation.

7. Use of CRRT removes middle molecules more effectively than IHD does, and therefore is of theoretical benefit in patients with sepsis and multiple organ failure.

8. Use of CRRT is believed by many clinicians to result in better outcomes; however, this point has not been conclusively demonstrated.

9. The choice of the type of CRRT depends on institutional factors and resources; however, in general, venovenous pump-driven systems (CVVH, CVVHD) are preferable to arteriovenous systems (CAVH, CAVHD) because they are more thorough and have a lower incidence of access complications.

Key Indications

- Use of CRRT provides excellent metabolic control and is particularly useful for managing volume status in critically ill patients.

- The CRRT alternative is preferable to IHD in hemodynamically unstable patients.

Overview, Supplies, and Procedures

A. Principles

1. Diffusion

a. Solutes diffuse across a semipermeable membrane down their concentration gradient.

b. Molecules move from the compartment with a higher concentration to the one with a lower concentration.

c. Diffusion is proportional to the concentration gradient, surface area, and diffusion coefficient of the solute.

2. Convection

a. Solutes are transported across a semipermeable membrane along with solvent ("solvent drag") by filtration in response to a transmembrane pressure gradient.

b. Convection is dependent on filtration rate, membrane permeability, and solute concentration.

c. Removes "middle" molecules more effectively than diffusion

3. Ultrafiltration is the separation of plasma water and solutes form whole blood across a semipermeable membrane in response to transmembrane pressure.

B. Vascular access

1. Two separate single-lumen catheters are used for arteriovenous access.

2. Double-lumen catheters are used for venovenous access.

3. Large-bore catheters are preferable.

4. Arterial access is associated with more complications.

5. Femoral access is preferred (especially for arterial access).

6. Femoral access is good in immobile patients.

7. Subclavian or internal jugular access allows the patient greater mobility.

8. Subclavian access should be avoided in patients with end-stage kidney disease or who are likely to develop chronic renal failure, since it may limit the ability to create an arteriovenous fistula for permanent access.

C. Membranes

1. Membranes for hemofiltration are designed to have low resistance to flow and a high ultrafiltration coefficient with a minimal tendency to clot.

2. Membranes are made of biocompatible materials to limit activation of complement and other humoral systems.

3. The optimal membrane may depend on the form of CRRT chosen.

4. The ultrafiltration rate of a membrane commonly decreases over time, partly because of clotting and partly because of other membrane factors.

D. Replacement fluid

1. The necessity for and volume of replacement

fluid and dialysate used during CRRT depends on the choice of CRRT technique employed.

2. Composition should aim to maintain normal electrolyte and acid-base status; the usual replacement fluid approximates the electrolyte composition of normal plasma.

   a. The sodium concentration is typically approximately 150 mmol/L.

   b. It may be necessary to add potassium to replacement fluid or dialysate to avoid hypokalemia.

   c. Supplemental calcium and magnesium are necessary.

   d. Either bicarbonate or lactate is added to buffer pH.

   e. Lactate should be avoided in patients with impaired lactate metabolism and lactic acidosis.

   f. If glucose is added to the replacement fluid, the carbohydrate load can be substantial and may lead to hyperglycemia.

3. Other fluids may be required—for example, to provide nutritional support.

4. *Pre-dilution* means the replacement fluid is added to the patient's blood prior to entry into the hemofilter; this may result in enhanced clearance and increased patency.

5. *Post-dilution* means the replacement fluid is added to the patient's blood after its exit from the hemofilter.

E. Anticoagulation options

   1. No anticoagulation

      a. Saline solution

      b. Thrombocytopenia ($<$80,000 platelets/μL) is associated with less risk of filter clotting.

   2. Unfractionated heparin

      a. Standard method

      b. 1,000 to 2,000 U are given as a loading dose.

      c. 5 to 10 U/kg per hour is the usual maintenance dose.

      d. Seek to maintain the activated clotting time at 200 to 250 seconds, or the partial thromboplastin time at 1.5 to 2 times the control value.

   3. Regional heparin

      a. Use standard heparin infused into the circuit prior to the filter.

      b. Infuse protamine (10 to 20 mg/hour) into the circuit after the filter.

   4. Low molecular weight heparin

      a. 40 mg is the initial dose.

   b. 10 to 40 mg every 6 hours is the usual maintenance dose.

   c. Monitor factor Xa levels (0.1 to 0.4 U/mL is desirable).

5. Citrate

   a. 4% trisodium citrate (150 to 180 mL/hour)

   b. Seek to maintain activated clotting time at 200 to 250 seconds.

   c. Seek to maintain serum ionized calcium at 0.96 to 1.2 mmol/L.

   d. Associated with development of citrate-induced alkalosis

6. Prostacyclin

   a. Give heparin (2 to 4 U/kg).

   b. Infuse prostacyclin (4 to 8 ng/kg per minute).

   c. Monitor platelet-aggregation time.

   d. The main problem with this approach is development of hypotension.

7. Nafamostat mesylate

   a. A serine protease inhibitor

   b. Dose: 0.1 mg/kg per hour

   c. Monitor activated clotting time.

F. Clearance

   1. Solute clearance

      a. Continuous removal of solute

      b. Diffusive clearance removes smaller molecules, whereas convective clearance more effectively removes middle molecules.

      c. Urea clearance with CVVH and CVVHD can reach 50 L/day, which is comparable to clearance rates obtained with daily IHD.

      d. Urea clearance with CAVHD is somewhat less than daily IHD but greater than every-other-day hemodialysis.

      e. Urea clearance with CAVH is 10 to 15 L/day.

   2. Volume removal

      a. Ultrafiltration

      b. Isotonic fluid removal

      c. The use of CRRT is associated with less hemodynamic instability than is intermittent hemodialysis.

      d. Fluid balance is the difference between ultrafiltration volume and replacement fluid volume.

      e. Requires frequent (at least hourly) monitoring and readjustment of fluid replacement rate

      f. With CRRT it is possible to target a specific net fluid balance.

      g. The large capability for removal of fluid

with CRRT allows for aggressive nutritional support.

3. Acid-base balance

  a. Replace both the bicarbonate used to buffer acid production and the bicarbonate removed by continuous therapy.

  b. The choice of the most appropriate replacement buffer in some forms of metabolic acidosis remains controversial.

  c. Bicarbonate-, lactate-, and citrate-based dialysate or replacement fluids all have been used.

  d. In general, 30 to 35 mmol/L of buffer base is sufficient.

  e. In severe lactic acidosis or liver failure, bicarbonate may be preferable.

  f. Monitor ionized calcium when using bicarbonate buffer.

  g. Acetate-containing buffers should be avoided to avoid negative hemodynamic effects that can occur with hyperacetatemia.

4. Cytokine removal

  a. Convective clearance permits removal of middle molecules (molecular weight 6,000 to 10,000 daltons), including mediators implicated in the pathogenesis of sepsis, the systemic inflammatory response, and multiple organ system failure.

  b. Several studies have demonstrated removal of mediators by continuous hemofiltration.

  c. Although some studies have shown a relationship between hemofiltration and clinical improvement, a clear clinical benefit has yet to be demonstrated.

  d. High-volume techniques may be more effective.

5. Drug clearance

  a. Determinants include

    (1) Delivery to filter: blood flow and volume distribution

    (2) The ultrafiltration properties of the drug: protein binding (sieving coefficient) and molecular weight

    (3) Ultrafiltration rate

  b. Convective clearance in CRRT allows for removal of larger molecular weight drugs than hemodialysis does (e.g., vancomycin).

  c. Clearance can be estimated by considering the filtration rate as equivalent to the glomerular filtration rate; however, many drugs have been specifically studied in CRRT and dosing guidelines are available.

  d. Use of CRRT may be advantageous in intoxications, if there is rapid rebound after intermittent removal.

6. Higher doses of CVVH may improve survival in critically ill patients with acute renal failure.

PEARL

Replacement fluid composition must be individualized for each patient and adjusted as needed.

Bibliography

Journois D, Silvester W. Continuous hemofiltration in patients with sepsis and multiorgan failure. Semin Dialysis 1996;9:173–178.

Kaplan AA. Continuous renal replacement therapy in the intensive care unit. J Intensive Care Med 1998;13:85–105.

Manns M, Sigler MH, Teehan BP. Continuous renal replacement therapies: an update. Am J Kidney Dis 1998; 32:185–207.

Ronco C. Continuous renal replacement therapies for the treatment of acute renal failure in the intensive care patient. Clin Nephrol 1993;40:187–198.

Ronco C, Bellomo R, Homel P, et al. Effects of different doses in continuous venovenous haemofiltration on outcomes of acute renal failure: a prospective randomised trial. Lancet 2000;356:26–30.

205 Intrahospital Transport

Sheila Sudhakar
Richard W. Carlson

Indications and Contraindications

Transport of the critically ill involves risk to the patient as well as clinical and logistical challenges to hospital personnel. Reasons for transport are to provide additional care or diagnostic or therapeutic procedures not available at the patient's current location. This includes the initial transport from the emergency department or from the operating suite as well as movement from the intensive care unit (ICU) to the operating suite, imaging center, or other specialized area within the facility. The interval of transport is a period of potential instability that may be life-threatening. Accordingly, if the diagnostic test, procedure or intervention is unlikely to significantly alter management or outcome, transport should be avoided. For essential services, risk may be minimized by careful planning and communication, use of appropriately qualified personnel, specialized equipment, and adherence to guidelines and protocols.

Key Principles of Safe Transport

- Experienced staff
- Prior clinical assessment
- Planning
- Uninterrupted monitoring
- Documentation
- Suitable equipment
- Stabilization prior to transport
- Communication
- Direct handover of patient

Special Considerations

A. Temporal features affecting transport: for disorders with progressive severity, delay increases mortality and morbidity
B. Level of care required during transport
   1. Related to severity of disorder and special care requirements
   2. Focus on requisite personnel and equipment rather than time.
C. Complications of transport
   1. Equipment failure or loss of electrical power for monitoring and therapy
   2. Disruption of airway or of vascular or other access

3. Infiltration of venous access; uncontrolled fluid therapy
4. Hemodynamic instabililty: hypotension or hypertension, dysrhythmias, myocardial ischemia
5. Respiratory instability: hypoxemia, hypocapnia or hypercapnia, mucus plugs, atelectasis, mainstem bronchial intubation, extubation, barotrauma, aspiration
6. Central nervous system instability
7. Loss or disruption of grafts, sutures, drains
8. Agitation, pain, sedation

> **PEARL**
>
> The highest risk of intrahospital transport occurs during physical movement of the patient.

Procedure

A. Coordination and communication
   1. Assure physician-to-physician and nurse-to-nurse communication of the patient's clinical status.
   2. Confirm that destination is ready to receive the patient.
   3. Alert ancillary services regarding timing and required equipment and personnel.
   4. Notify responsible physician to accompany patient or ensure physician availability.
   5. Document indications for transport and clinical status during transport.
B. Personnel required: at least two persons should accompany the patient
   1. One should be the bedside critical care nurse or a specifically trained transport critical care nurse.
   2. Additional personnel may include a respiratory therapist, a registered nurse, or a critical care technician.
   3. A physician should accompany patients with unstable physiology or those who may require interventions beyond the scope of standing orders or nursing practice.
C. Equipment
   1. Cardiac monitor and defibillator

2. Airway management equipment including a resuscitation bag

3. Oxygen source of adequate volume to meet the patient's needs during the interval of transport

4. Resuscitation drugs, such as epinephrine, atropine, and lidocaine

5. Sphygmomanometer

6. Intravenous fluids and continuous infusion drugs; battery-operated IV pump(s)

7. For mechanically ventilated patients a device capable of delivering the minute ventilation, inspiratory pressure, FIO_2, and positive end-expiratory pressure required by the patient

8. Additional drugs to meet anticipated needs (including scheduled intermittent drugs, sedation, and analgesia) with appropriate orders to provide for their administration if a physician is not present

9. Resuscitation cart and suction equipment should be readily available (within 4 minutes).

D. Monitoring during transport

1. Provide, if possible, the same physiologic monitoring required in the ICU.

2. Minimum level of monitoring

a. Continuous monitoring, with periodic documentation, of electrocardiogram and pulse oximetry

b. Intermittent measurement of recording of vital signs

3. For selected patients

a. Capnography

b. Continuous measurement of arterial, pulmonary artery, central venous, or intracranial pressure

c. Airway pressure

Key Procedure Points

- Plan and communicate fully.

- Provide appropriate personnel and equipment.

- Ensure uninterrupted monitoring.

- Document events and vital signs.

Bibliography

Clemmer TP, Thomas F. Transport of the critically ill. Crit Care Med 2000;28:265–266.

Guidelines Committee of the American College of Critical Care Medicine, Society of Critical Care Medicine and American Association of Critical Care Nurses Transfer Guidelines Task Force. Guidelines for the transfer of critically ill patients. Crit Care Med 1993;21:931–937.

Manji M, Bijon JF. Transporting critically ill patients. Intensive Care Med 1995;21:781–783.

Millman RP, Braman SS. Transporting Critically Ill Patients. In: Carlson RW, Geheb MA (eds). Principles and Practice of Intensive Care Medicine. Philadelphia: WB Saunders, 1992, pp 54–57.

Wallace PG, Ridley SA. ABC of intensive care: transport of critically ill patients. BMJ 1999;319:368–371.

Waydhas C, Schneck G, Duswald KH. Deterioration of respiratory function after intrahospital transport of critically ill surgical patients. Intensive Care Med 1995;21:784–789.

206 Do Not Resuscitate Orders
Margaret L. Campbell

"Do not resuscitate" (DNR) orders and other decisions to forgo life-sustaining treatments are made frequently in the intensive care unit by clinicians in conjunction with patients or their surrogates and supported by moral, professional, and legal standards. A growing body of evidence about the prognoses associated with critical illnesses and the undesirable outcomes of protracted life-sustaining treatments drives these decisions. Palliative strategies replace curative interventions after decisions have been made to forgo life-sustaining treatments if the goal of care is to focus on the patient's comfort.

Key Ethical Precepts and Legal Standards

Ethical Precepts	Legal Standards
• Autonomy	• Constitutional right to privacy
• Beneficence	• Common law right to self-determination
• Non-maleficence	• Patient Self-Determination Act of 1990
• Distributive justice	• State regulations or statutes

Decision-Making Process

A. Order of precedence for decision making
 1. Autonomous: capable patient able to make an informed decision
 2. Advance directive: i.e., patient has previously identified applicable preferences
  a. Durable power of attorney for health care: formalized proxy appointment
  b. Living will: instruction document
  c. Verbal statements to family members or significant others
 3. Court-appointed guardian (if any)
 4. Natural surrogate: family, significant others
B. Decision-making process
 1. Establish patient's capacity to make a decision.
  a. Understands relevant information
  b. Has insight into the situation and its consequences
  c. Manipulates information to compare benefits and risks
  d. Communicates choices
 2. Identify relevant surrogate(s) if the patient is incapable.
  a. Court-appointed guardian
  b. Family member(s)
  c. Significant other(s)
 3. Discuss options.
  a. Use a "face-to-face" approach.
  b. Ensure privacy during discussions.
  c. Provide comprehensive and comprehensible information.
  d. Demonstrate compassion and empathy.
  e. Offer relevant options.
 4. Document outcomes of the discussion.
  a. Who was present
  b. Patient's response or reason for nonparticipation
  c. Surrogate's response
  d. Treatment goals

Key Principles

- Capable patients have a common law and constitutional right to forgo treatment.
- Incapable patients have the same rights that must be exercised through a surrogate.
- The decision-making process should occur in the clinical setting.
- Recourse to the courts is reserved for unreconciled disputes.
- Hospital ethics committees provide consultation to resolve treatment disputes.

DNR Treatment Goals

A. Full support without resuscitation (DNR)
 1. Patient may have an equivocal prognosis.
 2. Resuscitation is to be withheld if cardiac arrest occurs.
 3. All relevant interventions, short of cardiopulmonary resuscitation (CPR), continue.

4. The patient remains in the intensive care unit (ICU).

B. Conservative treatment with specified limitations

1. The patient typically has a serious chronic illness that is potentially reversible.

2. Cardiopulmonary resuscitation and other specified patient-specified interventions (e.g. endotracheal intubation) will be withheld.

3. All other patient-specified interventions are provided.

4. Patient may or may not require treatment in an ICU.

C. Comfort measures only

1. Patient has an end-stage illness or a poor prognosis for survival.

2. Resuscitative strategies will be withheld.

3. Palliative strategies will be incorporated.

4. Patient generally does not require treatment in an ICU.

D. Withdrawal of life-sustaining treatment

1. Patient has an end-stage illness, a poor prognosis for survival, or brain death.

2. Resuscitative strategies will be withheld.

3. Life-sustaining treatment will be withdrawn.

4. Palliative strategies will be incorporated.

Palliative Care Considerations

A. Discontinue potentially uncomfortable or superfluous interventions.

1. Frequent vital sign assessments and electrocardiographic monitoring

2. Invasive monitors: e.g., arterial, pulmonary artery, and intracranial pressure monitoring catheters

3. Arterial and venous punctures for laboratory tests

4. Frequent turning and rotation/percussion beds

5. Wound debridement and frequent dressing changes

6. Pneumatic compression devices for venous thrombosis prophylaxis

7. Specialized hypothermia treatment devices

B. Discontinue superfluous drugs.

1. Prophylactic drugs: e.g., heparin, H_2-receptor antagonists, anticonvulsants

2. Drugs that confer no comfort benefit

a. Antimicrobial agents, unless infection is source of distress, such as tracheitis or perirectal herpes

b. Stool softeners and laxatives, unless patient is stable and eating

c. Intravenous hydration

C. Add palliative interventions.

1. Analgesia titrated to patient's responses, reported or observed

2. Sedation titrated to patient's responses

3. Food and water by mouth according to patient's appetite and thirst

4. Mouth and skin lubrication

5. Unrestricted visitation by family and friends

6. Reduction in lights and noise

Withdrawal of Life Support

A. Provisions before withdrawal of any form of life support

1. Determine the adequacy of the decision making.

2. Determine the time of day for withdrawal, considering.

a. Availability of hospital support personnel

b. Availability of family, if they intend to be present

3. Establish palliative care orders, including DNR order.

4. Establish IV access if not present.

5. Establish ready accessibility to analgesics and sedatives.

6. Discontinue neuromuscular blocking agents.

a. They provide no analgesia or sedation.

b. They mask signs of patient distress.

c. They produce suffocation in the conscious patient.

B. Vasopressor drug withdrawal

1. Hypotension produces no distress.

2. Turn off rather than wean.

3. Discontinue vasopressor drugs before ventilator withdrawal.

a. Hypotension will reduce cerebral perfusion.

b. Patient will experience less distress.

C. Ventilator withdrawal (Table 206–1)

1. Pre-sedation with midazolam, lorazepam, or morphine

a. Conscious patients who desire pre-sedation

b. Conscious patients who are likely to develop dyspnea

c. Patients with impaired consciousness but observable dyspnea

d. Patients with impaired consciousness who are likely to develop dyspnea

TABLE 206-1. CONSIDERATIONS FOR WITHDRAWAL OF MECHANICAL VENTILATION ACROSS DIFFERING LEVELS OF PATIENT CONSCIOUSNESS

	BRAIN DEATH	COMA (BRAINSTEM FUNCTION ONLY)	IMPAIRED LEVEL OF CONSCIOUSNESS	CONSCIOUS
Pre-sedation	Not indicated	Not indicated	If signs of dyspnea or if dyspnea likely	If patient desires or if dyspnea likely
Drugs	None	None	Lorazepam, midazolam, or morphine	Lorazepam, midazolam, or morphine
Method	Turn off ventilator	Rapid wean or T-piece without weaning	Rapid wean then T-piece	Rapid or slow wean then T-piece
Extubation	Yes	Yes, unless appearance of airway distress can be anticipated	Yes, unless airway compromise and distress can be anticipated	Yes, unless airway compromise and distress can be anticipated

e. Not indicated in patients with coma and only brainstem activity

f. Not indicated in patients with brain death

2. Maintain comfort during and after withdrawal.

a. Morphine infusion at 50% of pre-sedation dose

b. Titrate to patient's report or observed signs of distress.

3. Withdrawal methods

a. Terminal weaning performed over minutes to hours

b. Direct placement to T-piece without weaning of positive pressure ventilation

c. Direct extubation without weaning: applicable only in patients with brain death

4. Extubation considerations

a. The endotracheal tube is a potential source of discomfort.

b. Airway compromise in patients with coma may give the appearance of discomfort.

c. The decision to extubate balances consideration for comfort versus risks of airway compromise.

5. Indications for continued oxygen therapy

a. Patient report or signs that comfort level is improved

b. Not indicated if no distress

c. Decreasing oxygen saturation provides no evidence of distress.

Key Treatment

- Appropriate interventions are determined by the treatment goals and the patient's ability to experience discomfort.

- Many ICU interventions and treatments are sources of discomfort and should be evaluated for discontinuation or adjustment to avoid causing pain.

- Analgesics and sedatives are titrated to the patient's report of distress, if conscious, or to the patient's observable behaviors.

 Bibliography

Appelbaum PS, Grisso T. Assessing patients' capacities to consent to treatment. N Engl J Med 1988;319:1635–1638.

Brody H, Campbell ML, Faber-Langendoen K, et al. Withdrawing intensive life-sustaining treatments: recommendations for compassionate clinical management. N Engl J Med 1997;336:652–657.

Campbell ML. Forgoing life-sustaining therapy: how to care for the patient who is near death. Aliso Viejo, CA: American Association of Critical Care Nurses, 1998.

The Hastings Center. Guidelines on the termination of life-sustaining treatment and the care of the dying. Bloomington, IN: Indiana University Press, 1987.

President's Commission for the Study of Ethical Problems in Medicine and Biomedical and Behavioral Research. Deciding to forgo life-sustaining treatment: ethical, medical and legal issues in treatment decisions. Washington, DC: U.S. Government Printing Office, 1983.

207 Brain Death Determination

James A. Kruse

Definitions

A. Death: either (1) irreversible cessation of circulatory and respiratory functions, or (2) irreversible cessation of all functions of the entire brain, including the brain stem

1. Wording is from the Uniform Determination of Death Act.

2. Endorsed by the American Medical Association, the American Bar Association, and the President's Commission for the Study of Ethical Problems in Medicine and Biomedical and Behavioral Research

B. Brain death: irreversible cessation of all functions of the entire brain, including the brain stem

C. Brain death protocol

1. A formalized procedure used for determining whether an individual meets criteria-confirmed brain death

2. The guidelines given below conform to American Academy of Neurology recommendations; certain requirements may vary according to institution-specific policies or jurisdictional legalities.

D. Apnea test: a procedure employed during the evaluation of brain death to determine whether brain stem function affecting respiration is present

Key Indications for Considering Formal Brain Death Evaluation (All Must Be Present)

- Establishment of an etiology capable of causing brain death

- Absence of arousal, response, or brain stem reflexes in the absence of sedating or neuromuscular blocking drugs

- No evidence of spontaneous respiratory activity, including patient-initiated triggering of mechanical ventilation

- Exclusion of potentially reversible causes of brain dysfunction

Contraindications

A. Evidence of brain function; e.g., decerebrate or decorticate posturing, persistent vegetative state, locked-in syndrome, presence of brain stem reflexes, or spontaneous respiration

B. Hypothermia: core body temperature lower than 32°C

C. Overdose or intoxication with a drug or toxin having central nervous system depressant effects (e.g., sedative-hypnotic or narcotic drugs); toxicologic screening is necessary in some cases

D. Peripheral neuromuscular dysfunction due to disease or drug effect (e.g., neuromuscular blocking drugs)

E. Circulatory shock, as manifest by hypotension or a requirement for vasopressor therapy to maintain blood pressure

F. Severe hypoxemic or hypercapnic respiratory failure (prevents safe performance of apnea testing)

G. Severe electrolyte, fluid, acid-base, or endocrine disturbances (e.g., severe hyponatremia, hypernatremia, hypovolemia, acidemia, hypoglycemia, or hyperosmolar coma)

H. Special considerations and criteria apply to certain pediatric patients (not discussed here).

CAUTION

The term "brain death" should not be ascribed to a patient until a full brain death evaluation has been completed and the results unequivocally indicate that brain death has occurred.

Procedure

A. Confirm that an etiology has been established that is capable of explaining the coma and causing brain death.

1. Etiologic diagnosis is based on history, physical examination, laboratory tests, and imaging studies.

2. Etiology is often demonstrable by computed tomography or magnetic resonance imaging (e.g., intracranial hemorrhage, herniation, cerebral edema).

3. Process is sufficiently severe to cause brain death.

B. Confirm that no contraindications are present.

1. Confirm that body temperature is higher than 32°C.

2. Exclude presence of sedating, narcotic, or neuromuscular blocking drugs.

3. See above contraindications section.

C. Confirm absence of motor response to noxious sensory stimuli.

1. Confirm that the Glasgow coma scale score is 3.

   a. No spontaneous or stimulated eye movements

   b. No decerebrate or decorticate posturing

   c. Spinal reflexes may be present in the face of brain death.

2. Confirm absence of motor response to painful stimuli at both the cranial and the somatic distributions of sensory afferents.

   a. No grimacing response to bilateral noxious stimulation of supraorbital ridge or temporomandibular joint

   b. No grimacing or other cranial or somatic response to deep nail bed pressure stimulation in all extremities

D. Confirm bilateral absence of all brain stem reflexes.

1. Absent cranial motor activity (e.g., grimacing, lip smacking, tongue movements, eyelid movement, extraocular muscle movements, or accessory respiratory movements)

   a. No response to noxious tactile stimulation over cranial sensory afferent distribution, including supra-orbital pressure

   b. No response to noxious tactile stimulation over somatic sensory afferent distribution

   c. No jaw reflex

2. Absent pupillary constriction

   a. Pupils must be mid-size or dilated.

   b. Absent direct and consensual pupillary constriction to bright light exposure

   c. Ensure that atropine or other mydriatic drugs have not been administered.

3. Absent corneal reflexes: tested using a cotton-tipped swab to stimulate cornea

4. Absent oculocephalic reflex (Doll's-eyes reflex): cannot perform test if there is cervical spine fracture or instability

5. Absent oculovestibular reflexes

   a. Tested by cold caloric stimulation using at least 50 mL irrigation with ice water to each unobstructed ear canal with the head positioned at a 30 degree angle

   b. Allow at least 1 minute after injection and

at least 5 minutes between sequential testing of each ear.

   c. Tonic deviation toward the stimulated side occurs in unconscious patients with an intact reflex; no response occurs in brain death.

6. Absent pharyngeal (gag) reflex: tested by stimulation of posterior pharynx with tongue depressor

7. Absent tracheal (cough) reflex: tested by deep tracheal suctioning with stimulation of the carina and bronchus

8. The following clinical observations may be seen in patients with brain death.

   a. Segmental spinal activity

      (1) Spinal deep tendon reflexes

      (2) Babinski reflexes

      (3) Certain spine-mediated movements (e.g., shoulder adduction, back arching)

   b. Certain autonomic responses

      (1) Tachycardia

      (2) Normal blood pressure or sudden changes in blood pressure

      (3) Diaphoresis or blushing

      (4) Absence of diabetes insipidus

E. Perform apnea test

1. Do not perform unless all of the previous findings are consistent with brain death.

2. Its purpose is to demonstrate lack of respiration attributable to the absence of brain stem activity.

   a. Requires that there be a stimulus (i.e., hypercapnia) to provoke a brain stem respiratory response

   b. Targeted $PaCO_2$ at the conclusion of apnea testing is at least 60 torr (preferably with arterial blood pH <7.28), or at least 20 torr above baseline level if there is preexisting hypercapnia.

3. Ensure that the patient is not hypovolemic, hypotensive (systolic blood pressure <90 mm Hg), hypothermic (core temperature <36.5°F), or hypoxemic (must be able to achieve a PaO_2 greater than 200 torr using supplemental oxygen).

4. Assemble supplies needed for sampling arterial blood and performing tracheal oxygen insufflation; ensure a proper connection between the oxygen source and a suitable insufflation catheter.

5. If the patient is hypocapnic, adjust minute ventilation to achieve a $PaCO_2$ of 40 to 45 torr, and document this by arterial blood gas analysis.

6. Pre-oxygenate the patient using an FiO$_2$ of 1.00 for at least 5 minutes and ensure a PaO$_2$ higher than 200 torr.

7. Remove the ventilator circuit connection from the endotracheal or tracheostomy tube and insert the insufflation catheter, set to deliver 100% oxygen at 6 to 8 L/minute, into the trachea with its tip positioned at or above the carina.

8. Observe the patient for respiratory and other movements for approximately 8 minutes (conclude test immediately if spontaneous respirations or other signs of brain activity become evident during the test).

   a. The typical increase in PaCO$_2$ during apnea testing is 3 to 5 torr/minute.

   b. Higher rates (e.g., 6 torr/minute) are observed in some patients.

   c. Low rates (e.g., 3 torr/minute) are observed at lower body temperature and with lower baseline PaCO$_2$.

9. At the end of the observation period, obtain arterial blood gas expeditiously and immediately resume mechanical ventilation.

10. The apnea test is positive (i.e., consistent with brain death) if no respirations are observed during the apneic observation period and PaCO$_2$ obtained at the conclusion of the apneic period is at least 60 torr (preferably with arterial blood pH <7.28).

    a. Respiratory movements preclude a diagnosis of brain death.

    b. Certain respiratory-like movements, e.g., shoulder adduction or back arching (not associated with significant tidal volumes), can be seen in patients with brain death.

    c. Insufficient hypercapnia (PaCO$_2$ <60 torr) at the conclusion of the test renders the interpretation indeterminate.

       (1) After a period of ventilation, the apnea test may be repeated using a longer period of apnea (e.g., 10 minutes).

       (2) Additional confirmatory testing may be considered (see below).

    d. Excessively high PaCO$_2$ (>100 torr) theoretically could lead to false-positive results by CO$_2$ narcosis and risk adverse cardiac effects.

F. To confirm brain death, reevaluation is performed after passage of time.

   1. Retesting consists of repeating the entire protocol, including the apnea test.

   2. Appropriate time interval between evaluations

      a. Typically stipulated as at least 6 hours in cases of brain destruction that is obvious by imaging studies, or at least 24 hours in other cases (e.g., anoxic encephalopathy)

      b. Specification of the interval is often stipulated by institutional protocol.

      c. Retesting is considered optional by some authorities under certain circumstances.

G. Protocols may require independent confirmation by a second qualified physician.

Other Tests

A. Indications for selection of optional evaluation modalities

   1. Preexisting pupillary abnormalities, enucleation, severe chemosis, or trauma involving the eyes or ears that precludes evaluation of associated reflexes

   2. Basal skull fracture may disrupt the oculovestibular reflex.

   3. Other cranial neuropathies

   4. Severe pulmonary disease precluding apnea testing or its interpretation (i.e., hypoxemia or preexisting hypercapnia)

B. Modalities

   1. Electroencephalography (EEG)

      a. Absence of EEG activity for at least 30 minutes using a 16-channel device is consistent with brain death if accepted technical criteria are met.

      b. Although some institutional protocols may still require it, there is no necessity for EEG confirmation of brain death in routine cases.

      c. Both false-positive and false-negative interpretations can occur.

         (1) Electrical artifacts can imply brain activity when there is none.

         (2) Electrocerebral silence can be seen in cases of reversible drug overdose or hypothermia, and in the presence of brain stem activity.

   2. Imaging studies

      a. Selective four-vessel radiocontrast angiography of the brain: absence of intracranial perfusion or filling at the level of the carotid bifurcation and the circle of Willis is consistent with brain death

      b. Radionuclide angiography of the brain

         (1) Technetium 99m-labeled pertechnetate brain flow study does not allow adequate imaging of posterior fossa perfusion.

(2) Technetium 99m-labeled hexamethylpropylyeneamineoxime perfusion imaging has ability to better assess posterior fossa circulation.

c. Computed tomography scintillation methods

3. Transcranial Doppler ultrasonography

   a. Has been used to assess circulatory arrest of the cerebral, basilar, and vertebral arteries

   b. Interpretation requires considerable experience and absence of flow signals does not confirm brain death

4. Atropine test

   a. Performed by IV injection of 2 mg atropine; lack of increase in heart rate expected in brain death

   b. Insufficient, by itself, for confirmation of brain death

   c. Due to potential for interference with pupillary and EEG testing, atropine must not be administered until those assessments have been completed.

5. Other proposed modalities include brain stem auditory and somatosensory evoked potentials, magnetic resonance imaging and xenon computed tomography, N_2O brain flow studies, and examination of cerebral arteriovenous oxygen difference.

Complications of Apnea Testing

A. Hemodynamic compromise

   1. Do not perform apnea testing in patients with circulatory shock.

   2. Correct hypovolemia prior to apnea testing.

   3. Monitor blood pressure, preferably using an intra-arterial catheter, and electrocardiogram during apnea testing.

   4. Conclude test if hypotension or bradycardia or other dysrhythmia develops.

B. Hypoxemia

   1. Do not perform apnea testing in patients with uncorrected hypoxemia or requiring high levels of FIO_2.

   2. Monitor SaO_2, using pulse oximetry, and electrocardiogram continuously.

   3. Conclude apnea test if significant desaturation or dysrhythmia occurs.

C. Severe acidemia

   1. Do not perform apnea testing in patients with severe metabolic acidosis or preexisting severe hypercapnia.

   2. Monitor electrocardiogram and blood pressure.

   3. Conclude apnea test if significant dysrhythmia or hypotension occurs.

D. Barotrauma (due to oxygen insufflation): avoid excessive insufflation flow rates

E. Inability to obtain post-test confirmatory arterial blood gas sample in a timely manner

   1. Have heparinized sampling syringe and other needed supplies prepared in advance.

   2. Use of an indwelling arterial catheter is helpful.

Bibliography

Beresford HR. Brain death. Neurol Clin 1999;17:295–306.

Dominguez-Roldan JM, Barrera-Chacon JM, Murillo-Cabezas F, et al. Clinical factors influencing the increment of blood carbon dioxide during the apnea test for the diagnosis of brain death. Transplant Proc 1999;31:2599–2600.

Goudreau JL, Wijdicks EFM, Emery SF. Complications during apnea testing in the determination of brain death: predisposing factors. Neurology 2000;55:1045–1048.

President's Commission for the Study of Ethical Problems in Medicine and Biomedical and Behavioral Research. Defining death. A report on the medical, legal and ethical issues in the determination of death. Washington, D.C.: U.S. Government Printing Office, 1981.

Quality Standards Subcommittee of the American Academy of Neurology. Practice parameters for determining brain death in adults. Neurology 1995;45:1012–1014.

Wijdicks EFM. The diagnosis of brain death. N Engl J Med 2001;344:1215–1221.

208 Fluid Challenge

James A. Kruse

Key Definitions

- *Fluid challenge:* a diagnostic, and potentially therapeutic, maneuver used to assess the likelihood that oliguria or hemodynamic derangements are due to hypovolemia

- *Hypovolemia:* critically diminished intravascular volume

Pathophysiology

A. The Frank-Starling relationship governs the effect of fluid loading on cardiac function.

1. Normally, as ventricular end-diastolic volume is increased by intravascular fluid administration, stroke volume increases until a plateau value is reached.

2. If ventricular compliance remains constant, a change in end-diastolic volume is reflected by a proportional change in end-diastolic pressure.

   a. Central venous pressure (CVP) reflects right ventricular filling.

   b. Pulmonary artery occlusion pressure (PAOP) reflects left ventricular filling.

3. The end-diastolic pressure or volume at which stroke volume reaches a plateau varies, especially in critically ill patients, as a result of alterations in cardiac contractility, compliance, and afterload.

   a. For the average patient with sepsis, cardiac output plateaus at a PAOP of 12 to 15 mm Hg.

   b. For the average patient with cardiogenic shock, cardiac output typically reaches plateau levels at a PAOP of 18 to 20 mm Hg.

B. Starling's equation

1. Governs the relationship between variables that determine fluid flux from the capillary to the interstitium (see Chapter 7, Pulmonary Edema)

2. Largely dependent on capillary hydrostatic pressure, which increases with expansion of intravascular volume

3. Fluid loading beyond the Frank-Starling plateau does not benefit systemic perfusion but may lead to hydrostatic (cardiogenic) pulmonary or systemic edema.

Key Indications

- Suspected hypovolemia

- Low cardiac filling pressures and signs of hypoperfusion

- Hypotension or requirement for vasopressors to maintain blood pressure

- Low cardiac output with signs of hypoperfusion

- Acute oliguria

- Hyperlactatemia that may be due to hypoperfusion

Key Contraindications

- Fluid overload involving the intravascular space

- Pulmonary edema (fluid challenge may be indicated in some cases of pulmonary edema associated with hypotension or hypoperfusion, particularly permeability pulmonary edema)

Procedure

A. Select fluid type; always use isotonic (or near-isotonic) fluid.

1. Crystalloid solutions (most commonly used): normal saline, Ringer's lactate

2. Colloids: albumin, hetastarch

3. Blood products (e.g., packed red cells, fresh frozen plasma): used only if otherwise indicated (i.e., for anemia or coagulopathy) and available

B. Select desired total volume of the challenge.

1. Defines planned end point of challenge and minimizes risk of fluid overload

2. Typically selected volumes are between 200 and 1,000 mL.

3. The volume selected should reflect the physician's confidence that challenge can be carried out safely; e.g., a smaller volume is selected in patients with a higher likelihood of having an adverse effect from the challenge.

   a. Consider the probability that hypovolemia is present and the degree of hypovolemia (e.g., use smaller challenge volumes in patients with higher baseline filling pressures).

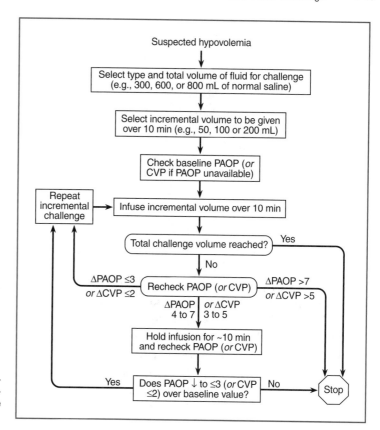

Figure 208-1 Fluid challenge algorithm. PAOP = pulmonary artery occlusion pressure (mm Hg); CVP = central venous pressure (mm Hg); Δ = signifies change (increase) from baseline filling pressure.

b. Consider left ventricular function (i.e., the propensity for developing hydrostatic pulmonary edema).

c. Consider the consequences of impairing pulmonary function (e.g., less worrisome in a patient who is already intubated and has good oxygenation on a low FIO₂, versus a patient who has respiratory distress while spontaneously breathing on a high FIO₂).

d. Consider renal function (i.e., the ability to excrete the infused volume, with or without the use of a diuretic).

C. Select infusion rate.

1. Determined in conjunction with the volume selected

2. A rapid infusion rate is generally preferable to a slow infusion rate.

a. A rapid infusion rate increases the likelihood that an effect (positive or negative) will be evident, thus indicating whether hypovolemia was present or not.

b. In the event that hypovolemia was not present and pulmonary capillary pressure increased to the point of having an effect on gas exchange, a small volume rapidly infused would be expected to dissipate (mainly into systemic interstitial tissues) in a short while, allowing pulmonary capillary pressure

and gas exchange to return almost to their previous levels.

c. If a much larger volume is infused over a much longer period, equilibration with the interstitial fluid space will occur, leading to "saturation" of the interstitium. Thus, when pulmonary capillary pressure is critically increased there is less chance that it will abate spontaneously, especially if renal function is substantially impaired.

D. If desired, the selected volume may be administered incrementally and a preemptive criterion used to determine whether the challenge will be interrupted or repeated one or more times (see Fig. 208-1)

1. Select the incremental volume: e.g., 200 mL over 10 minutes

2. For patients with a central venous catheter

a. If CVP increases by 2 mm Hg or less, repeat the incremental fluid challenge (unless the total challenge volume has been reached).

b. If CVP increases by more than 2 mm Hg but less than or equal to 5 mm Hg, hold infusion until CVP drops to within 2 mm Hg of baseline value (abort challenge if this does not occur in approximately 10 minutes).

c. If CVP increases by more than 5 mm Hg, discontinue the challenge.

3. For patients with a pulmonary artery catheter
   a. If PAOP increases by 3 mm Hg or less, repeat the bolus infusion (unless the total challenge volume has been reached).
   b. If PAOP increases by more than 3 mm Hg but less than or equal to 7 mm Hg, hold infusion until PAOP drops to within 3 mm Hg of the baseline value (abort the challenge if this does not occur in approximately 10 minutes).
   c. If PAOP increases by more than 7 mm Hg, discontinue the challenge.

Monitoring

A. If CVP or PAOP increase only a little or not at all during the fluid challenge, or if they increase but quickly return to near baseline, consider cautiously proceeding with an additional fluid challenge if signs of hypoperfusion remain.

B. Rapid increases in CVP or PAOP during the fluid challenge suggest that the plateau of the Frank-Starling relationship is near or has been reached.
   1. Further administration of fluid is less likely to benefit cardiac output and more likely to provoke pulmonary edema.
   2. Discontinue further fluid infusion and monitor additional physiologic variables.

C. Additional monitoring
   1. Tachycardia may improve if the fluid challenge is effective.
   2. Arterial blood pressure may improve in response to fluid challenge in patients with hypotension or in those requiring vasopressor drugs to support blood pressure.
   3. Continuous thermodilution monitoring of cardiac output can provide additional rapid feedback as to the effects of the fluid challenge (also see Chapter 214, Hemodynamic Monitoring).

4. Continuous fiberoptic $S\bar{v}O_2$ monitoring can provide similar feedback by its reciprocal relationship with cardiac output, which is typically seen when hypoperfusion is due to hypovolemia or left ventricular dysfunction.

5. Measurement of systemic oxygen consumption (VO_2) before and after a fluid challenge sufficient to appreciably raise oxygen delivery (DO_2) may demonstrate oxygen supply dependency, corroborating critical hypoperfusion (see Chapter 216, Monitoring Oxygen Transport).

6. Other physiologic variables require longer observational periods to assess the impact of a fluid challenge, but they can still be useful when monitored over time.
   a. Urine output
   b. Blood lactate concentration
   c. Gastric intramucosal PCO_2 or pH

Bibliography

Aeder MI, Crowe JP, Rhodes RS, et al. Technical limitations in the rapid infusion of intravenous fluids. Ann Emerg Med 1985;14:307–310.

Haupt MT. Therapy: effects of fluid resuscitation. In: Edward JD, Shoemaker WC, Vincent J-L (eds). Oxygen Transport: Principles and Practice. London: WB Saunders, 1993; pp 175–192.

Imm A, Carlson RW. Fluid resuscitation in circulatory shock. Crit Care Clin 1993;9:313–333.

Kaufman BS (ed). Fluid resuscitation of the critically ill. Crit Care Clin 1992;8(2):235–463.

Magder S, Lagonidis D. Effectiveness of albumin versus normal saline as a test of volume responsiveness in post-cardiac surgery patients. J Crit Care 1999;14:164–171.

Wagner JG, Leatherman JW. Right ventricular end-diastolic volume as a predictor of the hemodynamic response to a fluid challenge. Chest 1998;113:1048–1054.

209 Sengstaken-Blakemore Tube Placement

James A. Kruse

Definitions

A. Sengstaken-Blakemore (SB) tube (Fig. 209–1)
1. A three-lumen tube containing an intragastric balloon, esophageal balloon, and gastric aspiration port
2. Used to control bleeding varices at the level of the esophagus, gastroesophageal junction, or adjacent gastric fundus by balloon tamponade

B. Minnesota tube
1. A variant of the SB tube containing a fourth lumen that opens into the esophagus above the esophageal balloon
2. The fourth lumen provides a means of maintaining the esophagus clear of swallowed secretions during balloon tamponade.

C. Linton tube (not discussed further here): as originally described, a two-lumen tube containing a gastric sump drain and a gastric, but no esophageal, balloon

D. Linton-Nachlas tube (not discussed further here): a three-lumen modification of the Linton tube containing an esophageal sump orifice that opens just above the gastric balloon

Key Contraindications (Relative)

- Lack of adequate airway control
- Recent esophageal surgery
- Recent sclerotherapy
- Esophageal stricture

Procedure

A. Patient preparation
1. Explain procedure to patient.
2. Strong consideration should be given to endotracheal intubation, if not already instituted, especially in patients with an altered sensorium.
3. Positioning
   a. Position awake patients in a high Fowler's or semi-erect position, if possible.
   b. Otherwise, position the patient in the lateral decubitus position with the left side down.

4. Parenteral sedation or analgesia may be considered in patients who have a secure airway.
5. Topical anesthetic (e.g., a proprietary solution of 2% tetracaine, 2% butylaminobenzoate, and 14% benzocaine) may be sprayed onto the posterior oropharynx for 1 to 2 seconds while depressing the tongue with a tongue blade.
6. To minimize the risk of inducing vomiting during the procedure, use an oro- or nasogastric (NG) tube to aspirate the stomach contents; then remove the NG tube.
7. Transnasal insertion
   a. Not recommended in the face of thrombocytopenia or coagulopathy
   b. Determine appropriate naris for tube insertion.
      (1) Check for deviated septum and difference in size or patency of nares, selecting the larger passage.
      (2) Patency may be assessed in cooperative patients by instructing them to inhale through the nose while the clinician occludes the nares one at a time.
   c. Topical sympathomimetic agent (e.g., 0.5% phenylephrine) may optionally be sprayed or applied into nares, if no contraindication, to constrict turbinates.
   d. Topical anesthetic (e.g., 5 mL of 2% lidocaine jelly) or surgical lubricant may optionally be instilled into selected naris and allowed to flow posteriorly to the nasopharynx by gravity (head extended) and by encouraging the patient to sniff.

B. Tube preparation
1. Sengstaken-Blakemore tube
   a. Align a standard NG tube with the SB tube so that the distal end of the NG tube terminates at the proximal end of the esophageal balloon of the SB tube.
   b. Apply adhesive tape markers or permanent ink marks to the proximal portion of both tubes to serve as witness marks for maintaining the above alignment once the tubes are inserted.
   c. Once in its proper position, the NG tube will terminate in the mid-esophagus just

749

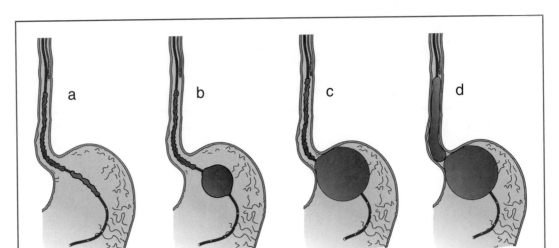

Figure 209–1 Sengstaken-Blakemore (SB) tube in (a) initial position after insertion (balloons deflated); (b) after partial inflation of gastric balloon, but before traction is applied (performed to allow radiographic confirmation of intragastric positioning); (c) after complete inflation of gastric balloon and application of traction; (d) after inflation of esophageal balloon. Note auxiliary esophageal sump tube positioned parallel to SB tube and with its tip located just above the esophageal balloon.

above the esophageal balloon of the SB tube; the NG tube will be connected to suction to keep the esophagus clear of swallowed secretions during balloon tamponade.

2. Minnesota tube: because the Minnesota tube has a fourth lumen leading to an esophageal aspiration port, the use of a secondary intraesophageal tube is obviated

3. Test the esophageal sump lumen (Minnesota tube) and gastric sump lumen (SB and Minnesota tubes) for patency.

4. Test the esophageal and gastric balloons by inflating their respective lumens with air using a syringe to ensure they are airtight.

5. Aspirate all air from both balloons to completely deflate them.

6. Lubricate the distal gastric portion of the SB or Minnesota tube, as well as the distal end of the NG tube (if an SB tube is used), and the esophageal and gastric balloons using water-soluble lubricating jelly containing 2% lidocaine.

C. Tube introduction
   1. Tube orientation
      a. Some tubes may be constructed asymmetrically for better anatomical conformity.
      b. Consult the manufacturer's package insert for proper orientation of the tube during and after insertion.
   2. Transnasal route
      a. Insert the tip of the SB or Minnesota tube into naris and direct it posteriorly (not supe-

riorly), parallel to both the nasal septum and the superior surface of the hard palate.
      b. If resistance is encountered, steady pressure should be gently applied. Forceful insertion can result in patient discomfort and epistaxis. Slight rotation of the tube may be helpful.
   3. Transoral route
      a. Insert the SB or Minnesota tube into the oral cavity and direct it posteriorly and then inferiorly.
      b. In anesthetized, paralyzed, or deeply sedated patient's, the operator can direct the tube with the index finger into the hypopharynx.
      c. In difficult cases a laryngoscope can be utilized to visualize the larynx and hypopharynx while directing the tube into the esophageal opening.
   4. Both routes
      a. Once the tip of the SB or Minnesota tube approaches the pharynx, slightly flex the patient's neck and advance the tube.
      b. Awake, cooperative patients: ask the patient to swallow as the tube is being advanced from the nasopharynx to the oropharynx and into the esophagus
      c. Advance tube through the esophagus and into the stomach, to at least the 50 cm mark (Fig. 209–1a).
      d. For the SB tube: insert the marked NG tube to a distance that allows it to be aligned

with the witness mark on the SB tube, and tape the two tubes together

---

WARNING

Inflation of the gastric balloon within the esophagus (tube not inserted far enough) or the duodenum (tube advanced too far) can cause potentially fatal rupture of the viscus.

D. Verification of intragastric placement

1. Auscultation and air insufflation

   a. Rapidly inject 20 to 50 mL of air into the gastric sump lumen (not the gastric balloon lumen) while auscultating over the left upper quadrant.

   b. Auscultation of the distinctive sound of air insufflating the stomach is traditionally accepted as denoting intragastric placement of tube (not 100% accurate).

2. Aspiration

   a. Apply negative pressure to the gastric sump lumen using a large syringe (excessive negative pressure may collapse the lumen).

   b. Examine aspirate to confirm the presence of blood (if active upper gastrointestinal hemorrhage) or typical gastric secretions.

3. Partial gastric balloon inflation (Fig. 209–1b)

   a. As a precaution to avoid excessive dilation of the esophagus in case the gastric balloon has not traversed the gastroesophageal junction, inject only 50 to 80 mL of air into the gastric balloon at this point.

   b. Cap and double clamp the gastric port, but do not apply traction (hemostat clamps may be used to occlude the tubing, but their jaws should be covered with plastic or rubber tubing).

   c. Obtain a low-chest, high-abdomen, portable x-ray.

   d. Confirm that the gastric balloon, visible as a round lucency on the x-ray, lies below the diaphragm, confirming its intragastric location.

E. Gastric balloon tamponade (Fig. 209–1c)

1. Unclamp and deflate the gastric balloon.

2. Slowly refill the gastric balloon, this time with 200 to 250 mL of air (check package insert for manufacturer's exact recommendation), double clamp it, and cap it.

3. Manually apply gentle but firm traction and secure the tube by any of various methods.

   a. For tubes inserted transnasally, a foam rubber sponge block (~4 × 4 × 4 cm) can be taped to both the tube and the patient's nose.

   b. A cord may be attached to the tube and led to a simple pulley mounted over the bed using orthopedic traction apparatus and terminating with an appropriate weight to supply the desired tension.

   c. A football helmet with a face guard (preferably one with a single bar to allow maximum access to the face) may be placed on the patient's head and the tube secured to the guard using the appropriate amount of traction.

   d. A padded baseball catcher's mask may be strapped to the patient's face and the tube secured to the front of the mask to maintain traction.

F. Test for ongoing bleeding

1. Lavage and aspirate from the gastric sump lumen.

   a. Continued return of blood from this lumen suggests that bleeding is coming from the stomach and will not be controlled by gastric balloon inflation and traction alone.

   b. Lack of continued blood return from gastric sump suggests that bleeding has either been controlled by the gastric balloon or that the bleeding is from an esophageal source.

2. Aspirate from the esophageal lumen (Minnesota tube) or the separate esophageal tube (SB tube).

   a. Lack of blood from this port argues against an esophageal source of bleeding.

   b. Continued aspiration of blood from this lumen suggests that bleeding is coming from the esophagus and that esophageal balloon inflation is necessary.

G. Inflation of esophageal balloon (Fig. 209–1d)

1. Not recommended if gastric balloon inflation alone controls bleeding

2. A trial using only gastric balloon inflation is recommended to ensure that esophageal bleeding is ongoing prior to initiating esophageal tamponade.

3. Tamponade is performed by inflating the esophageal balloon with a hand pump and manometer (similar to a manual sphygmomanometer) connected with a Y-adaptor to the esophageal balloon lumen.

4. Sufficient air is used to raise the pressure of the esophageal balloon to approximately 30 mm Hg.

5. Generally, the pressure may be adjusted be-

tween 25 and 45 mm Hg (consult package insert for manufacturer's recommendation), but use the lowest effective pressure necessary to control hemorrhage.

6. Once the desired pressure is determined and attained, the esophageal balloon lumen is double-clamped.

H. Sump drainage

1. The gastric sump lumen is connected to suction to monitor for ongoing gastric bleeding.

2. The esophageal sump lumen (Minnesota tube) or the separate tube terminating in the mid-esophagus (SB tube) is connected to suction to keep the esophagus clear of swallowed secretions.

3. Application of excessive negative pressure may collapse the soft drainage lumens.

4. Similarly, use of intermittent suction may be more effective than continuous suction.

I. Continued bleeding despite the above measures

1. For evidence of ongoing gastric bleeding

a. Consider the use of higher pressure in the gastric balloon; e.g., up to 300 mL or more (consult manufacturer's package insert for recommendation on maximum balloon volume).

b. Increased traction on the tube may then be warranted; use of 500 to 1,500 g of traction has been reported.

2. For evidence of continued esophageal bleeding

a. Consider increasing traction followed by use of higher pressure in the esophageal balloon (e.g., up to 60 mm Hg).

b. This entails an increased risk of chest pain, esophageal necrosis, and esophageal rupture.

3. Use of higher balloon volumes and increased traction should be time limited, because they can lead to serious pressure ulceration of the gastric and esophageal mucosa within a matter of hours.

4. Application of excessive traction is hazardous because it could result in displacement of the inflated balloon into the esophagus.

PEARL

Balloon tamponade of bleeding esophageal or gastric varices is a temporary measure. Once emergency hemostasis is achieved by this technique, plans for alternative therapy using pharmacologic, endoscopic, surgical, or radiologic intervention (e.g., band ligation, sclerotherapy, or transjugular intrahepatic portosystemic shunting) should be urgently considered.

Monitoring and Maintenance

A. Constant surveillance in an ICU or similarly monitored setting is necessary while the tube is in place.

1. Maintain the patient in a semirecumbent position.

2. Appropriate sedation is necessary; however, patients without a cannulating airway are at increased risk for aspiration or airway compromise.

3. Continuous electrocardiographic monitoring is employed.

4. Monitor the patient for signs of chest pain, aspiration, or respiratory distress.

5. Nursing personnel should be vigilant to recognize airway occlusion caused by retrograde tube displacement.

a. Management of this emergency entails firmly gripping the catheter at the level of the patient's mouth or nose, transecting the catheter with scissors between the grasping hand and the junction of the various ports, and rapidly withdrawing the tube.

b. Scissors should be prominently displayed at the bedside and labeled for emergency use only.

6. Surveillance radiographs should be performed daily while the tube is in place.

B. Flushing the gastric sump lumen

1. After initial insertion and whenever active bleeding is detected, sufficient lavage should be performed to clear blood from the patient's stomach.

2. The gastric sump lumen is at risk of clogging if blood is allowed to clot within it.

C. Balloon management

1. It is common practice to maintain balloon inflation (gastric, or if necessary, both gastric and esophageal) for the first 12 to 24 hours.

a. After 12 to 24 hours, the esophageal balloon is deflated and the esophageal sump aspirate noted.

b. If no bleeding manifests from the esophageal sump, the gastric balloon can subsequently be deflated to test for hemostasis.

c. Before deflating the gastric balloon, traction must first be released from the tube or else the tube will retract into the esophagus.

d. Prolonged esophageal balloon inflation, up to 36 or 48 hours, has been employed, but it is likely that the risk of serious esophageal complications or death is substantially increased.

2. While the esophageal balloon is inflated, the pressure should be monitored intermittently or continuously.

   a. One method of performing this is to keep the manometer and Y-adaptor connected to the esophageal balloon lumen and double-clamping the esophageal balloon port; periodic measurements (e.g., every 1 or 2 hours) are obtained by releasing the two clamps transiently.

   b. Continuous measurement may be performed by not clamping the tubes (or by clamping only the tube leading to the pressure pump bulb), thus allowing the manometer to be in constant connection with the esophageal lumen.

   c. If necessary, the pressure can be periodically readjusted to the desired level.

3. Some authors recommend periodic deflation (e.g., every 3 to 8 hours) of the gastric and esophageal balloon to reduce the risk of pressure necrosis.

   a. May reduce the risk of pressure necrosis

   b. Advisable if esophageal balloon tamponade is necessary for longer than 24 hours

4. The gastric balloon should not be deflated while the esophageal balloon is inflated.

5. Whenever the gastric balloon is deflated, even when traction has been released, there is a risk that its position will change and the gastric balloon may enter the esophagus.

6. Although radiocontrast solutions enhance the ability to visualize the balloon on radiographs, only air should be used to inflate the tube's balloons. Contrast or other liquids may result in inability to deflate the balloons.

7. After deflation of both balloons, the tube is allowed to remain in place for 24 hours as a precaution in case bleeding recurs.

8. Just prior to removal, transect the tube to minimize the prospect of incomplete deflation of the balloons.

CAUTION

To avoid esophageal pressure necrosis, the esophageal balloon should not remain inflated for more than 24 hours.

Complications (also see Chapter 210, Transnasal and Transoral Gastroenteric Intubation)

A. Failure to control hemorrhage

B. Aspiration pneumonitis

C. Chest pain

D. Airway obstruction

E. Tissue erosion, ulceration, or necrosis

   1. Naris (if transnasal insertion)

   2. Esophagus (due to inflated esophageal balloon)

   3. Gastroesophageal junction (due to inflated gastric balloon)

   4. Tracheoesophageal fistula

F. Ruptured viscus

   1. Esophagus

   2. Stomach

   3. Duodenum

   4. Jejunum (patients status post gastrojejunostomy)

   5. Tracheal rupture (if balloon is inflated while malpositioned within the trachea)

G. Impaction of balloon lumen preventing deflation

Key Outcome

- Balloon tamponade is effective for stopping variceal hemorrhage in approximately 80% of cases.

- Rebleeding after cessation of tamponade is common, occurring in approximately 50% of cases.

Bibliography

Crerar-Gilbert A. Oesophageal rupture in the course of conservative treatment of bleeding oesophageal varices. J Accid Emerg Med 1996;13:225–227.

Kelly DJ, Walsh F, Ahmed S, et al. Airway obstruction due to a Sengstaken-Blakemore tube. Anesth Analg 1997;85:219–221.

Roberts LR, Kamath PS. Pathophysiology and treatment of variceal hemorrhage. Mayo Clin Proc 1996;71:973–983.

Thomas P, Auge A, Lonjon T, et al. Rupture of the thoracic trachea with a Sengstaken-Blakemore tube. J Cardiovasc Surg (Torino) 1994;35:351–353.

210 Transnasal and Transoral Gastroenteric Intubation

James A. Kruse

Definitions

A. Nasogastric tube
   1. A flexible catheter of variable caliber (typically 14 to 18 Fr) containing one or more lumens and usually intended to be introduced transnasally into the stomach
   2. May also be inserted transorally (orogastric tube)
   3. Usually constructed of polyvinyl chloride
   4. Typically used for aspirating stomach contents or administering drugs or tube-feeding mixtures
   5. Variations
      a. Levin tube: a simple, single-lumen nasogastric tube
      b. Salem tube: contains one lumen for aspiration and a second lumen used as a vent to allow air return to the stomach, minimizing distal tube adherence to the mucosa during suctioning
      c. Ewald tube: an extra large diameter (e.g., 36 Fr) orogastric tube commonly used for gastric lavage to remove blood clots or pill fragments
      d. Balloon tonometry tube: see Chapter 219, Gastric Tonometry
      e. Sengstaken-Blakemore and Minnesota tubes: see Chapter 209, Sengstaken-Blakemore Tube Placement

B. Nasoenteric tube
   1. A flexible, usually single-lumen, small-bore (<12 Fr) catheter intended to be introduced through the nose and into the small intestine (usually the duodenum)
   2. May also be inserted transorally (oroenteric tube)
   3. Usually constructed of polyurethane or silicone, with or without a weighted distal end
   4. Typically used for delivering enteral nutrition
   5. Variations
      a. Weighted tubes
         (1) Contain an encased metallic weight, formerly mercury but now commonly tungsten, at the tip
         (2) Traditionally, assumed to facilitate passage through the esophagus and pylorus, although recent investigations have shown that unweighted tubes may have a higher frequency of achieving transpyloric placement
      b. Miller-Abbott and Cantor tubes
         (1) Extra-long, bag- or balloon-tipped (formerly filled with mercury) tubes with multiple side orifices along the distal portion
         (2) Traditionally used for intestinal decompression
      c. Tubes containing an inner stylet
         (1) Tube is marketed with a mating wire or filament stylet that is inserted through the tube prior to insertion, and removed immediately after insertion.
         (2) Purpose of the stylet is to stiffen tubes made from soft polymers to facilitate their insertion.
         (3) Caution: if the stylet is reinserted while the tube is within the patient there is a risk that the stylet may perforate the tube or exit a side hole, and puncture, perforate or otherwise injure the esophagus, stomach, or duodenum
      d. Combination gastroenteric tubes
         (1) Multilumen tube: intended to be positioned with its tip and distal orifice(s) in the duodenum or jejunum for enteral alimentation, and containing one or two additional lumens that open at the level of the stomach to allow gastric aspiration
         (2) Telescopic combination tube: a large-bore nasogastric tube with mating wire-guided, coaxial inner tube that can be advanced independently into the duodenum or jejunum to allow simultaneous gastric aspiration and intestinal feeding

Key Indications

- Gastric lavage, e.g., for active upper gastrointestinal hemorrhage or decontamination following toxic ingestion
- Emptying or decompression of stomach using continuous or intermittent aspiration
- Drug delivery, when patient unable to take drugs by mouth
- Gastric feeding or enteral nutrition

Key Contraindications to Transnasal Intubation (*transoral intubation not contraindicated*)

- Bilateral nasal obstruction
- Sinusitis
- Maxillofacial trauma
- Basal skull fracture
- Thrombocytopenia
- Coagulopathy
- Epistaxis
- Nasal telangiectasia

Procedure

A. Patient preparation

1. Explain the procedure to the patient and, if possible, enlist cooperation.

2. Position awake patients in high Fowler's or sitting position, if possible.

3. Parenteral sedation or analgesia may be considered in selected patients when the procedure is performed in a monitored setting and there are no contraindications.

4. Optionally, awake patients may be given a benzocaine throat lozenge prior to the procedure, if not contraindicated.

5. Transnasal insertion

   a. Determine appropriate naris for tube insertion.

      (1) Check for deviated septum and difference in size or patency of nares, and select the larger opening.

      (2) Patency may be assessed in cooperative patients by instructing them to inhale through the nose while the clinician occludes the nares one at a time.

   b. Topical sympathomimetic agent (e.g., 0.5% phenylephrine) may optionally be sprayed into nares, if there is no contraindication, to constrict turbinates.

   c. Topical anesthetic (e.g., 5 mL of 2% lidocaine jelly) or surgical lubricant may optionally be instilled into selected naris and allowed to flow posteriorly to the nasopharynx by gravity (head extended) and by encouraging the patient to sniff.

   d. Topical anesthetic (e.g., a proprietary mixture of 2% tetracaine, 2% butylaminobenzoate, and 14% benzocaine) may be sprayed onto the posterior oropharynx for 1 second while depressing tongue with a depressor blade.

B. Tube preparation

1. Estimate the appropriate insertion distance and mark the catheter.

   a. For nasogastric insertion, measure the distance from the tip of the patient's nose to the tip of the earlobe to the xiphoid process (typically 50 to 60 cm).

   b. For nasoenteric insertion, add 25 cm to the above distance.

2. Inspect the tube for defects.

3. Lubricate the distal 15 cm of tube using a liberal amount of water-soluble lubricant with or without 2% lidocaine.

4. Feeding tubes containing an inner stylet

   a. The stylet is removed, lubricated with a small amount of mineral oil (check manufacturer's recommendation for lubricant type), and replaced in the catheter prior to insertion.

   b. Some stylets contain a hygromer coating that is activated by water; other lubricants are not to be used with these stylets.

   c. Ensure that the stylet does not protrude from the end hole or any side holes in the tube, or perforate the tube.

C. Tube introduction

1. Transnasal route

   a. Insert tip of tube into naris and direct posteriorly (not superiorly), parallel to both the nasal septum and the superior surface of the hard palate.

   b. If resistance is encountered, steady pressure should be gently applied. Forceful insertion can result in patient discomfort and epistaxis. Slight rotation of the tube may be helpful.

CAUTION

Do not direct a nasogastric tube superiorly when introducing it into the naris. The tube should be directed posteriorly along the floor of the nasal cavity.

2. Transoral route: insert the tube into the oral cavity and direct it posteriorly and then inferiorly

3. Both routes

   a. Once the tip of the tube approaches the pharynx, slightly flex the patient's neck and advance the tube.

   b. Awake, cooperative patients

(1) Ask the patient to swallow as the tube is advanced from the nasopharynx to the oropharynx and into the esophagus.

(2) If able to take water orally, have patient sip water through a straw to facilitate swallowing as the tube is advanced.

c. Advance the tube through the esophagus and into the stomach.

d. Periodically inspect the patient's mouth to ensure that the (transnasal) tube has not been inadvertently directed into the oral cavity, or that the (transoral or transnasal) tube is not looping or coiling in the pharynx.

D. Alternative procedures

1. Gelatin capsule method for inserting small-caliber, highly compliant gastric feeding tubes

a. A small-bore, nonweighted feeding tube is placed alongside a standard nasogastric tube with their distal ends evenly aligned.

b. The distal ends of the two tubes are both wedged into one-half of a single, large gelatin capsule to fix them together.

c. The tubes are inserted through the nose or mouth, with the larger, stiffer tube serving to facilitate passage into the stomach.

d. Once in place, sufficient time is allowed for the capsule to dissolve and then the larger tube is carefully withdrawn.

2. Tube cooling

a. A standard polyvinyl chloride nasogastric tube is wrapped into a coil and cooled by refrigeration or immersion in ice until the time of insertion.

b. Without allowing the tube to warm, it is quickly inserted in the usual manner.

c. Low temperature stiffens the tube and facilitates insertion.

3. Direct laryngoscopy

a. Using a standard laryngoscope, as is used for endotracheal intubation, the hypopharynx, larynx, and esophageal opening are directly visualized as the tube is advanced transnasally or transorally into the hypopharynx.

b. The tip of the tube is grasped transorally using Magill forceps and directed into the esophageal opening as an assistant advances the tube.

c. A useful technique when difficulties are encountered using the standard procedure

E. Verification of intragastric placement

1. Auscultation and air insufflation

a. Routinely employed immediately after tube insertion

b. Rapidly inject 20 to 50 mL of air into the tube lumen using a suitable syringe while auscultating over the left upper quadrant.

c. Auscultation of the distinctive sound of air insufflating the stomach has traditionally been accepted as denoting intragastric placement of tube; however, false-positive results can occur with esophageal, intestinal, and respiratory tract placement.

2. Aspiration

a. Apply negative pressure to the tube lumen using a large (35 to 60 mL), Tuoy-tipped syringe.

b. Excessive negative pressure may collapse the lumen of tubes made from more flexible polymers, impairing ability to aspirate gastric contents.

c. Examine the aspirate to confirm typical gastric secretions, bile (if the tube is past the pylorus or there is reflux), or stomach contents.

3. pH testing

a. Aspirate fluid from the tube and determine pH using indicator test paper.

b. Gastric aspirates usually (~80% of patients) have a pH of 1.0 to 4.0.

(1) Use of antacids, H_2-receptor blocking agents, or proton pump inhibitors can result in substantially higher values, but frequently do not.

(2) Patients with achlorhydria can have substantially higher values in the absence of the above drug therapy.

c. Respiratory secretions usually show a pH over 7.0, signifying inadvertent intratracheal placement.

4. Water injection: provocation of coughing following injection of 2 to 3 mL of water through the tube suggests placement in the tracheobronchial tract

5. Water immersion

a. The proximal end of the tube is immersed into a container of tap water and inspected.

b. The appearance of bubbling from the tube, synchronous with respiration, suggests that the tube lies within the respiratory tract.

c. Bubbling can occasionally occur when the tube is properly positioned in the stomach.

6. Carbon dioxide detection

a. A commercially available, disposable, semiquantitative, colorimetric CO_2 detection device marketed for confirmation of endotracheal tube placement is adapted to the nasogastric tube after insertion.

b. Transtracheal insertion is denoted by color change indicative of the presence of exhaled CO_2 gas.

c. Lack of color change is consistent with gastric insertion.

d. Although preliminary investigation demonstrated 100% accuracy with this technique, further study is needed to confirm these findings.

e. Sidestream quantitative capnometry or capnography could also be used in this way.

7. Plain radiographic imaging

8. Direct laryngoscopy: a laryngoscope is used to assure that the tube enters the esophagus rather than the trachea (does not guarantee that the tube enters the stomach)

F. Transpyloric advancement of enteric tubes

1. Blind technique

a. The tube is simply advanced the estimated distance required to reach the dudenum or jejunum.

b. If subsequent radiographic imaging shows that the tube lies within the gastric lumen, spontaneous transpyloric migration may occur in some patients. This movement may be facilitated by positioning the patient in the lateral decubitus position with the right side down, and with the use of metoclopramide (see below).

2. Stylet technique

a. A tube containing a stylet is inserted into the stomach and then simply advanced to the estimated required distance.

b. The stylet is removed and correct placement is verified.

c. Optionally, the stylet may be allowed to remain in place until radiographic confirmation of correct placement is obtained; if the tube has not entered the duodenum, additional manipulation is possible without the risks associated with reinsertion of the stylet.

3. Air insufflation technique

a. After intragastric placement of the tube (with stylet) to the level of the fundus is achieved, 500 mL of air is insufflated into the stomach via repeated injection with a 50 or 60 mL syringe, and the tube is then advanced.

b. In one study, successful duodenal intubation was achieved nearly twice as often with this technique.

c. Not recommended after esophageal or gastric surgery, or in the face of active peptic ulcer disease or bleeding

4. "Corkscrew" technique

a. A 10 to 12 Fr feeding tube with an inner metal stylet is inserted into the stomach in the usual manner.

b. The stylet is removed, bent to a 30-degree angle approximately 2 to 3 cm from its distal tip, and reinserted into the tube.

c. By means of the air insufflation technique (see above), the tube is rotated and advanced in short bursts to the appropriate point beyond the pylorus.

d. Note that many authors advise against reinsertion of the stylet while the tube is in place to avoid potential injury (see earlier, under Definitions).

5. Pharmacologically assisted technique

a. Administer metoclopramide (10 to 20 mg intravenously over 2 minutes), 10 minutes prior to tube insertion to stimulate gastric peristalsis; erythromycin has also been used for this purpose.

b. Proceed as in the blind technique, then position the patient in the lateral decubitus position with the right side down.

6. Fluoroscopic placement

a. Intragastric position is confirmed under fluoroscopy.

b. The tube is manually advanced and manipulated through the pylorus under fluoroscopic observation.

c. The success rate for intraduodenal placement approaches 90%.

7. Endoscopic placement

a. A suture is tied to the distal end of the tube (some commercially available tubes have an attached string for this purpose), and the tube is inserted into stomach in the standard manner, usually transnasally.

b. The endoscope is inserted transorally into the stomach, and the stomach is insufflated with air.

c. The suture is grasped using forceps inserted through the biopsy channel of the endoscope.

d. The endoscope is advanced through the pylorus and past the ampulla of Vater, and the tube is released in the duodenum.

e. Alternatively, the endoscope may be positioned stationary at the pylorus and used simply to observe that the tube passes into the duodenum during manual advancement and manipulation.

f. The success rate for intraduodenal placement is over 90%.

8. Fluoroendoscopic placement of enteric feeding tube, or combination gastric-enteric tube, using the guidewire method

   a. The endoscope is advanced transorally to the distal duodenum.

   b. A flexible guidewire is introduced through the endoscope channel and advanced beyond the ligament of Treitz under fluoroscopic guidance.

   c. The endoscope is slowly removed while advancing the guidewire under fluoroscopy to maintain its position in the jejunum.

   d. The guidewire may be transferred from the mouth to the nose, if desired.

      (1) An 8 Fr pediatric Levin tube is inserted through the nose to the oropharynx, and the distal end is retrieved through the oral cavity.

      (2) The proximal end of the guidewire is inserted into the distal end of the Levin tube, and the wire is advanced and retrieved from the proximal end of the tube.

      (3) The Levin tube is removed from the nose without disturbing the position of the guidewire, and the wire is straightened in the pharynx.

   e. Lubricate the inner lumen of the feeding tube with the lubricant indicated by the manufacturer, and lubricate the outer tip of the tube with water-soluble lubricant.

   f. Insert the tube over the guidewire to the appropriate distance under fluoroscopic guidance.

   g. If a combination gastric-enteric tube is used, ensure that the radiopaque markers near the proximal opening(s) are within the stomach and the distal portion of the tube is in the duodenum or jejunum.

   h. Remove guidewire and confirm final placement using fluoroscopy.

G. Verification of enteric placement (for blind insertion techniques)

   1. Aspiration

      a. Bile aspiration suggests that the tube is past the pylorus.

      b. Ability to recover injected air by aspiration suggests that the tube is in the stomach rather than past the pylorus.

   2. Auscultation and air insufflation

      a. Performed as for verification of intragastric placement

      b. Air entering the pylorus tends to be loudest over the mid-epigastrium and radiates to the left upper quadrant.

      c. Air entering the proximal duodenum tends to be heard loudest over the right upper quadrant.

      d. Air entering the distal duodenum and jejunum tends to be of higher pitch and more distant amplitude, and localizes more to the left flank than to the stomach.

   3. pH testing

      a. See above under E. Verification of intragastric placement.

      b. Intestinal aspirate usually yields a pH of 5.0 to 8.0 (~90% show pH over 6.0), versus less than 4.0 for gastric aspirate.

   4. Injection of water and water-immersion methods: see above under E. Verification of intragastric placement

   5. Injection of blue food dye through a gastric tube

      a. Dye is injected into the feeding tube.

      b. Aspiration from a preexisting or newly placed gastric tube is performed.

      c. Recovery of dye from the gastric tube suggests that the feeding tube is not past the pylorus.

   6. Radiographic confirmation: recommended routinely after blind placement

H. Methods of securing the tube

   1. After cleaning and drying the skin, the tube may be taped to the skin of the nose, upper lip, or side of the face with adhesive tape or a transparent adhesive dressing.

   2. Avoid traction or pressure on naris (transnasal insertion), lips, or the corner of the mouth (transoral insertion).

   3. Proprietary devices are available that attach to the tube and to the patient's skin using an adhesive or a bridle-like device.

CAUTION

Choking, coughing, dysphonia, or distress during insertion may indicate that the tube has entered the trachea.

Complications

A. Specific to transnasal insertion

   1. Epistaxis

   2. Rhinitis

   3. Sinusitis

4. Otitis media

5. Injury to nasopharyngeal mucosa

6. Intracranial insertion (in the presence of a basal skull fracture)

7. Cutaneous breakdown, laceration or pressure necrosis at naris from tube or securing tape

B. Specific to transoral insertion

1. Injury to oropharyngeal mucosa

2. Parotitis

3. Tissue breakdown, laceration or pressure necrosis involving skin, lips, or oral structures from tube or securing tape

C. Physical complications common to both the transoral and the transnasal routes

1. Pharyngodynia and pharyngitis

2. Odynophagia, dysphagia, and vomiting

3. Occult dislodgement of tube from stomach to esophagus or pharynx

4. Inadvertent removal of tube

5. Submucosal pharyngeal placement or perforation

6. Clogging of tube (more common with small-bore feeding tubes)

7. Aspiration pneumonitis or pneumonia

8. Hoarseness, vocal cord paralysis

9. Gastroesophageal reflux

10. Esophageal stricture

11. Tracheal intubation (can occur even in the presence of a cuffed endotracheal tube)

   a. Intrapulmonary instillation of drugs or tube feeding

   b. Bronchial intubation

     (1) Coughing, bronchorrhea, respiratory distress

     (2) Pulmonary hemorrhage, hemoptysis

     (3) Transbronchial perforation

     (a) Pneumothorax, pneumomediastinum, subcutaneous emphysema

     (b) Hydrothorax

     (c) Pleural entry with possible bronchopulmonary fistula or empyema

12. Pulmonary atelectasis

13. Erosion or ulceration of esophagus, gastroesophageal junction, or stomach

14. Rupture of esophageal varix, or other esophageal or gastrointestinal bleeding

15. Esophageal perforation

   a. Mediastinitis

   b. Tracheoesophageal fistula

   c. Aortoesophageal fistula

16. Intestinal obstruction or perforation

17. Cardiac dysrhythmias

18. Knotting or breakage of tube in situ

D. Metabolic complications of gastric aspiration

1. Metabolic alkalosis

2. Hypokalemia

3. Disturbances of water and sodium balance

 ## Bibliography

Lord LM, Weiser-Maimone A, Pulhamus M, et al. Comparison of weighted vs unweighted enteral feeding tubes for efficacy of transpyloric intubation. JPEN 1993:17:271–273.

Metheny NA, Clouse RE. Bedside methods for detecting aspiration in tube-fed patients. Chest 1997;111:724–731.

Napolitano LM, Wagle M, Heard SO. Endoscopic placement of nasoenteric feeding tubes in critically ill patients: a reliable alternative. J Laparoendoscopic Adv Surg Tech 1998;8:395–400.

Singer AJ, Konia N. Comparison of topical anesthetics and vasoconstrictors vs lubricants prior to nasogastric intubation: a randomized, controlled trial. Acad Emerg Med 1999;6:184–190.

Snider RD, Kruse JA. Catheter breakage. An unusual complication of naso-enteric feeding tubes. Am J Gastroenterol 1995;90:1171–1172.

211 Enteral Feeding

Jorge A. Guzman

Malnutrition is common in hospitalized patients and is associated with nosocomial infection, prolonged hospital stay, and increased mortality. The immunologic function of the gastrointestinal (GI) tract plays a major role in the pathogenesis of infection in critically ill patients in the intensive care unit. Alteration of the immunocompetence of this barrier results in bacterial translocation, which may initiate the inflammatory cascade that leads to multiple organ dysfunction. Intestinal stimulation from enteral feedings helps maintain normal GI structural and functional integrity, thereby reducing infection-related morbidity.

Key Indications

- Critically ill patients with a functional gastrointestinal tract who are not expected to eat within 2 to 4 days

- Early enteral nutrition, within 48 to 72 hours of admission to the ICU, is recommended unless contraindicated.

Contraindications

A. Intractable vomiting

B. Intestinal obstruction

C. Paralytic ileus

D. Severe diarrhea

E. Peritonitis

F. Severe pancreatitis

G. Gastrointestinal ischemia

H. Persistent hemodynamic instability

I. Severe malabsorption

J. Early stages of short bowel syndrome

Key Advantages of Enteral Nutrition over Parenteral Nutrition

- Maintains gut structure and function

- Enhances nutrient utilization

- Safer administration

- Lower costs

Procedure

A. Perform nutritional assessment (see Chapter 213, Nutritional Assessment).

B. Ensure that there are no contraindications.

C. Select route for enteral feedings (see Fig. 211–1).

 1. Nasogastric intubation is the preferred route for patients expected to later resume oral feedings.

 2. Consider nasoduodenal or nasojejunal intubation for patients at risk of aspiration.

   a. Patients with abnormal sensorium

   b. Patients with impaired swallowing ability

 3. Percutaneous endoscopic gastrostomy (PEG) or surgically placed tube jejunostomy is indicated when long-term feeding is anticipated.

D. Select the method of administration.

 1. Nasoduodenal, nasojejunal, and surgical jejunostomy tubes necessitate continuous administration.

 2. Nasogastric or gastrostomy tube feedings may use continuous or intermittent (bolus) administration.

   a. Advantages of continuous administration

     (1) May provide better prophylaxis against stress ulceration

     (2) Fewer metabolic disturbances (postprandial hyperglycemia, increased oxygen consumption, thermogenesis)

     (3) May be preferable for gastric feedings in some critically ill patients (less gastric distension and aspiration, better tolerance)

   b. Disadvantages of continuous administration: elevated gastric pH may favor bacterial colonization and subsequent nosocomial infections

   c. Advantages of bolus administration: preferred for ambulatory or rehabilitation patients since they are not connected to an infusion pump

   d. Disadvantages of bolus administration

     (1) Fluctuating gastric pH may favor stress ulceration

     (2) Increased incidence of gastric distension

E. Select feeding formula

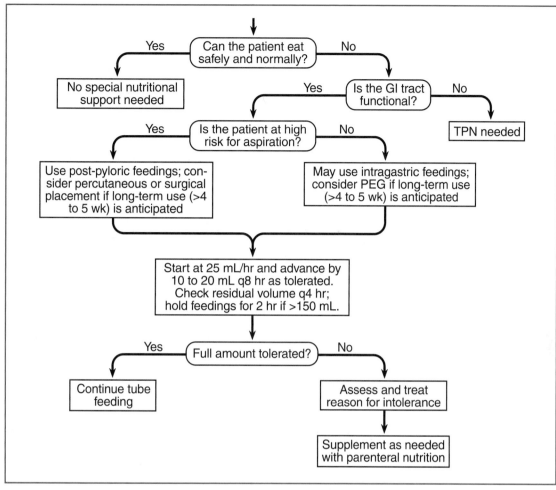

Figure 211–1 Proposed algorithm for initiation and dosing of continuous enteral nutrition therapy in critically ill patients. GI = gastrointestinal; PEG = percutaneous endoscopic gastrostomy; TPN = total parenteral nutrition.

1. Standard isotonic formulas
   a. Examples: Isocal, Osmolite, Nutren 1.0
   b. Balanced mix of carbohydrates, protein, and fat
   c. Nonprotein calories : nitrogen (kcal : N) ratio is typically around 150 : 1
   d. Typically 1 kcal/mL
   e. Recommended as routine starting formula

2. Standard fiber-containing formulas
   a. Examples: Jevity, Probalance, Ultracal
   b. Isotonic with added soy polysaccharide fiber
   c. Fiber increases transit time, improves intestinal architecture, and reduces diarrhea.

3. High caloric density
   a. Examples: TwoCal HN, NovaSource 2.0, Nutren 1.5
   b. For fluid-restricted or highly catabolic patients
   c. Typically contain 1.5 to 2 kcal/mL

4. High-protein
   a. Examples: Promote, Traumacal, Replete
   b. Contain higher protein content than standard formulations
   c. Typically have a kcal : N ratio of about 125 : 1
   d. Provides high-protein diet without excessive calories
   e. Well suited for critically ill patients with high-protein needs, e.g., wound healing

5. Elemental (free amino acid or peptide-based) products
   a. Examples: Vivonex, Perative, Alitrag
   b. Macronutrients are in simpler form than standard formulations (e.g., amino acids instead of protein).
   c. Facilitates digestion and absorption
   d. Advantageous for patients with malabsorption or stress-induced GI dysfunction

6. Pulmonary formulations

    a. Example: Pulmocare

    b. Have a lower proportion of calories as carbohydrates

    c. Generate less CO_2 than standard formulas

    d. Rationale for use is to minimize CO_2 generation in patients with hypercapnia or limited pulmonary reserve.

  7. Renal formulations

    a. Example: Nepro, RenalCal, Suplena

    b. High-calorie formulations with modified electrolyte and protein content useful for patients with renal insufficiency or failure and limited ability to eliminate water, nitrogen, and electrolytes

    c. High-calorie, moderate protein, low potassium content formulations for predialysis patients (e.g., Suplena, RenalCal)

    d. High-calorie, low protein, no potassium, no phosphate: for renal failure patients (e.g., RenalCal)

    e. High-calorie, moderate protein, low potassium, low phosphorus formulation for dialysis patients (e.g., Nepro)

  8. Branched-chain amino acid

    a. Example: NutriHep

    b. High in branched-chain amino acids, low in aromatic amino acids

    c. May minimize synthesis of false neurotransmitters involved in hepatic encephalopathy

    d. Rationale for use is to allow adequate nitrogen balance in patients prone to develop hepatic encephalopathy.

  9. Glucose intolerance formulations

    a. Example: Glucerna

    b. Low carbohydrate formula for patients with diabetes or glucose intolerance

  10. Immune enhancing formulations

    a. Contain supplemental L-arginine and nucleic acids

    b. May reduce the magnitude and duration of acute phase inflammatory response and the risk of infection

    c. Example: Impact

F. Select target dose based on estimated energy expenditure (see Chapter 213, Nutritional Assessment).

G. Initiating administration

  1. Continuous method

    a. Start infusion at 25 mL/hour.

    b. Advance rate by 10 to 20 mL/hour every 6 to 8 hours, as tolerated, to achieve goal.

    c. Check residual volume every 4 hours; hold feeding for 2 hours if more than 150 mL.

  2. Bolus method

    a. Initiate gastric feeding with 100 mL bolus of full-strength (1 kcal/mL) formula, followed by 50 mL water flush through feeding tube.

    b. Advance feedings by 50 mL every 4 hours if gastric residual volume is less than 100 mL or less than half the volume previously delivered.

    c. When the volume reaches 300 mL (250 mL of formula plus 50 mL water flush), change feeding intervals to every 3 hours or every 2 hours, as needed, to meet caloric needs.

H. Monitor progress with follow-up assessment (see Chapter 213, Nutritional Assessment).

Complications

A. High residual gastric volume

  1. Consider changing from bolus to continuous administration.

  2. Consider trial of metoclopramide to increase gastric motility.

  3. Discontinue narcotics or other motility-slowing drugs.

B. Diarrhea

  1. Review selected tube-feeding formulation and concomitant drugs for possible cause.

  2. Send stool sample for *Clostridium difficile* cytotoxin.

  3. If using hypertonic formula, dilute to 3/4 strength.

  4. If continuous feeding is used, consider decreasing administration rate.

  5. Eliminate or reduce possible problem nutrients: lactose, sucrose or maltose, gluten, complex fats.

  6. Reduce carbohydrate concentration in true osmotic diarrhea; may try formulation containing oligosaccharides or disaccharides.

  7. Consider administering a "stool-drying agent."

    a. Kaolin-pectin suspension: 15 to 30 mL after each loose stool, up to 8 doses per day

    b. Diphenoxylate (5 mg) and atropine (0.05 mg): equivalent to 4 tablets or 10 mL of Lomotil, up to every 6 hours

C. Abdominal distension or constipation

  1. Consider adding more water to GI feeding regimen.

  2. Discontinue narcotics or other motility-slowing drugs.

  3. Exclude fecal impaction.

4. Consider abdominal x-ray.

5. Consider laxative or suppository.

D. Aspiration

1. Elevate head of bed.

2. Check gastric residual volume before each bolus feed.

3. Use a small-bore feeding tube.

4. Consider continuous feeding.

E. Metabolic complications

1. Electrolyte imbalances

a. Monitor serum Na, K, Cl, total CO_2, Ca, Mg, and P concentrations.

b. Provide supplemental K, Mg and P, as needed.

2. Hypoglycemia or hyperglycemia

a. Monitor blood glucose.

b. Provide insulin or IV dextrose, as indicated.

3. Hyperosmolar state

a. Monitor serum Na concentration.

b. Adjust free water administration as needed to maintain normal sodium concentration.

F. Mechanical complications

1. Complications related to tube insertion (e.g., epistaxis, tracheobronchial placement)

2. Sinusitis: due to nasal tubes

3. Erosions or ulcerations

a. Cutaneous lesions at naris, from nasogastric or nasoenteric tube

b. Esophageal or gastric lesions

4. Feeding tube breakage, displacement, or migration

PEARLS

- Enteral nutrition is preferred over parenteral nutrition if gut function is intact.

- Begin enteral nutrition early, using standard isotonic formulas.

- Elevate head of bed and check gastric residual volumes periodically.

Bibliography

Beale RJ, Byrg DS, Bihari DJ. Immunonutrition in the critically ill: a systematic review of clinical outcome. Crit Care Med 1999;27:2799–2805.

Clevenger FW, Rodriguez DJ. Decision-making for enteral feeding administration: the why behind the where and how. Nutr Clin Pract 1995;10:104–113.

Guenter P, Jones S, Sweed MR, et al. Delivery systems and administration of enteral nutrition. In: Rombeau JL, Rolandelli RH (eds). Clinical Nutrition. Enteral and Tube Feeding, 3rd ed. Philadelphia: WB Saunders, 1997; pp 240–267.

Hernandez G, Velasco N, Wainstein C, et al. Gut mucosal atrophy after a short enteral fasting period in critically ill patients. J Crit Care 1999;14:73–77.

Jolliet P, Pichard C, Biolo G, et al. Enteral nutrition in intensive care patients: a practical approach. Clin Nutr 1999;18:47–56.

Metheney N. Minimizing respiratory complications of nasoenteric tube feedings: state of the science. Heart Lung 1993;22:213–223.

212 Parenteral Nutrition

Jorge A. Guzman

In spite of advantages of the gastrointestinal (GI) route over the IV route, parenteral nutrition is frequently prescribed in critically ill patients. In the intensive care unit setting, it is used mainly in patients in whom the GI tract cannot be utilized, or those in whom enteral nutrition alone cannot provide the desired caloric load. Parenteral nutrition can be administered centrally or peripherally, depending on the total caloric load desired and a risk–benefit analysis of central venous catheter placement.

Indications

A. Patients with inability to absorb nutrients via the GI tract
   1. Severe inflammatory bowel disease
   2. Peritonitis
   3. Gastrointestinal obstruction
   4. Uncontrollable diarrhea
   5. Severe pancreatitis
   6. Shock states
   7. Enterocutaneous fistulas
   8. Persistent ileus
   9. Massive abdominal distension
   10. Severe gastrointestinal bleeding

B. Severe malnutrition in the face of a nonfunctional GI tract

C. Severely catabolic patients who will be unable to use their GI tract within 5 to 7 days

D. Any patient undergoing major surgery or moderate stress and who will not resume an enteral diet for 7 to 10 days

---

PEARL

Parenteral nutrition is reserved for patients in whom the enteral route cannot be used.

Dosing and Administration

A. Components
   1. Dextrose
     a. The obligate substrate for brain, red and white blood cells, and renal medulla and the major energy substrate used in most parenteral nutrition formulations

     b. Available in stock concentrations ranging from 5% to 70%

     c. The monohydrate form of dextrose yields 3.4 kcal/g.

     d. Daily dose is based on estimation of energy requirements (see Chapter 213, Nutritional Assessment), usually split between dextrose and fat emulsion.

     e. Typically used to supply between 50% and 70% of the total caloric requirements, with the remainder supplied by lipid emulsion

     f. Parenteral solutions containing a final concentration of dextrose of 10% or more should be administered through a central venous access because of their high osmolality.

     g. Infusion rates should not exceed 5 mg/kg per minute.

   2. Intravenous fat emulsions
     a. Used as a source of essential fatty acids and to provide between 30% (typical) and 50% of the total caloric requirements, with the remainder supplied by dextrose

     b. Yields 9 kcal/g

     c. Fat emulsions are commercially available in 10%, 20%, and 30% concentrations, providing 1.1, 2.0, and 3.0 kcal/mL, respectively.

     d. Can be mixed with parenteral nutrition solution or infused separately via central or peripheral vein

     e. Maximum dose should not exceed 2.5 g/kg per day.

     f. Excessively rapid infusions may provoke pulmonary vasoconstriction.

     g. Triglyceride concentration should be measured post-infusion periodically to monitor fat clearance.

       (1) Particularly relevant in disease states associated with impaired fat metabolism (e.g., pancreatitis, hepatic failure, sepsis, hypermetabolic states)

(2) Triglyceride levels lower than 450 mg/dL during continuous lipid infusions are acceptable.

3. Amino acids

a. Crystalline amino acid solution take the place of dietary protein as a source of nitrogen for protein synthesis.

b. Standard amino acid solutions have a balanced profile of essential, semi-essential, and nonessential amino acids.

c. Solutions high in branched-chain amino acids have not been proven to confer special benefit.

d. 10% amino acid solutions are most commonly used, but they are commercially available in a range of concentrations from 3% to 15%.

e. Amino acid solutions are available with and without added electrolytes; those with added electrolytes are designed to meet typical requirements in the average patient, but they may not be satisfactory for all patients (e.g., those with renal failure), and formulation adjustment may be necessary after initiation.

f. Initiation of therapy can be estimated at 1.2 to 1.5 g/kg per day and adjusted with periodic monitoring of nitrogen balance to promote positive nitrogen balance (see Chapter 213, Nutritional Assessment).

g. Patients with chronic renal failure should be started at a lower dose; e.g., 0.8 g/kg per day.

h. Consider decreasing the administered dose if

(1) Serum urea nitrogen rises precipitously or to high levels.

(2) Blood ammonia level rises and is associated with encephalopathy.

(3) The patient has marked renal insufficiency, but is not receiving dialysis.

(4) Nitrogen balance study indicates excessive administration.

i. Consider increasing the administered dose if

(1) Nitrogen balance study indicates inadequate dose (nitrogen balance less than 2 g/day).

(2) Hemodialysis is initiated.

4. Electrolytes

a. Sodium

(1) Typical requirement: 70 to 100 mEq/day

(2) Typical final admixture concentration: 35 mEq/L; range 0 to 150 mEq/L

(3) Specific requirement varies with water requirements, body sodium balance, and renal and cardiac function.

b. Potassium

(1) Typical requirement: 70 to 100 mEq/day or 5 to 6 mEq/g nitrogen

(2) Typical final admixture concentration: 30 mEq/L; range 0 to 80 mEq/L

(3) Actual requirement may be greater than 200 mEq/day in some cases.

c. Chloride

(1) Typical requirement: 80 to 120 mEq/day

(2) Typical final admixture concentration: 40 mEq/L; range 0 to 150 mEq/L

(3) Anions are supplied chiefly as chloride and acetate, with the ratio dependent on acid-base balance.

d. Magnesium

(1) Typical requirement: 15 to 20 mEq/day, as magnesium sulfate

(2) Typical final admixture concentration: 8 mEq/L (4 mmol/L); range 0 to 16 mEq/L (0 to 8 mmol/L)

(3) Decreased requirement in renal failure

e. Calcium

(1) Typical requirement: 10 to 20 mEq/day, as calcium gluconate

(2) Typical final admixture concentration: 4 mEq/L (2 mmol/L); range 0 to 16 mEq/L (0 to 8 mmol/L)

(3) Increased requirement after multiple blood transfusions

f. Phosphorus

(1) Typical requirement: 20 to 30 mmol/day (7 to 9 μmol/nonprotein kcal), as sodium or potassium phosphate salt

(2) Typical final admixture concentration: 15 mmol/L (range 0 to 20 mmol/L)

(3) Lipid emulsions contain phosphorus (15 mmol/L) as phospholipid.

g. Acetate

(1) Typical provision: 0 to 60 mEq/day, as sodium or potassium salt

(2) Typical final admixture concentration: 14 mEq/L

(3) Increase if metabolic acidosis; decrease or discontinue if metabolic alkalosis.

5. Vitamins (some are contained in IV multivitamin preparations)

a. Vitamin A: daily dose: 3,300 IU/day (up to 5,000 IU/day)

b. Thiamine (vitamin B_1): daily dose: 1 to 5 mg/day (50 to 100 mg initially if possibility of deficiency state)

c. Riboflavin (vitamin B_2): daily dose: 3.6 (range 1.1 to 5) mg/day

d. Niacin: daily dose: 10 to 40 mg/day

e. Vitamin B_6 (pyridoxine): daily dose: 4 (range 1.6 to 4) mg/day

f. Vitamin B_{12} (cyanocobalamin): daily dose: 5 (range 3 to 12) μg/day, or 100 μg/week intramuscularly or intravenously

g. Folate: daily dose: 400 μg/day (up to 5 mg/day)

h. Vitamin C (ascorbic acid): daily dose: 100 (range 45 to 500) mg/day

i. Vitamin D: daily dose: 200 to 400 IU/day

j. Vitamin E: daily dose: 10 to 15 IU/day

k. Vitamin K_1 (phytonadione)

(1) Dose: 10 to 20 mg once per week

(2) Not included in standard multivitamin products and must be provided separately

(3) Maintenance phytonadione is preferably given by subcutaneous injection because of the risk of anaphylaxis if given intravenously.

l. Pantothenic acid: daily dose: 15 (range 5 to 15) mg/day

m. Biotin: daily dose: 60 (range 60 to 300) μg/day

6. Trace elements (standard preparations based on average requirements should be provided as an additive to the parenteral nutrition mixture)

a. Zinc

(1) Typical daily dose: 3 mg (range 2.5 to 4.0 mg)

(2) Consider increased requirements in patients with diarrhea, other GI fistula losses, ethanol abuse, or severe catabolic states.

b. Copper

(1) Typical daily dose: 1.2 mg (range 0.5 to 3.0 mg)

(2) Decrease dose in patients with biliary tract obstruction.

c. Manganese

(1) Typical daily dose: 300 μg (range 150 to 800 μg)

(2) Decrease dose in patients with biliary tract obstruction.

d. Selenium

(1) Typical daily dose: 100 μg (range 40 to 200 μg)

(2) Typically added after 4 weeks of parenteral nutrition

e. Iodine: typical daily dose: 100 μg (range 1 to 2 μg/kg)

f. Chromium

(1) Typical daily dose: 12 μg (range 5 to 15 μg)

(2) Decrease dose in patients with renal failure.

7. Iron

a. Not included in trace element admixtures

b. Supplementation is generally not required unless there is preexisting iron deficiency or the patient is receiving long-term parenteral nutrition.

c. Assessed by hemoglobin, hematocrit, erythrocyte indices, serum iron, total iron binding capacity and saturation, and ferritin levels

d. Iron dextran

(1) Can be given intravenously, if parenteral iron supplementation is necessary

(2) Fatal anaphylaxis has been reported.

(3) A test dose should be given before each administration.

8. Water

a. Sterile water is added to parenteral nutrition formula to adjust the total volume of fluid needed according to each individual patient.

b. Fluid requirements in critically ill patients are variable, therefore, fluid intake needs to be individualized.

c. Standard formulas may be used as a starting point for determining water requirements (L/day).

(1) From body weight: 30 to 35 mL/kg

(2) From body weight: 100 mL/kg for the first 10 kg + 50 mL/kg for the next 10 kg + 20 mL/kg for every 10 kg thereafter

(3) From body surface area: 1.5 L/m²

(a) Body surface area (BSA) may be derived using standard nomograms.

(b) Alternatively, BSA (m²) may be calculated from weight (kg) and height (inches) using:

$$BSA = weight^{0.425} \times (2.54 \times height)^{0.725} \times 0.007184)$$

B. Initiating and titrating administration

1. Begin infusion rate at 25 to 50 mL/hour and increase infusion by 25 to 50 mL/hour per day until targeted calorie and nitrogen doses are reached.

2. If hyperglycemia develops

   a. May temporarily decrease hourly infusion rate or decrease glucose concentration of solution; or,

   b. May begin sliding-scale coverage of regular insulin

   c. Once insulin requirements are determined, regular insulin may be added to the parenteral nutrition solution.

   d. Reconsider the dextrose : lipid calorie ratio.

3. If the triglyceride level is greater than 450 mg/dL, decrease lipid administration.

4. Periodic readjustment of admixture components may be required according to such factors as the patient's prevailing volume status, serum electrolyte values, and respiratory quotient, among others.

Monitoring

A. Prior to initiation of parenteral nutrition and multiple times daily until stability is achieved

1. Serum or blood glucose concentration, or

2. Semiquantitative urine glucose and ketone levels

B. Prior to initiation of parenteral nutrition and periodically thereafter

1. Serum sodium, potassium, chloride, total CO_2, glucose, urea nitrogen, creatinine, magnesium, calcium, and phosphate concentrations

   a. Obtain daily, at least initially.

   b. May decrease frequency (e.g., thrice weekly) thereafter in selected cases

2. Liver function tests: assessed at least weekly

3. Prothrombin and partial thromboplastin times: assessed at least weekly

4. Complete blood cell count including differential white cell and platelet counts: assessed at least weekly

5. Serum triglyceride level to assess lipid clearance

a. Intermittent lipid emulsion therapy

   (1) Obtain level 6 hours post–lipid infusion.

   (2) A level lower than 400 mg/dL is generally acceptable.

b. Continuous lipid emulsion therapy

   (1) Obtain random level.

   (2) A level lower than 500 mg/dL is generally acceptable.

6. Serum pre-albumin or transferrin concentration: weekly

7. Perform indirect calorimetry and revise caloric prescription if necessary.

   a. Assess weekly.

   b. Respiratory quotient higher than 1 generally indicates overfeeding.

8. Perform nitrogen balance study.

   a. Balance lower than 2 g/day indicates potential need for increased amino acid administration.

   b. Marked or precipitous increase in serum urea nitrogen indicates need to decrease amino acid administration.

C. Routine monitoring of vitamin and trace element levels is unnecessary (may be indicated if deficiency is suspected).

Key Complications

- Mechanical (related to central IV access): e.g., pneumothorax, catheter malposition, air embolism, hemorrhage

- Infectious: catheter site infection, infusion or catheter-related blood stream infection, or sepsis

- Metabolic: glucose intolerance, electrolyte imbalance, azotemia, excess CO_2 production, abnormal liver function tests, hepatic steatosis, hyperosmolar states, lipemia, underfeeding or overfeeding

Special Considerations

A. Hepatic failure

1. Indications for nutritional support are the same for patients with liver disease as for any other critically ill patient.

2. Patients without hepatic encephalopathy can tolerate formulas consisting of standard amino acids.

3. Formulations high in branched-chain amino acids and low in aromatic amino acids may have a role in patients with hepatic encephalopathy and those

a. Experiencing persistent encephalopathy despite adequate medical therapy

b. For whom it is difficult to supply adequate protein without worsening their encephalopathy

4. Patients may be at increased risk for deficiencies of vitamins and zinc.

B. Renal failure

1. Most patients with acute renal failure tolerate standard amino acid formulas that include a mixture of essential and nonessential amino acids.

2. When fluid restriction is necessary for patients with acute oligoanuric renal failure, the optimal quantity of non-protein calories should be provided using the higher concentrations of dextrose and lipid.

3. Decreased amino acid administration will avoid worsening azotemia in patients with renal failure who are not receiving dialysis.

4. Patients receiving hemodialysis require increased amounts of amino acid and water-soluble vitamins.

5. Trace elements can be withheld for the first 2 weeks, and then given every other (non-dialysis) day.

C. Respiratory failure

1. Provide nutritional support to meet energy and protein requirements and thereby limit wasting of respiratory muscles.

2. To prevent excess CO_2 production, monitor nutrient intake and respiratory quotient, and avoid overfeeding.

3. May be benefit in prescribing higher lipid-to-carbohydrate ratios to minimize CO_2 generation, but the utility of this strategy remains to be determined in controlled trials

D. Acute pancreatitis

1. Parenteral nutrition is generally indicated in patients with severe pancreatitis who have been unable to tolerate oral or enteral nutrition for longer than 1 week.

2. Enteral nutrition is preferred unless it exacerbates abdominal pain.

3. Lipid emulsions may be given as long as serum triglyceride levels do not exceed 400 mg/dL.

E. Diabetes mellitus or glucose intolerance

1. Limit dextrose to 200 g for the first 24 hours (e.g., 1 L of 20% dextrose).

2. Most patients will require insulin; a basal amount of regular insulin may be added to the formula (typically, 0.1 U/g dextrose, but will vary).

3. Supplemental regular insulin can be made available using every-6-hour sliding-scale coverage; typically:

a. 2 to 3 U for blood glucose level 200 to 250 mg/dL

b. 4 to 6 U for blood glucose level 251 to 300 mg/dL

c. 6 to 9 U for blood glucose level 301 to 350 mg/dL

d. 8 to 12 U for blood glucose level higher than 350 mg/dL

4. If blood glucose is consistently higher than 200 mg/dL, increase the regular insulin in the parenteral nutrition solution by 0.05 U/g dextrose per day.

5. A separate IV infusion of regular insulin may be necessary if there is unacceptable hyperglycemia despite having regular insulin of at least 0.2 U/g dextrose in the parenteral nutrition solution.

6. If hypoglycemia develops, give an injection of dextrose (12.5 to 25 g), monitor the blood glucose more closely, and decrease the content of insulin in the parenteral nutrition formula by 50%.

F. Peripheral parenteral nutrition

1. Used for short-term (<2 weeks) partial nutritional support when neither the enteral route nor central venous access is feasible

2. Not optimal for patients with marked malnutrition, fluid restriction, severe metabolic stress, or a need for prolonged nutritional support

3. Osmolality of the infusate limits total nutrient delivery.

a. Osmolality should not exceed 600 to 800 mOsm/kg H_2O.

b. Osmolality (mOsm/kg H_2O) may be approximated from the percentage of amino acid and dextrose in the infusate using:

$$\text{Osmolality} \approx (100 \times \%\text{amino acid}) + (50 \times \%\text{dextrose})$$

c. The above formula does not include added electrolytes.

4. Typical mixtures contain equal volumes of 3% to 5% amino acid solution and 5% to 10%

dextrose solution, plus added electrolytes, vitamins, and trace elements.

5. Lipid emulsion may be combined with the above or given via separate IV access.

Key Treatment

- If there are no specific contraindications, provide 70% of the total caloric requirements as carbohydrates and 30% as lipids to start.

- Include amino acids to deliver 1.5 g/kg per day.

- Include required electrolytes, vitamins, and trace elements.

- Intravenous parenteral nutrition is unlikely to benefit a patient who will be able to take enteral nutrition within 4 to 5 days after illness.

Bibliography

ASPEN Board of Directors. Guidelines for the use of parenteral and enteral nutrition in adult and pediatric patients. J Parenteral Enteral Nutr 1993;17(Suppl):1SA–52SA.

Cerra FB, Benitez MR, Blackburn GL, et al. Applied nutrition in ICU patients: a consensus statement of the American College of Chest Physicians. Chest 1997;111:769–778.

Dickerson RN, Brown RO, White KG. Parenteral nutrition solutions. In: Rombeau JL, Caldwell MD (eds). Clinical Nutrition. Parenteral Nutrition, 2nd ed. Philadelphia: WB Saunders, 1993; pp 310–333.

Heyland DK, MacDonald S, Keefe L, et al. Total parenteral nutrition in the critically ill patient. JAMA 1998; 280:2013–2019.

McMahon MM, Rizza RA. Nutrition support in hospitalized patients with diabetes mellitus. Mayo Clin Proc 1996;71:587–594.

Nakasaki H, Ohta M, Soeda J, et al. Clinical and biochemical aspects of thiamine treatment for metabolic acidosis during total parenteral nutrition. Nutrition 1997;13:110–117.

Sax HC. Complications of total parenteral nutrition and their prevention. In: Rombeau JL, Caldwell MD (eds). Clinical Nutrition. Parenteral Nutrition, 2nd ed. Philadelphia: WB Saunders, 1993; pp 310–333.

213 Nutritional Assessment

Jorge A. Guzman

Malnutrition is common in hospitalized patients, with a reported prevalence as high as 40%. It is associated with an increased incidence of infectious complications, compromised immunity, decreased wound healing, prolonged hospital stay, and increased mortality. Thus, evaluating nutritional status in hospitalized patients detects malnutrition and assesses prognosis.

 Key Definitions

- Energy expenditure (EE): the number of kilocalories expended over a 24-hour period

- Basal EE (BEE): resting EE in the healthy subject

History and Physical Findings

A. History
  1. Recent prehospital weight change
  2. Recent prehospital dietary intake and recent changes in intake
  3. Gastrointestinal symptoms
  4. Subjective functional capacity
  5. Alcohol or drug addiction
  6. Intentional, fad diets
B. Weight and height-based indices and nutritional requirement determination
  1. Obtain actual (current) body weight (ABW).
  2. Percentage of usual body weight
    a. Calculated as 100% × ABW/usual body weight
    b. 85% to 94% = mild weight loss
    c. 75% to 84% = moderate weight loss
    d. <75% = severe weight loss
  3. Ideal body weight (IBW)
    a. Determined from actuarial (e.g., Metropolitan Life Insurance) tables
    b. Alternatively, estimated by formula
      (1) Men: IBW (kg) = 48.2 + (2.3 × height in inches >5 feet)
      (2) Women: IBW (kg) = 45.5 + (2.3 × height in inches >5 feet)
  4. Adjusted body weight = 0.25 × (actual body weight − IBW) + IBW

5. Simple weight-based estimate of BEE
    a. BEE = 25 to 30 kcal/kg per day
    b. Use actual body weight if it is no more than 25% over IBW.
    c. Use adjusted body weight if actual body weight is more than 25% over IBW.
6. Percentage of ideal body weight
    a. Calculated as 100% × ABW/IBW
    b. 80% to 90% = mildly underweight
    c. 70% to 79% = moderately underweight
    d. <70% = severely underweight
7. Body mass index (BMI)
    a. Calculated as weight/height^2 (kg/m^2)
    b. ≤17.5 kg/m^2 = underweight
    c. ≤16 kg/m^2 = cachexia
    d. >30 kg/m^2 = obesity
8. Estimation of BEE using the Harris-Benedict equations
    a. Men: BEE = 66.47 + (13.75 × ABW) + (5.00 × height) − (6.76 × age)
    b. Women: BEE = 655.10 + (9.56 × ABW) + (1.85 × height) − (4.68 × age)
    c. Where BEE is in kcal/day, ABW is in kilograms, height is in centimeters, and age is in years
    d. If febrile patients, increase BEE by 10%/°C above 37°C.
    e. EE = BEE × F, where F is a factor to adjust for activity, stress, severely catabolic states, or injury (range for F is 1.1 to 2.0)
      (1) Out of bed: 1.3
      (2) Infection: 1.2 to 1.8
      (3) Surgery: 1.1 to 1.2
      (4) Trauma: 1.3 to 1.6
      (5) Burn injury: 1.5 to 2.0 (40% to 100% body surface area of burn)
9. Estimation of EE using the Ireton-Jones equations
    a. For spontaneously breathing patients:

    EE = 629 − (11 × age) + (25 × weight) − (609 × obesity factor)

    b. For mechanical ventilator-dependent patients:

$$EE = 1925 - (10 \times age) + (5 \times weight)$$
$$+ (281 \times sex\ factor)$$
$$+ (292 \times trauma\ factor)$$
$$+ (851 \times burn\ factor)$$

   c. Units and factor definitions

     (1) EE: kcal/day

     (2) Weight: kg

     (3) Age: years

     (4) Obestity factor: = 1 if weight is more than 30% over IBW; otherwise = 0

     (5) Sex factor: = 1 if male; 0 if female

     (6) Trauma factor: = 1 if present; 0 if absent

     (7) Burn factor: = 1 if burn injury present; 0 if absent

  10. Estimation of protein requirements

    a. Normal subjects: 1.0 to 1.5 g/kg IBW per day

    b. Exceptionally catabolic patients: 1.5 to 2.0 g/kg IBW per day

    c. Patients with hepatic failure: 0.8 to 1.4 g/kg IBW per day

    d. Patients with renal failure: 0.5 to 1.4 g/kg IBW per day

C. Routine physical examination

  1. Assess subcutaneous tissue over triceps and chest for loss of subcutaneous fat.

  2. Assess muscle mass (e.g., temporalis, quadriceps, deltoid, and intrinsic hand muscles) for signs of wasting.

  3. Assess voluntary grip strength.

  4. Assess for signs of specific nutritional deficiencies (examples):

    a. Alopecia: protein–calorie malnutrition

    b. Increased extracellular fluid (e.g., pedal or sacral edema, ascites): severe protein malnutrition

    c. Xerosis: vitamin A deficiency

    d. Dermatitis: zinc deficiency

    e. Petechiae or ecchymoses: vitamin C or K deficiency

    f. Keratomalacia: vitamin A deficiency

    g. Glossitis: pyridoxine, zinc, niacin, folate, vitamin B_{12} deficiency

    h. Confabulation: thiamine deficiency

    i. Neuropathy: thiamine, pyridoxine, vitamin B_{12} deficiency

D. Anthropometry

  1. Skinfold thickness

    a. Allows estimation of percentage body fat

    b. Assessed with skinfold calipers and reference tables

    c. Mid-arm skinfold thickness over the triceps muscle (TSF) is most common site for single measure assessment.

    d. Ideally determined from average of repeated measurements taken from multiple body sites

  2. Arm muscle circumference (AMC)

    a. Allows estimation of somatic protein stores

    b. Assessed by tape measurement of mid-upper arm circumference (MAC), caliper measurement of TSF, and reference tables

    c. Calculated as: $AMC = MAC - (\pi \times TSF)$

Laboratory Findings

A. Plasma protein assays

  1. Albumin

    a. Readily available test for assessing visceral protein stores

    b. 2.8 to 3.5 g/dL indicates mild depletion.

    c. 2.1 to 2.7 g/dL indicates significant depletion.

    d. <2.1 g/dL indicates severe depletion.

    e. Concentration correlates inversely with mortality.

    f. May not respond to rapid changes in nutritional status due to long half-life (2 to 3 weeks)

    g. Affected by other factors (e.g., renal loss in nephrosis, decreased synthesis in cirrhosis, marked transcapillary shifting in some disease states)

  2. Pre-albumin

    a. Sensitive indicator of short-term protein–calorie deficiency due to short (~2 day) half-life

    b. 10 to 15 mg/dL indicates mild malnutrition.

    c. 5 to 9 mg/dL indicates moderate malnutrition.

    d. <5 mg/dL indicates severe malnutrition.

    e. Responds within 3 days to refeeding

    f. Decreased in liver disease, cystic fibrosis, hyperthyroidism, and inflammation

  3. Transferrin

    a. A circulating β_2-globulin that reflects visceral protein stores

    b. Has a shorter half-life (4 to 10 days) than albumin

    c. 150 to 200 mg/dL indicates mild depletion.

    d. 100 to 150 mg/dL indicates moderate depletion.

    e. <100 mg/dL indicates severe depletion.

f. Level can be estimated from total iron-binding capacity if direct assay is unavailable, but each laboratory should develop its own regression formula for this estimate.

g. Other factors can result in increased transferrin (e.g., iron deficiency, pregnancy, exogenous estrogens).

4. Retinol-binding protein

a. Sensitive indicator of short-term protein deficiency due to short (10 to 12 hours) half-life

b. Normal plasma level: 3 to 6 mg/dL; less than 2.6 mg/dL indicates protein–calorie malnutrition

c. Responds within 3 days to refeeding

d. Altered in liver disease, renal failure, cystic fibrosis, hyperthyroidism, and inflammation

B. Nitrogen balance study

1. Assesses protein turnover

2. 1 g of nitrogen is equivalent to 30 g of lean tissue.

3. 1 g of average dietary protein contains 6.25 g of nitrogen.

4. Balance is calculated as: dietary nitrogen intake − urinary nitrogen excretion − stool nitrogen excretion − skin nitrogen loss − ΔBUN

a. All terms are in grams per day.

b. Dietary nitrogen intake (g/day) is calculated from dietary protein intake (g/day) by: nitrogen intake = protein intake / 6.25

c. Urinary nitrogen (UUN)

(1) Obtained from a 24-hour urine collection for urine urea nitrogen concentration and urinary volume

(2) UUN (g/day) can be derived from urinary urea (g/day) by: urinary urea/2.14

d. Combined stool and skin losses can be estimated as 4 g/day (can be higher in severe diarrhea).

e. ΔBUN term stands for the increase in nitrogen accumulation in body fluids.

(1) Applicable in patients with renal dysfunction and significant rises in BUN

(2) Determined from serum urea nitrogen (BUN, mg/dL) immediately before (pre) and after (post) 24-hour urine collection for balance study, and estimated total body water

(3) Calculated as: $(BUN_{post} - BUN_{pre}) \times (F \times Wt)$, where Wt is body weight (kg) and F is the estimated proportion of body weight that is water (0.6 for men, 0.55 for women)

f. Goal is positive balance of 2 g/day.

C. Creatinine–height index

1. Expressed as a percentage and calculated as:

$$\frac{100 \times \text{measured creatinine production}}{\text{expected creatinine production}}$$

2. Measured creatinine production is assessed in mg/day from a 24-hour urine collection.

3. Expected creatinine production is determined as

a. 23 mg/kg IBW per day for men

b. 18 mg/kg IBW per day for women

4. 61% to 80% indicates mild protein malnutrition.

5. 40% to 60% indicates moderate protein malnutrition.

6. <40% indicates severe protein malnutrition.

7. Invalid if significant renal dysfunction

D. Catabolic index

1. Calculated as: UUN − (0.08 × protein intake) − 3

2. UUN and protein intake are in grams per day.

3. Interpretation

a. ≤0: no catabolic stress

b. 0 to 5: moderate catabolic stress

c. >5: severe catabolic stress

E. Tests of immunologic function

1. Total (absolute) lymphocyte count

a. 1,201 to 1,800 cells/mm^3 associated with mild malnutrition

b. 900 to 1,200 cells/mm^3 associated with moderate malnutrition, and predicts higher complication and mortality rates

c. <900 cells/mm^3 associated with severe malnutrition

d. Drawback: stress and infection can independently alter circulating white blood cell counts

2. Delayed cutaneous hypersensitivity

a. Test for cutaneous reaction to intradermal injection of several common antigens (e.g., *Candida,* mumps, tetanus toxoid, streptokinase/streptodornase)

b. Anergy is correlated with malnutrition, susceptibility to sepsis, and mortality.

c. More than 5 mm induration indicates normal reaction and intact cellular immunity.

d. Indurations of 5 mm or less suggests malnutrition.

e. Stress, infection, and immunosuppression can also cause anergy.

F. Other serum biochemical tests

1. Electrolyte concentrations: assess for deficiencies of K, Ca, Mg, P
2. Vitamin levels
   a. Vitamin B_{12}: consider if circulating macrocytic erythrocytes detected
   b. Folate: consider if circulating macrocytic erythrocytes detected
   c. Other vitamins: not routinely assessed
3. Iron: consider measurement (serum iron, total iron-binding capacity, ferritin) if microcytic, hypochromic erythrocyte indices or anemia present
4. Trace elements: not routinely assessed

Key Laboratory Tests

- Serum electrolyte, urea nitrogen, and creatinine concentrations
- Serum albumin concentration
- Serum pre-albumin or transferrin concentration
- Total lymphocyte count
- Nitrogen balance study (requires 24-hour urine for urea nitrogen)

Other Tests

A. Reverse Fick method of EE determination
   1. EE (kcal /day) = VO_2 × 6.8 (fasting) or VO_2 × 7.1 (postprandial)
   2. Where VO_2 (mL/min) = cardiac output × $(CaO_2 - C\bar{v}O_2)$ × 10
   3. Cardiac output (L/min) is commonly determined by the thermodilution method.
   4. CaO_2 and $C\bar{v}O_2$ (mL/dL) determined from hemoglobin, arterial and mixed venous blood gas, and oximetry analysis (see Chapter 216, Monitoring Oxygen Transport)
   5. Limitation
      a. Requires pulmonary artery catheterization
      b. Result may not be representative of average EE throughout the day.
B. Energy expenditure determination by indirect calorimetry using expired gas analysis
   1. Derives EE from measurement of systemic oxygen consumption (VO_2) and carbon dioxide production (VCO_2).

2. Calculated using the Weir equation:
   a. EE = 5.67 × VO_2 + 1.60 × VCO_2 − 2.17 UUN
   b. Where EE is in kcal/day, and VO_2 and VCO_2 are in mL/min, and UUN is in g/day
3. Limitations
   a. Time consuming, labor intensive, requires special equipment
   b. Result may not be representative of average EE throughout the day.
   c. Accuracy is impaired when using high levels of FIO_2 due to limitations of on-line expired gas analyzers.

Key Monitoring

Daily (initially, at least)	Weekly
Measure body weight.	Review calorie and protein intake.
Assess fluid intake and output.	Perform indirect calorimetry.
Assay serum Na, K, Cl, Ca, Mg, P.	Perform nitrogen balance.
Assay serum total CO_2 content.	Assay serum pre-albumin or transferrin level.
Assay blood glucose concentration.	Assay serum triglyceride concentration.

Bibliography

Christman JW, McCain RW. A sensible approach to the nutritional support of mechanically ventilated patients. Intensive Care Med 1993;19:129–136.
Detsky AS, Smalley PS, Chang J. Is this patient malnourished? JAMA 1994;271:54–58.
Elia M. Assessment of nutritional status and body composition. In: Rombeau JL, Rolandelli RH (eds). Clinical Nutrition: Enteral and Tube Feeding, 3rd ed. Philadelphia: WB Saunders, 1997; pp 155–173.
Ireton-Jones CS, Turner Jr WW, Liepa GU, et al. Equations for the estimation of energy expenditures in patients with burns with special reference to ventilatory status. J Burn Care Rehabil 1992;13:330–333.
Lang CH, Abumrad NN (eds). Nutrition in the critically ill patient. Crit Care Clin 1995;11(3):569–790.
Manning EMC, Shenkin A. Nutrition assessment in the critically ill. Crit Care Clin 1995;11:603–634.

214 Hemodynamic Monitoring

James A. Kruse

This chapter summarizes measured and derived hemodynamic variables, methods of their determination, their normal ranges in resting adults, and key interpretations.

Hemodynamic Pressures

A. Mean arterial pressure (MAP)
1. The average blood pressure in systemic arteries
2. Determined by
   a. Indwelling arterial catheterization and electronic pressure transduction (highly accurate)
   b. In the absence of an indwelling arterial catheter it may be estimated from systolic (BP_s) and diastolic (BP_d) systemic arterial pressures by either of the following formulas.

   $$(1) \quad MAP = BP_d + \frac{BP_s - BP_d}{3}$$

   $$(2) \quad MAP = \frac{1}{3} \times BP_s + \frac{2}{3} \times BP_d$$

3. Normal range: 85 to 100 mm Hg
4. Abnormal values define hypotension and hypertension.
5. Acceptable range in a given patient is heavily dependent on the patient's chronic baseline range.

B. Systemic pulse pressure
1. Pressure responsible for force of palpable arterial pulsations
2. Equal to $BP_s - BP_d$
3. Normal range: 30 to 60 mm Hg
4. Increased in hyperdynamic states: e.g., sepsis, thyrotoxicosis, aortic insufficiency
5. Decreased in dilated cardiomyopathy, most forms of circulatory shock, other hypodynamic states, myxedema coma, cardiac tamponade

C. Mean systolic pressure (MSP)
1. The average arterial blood pressure during systole
2. Estimated by:

   $$MSP = BP_d + \frac{2}{3} \times (BP_s - BP_d)$$

3. Normal range: 95 to 125 mm Hg
4. Used to calculate left ventricular stroke work index (see below)

D. Central venous pressure (CVP)
1. Intraluminal pressure within proximal great veins of chest
2. Normal range: 1 to 7 mm Hg
3. Equivalent to right atrial pressure
4. Measured by central venous catheterization and manometry or electronic pressure transduction
5. Employed clinically to estimate right ventricular (RV) preload and relative intravascular volume
6. Increased in RV failure, tricuspid stenosis, tricuspid insufficiency, excessive intravascular volume, restrictive cardiomyopathy, constrictive pericarditis, pericardial tamponade
7. Decreased in absolute or relative hypovolemia

E. Right ventricular pressure
1. Intracavitary pressure within RV
2. Measured during pulmonary artery catheterization
3. Systolic RV pressure
   a. Normal range: 15 to 30 mm Hg
   b. Increased in pulmonary embolism and other causes of pulmonary hypertension
   c. Decreased in most forms of circulatory shock
4. Diastolic RV pressure
   a. Normal range: 1 to 7 mm Hg
   b. Increased in intravascular fluid overload, RV failure, cardiac tamponade, tricuspid or pulmonic insufficiency, restrictive cardiomyopathy, constrictive pericarditis
   c. Decreased in tricuspid stenosis, hypovolemia, most forms of circulatory shock

F. Pulmonary artery (PA) pressure
1. Intraluminal pressure within proximal PA
2. Normal range:
   a. Systolic PA pressure (PA_s): 15 to 30 mm Hg
   b. Diastolic PA pressure (PA_d): 5 to 13 mm Hg
   c. Mean PA pressure (MPA): 9 to 18 mm Hg
3. Increased values define pulmonary hypertension.
4. Low values seen in most forms of circulatory shock

G. Pulmonary artery occlusion pressure (PAOP)

1. Pressure measured at end-expiration from the tip of a flow-directed PA catheter when the balloon is inflated within and occluding the PA

2. Normal range: 4 to 12 mm Hg

3. Employed clinically to estimate left ventricular (LV) preload (i.e., LV end-diastolic pressure and volume), pulmonary capillary pressure, and relative intravascular volume

4. Usually 1 to 4 mm Hg lower than PA diastolic pressure, in the absence of pulmonary hypertension

5. Increased in LV failure, cardiogenic pulmonary edema, mitral stenosis or insufficiency, cardiac tamponade, fluid overload, decreased LV compliance and (spuriously) in West zone I or II conditions, and use of PEEP

6. Decreased in hypovolemia and increased LV compliance

Measures of Cardiac Function

A. Cardiac output (CO)

1. Volume of blood pumped by the heart into the systemic circulation each minute

2. Methods of determination

a. Thermodilution:

$$\frac{60 \times V_i \times C_i \times S_i \times K_{cal} \times K_{cor} \times (T_b - T_i)}{C_b \times S_b \times \int_0^t \Delta Tb(t)dt}$$

where

(1) V_i = injectate volume (mL)

(2) C_i and C_b = specific heat of injectate and blood (cal/g per °C), respectively

(3) S_i and S_b = specific gravity of injectate and blood, respectively

(4) K_{cal} = calibration constant

(5) K_{cor} = temperature loss correction constant

(6) T_b and T_i = baseline blood temperature and injectate temperature (°C), respectively

(7) Integral term = area under thermodilution curve (t = time)

b. Fick method:

$$CO = \frac{Vo_2}{10 \times a\bar{v}Do_2}$$

where $a\bar{v}Do_2$ obtained from arterial and mixed venous blood analysis and Vo_2 obtained by expired gas analysis (see Chapter 216, Monitoring Oxygen Transport)

c. Indocyanine green dye dilution method

d. Esophageal Doppler

e. CO_2 rebreathing method

f. Thoracic electrical impedance cardiography

3. Normal range: 4.5 to 6.0 L/minute

4. Determinants

a. Heart rate

b. Preload

c. Afterload

d. Contractility

B. Cardiac index (CI)

1. Normalizes cardiac output to body surface area (BSA)

2. Body surface area (m²) may be estimated by

$$BSA = 0.007184 \times Wt^{0.425} \times Ht^{0.725}$$

where Wt = weight (kg) and Ht = height (cm)

3. CI = CO/BSA; preferred over CO

4. Normal range: 2.6 to 4.0 L/minute per m²

5. Increased in hyperdynamic states; e.g., sepsis and other systemic inflammatory conditions, advanced hepatic disease, beriberi, thyrotoxicosis, pregnancy, exercise, fluid overload (in the absence of heart disease), inotropic pharmacotherapy, arteriovenous fistula

6. Decreased in most forms of cardiac failure, circulatory shock (except for some forms of septic shock), severe valvular heart disease, pulmonary embolism, cardiac tamponade

C. Stroke volume (SV)

1. Volume of blood ejected by cardiac ventricle with each heart beat

2. Normalizes cardiac output for heart rate

3. SV = 100 × CO/heart rate

4. Normal range: 60 to 85 mL

5. Reflects combined effects of preload, afterload, and contractility

D. Stroke index (SI)

1. SI = SV/BSA

2. Normal range: 35 to 50 mL/m²

3. Normalizes SV to body size

E. Left ventricular stroke work index (LVSWI)

1. LVSWI = 0.0136 × SI × (MSP − PAOP)

2. Normal range: 40 to 60 g·m/m²

3. A measure of physical work performed by the LV

4. Employed clinically as an indicator of overall LV function (cardiac output normalized for patient's body size, heart rate, and LV afterload)

Key Interpretations*

	MAP	CI	CVP	MPA	PAOP	SVRI	PVRI	RVEF	RVEDI
• Left ventricular failure	V	↓	N-↑	↑	↑	↑	↑	N	N
• Cardiogenic shock	↓	↓	↑	V	↑	↑	↑	↓	↑
• Massive pulmonary embolism	↓	↓	↑	↑	N	↑	↑	↓	↑
• Cor pulmonale	N	N-↓	↑	↑	N	N	↑	↓	↑
• Pericardial tamponade	↓	↓	↑	↑	↑	↑	↑	↓	↓
• Sepsis or septic shock	N-↓	↑	V	↑	V	↓	↑	↓	↑

*MAP = mean arterial pressure, CI = cardiac index, CVP = central venous pressure, MPA = mean pulmonary artery pressure, PAOP = pulmonary artery occlusion pressure, SVRI = systematic vascular resistance index, PVRI = pulmonary vascular resistance index, RVEF = right ventricular ejection fraction, RVEDI = right ventricular end-diastolic volume index, N = typically normal, ↓ = typically decreased, ↑ = typically increased, V = variable.

F. Right ventricular stroke work index (RVSWI)

1. A measure of physical work performed by RV

2. $RVSWI = 0.0136 \times SI \times [PA_d + \frac{2}{3}(PA_s - PA_d) - CVP]$

3. Normal range: 5 to 10 g·m/m²

4. Increased in pulmonary hypertension and hyperdynamic states

5. Decreased in hypotension and hypodynamic states

G. RV ejection fraction (RVEF)

1. An overall measure of RV function; also used as an indicator of RV contractility

2. Normal range: 0.45 to 0.60

3. Determined by thermodilution, echocardiography, or nuclear techniques

4. Increased in some hyperdynamic states

5. Decreased in pulmonary embolism, RV myocardial infarction, severe acute or chronic lung disease, global myocardial dysfunction

H. Right ventricular end-diastolic volume index (RVEDVI)

1. A direct measure of RV preload, normalized to body size

2. Estimated by

a. Echocardiography, by extrapolated planimetry

b. Thermodilution, by $RVEDVI = SI/RVEF$

3. Normal range: 70 to 120 mL/m²

4. Increased in RV failure, fluid overload, tricuspid or pulmonic insufficiency

5. Decreased in absolute or relative hypovolemia

Hemodynamic Resistances

A. Systemic vascular resistance (SVR)

1. Used to estimate the following

a. The overall degree of vasoconstriction or vasodilation of the systemic vasculature

b. Left ventricular afterload

c. Systemic vascular impedance

2. $SVR = 79.9 \times \dfrac{MAP - CVP}{CO}$

3. Normal range: 900 to 1400 dyne·sec/cm⁵

B. Systemic vascular resistance index (SVRI)

1. SVR normalized to body size; SVRI preferred over SVR

2. $SVRI = SVR \times BSA$

3. Normal range: 1600 to 2400 dyne·sec·m²/cm⁵

4. Increased in hypovolemia, low output states (including hypovolemic shock and cardiogenic shock), vasopressor administration

5. Decreased in most forms of sepsis and septic shock, neurogenic shock, advanced liver disease, arteriovenous fistula, vasodilator administration

C. Pulmonary vascular resistance (PVR)
1. Used to estimate the following
   a. The overall degree of vasoconstriction or vasodilation of the pulmonary vasculature
   b. Right ventricular afterload
   c. Pulmonary vascular impedance
2. $PVR = 79.9 \times \dfrac{MPA - PAOP}{CO}$
3. Normal range: 30 to 150 $dyne \cdot sec/cm^5$

D. Pulmonary vascular resistance index (PVRI)
1. Pulmonary vascular resistance normalized to body size; PVRI is preferred over PVR
2. $PVRI = PVR \times BSA$
3. Normal range: 50 to 270 $dyne \cdot sec \cdot m^2/cm^5$
4. Increased in acute lung injury, some types of chronic lung disease, hypoxemia of any etiology, other causes of pulmonary hypertension (including LV failure, mitral valve disease, pulmonary embolism, post–lung resection surgery, and primary pulmonary hypertension) and vasoconstrictor administration
5. Decreased in systemic vasodilator or inhaled nitric oxide administration

Bibliography

Ahrens TS, Taylor LA. Hemodynamic Waveform Analysis. Philadelphia: WB Saunders, 1992.

Clark VL, Kruse JA, Carlson RW. Altered cardiac physiology. In: Cerra FB, Abrams JH (eds). Essentials of Surgical Critical Care. St. Louis: Quality Medical Publishing, 1993, pp 220–231.

Daily EK, Schroeder JS. Techniques in Bedside Hemodynamic Monitoring, 5th ed. St. Louis: Mosby, 1994.

Kern MJ. Hemodynamic Rounds, 2nd ed. New York: Wiley-Liss, 1999.

Kruse JA, Armendariz E. Hemodynamic monitoring. In: Carlson RW, Geheb MA (eds). Principles & Practice of Medical Intensive Care. Philadelphia: WB Saunders, 1993, pp 1079–1103.

Vyskocil J, Kruse J. Hemodynamics and oxygen transport. J Crit Illness 1994;9:447–459.

215 Fast Flush Test

James A. Kruse

Fluid-filled catheter-transducer systems are employed commonly in the intensive care unit to assess intravascular and intracardiac pressures, including central venous, systemic arterial, and pulmonary arterial pressures. To ensure accurate measurements, the operator should be familiar with the particular equipment used and methods for calibrating these systems and evaluating their dynamic response at the bedside. Accurate systolic arterial pressure measurement by these methods is dependent on an adequate dynamic response. Diastolic pressure accuracy is less dependent, and mean arterial pressure (MAP) is immune from these effects. Mean central venous pressure (CVP) measurement is similarly immune; however, inaccurate CVP waveform appearance can result from poor dynamic response. This chapter reviews the proper system configuration for intravascular pressure monitoring using indwelling central venous or arterial catheters, and a bedside method of rapidly evaluating the system's dynamic response using the "fast flush test."

System Configuration

A. Ensure proper fluid-filled connection between catheter and transducer (Fig. 215–1).
   1. Low-compliance tubing must be used.
   2. Length of connecting tubing should not be unnecessarily long.
   3. A zeroing stopcock must be included.
      a. In a typical configuration the zeroing stopcock is mounted directly above the transducer, as shown.
      b. Connections to stopcocks should avoid right-angle path for pressure transmission during monitoring.
      c. Minimize the number of stopcocks and connections between catheter and transducer.
   4. Transducer, stopcocks, and connecting tubing must be filled with sterile saline before connecting to the catheter.
   5. All air bubbles must be flushed from connection tubing, stopcock(s), and transducer (caution: do not allow bubbles to enter catheter or patient).
   6. Ensure that any stopcocks are set to the correct position.
      a. Never allow an open path between the catheter lumen and the atmosphere, lest bleeding or air embolism result.
      b. Ensure a continuous unobstructed fluid path between transducer and catheter lumen during monitoring.
   7. Ensure that all stopcock hubs are either connected to tubing or capped.

B. Ensure that flush device is connected to system (Fig. 215–1).
   1. Device has a flow resistor that allows continuous slow flushing of the system.
   2. Device also allows intermittent high flow flushing when integral valve is manually actuated.
   3. The flush device is located between transducer and source of pressurized sterile flush solution.
   4. In vertical configurations, the flush device should be located below the level of the transducer, and a zeroing stopcock should be located above the level of transducer to facilitate removal of air bubbles from transducer.

C. Ensure that the flush source is connected to the system.
   1. Sterile normal saline contained in standard plastic IV bag is used as flush source.
   2. Intravenous bag must be placed within pressure cuff and inflated to well above patient's systolic pressure (typically 300 mm Hg), as indicated on pressure gauge.

D. Ensure that coupling electrical cable tightly mates to connections on the transducer and the monitor.

E. Test fluid and electrical portions of the system for proper configuration before connecting to the catheter.
   1. Ensure that the electronic monitor displays a flatline waveform and near-zero pressure.
   2. Flush the system to ensure that it is filled with fluid and to remove any remaining air bubbles.
   3. Shake the fluid-filled connecting tube and visualize an oscillating waveform on display to be sure that pressure transduction is taking place.
   4. Connect to catheter and observe appropriate waveform.
   5. May need to adjust display scale on monitor (e.g., 0 to 30 mm Hg range for CVP, or 0 to 300 mm Hg range for systemic arterial pressure)

F. Level system.
   1. Position the patient supine and determine the

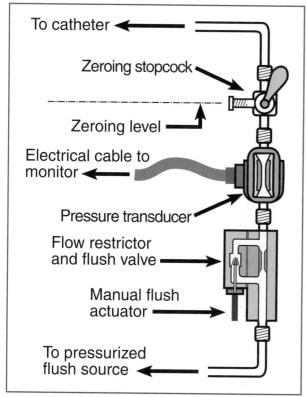

Figure 215-1 Typical vertical-arrangement configuration of pressure transducer, zeroing stopcock, flush device, and fluid-filled connection tubing. Stopcock position shown (closed to patient) allows zeroing of electronic monitor or flushing of residual air bubbles from transducer. In the normal monitoring position stopcock would be adjusted so it is closed to the atmosphere and allows a straight-through path from indwelling catheter to transducer. Midaxillary line of supine patient should be vertically aligned to level of dashed line.

reference level: mid-axillary line at fourth intercostal space

2. Level the air–fluid interface of the zeroing stopcock with the reference point on the patient.

3. If transducer and stopcock are mounted to IV pole, use a carpenter's level to ensure true horizontal alignment.

G. Zero system.

1. Adjust the stopcock valve so that the patient side is closed and the transducer side is open to the atmosphere.

2. Set the electronic monitor to register zero pressure.

   a. Analogous to taring a balance or scale

   b. Actual zeroing method depends on particular monitor.

3. Return stopcock valve to monitoring position.

Key Monitoring Points

- Level the system by aligning the air–fluid interface of the zeroing stopcock hub to level of supine patient's mid-chest.

- Zero the system by opening the zeroing stopcock to expose the transducer lumen to the atmosphere; then set the electronic monitor to zero.

- Perform the fast flush test to assess dynamic response.

- Maximize f_n (one period of oscillation completed in less than 2 mm) and optimize damping (amplitude ratio 0.1 to 0.5).

Fast Flush Test Procedure

A. Use the flush device to manually flush the system for approximately 0.5 to 1 second to raise the displayed pressure to that of the pressurized flush source.

B. Abruptly discontinue flushing and observe the waveform on the monitor.

C. A square wave will appear, terminated by a brief period of damped oscillation (Fig. 215-2).

D. Assess the resonant frequency (f_n) and damping characteristics of system.

   1. Quantitative approach

      a. Estimate f_n

         (1) Calculate reciprocal of oscillation period (peak-to-peak interval).

         (2) Read the waveform period (τ, in seconds) off the strip chart recording of pressure during the fast-flush test; e.g., if $\tau = 0.06$ s, then $f_n = 1 \div 0.06$ or ~17 Hz.

         (3) If using 25 mm/s recording speed, can alternatively calculate as $f_n = 25$ mm/s $\div$ distance (in mm) between oscillation peaks; e.g., if period is 1.5 mm, then $f_n = 25$ mm/s $\div 1.5$ mm ≈ 17 Hz

         (4) For accurate dynamic pressure measurements f_n should ideally be at least 25 Hz; values greater than 8 Hz may be acceptable if damping is optimized; values lower than 8 Hz are unacceptable.

      b. Estimate damping characteristics using ratio of waveform amplitude deviation over two successive deflections (A1 and A2) on fast-flush testing.

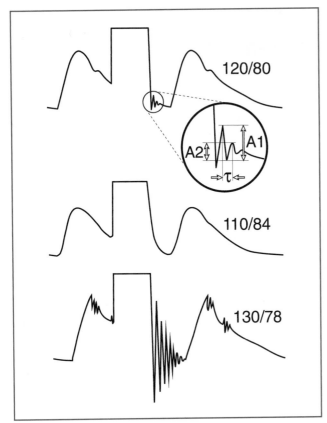

Figure 215-2 Pressure-time waveforms during fast-flush testing of dynamic response of arterial pressure monitoring systems. *Top:* optimal dynamic response showing true intra-arterial blood pressure. *Middle:* overdamped system showing spuriously low systolic pressure. *Bottom:* hyperresonant, underdamped system showing spuriously elevated systolic pressure. *Inset:* method of determining amplitude ratio (A2 ÷ A1) and resonant waveform period (τ). A1 and A2 = successive amplitudes.

(1) Ratio between 0.1 to 0.25 is adequate if f_n is greater than 10 Hz.

(2) Ratio between 0.05 to 0.35 is adequate if f_n is greater than 15 Hz

(3) Ratio below 0.5 is adequate if f_n is greater than 20 Hz.

(4) Ratio below 0.7 is adequate if f_n is greater than 25 Hz.

2. Qualitative approach

   a. Lack of oscillation indicates overdamping or low resonant frequency (Fig. 215-2, middle) and results in a spuriously lowered systolic pressure measurement.

   b. Ringing (excessive oscillation) indicates underdamping or low resonant frequency (Fig. 215-2, bottom) and results in a spuriously elevated systolic pressure measurement.

E. Correct the configuration problem of the fluid-filled portion of the system until an acceptable pattern (Fig. 215-2, top) is observed.

1. Causes of overdamping (amplitude ratio too low)

   a. Large air bubbles in transducer, stopcock(s), connection tubing, or catheter

   b. Kinking of catheter or connection tubing

   c. Blood clots or fibrin within catheter or tubing

   d. High-compliance connection tubing (e.g., regular IV tubing)

   e. Excessively long connection tubing

   f. Poorly fitting connections

   g. Small-bore catheters

   h. Inadequate pressure bag inflation

2. Causes of underdamping (amplitude ratio too high)

   a. Tiny air bubbles in transducer, stopcock(s), connection tubing, or catheter

   b. Large-bore catheters

   c. Excessive number of stopcocks or connections

   d. Short connecting tubing

3. Causes of low resonant frequency

   a. Air bubbles in transducer, stopcock(s), connection tubing, or catheter

   b. Excessively long connection tubing (1 meter or longer)

   c. Small-diameter tubing or catheter

   d. Increased system compliance

   e. Excessive numbers of stopcocks, connections, injection ports, etc.

PEARL

Target the titration of vasoactive drug infusions to MAP, which is unaffected by the monitoring system's dynamic response, rather than systolic pressure.

 Bibliography

Fessler HE, Shade D. Measurement of vascular pressure. In: Tobin MJ (ed). Principles and Practice of Intensive Care Monitoring. New York: McGraw-Hill, 1998, pp 91–106.

Gardner RM. Accuracy and reliability of disposable pressure transducers coupled with modern pressure monitors. Crit Care Med 1996;24:879–882.

Kleinman B, Frey K, Stevens R. The fast flush test—is the clinical comparison equivalent to its in vitro simulation? J Clin Monitoring 1998;14:485–489.

Kleinman B, Powell S, Gardner RM. Equivalence of fast flush and square wave testing of blood pressure monitoring systems. J Clin Monitoring 1996;12:149–154.

216 Monitoring Oxygen Transport

Jorge A. Guzman

The delivery and utilization of oxygen by systemic tissues requires integration of the respiratory, cardiovascular, and microvascular systems. Inadequate tissue oxygenation is relatively common in critically ill patients and reversal of tissue hypoxia remains a fundamental goal of resuscitation. Therefore, monitoring oxygen transport and utilization is potentially important for prevention and reversal of tissue hypoxia.

Indications for Oxygen Transport Monitoring

A. Circulatory shock of any etiology: e.g., cardiogenic or hypovolemic shock
B. Markedly decreased cardiac output: e.g., severe left ventricular dysfunction
C. Microcirculatory dysfunction: e.g., septic shock
D. States of high metabolic demand: e.g., sepsis, thyroid storm, severe burn injury
E. Severe anemia with concomitant critical illness or cardiopulmonary dysfunction
F. Severe hypoxemia: e.g., acute respiratory distress syndrome (ARDS) and respiratory insufficiency
G. Critically ill patients who have other indications for hemodynamic monitoring

Basic Measurements and Calculations

A. Arterial oxygen content (CaO_2)
1. The volume of oxygen (mL) contained in each deciliter of systemic arterial blood
    a. Includes oxygen bound to hemoglobin within erythrocytes
    b. Also includes oxygen physically dissolved in plasma, although this generally accounts for a nearly negligible fraction of the oxygen content
2. $CaO_2 = 1.39 \times Hb \times SaO_2 + 0.0031 \times PaO_2$ where
    a. Hb is blood hemoglobin concentration (g/dL).
    b. SaO_2 is fractional arterial blood oxyhemoglobin saturation measured by CO-oximetry.
    c. PaO_2 is arterial blood oxygen tension (torr) measured by blood gas analysis.
3. Normal range: 18 to 20 mL/dL
4. Decreased in arterial hypoxemia, anemia, carbon monoxide poisoning, and methemoglobinemia
5. Increased in polycythemia, excessive erythrocyte transfusion, hyperbaric oxygen therapy

B. Mixed venous oxygen saturation ($S\bar{v}O_2$)
1. The fractional oxyhemoglobin saturation of mixed venous (i.e., pulmonary artery) blood
2. Measurement methods
    a. In vitro oximetry by analysis of mixed venous blood samples intermittently obtained by way of an indwelling pulmonary artery catheter
    b. In vivo monitoring using a special pulmonary artery catheter that allows continuous fiberoptic oximetry
3. Normal range: 0.66 to 0.74
4. Decreased in arterial hypoxemia, low cardiac output or low systemic oxygen delivery states, and conditions associated with high oxygen demand
5. Increased in states of high cardiac output and high oxygen delivery, low oxygen demand, systemic shunting, and impaired oxygen extraction capability

C. Mixed venous oxygen content ($C\bar{v}O_2$)
1. The volume of oxygen (mL) contained in each deciliter of mixed venous blood
2. $C\bar{v}O_2 = 1.39 \times Hb \times S\bar{v}O_2 + 0.0031 \times P\bar{v}O_2$, where $P\bar{v}O_2$ is mixed venous blood oxygen tension (torr) measured by blood gas analysis
3. Normal range: 13 to 16 mL/dL
4. Decreased in states of decreased arterial oxygen content, increased oxygen consumption, and decreased oxygen delivery
5. Increased in states of high cardiac output and high oxygen delivery, low oxygen demand, systemic shunting, and decreased oxygen extraction capability

D. Arteriovenous oxygen content difference ($a\bar{v}DO_2$)
1. The volume of oxygen (mL) removed from each deciliter of arterial blood during passage through the systemic circulation
    a. Varies directly with peripheral oxygen extraction, often in response to changes in oxygen delivery
    b. Also influenced by CaO_2
2. $a\bar{v}DO_2 = CaO_2 - C\bar{v}O_2$
3. Normal range: 3.6 to 5.0 mL/dL
4. Decreased in severe sepsis, severe hepatic disease, large arteriovenous fistula, thiamine deficiency, Paget's disease, and cyanide poisoning; may also be decreased in severe anemia or hypoxemia

5. Increased in low cardiac output states and in mild to moderate anemia or hypoxemia

E. Systemic oxygen delivery (DO_2)

1. Volume of oxygen (mL) delivered to the systemic circulation each minute

    a. Commonly obtained by in vitro assays of hemoglobin, PaO_2 and SaO_2, plus thermodilution cardiac output (L/minute) measurement using a pulmonary artery catheter

    b. Varies directly with cardiac output and arterial oxygen content

2. $DO_2 = CaO_2 \times$ cardiac output $\times$ 10

3. Normal range: 900 to 1,100 mL/minute

F. Systemic oxygen delivery index (DO_2I)

1. DO_2 normalized to body surface area (BSA); preferred over DO_2

2. $DO_2I = DO_2/BSA$

3. BSA (m^2) may be estimated using commonly available nomograms or by:

$$BSA = 0.007184 \times Wt^{0.425} \times Ht^{0.725},$$

where Wt = weight (kg) and Ht = height (cm)

4. Normal range: 530 to 600 mL/minute per m^2

5. Decreased in states of low cardiac output and low arterial oxygen content

6. Increased in hyperdynamic states (e.g., sepsis, exercise, thyrotoxicosis)

G. Oxygen consumption (VO_2)

1. Volume of oxygen (mL) consumed by systemic tissues each minute

    a. Normally varies directly with systemic oxygen demand, i.e., metabolic rate

    b. VO_2 is less than systemic oxygen demand if there is oxygen supply dependency (see below).

2. Determined by

    a. Reverse Fick method

    (1) $VO_2 = 10 \times$ cardiac output $\times$ a$\bar{v}DO_2$

    (2) Requires pulmonary artery catheterization for sampling mixed venous blood and measuring cardiac output (L/minute)

    b. Expired gas analysis:

$$VO_2 = \frac{(VI \times FIO_2) - (VE \times FEO_2)}{t}$$

where

    (1) $VI = VE \times (1 - FEO_2 - FECO_2)/(1 - FIO_2 - FICO_2)$

    (2) VI and VE = inspired and expired gas volumes, respectively (mL)

    (3) t = sampling time interval (minutes)

    (4) Other terms represent inspired and expired gas fractions, determined by gas analysis

3. Normal range: 200 to 300 mL/minute

4. Normally determined by systemic oxygen demand, but can vary directly with DO_2 in circulatory shock

H. Oxygen consumption index (VO_2I)

1. VO_2 normalized to body surface area; preferred over VO_2

2. $VO_2I = VO_2/BSA$

3. Normal range: 110 to 160 mL/minute per m^2

4. Decreased in conditions associated with low oxygen demand, critically low DO_2, or severely impaired oxygen extraction

5. Increased in conditions associated with high oxygen demand or uncoupled oxidative phosphorylation

I. Oxygen extraction (O_2ex)

1. The fraction of systemically delivered oxygen that is consumed by peripheral tissues

2. Calculated by either of the following equations

    a. $O_2ex = VO_2/DO_2$

    b. $O_2ex = a\bar{v}DO_2/CaO_2$

Figure 216-1 Relationships between DO_2 versus VO_2 and O_2ex. *Solid black line* represents the physiologic relationship observed when DO_2 is independently varied, e.g., during hemorrhagic shock or imposed increases in cardiac output. *Dot* represents normal resting conditions. If DO_2 is independently varied over a wide range, VO_2 remains near constant due to compensatory changes in O_2ex (*dashed black line*). When DO_2 falls below the critical point of maximum O_2ex, VO_2 becomes dependent on DO_2, and anaerobic metabolism ensues. The slope ($\Delta VO_2/\Delta DO_2$) of the supply dependency portion of the curve corresponds to maximal O_2ex. *Gray lines* represent the DO_2 versus VO_2 (*solid*) and O_2ex (*dashed*) relationships observed in certain pathologic inflammatory conditions such as sepsis and acute respiratory distress syndrome. As DO_2 falls in these conditions, maximal O_2ex is diminished (pathologic supply-dependency).

TABLE 216–1. CHANGES IN OXYGEN TRANSPORT VARIABLES TYPICALLY OBSERVED IN VARIOUS CLINICAL CONDITIONS*

	CaO$_2$	S$\bar{v}$O$_2$	DO$_2$	VO$_2$	a$\bar{v}$DO$_2$	O$_2$ex
Heart failure	nl	↓	↓	nl	↑	↑
Cardiogenic shock	nl	↓↓	↓↓	nl	↑↑	↑
Hypovolemic shock	nl	↓↓	↓↓	↓	↑↑	↑↑
Hemorrhagic shock	nl or ↓	↓↓	↓↓	↓	↑↑	↑↑
Septic shock	nl	↓ or ↑	↓ or ↑	nl or ↓	↓ or ↑	↓ or ↑
Sepsis	nl	↑	↑	nl or ↑	↓	↓
Severe anemia	↓↓	↓↓	↓ or nl†	nl	↓	↑↑
Severe hypoxemia	↓↓	↓↓	↓ or nl†	nl	↓	↑↑

*CaO$_2$ = oxygen concentration, arterial; S$\bar{v}$O$_2$ = mixed venous oxygen saturation; DO$_2$ = systemic oxygen delivery; VO$_2$ = oxygen consumption; a$\bar{v}$DO$_2$ = arteriovenous oxygen content difference; O$_2$ex = oxygen extraction; nl = normal.
†Normal if adequate cardiac reserve.

3. Normal range: 0.22 to 0.28

4. Increased in most conditions associated with systemic hypoperfusion

5. Decreased in severe sepsis, severe hepatic disease, large arteriovenous fistula, thiamine deficiency, Paget disease, and cyanide poisoning

Relationship Between VO$_2$ and DO$_2$

A. The physiologic relationship between DO$_2$ and VO$_2$ (Fig. 216–1) is biphasic.

1. Compensation for decreased DO$_2$ occurs at the tissue level as an increase in O$_2$ex, which serves to maintain VO$_2$ to satisfy metabolic demands.

2. Critical reductions in DO$_2$, i.e., below the point of maximal O$_2$ex, lead to a decrease in VO$_2$ (supply-dependency) and partial reliance on anaerobic metabolism to meet prevailing metabolic demands.

3. Laboratory studies report critical DO$_2$ to be approximately 8 mL/kg per minute in animal models.

4. Critical DO$_2$ levels for critically ill patients are less well defined, varying with the level of underlying oxygen demand and the degree of systemic inflammation.

5. Increased arterial blood lactate concentration is generally observed when DO$_2$ falls below the critical level.

B. The VO$_2$ vs DO$_2$ relationship can be altered in patients with systemic inflammation (e.g., sepsis, ARDS, pancreatitis).

1. Oxygen extraction capabilities may be impaired, resulting in a decrease in the slope of the supply dependency portion of the VO$_2$ vs DO$_2$ relationship (so-called pathological supply dependency).

2. The plateau phase of the VO$_2$ vs DO$_2$ relationship may not be apparent; this may be due to marked increases in systemic oxygen demand unmet by prevailing oxygen availability at the tissue level.

3. VO$_2$ may be increased (due to increased oxygen demands) or decreased (due to inadequate DO$_2$ or impaired oxygen extraction).

PEARLS

- The presence of oxygen supply dependency can be a sign of tissue hypoxia and incomplete resuscitation.

- Careful interpretation of oxygen transport variables can provide important clues to the underlying disorder (Table 216–1).

- Although some clinical investigations have shown that resuscitation directed to set, supranormal end points of VO$_2$ and DO$_2$ may improve outcome, most data does not support this generalized approach.

Bibliography

Chittock DR, Ronco JJ, Russel JA. Monitoring of oxygen transport and oxygen consumption. In: Tobin MJ (ed). Principles and Practice of Intensive Care Monitoring. New York: McGraw-Hill, 1998; pp 317–343.

Gutierrez G, Arfeen QA. Oxygen transport and utilization. In: Dantzker DR, Scharf SM (eds). Cardiopulmonary Critical Care. Philadelphia: WB Saunders, 1999; pp 173–208.

Nelson D, Beyer C, Samsel R, et al. Pathologic supply dependency of systemic and intestinal O$_2$ uptake during bacteremia in dogs. J Appl Physiol 1987;63:1487–1489.

Nightingale P. Practical points in the application of oxygen transport principles. Intensive Care Med 1990;16:S173–S177.

Shumacker PT, Cain SM. The concept of critical oxygen delivery. Intensive Care Med 1987;13:223–229.

217 Capnography

Jorge A. Guzman

Definitions

A. Capnography: the measurement and graphic display of expired carbon dioxide tension (PCO_2) versus time; exhaled CO_2 is a reflection of CO_2 production (metabolism), transport (blood and circulation), and elimination (ventilation)

B. Capnograph: a device for performing capnography

C. Capnometry: the measurement and numeric display of end-tidal PCO_2 ($PetCO_2$); $PetCO_2$ is the PCO_2 at the end of exhalation

D. Capnogram: a graphic recording of expired PCO_2 versus time

Methods

A. Sampling methodology (Table 217–1)
  1. Mainstream capnography
     a. The CO_2 sensor resides within the breathing circuit close to the patient's airway.
     b. The sensor is connected by an electrical cable to a bedside analyzer.
  2. Sidestream devices
     a. Fine-bore tubing carries a gas sample from the patient to a distant CO_2 sensor and analyzer.
     b. The analyzer may be located at the bedside device or at a central location.
     c. An airway adaptor is used to attach the connecting tubing to the junction of the endotracheal tube and ventilator circuit in patients receiving mechanical ventilation.
     d. Specialized nasal prongs allow sidestream gas sampling from the nose in spontaneously breathing patients, with or without supplemental oxygen administration.
B. Analytic methodology
  1. Colorimetric capnometry
     a. Based on the color change of an indicator reagent (e.g., phenolsulfonphthalein) that occurs in the presence of CO_2 gas
     b. Used as a portable, non-electronic, single-patient-use device to differentiate endotracheal from esophageal intubation
     c. Advantages: inexpensive, easy availability, simplicity

d. Disadvantages: semiquantitative; does not allow time-based recordings

2. Mass spectroscopy
   a. Any gas bombarded with an electron beam yields characteristic ions of known mass that can be accelerated and deflected by an electromagnetic field to separate the ions according to their mass and produce an electrical current proportional to the concentration of the particular gas.
   b. Advantages: can be used to measure several gases simultaneously and can monitor several patients at once (e.g., to monitor multiple patients undergoing general anesthesia in a cluster of operating rooms)
   c. Disadvantages: long calibration times, expensive, and only practical as a sidestream device; does not provide continuous display when more than one patient is analyzed by a given instrument
3. Infrared spectroscopy
   a. CO_2 has a characteristic pattern of infrared light absorbance, maximal near a wavelength of 4.28 μm.
   b. Gas located between a focused beam of light and a photodetector results in an electronic signal that is proportional to the PCO_2 of the gas.
   c. Advantages: continuous display, rapid response, less expensive than mass spectroscopy
4. Raman spectroscopy
   a. When light strikes a gas molecule, energy is absorbed and re-emitted at the same wavelength (Rayleigh scattering); however, a small fraction of the absorbed energy is re-emitted at a different wavelength (Raman scattering).
   b. The change in wavelength and the amount of scattering are used to determine the constituents and concentration of the analyte.
   c. Can detect several gases simultaneously and can be used in operating rooms
   d. Disadvantages: although it is a clinically accepted method, it is not applied in most commercially available capnographs due to the expense, noise, and weight of the device

TABLE 217-1. ADVANTAGES AND DISADVANTAGES OF SIDESTREAM VERSUS MAINSTREAM CAPNOGRAPHS

CAPNOGRAPH	ADVANTAGES	DISADVANTAGES
Mainstream	Measurement occurs at point of interest (patient's airway)	Bulky sensor at patient's airway
	Fast response time	Not practical in non-intubated patients
	No aspiration-induced reduction of tidal volume	Secretions and condensation may block sensor
Sidestream	No bulky sensor at patient's airway	Secretions clog sample tubing
	Can be used in non-intubated patients	Water trap required and must be changed or emptied periodically
	Ability to measure gases other than CO_2	Slow response time
		Sampling may decrease tidal volume

Interpretation of the Capnogram

A. The normal capnogram (Fig. 217–1) consists of four phases.

1. Phase I: represents the beginning of exhalation, during which P_{CO_2} remains almost zero while gas from the anatomic dead space leaves the upper airway

2. Phase II: the waveform rises sharply as exiting alveolar gas mixes with dead-space gas

3. Phase III: the capnogram reaches a plateau representing gas from the alveolar space

   a. The terminal and highest portion of the plateau represents Pet_{CO_2}.

   b. The slope of phase III is determined by the ventilation/perfusion ($\dot{V}/\dot{Q}$) status of the lung.

   c. Patients with increased dead-space ventilation, e.g., those with chronic obstructive pulmonary disease, have a steeper phase III and may not reach a clear plateau.

4. Phase IV: the waveform sharply decays as inspiration begins

B. Causes of increased Pet_{CO_2}

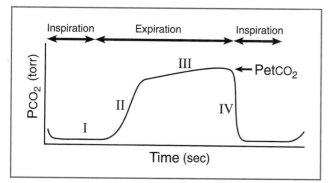

Figure 217–1 Normal pattern of expired P_{CO_2} versus time. Phase I = inspiration; phase II = beginning of expiration; phase III = alveolar plateau; phase IV = beginning of inspiration; Pet_{CO_2} = end-tidal P_{CO_2}.

1. Increased CO_2 production and delivery to the lungs
   a. Fever
   b. Sepsis
   c. Seizures
   d. Other causes of increased metabolic rate
   e. Bicarbonate administration

2. Decreased alveolar ventilation
   a. Respiratory depression
   b. Respiratory muscle weakness
   c. Other causes of hypoventilation

3. Equipment malfunction
   a. Leaks in ventilator circuit
   b. Rebreathing

C. Causes of decreased Pet_{CO_2}

1. Decreased CO_2 production and delivery to the lungs
   a. Hypothermia
   b. Other causes of decreased metabolic rate
   c. Pulmonary hypoperfusion
   d. Pulmonary embolism
   e. Cardiac arrest
   f. Hypotension
   g. Hemorrhage

2. Increased alveolar ventilation (hyperventilation)
   a. Increased minute volume
   b. Decreased dead space

3. Equipment malfunction
   a. Airway obstruction
   b. Ventilator disconnection
   c. Airway leaks (e.g., around endotracheal tube)

D. Causes of abnormal waveform patterns (Fig. 217–2)
1. Airway obstruction
2. Rebreathing
3. Recovery from neuromuscular blockade
4. Artifacts (e.g., cardiac oscillations, erratic breathing patterns)

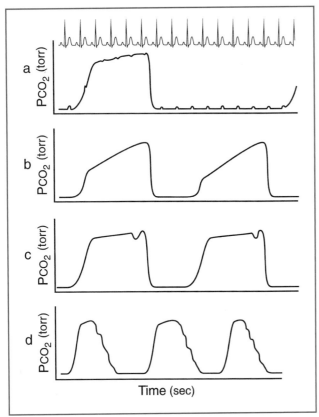

Figure 217–2 (*a*) Capnogram showing cardiac oscillations apparent during slow breathing. (*b*) Capnogram showing a slow rise in the alveolar component of the waveform, consistent with partial airway obstruction. (*c*) Capnogram characteristic of the early stage of recovery from neuromuscular blockade. (*d*) Capnogram showing incomplete alveolar plateaus as a consequence of air leakage (e.g., deflated endotracheal or tracheostomy cuff).

Clinical Applications

A. Assurance of pulmonary ventilation
   1. The most relevant indication for intensive care unit patients
   2. Monitors for the consistent presence of CO_2 in exhaled gases, thus affirming alveolar ventilation
   3. Does not assure that the endotracheal tube is correctly positioned: e.g., it may be located at the pharynx or in one of the mainstem bronchi

B. Noninvasive estimation of $PaCO_2$
   1. In healthy subjects, $PetCO_2$ is normally a few torr less than $PaCO_2$ (gradient <5 torr), but this relationship changes substantially with changes in the $\dot{V}/\dot{Q}$ relationship (increases in $\dot{V}/\dot{Q}$ are associated with decreased $PetCO_2$).
   2. Therefore, capnography is not a reliable means of estimating $PaCO_2$.

C. Detection of blood flow restoration during cardiopulmonary resuscitation (CPR)

   1. In experimental models, $PetCO_2$ monitored during CPR correlates with cardiac output, perfusion pressures, and successful resuscitation from cardiac arrest.
   2. Clinically, successfully resuscitated patients have higher $PetCO_2$ than those who cannot be resuscitated.
   3. Other factors commonly occurring during CPR can affect $PetCO_2$ independent of the effects of perfusion.
      a. Large changes in minute ventilation affect $PetCO_2$.
      b. Administration of bicarbonate increases $PetCO_2$ without necessarily changing pulmonary blood flow.
   4. Capnometry can be used as an supplemental noninvasive monitoring device during CPR, but its potential for routine use is evolving.

D. Assessment of ventilation during weaning from mechanical ventilation
   1. Changes in $PaCO_2$ do not correlate well with changes in $PetCO_2$ during weaning from mechanical ventilation.
   2. Thus, routine capnography is not currently recommended during weaning.

E. Titration of positive end-expiratory pressure (PEEP)
   1. Optimal levels of PEEP maximize alveolar recruitment and improve $\dot{V}/\dot{Q}$ matching, changes that can be reflected in lowered $PetCO_2$.
   2. However, changes in $PetCO_2$ in response to PEEP have not been clearly established; thus, capnography is not recommended for routine PEEP titration.

F. Uncommon situations specific to the operating room
   1. Because of the increased CO_2 production that occurs in this disorder, increasing $PetCO_2$ can be an early sign of malignant hyperthermia during anesthesia.
   2. $PetCO_2$ monitoring has been reported to be useful in detecting dangerous levels of arterial hypercarbia that can occur from intra-abdominal CO_2 insufflation during laparoscopic surgery.

G. Estimation of dead-space ventilation
   1. Ratio of respiratory dead space to tidal volume ratio (V_d/V_t) can be assessed by:

$$V_d/V_t = \frac{PaCO_2 - P\bar{e}CO_2}{PaCO_2}$$

   2. Where $P\bar{e}CO_2$ is mean expired PCO_2 (ideally obtained by integration under the expiratory portion of the capnogram)
   3. Dead space volume can be obtained from V_d/V_t and tidal volume (if known) by multiplication.
   4. V_d/V_t has been used as a weaning parameter, using <0.6 as the decision criterion.

PEARLS

- PetCO$_2$ is not recommended as a routine noninvasive monitor of PaCO$_2$.

- Capnometry is a helpful bedside tool to rapidly differentiate esophageal from tracheal intubation.

- PetCO$_2$ may have utility for monitoring circulatory adequacy during CPR or titration of PEEP.

Bibliography

Boysen PG. The technique of capnography. J Crit Illness 1989;4:53–59.

Falk JL, Rackow EC, Weil MH. End-tidal carbon dioxide concentration during cardiopulmonary resuscitation. N Engl J Med 1988;318:607–611.

Hess DR. Capnometry. In: Tobin MJ (ed). Principles and Practice of Intensive Care Monitoring. New York: McGraw-Hill, 1998; pp 377–400.

Rodriguez RM, Light RW. Capnography in the ICU. J Crit Illness 1998;13:372–378.

Stock MC. Capnography for adults. Crit Care Clin 1995; 11:219–232.

218 Blood Gas and Oximetry Monitoring

James A. Kruse

Indications

A. For in vitro arterial blood gas analysis and oximetry
   1. Assessment of arterial blood oxygenation and derivation of arterial oxygen content (CaO_2)
   2. Assessment of ventilation
   3. Detection, characterization, and quantification of acid-base imbalances
   4. Assessment of systemic oxygen delivery (DO_2)
   5. Detection and quantification of carboxyhemoglobin or methemoglobin

B. For in vitro mixed venous blood gas analysis and oximetry
   1. Assessment of mixed venous blood oxygenation and derivation of mixed venous blood oxygen content ($C\bar{v}O_2$)
   2. Inferring systemic perfusion (by $P\bar{v}O_2$ and $S\bar{v}O_2$)
   3. Assessment of tissue oxygen extraction (O_2ex)
   4. Measurement of venous admixture (shunt)
   5. Assessment of systemic oxygen consumption ($\dot{V}O_2$) by the Fick method

Procedure

A. Obtaining blood specimen
   1. General measures
      a. Ensure that all needed supplies are readily available, including ice for specimen transport.
      b. Don gloves and eye protection.
      c. When using liquid heparin solution to anticoagulate the syringe, ensure that heparin solution is dispersed throughout the syringe barrel and is entirely expelled, except for the heparin remaining in the dead space at the syringe tip.
   2. From radial artery using needle and syringe (see Chapter 191, Arterial Catheterization)
      a. Method is similar to initial portion of gaining access during arterial catheterization, using a heparinized syringe with 20- to 25-gauge needle.
      b. Evaluate collateral circulation using Allen test.
      c. Supinate and immobilize the patient's hand and forearm, and place a folded towel under the wrist to maintain dorsiflexion.
      d. Scrub site with suitable antiseptic.
      e. Locate radial artery pulsation 1 to 2 cm proximal to wrist crease by palpation.
      f. Puncture skin with needle at an angle 45° to 90° to the skin with the bevel directed upward.
      g. Advance needle slowly toward pulse until pulsatile arterial blood appears spontaneously in syringe; do not manually withdraw plunger of syringe.
      h. After obtaining the required volume of arterial blood, remove the needle and apply manual pressure to the site for at least 5 minutes.
      i. Femoral or brachial artery may also be used as access points using similar technique.
   3. From indwelling systemic arterial or pulmonary artery catheter with in-line 3-way stopcock
      a. Ensure that stopcock handle is adjusted so free hub is closed to system.
      b. Remove cap from free hub of stopcock, insert empty syringe onto hub, and adjust stopcock handle so free hub is open to arterial catheter (maintain sterility of stopcock hub and inner portion of removed stopcock hub cap).
      c. Aspirate all flush solution from catheter and any extension tubing, plus a sufficient volume of blood to assure that catheter, tubing, and stopcock dead space contain blood that is uncontaminated by residual flush solution.
      d. Adjust stopcock handle so that arterial catheter is closed to atmosphere and flush source.
      e. Remove and discard syringe containing aspirated fluid–blood mixture.
      f. Attach heparinized syringe to free hub of stopcock and adjust stopcock so syringe is open to artery.
      g. Allow blood to flow into sampling syringe.
      h. Adjust stopcock handle so hub with attached syringe is closed to system and catheter is open to flush source.

i. Flush catheter using the flush device (see Chapter 215, Fast Flush Test) and remove sampling syringe.

j. Adjust stopcock handle so that free hub is open to flush device and flush free hub of stopcock.

k. Replace cap onto stopcock hub (replace with new sterile cap if inner portion of old cap was contaminated).

l. Adjust stopcock handle so that catheter connects to pressure transducer.

4. From indwelling arterial catheter using in-line blood conservation device

a. Blood-conservation devices allow aspirated dead space volume blood to be reinfused.

b. Procedure varies somewhat among available devices.

B. Specimen handling

1. Within 10 seconds of obtaining sample, hold syringe vertically with tip directed upward and expel any dead space air, bubbles, or froth from syringe.

2. Immediately cap syringe tightly to ensure that sample is anaerobic.

3. Place sample syringe in ice water slush and transport to blood gas laboratory as soon as possible (sample should be analyzed within 30 minutes).

CAUTION

To avoid spurious results, blood gas analysis should be performed within 10 minutes for specimens maintained at ambient temperature, and within 30 minutes for specimens maintained in ice water.

Interpretation

A. Direct measurements of gas exchange

1. Arterial oxygen tension (PaO_2)

a. Normally greater than 90 torr breathing ambient air

b. Normal range varies with age (years) according to:

$$PaO_2 = -0.43 \times Age + 109 \pm 8$$

c. Normal range also varies with altitude.

d. Low values can occur as a result of ventilation–perfusion mismatch, intrapulmonary or right-to-left intracardiac shunting, hypoventilation, alveolar diffusion impairment, or low inspired oxygen concentration or pressure.

2. Arterial saturation (SaO_2) derived from PaO_2 or directly measured by oximetry

a. Oxyhemoglobin saturation of arterial blood

(1) Normally greater than 0.94 breathing ambient air

(2) Low values can occur for same reasons as low PaO_2, and (using CO-oximetry) due to carbon monoxide poisoning or methemoglobinemia.

b. Ideally measured by CO-oximetry

(1) An in vitro, multi-wavelength, spectrophotometric method that quantifies oxyhemoglobin (O_2Hb), deoxyhemoglobin (deoxyHb), carboxyhemoglobin (CO-Hb), and methemoglobin (metHb)

(2) Allows determination of fractional SaO_2 by

$$\text{Fractional } SaO_2 = \frac{O_2Hb}{deoxyHb + O_2Hb + CO\text{-}Hb + metHb}$$

c. Some blood gas laboratories use limited wavelength oximetry that only allows determination of functional SaO_2.

(1) Calculated as

$$\text{Functional } SaO_2 = \frac{O_2Hb}{deoxyHb + O_2Hb}$$

(2) Not valid in the face of carboxyhemoglobinemia or methemoglobinemia

d. Some blood gas laboratories do not have oximetry capabilities but may report a derived value for SaO_2.

(1) SaO_2 in this case is estimated from PaO_2 based on an assumed normal oxyhemoglobin dissociation curve.

(2) Not valid in the face of carboxyhemoglobinemia or methemoglobinemia

e. SaO_2 determined by pulse oximetry (SpO_2)

(1) Employs an optoelectronic probe typically affixed to the fingertip, toe, or pinna to estimate functional oxyhemoglobin saturation

(2) May be used as an alternative to conventional arterial blood sampling and in vitro oximetry and PaO_2 analysis

(3) Provides a simple, continuous, noninvasive, and generally reliable estimate of oxyhemoglobin saturation

(4) See also Chapter 5, Tachypnea and Hypoxemia.

3. Mixed venous oxygen tension ($P\bar{v}O_2$)

a. Oxygen tension of blood from pulmonary artery measured by in vitro gas analysis

b. Normal range is 36 to 44 torr.

c. Abnormal values interpreted as for $S\bar{v}O_2$

4. Mixed venous oxygen saturation ($S\bar{v}O_2$)

a. Oxyhemoglobin saturation of blood from pulmonary artery can be measured in vitro by transmission spectrophotometry, or in vivo by reflectance spectrophotometry using a fiberoptic pulmonary artery catheter.

b. Normal range is 0.66 to 0.74.

c. Decreased with arterial hypoxemia, low cardiac output, low DO_2, high oxygen demand and $\dot{V}O_2$

d. Increased with high cardiac output and DO_2, low oxygen demand and $\dot{V}O_2$, systemic shunting, and decreased oxygen extraction capability

5. Arterial carbon dioxide tension ($PaCO_2$)

a. Normal range is 36 to 44 torr.

b. Assesses adequacy of ventilation and assists in characterizing acid-base derangements

6. Mixed venous carbon dioxide tension ($P\bar{v}CO_2$)

a. CO_2 tension of blood from pulmonary artery

b. Normal range is 42 to 48 torr.

c. Increased with arterial hypercapnia (i.e., high $PaCO_2$) and hypoperfusion; decreased with arterial hypocapnia

7. Carboxyhemoglobin and methemoglobin saturations; see Chapter 71, Carbon Monoxide Poisoning, and Chapter 72 Methemoglobinemia

B. Derived variables

1. $PaO_2 : FIO_2$ ratio (PaO_2/FIO_2)

a. Provides an index of oxygenation normalized to the inspired oxygen fraction

b. PaO_2/FIO_2 over 400 torr is normal.

c. PaO_2/FIO_2 greater than 200 torr but less than 300 torr is often used as a criterion for acute lung injury.

d. PaO_2/FIO_2 of 200 torr or less is often used as a criterion for acute respiratory distress syndrome.

e. Advantage: simple to calculate, but threshold for normal varies somewhat with FIO_2

2. Alveolar oxygen tension (PAO_2)

a. Estimated average partial pressure of oxygen in alveolar gas

b. Calculated from simplified alveolar air equation by $PAO_2 = FIO_2 \times (P_{bar} - PH_2O) - PaCO_2/RQ$ where P_{bar} = prevailing barometric pressure, PH_2O = vapor pressure of water (47 torr at 37°C), and RQ = respiratory quotient

c. The RQ is calculated as $\dot{V}CO_2/\dot{V}O_2$ or assumed to be normal (0.8); $\dot{V}CO_2$ (CO_2 production) and $\dot{V}O_2$ can be determined by expired gas analysis.

d. Normal range: depends on FIO_2, P_{bar}, $PaCO_2$, and RQ

3. Alveolar–arterial oxygen tension gradient (A-aDO_2)

a. The average gradient of oxygen tension across the alveolar–capillary membrane, calculated as $PAO_2 - PaO_2$

b. Normally less than 20 torr while breathing ambient air near sea level

c. Increases with increasing FIO_2, intrapulmonary shunting, ventilation–perfusion mismatch

d. Remains normal in high-altitude hypoxemia and hypoxemia due entirely to hypoventilation

e. Also used to provide an index of oxygenation relative to the level of supplemental oxygen provided

f. Disadvantage: normal value varies with FIO_2, barometric pressure, body temperature, and respiratory quotient

4. Alveolar–arterial oxygen tension ratio (a/APO_2)

a. The average fraction of alveolar oxygen tension present in the pulmonary capillaries, calculated as PaO_2/PAO_2

b. Normally more than 0.90

c. Provides an index of oxygenation indexed to level of supplemental oxygen provided, and a measure of the efficiency of oxygenation

d. Advantage over A-aDO_2: normal range does not vary with FIO_2

PEARL

The FIO_2 required (newFIO_2) to achieve a desired PaO_2 (newPaO_2) can be estimated from the current a/APO_2 by the following equation:

$$\text{new}FIO_2 = \left(\frac{\text{new}PaO_2}{\text{a/}APO_2} + \frac{PaCO_2}{RQ} \right) \times \frac{1}{P_{bar} - PH_2O}$$

---

5. Arterial (CaO_2) and mixed venous ($C\bar{v}O_2$) blood oxygen content (see Chapter 216, Monitoring Oxygen Transport)

6. Pulmonary capillary oxygen content ($C\acute{c}O_2$)

a. The volume (mL) of oxygen per deciliter of pulmonary capillary blood

b. Normally: >19 mL/dL

c. Estimated by: $C\dot{c}O_2 = (1.39 \times Hb) + (0.0031 \times PaO_2)$, where Hb is blood hemoglobin concentration (g/dL)

d. Used to calculate venous admixture

7. Pulmonary venous admixture or shunt fraction ($\dot{Q}s/\dot{Q}t$)

a. The fraction of blood flow through the pulmonary vasculature that bypasses ventilated alveoli, calculated as:

$$\frac{\dot{Q}s}{\dot{Q}t} = \frac{C\dot{c}O_2 - CaO_2}{C\dot{c}O_2 - C\bar{v}O_2}$$

b. Normal range: < 0.07

c. Increased in many forms of acute lung disease (e.g., pulmonary edema and pneumonia) and with right-to-left intracardiac shunts

d. Marked elevations result in hypoxemia that is refractory to supplemental oxygen therapy.

8. Oxygen extraction (O_2ex) and oxygen consumption ($\dot{V}O_2$): see Chapter 216, Monitoring Oxygen Transport

9. Dead space to tidal volume ratio (V_d/V_t)

a. Ratio of respiratory dead space to tidal volume ratio (V_d/V_t) can be estimated using

$$V_d / V_t = \frac{PaCO_2 - P\bar{e}CO_2}{PaCO_2}$$

b. $P\bar{e}CO_2$ is mean expired PCO_2, which can be obtained by integration under the expiratory portion of the capnogram (see Chapter 217, Capnography).

c. Normal value is approximately 0.3; 0.6 has been used as a cut-off value for assessing readiness for weaning from mechanical ventilation.

d. Dead space volume (V_d) can be obtained from measurement of tidal volume (V_t) using $V_d = V_t \times V_d/V_t$

10. Alveolar ventilation ($\dot{V}_A$)

a. The effective portion of minute ventilation, normally 4 to 6 L/minute at rest

b. Estimated from systemic CO_2 production ($\dot{V}CO_2$) by

$$\dot{V}_A = 0.863 \times \dot{V}CO_2 / PaCO_2$$

c. May also be derived from V_d/V_t and minute volume ($\dot{V}_E$) using

$$\dot{V}_A = (1 - V_d/V_t) \times \dot{V}_E, \text{ where}$$
$$\dot{V}_E = V_t \times \text{respiratory rate}$$

PEARL

The $\dot{V}_E$ necessary (required $\dot{V}_E$) to yield a desired $PaCO_2$ (desired $PaCO_2$) can be estimated from the present $PaCO_2$ (current $PaCO_2$) and $\dot{V}_E$ (current $\dot{V}_E$) by the following equation:

$$_{required}\dot{V}_E = \frac{_{current}\dot{V}_E \times _{current}PaCO_2}{_{desired}PaCO_2}$$

Pitfalls

A. Pitfalls of obtaining blood specimens for blood gas analysis

1. Effect of puncturing peripheral vein instead of artery

a. Measured PO_2 and pH will be spuriously lower than actual arterial values.

b. Measured PCO_2 will be spuriously higher than $PaCO_2$.

2. Effect of not expelling excess heparin solution from sampling syringe

a. Heparin dilution will tend to spuriously decrease PCO_2.

b. Has little effect on PO_2, oxyhemoglobin saturation, or pH

3. Effect of aspirating insufficient dead space volume when obtaining sample from an indwelling arterial catheter

a. Sample will be contaminated with flush solution to a variable degree.

b. As with heparin dilution, the major effect will be a spurious decrease in PCO_2.

B. Blood gas specimen handling pitfalls

1. Effect of ambient air bubbles or froth in sample syringe

a. If patient's PO_2 exceeds room air PO_2 (typically approximately 150 torr at sea level) then the result will be spuriously lower than the true value.

b. If patient's PO_2 is less than room air PO_2 then the result will be spuriously increased.

c. Saturation values greater than 0.95 are usually not affected, but lower saturations can be spuriously affected in the same manner as PO_2.

2. Effect of delaying assay or not transporting sample on ice

a. PCO_2 will tend to be spuriously increased due to ongoing cellular metabolism by red and white blood cells.

b. PO_2 will tend to be spuriously decreased because of ongoing aerobic metabolism by white blood cells.

c. pH will tend to be spuriously decreased because of ongoing anaerobic metabolism by red blood cells.

3. Effect of extreme leukocytosis (e.g., from leukemia): spuriously low PO_2 results can occur, especially if analysis is delayed

C. Pitfalls of SaO_2 interpretation

1. Recognize that functional SaO_2 measurements and SaO_2 values derived from PaO_2 are invalid in the face of carboxyhemoglobinemia and methemoglobinemia.

2. Pitfalls of pulse oximetry

a. Detection of sudden arterial oxyhemoglobin desaturation may be delayed by approximately 1 minute when probe is placed on a toe rather than a finger or ear.

b. Unlike conventional blood gas analysis, pulse oximetry does not provide information on hypocapnia or hypercapnia or acid-base disturbances.

c. Unreliable in carbon monoxide poisoning and methemoglobinemia (see Chapters 71 and 72)

d. Signal may be unobtainable in patients with circulatory shock or suboptimal probe alignment.

PEARL

When using pulse oximetry, validate the signal quality by ensuring a typical waveform on the photoplethysmographic tracing, and check for concordance between electrocardiographic and pulse oximetry heart rate determinations.

 Bibliography

American Association of Respiratory Care. AARC clinical practice guideline: pulse oximetry. Respir Care 1991;36: 1406–1409.

Hamber EA, Bailey PL, James SW, et al. Delays in the detection of hypoxemia due to site of pulse oximetry probe placement. J Clin Anesthesia 1999;11:113–118.

Sasse SA, Jaffe MB, Chen PA, et al. Arterial oxygenation time after an FIO_2 increase in mechanically ventilated patients. Am J Respir Crit Care Med 1995;152:148–152.

Urbina LR, Kruse JA. Blood gas analysis and related techniques. In: Carlson RW, Geheb MA (eds). Principles & Practice of Medical Intensive Care. Philadelphia: WB Saunders, 1993:235–251.

219 Gastric Tonometry

Jorge A. Guzman

Gastrointestinal tonometry is a relatively noninvasive technique that measures gut intramucosal P_{CO_2} ($PiCO_2$) by allowing equilibration of CO_2 between a fluid-filled or gas-filled balloon and the gut mucosal layers. P_{CO_2} from the tonometry balloon can be assayed using a blood gas analyzer (if the sampling medium is fluid) or by infrared spectroscopy (if the sampling medium is gas). Gastric intramucosal pH (pH_i) can be derived from $PiCO_2$ using a modification of the Henderson-Hasselbalch equation. Although several gastrointestinal sites can be used to monitor intramucosal values, the stomach is most frequently chosen in the intensive care unit setting.

Physiologic Basis

A. Factors affecting tissue CO_2

1. Tissues generate CO_2 during normal oxidative metabolism at a rate reflected by the respiratory quotient.

2. CO_2 production increases during anaerobic metabolism as hydrogen ions are produced and buffered by tissue bicarbonate according to

$$H^+ + HCO_3^- \rightarrow H_2O + CO_2$$

3. CO_2 can also accumulate at the tissue level if regional perfusion slows, thereby delaying removal of CO_2 generated by the tissues (flow stagnation).

B. Gut mucosa is particularly susceptible to decreased perfusion and tissue oxygenation.

C. This vulnerability is related to anatomic features of the mucosal blood supply.

1. Right-angle branching patterns of capillaries from the supplying submucosal arterioles are responsible for a lower mucosal capillary hematocrit.

2. Countercurrent blood flow in the mucosa allows oxygen to shunt from arteriole to venule and CO_2 to recirculate at the villus tip.

D. These circulatory patterns make the splanchnic circulation a sensitive site for monitoring the adequacy of tissue perfusion since it manifests the harmful effects of decreased cardiac output and maldistribution of blood flow early in the evolution of circulatory shock.

- Detection of intestinal ischemia

- Prediction of stress ulceration

- Prediction of successful weaning from mechanical ventilation

- Outcome prediction in surgical or medical intensive care unit patients

- Assessment of adequacy of resuscitation from circulatory shock

- Intraoperative and postoperative monitoring

- As an adjunctive tool to invasive hemodynamic monitoring

Technical Considerations

A. The conventional gastric tonometry catheter is a standard vented nasogastric tube containing an extra lumen leading to a silicone balloon located near the tip (Fig. 219-1). Because the balloon membrane is highly permeable to CO_2, the P_{CO_2} of the fluid or gas inside the balloon will approximate the P_{CO_2} of the stomach lumen and surrounding mucosal tissue after allowing sufficient equilibration time.

1. Saline tonometry

a. The conventional fluid instilled into the silicone balloon is normal saline.

b. A timed equilibration period of 60 to 90 minutes is required.

c. Requires proper anaerobic handling of the aspirated sample and use of a blood gas analyzer to measure the saline P_{CO_2}

d. The technique is labor-intensive and time consuming.

e. Certain blood gas analyzers may yield spurious results (underestimation of true P_{CO_2} due to design characteristics of the instruments).

2. Gas tonometry

a. The balloon is filled with ambient air.

b. Gas in equilibrium with the surrounding mucosal P_{CO_2} is conducted past an extracor-

793

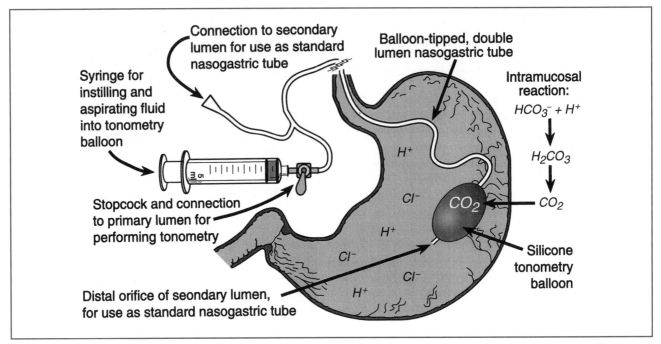

Figure 219–1 Schematic representation of a tonometry balloon lying in close proximity to the gastric mucosa. CO_2 generated as consequence of bicarbonate buffering of H^+ ions diffuses freely from the gut mucosa to the gastric lumen and from there to the lumen of the gas-filled or fluid-filled balloon.

poreal infrared sensor that allows PCO_2 reading.

c. This method eliminates sample handling and use of blood gas analyzers and provides frequent (if gas is automatically aspirated and analyzed, say, every 10 to 15 minutes) or continuous (if gas is recirculated continuously) measurements.

3. Irrespective of the technique used, pH_i can be calculated using the Henderson-Hasselbalch equation.

a. Henderson-Hasselbalch equation:

$$pH_i = 6.1 + \log\left(\frac{HCO_3^-}{0.03 \times PCO_2}\right)$$

b. Where 6.1 is the pK' of carbonic acid and 0.03 is the solubility coefficient for CO_2

c. Use of this calculation assumes that CO_2 diffuses freely in tissue, that luminal and mucosal PCO_2 are in equilibrium, and that arterial and gastric mucosal bicarbonate concentrations are identical.

d. pH_i values higher than 7.32 have been considered normal.

Procedure for Saline Tonometry

A. Prime the catheter prior to insertion.

B. Insert the catheter inside the stomach as with any nasogastric tube.

C. Instill the recommended volume of saline into the balloon.

D. Allow a timed equilibration period (20 minutes is the minimum recommended).

E. Aspirate the saline sample into a syringe, taking anaerobic handling precautions.

1. Expel gas bubbles.

2. Cap syringe.

3. Transport quickly to blood gas laboratory for stat analysis.

F. Assay sample PCO_2 using a blood gas analyzer.

G. Adjust measured PCO_2 to steady-state $PiCO_2$ using the manufacturer's correction factor according to: $PiCO_2$ = measured PCO_2 × correction factor

H. Calculate pH_i (if desired) using the Henderson-Hasselbalch equation.

Pitfalls

A. Because pH_i calculations are cumbersome and because arterial and mucosal bicarbonate concentrations have been shown to be different under some circumstances, monitoring $PiCO_2$ or the difference between $PiCO_2$ and $PaCO_2$ is commonly recommended.

B. Normal values for the PCO_2 difference range between 6 and 10 torr.

C. H_2-receptor blockade

1. Exocrine secretion of hydrogen ions by stomach parietal cells can increase luminal PCO_2 by reacting with bicarbonate ions and generating CO_2.

TABLE 219–1. POTENTIAL EXPLANATIONS FOR CHANGES IN GASTRIC INTRAMUCOSAL P_{CO_2} ($P_{I_{CO_2}}$)

	REAL	SPURIOUS
Increased $P_{I_{CO_2}}$	Reduced regional blood flow	Arterial hypercarbia
	Reduced regional tissue oxygenation	Enteral feedings
	Abnormal regional cellular energy metabolism	Low gastric pH
Decreased $P_{I_{CO_2}}$	Increased regional blood flow	Arterial hypocarbia
	Increased regional tissue oxygenation	
	Reduction in regional DO_2 with concomitant decrease in V_{CO_2}	

DO_2: oxygen delivery.
V_{CO_2}: carbon dioxide production.

2. In this case, elevated P_{CO_2}, as assessed by tonometry, will reflect this reaction rather than intramucosal acidosis (Table 219–1).

3. Use of H_2-receptor blockers minimizes release of hydrochloric acid and avoids misinterpretation of the tonometry findings.

D. Enteral feedings

1. Enteral feedings stimulate secretion of hydrogen ions, which are buffered by bicarbonate ions contained in the food or released by nonparietal gastric cells, thereby generating CO_2.

2. In this case elevated intraluminal P_{CO_2} will not reflect intramucosal acidosis and could lead to misinterpretation of tonometry results.

3. To avoid this interaction, duodenal feedings are preferred.

4. Alternatively, discontinuation of gastric feedings at least 1 hour prior to obtaining tonometric measurements is recommended.

E. Saline P_{CO_2} assay

1. Saline solution as a sampling medium induces significant biases in some blood gas analyzers.

2. Low stability of CO_2 because of low buffering capacity of saline solutions induce CO_2 loss yielding falsely low P_{CO_2} readings.

3. Low CO_2 stability can be improved with the use of phosphate-buffered solutions instead of normal saline.

4. Although the accuracy of most blood gas analyzers for P_{CO_2} assay is improved by the use of buffered solutions, the required equilibration time is longer and their routine use is not recommended.

F. Gastric suction: the use of nasogastric suction appears to have little effect on $P_{I_{CO_2}}$ and pH_i measurements.

Contraindications

A. Nasopharyngeal obstruction or maxillofacial trauma (orogastric catheter insertion is a potential option)

B. Esophageal disorders

1. Esophageal obstruction

2. Tracheoesophageal fistula

3. Large esophageal varices

C. Recent gastric hemorrhage (blood contains bicarbonate and may spuriously increase tonometric P_{CO_2})

D. Bleeding diathesis (orogastric catheter insertion is an option)

Key Points

- Gastric tonometry measures gut mucosal P_{CO_2}, a clinically useful variable that is sensitive to alterations in splanchnic perfusion and oxygenation.

- Gut intramucosal P_{CO_2} and the gradient between arterial and intramucosal P_{CO_2} are preferred monitoring variables over intramucosal pH.

- Gas tonometry provides automated measurements obviating the delays and inconveniences of the conventional saline technique.

Bibliography

Antonsson JB, Boyle III CC, Kruithoff KL, et al. Validation of tonometric measurement of gut intramural pH during endotoxemia and mesenteric occlusion in pigs. Am J Physiol 1990;259:G519–523.

Groeneveld ABJ, Kolkman JJ. Splanchnic tonometry: a review of physiology, methodology, and clinical application. J Crit Care 1994;9:198–210.

Gutierrez G, Palizas F, Doglio G, et al. Gastric intramucosal pH as a therapeutic index of tissue oxygenation in critically ill patients. Lancet 1992;339:195–199.

Guzman JA, Kruse JA. Development and validation of a technique for continuous monitoring of gastric intramucosal pH. Am J Respir Crit Care Med 1996;153:694–700.

Parviainen I, Vaisänen O, Ruokonen E. Effect of nasogastric suction and ranitidine on calculated gastric intramucosal pH. Intensive Care Med 1996;22:319–323.

Taylor DE, Gutierrez G. Tonometry. A review of clinical studies. Crit Care Clin 1996;12:1007–1029.

Temmesfeld-Wollbrück B, Szalay A, Olschewski, et al. Advantage of buffered solutions or automated capnometry in air-filled balloons for use in gastric tonometry. Intensive Care Med 1997;23:423–427.

220 Intracranial Pressure Monitoring

Daniel B. Michael

The diagnosis of elevated intracranial pressure (ICP) or intracranial hypertension, like that of arterial hypertension, may be inferred from the history and physical examination but can only be confirmed by measuring the pressure. At present the only reliable way to determine ICP is to place a pressure transmitting or sensing device (an ICP monitor) within the cranial cavity.

Indications

A. Considered in intensive care unit (ICU) patients with conditions associated with elevated ICP when frequent, accurate clinical examinations are not possible
B. Recommended for all traumatic brain injury patients in coma; i.e., Glasgow coma scale 8 or less (see Chapter 4, Coma)
C. May be withheld if the risks associated with monitoring are equal to or exceed the expected outcome of the disease
D. Use of ICP monitoring may achieve the following.
    1. Help in detecting mass lesions early
    2. Limit the indiscriminate use of therapies directed at lowering ICP, which can be harmful
    3. Reduce ICP by draining cerebrospinal fluid (CSF) and thus improving cerebral perfusion
    4. Improve outcome (however, there is no class I evidence for this)

Contraindications

A. Any condition in which the risks of ICP monitor insertion exceed the potential benefit (e.g., not indicated in cases of medical futility or comfort care only)
B. Relative contraindications
    1. Passing monitor through certain pathologic tissues (e.g., melanoma or empyema)
    2. Bleeding diathesis (correct before procedure is performed)

Procedure

A. Types of devices
    1. Ventriculostomy with external ventricular drainage device (Fig. 220–1)
        a. Historically, the first technique used; remains the preferred device
        b. Allows monitoring of ICP via fluid-filled manometer or transducer
        c. Elevated ICP can be treated by CSF drainage.
        d. Can be used to instill drugs (e.g., thrombolytic agents for intraventricular hemorrhage)
        e. Requires precise placement of catheter tip in lateral ventricle
        f. Use external auditory meatus as zero point to measure pressure.
        g. Control CSF drainage by adjusting drainage level (set chamber at 0 to 25 mm Hg above external auditory meatus; 1 mm Hg = 1.36 cm H_2O)
        h. Avoid excessive drainage of CSF: setting chamber below 0 mm (external auditory meatus) may cause a syphon effect, rupture of bridging veins, and fatal subdural hematoma
        i. Experienced nursing care is essential.
    2. Subarachnoid bolt
        a. A hollow bolt is inserted into the subarachnoid space and fluid-coupled to a transducer.
        b. Easily obstructed
        c. Does not allow CSF drainage
        d. Largely of historical interest
    3. Epidural pressure monitor
        a. A strain-gauge transducer inserted through a burr hole into the epidural space
        b. Can yield erroneous values at higher pressures
        c. Infrequently used
    4. Micro-implantable strain-gauge devices (may be placed in brain parenchyma, ventricle, or subdural space [postcraniotomy])
        a. Fiberoptic sensor
            (1) Camino catheter (NeuroCare Group, Pleasant Prairie, WI)
            (2) Subject to fracture of fiberoptic cable
        b. Piezoelectric sensor

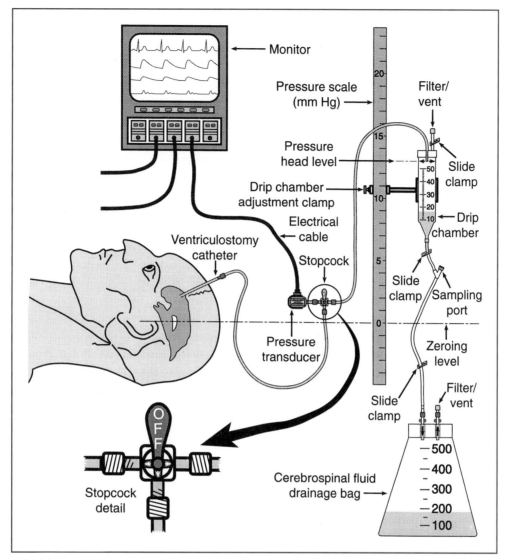

Figure 220–1 Ventriculostomy catheter in place and connected to pressure transducer, external drainage device, and electronic monitor. WIth stopcock handle turned upward, as shown, intracranial pressure (ICP) can be read electronically or by the manometer. If ICP exceeds the pressure head adjustment level, this configuration allows overflow drainage of cerebrospinal fluid and limits ICP to the set level of the pressure head (i.e., vertical distance between zero level and pressure head level, adjusted by raising or lowering drip chamber). Intracranial pressure can be monitored electronically without allowing drainage by turning the stopcock handle to the right. Turning the stopcock handle to the down position allows zeroing and calibration of the transducer. For zeroing, the drip chamber adjustment clamp is loosened and the chamber is temporarily lowered to align the pressure head level with the zero level of the scale and with the external auditory meatus. The electronic monitor is then set to read zero. With the stopcock handle in the down position, calibration can be checked by raising the pressure head level to the 20 mm Hg mark on the scale (27.2 cm H₂O) and confirming that the electronic monitor reads 20 mm Hg. (Adapted from Michael DB. *Intracranial Hypertension.* Grosse Pointe Shores, MI, Daniel B. Michael, 2000, with permission.)

(1) Codman Microsensor (Johnson & Johnson, New Brunswick, NJ)

(2) Subject to electronic drift and cannot be recalibrated

5. Combination or "hybrid" catheters (e.g., Codman Microsensor Ventricular Catheter Kit)

   a. A combination ventriculostomy catheter and piezoelectric strain gauge

   b. Has the advantage of redundant ICP monitoring

   c. Provides accurate pressure even if ventriculostomy tip placement is suboptimal

   d. May be prone to obstruction if ventriculostomy catheter and strain gauge are coaxial

   e. More expensive than simple ventriculostomy

B. Place in "silent" brain regions to minimize potential neurologic complications

   1. Ipsilateral to pathology

   2. Nondominant hemisphere (usually right side)

3. Position 1 cm anterior to the coronal suture in the midpupillary line.

C. Insertion (technique varies depending on type of monitor inserted)

1. May be performed in emergency department, ICU, or operating room with no significant differences in complication rate

2. Use aseptic technique.

3. Infiltrate scalp with local anesthetic (1% to 2% lidocaine) above galea.

4. Usual entrance site for ventriculostomy is 3 cm lateral to the midline and 1 cm anterior to the coronal suture.

5. Incise scalp, drill appropriate hole with twist drill and bit (mechanical stop device on bit is set to 0.1 to 1.5 cm to prevent accidental entry into brain).

6. Irrigate with sterile saline and place a monitoring catheter.

7. Ventriculostomy tube is inserted orthogonal to a plane tangent to the surface of the skull to a depth of 5 to 6 cm or less.

8. Tunnel the device (if appropriate).

9. Suture scalp, secure device with stay suture, and apply sterile dressing.

D. Use of antibiotics

1. No evidence that continuous use of antibiotic during course of ICP monitoring reduces infection risk

2. May consider single per-procedure antibiotic dose (e.g., 1 g cefazolin intravenously at the start of the procedure)

Postprocedure Management

A. Maintain dry sterile dressing; change carefully every 3 days or if it becomes wet or soiled.

B. Sample CSF from external ventricular drainage device for microbiological culture no more frequently than every 3 days.

C. Remove monitor as soon as ICP is normal for 24 hours without need for treatment.

1. "Wean" external ventricular drainage device by raising drainage chamber to 20 to 25 mm Hg.

2. Clamp when CSF drainage is less than 20 to 60 mL/day.

3. Remove after clamped for 24 hours without any change in neurologic examination.

Key Complications

- Malposition of monitoring device
- Obstruction of ventriculostomy
- Hemorrhage (0.9% to 3.3%)
- Infection (0 to 22%)
- Death (0.002%)

Interpretation

A. Record initial and hourly ICP readings.

1. Normal: 0 to 15 mm Hg (0 to 20 cm H_2O)

2. Treat if higher than 20 mm Hg.

3. Pressures lower than 0 mm Hg may be seen in postsurgical or open head injury cases.

4. Intracranial pressure data must be interpreted in the context of the patient's clinical condition and other relevant findings; e.g., an abrupt drop in ICP in a patient with severe traumatic brain injury may indicate brain death.

B. Waveform characteristics

1. Normal waveform

a. Percussion, tidal wave, and dicrotic waves

(1) Occur at the same frequency as the heart rate

(2) Correspond to transmitted arterial blood pressure fluctuations (see Fig. 220–2)

(3) Tall, peaked waves indicate patient is moving toward the right on the elastance curve (see Fig. 84–1).

b. Respiratory fluctuations

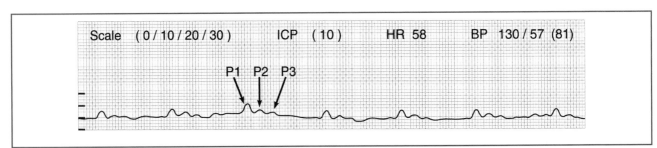

Figure 220–2 Normal ICP tracing (~10 mm Hg). P_1: percussion wave; P_2: tidal wave; P_3: dicrotic wave. (Adapted from Michael DB. *Intracranial Hypertension*. Grosse Pointe Shores, MI: Daniel B. Michael, 2000, with permission.)

(1) Occur at the same frequency as the respiratory rate

(2) Due to changes in intrathoracic pressure transmitted to the brain via the vasculature

2. Lundberg A waves

a. Abnormal plateau waves lasting from 5 to 20 minutes with pressures as high as 100 mm Hg recorded in awake patients with papilledema

b. Represent an early sign of worsening intracranial hypertension

3. Lundberg B waves

a. Abnormal waves of frequency up to 0.5 Hz and amplitude up to 50 mm Hg

b. Of uncertain clinical significance

4. Lundberg C waves

a. Abnormal waves of frequency of 0.125 to 0.250 Hz and normal amplitude

b. Thought to reflect the Traub-Hering-Mayer waves of transmitted systemic blood pressure, which may be caused by periodic changes in vasomotor tone

Bibliography

Bullock R, Chesnut RM, Clifton G, et al. Part 1: Guidelines for the management of severe head injury. J Neurotrauma 2000;17:451–553.

Guyot LL, Diaz FG, Dowling C, Michael DB. Cerebral monitoring devices: analysis of complications. Acta Neurochirg 1998;71:47–49.

Michael DB. Intracranial Hypertension. Grosse Pointe Shores, MI, Daniel B. Michael, 2000.

Ward JD. Intracranial pressure monitoring. In: Champion HR, Robbs JV, Trunkey DD (eds). Rob and Smiths' Operative Surgery: Trauma Surgery, Part I, 4th ed. London: Butterworths, 1989; pp 217–223.

221 Sedation Monitoring

M. Sherif Mokhtar
Richard W. Carlson

Most patients in intensive care units (ICUs) receive sedation to help control anxiety or fear; combat effects of toxic ingestions or withdrawal syndromes; promote sleep; decrease physical activity, metabolism, or oxygen consumption; provide amnesia during procedures and neuromuscular paralysis; as well as to facilitate management of mechanical ventilation. Sedation permits medical and nursing care of patients. A standard approach to monitoring sedation should be employed to evaluate the level of sedation and to allow appropriate dosing adjustments in sedative, analgesic, and paralytic agents to individualize their use according to the patient's condition, the specific setting, and the anticipated duration of use. Pain management should be considered separately from sedation. Specific sedative drugs, analgesic agents, and clinical conditions requiring their use (e.g., alcohol withdrawal) are treated elsewhere in this text.

Key Indications

- Anxiety or fear
- Agitation
- Bedside procedures
- Status epilepticus
- Tetanus
- Certain drug overdoses
- Inadequate or poor quality of sleep
- Facilitation of mechanical ventilation
- Neuromuscular blockade
- Drug-withdrawal syndromes
- Increased intracranial pressure
- Need to decrease oxygen consumption

Monitoring

A. Sedation and pain assessment
  1. No one scale or monitoring system meets all requirements.
  2. Separately identify and quantify pain versus agitation or anxiety.
  3. Most sedatives have little or no analgesic effect.
  4. Opiates are excellent analgesics, but they produce central nervous system depression.
  5. Centrally acting α-adrenergic agonists have both sedative and analgesic properties.
B. Pain evaluation
  1. A zero-to-ten visual-analog pain scale can be used for awake patients who are able to interact with bedside staff:

Worst pain		No pain
10	5	0

  2. Assessment of pain in sedated or obtunded patients
    a. Facial grimacing or jaw clenching
    b. Diaphoresis
    c. Hypertension
    d. Dilated pupils
    e. Withdrawal or movement during dressing changes or bedside procedures
    f. Increase in heart rate or respiratory rate
    g. Increase in cardiac output or oxygen consumption
C. Sedation scales (representative bedside instruments)
  1. Glasgow coma scale (see Table 4–1)
    a. Designed for assessment of neurologically injured patients
    b. Not a sedation scale, but useful to evaluate level of obtundation
  2. Ramsay sedation scale (see Table 69–3)
    a. Developed and commonly used for monitoring pharmacologically induced sedation in the ICU
    b. Usual goal is to achieve a score of 2 to 3.
  3. Observer's assessment of alertness sedation scale
    a. A more comprehensive scale (Table 221–1)
    b. Useful for agents such as benzodiazepines and for treatment of withdrawal syndromes (see Chapter 69, Alcohol Withdrawal Syndrome)
    c. Aim for a score of 4 to 5 for most patients.
  4. Riker sedation–agitation scale (Table 221–2)
    a. Developed for ICU use and validated prospectively
    b. For most patients the goal is level 0.
D. Electroencephalographic (EEG) monitoring
  1. Electroencephalographic and evoked potentials
  2. Processed EEG signals (e.g., bispectral analysis)

TABLE 221-1. OBSERVER'S ASSESSMENT OF ALERTNESS SEDATION SCALE*

RESPONSIVENESS	SPEECH	FACIAL EXPRESSION	EYES	SCORE
Readily responds to name spoken in normal tone	Normal	Normal	Clear, no ptosis	5
Lethargic response to name spoken in normal tone	Slowed or thickened	Mildly relaxed	Glazed, or mild ptosis	4
Responds only after name called loudly or repeatedly	Slurring or slowing	Markedly relaxed (slack jaw)	Glazed and ptosis (> ½ of the eye)	3
Responds only after mild prodding or shaking	Few recognizable words	—	—	2
Does not respond to mild prodding or shaking	—	—	—	1

* Adapted from Chernik DA, Gillings D, Laine H, et al. Validity and reliability of the observer's assessment of alertness/sedation scale: study with intravenous midazolam. J Clin Psychopharmacol 1990;10:244–251, with permission.

E. Imaging and physiologic monitoring methods that can provide additional information on central nervous system structure and function but that do not directly assess sedation

1. Jugular bulb oxygen monitoring

2. Computed tomography, positron emission tomography, or magnetic resonance imaging

3. Intracranial pressure monitoring

4. Cerebral blood flow monitoring

PEARL

Most sedatives have little or no analgesic properties. Co-administration of analgesic agents may be necessary.

Interactions

A. Withdrawal from or reduction of sedation for clinical assessment

1. Consider daily interruption of sedation to assess neurologic status and prospect for weaning from mechanical ventilation.

2. Evaluate cumulative effects of agents on duration of sedation.

B. Neuromuscular blockade

1. Occasionally used in the ICU setting

2. Requires adequate sedation

3. Special considerations in common with sedation

a. Protect from eye injury, cutaneous pressure necrosis, and ventilator disconnection.

b. Provide prophylaxis for deep vein thrombosis and range of motion therapy.

TABLE 221-2. RIKER SEDATION-AGITATION SCALE*

SCORE	AGITATION	DESCRIPTION
+3	Immediate threat to safety	Pulls at endotracheal tube, tries to remove catheters, climbs over bed rails, strikes at staff, violent thrashing
+2	Dangerously agitated	Does not calm despite frequent verbal reminders, requires physical restraints, bites endotracheal tube
+1	Agitated	Anxious or mildly agitated, tries to sit up, calms to verbal instructions
0	Calm and cooperative	Calm, awakens easily, follows commands
−1	Sedated	Difficult to arouse, awakens to verbal stimuli or gentle shaking, drifts off, follows simple commands
−2	Very sedated	Arouses to physical stimuli, does not communicate or follow commands, may move spontaneously
−3	Unarousable	Minimal or no response to noxious stimuli, does not communicate or follow commands

* Adapted from Riker RR, Fraser GL, Cox PM. Continuous infusion of haloperidol controls agitation in critically ill patients. Crit Care Med 1994;22:433–440 and Riker RR, Picard JT, Fraser GL. Prospective evaluation of the Sedation-Agitation Scale for adult critically ill patients. Crit Care Med 1999;27:1325–1329, with permission.

4. Also see Chapter 168, Neuromuscular Blocking Drugs.

CAUTIONS—Neuromuscular Blockade

- Does not produce sedation, amnesia, pain control, or anxiolysis

- Prolonged weakness or paralysis may occur.

- Must ensure adequate sedation and pain management

- Electrical status epilepticus may continue despite neuromuscular blockade.

- Increased risk of potentiated or prolonged weakness in combination with corticosteroids, local anesthetics, aminoglycosides, calcium channel blockers, furosemide, or β-adrenergic blockers

---

Bibliography

Avramov MN, White PF. Methods for monitoring the level of sedation. Crit Care Clin 1995;4:803–826.

Hall RI, Sandham D, Cardinal P, et al. Propofol vs. midazolam for ICU sedation: a Canadian multicenter randomized trial. Chest 2001;199:1151–1159.

Kress JP, Pohlman AS, O'Connor MF, Hall JB. Daily interruption of sedative infusions in critically ill patients undergoing mechanical ventilation. N Engl J Med 2000; 342:1471–1477.

Mirenda J, Broyles G. Propofol as used for sedation in the ICU. Chest 1995;108:539–548.

Prielipp RC, Coursin DB, Wood KE, et al. Complications associated with sedative and neuromuscular blocking drugs in critically ill patients. Crit Care Clin 1995;11: 983–1003.

Riker RR, Picard JT, Fraser GL. Prospective evaluation of the sedation-agitation scale for adult critically ill patients. Crit Care Med 1999;27:1325–1329.

Rosow C, Manberg PJ. Bispectral index monitoring. Anesth Clin North Am 1998;2:89–107.

Simmons LE, Riker RR, Prato BS, et al. Assessing sedation during intensive care unit mechanical ventilation with the bispectral index and the sedation-agitation scale. Crit Care Med 1999;27:1499–1504.

Talke P, Li J, Jain U, et al. Effects of perioperative dexmedetomidine infusion in patients undergoing vascular surgery. Anesthesiology 1995;82:620–633.

Young C, Knudsen N, Hilton A, Reves JG. Sedation in the intensive care unit. Crit Care Med 2000;28:854–866.

222   **Oxygen Therapy**

James A. Kruse

Key Definitions

- High-flow oxygen delivery devices: provide supplemental oxygen at a specified (fixed) FIO_2 and with sufficient flow to meet or exceed the patient's inspiratory flow rate

- Low-flow oxygen delivery devices: supply supplemental oxygen, but at a flow rate below the patient's peak inspiratory flow demand, resulting in variable entrainment of ambient air into the patient's airway and a variable FIO_2

Classification

A. Nasal cannula

1. A low-flow oxygen delivery device consisting of two hollow prongs that insert a short distance into the nares, connected by tubing to an oxygen source (typically regulated to 1 to 5 L/minute)

2. Commonly used when precise regulation of FIO_2 is not important and only low levels of supplemental oxygen are needed

3. Advantages: commonly available; more comfortable than an oxygen mask for most patients; not claustrophobic; allows patient to eat, speak, and expectorate

4. Disadvantages: drying to nasal mucosa and eyes; may be ineffective during mouth breathing; FIO_2 limited to low levels; FIO_2 varies with respiratory variables (e.g., rate and tidal volume)

B. Simple face mask

1. A low-flow oxygen delivery device consisting of a mask with open expiratory vents to minimize CO_2 accumulation, no external reservoir, and small-bore tubing allowing connection to an oxygen source

2. Advantages: simple and available; effective during mouth breathing; allows higher delivered flow rates and FIO_2 compared to nasal cannula; can provide higher humidification than nasal cannula; potentially less drying to nasal mucosa

3. Disadvantages: uncomfortable for some patients, especially for prolonged periods; interferes with eating, speaking, expectorating; FIO_2

varies with respiratory variables; aspiration possible if vomiting occurs; CO_2 rebreathing is possible; requires minimum flow rate to minimize CO_2 rebreathing

C. Simple air-entrainment mask

1. A high-flow device that uses a sized jet orifice in conjunction with an air entrainment port to deliver a specified (fixed) FIO_2

2. Commonly referred to as a "Venturi" mask; however, this is a misnomer

   a. No Venturi tube is employed.

   b. Entrainment is due to viscous shear forces created by the in-line oxygen jet, rather than by decreased lateral pressure by the Bernoulli effect.

3. Advantages: simple to use and readily available; FIO_2 does not vary appreciably with respiratory variables; particularly useful for acutely ill patients with hypercapnic chronic obstructive lung disease

4. Disadvantages: less comfortable than nasal cannula for most patients; moisture accumulation can obstruct tubing or entrainment ports and raise FIO_2; at higher FIO_2 settings, patients with high peak inspiratory flow rates may exceed the capacity of this device and actually receive a lower FIO_2; difficult to achieve expected FIO_2 reliably when set for FIO_2 levels higher than 0.40; drying effect due to high gas flows (for devices set to an FIO_2 higher than 0.28 that are used with only a bubble humidifier)

D. Aerosol mask

1. A mask connected via large-bore tubing to a nebulizer and oxygen source (alternatively, a large-volume humidifier system can be used, but it does not provide an aerosol mist)

2. FIO_2 of the delivered gas may be set using an air-entrainment device or an oxygen-air blender.

3. Advantages: high delivered flow rates possible; less drying to mucous membranes; analytic determination of FIO_2 can be performed relatively easily; the aerosol mist may be preferred by some patients, particularly those with nasal or pharyngeal irritation

4. Disadvantages: some patients do not tolerate

the aerosol mist, especially for prolonged periods; can provoke bronchospasm; FIO_2 may vary with physiologic variables if a sufficiently high-flow source is not employed (especially when attempting to achieve high FIO_2 levels); moisture accumulation can obstruct tubing or entrainment ports and raise FIO_2; actual FIO_2 often less than theoretically delivered value; associated equipment may be noisy

E. Face tent

1. A variation of the aerosol mask in which the device fits under and in front of the mouth, but is open at the top and does not cover the nose

2. Some patients who find masks uncomfortable tolerate this device.

F. Tracheostomy collar

1. A device that resembles a partial face mask and is positioned in front of tracheostomy and held in place with a neck strap

2. Usually connected to an aerosol source and air-entrainment oxygen system

G. Non-rebreather mask

1. A face mask incorporating one-way valve(s) allowing exhalation from the mask, and a reservoir bag with a one-way valve to prevent exhalation into the bag

2. One of the exhalation valve ports is frequently left open as a fail-safe to prevent suffocation in the event of exhalation valve failure or interruption of gas flow into the mask.

3. Advantages: able to achieve high levels of FIO_2 (but in practice never 1.00 using standard disposable masks); easy to use

4. Disadvantages: exact FIO_2 not determinable and can vary

H. Partial non-rebreather mask

1. A face mask incorporating an unvalved reservoir bag and open exhalation port(s) in the mask

2. A variable portion of exhaled gas enters the reservoir (mostly during the early phase of expiration, so it contains little CO_2).

3. Advantages: able to achieve higher levels of FIO_2 than simple face masks; easy to use

4. Disadvantages: delivers lower levels of FIO_2 than the non-rebreather mask; exact FIO_2 not determinable and can vary; CO_2 rebreathing is possible

I. Tusk mask

1. A mask having segments of wide-bore tubing attached to each of two exhalation ports on the mask, which serve as reservoirs

2. The device is often improvised from an aerosol mask, a non-rebreather mask, or a partial non-rebreather mask by attaching a 15-cm-long segment of 2.5-cm-diameter corrugated ventilator circuit tubing to each exhalation port (after removing any valves).

3. Advantage: demonstrated to achieve significantly higher FIO_2 levels than with standard disposable non-rebreather masks

4. Disadvantages: lack of commercial availability necessitates improvised construction, somewhat unwieldy

J. Tight-seal masks

1. Full facial tight-seal mask

   a. Typical device has an air-cushioned elastomeric edge that can form an airtight seal around the patient's nose and mouth if held firmly in place.

   b. Used for delivering inhalational anesthesia by face mask or for resuscitation or procedures (in conjunction with resuscitation bag and valve) or for delivering continuous positive airway pressure (CPAP) or bilevel CPAP by face mask

   c. Advantages: able to achieve FIO_2 of 1.00 (if completely leak free), can be used in conjunction with other devices (e.g., resuscitation bag or positive pressure generator) to noninvasively assist ventilation or provide CPAP

   d. Disadvantages: must be held in place by clinician or else using large elastic bands or tightly adjustable straps; requires special equipment; claustrophobic and uncomfortable for patient; aspiration risk

2. Nasal mask

   a. Has an air-cushioned elastomeric edge that can potentially form an airtight seal around the patient's nose, but the patient's mouth remains uncovered

   b. Used for delivering nasal CPAP or bilevel CPAP

   c. Advantages: can be used in conjunction with other equipment to noninvasively assist ventilation or provide CPAP

   d. Disadvantages: must be held in place using large elastic bands or tightly adjustable straps; requires special equipment; claustrophobic and uncomfortable for some patients; aspiration risk

K. Endotracheal (or tracheostomy) tube delivery connections

1. Wye-adaptor

a. Used to connect inspiratory and expiratory limbs of mechanical ventilator circuit to endotracheal tube

b. A short length of corrugated tubing may be inserted between the endotracheal tube and the wye-adaptor to lessen weight at the end of the endotracheal tube or to intentionally add extra dead-space.

2. Tee-adaptor

a. Also referred to as a tee-piece or Briggs adaptor

b. One of the in-line ports of the tee-piece is connected to a humidified or aerosolized oxygen source using wide-bore corrugated tubing; the other in-line port is connected to a short (e.g., 15 to 45 cm) segment of the same type of tubing, the other end of which is open to the atmosphere.

c. The third port of the tee-piece connects to the endotracheal or tracheostomy tube.

d. The short corrugated tubing segment serves as a reservoir.

e. Most often used during spontaneous breathing trials in patients being weaned from mechanical ventilation

Indications

A. Indications for supplemental oxygen therapy

1. Documented hypoxemia: PaO_2 lower than 60 torr or SaO_2 lower than 0.90

2. Suspected hypoxemia based on clinical scenario (includes most medical and surgical emergencies, such as the following)

a. Cardiopulmonary arrest

b. Cardiogenic or noncardiogenic pulmonary edema

c. Circulatory shock

d. Acute myocardial infarction

e. Acute asthma or other causes of bronchospasm

f. Acute pulmonary embolism

g. Pneumonitis resulting from aspiration, near drowning, severe pneumonia, etc.

h. Drug overdose

i. Acute seizure or post-ictal state

j. Severe trauma

3. Suspected hypoxemia based on clinical signs or symptoms of hypoxia (e.g., dyspnea, tachypnea, tachycardia, cyanosis, confusion, chest pain)

4. High propensity to develop hypoxemia; e.g.,

a. During and after anesthesia

b. Transport of unstable patients

c. Bronchoscopy and certain other procedures

5. Specific situations in which supplemental oxygen may be indicated despite normal or supranormal PaO_2

a. Carbon monoxide poisoning

b. Methemoglobinemia

c. Cyanide poisoning

d. Pneumothorax, pneumomediastinum, subcutaneous emphysema

e. Pneumoencephalus

f. Air embolism

B. Potential indications for low-flow oxygen delivery systems

1. FiO_2 requirement less than 0.45

2. Respiratory rate less than 25 breaths/minute

3. Normal or near-normal tidal volume

4. Regular respiratory pattern

C. Potential indications for high-flow oxygen delivery systems

1. FiO_2 requirement more than 0.45

2. Respiratory rate more than 25 breaths/minute

3. Shallow tidal volume

4. Irregular respiratory pattern (e.g., Cheyne-Stokes respirations)

5. Evidence of alveolar hypoventilation with CO_2 retention

Key Contraindications

- Oxygen therapy should not be used in the absence of a specific indication.

- Low-flow oxygen delivery devices are contraindicated in patients with unstable hypercapnia.

- Tight-seal masks are contraindicated in patients with an altered sensorium or impaired gag reflex (except in resuscitation or anesthesia settings).

Typical dosing (Estimating FiO_2)

A. Nasal cannula

1. Crude estimate of FiO_2 can be made using: $0.04 \times F + 0.2$, where F is oxygen flow (between 1 and 4 L/minute).

2. Lower FiO_2 levels are expected in patients with tachypnea or alterations in tidal volume.

3. Oxygen flow rates greater than 5 L/minute are not well tolerated.

B. Simple face mask

1. Crude estimate of FIO_2 is 0.40 to 0.60 using 5 to 12 L/minute oxygen flow.

2. Oxygen flow rates less than 5 L/minute are not recommended because of the risk of CO_2 rebreathing.

C. Air-entrainment mask

1. Requires use of a specific metering device in conjunction with a specific oxygen flow rate to supply the specified FIO_2

2. Entrainment devices are widely available with jet orifices sized to supply fixed FIO_2 levels of 0.24, 0.28, 0.31, 0.35, 0.40, and 0.50.

3. Variable air-entrainment devices allow FIO_2 to be manually adjusted (in conjunction with providing the specified oxygen flow rate) without substituting a new entrainment jet.

D. Aerosol mask, face tent, or tracheostomy collar

1. With dilution set to deliver FIO_2 of 0.40, 0.60, or 1.00, typical hypopharyngeal FIO_2 levels of approximately 0.40, 0.47, and 0.54 have been measured by some observers; actual performance can vary with flow rate provided and patient characteristics.

2. FIO_2 levels of 0.70 or higher may be achieved using a high-flow system in patients with low respiratory rates and tidal volumes.

E. Reservoir masks

1. Non-rebreathing mask

a. In theory can deliver an FIO_2 of 1.00, but only if the mask forms an airtight seal and all exhalation ports are valved

b. In practice, FIO_2 levels of 0.60 to 0.80 are typically achieved using oxygen flow rates of 8 to 15 L/minute with standard disposable devices.

2. Partial rebreathing mask: FIO_2 levels of 0.40 to 0.80 are typically achieved using oxygen flow rates of 6 to 15 L/minute

3. Oxygen flow rate should be sufficient to prevent reservoir bag from deflating during inspiration.

CAUTION

Except for certain high-flow oxygen delivery devices (e.g., air-entrainment masks), FIO_2 delivered to the airway can only be crudely estimated and will vary with the device flow rate and the patient's respiratory rate, tidal volume, inspiratory flow rate, anatomic dead space, and other factors.

Complications

A. Hypoxemia

1. Can occur with incorrect selection of delivery device, insufficient oxygen flow rate, worsening of pulmonary function while receiving a given type of oxygen therapy, an increase in inspiratory flow rate when using a low-flow device, etc.

2. Prevented by monitoring using pulse oximetry or arterial blood gas analysis

B. Oxygen toxicity

1. At high levels oxygen causes a form of acute cytotoxic lung injury leading to increased pulmonary capillary permeability and pulmonary edema, possibly secondary to altered leukocyte function, generation of free radicals (e.g., peroxide and superoxide), and ciliary dysfunction.

2. Onset and severity have been shown in animal studies to be related to both dose and duration of exposure, but there is wide interspecies variation.

3. FIO_2 levels of 0.50 or less appear to be safe, even if administered for prolonged periods.

4. FIO_2 levels of 0.60 or more administered for longer than 24 hours probably have toxic pulmonary effects in humans.

5. Retrolental fibroplasia (retinopathy of prematurity) can occur in neonates exposed to high concentrations of oxygen, but it does not occur in adults.

C. Hypercapnia

1. A concern in patients with chronic obstructive pulmonary disease, particularly those with chronic hypoxemia and hypercapnia receiving excessive levels of supplemental oxygen

2. This phenomenon may be due to loss of the normal hypoxic respiratory drive or increased inhomogeneity of ventilation–perfusion distribution.

3. Avoided by using controlled oxygen delivery devices (e.g., air-entrainment devices) and titrating the FIO_2 to the minimum level required to correct hypoxemia

4. Can also occur when using low oxygen flow rates with simple face masks, and partial non-rebreathing masks, leading to insufficient CO_2 washout from mask and consequent CO_2 rebreathing; sticking or malfunctioning expiratory valves on non-rebreather masks can have a similar effect

D. Denitrogenation atelectasis

1. Normally there is residual nitrogen in the alve-

oli that is in equilibrium with P_{N_2} of the blood, which maintains alveolar tension even if all oxygen is absorbed from these alveoli (and not replaced because of underventilation).

2. Steady-state administration of oxygen at an F_{IO_2} of 1.00 displaces all nitrogen from the alveoli and blood.

3. Oxygen absorbed into the blood from underventilated alveoli can lead to areas of microatelectasis from alveolar collapse in response to low gas tension (which would not have occurred if alveolar P_{N_2} were not zero).

E. Adverse effects to skin and mucous membranes

1. Drying effect of administered gas mixture if inadequately humidified

a. Irritation of nasal, nasopharyngeal, oral mucous membranes, conjunctiva, lips or facial skin can cause patient discomfort.

b. Uncommonly can result in chapped lips, dermatitis, or epistaxis

2. Pressure ulceration (e.g., on ears or face) due to edge of mask, tight fitting mask straps, or nasal cannula tubing

F. Aspiration

1. Can result from vomiting while wearing an oxygen mask

2. Risk is highest with tight-seal face masks, as used for CPAP delivered by mask.

3. Except in resuscitation or anesthesia situations, tight-seal masks are contraindicated in patients with an altered sensorium or impaired airway or gag reflexes.

G. Respiratory tract infection from microbial contamination of a humidifier or a nebulizer system

H. Burn injury from a realized fire hazard

PEARL

Because it is more difficult to prevent ambient air entrainment with face masks than with endotracheal delivery, the target F_{IO_2} after extubation should be 0.05 higher than the minimum requirement needed during intubation to assure acceptable oxygenation.

Bibliography

Bazuaye EA, Stone TN, Corris PA, et al. Variability of inspired oxygen concentration with nasal cannulas. Thorax 1992;47:509–511.

Capellier G, Beuret P, Clement G, et al. Oxygen tolerance in patients with acute respiratory failure. Intensive Care Med 1998;24:422–428.

DuPre JR, Davis WB. Pulmonary oxygen toxicity: does it make a difference? Clin Pulm Med 1997;4:213–220.

Gay PC, Edmonds LC. Severe hypercapnia after low-flow oxygen therapy in patients with neuromuscular disease and diaphragmatic dysfunction. Mayo Clin Proc 1995; 70:327–330.

Hnatiuk OW, Moores LK, Thompson JC, et al. Delivery of high concentrations of inspired oxygen via tusk mask. Crit Care Med 1998;26:1032–1035.

Mao C, Wong DT, Slutsky AS, et al. A quantitative assessment of how Canadian intensivists believe they utilize oxygen in the intensive care unit. Crit Care Med 1999; 27:2806–2811.

Small D, Duha A, Wieskopf B, et al. Uses and misuses of oxygen in hospitalized patients. Am J Med 1992;92:591–595.

223 Conventional Mechanical Ventilation

Alain Tremblay
Kalpalatha K. Guntupalli

Key Indications for Mechanical Ventilation

- Hypoxemic respiratory failure
- Hypercarbic respiratory failure
- Neuromuscular respiratory failure
- Requirement for general anesthesia or therapeutic muscle paralysis (e.g., surgery)

Terminology (Modes of Mechanical Ventilation)

A. Negative pressure modes
   1. Use an external device to apply negative pressure over the chest (cuirass vest) or whole body except head (iron lung) to decrease intrathoracic pressure below atmospheric pressure and effect lung inflation
   2. Chiefly of historical interest as positive pressure modes are almost universally used in intensive care units (ICUs) today.

B. Controlled mandatory ventilation
   1. A time-triggered mode (i.e., breath is initiated after a set time elapses), not a patient-triggered mode
   2. Most often used in a volume-controlled mode in which the operator sets tidal volume (Vt), respiratory rate (f), and inspiratory flow rate ($\dot{V}i$)
   3. Can be volume-cycled (i.e., inspiration normally ends when the set tidal volume is delivered) or pressure-cycled (i.e., inspiration normally ends when a set inspiratory pressure is reached)
   4. Almost exclusively applied in anesthetized and therapeutically paralyzed subjects
   5. Patient has no control of minute volume ($\dot{V}e$).

C. Assist-controlled ventilation
   1. A volume-controlled mode in which the operator sets Vt, $\dot{V}i$, and minimum f
   2. A time-triggered mode, but patient can trigger additional breaths above the operator set f
   3. Allows patient control of f and $\dot{V}e$ above baseline settings; patient has no control of Vt or $\dot{V}i$

   4. Commonly employed in the ICU, especially when initiating mechanical ventilation, for patients who require full or substantial ventilatory support

D. Synchronized intermittent mandatory ventilation (SIMV)
   1. A volume-controlled mode in which the operator sets Vt, $\dot{V}i$, and a mandatory minimum f
   2. Mandatory breaths are positive pressure breaths that provide full ventilatory assistance and deliver the set Vt; patient does not control Vt during these mandatory breaths.
   3. Mandatory breaths are either time-triggered (if patient does not initiate inspiration) or synchronized to patient triggering (if patient provides an inspiratory effort near the triggering time interval).
   4. Spontaneous breaths are allowable between mandatory breaths, but patient receives no positive pressure ventilatory assistance during these spontaneous breaths.
   5. Provides preset ventilatory backup to guarantee minimum $\dot{V}e$, but allows spontaneous breathing above this level of support
   6. Developed as a weaning mode (see Chapter 226, Discontinuing Mechanical Ventilation)

E. Pressure support
   1. Operator sets inspiratory support pressure.
   2. Patient triggers (initiates) each breath and determines f.
   3. Vt and $\dot{V}e$ are influenced by patient's interaction with ventilator and depend on the level of pressure support and the patient's inspiratory effort, airway resistance, total static respiratory system compliance (Crs), and other factors.
   4. Inspiration ends when $\dot{V}i$ drops below a set percentage (typically 25% to 33%) of peak $\dot{V}i$.
   5. Provides no backup Vt, $\dot{V}e$, or f (although some ventilators may have a fail-safe mechanism that provides mandatory positive pressure breaths in the event of apnea)
   6. Provides good patient–ventilator synchrony
   7. Useful for spontaneously breathing patients who can generate at least some degree of inspiratory effort

8. If necessary, high levels of pressure support may be selected to provide adequate Vt and V̇e.

9. Commonly used for weaning (see Chapter 226, Discontinuing Mechanical Ventilation)

10. Low pressure support levels (e.g., 5 cm H₂O) may be used to overcome circuit and endotracheal tube resistance in spontaneously breathing patients.

F. Pressure control

1. Operator sets inspiratory pressure, f, and either inspiratory to expiratory (I:E) ratio or inspiratory time (Ti).

2. Usually employed as a time-triggered mode, with time-cycled breaths provided at the set level of positive pressure (usually requires sedation and therapeutic paralysis)

3. If patient triggering is allowed, as f increases for a given Ti, expiratory time (Te) will decrease.

    a. This may lead to auto-positive end-expiratory pressure (auto-PEEP) and dynamic hyperinflation (see Chapter 225, Positive End-Expiratory Pressure).

    b. If I:E ratio is the set variable, Ti and Te will decrease as f increases, with a fall in Vt.

4. Vt and V̇e are affected by patient–ventilator interaction (e.g., will vary with Crs and airway resistance).

5. Commonly used for management of acute respiratory distress syndrome (ARDS), and often maintains lower inspiratory pressures for a given level of oxygenation

---

CAUTIONS

With Pressure Control Mode Ventilation

- Does not provide a guaranteed Vt or V̇e

- May lead to hemodynamic compromise due to higher mean airway pressure

- Has potential for causing auto-PEEP

G. Synchronized intermittent mandatory ventilation + pressure support (a hybrid mode)

1. Synchronized intermittent mandatory ventilation provides a mandatory number of fully assisted positive pressure breaths each minute, with pressure support providing partial assistance of any additional (spontaneous) breaths.

2. Low-level (e.g., approximately 5 cm H₂O) pressure support may be used to overcome endotracheal tube and circuit resistance during spontaneous breaths.

3. Low SIMV rates (e.g., approximately 4 breaths/min) may be used for patients with periodic breathing (e.g., Cheyne-Stokes respiration) to prevent triggering of apnea alarm.

4. May be used as a weaning mode

5. High-level pressure support used in conjunction with SIMV may be employed as a primary ventilatory mode, but this has no clear advantage over assist-controlled or pure pressure support modes.

H. Newer and investigational modes (see Chapter 224, Newer Modes of Mechanical Ventilation)

Procedure

A. Initiation of mechanical ventilation

1. Secure appropriate interface with ventilator (e.g., endotracheal tube or tracheostomy).

2. Select initial ventilator settings.

    a. Select mode (assist-controlled recommended as initial mode; typical settings that follow conform to assist-controlled mode).

    b. Select initial settings for Vt (typically 5 to 12 mL/kg) and f to achieve V̇e (typically 140 mL/kg per minute or 8 to 14 L/min).

    c. Select V̇i (typically 40 to 60 L/min).

    d. Set FIO₂ to 1.00.

    e. Select PEEP of 0 or, if no contraindication (see Chapter 225, Positive End-Expiratory Pressure), 5 cm H₂O.

    f. Select trigger mechanism.

        (1) Pressure trigger: patient generates negative airway pressure below a pre-set threshold (typically between 0.05 and 3 cm H₂O) to initiate mechanical breath

        (2) Flow trigger: constant gas flow is maintained across the ventilator circuit; inspiratory effort causes differential flow between inspiratory and expiratory limbs of the circuit which triggers a mechanical breath

---

CAUTION

Incorrect setting of triggering mode or thresholds may increase work of breathing and lead to patient–ventilator dysynchrony.

---

3. Observe peak inspiratory pressure (P_peak) and plateau pressure (P_plateau) and assess patient–ventilator synchrony (see below, under Monitoring).

4. Provide appropriate sedation, as necessary.

5. Obtain arterial blood gas after 15 to 30 minutes.

a. Assess adequacy of ventilation ($PaCO_2$) and adjust f or Vt as necessary, then reassess $PaCO_2$.

b. Assess adequacy of oxygenation (SaO_2) and titrate FIO_2 (between 0.21 and 1.00) as necessary to achieve targeted oxygen level (usually $SaO_2 \geq 0.90$ torr or $PaO_2 > 60$ torr); may use pulse oximetry for subsequent adjustments of FIO_2.

c. If FIO_2 requirement is greater than 0.50, a trial of higher PEEP (above 5 cm H_2O) should be considered if there is no contraindication (see Chapter 225, Positive End-Expiratory Pressure).

6. Assess hemodynamic status.

7. Subsequent settings are titrated according to clinical response and measurements of gas exchange.

Monitoring

A. Monitor ventilator alarms.

1. Available alarms include threshold minimum and maximum values for f, airway pressure, I:E, and exhaled Vt (typically set by respiratory therapist).

2. In volume-controlled modes, P_{peak} can serve to identify risk of barotrauma, especially in patients with abnormal Crs.

3. In pressure-controlled modes, alarms for minimum and maximum values of Vt and $\dot{V}e$ alert clinicians to inadequate ventilation.

4. Apnea alarm (low or zero f) signals disconnection from ventilator circuit or lack of patient triggering (in flow or pressure-triggered modes without an adequate mandatory back-up rate).

B. Monitor patient.

1. Monitor clinical status: close clinical monitoring by nursing and respiratory therapy personnel is essential for critically ill patients receiving mechanical ventilation

2. Employ continuous electrocardiographic monitoring.

3. Employ continuous intra-arterial or frequent intermittent noninvasive blood pressure monitoring.

4. Monitor oxygenation using continuous pulse oximetry or intermittent blood gas analysis.

5. Monitor adequacy of ventilation by assessing $PaCO_2$ using intermittent blood gas analysis; end-tidal CO_2 monitoring may be useful in selected patients (see Chapter 217, Capnography).

6. Obtain serial chest x-rays.

a. Typically obtained daily for acutely ill, mechanically ventilated ICU patients

b. Allows sequential assessment of cardiopulmonary pathology; position of catheters, endotracheal tubes, and other devices; and complications (e.g., pneumothorax, atelectasis, mainstem intubation).

C. Monitor patient–ventilator interaction.

1. Monitor airway pressure, airway flow, and tidal volume (Fig. 223–1).

a. P_{peak} is maximum inspiratory pressure during positive pressure ventilation and reflects the effects of both Crs and airway resistance.

b. Plateau pressure ($P_{plateau}$) is static airway pressure obtained during an end-inspiratory hold maneuver, allowing equilibration of pressure within the airways.

(1) May be obtained with patient on assist-controlled mode (with current settings for PEEP, rate and Vt) by setting an inspiratory pause of 0.5 to 1 second and observing airway pressure at end of pause

(2) May also be obtained by manually occluding exhalation port at end-inspiration and observing $P_{plateau}$ from airway pressure reading

(3) Use the average value from several breaths or use graph function (time versus pressure) on ventilator monitor to ensure that the inspiratory plateau is achieved.

c. Comparison of these variables can aid in distinguishing between increased airway resistance and decreased lung or thoracic compliance as the cause of high airway pressures.

(1) Elevated P_{peak} + normal $P_{plateau}$ suggests airway restriction (i.e., bronchospasm, secretions, tube occlusion).

(2) Elevated P_{peak} + high $P_{plateau}$ suggests abnormal Crs (e.g., ARDS).

(3) Goal is $P_{plateau}$ lower than 35 cm H_2O and minimal difference between P_{peak} and $P_{plateau}$.

2. Monitor Crs and dynamic compliance (Cd) in selected cases.

a. Crs is calculated as $Vt/(P_{plateau} - PEEP)$.

(1) Normal value is approximately 60 mL/cm H_2O.

(2) Increased in emphysema; decreased in conditions that decrease lung compliance (e.g., pulmonary edema or fibrosis) or extrapulmonary thoracic compliance (e.g., pleural effusion or kyphoscoliosis)

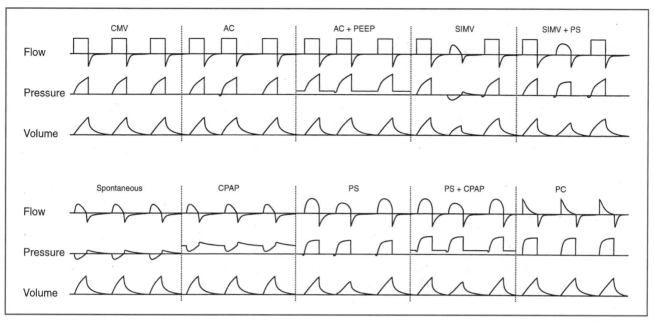

Figure 223–1. Typical time domain flow, volume, and pressure waveforms for controlled mandatory ventilation (CMV), assist-controlled mode (AC), synchronized intermittent mandatory ventilation (SIMV), spontaneous breathing, continuous positive airway pressure mode (CPAP), pressure support mode (PS), pressure control mode (PC), and certain hybrid modes. Negative deflections in pressure–time waveforms indicate patient-initiated inspiratory efforts, which in AC and PS modes may trigger a positive pressure mechanical breath. Note that some mechanical ventilators allow modification of the flow waveform patterns (not depicted). PEEP = positive end-expiratory pressure.

b. Cd is calculated as $Vt/(P_{peak} - PEEP)$.
   (1) Normal value is only marginally less than Crs.
   (2) Decreased in conditions associated with airway obstruction (e.g., mucous plugging or bronchospasm) and conditions that decrease Crs
c. Values may help assess underlying disorder and work of breathing; e.g., a wide gradient between Crs and Cd suggests airway obstruction; however, can be difficult to determine on awake patients with high f, and may require use of sedation.
3. Monitor airway resistance (Raw) in selected cases.
   a. Calculated as $(P_{peak} - P_{plateau})/\dot{V}i$
   b. Normal range is 2 to 8 cm $H_2O \cdot sec/L$.
   c. A measure of the dynamic impedance to air flow in the airways; quantifies airway obstruction
4. Monitor for auto-PEEP (see Chapter 225, Positive End-Expiratory Pressure).

Complications

A. Airway access complications (see Chapter 189, Endotracheal Intubation), including nosocomial pneumonia
B. Ventilator-induced lung injury

1. Oxygen toxicity: threshold for humans not known but toxicity is thought to be a risk at FIO_2 levels above 0.55
2. Barotrauma: high inflation pressures may induce barotrauma (e.g., pneumothorax, pneumomediastinum, or subcutaneous emphysema)
3. Volutrauma: high inflation volumes and repeated end-expiratory collapse, followed by re-opening during inspiration (cyclic recruitment–derecruitment), may induce inflammatory mediator release and acute lung injury
4. A recommended strategy for minimizing these complications in ARDS is the "open lung" approach using PEEP and targeting $P_{plateau}$ below 30 cm H_2O, FIO_2 <0.55, and Vt of 6 mL/kg (also see Chapter 8, Acute Respiratory Distress Syndrome, and Chapter 225, Positive End-Expiratory Pressure).
C. Auto-PEEP
   1. Presence of auto-PEEP can require greater patient effort to trigger breaths, independent of pressure or flow settings on mechanical ventilation.
   2. See Chapter 225, Positive End-Expiratory Pressure
D. Hemodynamic instability
   1. Increases in intrathoracic pressure reduce preload and can lead to hypotension and decreased cardiac output.

2. More likely to occur if patient is hypovolemic or if there are high levels of P_{peak}, extrinsic PEEP, or auto-PEEP

3. Often responds to fluid loading; may also respond to use of lower Vt or maneuvers that lower airway pressure

E. Patient–ventilator dysynchrony

1. Signs and symptoms may include agitation, diaphoresis, tachycardia, tachypnea, paradoxical thoracoabdominal breathing pattern (i.e., inward movement of abdomen during inspiration), increased P_{peak}.

2. Exclude malposition of endotracheal tube, airway obstruction, hypoxemia, pneumothorax, incorrect triggering threshold, etc.

3. May respond to adjustment of flow and pressure settings, or require sedation

Bibliography

The Acute Respiratory Distress Syndrome Network. Ventilation with lower tidal volumes as compared with traditional tidal volumes for acute lung injury and the acute respiratory distress syndrome. N Engl J Med 2000;342: 1301–1308.

Dreyfuss D, Saumon G. Ventilator-induced lung injury. Lessons from experimental studies. Am J Respir Crit Care Med 1998;157:294–323.

Jubran A, Tobin MJ. Monitoring during mechanical ventilation. Clin Chest Med 1996;17:453–474.

Lachman B. Open up the lung and keep the lung open. Intensive Care Med 1992;18:319–321.

Laghi F, Karamchandani K, Tobin MJ. Influence of ventilator settings in determining respiratory frequency during mechanical ventilation. Am J Respir Crit Care Med 1999;160:1766–1770.

McKibben AW, Ravenscraft SA. Pressure-controlled and volume-cycled mechanical ventilation. Clin Chest Med 1996;17:395–410.

Tobin MJ. Advances in mechanical ventilation. N Engl J Med 2001;334:1986–1996.

224 Newer Modes of Mechanical Ventilation

Alain Tremblay
Kalpalatha K. Guntupalli

Although the title implies that the following approaches to mechanical ventilation are new, some have been in use for decades, although they were not generally accepted as standard therapy or frequently used in the ICU. Nevertheless, some of these modes are now available on newer generation ventilators and are used for selected conditions. Some of the topics herein refer to specific modes of ventilation; others may be characterized as adjunctive measures. They are included as emerging modalities and as a review of the rationale underlying their use.

Definitions

A. Noninvasive positive pressure ventilation (NIPPV)
   1. Positive pressure ventilation without invasive airway access (endotracheal tube or tracheostomy)
   2. Ventilator–patient interface achieved using an airtight mask over nose or over nose and mouth
B. High-frequency ventilation (HFV)
   1. Modes of ventilation characterized by low Vt (at, near, or below deadspace volume) at frequencies beyond that used for conventional positive pressure ventilation (i.e., >1 Hz)
   2. Gas exchange occurs by bulk flow, coaxial flow, pendelluft, Taylor dispersion, or facilitated molecular diffusion.

Key Classification of HFV by Respiratory Frequency

- High-frequency positive pressure ventilation: 1 to 2 Hz

- High-frequency jet ventilation: approximately 1.5 to 10 Hz

- High-frequency oscillation: approximately 5 to 50 Hz

C. Inverse ratio ventilation
   1. Ventilatory mode with reversal of usual inspiratory:expiratory (I:E) ratio of 1:2 to as high as 4:1 or greater
   2. Increases mean alveolar pressure without increasing peak airway or plateau pressure

   3. Facilitates alveolar gas mixing by employing long time constants; improves ventilation–perfusion mismatch and hypoxemia
   4. Short expiratory times produce intrinsic (auto-) positive end-expiratory pressure (PEEP)
      a. May be a major mechanism of improving PaO_2
      b. Caution: risk of hyperinflation and barotrauma, especially in volume-controlled modes
D. Liquid ventilation
   1. Use of liquid as the medium for gas exchange
      a. Requisite media properties include low surface tension, high vapor pressure, and high solubility of O_2 and CO_2.
      b. Perfluorocarbon media are under evaluation.
   2. Full liquid ventilation: complete filling of lung with liquid medium (requires special ventilators)
   3. Partial liquid ventilation: partial filling of lung (usually to functional residual capacity) with superimposed gas ventilation using a conventional ventilator
   4. Putative advantages
      a. Recruitment of alveoli in dependent zones ("liquid PEEP")
      b. Improved lung compliance in regions of lung injury
      c. Enhanced gas exchange in regions of lung injury
      d. Possible anti-inflammatory properties
      e. Lavage of debris
E. Permissive hypercapnia
   1. Intentional production or tolerance of respiratory acidosis for the purpose of limiting airway pressures and hyperinflation
   2. $PaCO_2$ is allowed to rise and pH allowed to decrease.
   3. The maximum "safe" level of hypercapnia and role of buffering agents are controversial.
   4. Deep sedation is often required to decrease respiratory drive; neuromuscular blockade may be required in some cases.
F. Volume control + volume-assured pressure support

1. Dual-control mode that combines the beneficial effects of pressure support on synchrony and gas mixing to the full support provided by volume control ventilation

2. Ensures a guaranteed Vt in pressure support mode: if the set Vt is not delivered, a preset flow is applied until Vt is achieved

3. Guaranteed Vt back-up can be added during weaning with pressure support.

G. Proportional assist ventilation

1. Provides high levels of respiratory support while potentially enhancing patient–ventilator synchrony because the patient controls tidal volume and flow

2. Breath-by-breath patient-initiated flow is tracked using microprocessor technology, and the tracking is used to provide continuously adjusted inspiratory support of volume and flow.

H. Airway pressure-release ventilation

1. Spontaneous breathing mode with mechanical ventilatory assistance alternating between long period of set inspiratory pressure followed by a shorter "release" expiratory pressure

2. Patient's tidal breaths are supplemented by ventilator pressure cycling.

3. No patient–ventilator synchronization is required.

4. May allow ventilation with lower peak pressures, although transpulmonary pressures for given Vt are dependent on lung compliance

I. Other self-adaptive or dual-control modes

1. Pressure supplementation

2. Pressure-regulated volume control

3. Pressure augmentation

4. Variable pressure support, variable pressure control

5. Autoflow

6. Adaptive support ventilation

Indications

A. Noninvasive positive-pressure ventilation

1. Exacerbation of chronic obstructive pulmonary disease (COPD) with hypercarbic respiratory failure

   a. May decrease the need for endotracheal intubation and decrease length of stay

   b. Expiratory pressure improves oxygenation and may facilitate initiation of breaths by overcoming high inspiratory threshold imposed by auto-PEEP.

   c. Inspiratory pressure (when set to a level higher than expiratory pressure) improves ventilation.

   d. Currently a standard ventilatory method for this population if there are no contraindications

2. Acute cardiogenic pulmonary edema

   a. Continuous positive airway pressure (CPAP) improves hypoxemia, hypercarbia, and work of breathing with reduced requirement for intubation.

   b. Also reduces left ventricular preload and afterload, and redistributes edema fluid to non–gas-exchanging areas

   c. Bilevel CPAP may be associated with more chest pain and risk of myocardial ischemia compared to CPAP.

3. Other indications (selected cases)

   a. Acute respiratory distress syndrome

   b. Pneumonia

   c. Postoperative respiratory failure

   d. Failed extubation

   e. Asthma exacerbation

   f. Respiratory failure in "no intubation" patients

   g. Chronic use for treatment of obstructive sleep apnea (usually using CPAP)

   h. Chronic respiratory failure due to neuromuscular or restrictive thoracic disease

B. High-frequency ventilation

1. Acute respiratory distress syndrome

   a. May reduce ventilator-induced lung injury by minimizing hyperinflation and cyclic recruitment–derecruitment

   b. Studies suggest improved lung mechanics, alveolar gas mixing, and oxygenation, but survival is not altered.

   c. Use with concurrent interventions, such as recruitment maneuvers, is under study.

2. Bronchopleural fistula

   a. May reduce airway pressures and Vt, favoring fistula closure

   b. Case reports suggest efficacy.

3. Use during thoracic surgery to minimize tidal lung inflations

4. Ventilation during laryngeal surgery or bronchoscopy

C. Inverse ratio ventilation

1. Acute respiratory distress syndrome

2. Other causes of severe hypoxemic respiratory failure

D. Liquid ventilation
1. Demonstrated efficacy in neonatal respiratory distress syndrome
2. Ongoing studies in adults

E. Permissive hypercapnia
1. Status asthmaticus
   a. Employed in lieu of aggressive ventilation to normalize $PaCO_2$
   b. May limit risks of hyperinflation, barotrauma and death
2. Selected cases of COPD exacerbation
3. Acute respiratory distress sydrome

F. Proportional assist ventilation
1. Most commonly used for COPD patients with severe respiratory failure
2. May increase patient comfort, ameliorate hyperventilation, and decrease requirements for sedation

Procedure

A. Noninvasive positive pressure ventilation
1. Explain procedure and reassure patient.
2. Select mask and adjust fit.
   a. Availability of multiple mask sizes is necessary for optimal fit, patient tolerance, and avoidance of unnecessary dead space.
   b. Choice of nasal versus face mask is a matter of individual preference, fit, and patient tolerance.
   c. Consider wound dressing over bridge of nose and at pressure points.
   d. Ensure tight fit, but allow space for two fingers beneath head straps.
3. Position head of bed at a 45 degree, if possible.
4. Noninvasive CPAP application
   a. Not a mode of ventilation, but can improve oxygenation and lower the work of breathing
   b. May be configured using a conventional ventilator (e.g., using CPAP mode and 0 cm H_2O pressure support), generated via wall gas supply, or by use of a dedicated CPAP machine.
5. Bilevel CPAP using a NIPPV ventilator
   a. Compared to conventional ventilators, NIPPV ventilators are easy to use, more portable, less expensive, and usually have more sensitive trigger mechanisms incorporating leak compensation.
   b. Typical initial settings: respiratory rate (f) 12 to 16 breaths/minute, inspiratory pressure 12

to 15 cm H_2O, expiratory pressure 5 to 8 cm H_2O, and FIO_2 adjusted to achieve SaO_2 >0.90
   c. Set alarms.

CAUTION

Inspiratory pressure on bilevel CPAP ventilators are absolute pressures above atmospheric, whereas pressure support settings on conventional ventilators are pressures set above CPAP.

---

6. Bilevel CPAP using a conventional ventilator
   a. Noninvasive positive pressure ventilation using a traditional ventilator allows additional monitoring and alarm functions (although newer generation NIPPV ventilators have many of these features).
   b. Other modes, e.g., assist-controlled and pressure control, can also be selected.
   c. Silence ventilator alarms, set CPAP initially at 0 cm H_2O with pressure support at 10 cm H_2O, and titrate FIO_2 to achieve SaO_2 greater than 0.90.
   d. Increase CPAP to at least 5 cm H_2O and increase pressure support level to achieve exhaled tidal volume greater than 7 mL/kg, f lower than 25 breaths/minute, and patient comfort.
   e. Avoid peak pressures higher than 30 cm H_2O.
   f. Set alarms and apnea backup.
7. Observe for gastric distention, nausea, vomiting, agitation, and changes in sensorium.

B. High-frequency jet ventilation
1. Typical initial settings: driving pressure of 30 psi, rate of 100 "breaths"/minute, inspiratory time of 30%
2. Titration strategies
   a. To improve ventilation (decrease $PaCO_2$): increase driving pressure, increase inspiratory time, or decrease rate
   b. To improve oxygenation (increase PaO_2): increase FIO_2, or add or increase PEEP

C. Inverse ratio ventilation
1. Volume controlled mode: decrease inspiratory flow rates or add end-inspiratory plateau or pause
2. Pressure-controlled mode: adjust inspiratory time and f, or set I : E on ventilator

D. Permissive hypercapnia

1. Arterial blood pH levels to 7.15 to 7.20 may be tolerated in many patients without the use of buffering agents.
2. Role of NaHCO$_3$ is not well defined. High doses are required at low pH; and this may lead to paradoxical intracellular acidosis and increased intracellular CO_2 production.

E. Proportional assist ventilation
1. Set gain to desired level of support (0 to 100%) in proportion to patient effort.
2. Increasing patient effort automatically leads to immediate increase in machine output; when patient relaxes, machine decreases output.

Complications and Limitations

A. Noninvasive positive-pressure ventilation
1. Facial skin breakdown
2. Gastric distention, aspiration
3. Failure of face-mask seal
4. Patient intolerance
5. Nasal congestion
6. Cannot use on uncooperative or obtunded patients
7. Cannot use continuously; provide rest intervals every 4 to 8 hours

B. High-frequency ventilation
1. Humidification is difficult.
2. Airway injury, including necrotizing tracheobronchitis, can occur.
3. High potential for air trapping and auto-PEEP

C. Inverse ratio ventilation
1. Requirement for heavy sedation, occasionally with neuromuscular blockade
2. May lead to hypercapnia or unrecognized auto-PEEP
3. Benefit of auto-PEEP versus extrinsic PEEP is not well defined.

D. Liquid ventilation
1. Unable to assess lung parenchyma by chest x-ray during liquid ventilation
2. Potential adverse effects on preload
3. Increased work of breathing because of high-density fluid mandates superimposed mechanical ventilation.
4. Long-term toxicity is unknown.

5. Requires frequent "topping off" because of evaporation at body temperature

E. Permissive hypercapnia
1. Central nervous system depression
2. Increased intracranial pressure
3. Cardiac dysrhythmias or ischemia
4. Shift of oxyhemoglobin dissociation curve to right
5. Complex hemodynamic and autonomic effects, including pulmonary hypertension, alterations of cardiac output, and myocardial depression
6. Decreased renal blood flow
7. Cannot be employed if there is refractory hypoxemia or preexisting severe metabolic acidosis

F. Volume-assured pressure support, volume support
1. Ventilator determines flow pattern.
2. Inspiratory time may be prolonged.

G. Proportional assist ventilation
1. Requires spontaneous breathing
2. No back-up ventilation; apnea alarm or back-up mode required
3. Resistance and compliance information are required to adjust settings.
4. Auto-PEEP can occur.
5. Potential for "runaway effect" if overcompensation (volume and pressure alarms required)

Bibliography

Appendini L, Purro A, Gudjonsdottir M, et al. Physiologic response of ventilator-dependent patients with chronic obstructive pulmonary disease to proportional assist ventilation and continuous positive airway pressure. Am J Respir Crit Care Med 1999;159:1510–1517.

Feihl F, Perret C. Permissive hypercapnia: how permissive should we be? Am J Respir Crit Care Med 1994;150:1722–1737.

Froese AB, Bryan AC. High frequency ventilation. Am Rev Respir Dis 1987;135:1363–1374.

Hirschl RB, Conrad S, Kaiser R, et al. Partial liquid ventilation in adult patients with ARDS: a multicenter phase I-II trial. Ann Surg 1998;228:692–700.

Keenan SP, Gregor J, Sibbald WJ, et al. Noninvasive positive pressure ventilation in the setting of severe, acute exacerbations of chronic obstructive pulmonary disease: more effective and less expensive. Crit Care Med 2000;28:2094–2102.

Keenan SP, Kernerman PD, Cook DJ, et al. Effect of noninvasive positive pressure ventilation on mortality in patients admitted with acute respiratory failure: a meta-analysis. Crit Care Med 1997;25:1685–1692.

Wiedermann HP. Partial liquid ventilation for acute respiratory distress syndrome. Clin Chest Med 2000;21:543–554.

225 Positive End-Expiratory Pressure

Ali A. Hamdan
Peter J. Papadakos

Positive end-expiratory pressure (PEEP) refers to pressure in the airway at the end of passive expiration that exceeds atmospheric pressure. The term is applicable to patients receiving mechanical ventilation. For spontaneously breathing subjects, the term *continuous positive airway pressure* (CPAP) is used when inspiratory and expiratory portions of the circuit are pressurized above atmospheric pressure. Positive end-expiratory pressure is used mainly to recruit or stabilize lung units and improve oxygenation in patients with hypoxemic respiratory failure.

Key Indications

- Acute lung injury and acute respiratory distress syndrome

- Cardiogenic pulmonary edema

- Diffuse pneumonia requiring mechanical ventilation

- Atelectasis associated with severe hypoxemia

- Other forms of severe hypoxemic respiratory failure

Key Contraindications

- Pneumothorax without pleural catheter

- Intracranial hypertension

- Hypovolemia (unless concomitantly treated)

- Bronchopleural fistula

- Recent pulmonary resection surgery

Effects and Mechanisms

A. Gas exchange
   1. Redistributes fluid within the alveoli and reduces intrapulmonary shunting
   2. Improves arterial oxygenation (PaO_2)
   3. Reduces FIO_2 requirements and risk of oxygen toxicity
B. Lung mechanics
   1. Helps prevent alveolar collapse
   2. Stabilizes and recruits lung units
   3. Increases functional residual capacity
   4. Improves lung compliance
   5. Shifts tidal deflections to the right along the inspiratory pressure-volume curve (Fig. 225–1), minimizing potential for ventilator-induced lung injury by preventing repetitive collapse of lung units at end-expiration followed by re-opening during inspiration
   6. May decrease the inspiratory work of breathing due to auto-PEEP in patients with obstructive airway disease
C. Hemodynamic effects of PEEP-induced increases in intrathoracic pressure
   1. Increases intraluminal central venous pressure
   2. Decreases venous return
   3. Decreases left and right ventricular preload (end-diastolic volume)
   4. Increases right ventricular afterload
   5. Decreases cardiac output, as a result of the above effects
      a. Hypotension and organ hypoperfusion can occur.
      b. Reduction of both cardiac output and blood pressure is particularly likely in the presence of hypovolemia.
   6. Decreases left ventricular afterload
   7. Decreases ventricular compliance
   8. Increases intracranial pressure, by increasing central venous pressure

Key Effects of PEEP

Beneficial	Adverse
Usually improves oxygenation	May worsen gas exchange
Stabilizes and recruits lung units	Decreases cardiac output
Improves lung compliance	Can cause barotrauma
Minimizes potential for ventilator-induced lung injury	Interferes with assessment of hemodynamic pressures

817

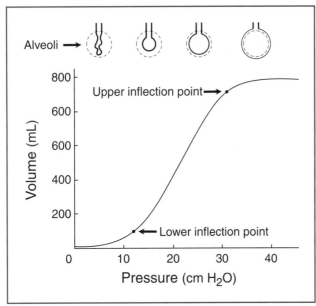

Figure 225-1. Lung inspiratory pressure–volume curve in a patient with acute respiratory distress syndrome. The outlines at the top of the graph indicate the state of alveolar inflation relative to maximum physiologic distention (dashed circles). The central linear portion of the curve demonstrates that large volume changes result when pressure changes occur between the two inflection points; i.e., when lung compliance, represented by the slope of the pressure–volume curve, is maximal. At airway pressures above the upper inflection point, compliance decreases, the limit of lung distention is approached, and the risk of barotrauma is high. Airway pressures below the lower inflection point are associated with low compliance, alveolar collapse, and atelectasis. A proposed strategy for optimizing mechanical ventilation and PEEP is to select a PEEP level just above the lower inflection point, and maintain plateau airway pressures below the upper inflexion point.

Procedure (Initiation and Titration of PEEP)

A. Begin PEEP at 5 cm H_2O.

B. Increase or decrease in increments of 2 or 3 cm H_2O.

C. After each adjustment of PEEP, assess effects on pulmonary function, pressure–volume relationships, oxygenation, and hemodynamics (see Monitoring section, below).

D. Goal of titration is to achieve optimal PEEP, which may be defined as the level of PEEP that allows the lowest FIO_2 (or FIO_2 less than 0.50, if achievable) while maintaining adequate oxygenation (PaO_2 greater than 60 torr, SaO_2 greater than 0.90) and avoiding uncorrectable adverse effects induced by PEEP.

E. Alternative proposed definitions of optimal PEEP

1. PEEP set to 2 cm H_2O above the lower inflection point of the inspiratory pressure–volume curve (see Fig. 225–1)

2. Level of PEEP associated with maximal lung compliance

3. Level of PEEP associated with maximal systemic oxygen delivery

4. Level of PEEP associated with minimum pulmonary venous admixture (intrapulmonary shunt)

Monitoring

A. Observe for development of barotrauma.

1. Manifestations include pneumothorax (including tension pneumothorax), subcutaneous emphysema, pneumomediastinum, interstitial emphysema, pneumoperitoneum, pneumopericardium, gas cysts, and systemic gas embolism.

2. Associated with plateau airway pressures greater than 35 cm H_2O, particularly in later stages of acute respiratory distress syndrome (ARDS) with lung remodeling

B. Monitor pulmonary function.

1. Monitor gas exchange by pulse oximetry or arterial blood gases.

2. Monitor airway plateau pressure and inspiratory:expiratory (I:E) ratio.

3. Assess effects on lung pressure–volume relationship (see Fig. 225–1).

C. Monitor hemodynamic effects of PEEP.

1. Assess for changes in heart rate, blood pressure, and indicators of organ perfusion (e.g., urine output, sensorium, and blood lactate concentration).

2. If available, monitor for changes in cardiac output and $S\bar{v}O_2$.

3. Consider fluid challenge if hypotension or signs of hypoperfusion manifest.

4. Positive end-expiratory pressure complicates interpretation of central venous pressure (CVP) and pulmonary artery occlusion pressure (PAOP).

   a. Positive end-expiratory pressure increases measured (i.e., intraluminal) values of CVP and PAOP by increasing intrathoracic pressure. Preload, however, is decreased.

   b. Right and left ventricular preload are dependent on transmural end-diastolic ventricular volumes (or corresponding pressures at a given level of ventricular compliance), and PEEP can increase the pressure on both sides of the cardiac chambers and intrathoracic veins.

   c. Increased intraluminal venous pressure opposes venous return to the right and left heart, resulting in decreased ventricular filling and preload.

d. The degree of transmission of PEEP to intrathoracic pressure varies with the degree of lung injury and its effect on lung compliance.

D. Monitor for auto-PEEP.

1. Auto-PEEP, or intrinsic PEEP, is due to inadequate time for lung emptying in the setting of increased airway resistance and expiratory flow limitation.

a. Can be caused by expiratory flow limitation (e.g., bronchospasm), severely decreased compliance (e.g., ARDS), and very high minute ventilation (e.g., hyperventilation or trauma)

b. Adverse effects include increased work of breathing, risk of barotrauma or volutrauma, and hemodynamic compromise.

2. Auto-PEEP is quantified as the difference between mean alveolar pressure and external airway pressure at end-expiration.

a. Newer generation ventilators can provide automated assessment of auto-PEEP.

b. May be manually determined by placing patient on assist-controlled mode, occluding airway at end-expiration, and observing passive increase in airway pressure

3. A goal of therapy should be to achieve the lowest practicable level of auto-PEEP.

Key Treatment Strategies for Minimizing Auto-PEEP

- Aggressive bronchodilator therapy

- Pain control and treatment of fever, to decrease minute volume

- Adequate sedation; consider selective use of neuromuscular blockade

- Minimize I:E; e.g., increase expiratory time and inspiratory flow rate, reduce tidal volume, reduce respiratory rate.

- In some cases, judicious application of (extrinsic) PEEP will counter intrinsic PEEP and decrease the work of breathing.

Bibliography

Lu Q, Vieira SRR, Richecoeur J, et al. A simple automated method for measuring pressure–volume curves during mechanical ventilation. Am J Respir Crit Care Med 1999;159:275–282.

Ranieri VM, Dambrosio M, Brienza N. Intrinsic PEEP and cardiopulmonary interaction in patients with COPD and acute ventilatory failure. Eur Respir J 1996;9:1283–1292.

Ranieri VM, Grasso S, Fiore T, Giuliani R. Auto-positive end-expiratory pressure and dynamic hyperinflation. Clin Chest Med 1996;:379–394.

Richard J-C, Maggiore, SM, Jonson B, et al. Influence of tidal volume on alveolar recruitment. Respective role of PEEP and a recruitment maneuver. Am J Respir Crit Care Med. 2001;163:1609–1613.

Vieira SRR, Puybasset L, Richecoeur J, et al. A lung computed tomographic assessment of positive end-expiratory pressure-induced lung overdistension. Am J Resp Crit Care Med 1998;158:1571–1577.

226 Discontinuing Mechanical Ventilation

Francisco J. Soto
Kalpalatha K. Guntupalli

The terms *discontinuing, liberating* or *weaning* from mechanical ventilation are commonly used to describe the process of removing a patient from ventilatory assistance and allowing resumption of spontaneous breathing. After general anesthesia, some drug overdoses, and certain other conditions, the duration of mechanical ventilation is typically short, and extubation is easily accomplished. When ventilatory assistance is required for cardiopulmonary insufficiency, especially in the setting of chronic obstructive lung disease or multiple organ system failure, weaning is usually more protracted, and may consume up to one-third of the total time on mechanical ventilation. The optimal method for weaning is controversial. Many physicians employ an empiric approach. Withdrawing ventilator support may involve periods of spontaneous breathing alternating with periods of ventilatory support, or a gradual reduction in the proportion of ventilation contributed by the ventilator. Weaning from mechanical support should be distinguished from the safe removal of an endotracheal tube or tracheostomy tube.

Indications

A. General considerations
  1. Improvement or resolution of the cause of respiratory failure
  2. Adequate level of consciousness
  3. Reduced sedative requirement (a daily "sedative holiday" reduces ventilator and intensive care unit [ICU] duration)
  4. Cardiopulmonary stability
B. Respiratory considerations
  1. PaO_2/FIO_2 at least 200 torr on positive end-expiratory pressure 5 cm H_2O or less
  2. Stable $PaCO_2$
  3. Spontaneous respiratory drive
  4. Adequate airway defense mechanisms and spontaneous clearance of secretions
C. Cardiovascular considerations
  1. Reduced or no requirement for vasoactive support
  2. Stabilization of myocardial ischemia, left ventricular failure, cardiac dysrhythmias
D. Other considerations
  1. Stable or improving nutritional status
  2. Stable and adequate hemoglobin concentration (generally more than 8 g/dL)
  3. Control of fluid, electrolyte, and renal status
  4. Sedation discontinued
  5. Address infections, ileus, constipation, ICU-associated myopathy, hypothyroidism, adrenal insufficiency

---

PEARL

Self-extubation: manage selected patients expectantly; many will not require reintubation

---

Procedure

A. Bedside weaning parameters (always obtained without mechanical assistance)
  1. Respiratory rate (f) should be less than 30 breaths/minute.
  2. Tidal volume should generally be greater than 5 mL/kg.
  3. Rapid shallow breathing index
     a. Calculated as f/Vt
     b. Quotient less than 105 breaths/minute per L predicts weaning success with good sensitivity and fair specificity.
     c. The single best, simple index of assessing readiness for weaning
  4. Maximum inspiratory pressure (negative inspiratory force)
     a. Difficult to perform; requires patient cooperation
     b. Absolute values greater than 20 cm H_2O are associated with weaning success.
     c. More predictive of weaning failure than success
  5. Vital capacity
     a. Assesses single breath muscle performance
     b. Values greater than 10 mL/kg suggest improved chances of weaning (but predictive value is poor).
  6. Minute ventilation ($\dot{V}e$)
     a. Calculated as f × Vt (poor predictive value)
     b. $\dot{V}e$ of 5 to 10 L/minute is favorable for successful weaning.

c. $\dot{V}e$ of 10 to 15 L/minute is less favorable.

d. $\dot{V}e > 15$ L/minute is least favorable for successful weaning.

7. Airway occlusion pressure ($P_{0.1}$)

a. The airway pressure 0.1 second after beginning of inspiration against an occluded airway; assesses respiratory drive

b. $P_{0.1}$ lower than 2 cm H_2O predicts successful weaning.

c. $P_{0.1}$ higher than 5 cm H_2O predicts weaning failure.

d. May be performed before and after CO_2 challenge

e. Technically difficult and requires special equipment

8. Other indices: work of breathing, oxygen cost of breathing, static compliance, airway resistance, tension–time index, dead-space (Vd), Vd/Vt, maximum voluntary ventilation, transdiaphragmatic pressure

B. Weaning methods

1. Spontaneous breathing trial

a. T-piece (Brigg's adaptor) circuitry is commonly employed, typically with approximately 5 cm H_2O continuous positive airway pressure, with humidified gas flow delivering at least twice $\dot{V}e$, at FIO_2 set to pre-trial level.

b. Performed for a 30-minute to 2-hour interval at least once daily

c. Consider extubation if trial is well tolerated by patient; if not, repeat next day unless contraindicated.

d. May be the most rapid method of weaning

2. Intermittent mandatory ventilation with stepwise reduction of mandatory breaths (typically in increments of 1 to 3 breaths/minute)

a. When the patient tolerates an intermittent mandatory ventilation rate below 5 or 6 breaths/minute, consider extubation.

b. May be used in conjunction with pressure support

c. May be the slowest method of weaning

3. Pressure support

a. Positive inspiratory pressure assists spontaneous ventilation, overcomes circuit resistance, and decreases the work of breathing.

b. May be combined with intermittent mandatory ventilation

c. Typically initiated at pressure support levels of approximately 15 cm H_2O to achieve acceptable Vt, and incrementally reduced by 2

to 5 cm H_2O until a level of approximately 5 to 7 cm H_2O is reached

d. Once the patient tolerates minimal pressure support settings (~5 to 7 cm H_2O), a 2-hour trial on these settings should be attempted at least daily. If the trial is well tolerated, consider extubation.

e. Pressure support weaning is usually faster than intermittent mandatory ventilation.

4. Criteria indicative of intolerance to weaning trial

a. Dyspnea or f greater than 35 breaths/minute

b. Heart rate or systolic blood pressure increase by more than 20% over baseline

c. Agitation, diminished sensorium, or diaphoresis

d. Cardiac dysrhythmias

e. Hypoxemia (PaO_2 less than 60 torr or SpO_2 less than 0.90)

f. Respiratory acidosis (arterial pH 7.30 or less)

Key Parameters Predictive of Successful Weaning

- f/Vt less than 100 breaths/minute per L

- Maximum inspiratory force greater than 20 cm H_2O

- Vital capacity greater than 10 mL/kg

- Minute ventilation less than 10 L/minute

Special Considerations

A. Ensure adequate treatment of bronchospasm.

B. Correct sleep deprivation, anxiety, and pain.

C. Post-extubation management

1. Discontinue respiratory depressants.

2. Monitor for at least 4 hours in ICU to detect intolerance to extubation.

3. Observe for post-extubation stridor.

4. Provide tracheal toilet.

5. Elevate head of bed, if possible.

6. Delay resumption of enteral feeding for at least 4 hours.

7. Reintubation rate may be as high as 20% and is not affected by weaning method.

D. Treatment of post-extubation stridor (may be due to glottic edema, tracheal stenosis, or laryngospasm)

1. Bronchodilators, aerosolized racemic epinephrine, parenteral corticosteroids

2. Noninvasive continuous positive airway pressure or positive pressure ventilation

3. Heliox

E. Tracheostomy

1. Indication is prolonged mechanical ventilation (more than 14 days or obvious need for prolonged ventilation).

2. Improves patient comfort, facilitates suctioning, and may enable speech

3. Less risk of laryngeal injury compared to prolonged endotracheal intubation

4. Complications include hemorrhage, pneumothorax, unintended decannulation, tracheal stenosis, death (mortality rate up to 2%).

PEARL

There is no clear evidence that weaning techniques improve respiratory muscle endurance.

Bibliography

Brochard L, Rauss A, Benito S, et al. Comparison of three methods of gradual withdrawal from ventilatory support during weaning from mechanical ventilation. Am J Respir Crit Care Med 1994;150:896–903.

Epstein SK. Etiology of extubation failure and the predictive value of the rapid shallow breathing index. Am J Respir Crit Care Med 1995;152:545–549.

Epstein SK, Ciubotaru RL, Wong JB. Effect of failed extubation on the outcome of mechanical ventilation. Chest 1997;112:186–192.

Esteban A, Alia I, Tobin MJ, et al. Effect of spontaneous breathing trial duration on outcome of attempts to discontinue mechanical ventilation. Am J Respir Crit Care Med 1999;159:512–518.

Esteban A, Frutos F, Tobin MJ, et al. A comparison of four methods of weaning patients from mechanical ventilation. N Engl J Med 1995;332:345–350.

Fisher MM, Raper RF. The "cuff-leak" test for extubation. Anaesthesia 1992;47:10–12.

Kress JP, Pohlman AS, O'Connor MF, et al. Daily interruption of sedative infusions in critically ill patients undergoing mechanical ventilation. N Engl J Med 2000;342: 1471–1477.

Vallverdu I, Calaf N, Subirana M, et al. Clinical characteristics, respiratory functional parameters, and outcome of a two-hour T-piece trial in patients weaning from mechanical ventilation. Am J Respir Crit Care Med 1998; 158:1855–1862.

Index

Note: Page numbers followed by the letter f refer to figures and those followed by t refer to tables.

A

AAA (abdominal aortic aneurysm), 444, 509–511
A-aDO$_2$ (alveolar–arterial oxygen tension gradient), 790
a/APO$_2$ (alveolar–arterial oxygen tension ratio), 790
ABCD (amphotericin B colloidal dispersion), 672t
Abciximab, 624–625
Abdominal aortic aneurysm (AAA), 444, 509–511
Abdominal auscultation, 440
Abdominal pain, acute, 439–445
in pancreatitis, 439, 441, 443, 446–449
Abdominal paracentesis, 716–718
Abdominal radiography
in abdominal trauma, 491–493
in acute abdominal pain, 442
in acute pancreatitis, 447
in diarrhea, 472
in toxic megacolon, 475
Abdominal trauma, 491–493
Abelcet. See Amphotericin B lipid complex (ABLC).
ABLC (amphotericin B lipid complex), 672t
ABO incompatibility, 3, 429
Abortion, septic, 553–554
Abruptio placentae, 554–555
Abscess
brain, 328, 333, 336
hepatic, 334–335, 337
intraperitoneal, 335–336
pancreatic, 335, 337, 446
paravertebral, 374
perinephric, 386
renal, 386
spinal epidural, 298–300, 328
splenic, 335, 337
tubo-ovarian, 439
ACE inhibitors. See Angiotensin converting enzyme (ACE) inhibitors.
Acebutolol, 576, 629
Acetaminophen
before intravenous HBIG, 373
drug interactions with, 201
for fever, 2
hepatic failure induced by, 202, 459, 461
overdose of, 201–204, 264–265
N-acetylcysteine for, 202–204, 459
Acetate, in parenteral nutrition solutions, 765
Acetazolamide, 589–591
Acetoacetate
in alcoholic ketoacidosis, 161–162
in diabetic ketoacidosis, 164–165
Acetonitrile ingestion, 247–248
Acetylcholine, 269
in myasthenia gravis, 304

N-Acetylcysteine (NAC)
for acetaminophen overdose, 202–204, 459
in methemoglobinemia, 255
Acetylsalicylic acid. See Aspirin.
Acid-base balance, 154–157, 155f
for continuous renal replacement therapy, 736
in rhabdomyolysis, 544, 545
Acidemia, 154
apnea test in, 745
Acid-inhibiting agents, 593–596
drug interactions with, 594–595
hypophosphatemia induced by, 147
in acute pancreatitis, 448
preoperative, 487
to prevent aspiration, 43
Acidosis, 154. See also Ketoacidosis.
lactic, 158–160
metabolic, 155–157, 155f
pulseless electrical activity due to, 112t, 113t
respiratory, 154–157, 155f
Acinetobacter baumanii infection, 333
Aciphex. See Rabeprazole.
Acquired immune deficiency syndrome (AIDS), 356–358, 357f
acute abdominal pain in, 445
cytomegalovirus infection in, 354
Pneumocystis carinii pneumonia in, 2–3, 38–39, 356, 359–361
transfusion-associated, 429
Acticoat, for burns, 514
Activated charcoal for drug overdose, 198
acetaminophen, 202, 204
alcohols and glycols, 237
calcium channel blockers or β-blockers, 226
cocaine, 221
cyanide, 246
cyclic antidepressants, 260
digoxin, 230
neuroleptics, 258
organophosphates, 270
salicylate, 207
sedative-hypnotics or narcotics, 211
theophylline, 214
Activated protein C, human recombinant. See Drotrecogin alfa activated.
Acute autonomic neuropathy, 307
Acute chest syndrome
chemotherapy-induced, 641, 642
in sickle cell disease, 433–434
Acute inflammatory demyelinating polyradiculoneuropathy (AIDP), 307
Acute motor axonal neuropathy (AMAN), 307
Acute motor sensory axonal neuropathy (AMSAN), 307
Acute renal failure (ARF), 477–480, 479t

Acute respiratory distress syndrome (ARDS), 23–26
chemotherapy-induced, 641
fat embolism with, 540, 541
high-frequency ventilation for, 814
in fulminant hepatic failure, 460
lung-protective ventilator strategy in, 24, 29
Acute sensory axonal neuropathy (ASAN), 307
Acute sequestration crisis in sickle cell disease, 433–434
Acyclovir
for bone marrow transplant recipients, 367
for herpes simplex virus infection, 351, 368, 373, 393
for organ transplant recipients, 373, 522
for varicella-zoster virus infection, 352
for viral pneumonia, 41
Adalat. See Nifedipine.
Adapin. See Doxepin.
Addison's disease, 132, 139, 191–193
Adenosine, 629–633
in atrial fibrillation, 104
in supraventricular tachycardia, 108–110
ADH (antidiuretic hormone)
in diabetes insipidus, 174–177
in syndrome of inappropriate antidiuresis, 178–180
Adrenal insufficiency, 191–193
preoperative evaluation in, 485
Adrenergic agonists, centrally acting, 575
for alcohol withdrawal syndrome, 242, 243
β$_1$-Adrenergic myocardial receptors, 571
β$_2$-Adrenergic receptor agonists, 636–638, 637t
for COPD, 46
for status asthmaticus, 34–35
α$_1$-Adrenergic receptor blockers, peripheral, 575
β-Adrenergic receptor blockers, 224–225, 224t, 576–581, 629
after peripheral vascular bypass, 505
classification of, 223
conduction disturbances induced by, 116
contraindications to, 61, 67, 577
cocaine intoxication, 220
tetanus, 315
for acute MI, 66–67
for alcohol withdrawal syndrome, 242, 243
for aortic dissection, 103, 576
for atrial fibrillation, 105
for mitral valve dysfunction, 72, 94
for monoamine oxidase inhibitor-tyramine interaction, 576
for pheochromocytoma, 189, 190

β-Adrenergic receptor blockers (Continued)
  for supraventricular tachycardia, 110
  for unstable angina, 61
  in cyclic antidepressant overdose, 261
  in intracerebral hemorrhage, 285
  in subarachnoid hemorrhage, 289
  in theophylline overdose, 215
  overdose of, 225–228
α_1-Adrenergic receptors, 571
α_2-Adrenergic receptors, 571
β_2-Adrenergic receptors, 571
Aerosol mask, 803–804, 806
AFB stain and culture, 375–376
Afterload, 5
Afterload reduction
  for cardiogenic pulmonary edema, 22, 78
  for mitral valve dysfunction, 72
Aggrastat. See Tirofiban.
Agranulocytosis, neuroleptic-induced, 257
AIDP (acute inflammatory demyelinating polyradiculoneuropathy), 307
AIDS. See Acquired immune deficiency syndrome (AIDS).
AIHA (warm autoimmune hemolytic anemia), 425–427
Air embolism, 561–563
Air-entrainment mask, 803, 806
Air-fluidized bed, 558
Airway management. See also Mechanical ventilation.
  endotracheal intubation, 677–682
  for COPD, 46
  for epiglottitis, 403
  for hemoptysis, 55
  for inhalation injury, 52, 513, 514
  for pneumonia, 41
    aspiration, 44
  for status asthmaticus, 34–35
  for tachypnea, 16
  in head trauma patients, 495
  in spinal cord-injured patients, 299
Airway pressure-release ventilation, 814
Airway stents, 711
AKA (alcoholic ketoacidosis), 161–163
Akathisia
  neuroleptic-induced, 257
  treatment of, 258
Albright's hereditary osteodystrophy, 135
Albumin, 566
  plasma assay of, 771
Albuterol, 637t, 638
  for COPD, 46
  for hyperkalemia, 133
  for status asthmaticus, 34
Alcohol, interaction with benzodiazepines, 608t
Alcohol abuse, 452
Alcohol intoxication, 12, 13, 209, 233–235, 237, 240, 452
Alcohol withdrawal syndrome (AWS), 240–243, 241t, 242t
  antihypertensives for, 576
Alcoholic hepatitis, acute, 452–454
Alcoholic ketoacidosis (AKA), 161–163
Alfenta. See Alfentanil.
Alfentanil, 604t
Alitrag, 761
Alkalemia, 154
Alkaline phosphatase serum activity, 441
Alkalosis, 154
  metabolic, 155, 155f, 157
  respiratory, 154, 155f, 156, 157
Allen test, 687
Allergic reactions
  anaphylaxis, 534–536

Allergic reactions (Continued)
  to hemodialysis, 732
  to transfusion, 429–430, 432
Allopurinol, for tumor lysis syndrome, 547
All-trans-retinoic acid, 641
Alopecia, toxin-induced, 195
Alteplase, 622
Alternating-pressure air mattress, 558
Aluminum hydroxide or carbonate, for hyperphosphatemia, 152
Alupent. See Metaproterenol.
Alveolar oxygen tension (PAO_2), 790
Alveolar ventilation ($\dot{V}_A$), 791
Alveolar–arterial oxygen tension gradient (A-aDO_2), 790
Alveolar–arterial oxygen tension ratio (a/APO_2), 790
AMAN (acute motor axonal neuropathy), 307
Amantadine
  for parkinsonism, 258
  for viral pneumonia, 41
  prophylaxis for influenza, 47
AmBisome. See Liposomal amphotericin B.
AMC (arm muscle circumference), 771
Amikacin, 650–652
  for tuberculosis, 661–663
Amiloride, 589–591
  for diabetes insipidus, 177
Amino acids, in parenteral nutrition solutions, 765
γ-Aminobutyric acid (GABA) receptors, 605
ϵ-Aminocaproic acid, for coagulopathy in fulminant hepatic failure, 460
Aminoglycoside antibiotics, 650–652
Aminophylline
  for COPD, 46
  for status asthmaticus, 35
4-Aminopyridine, for calcium channel blocker overdose, 227
Amiodarone, 629–633
  for atrial fibrillation, 105
  for atrial flutter, 106
  for supraventricular tachycardia, 110
  for ventricular tachydysrhythmias, 115
  in neuroleptic overdose, 257
Amitriptyline, 259
Amlodipine, 224t, 576
Amniotic fluid embolism, 553
Amoxacillin, 645, 648
Amoxapine, 259
Amoxicillin, 645, 646, 648
  for COPD, 47
Amoxicillin-clavulanate, 645, 646, 648
Amphotec. See Amphotericin B colloidal dispersion.
Amphotericin B, 671, 672t, 673–676, 674t
  drug interactions with, 676
  for aspergillosis, 349
  for blastomycosis, 348–349
  for candidal infection, 341–342, 368
  for catheter-related bloodstream infection, 405
  for coccidioidomycosis, 348
  for cryptococcosis, 348
  for histoplasmosis, 348
  for Malassezia furfur, 348
  for mucormycosis, 349
  for neutropenic cancer patients, 364
  for organ transplant recipients, 372
Amphotericin B colloidal dispersion (ABCD), 672t
Amphotericin B lipid complex (ABLC), 672t
Ampicillin, 645, 646, 648
Ampicillin-sulbactam, 645, 648
  for acute cholecystitis, 451

Ampicillian-sulbactam (Continued)
  for epiglottitis, 403
  for intra-abdominal infection, 338
  for organ transplant recipients, 372
  for sinusitis, 337
  for urosepsis, 385
Amprenavir, interaction with benzodiazepines, 608t
Amrinone, 568–570, 572t
  for calcium channel blocker or b-blocker overdose, 227
  for left ventricular systolic dysfunction, 7
Amsacrine, 642
AMSAN (acute motor sensory axonal neuropathy), 307
Amyl nitrite, for cyanide poisoning, 246
Amylase serum level, 441
  in pancreatitis, 446
Anafranil. See Clomipramine.
Analgesics
  after cardiac surgery, 501
  epidural, after peripheral vascular bypass, 505
  for burn injury, 514
  for delivery of infant in preeclampsia, 86
  for pressure ulcers, 557
  for rib fractures, 490
  for subarachnoid hemorrhage, 289
  for vaso-occlusive crisis in sickle cell disease, 433–434
  narcotic agonists, 602–604, 604t
  opiate overdose, 12, 13, 209–212
  preoperative, 487
Anaphylactoid syndrome of pregnancy, 553
Anaphylaxis, 534–536
  epinephrine for, 572–573
  transfusion reaction, 429–430, 432, 534
Ancobon. See 5-Flucytosine (5-FC).
Anectine. See Succinylcholine.
Anemia, 421–424, 422f
  oxygen transport variables in, 783t
  preoperative evaluation in, 485
Anesthesia
  anaphylactic reactions to, 534
  for cardioversion and defibrillation, 701–703
  for central venous catheterization, 683
  for chest tube thoracostomy, 724
  for endotracheal intubation, 678
  for fiberoptic bronchoscopy, 710
  for paracentesis, 716
  for Sengstaken-Blakemore tube placement, 749
  for thoracentesis, 719
  for transnasal intubation, 755
  malignant hyperthermia precipitated by, 301–303
Aneurysm, abdominal aortic, 444, 509–511
Angina
  grading of, 60t
  unstable, 59–63
Angiography
  abdominal, 442
  aortic, 102, 489
  bronchial, 55
  cerebral, 284
  for brain death determination, 744
  for lower gastrointestinal bleeding, 468
  for peripheral arterial occlusion, 507–508
  in abdominal aortic aneurysm, 509
  in endocarditis, 381–382
  pulmonary, 32
  upper gastrointestinal, 463
Angioplasty, carotid, 283
Angiotensin converting enzyme (ACE) inhibitors, 575–581

Angiotensin converting enzyme (ACE) inhibitors (Continued)
  contraindicated in pregnancy, 87, 552
  for acute MI, 67
  for cardiogenic pulmonary edema, 22, 78
  for cerebral infarction, 576
  for hypertensive nephropathy, 576
  for unstable angina, 62
  in intracerebral hemorrhage, 285
Anion gap. See Serum anion gap; Urine anion gap.
Anisoylated plasminogen-streptokinase activator complex (APSAC), 622–623
Anistreplase, 622
Anorectal bleeding, 466
Anorexia, abdominal pain with, 440
Antacids. See Acid-inhibiting agents.
Anterior cord syndrome, 298
Anthracyclines, cardiotoxicity of, 642–643
Anthropometry, 771
Antibiotics. See also specific drugs.
  aminoglycosides, 650–652
  anaphylactic reactions to, 534
  antituberculosis, 660–664
  carbapenems, 665–669
  cephalosporins, 645–649
  clindamycin, 665–669
  colitis associated with, 3
  during intracranial pressure monitoring, 798
  fluoroquinolones, 653–654
  for acute cholecystitis, 451
  for acute pancreatitis, 448
  for bone marrow transplant recipients, 367–368
  for catheter-related bloodstream infection, 405
  for clostridial gas gangrene, 332
  for COPD, 47
  for corynebacterial infection, 331
  for craniotomy patients, 499
  for deep space infections of neck, 389
  for endocarditis, 382–383
  for enterococcal infection, 331
  for epiglottitis, 403
  for Gram-negative infections, 337–338
  for head trauma patients, 495
  for infections in neutropenic cancer patients, 362–364
  for infectious diarrhea, 472–473
  for inhalation injury, 52, 514
  for Listeria monocytogenes infection, 331–332
  for meningitis, 337, 390
  for necrotizing soft-tissue infections, 400
  for organ transplant recipients, 372
  for pharyngeal diphtheria, 389
  for pneumonia, 40
    aspiration, 44
    Pneumocystis carinii, 360t
  for pressure ulcers, 557–558
  for Rhodococcus equi infection, 332
  for septic abortion, 554
  for septic shock, 325
  for spinal epidural abscess, 300
  for staphylococcal infections, 329
  for streptococcal infections, 330
  for tetanus, 315
  for toxic megacolon, 475
  for toxic shock syndrome, 396
  for urosepsis, 385
  for wound botulism, 313
  in ARDS, 26
  in status asthmaticus, 35
  interaction with benzodiazepines, 608t
  linezolid, 665–669

Antibiotics (Continued)
  macrolides, 655–659, 656t
  methemoglobinemia induced by, 253
  metronidazole, 665–670
  penicillins, 645–649
  preoperative, 487
  QT interval prolongation induced by, 114
  vancomycin, 663–667
Anticholinergic drugs
  for COPD, 46
  for fiberoptic bronchoscopy, 710
Anticholinergic poisoning, 263–266
Anticoagulants, 617–621. See also specific drugs.
  complications of, 419
  drug interactions with, 619
  for continuous renal replacement therapy, 735
  for deep venous thrombosis, 418
  for hypercoagulable states, 414–415
  for patients with prosthetic heart valves, 93t
  for peripheral arterial occlusion, 508
  in acute MI, 67
  in cor pulmonale, 49
  in pulmonary embolism, 32
  in unstable angina, 62
  post-craniotomy, 499
  prothrombotic state induced by, 413
  to prevent cerebral infarction, 282–283
Anticonvulsants, 611–616. See also specific drugs.
  drug interactions with, 612–613
  for post-cardiac arrest myoclonic seizures, 280
  for preeclampsia during labor and delivery, 86
  for status epilepticus, 13, 278–279
  for theophylline overdose, 215
  in alcohol withdrawal syndrome, 242, 243
  in anticholinergic poisoning, 265
  in calcium channel blocker or β-blocker overdose, 226
  in cyclic antidepressant overdose, 261
  in intracerebral hemorrhage, 285
  in neuroleptic overdose, 258
  in organophosphate poisoning, 270
  in salicylate intoxication, 207
  in serotonin syndrome, 268
  in theophylline overdose, 215
  post-craniotomy, 498
Antidepressants, 259
  cyclic, overdose of, 259–262
  serotonin syndrome induced by, 267–268
Antidiarrheal agents, 472
Antidiuretic hormone (ADH)
  in diabetes insipidus, 174–177
  in syndrome of inappropriate antidiuresis, 178–180
Antidotes, 199t
  for acetaminophen overdose, 202–204
Antidysrhythmic agents, 629–633. See also specific drugs.
  conduction disturbances induced by, 116
  for atrial fibrillation, 105
  for atrial flutter, 106
  for supraventricular tachycardia, 109–110
  in anticholinergic poisoning, 265
  in cyclic antidepressant overdose, 261
  in digoxin overdose, 232
  in neuroleptic overdose, 257–258
  in theophylline overdose, 215
  QT interval prolongation induced by, 114

Anti-emetics
  after N-acetylcysteine for acetaminophen overdose, 203
  to prevent aspiration, 44
Antifibrinolytic therapy, 411
Antifungal drugs, 671–676, 672t, 674t. See also specific drugs.
  drug interactions with, 676
  for aspergillosis, 349
  for blastomycosis, 348–349
  for bone marrow transplant recipients, 368
  for candidal infection, 341–342
  for coccidioidomycosis, 348
  for cryptococcosis, 348
  for histoplasmosis, 348
  for Malassezia furfur, 348
  for mucormycosis, 349
  for neutropenic cancer patients, 364
  for organ transplant recipients, 372
  for Trichosporon beigelii, 348
  interaction with benzodiazepines, 608t
  resistance to, 675
Antihistamines
  for anaphylaxis, 535
  QT interval prolongation induced by, 114
Antihypertensives, 575–581. See also specific drugs.
  cautions in head trauma patients, 496
  for aortic dissection, 103, 576
  for hypertensive crisis, 82, 577
  for pheochromocytoma, 189–190, 577
  in cocaine intoxication, 221
  in Guillain-Barré syndrome, 309
  in intracerebral hemorrhage, 285
  in pregnancy, 85, 87, 576
  in subarachnoid hemorrhage, 289
  preoperative, 487
Antilymphocyte immunoglobulin, for kidney transplantation, 521
Antiparkinsonian drugs, 258
Antiplatelet agents, to prevent cerebral infarction, 282
Antipyretics, 2, 532
Antithrombin III, 406, 413–414, 416–417
Antituberculosis drugs, 660–664
Antivenin
  for Centruroides exilicauda sting, 275
  for Latrodectus bite, 275
  for snakebites, 274–275, 274t
Antiviral drugs. See also specific drugs.
  for cytomegalovirus infection, 355
  for herpes simplex virus infection, 351
  for varicella-zoster virus infection, 352
Aortic aneurysm, abdominal (AAA), 444, 509–511
Aortic dissection, 102–103, 103f
  antihypertensives for, 576
  hypertension in, 82
  vs. acute MI, 65
  vs. angina, 60
Aortic injuries, 489, 490
Aortic regurgitation (AR), 90–92, 94
Aortic stenosis (AS), 90–93
Aortic valve replacement (AVR), 93–94
Aortoenteric fistula, 465, 468, 510
Aortography, 509
Apical approach for pericardiocentesis, 705
Aplastic anemia, 421
Aplastic crisis in sickle cell disease, 433–434
Apnea test, 742–745
Appendicitis, 440, 441, 443
APSAC (anisoylated plasminogen-streptokinase activator complex), 622–623
AR (aortic regurgitation), 90–92, 94

Arachnid bites, 272–275
Ardeparin, 620t
ARDS. *See* Acute respiratory distress syndrome (ARDS).
Arduan. *See* Pipercuronium.
ARF (acute renal failure), 477–480
Argatroban, 418, 617, 619–621
Arizona coral snakebite, 272
Arm muscle circumference (AMC), 771
Arterial air embolism, 561
Arterial blood gases
    acid-base disturbances, 154–157, 155f
    in alcohol withdrawal syndrome, 241
    in ARDS, 24
    in burn patients, 515
    in carbon monoxide poisoning, 250
    in cardiogenic shock, 89
    in cor pulmonale, 49
    in cyanide poisoning, 245
    in hypothermia, 526
    in lactic acidosis, 159
    in myasthenia gravis, 305–306
    in *Pneumocystis carinii* pneumonia, 360
    in pulmonary edema, 21
    in pulmonary embolism, 30
    in status asthmaticus, 34
    monitoring of, 788–792
Arterial carbon dioxide tension ($PaCO_2$), 790
Arterial catheterization, 687–689, 688f, 689f
Arterial oxygen content (CaO_2), 781, 783t, 790
Arterial oxygen saturation (SaO_2), 789, 792
Arterial oxygen tension (PaO_2), 789
Arteriography. *See* Angiography.
Arteriovenous oxygen content difference ($a\bar{v}DO_2$), 781–782, 783t
Arthritis, tuberculous, 374
Arthropod bites, 272–275
AS (aortic stenosis), 90–93
ASAN (acute sensory axonal neuropathy), 307
Ascites
    laboratory findings in, 718t
    paracentesis for, 716–718
Ascorbic acid, for methemoglobinemia, 255
Asendin. *See* Amoxapine.
L-Asparaginase, 642–644
Aspergillus infection, 344, 346, 347, 349
    antifungal therapy for, 671–676
    in bone marrow transplant patients, 366–368
    in organ transplant recipients, 370, 372, 523
Aspiration
    during oxygen therapy, 807
    enteral feeding-associated, 763
    pneumonitis/pneumonia, 37, 40, 42–45
    preoperative prophylaxis for, 487
Aspirin
    for acute MI, 66, 69
    for cerebral infarction, 282
    for fever, 2
    for hypercalcemia, 141
    for pericarditis, 98
    for unstable angina, 61
    intoxication with, 205–208
Assist-controlled ventilation, 808, 811f
Asthma, 34, 485
Atelectasis, 57–58
    denitrogenation, 806–807
Atenolol, 224t, 576, 579t
    before peripheral vascular bypass, 505
    for acute MI, 66–67

Atovaquone, for *Pneumocystis carinii* pneumonia, 360t
Atracurium, 599, 599t, 600
    for endotracheal intubation, 678
Atrial fibrillation and flutter, 104–106, 107
    after cardiac surgery, 502
    digoxin for, 626
    in angina, 60
    in myocardial contusion, 73
Atrial tachycardia, 107
Atrioventricular (AV) block, 116–118
    after cardiac surgery, 502
    cardiac pacing for, 67, 117
    in acute MI, 65
    in angina, 60
    in cyclic antidepressant overdose, 261
    in digoxin overdose, 229, 230, 232
Atrioventricular node re-entry, 107
Atropine
    for acute MI, 67
    for bradycardia, 6, 226
    for conduction disturbances, 117
    for organophosphate poisoning, 270–271
    for pulseless electrical activity, 111
    in cyclic antidepressant overdose, 261
    in digoxin toxicity, 232
Atropine test, 745
Atrovent. *See* Ipratropium bromide.
Aurorix. *See* Moclobemide.
Autoimmune hemolytic anemia (AIHA), warm, 425–427
Autonomic hyperreflexia, 577
Autonomic nervous system dysfunction, in chronic renal failure, 482–483
Auto-PEEP, 811, 819
AV block. *See* Atrioventricular (AV) block.
Aventyl. *See* Nortriptyline.
AVR (aortic valve replacement), 93–94
AWS (alcohol withdrawal syndrome), 240–243, 241t, 242t
$a\bar{v}DO_2$ (arteriovenous oxygen content difference), 781–782, 783t
Axillary vein thrombosis, 420
Azathioprine, 641
    for kidney transplantation, 521
    for myasthenia gravis, 306
Azithromycin, 655, 656t, 657, 658
    for pneumonia, 40, 41
Azotemia
    in diabetic ketoacidosis, 165
    in hyperosmolar nonketotic coma, 168
Aztreonam
    for intra-abdominal infection, 338
    for pneumonia, 40
    for urosepsis, 385

B

Babinski sign, 267
Bacillus cereus infection, 328, 332
Bacteremia, 322
    catheter-related, 404–405
    enterococcal, 330–331
    group B streptococcal, 330
    Staphylococcus aureus, 328, 329
Bacteriuria, 3, 384, 385
BAL. *See* Bronchoalveolar lavage (BAL).
Balloon valvuloplasty
    for aortic stenosis, 93
    for mitral stenosis, 94
Barbiturate coma, 285, 297
Barbiturates
    as anticonvulsants, 611–616
    drug interactions with, 608t, 613

Barbiturates *(Continued)*
    for alcohol withdrawal syndrome, 242, 243
    overdose of, 209–212
Barotrauma, 28–29, 36
    apnea test in patient with, 745
    in ARDS, 24, 28–29
    mechanical ventilation-induced, 28–29, 36, 811, 818
Basal energy expenditure (BEE), 770
Battle's sign, 12
BCNU (carmustine), 641–644
Becaplermin gel, for pressure ulcers, 558
BEE (basal energy expenditure), 770
Benazepril, 575
Benzathine penicillin G, 645
Benzocaine, for endotracheal intubation, 678
Benzodiazepines (BZDs), 605–608
    as anticonvulsants, 611–616
    drug interactions with, 608, 608t, 613
    for akathisia, 258
    for alcohol withdrawal syndrome, 242, 242t, 243
    for anticholinergic poisoning, 265
    for cocaine intoxication, 221
    for endotracheal intubation, 678
    for serotonin syndrome, 268
    for status epilepticus, 278
    in organophosphate poisoning, 270
    overdose of, 209–212
Benztropine, for extrapyramidal symptoms, 258
Benzylpenicillin, 645
Bepridil, 224t
    overdose of, 223
Bernard-Soulier syndrome, 410
Biliary colic, 439
Bilirubin serum concentration, 441
Bio-artificial liver support, 460–461
Biobrane skin substitute, 514
Biopsy
    brain, 392
    bronchial, 711
    open lung, 371
    renal, 9, 478
Bismuth subsalicylate overdose, 205
Bisphosphonates, for hypercalcemia, 141, 142
Bitolterol, 637t, 638
Bivalirudin, 617, 619, 620
BK virus infection, in organ transplant recipients, 370
Black widow spider bite, 272, 273, 275
Bladder obstruction, oliguria due to, 8
Blastomyces dermatitidis infection, 344–349
    antifungal therapy for, 671–676
Bleeding. *See* Hemorrhage.
Bleeding time, 409
Bleomycin, 641
Blood culture, 2
Blood pressure (BP)
    control in intracerebral hemorrhage, 285
    hypertensive crisis, 80–82
    hypokalemia and, 130
    hypotension, 5–7
    measurement of, 5
    pregnancy-induced hypertension, 83–87
    toxin-induced changes in, 195t
Blood substitutes, 424
Blood tests, preoperative, 486
Blood transfusion
    dilutional thrombocytopenia after, 410, 412
    for anemia, 424

Blood transfusion *(Continued)*
for coagulopathy, 407–408
for hemolytic-uremic syndrome, 428
for septic shock, 324
for sickle cell crises, 434
for thrombotic thrombocytopenic purpura, 428
for upper gastrointestinal hemorrhage, 463–464
for warm autoimmune hemolytic anemia, 427
transfusion reactions, 1, 3, 429–432, 534
Bloodstream infection, catheter-related (CRBSI), 404–405
Blue toe syndrome, 507
BMT. *See* Bone marrow transplantation (BMT).
"Body packing"
with cocaine, 220, 221
with narcotics, 211
Body surface area (BSA) estimation, 766–767
Body temperature
fever, 1–4
hypothermia, 525–529, 526t
measurement of, 2
Body weight, 770
Bone marrow transplantation (BMT)
autologous vs. allogeneic, 365
graft-versus-host disease after, 365, 436–438
infections after, 365–368
minitransplantation, 365
thrombotic thrombocytopenic purpura after, 409
Botulinum immunoglobulin, 313
Botulinum toxoid, 313
Botulism, 311–313
Bowel obstruction, 439, 440
BP. *See* Blood pressure (BP).
Bradycardia, 6
after cardiac surgery, 502
in calcium channel blocker or b-blocker overdose, 226
in cardiogenic shock, 88
toxin-induced, 195t
Brain abscess
empiric antibiotic therapy for, 337
Gram-negative, 333, 336, 337
Staphylococcus aureus, 328
Brain biopsy, 392
Brain death, 11
determination of, 742–745
withdrawal of mechanical ventilation in, 741t
Brain herniation, 295–296
Brain injury, traumatic (TBI), 484, 494–497, 497t
diabetes insipidus after, 174
intracranial hypertension and, 293–297
Brain stem reflexes, 11
confirming absence of, 743
Branched-chain amino acids in feeding formulas, 762
Brethaire. *See* Terbutaline.
Brethine. *See* Terbutaline.
Bretylium, 629–633
Bromocriptine, for malignant hyperthermia, 302
Bronchial biopsy, 711
Bronchial injuries, 488, 489
Bronchiectasis, 53
Bronchiolitis obliterans, chemotherapy-induced, 641, 642
Bronchoalveolar lavage (BAL), 711
fluid analysis, 712

Bronchoalveolar lavage (BAL) *(Continued)*
in ARDS, 24, 26
in fat embolism syndrome, 540
in pneumonia, 40
Bronchodilators
for aspiration pneumonia, 44
for atelectasis, 58
for chemotherapy-induced bronchiolitis obliterans, 642
for COPD, 46
for pneumonia, 41
for smoke inhalation, 52
for status asthmaticus, 34–35
inhaled, 636–638
preoperative, 487
Bronchopleural fistula, 489
high-frequency ventilation for, 814
Bronchoscopy, 2, 40
fiberoptic, 709–712
for hemoptysis, 55
in aspiration pneumonia, 44
in atelectasis, 58
in post-transplant pulmonary infections, 371
in smoke inhalation, 51
Bronkometer. *See* Isoetharine.
Brown recluse spider bite, 272–275
Brown-Sequard syndrome, 298
Brugada syndrome, 114
BSA (body surface area) estimation, 766–767
Bullae, toxin-induced, 194
Bumetanide, 589–591, 590t, 591t
for pulmonary edema, 77
Bundle branch block, 115
cardiac pacing for, 67
in acute MI, 65
in myocardial contusion, 73
Buprenex. *See* Buprenorphine.
Buprenorphine, 604t
Bupropion, 259, 267
Burn injury
electrical or lightning, 517–520
estimating size of, 512, 513f
inhalation injury and, 51–52, 513, 514
preoperative evaluation of, 485
thermal, 512–516
Busulfan, 641, 642, 644
Butorphanol, 604t
BZDs. *See* Benzodiazepines (BZDs).

C

C-1009, for intracranial hypertension, 297
CA (capreomycin), 661–663
CABG (coronary artery bypass grafting)
for acute MI, 66f
for aortic stenosis, 92
"Cafe coronary," 42
Calan. *See* Verapamil.
Calcifediol, for hypocalcemia, 137
Calcitonin, for hypercalcemia, 140–142
Calcitriol, for hypocalcemia, 137
Calcium balance
conversion factors for measuring concentration, 136t
hypercalcemia, 139–142
hypocalcemia, 135–138
in rhabdomyolysis, 543, 545
Calcium carbonate, 137, 138
Calcium channel blockers, 223, 224t, 576–581
classification of, 223
conduction disturbances induced by, 116
for acute MI, 67
for atrial fibrillation, 105

Calcium channel blockers *(Continued)*
for cor pulmonale, 49
for kidney transplant recipients, 522
for unstable angina, 62
in cyclic antidepressant overdose, 261
in thyroid storm, 183
indications for, 223–224
interaction with benzodiazepines, 608t
overdose of, 225–228
Calcium chloride, 137, 137t
Calcium gluceptate, 137, 137t
Calcium gluconate, 137, 137t
Calcium supplementation
contraindicated in digoxin toxicity, 138, 227, 231
for calcium channel blocker overdose, 227
for hypermagnesemia, 146
for hyperphosphatemia, 152
for hypocalcemia, 137–138, 137t
for salicylate intoxication, 208
hypophosphatemia induced by, 147
in ethylene glycol intoxication, 238
in parenteral nutrition solutions, 765
ventricular dysrhythmias induced by, 138
Calorimetric capnography, 784
Camino catheter, 796
Cancer patients
complications of chemotherapeutic agents in, 641–644
diarrhea in, 471, 473
hypoglycemia in, 171
infections in neutropenic patients, 362–364
toxic megacolon in, 474
Candidal infection, 339–342
antifungal therapy for, 671–676
in bone marrow transplant recipients, 366–368
in neutropenic cancer patients, 362–363
in organ transplant patients, 369, 370, 372, 523
Cantor tube, 754
CaO_2 (arterial oxygen content), 781, 783t, 790
Capnography, 784–787, 785f, 785t, 786f
Capnometry, 784
Capreomycin (CA), 661–663
Captopril, 575, 578, 579
for acute MI, 67
for left ventricular dysfunction, 78
for unstable angina, 62
Carafate. *See* Sucralfate.
Carbamazepine (CBZ), 611–616
for diabetes insipidus, 177
interaction with benzodiazepines, 608t
Carbapenems, 665–669
Carbenicillin, 645
Carbicarb, for lactic acidosis, 160
Carbon dioxide
capnography for measurement of, 784–787, 785f, 785t, 786f
factors affecting tissue level of, 793
increased production of, 18
total content of, 154
Carbon dioxide tension (PCO_2), 784
Carbon Monoxide Neuropsychiatric Screening Battery (CONSB), 249
Carbon monoxide poisoning, 249–252, 513
cyanide poisoning with, 246, 247, 252
Carboplatin, 642
Carboxyhemoglobin, 51, 247, 249, 250, 513, 790
Cardene. *See* Nicardipine.
Cardiac arrest, epinephrine for, 572–573

Cardiac catheterization
  in aortic stenosis, 92
  in mitral valve dysfunction, 72
  in pericardial tamponade, 100, 100f
  in pericarditis, 97
  indications for, 62–63
Cardiac index (CI), 76, 500, 775, 776
Cardiac injuries, 488, 490
Cardiac output (CO), 775
  after cardiac surgery, 500–501
  low, 76–78
Cardiac pacing
  for acute MI, 67
    right ventricular, 70
  for conduction disturbances, 67, 117
  in cyclic antidepressant overdose, 261
  in digoxin toxicity, 232
  in neuroleptic overdose, 257
  temporary transvenous pacemaker for,
    694–698, 695f
  transcutaneous, 699–700
Cardiac stress testing, 61, 62
Cardiac surgery, patient management after,
  500–503
Cardiac troponin, 61, 64, 66, 73
Cardilate. See Erythrityl tetranitrate.
Cardiogenic pulmonary edema, 20–22, 76–
  77
  noninvasive positive-pressure ventilation
    for, 814
Cardiogenic renal failure, 477
Cardiogenic shock, 88–89, 322
  after cardiac surgery, 501
  chemotherapy-induced, 642
  digoxin in, 628
  due to left ventricular failure, 75–79, 88
  hemodynamic monitoring in, 776
  oxygen transport variables in, 783t
Cardiomyopathy
  dilated, vs. pericardial tamponade, 100
  peripartum, 552
Cardiopulmonary bypass (CPB), thrombocytopenia due to, 410–412
Cardiopulmonary resuscitation (CPR)
  do-not-resuscitate orders, 739–741
  for air embolism, 562
  for anaphylaxis, 535
  for electrical or lightning injury, 519–520
  for near drowning, 537
  for pulseless electrical activity, 111
Cardiotoxicity, of chemotherapeutic agents,
  642–643
Cardiovascular evaluation, preoperative,
  486
Cardioversion, 701–703, 702t
  in cyclic antidepressant overdose, 261
  of atrial fibrillation, 105–106
  of atrial flutter, 106
  of supraventricular tachycardia, 110
Cardizem. See Diltiazem.
Carmustine (BCNU), 641–644
Carotid distribution ischemia, 281
Carotid endarterectomy, 283
Carotid sinus massage
  in atrial fibrillation and flutter, 104
  in conduction disturbances, 117
  in supraventricular tachycardia, 109
Caspofungin, 673
  for aspergillosis, 368
Catabolic index, 772
Catecholamines
  for calcium channel blocker or b-blocker
    overdose, 227
  in pheochromocytoma, 187–188
  vasoactive, 571–574, 572t
Cathartics, for drug overdose, 198

Catheter-related infection
  urinary, 386
  vascular, 2, 327, 404–405
    in bone marrow transplant recipients,
      366
    in neutropenic cancer patients, 362–
      364
Cauda equina syndrome, 298
CAVH (continuous arteriovenous hemofiltration), 733
CAVHDF (continuous arteriovenous hemodiafiltration), 733
CBF (cerebral blood flow), 293
  monitoring in fulminant hepatic failure,
    293
CBZ (carbamazepine), 611–616
  for diabetes insipidus, 177
  interaction with benzodiazepines, 608t
$C\dot{c}O_2$ (pulmonary capillary oxygen content),
  790–791
Cefaclor, 645
Cefazolin, 645, 647, 648
  for heart transplant recipients, 372
  for staphylococcal infection, 329
  for streptococcal infection, 330
Cefdinir, 645
Cefepime, 645, 647–649
  for bone marrow transplant recipients,
    367
  for Gram-negative infection, 337, 338
  for infections in neutropenic cancer pa-
    tients, 363
  for lung transplant recipients, 372
  for pneumonia, 40
Cefixime, 645, 647
Cefoperazone, 645
  for pneumonia, 40
Cefotaxime, 645, 647–649
  for epiglottitis, 403
  for Gram-negative infection, 337, 338
  for meningitis, 337, 390, 391
  for necrotizing soft-tissue infections, 400
  for organ transplant recipients, 372
  for pneumonia, 40
Cefotetan, 645
Cefoxitin, 645
Cefpodoxime proxetil, 645
Cefprozil, 645
Ceftazidime, 645, 647–649
  for aspiration pneumonia, 44
  for bone marrow transplant recipients,
    367
  for Gram-negative infection, 337, 338
  for infections in neutropenic cancer pa-
    tients, 363
  for meningitis, 390, 391
Ceftibuten, 645
Ceftizoxime, 645
  for Gram-negative infection, 338
Ceftriaxone, 645, 647–649
  for endocarditis, 382, 383
  for epiglottitis, 403
  for Gram-negative infection, 337, 338
  for meningitis, 337, 390, 391
  for pneumonia, 40
    aspiration, 44
Cefuroxime, 645, 647, 648
  for epiglottitis, 403
  for pneumonia, 40
Cefuroxime axetil, 645
Celexa. See Citalopram.
Celiac sprue, 473
Cellulitis, 399–401
Central cord syndrome, 298
Central venous catheter, 683–686, 684f
  thrombosis of, 551

Central venous pressure (CVP), 6, 746–748,
  747f, 774, 776
Centruroides exilicauda envenomation,
  272–275, 274t
Cephadroxil, 645
Cephalexin, 645, 648
Cephalosporins, 645–649
Cerebral aneurysms, 287, 289
Cerebral angiography, 284
Cerebral arterial-venous oxygen content dif-
  ference, 293–294
Cerebral autoregulation, 293
Cerebral blood flow (CBF), 293
  monitoring in fulminant hepatic failure,
    293
Cerebral edema, in fulminant hepatic fail-
  ure, 459, 461
Cerebral hyperemia, 295
Cerebral infarction, 82, 281–283
  antihypertensives for, 576
  in sickle cell disease, 433–435
Cerebral ischemia, 295
Cerebral metabolic rate of oxygen utiliza-
  tion, 294
Cerebral perfusion pressure (CPP), 293, 494
Cerebral salt wasting, 120
Cerebral vascular resistance (CVR), 293
Cerebral vasospasm, 287–289
Cerebrospinal fluid (CSF)
  drainage for intracranial hypertension,
    296
  lumbar puncture for examination of,
    713–715
Cervical root levels, 298
Cesarean delivery, for preeclampsia, 86
Charcot's triad, 334
Chemotherapeutic agent complications,
  641–644
Chest pain
  due to myocardial supply-demand mis-
    match, 65
  in acute MI, 64
  in aortic dissection, 102
  in pericarditis, 96
  in unstable angina, 59–63
  ischemic, risk stratification for, 61
  nonischemic, 59
Chest radiography
  in acute abdominal pain, 442
  in acute MI, 65
  in acute pancreatitis, 447
  in angina, 60
  in aortic dissection, 102
  in aortic injuries, 489
  in aortic regurgitation, 92
  in aortic stenosis, 92
  in ARDS, 24
  in aspiration, 44
  in atelectasis, 57
  in carbon monoxide poisoning, 250
  in cardiogenic shock, 88
  in COPD, 46
  in cor pulmonale, 49
  in deep space infections of neck, 388
  in endocarditis, 381
  in fat embolism, 540
  in hemoptysis, 54
  in hypotension, 6
  in left ventricular failure, 76
  in lung contusion, 488
  in mitral regurgitation, 92
  in myasthenia gravis, 305
  in pericardial tamponade, 101, 101f
  in pericarditis, 97
  in pneumonia, 40
    Pneumocystis carinii, 359–360

Chest radiography (Continued)
in pneumothorax, 28, 488
in post-transplant pulmonary infections, 370–371
in pulmonary edema, 21
in pulmonary embolism, 31
in pulmonic regurgitation, 93
in smoke inhalation, 51
in status asthmaticus, 34
in superior vena cava syndrome, 549
in tuberculosis, 377
Chest trauma, 488–490
Chest tube thoracostomy, 29, 40, 489–490, 724–728, 726f
Chickenpox, 351–352
CHIPES mnemonic, 196
Chlamydia diagnostic tests, 39
Chlorambucil, 641
Chloramphenicol, for clostridial gas gangrene, 332
Chlordiazepoxide, 605–607
for alcohol withdrawal syndrome, 242t
Chloride, in parenteral nutrition solutions, 765
Chloroquine, for hypercalcemia, 141
Chlorothiazide, 591
Chlorpromazine, 256
for serotonin syndrome, 268
Chlorpropamide, for diabetes insipidus, 177
Cholangitis, Gram-negative ascending, 334, 337
Cholecystectomy, 451
Cholecystitis, acute, 439, 441, 443, 450–451
acalculous, 334, 450–451
after abdominal aortic aneurysm repair, 510
after kidney transplantation, 524
calculous, 450–451
emphysematous, 451
Gram-negative, 334, 337
vs. acute hepatitis, 456
Cholestasis, 441
Cholesterol emboli syndrome, 507
Cholestyramine, for digoxin overdose, 230
Cholinergic crisis, 269
Cholinergic processes, 269
Chronic inflammatory demyelinating polyneuropathy (CIDP), 307
Chronic obstructive pulmonary disease (COPD), 46–47
cor pulmonale in, 48–49
noninvasive positive-pressure ventilation for, 814
Chronic renal failure, 481–483
CI (cardiac index), 76, 500, 775, 776
CIDP (chronic inflammatory demyelinating polyneuropathy), 307
Cimetidine, 594, 595t
conduction disturbances induced by, 116
for anaphylaxis, 536
for dapsone-induced methemoglobinemia, 255
interaction with benzodiazepines, 608t
to prevent aspiration, 43
Ciprofloxacin, 653–654
for aspiration pneumonia, 44
for bone marrow transplant patients, 368
for bone marrow transplant recipients, 367
for necrotizing soft-tissue infections, 400
for tuberculosis, 662
Circulation
bronchial, 53
pulmonary, 54

Circulatory shock
chemotherapy-induced, 642
epinephrine for, 572
Cirrhosis
alcohol-induced, 452, 454
ascites laboratory findings in, 718t
Cisatracurium, 597, 599, 599t, 600
for endotracheal intubation, 678
Cisplatin, 642–644
Citalopram, 259, 267
Citrate, for continuous renal replacement therapy, 735
Citrobacter infection, 333
Clarithromycin, 655–658, 656t
interaction with benzodiazepines, 608t
Clindamycin, 665–669
for bone marrow transplant recipients, 367
for clostridial gas gangrene, 332
for deep space infections of neck, 389
for Gram-negative infection, 338
for infections in neutropenic cancer patients, 364
for lung transplant recipients, 372
for necrotizing soft-tissue infections, 400
for Pneumocystis carinii pneumonia, 360t
for pneumonia, 40
aspiration, 44
for streptococcal infection, 330
for tetanus, 315
for toxic shock syndrome, 396
Clofibrate, for diabetes insipidus, 177
Clomipramine, 259
Clonazepam
for post-cardiac arrest myoclonic seizures, 280
for serotonin syndrome, 268
Clonidine, 575–581
conduction disturbances induced by, 116
Clonidine suppression test, in pheochromocytoma, 188
Clopidogrel
for unstable angina, 61
to prevent cerebral infarction, 282
Clostridium infection
C. botulinum, 311–313
C. difficile colitis, 3, 472, 473
in bone marrow transplant patients, 366, 367
in neutropenic cancer patients, 362–363
in organ transplant patients, 369, 523, 524
metronidazole for, 670
C. perfringens, 328, 332
C. perfringens necrotizing soft-tissue infections, 399–401
C. tetani, 314–316
Clotrimazole, for candidal infection, 341
Clotting factors, 406
Cloxacillin, 645, 646, 648
Clozapine, 256
CMV (cytomegalovirus) infection, 351t, 354–355
post-transplant, 354–355, 366–368, 369–370, 373, 523
prophylaxis for, 522
transfusion-associated, 429
CO (cardiac output), 775
after cardiac surgery, 500–501
low, 76–78
Coagulase-negative staphylococci, 327, 329
Coagulopathy, 406–408
hypercoagulable states, 413–415
in fulminant hepatic failure, 458–460
in heat stroke, 531, 533

Coagulopathy (Continued)
thrombocytopenia due to, 409–412
uremic, 522–523
Cocaine intoxication, 219–222
Coccidioides immitis infection, 344, 345, 347, 348
antifungal therapy for, 671–676
Codeine, 604t
Cold hemagglutinin disease, 425–427
Colestipol, for digoxin overdose, 230
Colitis
antibiotic-associated, 3
Clostridium difficile, 3, 472, 473
in bone marrow transplant patients, 366, 367
in neutropenic cancer patients, 362–363
in organ transplant patients, 369, 523, 524
metronidazole for, 670
ischemic, 510
Colloid fluids, 565t, 566
"Colon cutoff sign," 447
Colonic bleeding, 466
Colonoscopy, 467–468
CoLyte. See Polyethylene glycol (GoLytely, CoLyte) for drug overdose.
Coma, 11–13, 11t, 494
barbiturate, 285, 297
hyperosmolar nonketotic, 168–170
myxedema, 184–186
withdrawal of mechanical ventilation in, 741t
Combivent. See Ipratropium–albuterol combination metered dose inhaler.
Compartment syndrome
after electrical or lightning injury, 520
after peripheral vascular bypass, 504, 506
due to peripheral arterial occlusion, 508
in rhabdomyolysis, 545
Computed tomography (CT)
in abdominal aortic aneurysm, 509, 511
in abdominal trauma, 492
in acute abdominal pain, 442
in acute cholecystitis, 450
in acute pancreatitis, 447, 447t
in aortic dissection, 102
in aortic injuries, 489
in ARDS, 24
in carbon monoxide poisoning, 250
in cerebral infarction, 281
in comatose patient, 12
in COPD, 46
in cor pulmonale, 49
in deep space infections of neck, 388
in endocarditis, 381–382
in head trauma, 495, 497t
in hemoptysis, 54
in intracerebral hemorrhage, 284
in lower gastrointestinal bleeding, 468
in meningitis, 336
in patient with urinary catheter, 9
in pericarditis, 97
in pheochromocytoma, 188
in post-transplant pulmonary infections, 371
in pulmonary embolism, 31
in smoke inhalation, 51
in spinal cord compression, 299
in subarachnoid hemorrhage, 288
in subdural hematoma, 292
in superior vena cava syndrome, 549
in toxic megacolon, 475
in tuberculosis, 377–378
post-craniotomy, 498

Conduction disturbances, 116–118
cardiac pacing for, 67, 117
in acute MI, 65
in angina, 60
Congestive heart failure (CHF)
amrinone and milrinone for, 568
angina with, 60, 61
ascites laboratory findings in, 718t
chemotherapy-induced, 642
continuous renal replacement therapy for, 733–736
digoxin for, 626
in myxedema coma, 184
in valvular heart disease, 90
oxygen transport variables in, 783t
Conn's syndrome, 125, 129
CONSB (Carbon Monoxide Neuropsychiatric Screening Battery), 249
Constipation, enteral feeding-associated, 762–763
Continuous arteriovenous hemodiafiltration (CAVHDF), 733
Continuous arteriovenous hemofiltration (CAVH), 733
Continuous positive airway pressure (CPAP), 811f, 817
for aspiration pneumonia, 44, 45
for cardiogenic pulmonary edema, 22
for COPD, 47
in Guillain-Barré syndrome, 309
noninvasive, 815
Continuous renal replacement therapy (CRRT), 10, 733–736
for acute renal failure, 480
in fulminant hepatic failure, 460
Continuous venovenous hemofiltration (CVVH), 733
Controlled mandatory ventilation, 808, 811f
Cooling procedures, 532
COPD (chronic obstructive pulmonary disease), 46–47
cor pulmonale in, 48–49
noninvasive positive-pressure ventilation for, 814
Copper, in parenteral nutrition solutions, 766
Copperhead snakebite, 272
Cor pulmonale, 48–49
hemodynamic monitoring in, 776
Coral snake envenomation, 272–274
"Corkscrew" technique for transpyloric advancement of enteric tubes, 757
Corneal reflex, 11
confirming absence of, 743
Coronary artery bypass grafting (CABG)
for acute MI, 66f
for aortic stenosis, 92
Coronary artery disease
glycoprotein IIb/IIIa receptor antagonists for, 624–625
preoperative evaluation of, 484
risk factors for, 59
Coronary ischemia, 505
Coronary revascularization, 66f, 69, 89
Corticosteroids. See also specific drugs.
for acute alcoholic hepatitis, 453
for air embolism, 563
for ARDS, 26
for chemotherapy-induced lung toxicity, 642
for COPD, 47
for epiglottitis, 403
for Epstein-Barr virus infection, 353
for graft-versus-host disease, 436, 437
for hypercalcemia, 141

Corticosteroids (Continued)
for intracranial hypertension, 297
for kidney transplantation, 521
for laryngotracheobronchitis, 389
for myxedema coma, 186
for radiation-induced lung toxicity, 642
for septic shock, 325
for smoke inhalation, 52
for status asthmaticus, 35
for subdural hematoma, 292
for thyroid storm, 183
for toxic megacolon, 475
in aspiration pneumonia, 44
in tuberculosis, 663
preoperative, 487
Corynebacterium infection
C. jeikeium, 327, 331
C. peudodiphtheriticum, 327, 331
C. striatum, 327, 331
Cosyntropin stimulation test
for adrenal insufficiency, 192
in myxedema coma, 186
Cotrimoxazole, for COPD, 47
Cottonmouth snakebite, 272
Cough reflex, confirming absence of, 743
CPAP. See Continuous positive airway pressure (CPAP).
CPB (cardiopulmonary bypass), thrombocytopenia due to, 410–412
CPP (cerebral perfusion pressure), 293, 494
CPR. See Cardiopulmonary resuscitation (CPR).
Cranial nerve dysfunction, in myasthenia gravis, 304
Craniotomy
for subdural hematoma, 292
patient management after, 498–499
CRBSI (catheter-related bloodstream infection), 404–405
Creatine phosphokinase
in chronic renal failure, 482
in rhabdomyolysis, 543
MB isoenzymes, 61, 64, 66, 73
Creatinine serum concentration, 481
Creatinine–height index, 772
Crigler-Najjar syndrome, 441
Crotalid envenomation, 272–275, 274t
Crotalid Polyvalent Antivenin, 274, 274t, 275
Croup, 387–389
CRRT (continuous renal replacement therapy), 10, 733–736
for acute renal failure, 480
in fulminant hepatic failure, 460
Cryoprecipitate, 407, 411
Cryptococcus neoformans infection, 344–348
antifungal therapy for, 671–676
in organ transplant recipients, 370, 523
Crystalloid fluids, 564, 565t
Crystalluria, in ethylene glycol intoxication, 236, 236t
CS (cycloserine), 661–663
CSF (cerebrospinal fluid)
drainage for intracranial hypertension, 296
lumbar puncture for examination of, 713–715
CT. See Computed tomography (CT).
Cullen's sign, 407
Current, electrical, 517
Cushing's syndrome, 125, 129
Cushing's triad, 295
CVP (central venous pressure), 6, 746–748, 747f, 774, 776
CVR (cerebral vascular resistance), 293

CVVH (continuous venovenous hemofiltration), 733
CVVHDF (continuous venovenous hemodiafiltration), 733
C$\bar{v}$O$_2$ (mixed venous oxygen content), 781, 790
Cyanide binding agents, 247
Cyanide poisoning, 244–248, 513
Cyanmethemoglobin, 244
Cyanosis, toxin-induced, 194
Cyclic antidepressant overdose, 259–262
Cyclo-oxygenase inhibitors, 2
Cyclophosphamide, 641–644
for myasthenia gravis, 306
Cycloserine (CS), 661–663
Cyclosporin A, 643
for kidney transplantation, 521
for myasthenia gravis, 306
for toxic megacolon, 475
Cyproheptadine, for serotonin syndrome, 268
Cystitis
candidal, 339–341
hemorrhagic, in bone marrow transplant recipients, 366
Cysts, subpleural air, 28, 29
Cytarabine, 641–644
Cytokines
pyrogenic, 1
removal by continuous renal replacement therapy, 736
Cytomegalovirus (CMV) infection, 351t, 354–355
post-transplant, 354–355, 366–368, 369–370, 373, 523
prophylaxis for, 522
transfusion-associated, 429

D

Dactinomycin, 644
Dalteparin, 620t
Danaparoid, 617–621
Dantrolene, 634–635
for malignant hyperthermia, 302, 634–635
for neuroleptic malignant syndrome, 635
for tetanus, 315
Dapsone, for Pneumocystis carinii pneumonia, 360t, 372, 522
Daunorubicin, 642
D-dimer tests, 31, 417
Dead space to tidal volume ratio (V$_d$/V$_t$), 791
Dead-space ventilation, 786
Decarbazine, 644
Decerebrate posturing, 12
Decompressive fasciotomy, 545
Decorticate posturing, 11
Decubitus ulcers, 557–560
Deep sulcus sign, 28
Deep venous thrombosis (DVT), 416–420, 418f, 419t
anticoagulants for, 617–621
prophylaxis for
in craniotomy patients, 499
preoperative, 487
thrombolytic agents for, 622–623
Defibrillation, 701–703, 702t
Dehydration
hypernatremia due to, 124
in head trauma patients, 496
Delavirdine, interaction with benzodiazepines, 608t
Delayed cutaneous hypersensitivity test, 772

Delivery of infant, for preeclampsia, 85–86
Delta gap, 154, 156
Demeclocycline, for syndrome of inappropriate antidiuresis, 179
Dementia, dialysis-associated, 483
Demerol. See Meperidine.
Demoxepam, 605
Denitrogenation atelectasis, 806–807
Depolarizing neuromuscular blocking drugs, 597–601
Deponit. See Nitroglycerin (NTG).
Dermatitis, candidal, 339, 341
Desipramine, 259
Desmethylchlordiazepoxide, 605
Desmethyldiazepam, 605
Desmopressin
    for coagulopathies, 407, 411, 522
    for diabetes insipidus, 177
Desyrel. See Trazodone.
Dexamethasone
    for pneumococcal pneumonia, 390
    for spinal cord compression, 300
Dextran preparations, 566
Dextrose, 565
    for adrenal insufficiency, 193
    for alcoholic ketoacidosis, 162–163
    for diabetic ketoacidosis, 166–167
    for ethanol intoxication, 237
    for hypoglycemia, 172–173
    for salicylate intoxication, 207
    for unexplained coma, 12
    in parenteral nutrition solutions, 764
Diabetes insipidus (DI), 124, 174–177
    hypercalcemia and, 140
    post-craniotomy, 499
    psychogenic, 120
Diabetes mellitus
    diarrhea in, 473
    parenteral nutrition-associated, 768
    preoperative evaluation in, 485
Diabetic ketoacidosis (DKA), 161, 164–167
Dialysis
    dementia associated with, 482
    for acute renal failure, 480
    for alcohol or glycol intoxication
        diethylene glycol, 239
        ethanol, 237
        ethylene glycol, 238–239
        isopropanol, 238
        methanol, 238
        propylene glycol, 239
    for cyanide poisoning, 247
    for drug overdose, 198
        calcium channel blockers or b-blockers, 226
        lithium, 217
        salicylates, 208
    for hypercalcemia, 141
    for hyperkalemia, 134
    for hypermagnesemia, 146
    for hyperphosphatemia, 153
    for hypervolemic hypernatremia, 128
    for oliguria, 10
    for tumor lysis syndrome, 547
    hemodialysis, 729–732, 730t
    infection of access sites and devices for, 482
    permanent arteriovenous access for, 481
Diamond-Blackfan syndrome, 421
Diaphragmatic laceration, 488, 490
Diarrhea, 470–473
    abdominal pain with, 440
    chemotherapy-induced, 644
    Clostridium difficile, 3, 472, 473
        in bone marrow transplant patients, 366, 367

Diarrhea (Continued)
        in neutropenic cancer patients, 362–363
        in organ transplant patients, 369, 523, 524
        metronidazole for, 670
    enteral feeding-associated, 762
    in bone marrow transplant recipients, 366
    in neutropenic cancer patients, 362, 363
    in organ transplant recipients, 371
Diazepam, 605–607
    for alcohol withdrawal syndrome, 242t
    for cocaine intoxication, 221
    for status epilepticus/seizures, 278, 611, 612, 614–615
    for tetanus, 315
    in organophosphate poisoning, 270
Diazoxide, 575–581
DIC (disseminated intravascular coagulation), 406–407, 413–414
    in rhabdomyolysis, 544
    thrombocytopenia due to, 409–411
Dichloroacetate, for lactic acidosis, 160
Dicloxacillin, 645, 646, 648
Dicobalt ethylenediaminetetraacetate, for cyanide poisoning, 247
Diethylene glycol intoxication, 233–235, 238
Dieulafoy's lesion, 465
Diflucan. See Fluconazole.
Digibind. See Digoxin-specific antibody fragments.
Digitalis, in cor pulmonale, 49
Digoxin, 626–628
    drug interactions with, 626–627
    for atrial fibrillation and flutter, 105, 106, 626
    for cardiogenic pulmonary edema, 22
    for mitral valve dysfunction, 94
    for supraventricular tachycardia, 110
    interaction with amrinone and milrinone, 570
    therapeutic range for, 230
Digoxin overdose, 229–232
    calcium supplementation contraindicated in, 138, 227, 231
    hyperkalemia in, 133, 134, 229–231
Digoxin-specific antibody fragments, 230–231
Dihydrotachysterol, for hypocalcemia, 137
Dilacor. See Diltiazem.
Dilaudid. See Hydromorphone.
Diltiazem, 224t, 576, 579t, 629
    for atrial fibrillation, 105
    for atrial flutter, 106
    for cor pulmonale, 49
    for supraventricular tachycardia, 110
    for unstable angina, 62
    interaction with benzodiazepines, 608t
    overdose of, 223, 228
4-Dimethylaminophenol, for cyanide poisoning, 247
Diphenhydramine
    after N-acetylcysteine for acetaminophen overdose, 203
    before intravenous HBIG, 373
    for anaphylaxis, 535
    for extrapyramidal symptoms, 258
Diphtheria, pharyngeal, 387–389
Dipyridamole, to prevent cerebral infarction, 282
Direct Coombs test, 427
Disequilibrium syndrome, in chronic renal failure, 483
Disopyramide, 629
    interaction with amrinone and milrinone, 569

Disseminated intravascular coagulation (DIC), 406–407, 413–414
    in rhabdomyolysis, 544
    thrombocytopenia due to, 409–411
Distributive shock, 322
Diuretics, 589–592, 590t, 591t
    cautions in head trauma patients, 496
    for cardiogenic shock, 89
    for diabetes insipidus, 177
    for hypercalcemia, 140
    for hyperkalemia, 134
    for hypermagnesemia, 146
    for hypertension in pregnancy, 85
    for hypertensive nephropathy, 578
    for hypervolemic hypernatremia, 128
    for mitral valve dysfunction, 72
    for oliguria, 10
    for preload reduction, 21
    for pulmonary edema, 77
    hyponatremia and, 120
    hypophosphatemia induced by, 147
    in cor pulmonale, 49
    interaction with amrinone and milrinone, 569
    preoperative, 487
Diverticulitis, 443
Diverticulosis, 468
DKA (diabetic ketoacidosis), 161, 164–167
DNR (do-not-resuscitate) orders, 739–741
DO₂ (systemic oxygen delivery), 782, 782f, 783, 783t
DO₂I (systemic oxygen delivery index), 782
Dobutamine, 571, 572t, 573
    for cardiogenic pulmonary edema, 22, 78
    for cardiogenic shock, 89
    for left ventricular systolic dysfunction, 7
    for septic shock, 324
    interaction with amrinone and milrinone, 570
Dofetilide, 629–633
Doll's-eyes reflex, 11
    confirming absence of, 743
Dolophine. See Methadone.
Domperidone, to prevent aspiration, 43
Do-not-resuscitate (DNR) orders, 739–741
Dopamine, 571, 572t, 573
    as diuretic, 589, 590, 592
    for calcium channel blocker overdose, 227
    for cardiogenic pulmonary edema, 22
    for cardiogenic shock, 89
    for conduction disturbances, 117
    for low cardiac output, 78
    for low systemic vascular resistance, 6
    for oliguria, 10
    for septic shock, 324
    for spinal cord compression, 300
    in theophylline overdose, 215
    interaction with amrinone and milrinone, 570
Dopamine DA₁ receptors, 571
Dopexamine, 572, 572t
Doxacurium, 599t
Doxazosin, 575
    for pheochromocytoma, 189
Doxepin, 259
Doxorubicin, 642, 644
Doxycycline
    for COPD, 47
    for pneumonia, 41
Dressings, for pressure ulcers, 559–560
Droperidol, 256
    after N-acetylcysteine for acetaminophen overdose, 203
    to prevent aspiration, 44
Drotrecogin alfa activated, 319, 325
Drowning, 537–538

Drowsiness, 11
Drug extravasation, of vasoactive catechol-
amines, 573
Drug fever, 1, 3
Drug overdose, 13, 194–200. See also Poi-
soning.
    acetaminophen, 201–204, 264–265
    agents that may cause delayed toxicity,
        197t
    antidotes for, 199t
    calcium channel blockers and b-blockers,
        223–228
    clinical toxidromes caused by, 196t
    cocaine, 219–222
    coma due to, 11
    continuous renal replacement therapy for,
        733–736
    digoxin, 229–232
    hemodialysis for, 729–732
    lithium, 216–218
    neuroleptics, 256–258
    pulseless electrical activity due to, 112t,
        113t
    salicylates, 205–208
    sedative-hypnotics and narcotics, 209–212
    theophylline, 213–215
    toxins for which 24-hour monitoring is
        recommended, 197t
    toxins that alter vital signs, 195t
Drug withdrawal syndromes, antihyperten-
    sives in, 576
Drug-induced disorders
    acute renal failure, 477–478
    anaphylaxis, 534
    anticholinergic toxicity, 263–266
    coagulopathy, 407–408
    conduction disturbances, 116
    diarrhea, 470
    fulminant hepatic failure, 458
    gastrointestinal bleeding
        lower, 466
        upper, 463, 464
    Guillain-Barré syndrome-like neuropathy,
        307
    hypercalcemia, 139
    hypercoagulable states, 413
    hyperkalemia, 132
    hypermagnesemia, 146
    hypocalcemia, 135–136
    hypoglycemia, 171
    hypokalemia, 129
    hypomagnesemia, 143
    hypophosphatemia, 147
    hypothyroidism, 184
    impaired heat dissipation, 530
    lactic acidosis, 158
    malignant hyperthermia, 1, 3–4, 301–
        303
    mental status changes, 251
    methemoglobinemia, 253–254
    nephrogenic diabetes insipidus, 175
    neuroleptic malignant syndrome, 2, 4,
        257, 301–303
    QT interval prolongation, 114
    rhabdomyolysis, 542
    syndrome of inappropriate antidiuresis,
        178–179
    thrombocytopenia, 409, 411
    thyrotoxicosis, 181
    toxic megacolon, 474
Dubin-Johnson syndrome, 441
DVT. See Deep venous thrombosis (DVT).
Dysphagia, in cancer patients, 362
Dysrhythmias. See also Electrocardiography
    (ECG); specific dysrhythmias.
    after cardiac surgery, 501, 502

Dysrhythmias (Continued)
    antidysrhythmic agents for, 629–633
    atrial fibrillation and flutter, 104–106
    cardioversion and defibrillation for, 701–
        703, 702t
    chemotherapy-induced, 642–643
    due to electrical injury, 519
    in acute MI, 65
    in angina, 60
    in anticholinergic poisoning, 265
    in cardiogenic shock, 88
    in drug overdose
        cyclic antidepressants, 261
        digoxin, 229, 230, 232, 628
        neuroleptics, 257–258
        theophylline, 215
    in fulminant hepatic failure, 459
    in Guillain-Barré syndrome, 308
    in myocardial contusion, 73
    macrolide antibiotic-induced, 659
    supraventricular tachycardia, 107–110
    temporary transvenous pacemaker for,
        694–698
    transcutaneous pacing for, 699–700
    ventricular tachycardia and fibrillation,
        114–115
Dystonia, neuroleptic-induced, 257, 258

E

Eastern coral snakebite, 272, 274
Ebstein's anomaly, 91, 95
EBV (Epstein-Barr virus) infection, 351t
    in bone marrow transplant patients, 366
    in organ transplant patients, 370
    infectious mononucleosis, 352–353
ECG. See Electrocardiography (ECG).
Echocardiography
    after cardiac surgery, 501
    in acute MI, 65, 66
        right ventricular, 69
    in air embolism, 562
    in angina, 60
    in aortic dissection, 102
    in aortic injuries, 489
    in aortic regurgitation, 92
    in cardiogenic shock, 88
    in cor pulmonale, 49
    in endocarditis, 381
    in fat embolism, 540
    in fulminant hepatic failure, 459
    in hypotension, 6
    in infective endocarditis, 337
    in left ventricular failure, 76
    in mitral regurgitation, 92
    in mitral valve dysfunction, 72
    in myocardial contusion, 73
    in pericardial tamponade, 101
    in pericarditis, 97, 98f
    in peripheral arterial occlusion, 508
    in pulmonary edema, 21
    in pulmonary embolism, 31–32
    in pulmonic regurgitation, 93
    in supraventricular tachycardia, 108
    in tricuspid valve disease, 92–93
Eclampsia, 83, 84
    antihypertensives for, 576
Ectopic pregnancy, ruptured, 444–445
Edrophonium test for myasthenia gravis,
    305
EE (energy expenditure) determination, 770,
    773
EEG. See Electroencephalography (EEG).
Efavirenz, interaction with benzodiazepines,
    608t

Effexor. See Venlafaxine.
EGD (esophagogastroduodenoscopy), 467
Ehlers-Danlos syndrome, 90, 91
Elavil. See Amitriptyline.
Electrical impedance plethysmography, 31
Electrical injuries, 517–520
Electrical power, 517
Electrocardiography (ECG). See also Dys-
    rhythmias.
    after cardiac surgery, 500
    conduction disturbances on, 116–117,
        117t
    during fiberoptic bronchoscopy, 710
    during insertion of temporary transvenous
        pacemaker, 694–697
    for hypotension, 6
    in acute abdominal pain, 442
    in acute MI, 64–66
        right ventricular, 69, 70f
    in aortic dissection, 102
    in aortic regurgitation, 92
    in aortic stenosis, 92
    in atrial fibrillation, 104
    in atrial flutter, 104
    in burn patients, 515
    in cardiogenic shock, 88–89
    in cor pulmonale, 49
    in cyanide poisoning, 246
    in drug overdose
        anticholinergic agents, 265
        cyclic antidepressants, 260
        digoxin, 229, 628
        lithium, 216
        neuroleptics, 257
    in electrical injury, 519
    in Guillain-Barré syndrome, 308
    in hypercalcemia, 140
    in hyperkalemia, 132, 133f
    in hypocalcemia, 136
    in hypokalemia, 129, 130f
    in hypomagnesemia, 144
    in hypothermia, 526
    in mitral regurgitation, 92
    in myocardial contusion, 73
    in myxedema coma, 185
    in pericardial tamponade, 101
    in pericarditis, 97, 98f
    in pulmonary edema, 21
    in pulmonary embolism, 31
    in pulmonic regurgitation, 93
    in subarachnoid hemorrhage, 288
    in supraventricular tachycardia, 108
    in tricuspid valve disease, 92
    in unstable angina, 59–61
    in Wolff-Parkinson-White syndrome,
        108
    preoperative, 486
    pulseless electrical activity on, 111
Electroencephalography (EEG)
    for brain death determination, 744
    for monitoring sedation, 800
    in encephalitis, 392
    in status epilepticus, 279
    in subdural hematoma, 292
Electromyography (EMG)
    in Guillain-Barré syndrome, 308–309
    in myasthenia gravis, 305
Elemental feeding formulas, 761
EMB (ethambutol), 661–663
Embolism. See also Thromboembolic disor-
    ders.
    air, 561–563
    amniotic fluid, 553
    fat, 539–541
    pulmonary, 30–33, 32f–33f
    thrombolytic therapy-induced, 623

Embolization
  bronchial, 55
  for bleeding peptic ulcer, 465
EMG (electromyography)
  in Guillain-Barré syndrome, 308–309
  in myasthenia gravis, 305
Emphysema
  pulmonary interstitial, 29
  subcutaneous, 28, 29
Empyema
  gallbladder, 451
  Staphylococcus aureus, 328, 329
  subdural, 329
Enalapril, 575
  for acute MI, 67
  for unstable angina, 62
Enalaprilat, 578
Encephalitis, 392–393
  cytomegalovirus, 354
  herpes simplex, 350–351, 392, 393
  in bone marrow transplant recipients, 366
Encephalopathy
  hepatic, 458–462
  hypertensive, 82
  uremic, 482
  Wernicke's, 483
Endep. *See* Amitriptyline.
Endocarditis, infective, 379–383, 380t
  candidal, 342
  coagulase-negative staphylococcal, 329
  empiric antibiotic therapy for, 338
  enterococcal, 331
  Gram-negative, 334, 337, 338
  preoperative prophylaxis for, 487
  Streptococcus viridans, 330
Endoscopic retrograde cholangiopancreatog-
    raphy (ERCP), 448
Endoscopy
  for toxic megacolon, 475
  for transpyloric advancement of enteric
    tube, 757–758
  for upper gastrointestinal hemorrhage,
    463, 464
Endotracheal intubation, 677–682, 679f,
    680f
  fiberoptic bronchoscopy for, 709–712
  for cardiogenic shock, 89
  for pulmonary edema, 77
  for status asthmaticus, 35
  for tracheal injuries, 489
  in hemoptysis, 55
  in intracerebral hemorrhage, 285
  in myasthenia gravis, 306
  in smoke inhalation, 52
  in spinal cord-injured patients, 299
  indications for, 18
  neuromuscular blocking drugs for, 597–
    601
  rapid-sequence, to prevent aspiration, 43
Endotracheal tube delivery connections,
    804–805
Energy expenditure (EE) determination,
    770, 773
Enovil. *See* Amitriptyline.
Enoxaparin, 620t
  for pulmonary embolism, 32
  for unstable angina, 62
Enteral feeding, 760–763, 761f
Enteritis, tuberculous, 374
Enterobacter infection, 333
  urosepsis, 384
Enterococcus infection, 327, 330–331
  antibiotics for, 331
  endocarditis, 379, 382
  urosepsis, 384
  vancomycin-resistant, 331, 369, 666–667

Epidural abscess, spinal, 298–300
  Staphylococcus aureus, 328
Epidural pressure monitor, 796
Epigastric pain, 439
Epiglottitis, 402–403
Epinephrine, 571–573, 572t
  for anaphylactoid reaction to intravenous
    HBIG, 373
  for anaphylaxis, 535
  for bradycardia, 6
  for calcium channel blocker or β-blocker
    overdose, 227
  for conduction disturbances, 117
  for hemoptysis, 55
  for left ventricular dysfunction, 7, 78
  for pulseless electrical activity, 111
  for septic shock, 324
  racemic, for smoke inhalation, 52
Epirubicin, 642
Epoprostenol, for cor pulmonale, 49
Epstein-Barr virus (EBV) infection, 351t
  in bone marrow transplant patients, 366
  in organ transplant patients, 370, 523
  infectious mononucleosis, 352–353
Eptifibatide, 625
ERCP (endoscopic retrograde cholangiopan-
    creatography), 448
Ergocalciferol, for hypocalcemia, 137
Erythema, toxin-induced, 195
Erythema multiforme, 351
Erythrityl tetranitrate, 586
Erythromycin, 655–658, 656t
  for diphtheria, 389
  for pneumonia, 40, 41
  for *Rhodococcus equi* infection, 332
  for tetanus, 315
  interaction with benzodiazepines, 608t
  to prevent aspiration, 43
Erythropoietin, 424
Escharotomy, 515
Escherichia coli infection, 333, 384
Esmolol, 224t, 576, 579, 629
  for aortic dissection, 103
  for atrial fibrillation, 105
  for atrial flutter, 106
  for pheochromocytoma, 189
  in intracerebral hemorrhage, 285
  in subarachnoid hemorrhage, 289
  in theophylline overdose, 215
  in thyroid storm, 183
Esomeprazole, 595t
Esophageal balloon tamponade, 750f, 751–
    753
Esophageal injuries, 489, 490
Esophageal variceal bleeding, 464
  balloon tamponade for, 750f, 751–753
Esophagitis
  candidal, 339, 340
  herpes simplex, 351
  upper gastrointestinal hemorrhage due to,
    464
Esophagogastroduodenoscopy (EGD), 467
Estrogens, for hypercalcemia, 141
ETA (ethionamide), 661–663
Ethacrynic acid, 589–591
Ethambutol (EMB), 661–663
Ethanol
  for ethylene glycol intoxication, 238
  for methanol intoxication, 237–238
Ethanol intoxication, 12, 13, 233–235, 237
  vs. alcohol withdrawal syndrome, 240
Ethionamide (ETA), 661–663
Ethylene glycol intoxication, 233–236,
    238–239
Etidronate disodium, for hypercalcemia,
    141

Etoposide, 642
Euglobulin clot lysis time, 414
Euthyroid sick syndrome, 185
Ewart's sign, 100
Excretory urogram, 442
Expired gas analysis, 782
Extrapyramidal symptoms, neuroleptic-in-
    duced, 257, 258
Extravasation, of vasoactive catecholamines,
    573
Eye irrigation, 197

F

Fab (digoxin-specific antibody fragments),
    230–231
Face tent, 804, 806
Factor V Leiden, 413, 416–417
Factor VIII deficiency, 407
Famciclovir
  for bone marrow transplant recipients,
    367
  for herpes simplex virus infection, 351
  for herpes zoster, 352
Famotidine, 594, 595t
  to prevent aspiration, 43
Fasciitis, necrotizing, 399–401
  Gram-negative, 336, 337
  group A streptococcal, 329, 330
Fasciotomy, decompressive, 545
FAST (focused abdominal sonogram for
    trauma), 491–492
Fast flush test, 778–780, 779f, 780f
Fat embolism, 539–541
Fat embolism syndrome (FES), 539
Fat emulsions, intravenous, 764–765
5-FC (5-flucytosine), 672–676
  for cryptococcosis, 348
Fecal impaction, 444
Feeding formulas
  enteral, 760–762
  parenteral, 764–767
Felbamate, 612
Felodipine, 224t, 576
Femoral artery catheterization, 688, 689f
Femoral vein approach
  for central venous catheterization, 684–
    685
  for hemodialysis, 730–731
FENa (fractional excretion of sodium), 478
Fenoldopam mesylate, 572t, 575, 583–584
Fentanyl, 602, 603, 604t
  after cardiac surgery, 501
  for burn injury, 514
FES (fat embolism syndrome), 539
Fetal monitoring, 85
Fever, 1–4
  in anticholinergic poisoning, 265
  in bone marrow transplant recipients, 366
  in cocaine intoxication, 222
  in head trauma patients, 496
  in neuroleptic malignant syndrome, 257,
    301
  in neutropenic cancer patients, 362–364
  malignant hyperthermia, 1, 3–4, 301–
    303
  toxin-induced, 195t
FHF (fulminant hepatic failure), 455, 458–
    462
Fiber-containing feeding formulas, 761
Fiberoptic bronchoscopy, 709–712
Fibrinogen, 407, 414
Fibrinolysis, 407
Fick method to determine cardiac output,
    775

Fiddle-back spider bite, 272–275
Filgrastim, 639–640
"First use syndrome" with hemodialysis, 732
Fistula
    aortoenteric, 465, 468, 510
    bronchopleural, 489
        high-frequency ventilation for, 814
"Flail segment," 488
Flecainide, 629
Fluconazole, 671–676
    for blastomycosis, 348
    for candidal infection, 341–342, 368
    for catheter-related bloodstream infection, 405
    for coccidioidomycosis, 348
    for cryptococcosis, 348
    for organ transplant recipients, 372
    interaction with benzodiazepines, 608t
5-Flucytosine (5-FC), 672–676
    for cryptococcosis, 348
Fludarabine, 642, 643
Fluid challenge, 746–748, 747f
Fluid management
    composition of crystalloid and colloid-based fluids, 565t
    for acute renal failure, 479
    for adrenal insufficiency, 193
    for anaphylaxis, 535
    for ARDS, 25
    for aspiration pneumonia, 44
    for burn injury, 514
    for cerebral vasospasm prophylaxis, 289
    for diabetic ketoacidosis, 166
    for diarrhea, 472
    for electrical or lightning injury, 520
    for gastrointestinal bleeding
        lower, 468
        upper, 463
    for head trauma patients, 495, 496
    for heat stroke, 532
    for hypercalcemia, 140
    for hypermagnesemia, 146
    for hypernatremia, 127–128
    for hyperosmolar nonketotic coma, 169
    for hyponatremia, 121–122
    for hypotension in toxic shock syndrome, 396
    for hypothermia, 526
    for hypovolemia, 6–7
    for lactic acidosis, 160
    for lithium overdose, 217
    for low cardiac output, 78
    for rhabdomyolysis, 544
    for ruptured abdominal aortic aneurysm, 510
    for salicylate intoxication, 207
    for sepsis and systemic inflammatory response syndrome, 319
    for septic shock, 323–324
    for tumor lysis syndrome, 547
    hyponatremia induced by, 120, 121
    in alcoholic ketoacidosis, 162–163
    intravenous fluids, 564–567
Flumazenil, 605–608
    contraindicated in anticholinergic toxicity, 265
    for benzodiazepine overdose, 210
    for benzodiazepine reversal, 297t
    precautions for, 196, 212
Fluoroquinolone antibiotics, 653–654
    for tuberculosis, 662, 663
5-Fluorouracil, 642, 644
Fluoxetine, 259, 267
Fluphenazine, 256
Flushing, toxin-induced, 195

Fluvoxamine, 259, 267
    interaction with benzodiazepines, 608t
Focused abdominal sonogram for trauma (FAST), 491–492
Folic acid
    for alcohol withdrawal syndrome, 242
    for ethylene glycol intoxication, 238
    for methanol intoxication, 238
Fomepizole
    for ethylene glycol intoxication, 238, 239
    for methanol intoxication, 238
Food poisoning, 470
Food-borne botulism, 311–312
Foods, anaphylactic reactions to, 534
Foradil. See Formoterol.
Foramen ovale, patent, 561
Foreign body aspiration, 42
Formoterol, 637t, 638
Foscarnet
    for acyclovir-resistant herpes simplex virus, 351
    for bone marrow transplant recipients, 367, 368
    for cytomegalovirus infection, 355
    for varicella-zoster virus infection, 352
Fosinopril, 575
Fosphenytoin, 612, 614, 615
    for status epilepticus, 13, 278–279
    in organophosphate poisoning, 270
    interaction with benzodiazepines, 608t
Fractional excretion of sodium (FENa), 478
Fractures
    fat embolism associated with, 539
    pelvic, 491
    rib, 488, 490
Fragmin. See Dalteparin.
Frank-Starling relationship, 746
Free thyroxine index (FTI)
    in hypothyroidism, 185
    in thyroid storm, 182, 183
Free-radical scavengers, for intracranial hypertension, 297
Fresh-frozen plasma, 407
FTI (free thyroxine index)
    in hypothyroidism, 185
    in thyroid storm, 182, 183
Fulminant hepatic failure (FHF), 455, 458–462
Funduscopy, in hypertensive crisis, 81
Fungal infections
    candidal, 339–342
    catheter-related bloodstream infection, 405
    drug therapy for, 671–676, 672t, 674t
    in bone marrow transplant recipients, 365–368
    in neutropenic cancer patients, 342, 362
    in organ transplant recipients, 370, 372, 523
    non-candidal, 344–349
    sinusitis, 398
Fungizone. See Amphotericin B.
Fungoides cerebri, 296
Furosemide, 589–591, 590t, 591t
    for hypercalcemia, 140
    for hyperkalemia, 134
    for hypermagnesemia, 146
    for oliguria, 10
    for pulmonary edema, 77

G

G6PD (glucose 6-phosphate dehydrogenase) deficiency, 421, 423
GABA (γ-aminobutyric acid) receptors, 605

Gabapentin, 612
Gag reflex, 11
    aspiration due to impairments of, 42
    confirming absence of, 743
Gallbladder
    empyema of, 451
    gas within, 451
    ischemia of, 450
    perforation of, 451
Gallium nitrate, for hypercalcemia, 141
Gallstones
    acute cholecystitis due to, 450–451
    acute pancreatitis due to, 446–449
Ganciclovir
    for bone marrow transplant recipients, 368
    for cytomegalovirus infection, 355, 373
    for organ transplant recipients, 373, 522
    for viral pneumonia, 41
Gas gangrene, 332, 400
Gas tonometry, 793–794
Gastric balloon tamponade, 750f, 751
Gastric lavage for drug overdose, 197
    acetaminophen, 202
    alcohols and glycols, 237
    anticholinergic agents, 265
    calcium channel blockers or b-blockers, 226
    cocaine, 221
    cyanide, 246
    cyclic antidepressants, 260
    digoxin, 230
    lithium, 217
    neuroleptics, 258
    salicylate, 207
    sedative-hypnotics or narcotics, 210
    theophylline, 214
Gastric tonometry, 793–795, 794f, 795t
Gastric variceal bleeding, 464
    balloon tamponade for, 750f, 751–753
Gastroenteric intubation, 754–759
Gastrointestinal hemorrhage
    lower, 466–469
    Sengstaken-Blakemore tube placement for, 749–753, 750f
    upper, 463–465
Gastrostomy tube feedings, 42, 760–763
Gatifloxacin, for pneumonia, 41
GBS (Guillain-Barré syndrome), 307–310
    vs. botulism, 312
GCS (Glasgow Coma Scale), 11t, 288, 393, 494, 800
G-CSF (granulocyte colony-stimulating factor), 639–640
Gelatin preparations, 566
Genital herpes infection, 350–351
Genitourinary infection
    tuberculous, 374, 377
    urosepsis, 384–386
Gentamicin, 650–652
    for endocarditis, 382, 383
    for enterococcal infection, 331
    for Gram-negative infection, 337, 338
    for staphylococcal infection, 329, 382
Gestational hypertension, 83
GFR (glomerular filtration rate)
    in acute renal failure, 477
    in chronic renal failure, 481
Gilbert's syndrome, 441
Gingivostomatitis, herpes simplex, 350–351
Glanzmann's disease, 410
Glasgow Coma Scale (GCS), 11t, 288, 393, 494, 800
Glomerular filtration rate (GFR)
    in acute renal failure, 477
    in chronic renal failure, 481

Glucagon
for β-blocker overdose, 226–227
for hypoglycemia, 172
in cyclic antidepressant overdose, 261
Glucerna, 762
Glucose
for calcium channel blocker overdose, 227
for hyperkalemia, 133, 231
for hypermagnesemia, 146
for hyperphosphatemia, 152
for hypoglycemia, 172
Glucose 6-phosphate dehydrogenase (G6PD) deficiency, 421, 423
Glucose intolerance, parenteral nutrition-associated, 768
Glucose intolerance feeding formulations, 762
Glycol intoxication, 233–239
Glycoprotein IIb/IIIa receptor antagonists, 624–625
for unstable angina, 62
GoLytely. See Polyethylene glycol (Go-Lytely, CoLyte) for drug overdose.
Goodpasture's syndrome, 478
Graft-versus-host disease (GVHD), 436–438, 437t
after bone marrow transplantation, 365
transfusion-associated, 430–432, 437
Gram-negative infections, 333–338
aminoglycosides for, 650–652
in bone marrow transplant recipients, 365–368
in neutropenic cancer patients, 362
macrolides for, 655–657, 656t
nosocomial sinusitis, 397
urosepsis, 384
Gram-positive infections, 327–332
Granulocyte colony-stimulating factor (G-CSF), 639–640
Graves' disease, 181, 182
Grey Turner's sign, 407
Guanabenz, 577
Guanfacine, 577
Guillain-Barré syndrome (GBS), 307–310
vs. botulism, 312
Gunshot wounds
to abdomen, 491–493
to head, 494, 497
GVHD (graft-versus-host disease), 436–438, 437t
after bone marrow transplantation, 365
transfusion-associated, 430–432, 437

H

H2RAs. See Histamine-2 receptor antagonists (H2RAs).
HACEK group organisms
antibiotics for, 383
endocarditis due to, 379, 383
Haemophilus influenzae infection, 333
epiglottitis, 402–403
Haloperidol, 256, 303
Harris-Benedict equations, 770
Hashimoto's thyroiditis, 184
Hb (hemoglobin), 422
hemoglobin M, 253
in upper gastrointestinal hemorrhage, 463
HBIG (hepatitis B immunoglobulin), for liver transplant recipients, 373
HBO. See Hyperbaric oxygen (HBO) therapy.
Head injury, 484, 494–497, 497t
diabetes insipidus after, 174
intracranial hypertension and, 293–297

Headache, due to subarachnoid hemorrhage, 287
Health care workers, exposure to viral hepatitis, 457
Hearing loss
aminoglycoside-induced, 652
macrolide-induced, 659
Heart sounds
assessment of, 93
in acute MI, 64
in aortic regurgitation, 92
in cor pulmonale, 48
in endocarditis, 380
in mitral regurgitation, 92
in mitral valve prolapse, 92
in pericarditis, 96
in unstable angina, 59
Heart transplantation, 372
Heat exhaustion, 530, 531
Heat stroke, 530–533
Helicobacter pylori infection, 593
HELLP syndrome, 409
Hematemesis, 463
Hematochezia, 463, 466–467
Hematocrit, 422
in burn patients, 515
in upper gastrointestinal hemorrhage, 463
Hematoma, subdural, 13, 291–292
Hematuria, 441
Hemispheric ischemia, 281
Hemochromatosis, 135
Hemodialysis
compared with hemofiltration and CRRT, hemoperfusion, and peritoneal dialysis, 730t, 734
for acute renal failure, 480
for alcohol or glycol intoxication
diethylene glycol, 239
ethanol, 237
ethylene glycol, 238–239
isopropanol, 238
methanol, 238
propylene glycol, 239
for cyanide poisoning, 247
for drug overdose, 198
lithium, 217
salicylate, 208
theophylline, 215
for hypermagnesemia, 146
for hypervolemic hypernatremia, 128
for oliguria, 10
for tumor lysis syndrome, 547
Hemodynamic monitoring, 774–777
Hemofiltration
compared with hemodialysis, hemoperfusion, and peritoneal dialysis, 730t
for oliguria, 10
Hemoglobin (Hb), 422
hemoglobin M, 253
in upper gastrointestinal hemorrhage, 463
Hemoglobinopathies, 421, 423
Hemoglobinuria, 520
Hemolysis tests, 423
Hemolytic anemias, 421, 423, 425–428
Hemolytic transfusion reactions, 429–431
Hemolytic-uremic syndrome, 409, 411, 413, 427–428, 478
Hemoperfusion
compared with hemofiltration, hemodialysis, and peritoneal dialysis, 730t
for drug overdose, 198–199
calcium channel blockers or b-blockers, 226
sedative-hypnotics, 211
theophylline, 214–215
Hemoperitoneum, 492

Hemophilia, 406
Hemoptysis, massive, 53–56
Hemorrhage
after cardiac surgery, 502–503
after kidney transplantation, 522
after peripheral vascular bypass, 504–506
alveolar, 53
anemia due to, 421, 423
anticoagulant-induced, 617–619
gastrointestinal
lower, 466–469
upper, 463–465
glycoprotein IIb/IIIa receptor antagonist-induced, 624
in coagulopathies, 406–408
in salicylate intoxication, 208
in thrombocytopenia, 409–412
intracerebral, 284–286
management of, 407–408
pontine, 12
postpartum, 555–556
preretinal, 12
retinal, 295
subarachnoid, 12, 82, 287–290
Hemostasis
defects of, 406–408, 412
normal, 406, 409
surgical, 407
Hemothorax, 488, 490
Henderson-Hasselbalch equation, 793, 794
Henoch-Schönlein purpura, 478
Heparin, 617–621
complications of, 419
for acute MI, 67
for air embolism, 563
for central venous catheter thrombosis, 551
for cerebral infarction, 282
for continuous renal replacement therapy, 735
for deep venous thrombosis, 418
for hypercoagulable states, 414–415
for mitral valve dysfunction, 72
for pulmonary embolism, 32, 33
for unstable angina, 62
low molecular weight, 415, 418, 419, 617–621, 620t
post-craniotomy, 499
unfractionated, 617–621, 619t
Heparin-induced thrombocytopenia, 409–411, 413, 419, 617–619
Hepatic abscess, Gram-negative, 334–335, 337
Hepatic encephalopathy, 458–462
Hepatic failure
acetaminophen-induced, 202, 459, 461
continuous renal replacement therapy for, 733–736
fulminant, 455, 458–462
parenteral nutrition-associated, 767–768
Hepatic metastasis, ascites laboratory findings in, 718t
Hepatic transplantation, 371–372
for acetaminophen-induced hepatic failure, 203, 204
for acute alcoholic hepatitis, 453
for fulminant hepatic failure, 460–461
Hepatitis
acute alcoholic, 452–454
fulminant hepatic failure due to, 458, 460
in bone marrow transplant recipients, 366–368
in organ transplant recipients, 370, 523
macrolide antibiotic-induced, 659
transfusion-associated, 429
viral, 455–457

Hepatitis A infection, 455–457
Hepatitis A vaccine, 457
Hepatitis B immunoglobulin (HBIG), for liver transplant recipients, 373
Hepatitis B infection, 455–457
Hepatitis B vaccine, 457
  for liver transplant recipients, 373
Hepatitis C infection, 455–457
  alcoholic liver injury and, 452
Hepatorenal syndrome, 477
Hepatotoxicity, of chemotherapeutic agents, 644
Herpes labialis, 350–351
Herpes simplex virus (HSV) infection, 350–351, 351t
  in bone marrow transplant patients, 366, 367
  in kidney transplant patients, 523
  in neutropenic cancer patients, 362
Herpes zoster, 351–352
Herpetic whitlow, 350, 351
Hetastarch 6%, 566
HFV (high-frequency ventilation), 813–816
"HH" therapy for cerebral vasospasm, 289
"HHH" therapy for cerebral vasospasm, 289
High caloric density feeding formulas, 761
High-frequency ventilation (HFV), 813–816
High-protein feeding formulas, 761
Hirudin, 617
Histamine-2 receptor antagonists (H2RAs), 593–596, 595t
  for anaphylaxis, 536
  for bleeding duodenal ulcer, 465
  for stress ulcer prophylaxis, 285, 289
  in acute pancreatitis, 448
  preoperative, 487
  to prevent aspiration, 43
Histoplasma capsulatum infection, 344, 345, 347, 348
  antifungal therapy for, 671–676
History taking, preoperative, 484–485
HIV infection. See Human immunodeficiency virus (HIV) infection.
HSV (herpes simplex virus) infection, 350–351, 351t
  in bone marrow transplant patients, 366, 367
  in kidney transplant patients, 523
  in neutropenic cancer patients, 362
hTIG (human tetanus immunoglobulin), 315, 316
Human botulinum antitoxin, 313
Human herpes virus 6, 351t, 370
Human herpes virus 7, 351t, 370
Human herpes virus 8, 351t, 370
Human immunodeficiency virus (HIV) infection, 356–358, 357t
  acute abdominal pain in, 445
  cytomegalovirus infection in, 354
  Pneumocystis carinii pneumonia in, 2–3, 38–39, 356, 359–361
  transfusion-associated, 429
Human tetanus immunoglobulin (hTIG), 315, 316
Hydralazine, 575–581
Hydrochlorothiazide, 590
Hydrocodone, 604t
Hydrocortisone
  for adrenal insufficiency, 192–193
  for anaphylactoid reaction to intravenous HBIG, 373
  for anaphylaxis, 535
  for hypercalcemia, 141
  for myxedema coma, 186

Hydrocortisone (Continued)
  for thyroid storm, 183
  for toxic megacolon, 475
  preoperative, 487
Hydromorphone, 603, 604t
  for vaso-occlusive crisis in sickle cell disease, 434
Hydroxocobalamin, for cyanide poisoning, 247
β-Hydroxybutyrate
  in alcoholic ketoacidosis, 161–162
  in diabetic ketoacidosis, 164–165
Hydroxyurea, 644
  for acute chest syndrome in sickle cell disease, 434
Hyperbaric oxygen (HBO) therapy, 199
  for air embolism, 562
  for carbon monoxide poisoning, 251
  for clostridial gas gangrene, 332
  for cyanide poisoning, 247
  for methemoglobinemia, 255
  for necrotizing soft-tissue infections, 401
  for pressure ulcers, 560
  in pregnancy, 251
Hyperbilirubinemia, 441
Hypercalcemia, 139–142
  in rhabdomyolysis, 543, 545
Hypercapnia, 806
  permissive, 813, 815–816
    for ARDS, 24–25
    for COPD, 47
    for pulmonary edema, 22
Hypercoagulable states, 413–415
Hyperglycemia
  enteral feeding-associated, 763
  hyponatremia due to, 119, 121
  in diabetic ketoacidosis, 164
  in hyperosmolar nonketotic coma, 168
  post-craniotomy, 499
Hyperkalemia, 132–134, 133f
  heparin-induced, 618
  in acute renal failure, 479–480
  in diabetic ketoacidosis, 165
  in digoxin overdose, 133, 134, 229–231
  in heat stroke, 533
  in kidney transplant recipients, 522
  in rhabdomyolysis, 543, 545
  in tumor lysis syndrome, 546, 547
  induced by neuromuscular blocking drugs, 598
  pulseless electrical activity due to, 112t, 113t
Hyperlactemia, 158–160
Hypermagnesemia, 146
Hypernatremia, 124–128, 126f
  in diabetes insipidus, 174, 176
  in diabetic ketoacidosis, 165
  in head trauma patients, 496
  in hyperosmolar nonketotic coma, 168
Hyperosmolar nonketotic coma, 168–170
Hyperparathyroidism, 139
Hyperphosphatemia, 151–153
  in rhabdomyolysis, 543
Hyperproteinemia, 119
Hypersensitivity, delayed cutaneous, 772
Hypersensitivity pneumonitis, chemotherapy-induced, 641, 642
Hypertension
  aortic dissection due to, 102–103
  as risk factor for intracerebral hemorrhage, 284
  hypokalemia with, 130
  in cocaine intoxication, 221
  in Guillain-Barré syndrome, 308, 309
  in kidney transplant patients, 523
  in pheochromocytoma, 187

Hypertension (Continued)
  pregnancy-induced, 83–87
  toxin-induced, 195t
  vasoconstrictive catecholamine-induced, 573
Hypertensive crisis, 80–82
Hypertensive nephropathy, 576
Hyperthermia. See also Fever.
  heat stroke, 530–533
  malignant, 1, 3–4, 301–303
Hyperthyroidism, thyroid storm, 181–183
Hypertonic bicarbonate, for calcium channel blocker overdose, 227
Hypertonic saline, 565–566
Hypertonic sodium chloride, for calcium channel blocker overdose, 227
Hyperuricemia, 544
Hyperventilation
  for intracranial hypertension, 285, 297
  in head trauma patients, 496
  toxin-induced, 195t
Hypoalbuminemia, 136
Hypocalcemia, 135–138, 136t, 137t
  in ethylene glycol intoxication, 236
  in heat stroke, 533
  in rhabdomyolysis, 543, 545
Hypocoagulable states, 406
Hypoglycemia, 171–173
  enteral feeding-associated, 763
  seizures due to, 278
Hypokalemia, 129–131, 130f
  in diabetic ketoacidosis, 165
  in digoxin overdose, 229, 230, 232
  in heat stroke, 533
  in hyperosmolar nonketotic coma, 169, 170
  in rhabdomyolysis, 543, 545
Hypomagnesemia, 143–145
  in diabetic ketoacidosis, 165
  in digoxin overdose, 230, 232
  in hyperosmolar nonketotic coma, 169, 170
Hyponatremia, 119–123
  after subarachnoid hemorrhage surgery, 289
  in cardiogenic shock, 89
  in diabetic ketoacidosis, 165
  in head trauma patients, 496
  in hyperosmolar nonketotic coma, 168
  in syndrome of inappropriate antidiuresis, 178–180
  post-craniotomy, 498
Hypoparathyroidism
  hyperphosphatemia in, 153
  hypocalcemia due to, 135
Hypophosphatemia, 147–150
  in diabetic ketoacidosis, 165
  in hyperosmolar nonketotic coma, 169, 170
  in rhabdomyolysis, 543
Hypotension, 5–7
  in cardiogenic shock, 88
  in chronic renal failure, 482
  in cyclic antidepressant overdose, 261
  in fulminant hepatic failure, 459, 460
  in Guillain-Barré syndrome, 308, 309
  in neuroleptic overdose, 258
  in pericardial tamponade, 100
  in status asthmaticus, 36
  in theophylline overdose, 215
  in toxic shock syndrome, 396
  norepinephrine for, 572
  toxin-induced, 195t
  upper gastrointestinal hemorrhage with, 463
  vasodilatory catecholamine-induced, 573

Hypothermia, 525–529, 526t
due to near drowning, 537–538
in burn patients, 515
pulseless electrical activity due to, 112t, 113t
therapeutic, for intracranial hypertension, 297
toxin-induced, 195t
Hypotonic saline, 564–565
Hypoventilation
cor pulmonale due to, 48
hypoxemia due to, 14
mechanisms of, 17
toxin-induced, 195t
Hypovolemia, 746
chemotherapy-induced, 642
fluid therapy for, 6–7
low stroke volume due to, 5
oliguria due to, 8
pulseless electrical activity due to, 112t, 113t
Hypovolemic shock, 88, 322
oxygen transport variables in, 783t
Hypoxemia, 14–15
apnea test in patient with, 745
due to carboxyhemoglobinemia, 51
in aspiration pneumonia, 43
in carbon monoxide poisoning, 250
in cor pulmonale, 48, 49
in cyanide poisoning, 245
in status asthmaticus, 35
mechanisms of, 17
oxygen therapy for, 803–807
oxygen transport variables in, 783t
pulseless electrical activity due to, 112t, 113t
toxin-induced, 195

I

IABP. See Intra-aortic balloon conterpulsation (IABP).
IBD (inflammatory bowel disease), 473, 474
Ibuprofen, 2
Ibutelide, for atrial fibrillation, 105
Ibutilide, 629–633
IBW (ideal body weight), 770
ICH (intracerebral hemorrhage), 284–286
ICP (intracranial pressure), 293, 494
ICP (intracranial pressure) monitoring, 285, 288, 296
in head trauma patients, 495
post-craniotomy, 498
Idarubicin, 642
Ideal body weight (IBW), 770
Idiopathic thrombocytopenic purpura (ITP), 409–411
Ifosfamide, 642, 643
Imdur. See Isosorbide mononitrate.
Imipenem, 665–669
for bone marrow transplant recipients, 367
for clostridial gas gangrene, 332
for Gram-negative infection, 338
for infections in neutropenic cancer patients, 363
Imipenem cilastatin, 665, 669
for necrotizing soft-tissue infections, 400
for pneumonia, 40
for urosepsis, 385
Imipramine, 259
Immune enhancing feeding formulations, 762
Immune-mediated transfusion reactions, 429–431
Immunoglobulin A nephropathy, 478

Immunologic function tests, 772
Immunosuppression
for graft-versus-host disease, 436, 437
for kidney transplantation, 521
for myasthenia gravis, 306
Impedance plethysmography, 417
Implantable cardioverter-defibrillator, 115
Indapamide, 589–591
Indinavir, interaction with benzodiazepines, 608t
Indirect calorimetry, 773
Indomethacin
for diabetes insipidus, 177
for hypercalcemia, 141
for pericarditis, 98
Infantile botulism, 311, 312
Infections
antibiotics for
aminoglycosides, 650–652
antituberculosis drugs, 660–664
fluoroquinolones, 653–654
macrolides, 655–659, 656t
miscellaneous drugs, 665–670
penicillins and cephalosporins, 645–649
coma due to, 11
COPD due to, 46
diarrhea in, 470
due to smoke inhalation, 52
encephalitis, 392–393
epiglottitis, 402–403
fever due to, 1
fungal
candidal, 339–342
non-candidal, 344–349
Gram-negative, 333–338
Gram-positive, 327–332
Guillain-Barré syndrome associated with, 307
in acute pancreatitis, 448
in aspiration pneumonia, 43, 44
in craniotomy patients, 499
in fulminant hepatic failure, 460
in neutropenic cancer patients, 362–364
in renal failure
acute, 480
chronic, 482
in transplant recipients
bone marrow, 365–368
solid organs, 369–373, 522–524
life-threatening oropharyngeal, 387–389
meningitis, 390–391
necrotizing soft-tissue, 399–401
nosocomial sinusitis, 397–398
of dialysis access sites and devices, 482
of pressure ulcers, 557
opportunistic, in AIDS, 356–358, 357t
pneumonia in adults, 37–41
prophylaxis for burn injury, 514
rhabdomyolysis in, 542
sepsis and systemic inflammatory response syndrome, 317–319, 384
septic abortion, 553–554
septic shock, 88, 317, 319, 321–325, 323f
spinal epidural abscess, 298–300, 328
tetanus, 314–316
toxic megacolon due to, 474
toxic shock syndrome, 394–396
transfusion-associated, 429–432
viral
cytomegalovirus, 354–355
herpes, 350–353
human immunodeficiency virus, 356–358
wound botulism, 311–313

Infectious mononucleosis, 352–353
Infective endocarditis, 379–383, 380t
candidal, 342
coagulase-negative staphylococcal, 329
empiric antibiotic therapy for, 338
enterococcal, 331
Gram-negative, 334, 337, 338
preoperative prophylaxis for, 487
Streptococcus viridans, 330
Inferior vena caval filter, 33
Inflammatory bowel disease (IBD), 473, 474
Influenza, in organ transplant recipients, 370
Influenza vaccine, 373
Infrared spectroscopy capnography, 784
INH (isoniazid), 373, 660–663
Inhalation injury, 51–52, 513, 514
carbon monoxide poisoning, 249–252, 513
cyanide poisoning, 247, 513
Injuries
abdominal, 491–493
chest, 488–490
electrical and lightning, 517–520
envenomations, 272–275
myocardial contusion, 73–74
spinal cord compression due to, 298–300
subdural hematoma due to, 291–292
thermal burns, 512–516
Innohep. See Tinzaparin.
Inotropic agents. See also specific drugs.
for calcium channel blocker or β-blocker overdose, 227
for cardiogenic pulmonary edema, 22, 78
for mitral valve dysfunction, 72
for right ventricular MI, 70
for septic shock, 324
for systolic dysfunction, 7
precautions for, 227
Insulin
for alcoholic ketoacidosis, 163
for calcium channel blocker overdose, 227
for diabetic ketoacidosis, 166
for hyperkalemia, 133, 231
for hypermagnesemia, 146
for hyperosmolar nonketotic coma, 169–170
for hyperphosphatemia, 152
preoperative, 487
Integrelin. See Eptifibatide.
α-Interferon, for viral hepatitis, 457
Interleukin-2, 641
Internal jugular approach
for central venous catheterization, 684, 684f
for hemodialysis, 731
Interstitial nephritis, 477
Intra-abdominal infection
empiric antibiotic therapy for, 338
Gram-negative, 334–338
Intra-aortic balloon counterpulsation (IABP), 706–708, 707f
contraindications to, 62
for cardiogenic shock, 89
for left ventricular dysfunction, 7, 78
for mitral valve dysfunction, 72
for right ventricular MI, 70
for unstable angina, 62
Intracerebral hemorrhage (ICH), 284–286
Intracranial hypertension, 285, 293–297, 296f, 297t, 494
in fulminant hepatic failure, 460

Intracranial pressure (ICP), 293, 494
Intracranial pressure (ICP) monitoring, 285, 288, 296, 796–799, 797f, 798f
  in head trauma patients, 495
  post-craniotomy, 498
Intracranial pressure–volume curve, 293, 294, 294f
Intracranial pressure–volume index
Intracranial volume, 293
Intrahospital transport, 737–738
Intraperitoneal abscess, Gram-negative, 335–337
Intravenous fluids, 564–567
Intravenous immunoglobulin (IVIG)
  for cytomegalovirus infection, 355
  for Guillain-Barré syndrome, 309
  for idiopathic thrombocytopenic purpura, 411
  for myasthenia gravis, 306
  for toxic shock syndrome, 396
  for warm autoimmune hemolytic anemia, 427
Intravenous pyelography, 9
Inverse ratio ventilation, 813–816
  for ARDS, 25
Iodide salts, for thyroid storm, 183
Iodine
  in parenteral nutrition solutions, 766
  radioactive, 183
Iopanoic acid, for thyroid storm, 183
Ipratropium bromide, 636–638
  for COPD, 46
  for status asthmaticus, 35
Ipratropium–albuterol combination metered dose inhaler, 638
Ireton-Jones equations, 770–771
Iron, in parenteral nutrition solutions, 766
Iron deficiency anemia, 421, 423
Ischemia
  carotid distribution, 281
  cerebral, 295
  colonic, 510
  coronary, 505
  due to peripheral arterial occlusion, 507–508
  gallbladder, 450
  hemispheric, 281
  renal, 510
  retinal, 281
  vasoactive catecholamine-induced, 573
  vertebrobasilar, 281
Isocal, 761
Isocarboxazid, 267
Isoetharine, 637t, 638
Isoniazid (INH), 373, 660–663
Isopropanol intoxication, 233–235, 238
Isoproterenol, 571–573, 572t
  for bradycardia, 6
  for calcium channel blocker or b-blocker overdose, 227
  for neuroleptic-induced ventricular tachy-dysrhythmias, 257
Isoptin. See Verapamil.
Isordil. See Isosorbide dinitrate.
Isosorbide dinitrate, 586
  for preload reduction, 22
Isosorbide mononitrate, 586
  for preload reduction, 22
Isotonic feeding formulas, 761
Israpidine, 576
ITP (idiopathic thrombocytopenic purpura), 409–411
Itraconazole, 671–674, 676
  for aspergillosis, 349, 368
  for blastomycosis, 348–349
  for coccidioidomycosis, 348
  for histoplasmosis, 348

Itraconazole (Continued)
  for organ transplant recipients, 372
  interaction with benzodiazepines, 608t
IVIG. See Intravenous immunoglobulin (IVIG).

J
Janimine. See Imipramine.
JC virus infection, in organ transplant recipients, 370
Jervell and Lange-Nielsen syndrome, 114
Jevity, 761
Jugular venous oximetry, 495
Jugular venous oxyhemoglobin saturation, 293
Junctional tachycardia, 107

K
Kanamycin, 661–663
Kayexalate. See Sodium polystyrene sulfonate (Kayexalate).
Kayser-Fleischer rings, 136
Keratoconjunctivitis, herpes simplex, 350
Ketoacidosis
  alcoholic, 161–163
  diabetic, 161, 164–167
Ketoconazole, 671–674
  for histoplasmosis, 348
  interaction with benzodiazepines, 608t
α-Ketogluraric acid, for cyanide poisoning, 247
Ketorolac, for rib fractures, 490
Ketosis
  in alcoholic ketoacidosis, 161–162
  in diabetic ketoacidosis, 164–165
Kidney disease
  acute renal failure, 477–480, 479t
  chronic renal failure, 481–483
  history of, 485
  in fulminant hepatic failure, 460
Kidney transplantation, 371, 372, 521–524
Klebsiella infection, 333, 384

L
Labetalol, 224t, 579, 580
  for aortic dissection, 103, 576
  for cerebral infarction, 576
  for hypertension in pregnancy, 85, 87
  for pheochromocytoma, 189
  for preeclampsia-eclampsia, 576
  in cocaine intoxication, 221
  in intracerebral hemorrhage, 285
  in subarachnoid hemorrhage, 289
Lactic acidosis, 158–160
  in acetaminophen overdose, 202
  in cyanide poisoning, 245
  in isopropanol intoxication, 235
  in methanol intoxication, 235
  in propylene glycol intoxication, 236
  vs. alcoholic ketoacidosis, 161
Lambert-Eaton syndrome, 312
Lamifiban, 625
Lamistat. See Lamifiban.
Lamivudine, for hepatitis B infection, 457
Lamotrigine, 612
Langfitt pressure–volume curve, 293, 294, 294f
Lanoteplase (nPA), 622
Lansoprazole, 595, 595t
Laparoscopy, diagnostic, 492

Laparotomy, in abdominal trauma, 493
Large intestinal obstruction, 444
Laryngeal edema, epinephrine for, 572
Laryngotracheobronchitis, 387–389
Latex allergy, 534
Latrodectus spider bites, 272, 273, 275
Lead poisoning, 421, 423
Left ventricular (LV) failure, 7, 75–79
  hemodynamic monitoring in, 774
Left ventricular stroke work index (LVSWI), 775
Legionella infection
  diagnostic tests for, 39
  in organ transplant recipients, 370, 523
Lepirudin, 617–621
Levalbuterol, 637t, 638
Level of consciousness alterations, 11
  aspiration in, 42
  coma, 11–13, 11t
  Ramsay sedation scale, 242t
  withdrawal of mechanical ventilation in, 741t
Levo-Dromoran. See Levorphanol.
Levofloxacin, 653–654
  for aspiration pneumonia, 44
  for pneumonia, 41
  for streptococcal infection, 330
  for tuberculosis, 662
Levorphanol, 604t
LGIB (lower gastrointestinal bleeding), 466–469
Lidocaine
  as antidysrhythmic agent, 629–633
  for air embolism, 563
  for central venous catheterization, 683
  for chest tube thoracostomy, 724
  for endotracheal intubation, 678
  for paracentesis, 716
  for radial artery catheterization, 687
  for Sengstaken-Blakemore tube placement, 749
  for supraventricular tachycardia, 110
  for thoracentesis, 719
  for transnasal intubation, 755
  for ventricular dysrhythmias
    in digoxin overdose, 232
    in neuroleptic overdose, 257
  in anticholinergic poisoning, 265
  in cyclic antidepressant overdose, 261
  in theophylline overdose, 215
Life support withdrawal, 740–741, 741t
Lightning injuries, 517–520
Linezolid, 665–669
Linton tube, 749
Linton-Nachlas tube, 749
Lipase serum activity, 441
  in pancreatitis, 446
Liposomal amphotericin B, 672t
Liquid ventilation, 813, 815, 816
Lisinopril, 575
  for acute MI, 67
  for unstable angina, 62
Listeria monocytogenes infection, 327, 331–332
  in organ transplant recipients, 370, 523
Lithium, 259
  conduction disturbances induced by, 116
  for syndrome of inappropriate antidiuresis, 179
  for thyroid storm, 183
  overdose of, 216–218
Liver dysfunction
  acetaminophen-induced, 202, 459, 461
  acute alcoholic hepatitis, 452–454
  anticoagulants in, 620
  chemotherapy-induced, 644

Liver dysfunction *(Continued)*
  fulminant hepatic failure, 455, 458–462
  Gram-negative abscess, 334–335, 337
  history of, 485
  in bone marrow transplant recipients,
    366, 367
  in heat stroke, 533
  in neutropenic cancer patients, 363
  in organ transplant recipients, 370
  macrolides in, 659
  neuromuscular blocking drugs in, 599
  viral hepatitis, 455–457
Liver metastasis, ascites laboratory findings
  in, 718t
Liver transplantation, 371–372
  for acetaminophen-induced hepatic fail-
    ure, 203, 204
  for acute alcoholic hepatitis, 453
  for fulminant hepatic failure, 460–461
LMWH (low molecular weight heparin),
  415, 418, 419, 617–621, 620t
Local anesthesia
  anaphylactic reactions to, 534
  for central venous catheterization, 683
  for chest tube thoracostomy, 724
  for endotracheal intubation, 678
  for fiberoptic bronchoscopy, 710
  for paracentesis, 716
  for radial artery catheterization, 687
  for thoracentesis, 719
Lomustine, 643
Long QT syndromes, 114–115
Loop diuretics, 589–591
Loracarbef, 645
Lorazepam, 605–607
  for acute MI, 67
  for alcohol withdrawal syndrome, 242t
  for cocaine intoxication, 221
  for intracranial hypertension, 297t
  for seizures/status epilepticus, 13, 278,
    611, 612, 614
  for unstable angina, 62
  in calcium channel blocker or β-blocker
    overdose, 226
  in neuroleptic overdose, 258
  in organophosphate poisoning, 270
Lovenox. *See* Enoxaparin.
Low air loss bed, 558
Low cardiac output syndrome, 76–78
Low molecular weight heparin (LMWH),
  415, 418, 419, 617–621, 620t
Lower gastrointestinal bleeding (LGIB),
  466–469
Loxapine, 256
Loxosceles spider bites, 272–275
Ludiomil. *See* Maprotiline.
Ludwig's angina, 387
Lugol's solution, for thyroid storm, 183
Lumbar plexopathy, 507
Lumbar puncture, 713–715, 714f
  in subarachnoid hemorrhage, 288
Lundberg A, B, and C waves, 799
Lung biopsy, 371
Lung injury
  chemotherapy-induced, 641–642
  inhalation injury, 513
  transfusion-associated, 429–430, 432
  traumatic, 488, 489
Lung transplantation, 372
Lupus anticoagulant, 413, 414
Luvox. *See* Fluvoxamine.
LV (left ventricular) failure, 7, 75–79
  hemodynamic monitoring in, 776
LVSWI (left ventricular stroke work index),
  775
Lymphocyte count, total, 772

M

Macrolide antibiotics, 655–659, 656t
Mafenide acetate, for burns, 514
Magnesium balance
  hypermagnesemia, 146
  hypomagnesemia, 143–145
Magnesium chloride hexahydrate tablets,
  144
Magnesium gluconate dihydrate tablets, 145
Magnesium lactate, 145
Magnesium oxide tablets, 144
Magnesium sulfate
  for digoxin toxicity with hyperkalemia,
    134
  for hypomagnesemia, 144
  for preeclampsia during labor and deliv-
    ery, 86
  for status asthmaticus, 35
  for tetanus, 315
  for ventricular dysrhythmias
    in digoxin overdose, 232
    in neuroleptic overdose, 257
  specifying dosage of, 144
Magnesium supplementation
  for hyperosmolar nonketotic coma, 170
  for hypocalcemia, 137
  for hypomagnesemia, 144–145
  in parenteral nutrition solutions, 765
Magnetic resonance imaging (MRI)
  in abdominal aortic aneurysm, 509
  in aortic dissection, 102
  in carbon monoxide poisoning, 250
  in cerebral infarction, 281–282
  in comatose patient, 12
  in cor pulmonale, 49
  in deep venous thrombosis, 417
  in intracerebral hemorrhage, 284
  in meningitis, 336
  in pericarditis, 97
  in pulmonary embolism, 31
  in spinal cord compression, 299
  in subdural hematoma, 292
  in tuberculosis, 377
  of pheochromocytoma, 188
Malassezia furfur infection, 344, 348
Malignant hyperthermia, 1, 3–4, 301–303
  dantrolene for, 302, 634–635
Mallory-Weiss tears, 464
Manerix. *See* Moclobemide.
Manganese, in parenteral nutrition solutions, 766
Mannitol, 589–591
  in hyponatremia, 121
  for intracranial hypertension, 285, 296
  in rhabdomyolysis, 544
MAP (mean arterial pressure), 5, 774, 776
Maprotiline, 259
Marfan's syndrome, 90, 91
Mass spectroscopy capnography, 784
Massasaugas snakebite, 272
MAT (multifocal atrial tachycardia), 107,
  110
Maxair. *See* Pirbuterol.
Mean arterial pressure (MAP), 5, 774, 776
Mean systolic pressure (MSP), 774
Mechanical ventilation, 808–816. *See also*
  specific modes.
  after cardiac surgery, 500–502
  barotrauma induced by, 28–29, 36, 811,
    818
  complications of, 811–812
  conventional, 808–812, 811f
  for ARDS, 24–26
  for atelectasis, 58
  for cardiogenic shock, 89

Mechanical ventilation *(Continued)*
  for COPD, 47
  for head trauma patients, 495, 496
  for left ventricular dysfunction, 78
  for lung parenchymal injuries, 489
  for malignant hyperthermia, 302
  for *Pneumocystis carinii* pneumonia, 360
  for pulmonary edema, 22, 77
  for septic shock, 325
  for smoke inhalation, 52
  for status asthmaticus, 35
  in Guillain-Barré syndrome, 309
  in intracerebral hemorrhage, 285
  in myasthenia gravis, 306
  indications for, 18
  initiation of, 809–810
  lung-protective strategy for, 24, 29
  monitoring of, 810–811
  neuromuscular blocking drugs for, 597–
    601
  newer modes of, 813–816
  pneumonia associated with, 38, 39, 41
  positive end-expiratory pressure, 817–
    819, 818f
  respiratory acidosis or alkalosis in pa-
    tients on, 157
  survival of adults on, 19
  weaning from, 820–822
  withdrawal of life support, 740–741,
    741t
Meckel's diverticulitis, 443
Mediastinal tumors, superior vena cava syndrome due to, 549
Medicolegal issues
  brain death determination, 742–745
  do-not-resuscitate orders, 739–741
Megaloblastic anemia, 421, 423
Melena, 463
Melphalan, 641, 642
Mendelson's syndrome, 42
Meningitis, 390–391
  coma in, 12
  cryptococcal, 345–348
  empiric antibiotic therapy for, 337, 390
  fever in, 2
  Gram-negative, 333, 336, 337
  herpes simplex, 351
  in AIDS, 356
  in coccidioidomycosis, 345, 348
  Listeria monocytogenes, 331
  pneumococcal, 330
  tuberculous, 374, 663
Mental status alterations
  in carbon monoxide poisoning, 249–250
  in encephalitis, 392
  in organ transplant recipients, 371
  in serotonin syndrome, 267
Meperidine, 602, 604t
  before intravenous HBIG, 373
  contraindicated in sickle cell disease, 434
6-Mercaptopurine, 642, 644
Meropenem, 665–669
  for Gram-negative infection, 338
  for infections in neutropenic cancer pa-
    tients, 363
  for pneumonia, 40
Mesoridazine, 256
Metabolic acidosis, 155–157, 155f
  alcoholic ketoacidosis and, 161
  diabetic ketoacidosis and, 164
  in alcohol and glycol intoxications, 236t
    diethylene glycol, 237
    ethylene glycol, 236
    methanol, 235
    propylene glycol, 236
  in cyanide poisoning, 245

Metabolic acidosis *(Continued)*
  in rhabdomyolysis, 544
  in salicylate intoxication, 207
  lactic acidosis and, 159
  toxin-induced, 195
Metabolic alkalosis, 155, 155f, 157
  alcoholic ketoacidosis and, 161
  in rhabdomyolysis, 544
Metaproterenol, 637t, 638
  for COPD, 46
  for status asthmaticus, 34
Metastatic disease, spinal cord compression
    due to, 298, 299
Methadone, 604t
Methanol intoxication, 233–235, 237–238
Methemoglobin, 790
  stroma-free, for cyanide poisoning, 247
Methemoglobinemia, 253–255
  in cyanide poisoning, 245, 246
Methicillin, 645
Methicillin-resistant *Staphylococcus aureus*
  endocarditis due to, 382–383
  in organ transplant recipients, 369
Methimazole, for thyroid storm, 183
Methotrexate, 641–644
Methyl cyanide ingestion, 247–248
Methyl salicylate overdose, 205
L-N^G-Methylarginine, for septic shock, 324
N-Methyl-D-aspartate receptor antagonists,
    for intracranial hypertension, 297
α-Methyldopa, 575
  conduction disturbances induced by, 116
  for hypertension in pregnancy, 85
Methylene blue, for methemoglobinemia,
    255
Methylergonovine, for postpartum hemor-
    rhage, 555
Methylprednisolone
  for acute alcoholic hepatitis, 453
  for ARDS, 26
  for COPD, 47
  for graft-versus-host disease, 436, 437
  for kidney transplantation, 521
  for *Pneumocystis carinii* pneumonia, 360t
  for smoke inhalation, 52
  for spinal cord compression, 300
  for status asthmaticus, 35
  for thrombotic thrombocytopenic pur-
    pura, 428
  for toxic megacolon, 475
15-Methylprostaglandin F, for postpartum
    hemorrhage, 555
Methysergide, for serotonin syndrome, 268
Metoclopramide
  after N-acetylcysteine for acetaminophen
    overdose, 203
  to prevent aspiration, 43
Metolazone, 589–591
  for pulmonary edema, 77
Metoprolol, 224t, 576, 579t, 629
  after peripheral vascular bypass, 505
  for acute MI, 66
  for atrial fibrillation, 105
  for atrial flutter, 106
  for unstable angina, 61
Metronidazole, 665–670
  for acute cholecystitis, 451
  for aspiration pneumonia, 44
  for bone marrow transplant recipients,
    367
  for brain abscess, 337
  for clostridial gas gangrene, 332
  for *Clostridium difficile* colitis, 3
  for deep space infections of neck, 389
  for infections in neutropenic cancer pa-
    tients, 364

Metronidazole *(Continued)*
  for necrotizing soft-tissue infections, 400
  for tetanus, 315
  for toxic megacolon, 475
  for wound botulism, 313
Metyrosine, for pheochromocytoma, 189
Mexiletine, 629
Mezlocillin, 645, 646, 648
MFS (Miller-Fisher syndrome), 307, 308
MG (myasthenia gravis), 304–306, 312
MI. *See* Myocardial infarction (MI), acute.
MIBG (radioiodinated meta-iodobenzyl-
    guanidine) scintigraphy, 189
Miconazole, 673, 675
  for candidal infection, 341
Microangiopathic hemolytic anemia, 425,
    426
Microangiopathy, 413, 414
Microembolism, 406
Midazolam, 605–607
  for alcohol withdrawal syndrome, 242t
  for status epilepticus, 279
Miller-Abbott tube, 754
Miller-Fisher syndrome (MFS), 307, 308
Milrinone, 568–570
  for calcium channel blocker or b-blocker
    overdose, 227
  for cardiogenic pulmonary edema, 22
  for left ventricular dysfunction, 7, 78
Minnesota tube, 749, 750
Minoxidil, 575–581
Miosis, in drug overdose, 194
Mirtazapine, 259, 267
Mitomycin C, 641–644
Mitoxantrone, 642
Mitral regurgitation (MR), 90–92, 94–95
Mitral stenosis (MS), 90–92, 94
Mitral valve dysfunction in acute MI, 72
Mitral valve prolapse (MVP), 92
Mitral valve replacement (MVR), 94–95
Mivacron. *See* Mivacurium.
Mivacurium, 599t
Mixed venous carbon dioxide tension
    (PXCO_2), 790
Mixed venous oxygen content (C$\bar{v}O_2$), 781,
    790
Mixed venous oxygen saturation (S$\bar{v}O_2$),
    781, 783t, 790
Mixed venous oxygen tension (P$\bar{v}O_2$), 789–
    790
MK 801, for intracranial hypertension, 297
Mobitz types I and II AV block, 116
Moclobemide, 259, 267
Modified Allen test, 687
Moexipril, 577
Molindone, 256
Monoamine oxidase (MAO) inhibitors,
    259
  antihypertensives for interaction between
    tyramines and, 577
  serotonin syndrome and, 267–268
Monoket. *See* Isosorbide mononitrate.
Monro-Kellie doctrine, 293
Moraxella catarrhalis infection, 333
Moricizine, 629
Morphine, 602–604, 604t
  for acute MI, 69
  for burn injury, 514
  for intracranial hypertension, 297t
  for preload reduction, 21
  for tetanus, 315
  for unstable angina, 61
  for vaso-occlusive crisis in sickle cell dis-
    ease, 434
Moxifloxacin, for pneumonia, 41
MR (mitral regurgitation), 90–92, 94–95

MRI. *See* Magnetic resonance imaging
    (MRI).
MS (mitral stenosis), 90–92, 94
MSP (mean systolic pressure), 774
Mucormycosis, 344–349
  antifungal therapy for, 671–676
  in kidney transplant patients, 523
  vs. bacterial sinusitis, 398
Mucositis
  chemotherapy-induced, 644
  in bone marrow transplant recipients, 366
  in neutropenic cancer patients, 362
Multifocal atrial tachycardia (MAT), 107,
    110
Multiple myeloma, 411, 478
Murphy's sign, 450
Muscarinic receptors, 263
Muscle injury, 542
MVP (mitral valve prolapse), 92
MVR (mitral valve replacement), 94–95
Myasthenia gravis (MG), 304–306, 312
Mycobacterial infection, nontuberculous,
    374, 375
Mycobacterium tuberculosis infection, 374–
    378
  drug therapy for, 660–664
  drug-resistant, 660, 662
  hemoptysis in, 53
  in organ transplant recipients, 370, 373,
    523
Mycophenolate mofetil
  for kidney transplantation, 521
  for myasthenia gravis, 306
Mycoplasma diagnostic tests, 39
Mycostatin
  for candidal infection, 341
  for organ transplant recipients, 372
Mydriasis, in drug overdose, 194
Myeloproliferative disorders, 416
Myocardial contusion, 73–74
Myocardial infarction (MI), acute, 64–68
  in aortic dissection, 102
  in chronic renal failure, 482
  mechanical complications of, 71–72
    mitral valve dysfunction, 72
    ventricular free wall rupture, 71
    ventricular septal rupture, 71–72
  minimizing risk in abdominal aortic aneu-
    rysm, 509–510
  pulseless electrical activity due to, 112t,
    113t
  right ventricular, 69–70
  thrombolytic agents for, 622–623
Myocardial ischemia or necrosis, chemo-
    therapy-induced, 642
Myocardial oxygen supply-demand mis-
    match, 59, 65
Myoglobinemia, 543
Myoglobinuria, 520, 544
Myonecrosis, 399–401
Myxedema, pretibial, 182
Myxedema coma, 184–186

N

NAC (N-acetylcysteine)
  for acetaminophen overdose, 202–204,
    459
  in methemoglobinemia, 255
Nadolol, 224t, 576
Nafamostat mesylate, for continuous renal
    replacement therapy, 735
Nafcillin, 645, 646, 648
  for bone marrow transplant recipients,
    367

Nafcillin (Continued)
  for staphylococcal infection, 329, 382, 383, 396
Nalbuphine, 604t
Naloxone, 602–604
  for morphine reversal, 297t
  for opioid overdose, 210
  for unexplained coma, 12
Narcotic agonists, 602–604, 604t
Narcotic antagonists, 602
Narcotics, 602–604
  interaction with benzodiazepines, 608t
  overdose of, 209–212
Nardil. See Phenelzine.
Nasal cannula, 803, 805
Nasal mask, 804
Nasoenteric tube, 754
Nasogastric (NG) tube, 754, 760
Nausea and vomiting
  abdominal pain with, 439–440
  chemotherapy-induced, 644
NBDs. See Neuromuscular blocking drugs (NBDs).
Near drowning, 537–538
Neck, deep space infections of, 387–389
Necrotizing fasciitis, 399–401
  Gram-negative, 336, 337
  group A streptococcal, 329, 330
Necrotizing soft-tissue infections, 399–401
Needle thoracostomy, 490
Nefazodone, 259, 267
Negative pressure ventilation, 808
Neisseria meningitidis infection, 333
  meningitis, 390–391
Nelfinavir, interaction with benzodiazepines, 608t
Nephrosis, ascites laboratory findings in, 718t
Nepro, 762
Netilmicin, 650–652
Neuroleptic malignant syndrome, 2, 4, 257, 301–303
  dantrolene for, 635
  vs. serotonin syndrome, 268t
Neuroleptics
  for cocaine intoxication, 221
  for heat stroke, 532
  overdose of, 256–258
Neurologic evaluation
  post-craniotomy, 498
  preoperative, 484
Neuromuscular blocking drugs (NBDs), 597–601, 599t
  anaphylactic reactions to, 534
  drug interactions with, 598, 599
  for endotracheal intubation, 678
  for tetanus, 315
  in ARDS, 26
  malignant hyperthermia precipitated by, 301–303
  sedation and, 801–802
Neuroprotection, 495–496
Neurotoxicity, of chemotherapeutic agents, 643–644
Neutropenia
  filgrastim for, 639–640
  infections in cancer patients with, 362–364
Nexium. See Esomeprazole.
NG (nasogastric) tube, 754, 760
Nicardipine, 224t, 576, 579
  for preeclampsia-eclampsia, 576
Nifedipine, 224t, 579, 579t
  for cor pulmonale, 49
  for hypertension in pregnancy, 85
  overdose of, 223, 228

Nimbex. See Cisatracurium.
Nimodipine, for cerebral vasospasm, 289
NIPPV (noninvasive positive pressure ventilation), 813–816
Nisoldipine, 224t
Nitric oxide, inhaled
  for ARDS, 26
  for cor pulmonale, 49
Nitro-bid. See Nitroglycerin (NTG).
Nitro-Dur. See Nitroglycerin (NTG).
Nitrogard. See Nitroglycerin (NTG).
Nitrogen balance study, 772
Nitroglycerin (NTG), 572t, 575, 585–586
  for acute MI, 66
  for angina, 59
  for cardiogenic pulmonary edema, 21, 77
  for mitral valve dysfunction, 72
  for unstable angina, 61
  in cocaine intoxication, 221
Nitrol. See Nitroglycerin (NTG).
Nitrolingual. See Nitroglycerin (NTG).
Nitrong. See Nitroglycerin (NTG).
Nitroprusside. See Sodium nitroprusside (SNP).
Nitrosoureas, 644
Nitrostat. See Nitroglycerin (NTG).
Nizoral. See Ketoconazole.
Nocardia asteroides infection, in organ transplant recipients, 370, 523
Nondepolarizing neuromuscular blocking drugs, 597–601, 599t
Noninvasive positive pressure ventilation (NIPPV), 813–816
Non-rebreather mask, 804, 806
Nonsteroidal anti-inflammatory drugs (NSAIDs)
  anaphylactic reactions to, 534
  for pericarditis, 98
  for rib fractures, 490
  upper gastrointestinal hemorrhage induced by, 463, 464
Norcuron. See Vecuronium.
Norepinephrine, 571, 572, 572t
  for calcium channel blocker or b-blocker overdose, 227
  for low cardiac output, 78
  for low systemic vascular resistance, 6
  for neuroleptic overdose, 258
  for septic shock, 324
  for spinal cord compression, 300
  in cyclic antidepressant overdose, 261
  in theophylline overdose, 215
Norfloxacin, for bone marrow transplant patients, 368
Normal saline (NS), 564
Normiflo. See Ardeparin.
Norpramin. See Desipramine.
Nortriptyline, 259
Norvasc. See Amlodipine.
NovaSource 2.0, 761
nPA (lanoteplase), 622
NS (normal saline), 564
NSAIDs (nonsteroidal anti-inflammatory drugs)
  anaphylactic reactions to, 534
  for pericarditis, 98
  for rib fractures, 490
  upper gastrointestinal hemorrhage induced by, 463, 464
NTG. See Nitroglycerin (NTG).
Nubain. See Nalbuphine.
Nuchal rigidity, 12, 390
Nuclear cardiac imaging
  in acute MI, 65
  in unstable angina, 60
Nuromax. See Doxacurium.

Nutren 1.0, 761
Nutren 1.5, 761
NutriHep, 762
Nutritional assessment, 770–773
Nutritional support
  enteral feeding, 760–763, 761f
  for burn injury, 515
  in acute pancreatitis, 448
  in ARDS, 26
  parenteral nutrition, 764–769
Nystagmus
  in drug overdose, 194
  persistent, 12
Nystatin, 671, 673, 674, 676
  for candidal infection, 341

O

O₂ex (oxygen extraction index), 782–783, 782f, 783t, 791
Observer's assessment of alertness sedation scale, 800, 801t
Obstetric crises, 552–556
Obstructive airway disease
  respiratory failure due to, 17
  tachypnea due to, 15
Obstructive shock, 322
Occupational exposure to viral hepatitis, 457
Octreotide, for gastrointestinal bleeding, 464, 465, 468
Oculocephalic reflex, 11
  confirming absence of, 743
Oculovestibular reflexes, confirming absence of, 743
Ofloxacin, 653–654
  for tuberculosis, 662
Ogilvie's syndrome, 444
  after kidney transplantation, 524
Ohm's law, 5, 517
Olanzapine, 256
Oliguria, 8–10, 477
Omeprazole, 595, 595t
  for bleeding duodenal ulcer, 465
  to prevent aspiration, 43
Ondansetron
  after N-acetylcysteine for acetaminophen overdose, 203
  to prevent aspiration, 44
OP (organophosphate) poisoning, 269–271
Opiates, 602–604, 604t
  interaction with benzodiazepines, 608t
  overdose of, 12, 13, 209–212
Organophosphate (OP) poisoning, 269–271
Oropharyngeal infections
  candidiasis, 339–341
  life-threatening, 387–389
Osmolite, 761
Osmotic demyelination syndrome, 122, 123, 180
Osmotic diuretic, 589–591
Ovarian tumor, 444
Oxacillin, 645, 646, 648
  for staphylococcal infection, 329, 382, 383, 396
Oxazepam, 605
  for alcohol withdrawal syndrome, 242t
Oxcarbazepine, 612
Oximetry, 788–792
  CO-oximetry, 789
  jugular venous, 495
  pulse, 14, 15
    during fiberoptic bronchoscopy, 710
    in burn patients, 515
    in carbon monoxide poisoning, 250

Oximetry (Continued)
  in methemoglobinemia, 254
  pitfalls of, 792
Oxycodone, 604t
Oxygen consumption (VO_2), 782, 782f, 783, 783t
Oxygen consumption index (VO_2I), 782
Oxygen extraction (O_2ex), 782–783, 782f, 783t, 791
Oxygen therapy, 803–807
  for acute MI, 66, 69
  for air embolism, 562
  for anticholinergic toxicity, 265
  for atelectasis, 57
  for carbon monoxide poisoning, 251
  for COPD, 47
  for hemoptysis, 54
  for methemoglobinemia, 255
  for pneumonia, 41
  for pulmonary edema, 21, 22, 77
  for respiratory failure, 18
  for smoke inhalation, 52
  for status asthmaticus, 35
  for unstable angina, 61
  hyperbaric, 199
    for air embolism, 562
    for carbon monoxide poisoning, 251
    for clostridial gas gangrene, 332
    for cyanide poisoning, 247
    for methemoglobinemia, 255
    for necrotizing soft-tissue infections, 401
    for pressure ulcers, 560
    in pregnancy, 251
Oxygen toxicity, 806, 811
Oxygen transport monitoring, 781–783, 782f, 783t
Oxyhemoglobin concentration, 789
Oxytocin, for postpartum hemorrhage, 555

P

PA catheterization. See Pulmonary artery (PA) catheterization.
PA (pulmonary artery) pressure, 774, 776
Pacing. See Cardiac pacing.
$PaCO_2$ (arterial carbon dioxide tension), 790
PAE (paradoxical arterial embolism), 561
Paget's disease of bone, 139
Pain
  acute abdominal, 439–445
  evaluation of, 800
  vaso-occlusive crisis in sickle cell disease, 433–434
Pamelor. See Nortriptyline.
Pamidronate disodium, for hypercalcemia, 141
Pancreas transplantation, 372
Pancreatic abscess, 335, 337, 446
Pancreatic ascites, 718t
Pancreatic necrosis, 446, 448–449
Pancreatic pseudocyst, 446
Pancreatitis
  acute, 439, 441, 443, 446–449, 447t
    in kidney transplant patients, 523
    parenteral nutrition-associated, 768
Pancuronium, 597, 599, 599t
  for endotracheal intubation, 678
Panto. See Pantoprazole.
Pantoprazole, 595t
PAO_2 (alveolar oxygen tension), 790
PaO_2 (arterial oxygen tension), 789
PaO_2:FIO_2 ratio, 790
PAOP (pulmonary artery occlusion pressure), 692–693, 692f, 746, 747f, 748, 775, 776

Papilledema, 295
Para-aminosalicylic acid (PAS), 661–663
Paracentesis, 716–718
Paradoxical arterial embolism (PAE), 561
Paraproteinemias, malignant, 411
Parathormone (PTH)
  in hypercalcemia, 139
  in hyperphosphatemia, 152
  in hypocalcemia, 135
Parathyroidectomy, 141
Parenteral nutrition, 764–769
  in acute pancreatitis, 448
  phosphate in, 149
Parkinsonism, neuroleptic-induced, 257, 258
Parnate. See Tranylcypromine.
Paroxetine, 259, 267
Paroxysmal atrial tachycardia, 107
  digoxin for, 626
Paroxysmal cold hemoglobinuria, 425–428
Paroxysmal nocturnal hemoglobinuria, 423, 426
Partial non-rebreather mask, 804
Partial thromboplastin time (PTT), 414, 417
PAS (para-aminosalicylic acid), 661–663
Patent foramen ovale, 561
Patient positioning
  for central venous catheterization, 683
  for chest tube thoracostomy, 724
  for endotracheal intubation, 678
  for lumbar puncture, 713, 714f
  for Sengstaken-Blakemore tube placement, 749
  for thoracentesis, 719
  in ARDS, 25
  in atelectasis, 57, 58
  in intracranial hypertension, 296
  pressure ulcers associated with, 558
  to prevent aspiration, 43
Patient transport, intrahospital, 737–738
Pavulon. See Pancuronium.
Paxil. See Paroxetine.
PCO_2 (carbon dioxide tension), 784
PDE (phosphodiesterase) inhibitors
  amrinone and milrinone, 568–570
  for calcium channel blocker or b-blocker overdose, 227
PE. See Pulmonary embolism (PE).
PEA (pulseless electrical activity), 111, 112t, 113t
PEEP. See Positive end-expiratory pressure (PEEP).
Pelvic fractures, 491
Penciclovir, for herpes simplex virus infection, 351
Penicillin(s), 645–649
  for bone marrow transplant recipients, 367
  for clostridial gas gangrene, 332
  for deep space infections of neck, 389
  for diphtheria, 389
  for endocarditis, 382
  for enterococcal infection, 331
  for Listeria monocytogenes infection, 332
  for necrotizing soft-tissue infections, 400
  for staphylococcal infection, 329
  for streptococcal infection, 330, 396
  for tetanus, 315
  for wound botulism, 313
Penicillin G, 645–648
Penicillin V, 645, 647
Pentamidine, for Pneumocystis carinii pneumonia, 360t, 368, 372, 522
Pentastarch 10%, 566
Pentazocine, 604t

Pentobarbital
  for intracranial hypertension, 297
  for seizures, 614, 615
Pentostatin, 642–644
Pepcid. See Famotidine.
Peptic ulcer
  perforated, 442
  upper gastrointestinal hemorrhage due to, 464
Perative, 761
Percocet. See Oxycodone.
Percutaneous transluminal angioplasty, 289
Pericardial constriction, 96–99
  vs. pericardial tamponade, 100
  vs. right ventricular MI, 69, 101
Pericardial effusion, 96, 99
  in myxedema coma, 185
Pericardial friction rub, 96, 100
Pericardial knock, 96
Pericardial resection, 98–99
Pericardial tamponade, 7, 100–101
  after cardiac surgery, 502
  chest trauma with, 488–490
  due to pericarditis, 96, 97, 99
  hemodynamic monitoring in, 776
  pulseless electrical activity due to, 112t, 113t
  vs. right ventricular MI, 69
Pericardial tuberculosis, 375
Pericardial window, 98, 490
Pericardiectomy, 98
Pericardiocentesis, 98–99, 490, 704–705, 705f
Pericarditis, 96–99
  chemotherapy-induced, 642
  dialysis-associated, 481
  radiation-induced, 642
  tuberculous, 663
  uremic, 481
  vs. acute MI, 65
  vs. angina, 60
Perinephric abscess, 386
Peripartum cardiomyopathy, 552
Peripheral arterial occlusion, acute, 507–508
Peripheral parenteral nutrition, 768–769
Peripheral vascular bypass, patient management after, 504–506
Peritoneal carcinomatosis, 718t
Peritoneal dialysis. See also Dialysis; Hemodialysis.
  compared with hemodialysis, hemofiltration, and hemoperfusion, 730t
  for hypervolemic hypernatremia, 128
  for isopropanol intoxication, 238
Peritoneal lavage, 492
Peritonitis, 440, 442
  ascites laboratory findings in, 718t
  candidal, 340
  Gram-negative, 335, 337
  tuberculous, 374
Periumbilical pain, 439
Permissive hypercapnia, 813, 815–816
  for ARDS, 24–25
  for COPD, 47
  for pulmonary edema, 22
Perphenazine, 256
Persistent vegetative state, 11
Pertofane. See Desipramine.
Phenelzine, 259, 267
Phenobarbital, 611–615
  for status epilepticus, 13, 279
  in neuroleptic overdose, 258
  in organophosphate poisoning, 270
Phenoxybenzamine hydrochloride, for pheochromocytoma, 189, 577

Phenoxymethyl penicillin, 645
Phentolamine mesylate, 576–581
    for drug and ethanol withdrawal syn-
        dromes, 576
    for monoamine oxidase inhibitor-tyra-
        mine interaction, 576
    for pheochromocytoma, 189, 190, 577
    in cocaine intoxication, 221
Phentolamine provocation test, 188
Phenylephrine, 572, 572t, 573
    for calcium channel blocker overdose,
        227
    for low systemic vascular resistance, 6
    for neuroleptic overdose, 258
    for Sengstaken-Blakemore tube place-
        ment, 749
    for septic shock, 324
    for transnasal intubation, 755
    in cyclic antidepressant overdose, 261
    in theophylline overdose, 215
Phenytoin, 611–616, 629
    for head trauma patients, 495
    for status epilepticus, 13, 278
    for syndrome of inappropriate antidi-
        uresis, 179
    for ventricular dysrhythmias in digoxin
        overdose, 232
    in cyclic antidepressant overdose, 261
    in intracerebral hemorrhage, 285
    in organophosphate poisoning, 270
    in subarachnoid hemorrhage, 289
    in theophylline overdose, 215
    interaction with benzodiazepines, 608t
    post-craniotomy, 498
Pheochromocytoma, 187–190
    antihypertensives for, 577
Phlegmasia cerulea dolens, 507
Phosphate supplementation
    complications of, 149
    for diabetic ketoacidosis, 167
    for hypercalcemia, 141
    for hyperosmolar nonketotic coma, 170
    for hypophosphatemia, 149
    in parenteral nutrition solutions, 765
    specifying dosage for, 149
Phosphodiesterase (PDE) inhibitors
    amrinone and milrinone, 568–570
    for calcium channel blocker or b-blocker
        overdose, 227
Phosphorus balance
    hyperphosphatemia, 151–153
    hypophosphatemia, 147–150
    in rhabdomyolysis, 543
Physical examination, preoperative, 485–486
Physostigmine
    for anticholinergic poisoning, 265–266
    for cyclic antidepressant overdose, 261
Piezoelectric strain gauge, 796
Pindolol, 224t, 576
Piperacillin, 645, 646, 648
Piperacillin-tazobactam, 645, 646, 648
    for acute cholecystitis, 451
    for aspiration pneumonia, 44
    for Gram-negative infection, 337, 338
    for necrotizing soft-tissue infections, 400
Pipercuronium, 599t
Pirbuterol, 637t, 638
Pit viper envenomation, 272–275, 274t
Placental abruption, 554–555
Plasma protein assays, 771–772
Plasmapheresis
    for botulism, 313
    for Guillain-Barré syndrome, 309
    for myasthenia gravis, 306
    for thrombotic thrombocytopenic pur-
        pura, 411, 428

Plasminogen activator inhibitor 1, 406
Platelet dysfunction, uremic, 482
Platelet number and function, 409
Platelet transfusion, 407, 411, 412, 413
Plendil. See Felodipine.
Pleural decompression, 489–490
Pleural effusion, thoracentesis for, 3, 719–
    723
Pleural tuberculosis, 375
Plicamycin, 643, 644
    for hypercalcemia, 141
Plummer's syndrome, 181
Pneumocandins, for aspergillosis, 349
Pneumococcal antigen tests, 39
Pneumococcal infection, 327, 330
Pneumocystis carinii pneumonia, 2–3, 38–
    39, 356, 359–361, 360t
    in bone marrow transplant patients, 366–
        368
    in organ transplant recipients, 370, 372,
        523
    prophylaxis for, 522
Pneumomediastinum, 28
Pneumonia
    ARDS due to, 26
    aspiration, 37, 40, 42–45
    community-acquired, 37–40
    empiric antibiotic therapy for, 337
    Gram-negative, 333–334, 336–337
    group A streptococcal, 329–330
    herpes simplex, 351
    hospital-acquired, 37, 38, 40, 41
    in adults, 37–41
    in AIDS, 356
    in blastomycosis, 345–346
    in bone marrow transplant recipients,
        366, 367
    in neutropenic cancer patients, 362, 363
    pneumococcal, 330
    Pneumocystis carinii, 2–3, 38–39, 356,
        359–361, 360t
        in bone marrow transplant patients,
            366–368
        in organ transplant recipients, 370,
            372, 523
        prophylaxis for, 522
    Staphylococcus aureus, 328, 329
    ventilator-associated, 38, 39, 41
Pneumonitis
    aspiration, 37, 40, 42–45
    chemotherapy-induced, 641–642
    hypersensitivity, 641, 642
Pneumothorax, 488–490
    chest tube thoracostomy for, 724–728
    tension, 7, 28, 29, 112t, 113t, 488–490
Poisoning, 194–200. See also Drug over-
    dose.
    agents that may cause delayed toxicity,
        197t
    alcohols and glycols, 233–239
    anticholinergic, 263–266
    antidotes for, 199t
    carbon monoxide, 249–252, 513
    clinical toxidromes caused by, 196t
    cyanide, 244–248, 513
    methemoglobinemia, 253–255
    organophosphate, 269–271
    rhabdomyolysis due to, 542
    serotonin syndrome, 267–268
    toxins for which 24-hour monitoring is
        recommended, 197t
    toxins that alter vital signs, 195t
Polyarteritis nodosa, 478
Polycythemia, 478
Polydipsia
    dipsogenic, 120, 174

Polydipsia (Continued)
    in diabetes insipidus, 174
    psychogenic, 120, 174, 175
Polyethylene glycol conjugated supra oxide
    dismutase, for intracranial hyperten-
    sion, 297
Polyethylene glycol (GoLytely, CoLyte) for
    drug overdose, 198
    anticholinergic agents, 265
    calcium channel blockers or b-blockers,
        226
    digoxin, 230
    lithium, 217
Polyomavirus infection, in organ transplant
    recipients, 370
Polyuria
    after cardiac surgery, 501
    differential diagnosis of, 174–175
    in diabetes insipidus, 174
Positive end-expiratory pressure (PEEP),
    817–819, 818f
    assist-controlled mode with, 809f
    auto-PEEP, 811, 819
    barotrauma due to, 24, 28–29
    for ARDS, 24–26
    for aspiration pneumonia, 44, 45
    for atelectasis, 58
    for head trauma patients, 495, 496
    for pulmonary edema, 22
    for smoke inhalation, 52
Positive pressure ventilation
    for COPD, 47
    for pneumonia, 41
    for pulmonary edema, 21, 77
    for respiratory failure, 18
    for status asthmaticus, 35
    noninvasive, 813–816
Post-cardiac surgery management, 500–503
Post-craniotomy management, 498–499
Postpartum hemorrhage, 555–556
Post-peripheral vascular bypass manage-
    ment, 504–506
Potassium balance
    hyperkalemia, 132–134, 133f
    hypokalemia, 129–131, 130f
    in diabetic ketoacidosis, 165
    in digoxin overdose, 133, 134, 229
    in rhabdomyolysis, 543, 545
Potassium phosphate, 149
Potassium supplementation
    for diabetic ketoacidosis, 167
    for hyperosmolar nonketotic coma, 170
    for hypokalemia, 130–131, 232
    in adrenal insufficiency, 193
    in parenteral nutrition solutions, 765
Potassium-sparing diuretics, 589–591
Pott's disease, 374
PPD (purified protein derivative) test, 376
PPIs. See Proton-pump inhibitors (PPIs).
Pralidoxime, for organophosphate poison-
    ing, 271
Prazosin, 575–581
    for pheochromocytoma, 189, 577
Pre-albumin plasma assay, 771
Prednisone
    for hypercalcemia, 141
    for kidney transplantation, 521
    for Pneumocystis carinii pneumonia, 360t
    for thrombocytopenia, 411
    for warm autoimmune hemolytic anemia,
        427
Preeclampsia, 83–87
    antihypertensives for, 576
Pregnancy
    abruptio placentae, 554–555
    anaphylactoid syndrome of, 553

Pregnancy (Continued)
  anticoagulants in, 620
  hyperbaric oxygen therapy in, 251
  Listeria monocytogenes sepsis in, 331–332
  peripartum cardiomyopathy, 552
  postpartum hemorrhage, 555–556
  preoperative evaluation in, 485
  renal failure in, 477
  ruptured ectopic, 444–445
  septic abortion, 553–554
  tests for, 441–442
  thromboembolism in, 420
  uterine rupture in, 554
Pregnancy-induced hypertension, 83–87
Preload, 5, 6
  reduction of, 21–22
Premature atrial contractions
  in acute MI, 65
  in angina, 60
  in myocardial contusion, 73
Premature ventricular contractions (PVCs)
  after cardiac surgery, 502
  in acute MI, 65
  in angina, 60
  in myocardial contusion, 73
Preoperative evaluation, 484–487
Pressure control ventilation, 809, 811f
Pressure support ventilation, 808–809, 811f
Pressure ulcers, 557–560
Prevacid. See Lansoprazole.
Priapism, in sickle cell disease, 434, 435
Prilosec. See Omeprazole.
Primaquine, for Pneumocystis carinii pneumonia, 360t
Probalance, 761
Probenecid, interaction with benzodiazepines, 608t
Procainamide, 629–632
  for atrial fibrillation, 105
  for atrial flutter, 106
  for supraventricular tachycardia, 110
  for Wolff-Parkinson-White syndrome, 115
Procaine penicillin G, 645
Procarbazine, 641, 642
Procardia. See Nifedipine.
Prochlorperazine, 256
  after N-acetylcysteine for acetaminophen overdose, 203
Proctitis, herpes simplex, 350
Promethazine, 256
Promote, 761
Pronator drift, 498
Propafenone, 629–633
Propofol, 609–610
  for alcohol withdrawal syndrome, 242, 242t
  for intracranial hypertension, 297t
  for status epilepticus, 279
  in cyclic antidepressant overdose, 261
  in neuroleptic overdose, 258
Proportional assist ventilation, 814–816
Propranolol, 224t, 576
  for akathisia, 258
  for aortic dissection, 103
  for pheochromocytoma, 189
  in theophylline overdose, 215
  in thyroid storm, 183
Propylene glycol intoxication, 233–236, 238
Propylthiouracil, for thyroid storm, 183
Prostacyclin, for continuous renal replacement therapy, 735
Prosthetic heart valves, 93–95
  anticoagulation for patients with, 93t

Prosthetic heart valves (Continued)
  endocarditis in patients with, 379, 382, 383
Protein
  estimating requirements for, 771
  plasma assays for, 771–772
Protein C, 319, 406, 413–414, 416–417
Protein S, 406, 413–414, 416–417
Proteinuria, in pregnancy-induced hypertension, 83–84
Proteus infection, 333, 384
Prothrombin time (PT), 414, 417
Proton-pump inhibitors (PPIs), 593–596, 595t
  for bleeding duodenal ulcer, 465
  for stress ulcer prophylaxis, 285, 289
  preoperative, 487
  to prevent aspiration, 43
Protriptyline, 259
Prourokinase, 622
Prozac. See Fluoxetine.
Pseudohyperkalemia, 132
Pseudohypoglycemia, 172
Pseudohyponatremia, 119, 121
Pseudohypoparathyriodism, 135
Pseudomonas aeruginosa infection, 333
  in organ transplant patients, 369
  necrotizing, of soft tissue, 399–400
  urosepsis, 384
"Pseudothrombocytopenia," 409
Psychoactive drugs, 267
  cyclic antidepressant overdose, 259–262
  neuroleptic drug overdose, 256–258
  QT interval prolongation induced by, 114
  serotonin syndrome and, 267–268
PT (prothrombin time), 414, 417
PTH (parathormone)
  in hypercalcemia, 139
  in hyperphosphatemia, 152
  in hypocalcemia, 135
PTT (partial thromboplastin time), 414, 417
Pulmocare, 762
Pulmonary angiography, 32
Pulmonary artery (PA) catheterization, 690–693, 691f, 692f
  during barbiturate coma, 297
  for anaphylactoid syndrome of pregnancy, 553
  for hypotension, 6
  for left ventricular failure, 76
  for pulmonary edema, 21, 77
  in acute MI, 66
    right ventricular, 69
  in burn patients, 515
  in diabetic ketoacidosis, 166
  in hypernatremia, 127
  in hyperosmolar nonketotic coma, 169
  in rhabdomyolysis, 544
  in salicylate intoxication, 208
  in tricuspid valve disease, 93
  preoperative, 486
Pulmonary artery occlusion pressure (PAOP), 692–693, 692f, 746, 747f, 748, 775, 776
Pulmonary artery (PA) pressure, 774, 776
Pulmonary capillary oxygen content (CċO$_2$), 790–791
Pulmonary edema, 17, 20–22
  cardiogenic, 20–22, 76–77
  chemotherapy-induced, 642
  in fulminant hepatic failure, 459
  in kidney transplant recipients, 522
  neurogenic, 295
  uremic, 481, 483

Pulmonary embolectomy, 33
Pulmonary embolism (PE), 30–33, 32f–33f
  anticoagulants for, 617–621
  hemodynamic monitoring in, 776
  hemoptysis due to, 53
  pulseless electrical activity due to, 112t, 113t
  thrombolytic agents for, 622–623
  vs. right ventricular MI, 69
Pulmonary feeding formulations, 761–762
Pulmonary fibrosis, chemotherapy-induced, 641
Pulmonary function tests, in status asthmaticus, 34
Pulmonary hypertension
  aspiration in, 43
  cor pulmonale in, 48, 49
Pulmonary infection. See also Pneumonia.
  fever in, 2–3
  fungal, 344–349
  hemoptysis in, 53
  in bone marrow transplant recipients, 366–368
  in organ transplant recipients, 369–371
  pneumonia in adults, 37–41
  tuberculosis, 374–378
Pulmonary vascular resistance (PVR), 777
Pulmonary vascular resistance index (PVRI), 776, 777
Pulmonary venous admixture or shunt fraction (Q̇s/Q̇t), 791
Pulmonary–renal syndromes, 483
Pulmonic valve disease, 91, 93, 95
Pulse oximetry, 14, 15
  during fiberoptic bronchoscopy, 710
  in burn patients, 515
  in carbon monoxide poisoning, 250
  in methemoglobinemia, 254
  pitfalls of, 792
  to measure arterial oxygen saturation, 789
Pulseless electrical activity (PEA), 111, 112t, 113t
Pulsus paradoxus, 34, 96, 100
Pupillary reflexes, 11, 12, 498
  confirming absence of, 743
Purified protein derivative (PPD) test, 376
Purpura
  Henoch-Schönlein, 478
  idiopathic thrombocytopenic, 409–411
  post-transfusion, 429–432
  thrombotic thrombocytopenic, 409, 411, 413, 425–428
PVCs (premature ventricular contractions)
  after cardiac surgery, 502
  in acute MI, 65
  in angina, 60
  in myocardial contusion, 73
PVR (pulmonary vascular resistance), 777
PVRI (pulmonary vascular resistance index), 776, 777
PV̄CO$_2$ (mixed venous carbon dioxide tension), 790
PV̄O$_2$ (mixed venous oxygen tension), 789–790
Pyrazinamide (PZA), 661–663
Pyridixone, for ethylene glycol intoxication, 238
Pyridostigmine, for myasthenia gravis, 306
Pyrimethamine, for toxoplasmosis, 373
Pyrogens, endogenous, 1
Pyuria, 3, 384
PZA (pyrazinamide), 661–663

Q

Q fever, 39, 379
Qs/Qt (pulmonary venous admixture or shunt fraction), 791
QT interval prolongation, 114–115
Quelicin. *See* Succinylcholine.
Quetiapine, 256
Quinapril, 575
Quinidine, 629–631, 633
Quinupristin-dalfopristin, 665–669

R

Rabeprazole, 595t
Radial artery catheterization, 687–688, 688f
Radiation therapy
    diarrhea associated with, 473
    for neoplasms causing spinal cord compression, 300
    for tumor-related superior vena cava syndrome, 551
    lung toxicity of, 641, 642
    pericarditis induced by, 642
Radioiodinated meta-iodobenzylguanidine (MIBG) scintigraphy, 189
Raman spectroscopy capnography, 784
Ramipril, 575
    for acute MI, 67
    for unstable angina, 62
Ramsay sedation scale, 242t
Ranitidine, 594, 595t
    to prevent aspiration, 43
Rapacuronium, 599t
Raplon. *See* Rapacuronium.
Rash
    in bone marrow transplant recipients, 366, 367
    in neutropenic cancer patients, 362, 363
Rattlesnakes, 272
RBCs. *See* Red blood cells (RBCs).
Rebound tenderness, 439, 440
Recombinant single chain urokinase plasminogen activator, 622
Recombinant staphylokinase, 622–623
Recombinant tissue plasminogen activator (rt-PA), 622–623
    for pulmonary embolism, 33
Red blood cells (RBCs)
    acute hemolytic disorders, 425–428
    anemia due to intrinsic defects of, 421
    indices of, 422
    normal count of, 422
    sickle, 433
    transfusion of, 423
Red man syndrome, vancomycin-induced, 668
Regranex. *See* Becaplermin gel.
Remeron. *See* Mirtazapine.
Remifentanil, 604t
Renal abscess, 386
Renal biopsy, 9, 478
Renal dysfunction
    after abdominal aortic aneurysm repair, 510
    after peripheral vascular bypass, 504–506
    antibiotics in
        aminoglycosides, 651
        macrolides, 659
        penicillins and cephalosporins, 648–649
    anticoagulants in, 620
    chemotherapy-induced, 643
    digoxin in, 622

Renal dysfunction *(Continued)*
    in fulminant hepatic failure, 460
    in heat stroke, 531
    neuromuscular blocking drugs in, 599
Renal failure
    acute, 477–480, 479t
    chronic, 481–483
    due to heat stroke, 533
    nonoliguric, 477
    oliguric, 8, 477
    parenteral nutrition-associated, 768
Renal feeding formulations, 762
Renal function evaluation, 485
Renal ischemia, 510
Renal transplantation, 371, 372, 521–524
Renal vascular disorders, 477
RenalCal, 762
ReoPro. *See* Abciximab.
Reperfusion therapy, in acute MI, 66f, 69, 89
Replete, 761
Reserpine, in thyroid storm, 183
Respiratory acidosis, 154–157, 155f
    in cyanide poisoning, 245
Respiratory alkalosis, 154, 155f, 156, 157
    in salicylate intoxication, 206
Respiratory failure, 17–19
    in Guillain-Barré syndrome, 309
    parenteral nutrition-associated, 768
Reteplase (rPA), 622
Reticulocyte count, 422
Reticulocyte production index, 422–423
Retinal hemorrhage, 295
Retinal ischemia, 281
Retinitis, cytomegalovirus, 354
Retinol-binding protein plasma assay, 772
Reverse Fick method, 773, 782
Rewarming procedures, 527–528, 538
Rhabdomyolysis, 520, 542–545
    with hyperphosphatemia, 153
Rheumatic heart disease, 90–95
Rhizomucor infection, 344
    antifungal therapy for, 671–676
Rhizopus infection, 344
    antifungal therapy for, 671–676
Rhodococcus equi infection, 327, 332
Rhodotorula rubra infection, 344
Rib fractures, 488, 490
Ribavirin
    for respiratory syncytial virus, 368
    for viral hepatitis, 457
    for viral pneumonia, 41
Rickets, vitamin D dependent, 135
RIF. *See* Rifampin (RIF).
Rifabutin, 662
Rifamate, 661
Rifampin (RIF)
    for *Legionella* infection, 40
    for pneumonia, 40, 41
    for *Rhodococcus equi* infection, 332
    for staphylococcal infection, 329, 383
    for tuberculosis, 661–663
    prophylaxis for meningococcal meningitis, 391
Rifater, 661
Right ventricular ejection fraction (RVEF), 776
Right ventricular end-diastolic volume index (RVEDVI), 776
Right ventricular myocardial infarction, 69–70
Right ventricular pressure, 774
Right-to-left shunt, hypoxemia due to, 14
Riker sedation–agitation scale, 800, 801t
Ringer's lactate, 564
Risperidone, 256

Ritonavir, interaction with benzodiazepines, 608t
Rocuronium, 599, 599t
Romano-Ward syndrome, 114
Rotor syndrome, 441
rPA (reteplase), 622
rt-PA (recombinant tissue plasminogen activator), 622–623
    for pulmonary embolism, 33
Rule-of-nines, 512, 513f
Ruptured abdominal aortic aneurysm, 510–511
RVEDVI (right ventricular end-diastolic volume index), 776
RVEF (right ventricular ejection fraction), 776

S

Saccharomyces infection, 344
SAH (subarachnoid hemorrhage), 12, 82, 287–290
Salicylate intoxication, 205–208
Saline
    hypertonic, 565–566
    hypotonic, 564–565
    normal, 564
Saline tonometry, 793–795
Salmeterol, 637t, 638
Salmonella infection, 333
    in kidney transplant patients, 523
Salpingitis, 444
SaO₂ (arterial oxygen saturation), 789, 792
Saquinavir, interaction with benzodiazepines, 608t
Saruplase, 622
SB (Sengstaken-Blakemore) tube placement, 749–753, 750f
Sclerotherapy, for gastric and esophageal variceal bleeding, 464
Scorpion envenomation, 272–275, 274t
Scribner shunt, 730
SCUF (slow continuous ultrafiltration), 733
SE (status epilepticus), 11–13, 277–280
Sedation
    after cardiac surgery, 501
    benzodiazepines for, 605–608
    for alcohol withdrawal syndrome, 242, 242t
    for endotracheal intubation, 678
    for fiberoptic bronchoscopy, 710
    for intracranial hypertension, 296, 297t
    monitoring of, 800–802, 801t
    preoperative, 487
    propofol for, 609–610
Sedation scales, 800
Sedative-hypnotic overdose, 209–212
Seizures
    anticonvulsants for, 611–616
    in alcohol withdrawal syndrome, 242, 243
    in anticholinergic poisoning, 265
    in calcium channel blocker or β-blocker overdose, 226
    in cyclic antidepressant overdose, 261
    in eclampsia, 83, 84
    in hypoglycemia, 278
    in intracerebral hemorrhage, 285
    in neuroleptic overdose, 258
    in organophosphate poisoning, 270
    in salicylate intoxication, 207
    in serotonin syndrome, 268
    in theophylline overdose, 215
    induced by neuromuscular blocking drugs, 600

Seizures *(Continued)*
  myoclonic, after cardiac arrest, 280
  prophylaxis for
    in head trauma patients, 495
    post-craniotomy, 498
  status epilepticus, 11–13, 277–280
  types of, 277
Seldinger catheterization technique, 685, 688, 688f
Selective serotonin reuptake inhibitors (SSRIs), 259
  serotonin syndrome and, 267–268
Selegiline, 267
Selenium, in parenteral nutrition solutions, 766
Sellick maneuver, 43, 679
Sengstaken-Blakemore (SB) tube placement, 749–753, 750f
"Sentinel loop," 447
Sepsis, 317–319
  coagulation in, 406
  continuous renal replacement therapy for, 733–736
  hemodynamic monitoring in, 776
  in AIDS, 357
  oxygen transport variables in, 783t
  urosepsis, 384–386
Septic abortion, 553–554
Septic shock, 88, 317, 319, 321–325, 323f
  hemodynamic monitoring in, 776
  oxygen transport variables in, 783t
Septic thrombophlebitis, intracranial, 329
Serevent. *See* Salmeterol.
Serotonin syndrome (SS), 2, 4, 267–268
  vs. neuroleptic malignant syndrome, 268t
Serratia infection, 333, 384
Sertraline, 259, 267
Serum anion gap, 154, 156
  in alcohol and glycol intoxications, 236t
    diethylene glycol, 237
    ethylene glycol, 236
    methanol, 235
    propylene glycol, 236
  in cyanide poisoning, 246
  in diabetic ketoacidosis, 164
  in lactic acidosis, 159
  in rhabdomyolysis, 544
Serum osmole gap, 154, 156
  in alcohol and glycol intoxications, 236t
    diethylene glycol, 237
    ethylene glycol, 236
    isopropanol, 236
    methanol, 235
    propylene glycol, 236
  in alcoholic ketoacidosis, 162
  toxin effects on, 195–196
Serzone. *See* Nefazodone.
Sevelamer, for hyperphosphatemia, 152
Shigella infection, 333
Shock
  cardiogenic, 75–79, 88–89, 322
  chemotherapy-induced, 642
  distributive, 322
  epinephrine for, 572
  hypovolemic, 88, 322
  lactic acidosis due to, 158, 159
  obstructive, 322
  oxygen transport variables in, 783t
  septic, 88, 317, 319, 321–325, 323f
SI (stroke index), 775
SIAD (syndrome of inappropriate antidiuresis), 120, 178–180
  post-craniotomy, 499
Sick cell syndrome, 120
Sick sinus syndrome, 116
Sickle cell crises, 433–435

Silver sulfadiazine (Silvadene), for burns, 514
Simple face mask, 803, 805–806
SIMV (synchronized intermittent mandatory ventilation), 808, 811f
  with pressure support, 808, 811f
Sinemet, for parkinsonism, 258
Sinequan. *See* Doxepin.
Single chain urokinase plasminogen activator, recombinant, 622
Sinus tachycardia, 107
  after cardiac surgery, 502
  in acute MI, 65
  in cardiogenic shock, 88
  in cyclic antidepressant overdose, 261
  in myocardial contusion, 73
Sinusitis, 3
  empiric antibiotic therapy for, 337
  Gram-negative, 334, 336, 337
  in neutropenic cancer patients, 362, 363
  nosocomial, 397–398
SIRS (systemic inflammatory response syndrome), 317–319, 322, 384
Skin contamination, 197
Skin substitutes, 514
Skinfold thickness, 771
Slow continuous ultrafiltration (SCUF), 733
SM (streptomycin), 661–663
Small intestinal bleeding, 466
Small intestinal obstruction, 439, 443–444
Smoke inhalation, 51–52, 513, 514
  carbon monoxide poisoning from, 249–252, 513
  cyanide poisoning from, 247, 513
Snakebites, 272–275
SNP. *See* Sodium nitroprusside (SNP).
Sodium
  fractional excretion of, 478
  in parenteral nutrition solutions, 765
Sodium balance
  hypernatremia, 124–128
  hyponatremia, 119–123
  in diabetic ketoacidosis, 165
  in hyperosmolar nonketotic coma, 168
Sodium bicarbonate
  for alcoholic ketoacidosis, 163
  for drug overdose
    cyanide, 247
    cyclic antidepressants, 261
    ethylene glycol, 238
    methanol, 238
    neuroleptics, 258
    phenobarbital, 211
    salicylate, 207–208
  for hyperkalemia, 133, 231
  for lactic acidosis, 160
  for metabolic acidosis, 156–157
  for pulseless electrical activity, 111
  for rhabdomyolysis, 544–545
  for tumor lysis syndrome, 547
  in anticholinergic poisoning, 265
  in diabetic ketoacidosis, 167
Sodium citrate, to prevent aspiration, 43
Sodium iodide, for thyroid storm, 183
Sodium nitrite, for cyanide poisoning, 246
Sodium nitroprusside (SNP), 572t, 575, 587–588
  cyanide intoxication induced by, 244, 246, 247
  for aortic dissection, 103, 576
  for cardiogenic pulmonary edema, 22, 78
  for cerebral infarction, 576
  for drug and ethanol withdrawal syndromes, 576
  for pheochromocytoma, 189, 577
  for preeclampsia-eclampsia, 87, 576

Sodium nitroprusside (SNP) *(Continued)*
  for tetanus, 315
  in cocaine intoxication, 221
  in intracerebral hemorrhage, 285
  in subarachnoid hemorrhage, 289
Sodium phosphate, 149
Sodium polystyrene sulfonate (Kayexalate)
  for hyperkalemia, 133–134
    contraindicated in digoxin overdose, 231
  for lithium overdose, 217
Sodium thiosulfate, for cyanide poisoning, 246, 247
Soft-tissue infections, necrotizing, 399–401
Solfotel, for intracranial hypertension, 297
Sonography. *See* Ultrasonography (US).
Sonoran coral snakebite, 272
Sorbitol, for drug overdose, 198
Sorbitrate. *See* Isosorbide dinitrate.
Sotalol, 224t, 576, 629–633
  for atrial fibrillation, 105
  for atrial flutter, 106
  overdose of, 223
Spasticity, in patients with pressure ulcers, 558
Spherocytosis, 421
Spider bites, 272–275
Spinal cord compression, 298–300
Spinal epidural abscess, 298–300
  Staphylococcus aureus, 328
Spirometry, preoperative, 486
Spironolactone, 589–591
Splenic abscess, Gram-negative, 335, 337
Spondylitis, tuberculous, 374
Sporanox. *See* Itraconazole.
Sputum microbiological analysis, 39
SS (serotonin syndrome), 2, 4, 267–268
  vs. neuroleptic malignant syndrome, 268t
SSKI, for thyroid storm, 183
SSRIs (selective serotonin reuptake inhibitors), 259
  serotonin syndrome and, 267–268
St. Jude mechanical valve in aortic position, 90
Stab wounds, abdominal, 491, 493
Stadol. *See* Butorphanol.
Staphylococcus infection
  antibiotics for, 329
  cellulitis, 399
  coagulase-negative, 327, 329
  endocarditis, 379, 382–383
  in bone marrow transplant patients, 366
  in organ transplant recipients, 369
  nosocomial sinusitis, 397
  S. aureus, 327–329
    methicillin-resistant, 369, 382–383
    toxic shock syndrome, 328, 394–396
    urosepsis, 384
    vancomycin-resistant, 667
Staphylokinase, recombinant, 622–623
Starch preparations, 566
Starling's equation, 20, 746
Status asthmaticus, 34–36
Status epilepticus (SE), 11–13, 277–280
Stem cell transplantation, 365
Stenotrophomonas maltophilia infection, 333
Stomatitis, candidal, 339
Stool tests
  in diarrhea, 471–472
  in toxic megacolon, 475
Streptococcus infection
  antibiotics for, 330
  endocarditis, 379, 382
  group A, 327, 329–330
  group B, 327, 330

Streptococcus infection *(Continued)*
  necrotizing, of soft tissue, 399
  nosocomial sinusitis, 397
  S. pneumoniae, 327, 330
    in bone marrow transplant patients, 366, 367
    in organ transplant patients, 370, 373
  S. viridans, 327, 330
  toxic shock syndrome, 329, 395
  urosepsis, 384
Streptokinase, 622–623
  for central venous catheter thrombosis, 551
  for pulmonary embolism, 33
Streptomycin (SM), 661–663
Streptozotocin, 643
Stress ulcers, 465
  prophylaxis for, 285, 289, 499, 593–596
Stroke, 82, 281–283
  in sickle cell disease, 433–435
Stroke index (SI), 775
Stroke volume (SV), 5, 775
  low, 5–7
Stupor, 11
Subarachnoid bolt, 796
Subarachnoid hemorrhage (SAH), 12, 82, 287–290
Subclavian vein approach
  for central venous catheterization, 684, 684f
  for hemodialysis, 731
Subclavian vein thrombosis, 420
Subdural empyema, 329
Subdural hematoma, 13, 291–292
Sub-falcine brain herniation, 295
Sublimaze. *See* Fentanyl.
Subxiphoid approach for pericardiocentesis, 704–705, 705f
Succinylcholine, 597, 599
  contraindicated in spinal cord-injured patients, 299, 300
  for endotracheal intubation, 678
Sucralfate, 593–595
  for hyperphosphatemia, 152
  for stress ulcer prophylaxis, 285, 289
  in acute pancreatitis, 448
Sufenta. *See* Sufentanil.
Sufentanil, 604t
Sular. *See* Nisoldipine.
Sulfamylon. *See* Mafenide acetate.
Sulfosalicylic acid precipitation test, 9
Superior vena cava (SVC) syndrome, 549–551
Suplena, 762
Supraventricular tachycardia (SVT), 107–110, 109t
  in cocaine intoxication, 221
  in cyclic antidepressant overdose, 261
Suramin, 643
Surfactant therapy, for ARDS, 26
Surgical wound infections, 3, 399–401
  preoperative prophylaxis for, 487
Surmontil. *See* Trimipramine.
SV (stroke volume), 5, 775
  low, 5–7
SVC (superior vena cava) syndrome, 549–551
SVR (systemic vascular resistance), 5, 776
  decreased, 5–6
  increased, 80
SVRI (systemic vascular resistance index), 776
SVT (supraventricular tachycardia), 107–110, 109t
  in cyclic antidepressant overdose, 261

S̄vO₂ (mixed venous oxygen saturation), 781, 783t, 790
Synchronized intermittent mandatory ventilation (SIMV), 808, 811f
  with pressure support, 808, 811f
Syndrome of inappropriate antidiuresis (SIAD), 120, 178–180
  post-craniotomy, 499
Synercid. *See* Quinupristin-dalfopristin.
Syrup of ipecac, 197, 226
  for organophosphate poisoning, 270
Systemic inflammatory response syndrome (SIRS), 317–319, 322, 384
Systemic oxygen delivery (DO₂), 782, 782f, 783, 783t
Systemic pulse pressure, 774
Systemic vascular resistance (SVR), 5, 776
  decreased, 5–6
  increased, 80, 88
Systemic vascular resistance index (SVRI), 776

T

Tachycardia
  atrial fibrillation and flutter, 104–106
  supraventricular, 107–110
  toxin-induced, 195t
  vasoactive catecholamine-induced, 573
  ventricular, 114–115
Tachypnea, 14–16
Tacrolimus, for kidney transplantation, 521
Tagamet. *See* Cimetidine.
Talwin. *See* Pentazocine.
Tampon-associated toxic shock syndrome, 394–396
Tardive dyskinesia, 257
Taxol, 642
TB (tuberculosis), 374–378
  drug therapy for, 660–664
  drug-resistant, 660
  hemoptysis in, 53
  in organ transplant recipients, 370, 373
TBI (traumatic brain injury), 484, 494–497, 497t
  diabetes insipidus after, 174
  intracranial hypertension and, 293–297
TBW (total body water), 121, 127
Technetium 99m-hepato-iminodiacetic acid (HIDA) radionuclide scan, in acute cholecystitis, 450
Temperature measurement, 2
Temporary transvenous pacemaker, 694–698, 695f
Tenecteplase (TNK-rt-PA), 622
Teniposide, 641, 642
Tension pneumothorax, 7, 28, 29, 488–490
  chest tube thoracostomy for, 724–725
  pulseless electrical activity due to, 112t, 113t
Terazosin, 575
  for pheochromocytoma, 189
Terbutaline, 637t, 638
  for COPD, 46
Tetanus, 314–316
Tetanus/diphtheria vaccine, 315–316
Tetany, 136
Tetracycline
  for clostridial gas gangrene, 332
  for tetanus, 315
Texas coral snakebite, 272, 274
Thalassemia, 421, 423
Theophylline
  for COPD, 46

Theophylline *(Continued)*
  for status asthmaticus, 35
  interaction with benzodiazepines, 608t
  interaction with ciprofloxacin, 654
  overdose of, 213–215
Thermal burn injury, 512–516
  estimating size of, 512, 513f
  inhalation injury and, 51–52, 513
  preoperative evaluation of, 485
Thermodilution method to determine cardiac output, 775
Thermoregulatory impairment, 525
Thiamine
  for alcohol withdrawal syndrome, 242
  for alcoholic ketoacidosis, 163
  for anticholinergic toxicity, 265
  for ethanol intoxication, 237
  for ethylene glycol intoxication, 238
  for lactic acidosis, 160
  for unexplained coma, 12
Thiazide diuretics, 589–591
Thiocyanate, 244, 245
Thioridazine, 256
Thiotepa, 642
Thiothixene, 256
Third space fluid sequestration, 120
  pre-renal failure due to, 477
Thoracentesis, 3, 719–723, 720f, 721f
  in pneumonia, 40
Thoracic injuries, 488–490
Thoracostomy
  chest tube, 29, 40, 489–490
  needle, 490
Thrombin inhibitors, 617–621
Thrombocytopathy, 410–411
Thrombocytopenia, 409–412
  coagulopathy and, 406
  glycoprotein IIb/IIIa receptor antagonist-induced, 624
  heparin-induced, 409–411, 413, 419, 617, 618
  preoperative evaluation in, 485
Thrombocytosis, 413
Thromboembolic disorders, 15
  acute peripheral arterial occlusion, 507–508
  after peripheral vascular bypass, 504, 506
  anticoagulants for, 617–621
  coagulopathy, 406–408
  deep venous thrombosis, 416–420
  glycoprotein IIb/IIIa receptor antagonists for, 624–625
  hypercoagulable states, 413–415
  in pregnancy, 420
  preoperative prophylaxis for, 487
  pulmonary embolism, 30–33
  thrombolytic agents for, 622–623
Thrombolytic agents, 418, 622–623
  for acute MI, 66f, 89
  for central venous catheter thrombosis, 551
  for cerebral infarction, 282
  for peripheral arterial occlusion, 508
  for pulmonary embolism, 32–33
  intra-arterial, 282
Thrombophilia, 416
Thrombophlebitis
  Gram-negative suppurative, 334, 337, 338
  intracranial septic, 329
Thrombotic thrombocytopenic purpura (TTP), 409, 411, 413, 425–428
Thrush, 339, 340
Thymectomy, 306
Thyroid function tests
  in euthyroid sick syndrome, 185

Thyroid function tests (Continued)
  in hypothyroidism, 185
  in thyroid storm, 182–183
Thyroid storm, 181–183
Thyroidectomy, 183
Thyroid-stimulating hormone (TSH), 182, 183
Thyroxine (T₄)
  in euthyroid sick syndrome, 185
  in hypothyroidism, 185
  in thyroid storm, 182
Thyroxine supplementation, for myxedema coma, 186
Tiagabine, 612
Tiazac. See Diltiazem.
Ticarcillin, 645, 646, 648
Ticarcillin-clavulanate, 645, 646, 648
  for Gram-negative infection, 338
  for urosepsis, 385
Ticlopidine
  for unstable angina, 61
  to prevent cerebral infarction, 282
Tight-seal masks, 804
Tinzaparin, 620t
TIPS (transjugular intrahepatic portosystemic shunt), 464
Tirofiban, 625
Tissue complex urokinase plasminogen activator, 622
Tissue plasminogen activator, recombinant (rt-PA), 622–623
  for pulmonary embolism, 33
TMP-SMX. See Trimethoprim-sulfamethoxazole (TMP-SMX).
TNK-rt-PA (tenecteplase), 622
Tobramycin, 650–652
  for Gram-negative infection, 337, 338
Tocainide, 629
Tofranil. See Imipramine.
Tonometry, gastric, 793–795, 794f, 795t
Topiramate, 612
Topotecan, 642
Tornalate. See Bitolterol.
Torsemide, 589–591
  for pulmonary edema, 77
Total body water (TBW), 121, 127
Total lymphocyte count, 772
Total parenteral nutrition (TPN). See Parenteral nutrition.
Toxic megacolon, 474–476
Toxic shock syndrome (TSS), 394–396
  staphylococcal, 328, 394–396
  streptococcal, 329, 395
Toxidromes, 196t. See also Drug overdose; Poisoning.
Toxin identification, 196
Toxoplasma gondii infection, prophylaxis for heart transplant recipients, 373
TPN (total parenteral nutrition). See Parenteral nutrition.
Trace elements, in parenteral nutrition solutions, 766
Tracheal injuries, 488, 489
Tracheal reflex, confirming absence of, 743
Tracheobronchitis
  Aspergillus, 346
  candidal, 339–341
  empiric antibiotic therapy for, 337
  Gram-negative, 334, 336–337
  herpes simplex, 350
Tracheostomy, 822
  for ARDS, 25
  for Guillain-Barré syndrome, 309
  for head trauma patients, 496
  for spinal cord-injured patients, 299

Tracheostomy collar, 804, 806
Tracheostomy tube delivery connections, 804–805
Tracrium. See Atracurium.
Trandolapril, 575
Transcutaneous pacing, 699–700
Transcyte skin substitute, 514
Transferrin plasma assay, 771–772
Trans–foramen magnum brain herniation, 296
Transfusion reactions, 1, 3, 429–432, 534
Transjugular intrahepatic portosystemic shunt (TIPS), 464
Transnasal and transoral gastroenteric intubation, 754–759
Transplantation
  graft-versus-host disease after, 365, 436–438
  hepatic, 371–372
  infections after
    bone marrow transplant, 365–368
    solid organ transplant, 369–373
  kidney, 371, 372, 521–524
Transport, intrahospital, 737–738
Transpyloric advancement of enteric tubes, 757–758
Transtentorial brain herniation, 295–296
Tranylcypromine, 259, 267
Trauma
  abdominal, 491–493
  chest, 488–490
  electrical and lightning injuries, 517–520
  myocardial contusion, 73–74
  spinal cord compression due to, 298–300
  subdural hematoma due to, 291–292
  thermal burn injury, 512–516
  venom injuries, 272–275
Traumacal, 761
Traumatic brain injury (TBI), 484, 494–497, 497t
  diabetes insipidus after, 174
  intracranial hypertension and, 293–297
Trazodone, 259, 267
Triamterene, 589–591
Trichosporon beigelii infection, 344, 348
Tricuspid valve disease, 90–93, 95
Tricuspid valve replacement, 95
Tricyclic antidepressant overdose, 259–262
Triiodothyronine (T₃)
  in euthyroid sick syndrome, 185
  in hypothyroidism, 185
  in thyroid storm, 182, 183
Trimethaphan camsylate, 575–581
  for aortic dissection, 103, 576
Trimethoprim-sulfamethoxazole (TMP-SMX)
  for epiglottitis, 403
  for kidney transplant recipients, 372, 522
  for Listeria monocytogenes infection, 332
  for Pneumocystis carinii pneumonia, 360t, 368, 372
  for toxoplasmosis, 373
Trimetrexate, for Pneumocystis carinii pneumonia, 360t
Trimipramine, 259
Troleandomycin, interaction with benzodiazepines, 608t
Tromethamine, for lactic acidosis, 160
Tropical sprue, 473
TSH (thyroid-stimulating hormone), 182, 183

TSS (toxic shock syndrome), 394–396
  staphylococcal, 328, 394–396
  streptococcal, 329, 395
TTP (thrombotic thrombocytopenic purpura), 409, 411, 413, 425–428
Tuberculin skin testing, 376
Tuberculosis (TB), 374–378
  drug therapy for, 660–664
  drug-resistant, 660, 662
  hemoptysis in, 53
  in organ transplant recipients, 370, 373, 523
Tumor lysis syndrome, 153, 546–548
Tumors
  diarrhea associated with, 471, 473
  hypoglycemia induced by, 171
  pheochromocytoma, 187–190
  toxic megacolon associated with, 474
Tusk mask, 804
TwoCal HN, 761
Typhlitis, Gram-negative, 336

U

UGIB (upper gastrointestinal bleeding), 463–465
Ultiva. See Remifentanil.
Ultracal, 761
Ultrasonography (US)
  focused abdominal sonogram for trauma, 491–492
  for brain death determination, 745
  in abdominal aortic aneurysm, 509
  in acute abdominal pain, 442
  in acute cholecystitis, 450
  in acute pancreatitis, 447
  in air embolism, 562
  in pulmonary embolism, 31
  renal, 9, 10
  venous, 417
u-PA (urokinase plasminogen activator), 622
Upper gastrointestinal bleeding (UGIB), 463–465
Urea, for syndrome of inappropriate antidiuresis, 179
Uremia, 481–483
  hemodialysis for, 729–732
Uremic coagulopathy, 522–523
Ureteral disorders, pain of, 439
Ureteral obstruction, 8
Urethral obstruction, 8
Urinalysis, 385
  for acute abdominal pain, 441
  for oliguria, 8–9
  in rhabdomyolysis, 544
Urinary acidification, for drug overdose, 198
Urinary alkalinization
  for drug overdose, 198
  for rhabdomyolysis, 544–545
Urinary catheter-related infection, 386
Urinary tract infection (UTI)
  empiric antibiotic therapy for, 338
  enterococcal, 331
  fever in, 3
  Gram-negative, 336–338
  urosepsis, 384–386
Urine anion gap, 154, 156
Urine culture, 385
Urine diagnostic indices, 9
Urine fluorescence, in ethylene glycol intoxication, 236
Urine osmolality
  in diabetes insipidus, 174, 176

Urine osmolality *(Continued)*
  in hypernatremia, 125, 126f
  in syndrome of inappropriate antidiuresis, 179
Urokinase, 622–623
  for pulmonary embolism, 33
Urokinase plasminogen activator (u-PA), 622
US. *See* Ultrasonography.
Uterine atony, 555
Uterine rupture, 554
Uterotonic agents, 555
UTI. *See* Urinary tract infection (UTI).

V

VAE (venous air embolism), 561
Vaginitis, candidal, 339, 340
Valacyclovir
  for bone marrow transplant recipients, 367
  for herpes simplex virus infection, 351
  for herpes zoster, 352
Valproic acid, 611–615
  for post-cardiac arrest myoclonic seizures, 280
Valvular heart disease, 90–95
Vancomycin, 665–669
  for bone marrow transplant recipients, 367
  for brain abscess, 337
  for corynebacterial infection, 331
  for endocarditis, 382
  for enterococcal infection, 331
  for infections in neutropenic cancer patients, 364
  for meningitis, 390, 391
  for pneumonia, 40, 41
  for *Rhodococcus equi* infection, 332
  for staphylococcal infection, 329, 382–383
  for streptococcal infection, 330, 337
Vancomycin-resistant enterococci, 331, 369, 666–667
Variceal bleeding, upper gastrointestinal, 464
  balloon tamponade for, 750f, 751–753
Varicella-zoster immune globulin, 373
Varicella-zoster virus infection, 351–352, 351t
  in bone marrow transplant patients, 366, 367
  in organ transplant recipients, 370, 373, 523
Vascor. *See* Bepridil.
Vascular catheter-related infection, 2, 327, 404–405
  in bone marrow transplant recipients, 366
  in neutropenic cancer patients, 362–364
Vasoactive catecholamines, 571–574, 572t
Vasoconstrictors, 6
Vasodilators, 575. *See also* specific drugs.
  for cor pulmonale, 49
Vaso-occlusive crisis in sickle cell disease, 433–434
Vasopressin
  for diabetes insipidus, 176–177
  for septic shock, 324
Vasopressors
  for cardiogenic shock, 89
  in theophylline overdose, 215
V_d/V_t (dead space to tidal volume ratio), 791

Vecuronium, 599, 599t
  for endotracheal intubation, 678
Vena cava filters, 419
Venlafaxine, 259, 267
Venography
  contrast, 417
  in pulmonary embolism, 31
Venom injuries, 272–275
Venoms, anaphylactic reactions to, 534
Veno-occlusive disease, chemotherapy-induced, 644
Venous air embolism (VAE), 561
Venous thromboembolism (VTE), 416
Ventilation-perfusion ratio, 14
Ventilation-perfusion (V/Q) scan
  in cor pulmonale, 49
  in deep venous thrombosis, 417
  in pulmonary embolism, 31
  in smoke inhalation, 51
Ventilator-associated pneumonia, 38, 39, 41
Ventricular assist device, 7, 78, 89
Ventricular dysfunction
  diastolic, 20
  systolic, 7
Ventricular dysrhythmias, 114–115
  cardioversion and defibrillation for, 701–703
  in drug overdose
    cyclic antidepressants, 261
    digoxin, 229, 230, 232
    neuroleptics, 257–258
  in hypomagnesemia, 144
  induced by calcium supplementation, 138
  vs. supraventricular tachycardia, 109t
Ventricular fibrillation (VF), 114–115
  after cardiac surgery, 502
Ventricular free wall rupture, 71
  pericardial tamponade due to, 100
Ventricular septal rupture, 71–72
Ventricular tachycardia (VT), 114–115
  after cardiac surgery, 502
  in cocaine intoxication, 221
Ventriculostomy catheter, 796, 797f
  detecting infection in patients with, 499
  for head trauma patients, 495
Verapamil, 224t, 576, 579t, 629
  for atrial fibrillation, 105
  for atrial flutter, 106
  for multifocal atrial tachycardia, 110
  for unstable angina, 62
  interaction with benzodiazepines, 608t
  overdose of, 223, 228
Verelan. *See* Verapamil.
Vertebrobasilar ischemia, 281
VF (ventricular fibrillation), 114–115
  after cardiac surgery, 502
Vibrio vulnificus cellulitis, 399
Vicodin. *See* Hydrocodone.
Vigabatrin, 612
Violin spider bite, 272–275
Viral infections
  cytomegalovirus, 354–355
  encephalitis, 392–393
  herpes, 350–353
  human immunodeficiency virus, 356–358
  in bone marrow transplant recipients, 365–368
  in organ transplant patients, 369–370, 373
Virchow's triad, 30
Vitamins
  for alcohol withdrawal syndrome, 242
  for alcoholic ketoacidosis, 163

Vitamins *(Continued)*
  for ethanol intoxication, 237
  for ethylene glycol intoxication, 238
  for hypocalcemia, 137
  for intracranial hypertension, 297
  in parenteral nutrition solutions, 766
  vitamin D in hypocalcemia, 135, 137
Vivactil. *See* Protriptyline.
Vivonex, 761
VO₂ (oxygen consumption), 782, 782f, 783, 783t
VO₂I (oxygen consumption index), 782
Voltage, 517
Volume control plus volume-assured pressure support, 813–814, 816
Volutrauma, 29, 811
Vomiting
  abdominal pain with, 439–440
  chemotherapy-induced, 644
von Willebrand factor (vWF), 409
von Willebrand's disease, 406, 407
Voriconazole, 673
  for aspergillosis, 349
V/Q (ventilation-perfusion) scan
  in cor pulmonale, 49
  in deep venous thrombosis, 417
  in pulmonary embolism, 31
  in smoke inhalation, 51
VT (ventricular tachycardia), 114–115
  after cardiac surgery, 502
  in cocaine intoxication, 221
VTE (venous thromboembolism), 416
vWF (von Willebrand factor), 409

W

Waldenström's macroglobulinemia, 411, 416, 478
Warfarin, 617
  complications of, 419
  for deep venous thrombosis, 418
  for hypercoagulable states, 414–415
  for peripheral arterial occlusion, 508
  for pulmonary embolism, 32
  prothrombotic state induced by, 413
  to prevent cerebral infarction, 282–283
Warm autoimmune hemolytic anemia (AIHA), 425–427
Water, in parenteral nutrition solutions, 766
Water intoxication, 120
Water loading test, 179
"Water-bottle" heart, 97, 101
Water-deprivation test, 175–176
Weaning from mechanical ventilation, 820–822
Wegener's granulomatosis, 478
Weir equation, 773
Wellbutrin. *See* Bupropion.
Wenckebach phenomenon, 116
Wernicke's encephalopathy, 483
Western coral snakebite, 272
Wheezing, 34
Whole bowel irrigation for drug overdose
  anticholinergic agents, 265
  calcium channel blockers or b-blockers, 226
  digoxin, 230
  lithium, 217
  narcotics or sedative-hypnotics, 210, 211
Wilson's disease, 135, 136
Wiskott-Aldrich syndrome, 437
Withdrawal of life support, 740–741, 741t

Withdrawal syndromes, 2
Wolff-Parkinson-White (WPW) syndrome,
    107, 108, 114–115
Wolfram's disease, 175
Wood alcohol intoxication, 233–235, 237–
    238
Wound botulism, 311–313
Wound care
    for burns, 514–515
    for pressure ulcers, 559
WPW (Wolff-Parkinson-White) syndrome,
    107, 108, 114–115

Wye-adaptor for endotracheal tube, 802–
    805

X

Xopenex. *See* Levalbuterol.

Y

Yeast infection
    candidal, 339–342
    non-candidal, 344–349

Z

Zantac. *See* Ranitidine.
Zemuron. *See* Rocuronium.
Zinc, in parenteral nutrition solutions,
    766
Zoloft. *See* Sertraline.
Zonisamide, 612
Zyban. *See* Bupropion.

ISBN 0–7216–9419–5

Drugs

α- Methyldopa, 26, 162
Abciximab, 175
Acebutolol, 66, 162, 177
Acetazolamide, 166
Acid-inhibiting agents, 167
Activated charcoal, 59
Adenosine, 177
Albumin, 159, 208
Albuterol, 11, 14, 40, 179
Alfentanil, 169
Alteplase, 174
Aluminum hydroxide, 46
Amikacin , 183
Amiloride, 53, 166
Aminoglycosides, 183
Aminophylline, 11
Amiodarone, 177
Amlodipine, 66, 162
Amoxicillin, 182
Amoxicillin/clavulanate, 182
Amphotericin B, 188
Ampicillin, 182
Ampicillin-sulbactam, 182
Amrinone, 160, 161
Angiotensin converting enzyme inhibitors, 19, 20, 24, 162
Anistreplase, 174
Antiarrhythmic drugs, 177
Antibiotics, 182-188
Anticoagulants, 173
Anticonvulsants, 26, 172
Antidepressants, 59, 74
Antidysrhythmic agents, 177
Antifungal agents, 188
Antihypertensives, 162
Anti-pseudomonal penicillins, 182
Antituberculosis drugs, 186
Ardeparin, 173
Argatroban, 173
Aspirin, 19, 20
Atenolol, 66, 162, 177
Atracurium, 168
Atropine, 36, 75
Azithromycin, 185

β- Adrenergic blockers, 26, 162, 177
β- Lactam/β- lactamase antibiotics, 182
Barbiturates, 62, 79, 84, 172
Benazepril, 162
Benzathine penicillin G, 182
Benzodiazepines, 62, 79, 170
Bisphosphonates, 42
Bitolterol, 179
Bretylium, 177
Bronchodilators, 179
Buprenorphine, 169
Butorphanol, 169

Calcitonin, 42
Calcium carbonate, 41, 46
Calcium chloride, 40, 41
Calcium gluceptate, 41
Calcium gluconate, 40, 41
Captopril, 19, 20, 24, 162
Carbamazepine, 172
Carbenicillin, 182
Catecholamines, vasoactive, 161
Cefaclor, 182
Cefazolin, 182
Cefepime, 182

Cefotaxime, 182
Cefotetan, 182
Cefoxitin, 182
Cefpodoxime proxetil, 182
Cefoperazone, 182
Ceftazidime, 182
Ceftizoxime, 182
Ceftriaxone, 182
Cefuroxime, 182
Cephalexin, 182
Cephalosporins, 182
Charcoal, 59
Chemotherapy, 181
Chlorambucil, 181
Chlordiazepoxide, 69, 170
Chlorothiazide, 166
Cimetidine, 167
Ciprofloxacin, 184
Cisatracurium, 168
Cisplatin, 181
Clarithromycin, 185
Clindamycin, 187
Clonidine, 57, 162
Clopidigrel, 19
Cloxacillin, 182
Codeine, 169
Colloids, 159, 208
Corticosteroids, 11, 14, 42, 58
Cosyntropin, 58
Cyclic antidepressants, 59, 74

Dalteparin, 173
Danaparoid, 173
Dantrolene, 170
Desmopressin, 53
Dexamethasone, 58
Dextran, 159
Dextrose, 52, 159, 212
Diazepam, 69, 170
Diazoxide, 52, 162
Dicloxacillin, 182
Digoxin, 67, 176
Digoxin-specific antibodies, 59, 67
Diltiazem, 66, 162, 177
Diuretics, 3, 26, 166
Dofetilide, 177
Dobutamine, 161
Dopamine, 3, 161
Dopexamine, 161
Doxacurium, 168

Enalapril, 19, 162
Enoxaparin, 173
Epinephrine, 150, 161
Eptifibatide, 175
Erythromycin, 185
Esmolol, 31, 55, 66, 162, 177
Ethacrynic acid, 166
Ethambutol, 186
Ethionamide, 186
Etidronate disodium, 42

Famotidine, 167
Felodipine, 66, 162
Fenoldopam, 161, 163
Fentanyl, 169
Filgrastim, 180
Flecainide, 177
Fluconazole, 188
5-Flucytosine, 188
Fludrocortisone, 58

Fluids, intravenous fluids, 159
Flumazenil, 170
Fluoroquinolones, 184
Fomepizole, 68
Fosinopril, 162
Furosemide, 3, 40, 42, 166

γ- Hydroxybutyrate (GHB), 59
Gallium nitrate, 42
Gentamicin, 183
Glucagon, 52, 59
Glycoprotein IIb/IIIa receptor antagonists, 175
Granulocyte colony-stimulating factor, 180
Guanabenz, 162
Guanfacine, 162

H2-Blockers, 167
Heparin, 10, 19, 20, 118, 173
Hetastarch, 159, 208
Hydralazine, 26, 162
Hydrochlorothiazide, 166
Hydrocodone, 169
Hydrocortisone, 56, 58
Hydromorphone, 169
Hydroxyethyl starch, 159, 208

Ibutilide, 177
Imipenem cilistatin, 187
Inhaled bronchodilators, 11, 14, 179
Intravenous fluids, 159, 208
Iopanoic acid, 55
Ipodate, 55
Ipratropium bromide, 11, 14, 75, 179
Isoetharine, 179
Isoniazid, 48, 59, 186
Isoproterenol, 161
Israpidine, 66, 162
Itraconazole, 188

Kanamycin, 186
Ketoconazole, 188

Labetalol, 26, 66, 162, 177
Lamifiban, 175
Lansoprazole, 167
Lepirudin, 173
Levalbuterol, 179
Levofloxacin, 184
Levorphanol, 169
Lidocaine, 177
Linezolid, 187
Lisinopril, 162
Lorazepam, 69, 170
Low molecular weight heparin, 19, 20, 118, 173
Lugol's solution, 55

Macrolides, 185
Magnesium chloride, 43
Magnesium gluconate, 43
Magnesium lactate, 43
Magnesium oxide, 43
Magnesium sulfate, 26, 40, 43
Mannitol, 3, 84, 166
Meperidine, 169
Meropenem, 187
Metaproterenol, 179
Methadone, 169
Methicillin, 182
Methimazole, 55